Clay's Handbook of
Environmental Health

Clay's Handbook of Environmental Health

Seventeenth edition

EDITED BY

W.H. Bassett
DMA, FCIEH

*Director of Housing and Environmental Health
and Deputy Chief Executive, Exeter City Council*

CHAPMAN & HALL

London · Glasgow · Weinheim · New York · Tokyo · Melbourne · Madras

Published by Chapman & Hall, 2–6 Boundary Row, London SE1 8HN, UK

Chapman & Hall, 2–6 Boundary Row, London SE1 8HN, UK
Blackie Academic & Professional, Wester Cleddens Road, Bishopbriggs, Glasgow G64 2NZ, UK
Chapman & Hall GmbH, Pappelallee 3, 69469 Weinheim, Germany
Chapman & Hall USA, 115 Fifth Avenue, 41st Floor, New York, NY 10003, USA
Chapman & Hall Japan, ITP-Japan, Kyowa Building, 3F, 2–2–1 Hirakawacho, Chiyoda-ku, Tokyo 102, Japan
Chapman & Hall Australia, 102 Dodds Street, South Melbourne, Victoria 3205, Australia
Chapman & Hall India, R. Seshadri, 32 Second Main Road, CIT East, Madras 600 035, India

First edition 1933
Seventeenth edition 1995

©1995 Chapman & Hall

Typeset in 10/12 Times by Photoprint, Torquay, Devon
Printed in Great Britain at The Alden Press, Oxford.

ISBN 0 412 54870 4

A catalogue record for this book is available from the British Library

Library of Congress Catalog Card Number: 94–74695

This edition of Clays is dedicated
to F. Gerald Davies FCIEH, FRSH,
formerly Chief Public Health Inspector to
Exeter City Council before retirement in 1971.

Gerry Davies was the editor responsible for
several editions of this Handbook
between 1965 and 1977.

He died peacefully on 19 March 1994.

Contents

Contributors

Peter F. Allen BA, DMA, DMS, FCIEH, FRSH
  Head of Environmental Health Services,
  Oxford City Council

Peter E. Beeching BA, FCIEH
  Assistant Director of Housing and
  Environmental Health, Exeter City Council

Paul C. Belcher BA, MSc, MCIEH
  Principal Lecturer in Environmental
  Sciences, Cardiff Institute of Higher
  Education

Alan Blythe FCIEH, M.Inst, WM, DMS, FBIM
  Director of Environmental Services,
  Woodspring District Council, Avon

Hazel O. Carter BSc (Hons), MSc, CBiol,
  FCIEH
  Director of Education and Membership,
  Chartered Institute of Environmental
  Health, London

James Connelly MBBS, MSc, MRC Psych.,
  MFPHM
  Senior Lecturer in Public Health Medicine,
  School of Medicine, University of Leeds

Jeff Cooper MSc, BSc, M.Inst, WM, FRGS
  Waste Reduction Officer, London Waste
  Regulation Authority

John Cruickshank MA, MD, FRCPath
  Director, Public Health Laboratory, Exeter

Eric W. Foskett BSc (Econ), DPA, FCIEH, FRSH
  Formerly Director of Environmental
  Health, City of Manchester and Past
  President, Institution of Environmental
  Health Officers, London

Charles Gibson FREHIS
  Director of Professional Development,
  Royal Environmental Health Institute of
  Scotland, Edinburgh

Michael J. Gittins C.Eng, FCIEH, M.InstE,
  FRSH, MIOH
  Chief Environmental Health Officer,
  Leeds City Council

Brian P. Hanna FCIEH
  DMS
  Chief Executive, Belfast City Council

Veronica Habgood MSc, BSc, MCIEH
  Associate Head of School of Environmental
  Sciences, University of Greenwich, London

Neville Hobday DMA, FCIEH
  Director of Environmental Health and
  Housing Officer, Bedford Borough Council

M.L. Jassi BSc (Hons), DMS, MCIEH, MBIM,
  FRSH
  Environmental and Consumer Service
  Manager, City of Salford

Mike Jacob LLB, FCIEH, FRIPHH
Food Safety, Food Law Consultant,
Rickmansworth, Herts (formerly Chief
Environmental Health Officer, Department
of Health, London)

Maurice Jones FCIEH
Borough Environmental Health Officer,
Wellingborough

Martin J. Key MICEH, FRSH
Environmental Management Consultant,
Evesham

John G.W. Kirk FCIEH
Chief Environmental Health Officer,
Warwick District Council

John F. Leech, BSc (Hons), MCIEH
Assistant Principal Environmental Health
Officer, Exeter City Council

Richard T. Mayon-White MB, MRCP, FFCM
Consultant Public Health Physician,
Oxfordshire Health Authority

Frank Oliver MA, D.Phil
Lecturer in Statistics and Econmetrics,
University of Exeter

Paul P. Paddock BSc (Jt Hons), BSc (Hons),
MPhil., MCIEH, MIOSH
Principal Lecturer in Environmental
Health, The Nottingham Trent University

Richard J. Palfrey MCIEH
Principal Environmental Health Officer,
Exeter City Council

Stephen R. Palmer MA, MB, BChir, FFPHM
Director, Welsh Combined Centres for
Public Health, University of Wales, College
of Medicine, Cardiff

Nevil H. Parkinson FCIEH, M. Inst. WM
Director of Environmental Sciences, Selby
District Council

Ray Ranson MA, MRSH, MIH, MCIEH
Consultant in Environmental Health,
World Health Organization, London

Edward Ramsden FRSH, MCIEH, DBA, FCIS
Director of Environmental Health Services,
Swansea City Council

Peter Rotheram BA, FCIEH, FRSH
Executive Secretary, Association of Port
Health Authorities, Runcorn

Michael Squires, MIOH
Senior Environmental Health Technician,
Exeter City Council

John D. Wildsmith BSc (Hons), MCIEH,
FRSH
Senior Lecturer in Environmental Sciences,
Cardiff Institute of Higher Education

Frank B. Wright LLB (Leeds), LLM
(Leicester), FCIEH, FRSH, FRIPHH
Director of the European Health and
Safety Law Unit, University of Salford

Preface

The new framework introduced in the 16th edition has been widely welcomed and is therefore used again. This edition seeks to build upon that foundation by:

(a) updating in accordance with new legislation and professional practice;
(b) developing areas where interest has emerged or intensified; and
(c) introducing new material.

The legislative programme for each parliamentary year contains environmental legislation in abundance and throughout every parliamentary session there is a stream of secondary legislation affecting environmental health work. The deregulation initiative itself creates a need for a substantial amount of new, amending law. This is reflected in this edition up to early 1995 with indications in appropriate chapters about the way in which the relevant law is likely to be developed.

The areas where the content has been revised to reflect heightened concerns or new practice include:

1. The inclusion in the introductory chapter of information which is emerging from a WHO study of environmental health systems in Europe following the massive political changes which have taken place there.
2. The chapter on pest control has been re-written to reflect current approach and practice as has the chapter on environmental health law which now contains the section on statutory nuisances.
3. The Health of the Nation initiative as it relates to environmental health has been covered more extensively.
4. In the chapters on food safety the major changes to the function brought about by the single market, deregulation and the alteration in responsibilities with the advent of the national meat hygiene service are all included in this edition.
5. Issues about radon in water are now dealt with more thoroughly.
6. The chapter on waste management has been amended in relation to recycling and now includes information about recent developments in waste to energy plants. It also contains information on the new regime of waste management licensing.
7. More information is included concerning the pollution of rivers and seas with a review of recent studies into the health effects of contamination of bathing waters by sewage.

There are three new chapters:

(a) the enforcement of environmental health laws which includes discussion of current areas of concern involving risk assessment, inspection programming and consistency both in approach and interpretation;
(b) the effects of bad housing conditions on the health of the occupants; and
(c) a review of information technology systems and their use in the environmental health service.

In addition, there are three new case studies to reflect environmental health organizations, i.e. Salford, Selby and Warwick, each contributed by the Director of Environmental Health or equivalent.

I am very fortunate to have had continuing contributions from authors in the last edition, with the exception of Clarence Phenix who has sadly passed away. His chapter on environmental health in Northern Ireland has been revised by Brian Hanna of Belfast City Council and other new authors are Hazel Carter from the Chartered Institute of Environmental Health, Dr Jim Connelly from the University of Leeds Department of Public Health Medicine, Veronica Habgood of the University of Greenwich, Mike Jacob now Food and Safety Consultant and previously Chief Environmental Health Officer at the Department of Health, Paul Paddock of the Nottingham Trent University and Frank Wright, the Director of the European Health and Safety Law Unit at Salford University. I am extremely grateful to all authors for their efforts.

I am confident that this new edition will be even more useful than its predecessor to all those involved in environmental health work but I am always pleased to receive comments about the way in which future editions might be developed.

Finally, it should be noted that the male pronoun is used throughout for ease of reading. It should be taken to mean both male and female individuals.

W.H. Bassett
1995

Extract from the preface to the first edition

Under the ever-widening scope of public health administration, and in view of the high standard demanded of students presenting themselves for the examination of the Royal Sanitary Institute and Sanitary Inspectors' Examination Joint Board, the need has arisen for a handbook, more comprehensive and more in accord with the progressive demands of modern times, than has been available hitherto. At the request of the publishers, this volume has been prepared to meet that need.

Despite the number and variety of the subjects necessarily included in a book of this character, the author has endeavoured, as far as is practicable within the limits of a single volume of convenient size, to cover the whole range of the duties of a sanitary inspector, observing due proportion in the attention given to each subject, and while dealing fully and in detail with some subjects, omitting none that is of real importance.

The author has always felt that the subjects to be studied by sanitary inspectors are by no means of an uninteresting character. It has been his endeavour to make this book 'readable' and such as to rob systematic study of much of its inherent drudgery.

Few things are of more practical value to executive public health officers, either in examination or in practice, than the ability to illustrate answers or suggestions by sketches. In order to assist readers in this direction, the liberal illustration of technical matters has been made a special feature of the book; every illustration being from an original line drawing in which sectional details are shown, and which the reader may reproduce or develop for himself.

H.H.C

London, *April 1933*.

Introduction to environmental health

William H. Bassett

DEFINITION OF ENVIRONMENTAL HEALTH

Environmental health is defined by the World Health Organization (WHO) as being 'the control of all those factors in man's physical environment which exercise, or may exercise, a deleterious effect on his physical development, health or survival', and 'health' in this context is said to mean 'a state of complete physical, mental and social well-being'.* Environmental health is a broad concept but is, nevertheless, only one facet of public health which is 'the science and art of preventing disease, prolonging life and promoting health through organized efforts of society [1].

OBJECTIVES AND FUNCTIONS

The essence of an environmental health organization is the prevention, detection and control of environmental hazards which affect human health and will include the following considerations as an integral part of that process:

1. waste management;
2. food control;
3. housing;
4. epidemiological control;
5. air quality management;
6. occupational health and safety;
7. water resources management;
8. noise control;
9. protection of the recreational environment;
10. radiation health;
11. control of frontiers, air and sea ports and border crossings;
12. educational activities;
13. promotion and enforcement of environmental health quality standards;
14. collaborative efforts to study the effects of environmental hazards;
15. environmental impact assessment.

The last three considerations overlap with one another, and involve all 12 functions listed above them.

CURRENT WORLD-WIDE ISSUES

Environmental health standards are currently high on the political agendas of most developed countries as public concern over environmental issues increases. Dr Wilfried Kreisel, Director of the Environmental Health Division at WHO Headquarters in Geneva, has addressed the situation [2] and identifies two critical issues:

1. How environmental health can become a more potent force to serve people facing growing threats to their health.
2. How our improving environmental health technology can be better used to foster positive health.

* A further definition is found in the European Charter on Environment and Health – ". . . includes both the direct pathological effects of chemicals, radiation and some biological agents, and the effects (often indirect) on health and well being of the broad physical, physiological, social and aesthetic environment, which includes farming, urban development, land use and transport."

Kreisel says: 'Several aspects of this issue are being debated vigorously in the US whose current dialogue on human interactions with the environment is active and continuing. The country's resurgent public concern with the environment and its effects on human health has a remarkably wide range. It includes the international problems of acid rain, the greenhouse effect and depletion of the planet's ozone layer; national concerns with medical waste disposal, radioactive and toxic waste management, transportation accidents, health aspects of urbanization and traffic, occupational health and safety, air and water pollution, and sustaining the ecological balance of the coasts, wetlands, forests and farmlands; as well as local concerns over water quality, clean air, solid waste management and finding a balance between the economic incentives of development and a decent quality of life – issues that are fought out in counties and cities throughout the country.'

Such a statement could, of course, be made about the present situation in the UK. Kreisel goes on: 'This broad range of concerns applies not only to other industrialized countries, but also to most developing countries. The World Commission on Environment and Development has pointed out that developing countries face both the public health problems that have largely been solved over the last century and many of the problems that are being faced now.

'Such countries as Thailand, Nigeria and Brazil have yet to ensure safe water, basic sanitation and protection against communicable diseases for many of their people. At the same time they must deal with the health impacts of rapid, large-scale industrialization, urbanization and technological development. Massive population growth makes it even more difficult to solve this double load of problems. Growth outstrips many countries' economic development; it retards their social development and makes crushing demands on services, resources and the bearing capacity of the environment.

'Environmental health is, thus, a global problem. Though each country has its own profile of needs and problems and though some have stronger scientific, technical, economic and social resources to apply to the problems, no country has the situation fully under control.

'To put it another way, in every country on this planet, man-made environmental problems are being generated faster than we can solve or prevent them. In every country, environmental health capacity is inadequate to meet human needs, even as the problems themselves change, becoming more complex, more critical, more urgent.'

Kreisel identifies the need for changes in six aspects of environmental health if these issues are to be tackled successfully:

1. Continued technological advances for the detection and elimination of environmental hazards, including nuclear radiation and waste disposal, and improvements in the techniques of risk assessment.
2. The environmental health professions must broaden their understanding of environmental health, be more aware of the social environment, and be more prepared to advocate for that broader range of concerns.
3. An improvement in the quality of information upon which environmental health policies and programmes can be based, e.g. enhanced basic health information systems and comprehensive environmental monitoring statistics, and in the quantitative and qualitative elements of the manpower resources available to the service.
4. The development of the organizational concept of the extended environmental health unit, i.e. organizing environmental health as a broader system in which the environmental health unit is a key element. This is necessary to counter the segregation of core environmental health work which exists in many countries.
5. An improvement in intersectoral and inter-government relationships on environmental health matters. Co-ordination must be improved both vertically, i.e. between governments and national, regional and local organizations, and horizontally, i.e. different sectoral agencies dealing with aspects of environmental health at the same level of administration.
6. Better links with communities and more effective lobbying of those who determine, or

assist in the determination of, environmental health policies and levels of resource.

Kreisel completes his analysis by identifying how changes can be advanced by the attitudes of the environmental health profession:

1. We need a renewed sense of mission that is open to change and welcomes it.
2. We need to look beyond today's work, to invest part of our energies in building for the future.
3. We need to understand environmental health as a large system, in which we are a small but strategic element, one that can be made more effective through collaborative processes of system-building.
4. We need to see health as a function of society, not as the territory of an organization.
5. We need to function more and more co-operatively, to encourage the co-operation of others, and to support such co-operation.
6. We need to take a learning approach to our problem – learning from errors and communicating our experiences.
7. We need to upgrade our insights and skills in planning, developing our capabilities to programme for the large, complex system that is environmental health.
8. We need to recognize how little we can do by ourselves, to make alliances, and to improve communications outside our formal organizations.
9. We need to become more informed and effective advocates for health, not merely to make the arguments and share the information, but also to be of practical help to those we seek to influence.
10. We need to be patient, because the changes we seek will not come quickly; and we need to be determined, because those changes will not come easily.

Such attitudes are required just as much from the environmental health profession in the UK. as they are anywhere else in the world.

In 1990 the Director General of WHO established an independent Commission on Health and the Environment composed of internationally recognized experts in the scientific, social and political fields.

The Commission undertook an assessment of the relationship between health and the environment in the context of development. The conclusions and recommendations are set out in its report 'Our Planet, our Health' [5] and will help to shape future WHO programmes of co-operation and will provide the basis for a new global strategy for environmental health.

The Commission's study and report is recommended as essential reading to all students of environmental health. It provides confirmation that, despite the fact that the quality of the environment and the nature of development are major determinants of health, health rarely receives high priority in environmental policies and development plans. Health depends upon our ability to understand and manage the interaction between human activities and the physical environment but, although we have that knowledge, we have failed to act upon it. The report considers health and the environment in a global context and makes a large number of general recommendations which include:

1. All governments and international agencies should give a higher priority to developing a sustainable basis for the health of their people.
2. Priority should be given to reducing population growth, over-consumption and waste generation.
3. More effective action is required to deal with the health and environment problems that have most effect on poorer groups and to engender more participatory ways of working with those groups.
4. Each country should develop and implement an action programme to address its immediate and pressing health and environment problems. (For UK see Cmnd. 2426 1994 HMSO.)

There follows a series of sectoral recommendations dealing with food and agriculture, water, energy, industry, human settlements and urbanization and transboundary and international problems.

The nature of environmental health is clearly global, international, national, regional and local and needs to be vigorously pursued at all levels.

Article 129 of the 1992 Treaty on European Union (Maastricht) requires the Community to contribute towards ensuring a high level of human health protection and to direct action towards the prevention of diseases, in particular the major health scourges. The Commission has published a detailed communication on the framework for action in the field of public health.

The communication sets out the major health problems which confront the community and explains how priorities for action can be established. It examines possible actions and proposes a number of specific programmes.

The areas which have emerged as priority areas for future Community action are:

1. health promotion, education and training;
2. health data and indicators, and monitoring and surveillance of diseases;
3. cancer;
4. drugs;
5. AIDS and other communicable diseases;
6. accidents and injuries;
7. pollution-related diseases;
8. rare diseases.

These areas will be the subject of Commission proposals for action programmes, to be introduced over a 3-year period, to last for 5 years.*

ORGANIZATION

The organizational approach to the environmental health function differs widely throughout the world despite the fact that the tasks to be performed, particularly in the more industrialized countries, have a large measure of uniformity. Even within the European Region a marked variation can be seen. The countries of the 'new' Europe are incredibly diverse. Their diversity relates not only to their geographical and cultural differences but also, and perhaps more importantly, to the range of social and economic conditions that prevail in these countries. As a result, the perspectives and priorities which are adopted on environmental health issues, and particularly how environmental health services are delivered,

demonstrate a wide degree of variance throughout Europe. Some countries have well-established environmental health services which can trace their origins back one hundred years or more, whilst others are only now developing services for environmental health work.

Since the demise of the former Soviet Union, and the subsequent removal of Moscow's control over some of the countries in central and eastern Europe, the international community has focused largely on the environmental damage which the former administrations had bequeathed to the newly independent states and the other countries of central and eastern Europe. This work to date has concentrated mainly on the assessment of the actual physical environmental damage and the prioritization of direct capital investment. Economic reforms in eastern Europe will have a direct effect on the environment. The transition to a market economy from one of central control planning leads to a broad change of attitude and will give countries of eastern Europe the opportunity to begin to reform business practices. The wasting of resources which was common place in previous industrial practice should now be heavily resisted. The removal of subsidies on the various natural resource commodities will provide a sufficiently large financial incentive for the introduction of good housekeeping practices and the implementation of pollution control strategies.

The creation of a market economy cannot however, on its own, be left to ensure environmental improvement. A mixture of economic, social and regulatory reforms are required to create a comprehensive strategy of control which can be balanced, adaptable to changing circumstances, recognize the important need of economic growth and yet be truly effective in controlling environmental health problems. To develop such strategies it will be necessary for investments to be made in areas other than direct financing of capital intensive programmes. Investments also have to be made in the areas of education and institution building. Environmental health policies and strategies are of no value

---

* Also see the European Charter on Environment and Health (Dec. 1989), adopted by the first European Conference on Environment and Health in Frankfurt, and the Declaration on Action for Environment and Health in Europe adopted at the second Conference in Helsinki in 1994.

unless they can be implemented and monitored by suitably qualified and motivated personnel, situated in appropriate institutions with the necessary capacities. Environmental health services are primarily charged with these tasks. Environmental health services act as the interface between policy makers and those who are the subject of the policy control. Environmental health services also have a direct relationship with the general public in dealing with their complaints and concerns relating to environmental health issues. There is a need therefore for services to be appropriately targeted and sympathetically responsive to public needs whilst at the same time represent the views of the controlling authority, be that at local, regional or national level.

In recognition of the current trends, and rather than concentrating on individual hazards, the European Regional Office of the World Health Organization (WHO EURO) is carrying out work to support the reorganization and development of infrastructures for environmental health services throughout Europe.* A survey was carried out between March 1993 and March 1994 of some 26 countries from all over the European Region to ascertain how environmental health services were organized and delivered. Through this work it has become apparent that every country has established or is developing it own unique systems for the administration of environmental health. Their individuality reflects the different cultural, social and historical perspectives which mould any arm of government, and it is dangerous therefore to draw conclusions as to their suitability or comparisons against 'model' systems. Nevertheless some common elements can be identified, analysed and grouped into four main types of system.

First, a system of services delivery which is common in many countries of central and eastern Europe is where strong central and vertical controls are retained (Fig. A). Typically the Ministries of Health and Environment have weak links at national level and are concerned mainly with their own particular area of expertise. The actual services are provided at regional level within the country through their respective regional inspectorates of hygiene and epidemio-

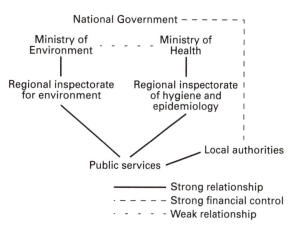

Fig. A European Environmental Health Service Organization – Approach 1.

logy and environment. These units have little or no autonomy and are staffed by public health doctors and engineers as appropriate. Normally in such systems local authorities of communes have little or no statutory control in respect of environmental health.

The second system for the delivery of environmental health services can be found in many of the southern European countries. This system has a level of co-ordination at a regional level before services are delivered to the public. Individual ministries still set their own agendas with weak communication and dialogue between them. They are then represented at a regional office. However in this instance the regional office is representative of all the relevant ministries. They are then co-ordinated to fit in with the needs of the locality through a government appointee commonly known as the 'Prefect' or through a 'Prefectual Council'. Once more local municipal and commune authorities have little or no involvement in service delivery (Fig. B).

The third system of control for environmental health service delivery is formed by both local and nationally controlled regional offices. Local authorities are used to deliver services relating to local environmental health problems, working within national guidelines and legislation. Regional offices of national ministries deal with strategic matters of national importance and where the

* See 'Concerns for Europe's Tomorrow', WHO Regional Publications: European series No. 53, WHO, Copenhagen.

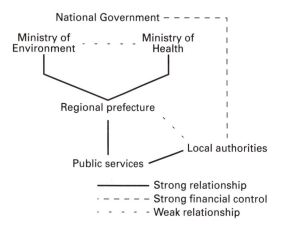

Fig. B European Environmental Health Service Organization – Approach 2.

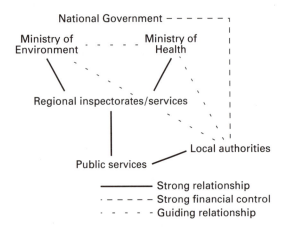

Fig. C European Environmental Health Service Organization – Approach 3.

technical expertise does not exist at the local level (Fig. C).

The fourth and final system which can be found in Europe for the delivery of environmental health services is based upon a system of federal government. In this situation a country is subdivided into different states which are bound by a few national statutes, but generally each state can set its own legislation, and systems of control and administration for environmental health control.

A useful publication to assist further study of the variations in European organization for environmental health is the *European Environmental Yearbook* [6]. This presents a summary of in-

formation on a wide range of environmental issues in the then 12 EU member states and provides a comparative study of the way in which organizations have been developed to deal with, for example, waste energy, pollution, etc.

THE ENVIRONMENTAL HEALTH OFFICER

Following a consultation by WHO on the 'Role, Functions and Training Requirements of Environmental Health Officers (Sanitarians) in Europe' in 1978 it was concluded that, 'Experience of those countries in the Region which have officers with specialized training in environmental health who are recognized as constituting a specific profession clearly demonstrates their value. Thus it would be to the advantage of all Member states to introduce into their environmental health service staff of this kind whom the consultation called in English 'environmental health officers'. Thus WHO favours the UK system of environmental health control based on a total environmental management system by environmental health officers.

That conclusion was followed by a further series of considerations by WHO, one of which looked at the development of environmental health manpower [4], and contained the following professional profile of the environmental health officer:

1. The environmental health officer is concerned with administration, inspection, education and regulations in respect of environmental health.
2. The numbers of environmental health officers should be sufficient to exercise adequate surveillance over health-related environmental conditions; this surveillance should include necessary monitoring activities. They must have a close association with the people in their area and be readily accessible to them, providing professional advice and guidance, and thereby gaining the community's confidence and encouraging its participation in improving environmental health. They should be members of multidisciplinary prim-

ary health care teams delivering comprehensive health care at community level.

3. The environmental health officer acts as a public arbiter of environmental health standards, maintaining close contact with the community. He must at all times be aware of the general environmental circumstances in his district, and must know what industrial hazards to health may arise there and what resources are available to him in the event of emergency.

4. He is a professional officer capable of developing professional standards and applying them in his own work in relation to that of non-professionals involved in environmental health. Also, his role will obviously touch on aspects with which the physician, veterinarian, toxicologist, engineer, nurse and others deal in a more specialized manner.

5. One of his vital functions is to maintain effective liaison with other professional officers who have a contribution to make in the promotion of environmental health, e.g. with regard to water resources management, waste management, housing, rodent, insect and other pest control, and protection of the recreational environment.

6. Environmental health officers would carry out the well-established duties of sanitarians/ sanitary inspectors, including inspection of housing and food hygiene, and also monitor and control the new hazards arising from intensive industrialization, e.g. pollution by chemical and physical agents, which could harm the health of a community.

7. Even greater emphasis than in the past should be placed on the preventive role of the environmental health officer in relation to environmental hazards to health.

8. He will obviously not possess the expertise of the physician in personal health, of the veterinarian in animal health, of the microbiologist in microbiology or of the sanitary engineer in the provision of water supplies. However, he will have background and practical knowledge of these areas sufficient for him to understand the principles involved, and he may develop some specialist expertise. He will be able to work easily with the other professionals. His wider experience will enable him to formulate an approach on a broader base, to contribute to the decisions to be made, or to make these decisions alone in cases where he has the necessary authority. He must understand the environmental aspects of the problems which are the concern of other professionals, so that he may contribute to their solution.

9. He must be able to plan and co-ordinate activities between different professional disciplines, official agencies and authorities. He needs to have continuing links with other professionals involved in environmental and health-related work. The other professionals with whom liaison will be appropriate include physicians, physicists, microbiologists, chemists, civil/building/sanitary engineers, veterinarians and lawyers.

10. In some countries and situations, the environmental health officer will initiate the collaboration; in others, he will provide the information and advice which are sought. His liaison role will extend beyond the other professionals to technicians and a range of other specialists, including those concerned with the public health laboratory services. While being able to act independently in both advisory and enforcement capacities, exercising self-reliance and initiative, he should be able also to function as a member of a team with other professionals in implementing environmental health programmes.

11. In industry and commerce, environmental control specialists interpret legislation, promote and maintain standards, and solve the problems which may come to light through, for example, a system of internal control or 'self-inspection'.

12. An important part of his functions must be to acquaint himself with actual or potential environmental hazards and to ensure that appropriate action is taken to deal with them, e.g. to safeguard the public from the hazards associated with microbiological contamination of food and with chemical residues in food substances, and to monitor and control potential and existing environmental hazards, with the backing of strong legislation.

13. A combination of training in public health and toxicology should enable him to cope with such problems as soil pollution due to degradation-resistant agricultural pesticides, leachates from industrial wastes, fall-out from the plumes of chemical works, liquid radioactive wastes from industry and research; chemical pollution of the work environment from solvents and from dust arising from processes using silica, asbestos and lead; pollution of the home environment due to such products as cosmetics, detergents, paints, pesticides and gas used as fuel; heavy contamination of water resources by mercury, antimony, barium, cobalt and other metals due to industrial wastes, pesticides used in agriculture, etc.; and new problems in food safety such as the irradiation of food.

14. An environmental health officer within the public service should have the following basic functions:
    (a) improving human health and protecting it from environmental hazards:
    (b) enforcing environmental legislation;
    (c) developing liaison between the inhabitants and the local authority, and between the local and higher levels of administration;
    (d) acting independently to provide advice on environmental matters:
    (e) initiating and implementing health education programmes to promote an understanding of environmental principles.

15. Because of the range of his functions, the environmental health officer will operate in a managerial capacity and in collaboration with other environmental agencies and services.

The increasing complexities of environmental health problems require a continuing development of expertise and an updating of knowledge. To maintain a leading role in dealing with environmentally related health problems, the environmental health officer must be in a position to respond to challenges presented by new hazards in the environment, and exercise influence in promoting and regulating environmental health activities. The environmental health officer's training should equip him with the necessary expertise to act at any level – national, provincial (or intermediate) or local – or within any sector, private or public.

Thus the environmental health officer is trained as a generalist across the range of the 15 basic environmental health activities identified above and therefore occupies a key position in the environmental health service. An important part of his functions must be to acquaint himself with actual or potential environmental hazards, and to ensure that appropriate action is taken to deal with them. In some cases, he may have the required authority and expertise. In others, he may need to press particular agencies to take appropriate action. There will also be occasions when he will need to consult other professional officers, and to make use of laboratory and other expert scientific services. A vital part of his functions will, therefore, be to maintain effective liaison with other relevant professional officers who have a contribution to make in the promotion of environmental health. Environmental health is very much a team concept, and this must be recognized in any organizational arrangements.

REFERENCES

1. *Report of the Committee of Enquiry into the Future Development of the Public Health Function* (1988) HMSO. Cmnd 289, London
2. Kreisel Wilfried (1990) Environmental health in the 1990s – affecting change. *Environmental Health*, **98** (3).
3. WHO (1980) *The environmental health officer in an industrial society*. Reports and Studies 29, Report on a WHO Consultation, WHO Regional Office for Europe. Copenhagen.
4. WHO (1987) *Development of Environmental Health Manpower*, Environmental Health Series 18 1987. WHO Regional Office for Europe. Copenhagen.
5. *Our Planet, Our Health: Report of the WHO Commission on Health and the Environment* (1992), WHO, Geneva.
6. *European Environmental Yearbook* (1991) Institute for Environmental Studies, Doc Ter International UK, London.

Part One
The Organization of
Environmental Health

1 Historical development of environmental health in the UK

Eric W. Foskett

INTRODUCTION

The history of the development of environmental health control in the UK is long and complex. Any brief version cannot contain the wealth of detail which is available, and so the course traced here is that of streams of developments and important landmarks.

Environmental health is concerned with any effect by any environmental factor on human or animal health. Initially, concern was limited to those factors which were easily discernible as affecting human health but, as the environment became better understood, it was recognized that the role of environmental health should be expanded.

It is not possible to assign a specific date from which problems relating to environmental health emerged. While this study has to have a beginning in time, it must be understood that the need to control the environment in the interests of health has been evolving for a long time, and it continues to evolve as a consequence of man's occupation of the planet.

For the purpose of this study, it is possible to divide the evolution of environmental health control into four time zones to which it is possible to assign some dates. These are no more than convenient, relatively imprecise, time boundaries because many important events straddled those boundaries and, in many cases, there were parallel streams of different activities in the same time scale.

The first of these periods may be regarded as being about 1750–1850; the second 1850–1900; the third 1900–45; and the fourth 1945 to the present day.

An historical perspective is important. A knowledge of what has happened in the past, and how and why changes came about, will make it easier to understand the present position. If the present position can be understood, it may be possible to make some intelligent forecasts of future developments.

In attempting to understand what has happened, and why it occurred, it is important not to make value judgements of past events based on present day knowledge and attitudes, for, in the last two centuries, social philosophies and scientific and technological knowledge have undergone many changes. What is common knowledge or practice today was largely unknown or unacceptable 150 years ago. Indeed, it may well be that the fourth boundary may prove to be inaccurate, and that boundary may, at some time in the future, be understood to have been drawn sometime in the 1980s, and that this study is being written at the beginning of the fifth period.

An understanding of the conditions which have, in Britain, led to a system of environmental health control may be thought to be exaggerated or over emphasized, but the entire period is very well documented with numerous literary sources to be consulted. These sources are to be found in the reports of numerous inquiries, in political writings, in newspaper reports, and in contemporary literature.

THE AGRICULTURAL REVOLUTION (1700–75)

It is common to associate the increasing need for intervention in the environment in the interests of health with the onset of industrialization. There is truth in this except what is usually termed 'the Industrial Revolution' was preceded by an 'agricultural revolution', which contributed greatly to the movement of population from the country to the towns.

Agricultural improvements, introduced by Charles Townshend, Thomas Coke, Jethro Tull, Robert Bakewell and others, in husbandry, the breeding of better livestock, the introduction of farm machinery, and the enclosure of land, reduced the demand for agricultural labour and the dispossessed workers migrated mainly to the towns.

For those who remained as farm workers, their lot was usually a very low living standard characterized by housing within a damp, overcrowded, cottage with few amenities. The greater productivity due to the agricultural revolution improved workers' diet a little, and made some contribution to a slowly declining rural death rate. Nevertheless, work on the land, often in bad weather, was unremitting toil for scant wages. Disease ravaged the family. The children were especially vulnerable but, for the adults, poor nutrition, excessive child bearing, a poor domestic environment, and exposure to the elements while working, contributed to a low life expectancy.

As towns expanded, it became increasingly difficult to provide a satisfactory food supply as they became more remote from their supply hinterland. The situation was ripe for fraudulent substitution, and for food to be adulterated. Doubtless most of the rural population would have preferred to remain in the hamlets and villages, but when they had to move they had few options. They could go to the small, often remote, villages in the hills where the presence of water power had induced the establishment of a textile mill, or to other villages which grew up around a mill, or they could retreat to the growing towns.

THE INDUSTRIAL REVOLUTION

The documentary evidence of environmental conditions is graphic. Accounts written in the first third of the nineteenth century relate to conditions created to cope with urban population increases due to the very high birth rates, and the influx of people into the towns during the preceding 50 or so years.

The pace of industrialization quickened with the development of the steam engine which enabled factories, and especially textile mills, to be set up in more favourable locations than villages on hillsides adjoining swift running water. With this transition came many environmental evils.

Machinery enabled production to be vastly increased with economies of scale to be grasped. As factories increased in size and complexity, they needed more workers who had to be housed nearby because, in the absence of public transport, they had to be able to walk to work.

The need to house workers close to the factories resulted in street after street of small, ill-constructed houses. There was little provision for drainage or refuse disposal; water supplies were inadequate and usually grossly polluted. To add to these unfavourable conditions, the houses were overshadowed by the tall factories and they were polluted by smoke, grit, and dust from both the factory furnaces and from domestic fires emitting low level smoke.

The bad environmental conditions were matched by the poor social conditions. Even though the working hours were very long, wages were low. As a result, workers suffered from malnutrition, and their poor physical condition was made worse by the ill-ventilated factories and, in some textile mills, the high temperatures and humidity. In addition to the adverse working conditions, there were few sanitary amenities within the factories.

For many workers, factory practices involved working with dangerous machinery, and fatal or disabling accidents to workers were common. If the adult workers suffered from bad working conditions the lot of the children was even worse.

Child labour was often considered an essential factor in production. There was always work a child could do and there was a place for them in the mines and in the mills. Indeed, children in textile mills and pottery factories often worked longer hours than the adults as they stayed to clean the machinery at the end of the day, or arrived earlier than the adult workers to ensure that they could start full production as soon as possible.

Children started to work at an early age and, in textiles especially, they formed part of a team. Adults who could not take a child with them might find work hard to get and, where the shortage of children was acute, mill owners imported children from poor law institutions as apprentices.

The general social and economic conditions in the early nineteenth century have to be viewed against a background of, initially, an unreformed parliament, an inadequate local government system, and a political philosophy which permitted, in the name of individual liberty, all manner of what would now be considered to be social abuses. Because of the current political and economic views, there was no political will to make deliberate attempts to ameliorate the conditions endured by most urban workers and their families.

In the first decades of the nineteenth century there was a considerable political ferment urging change, but almost always in vain. The people whose lot warranted improvement had little individual political influence, and the ability to organize to bring political pressure was a skill still to be learned.

Nevertheless, their plight was noticed, and many politicians and philanthropists adopted causes with which they sympathized, and fought for changes using their social and political connections to that end. In the more populous areas, groups of people emerged who became interested in the welfare of their fellows, and they supported inquiries and investigations. Physicians, such as Thomas Perceval of Manchester and James Currie of Liverpool, visited slum areas and reported what they had found.

Environmental disadvantage was not uniformly spread. There were many districts which were comparatively salubrious, even though few adequate sanitary amenities were available. Some of the more prosperous boroughs spent money improving parts of their areas but, in many instances, improvements were carried out by improvement commissioners appointed to implement, in a defined locality, environmental improvements specifically authorized by a private Act of Parliament, the cost being defrayed by a 'rate' levied on the householders in that area.

In 1795, a contagious disease swept through children working at a mill near Manchester, and the local Justices of the Peace took what action they could to prevent a recurrence.

Early in the nineteenth century there was the first move towards improving the conditions of some juvenile workers. Sir Robert Peel, himself a mill owner, introduced a Bill which became the **Health and Morals of Apprentices Act 1802**,

which passed with little or no opposition. Its chief provisions may be summarized as follows. The working hours of apprentices were limited to twelve a day. Night work (by apprentices) was to be gradually discontinued and to cease entirely by June 1804. Apprentices were to be instructed in reading, writing and arithmetic, and a suit of clothing was to be given yearly to each apprentice. Factories were to be white washed twice a year, and at all times properly ventilated; separate sleeping apartments were to be provided for apprentices of different sexes, and not more than two were to share a bed. Apprentices were to attend Church at least once a month . . . All mills and factories were to be registered annually with the Clerk of the Peace. The Justices had power to inflict fines of £2 to £5 for neglect to observe the above regulations. [1]

That summary indicates clearly the nature of the environmental conditions in textile mills. To enforce the Act the local bench of magistrates had to appoint two of their number, one of whom had to be a clergyman, to inspect mills. This Act was of little value. Strictly, it only applied to 'apprentices' and not to children whose parents consented to them working in the mills, and, in effect, the Act was an extension of the still existing Elizabethan Poor Law system.

Sadly, at that time, the forces pressing for change realized that they could not hope to improve working conditions, especially hours of work, for adult workers, and their best chance lay in an improvement in the terms of child labour. At least Peel's Bill showed that some of the worst environmental conditions had been recognized.

Although the first census was taken in 1801, the statistical picture of the times could only be achieved by analysing data derived from Bills of mortality and the register of baptisms, neither of which were very good data sources, While the compulsory registration of births, marriages and deaths was started after 1836, it was to take 50 more years to secure the notification of some communicable diseases.

An attempt was made in about 1835, using the above sources to compare infantile mortality. Over a century, there appears to have been some improvement in the mortality rate, but in 1829 disease was still killing children under five equivalent to about 30% of the number of children born that year. The 'diseases of infancy' were, for many years, to take a great toll of young people.

The social conditions, especially of poorer people, left most of the population vulnerable to the ravages of communicable diseases, especially tuberculosis, scarlet fever and smallpox.

By the beginning of the 1830s, there was a great deal of social unrest, especially over long working hours, the insanitary and dangerous conditions in work places, poverty and bad living conditions. The pressures that had led to the **Health and Morals of Apprentices Act 1802** were supplemented by other forces but, in the then economic and political climate, rapid change was unlikely. In 1819, the Factory Act was amended, but in a short period of time there were moves to change that too.

The agitations for the reform of Parliament and local government were close to bearing fruit. **The Reform Act 1832** changed the composition of Parliament, and this was followed by the reform of the existing municipal corporations in 1835. Unfortunately, there was no perceived need to provide a comprehensive local government system.

In late 1831, cholera was introduced to Britain, the disease being imported from Europe through the port of Sunderland. By the spring of 1832, cholera had spread to many towns and cities. In London, 5275 people died with a mortality rate of almost 50%, and there was a total of about 22 000 deaths out of a population of 14 million people.

Cholera is usually thought of as a tropical disase, but here the disease was manifesting itself in the cooler months of a temperate climate:

> Conditions in all the large towns were, at this time, very favourable to the spread of cholera. Much of the drinking water came from wells in the towns themselves in close proximity to cesspools. Even when piped water supplies existed, the water was often taken from rivers grossly polluted by human sewage . . . No-one realized that the drinking of polluted water was dangerous, and indeed even at the end of the century there were still a few die hards . . . who refused to believe that drinking water was an important vehicle of infection. [2, p. 67]

While this comment describes the state of the country's towns and the standard of scientific knowledge, it can also be emphasized that there was no adequate government machinery to deal with such an outbreak.

THE ROYAL COMMISSION ON CHILD LABOUR

The major social issue of the 1830s related to factory work, and the crucial aspects were hours of work and safety. There was general support for the reduction of children's hours and for a 10 hour day for adults. When a parliamentary bill to secure this was narrowly defeated, a 'Royal Commission on Child Labour' was set up to enquire quickly into the national position so as to assuage the anger of the working people.

Edwin Chadwick, recently appointed to public office as an Assistant Poor Law Commissioner, and rapidly promoted to be a commissioner by virtue of the excellence of his work, was seconded temporarily in 1833 to be Chief Commissioner for this Royal Commission. Chadwick and a small number of close colleagues steered this enquiry, but the field work was done inadequately by Assistant Commissioners appointed through political patronage.

Because the government demanded early action, Chadwick wrote the report personally. The report's recommendations pointed to fundamental changes in the industrial health and safety scene, and laid down important principles followed in later legislation.

Central to the problem were reducing the hours children could work and those hours which adults did work, and in promoting a solution which enabled adults to work long periods of time while reducing the hours allowed for a juvenile. Chadwick argued:

> Why not reduce the hours of children even more drastically than the ten hours' limitation suggested by the operatives – so drastically that two sets of children could be used to work against the normal adult day. In this way child labour would be used but not overworked: at the same time no reduction in the adult hours need take place. [3, p. 80]

Chadwick proposed that the Act should be enforced by a centralized inspectorate, the members of which would have wide powers, be salaried, and would act as a Board and, by meeting at intervals, would produce some degree of uniformity of action. **The Factory Act 1833** empowered the inspectors to enter premises and to require the fencing, etc. of dangerous machinery and the provision of sanitary conveniences. The inspectors had powers to require a satisfactory system of schooling for all children employed in the mills, and this was the first compulsory school system.

Chadwick's report was, generally, accepted, but he was never consulted about its implementation.

EDWIN CHADWICK

Chadwick, born in Manchester in 1800, went to London at an early age, there trained as a lawyer, and became involved with the followers of Jeremy Bentham who was a radical thinker and the father of the 'utilitarian' school of philosophy. Chadwick became a major exponent of Bentham's theories, and came to know others in Bentham's circle, some of whom became close working colleagues.

The work done on **The Factory Act 1833** was a diversion from the task which was to result in Chadwick being a major influence in the development of environmental health administration.

THE ROYAL COMMISSION ON THE POOR LAWS

The poor law administration in Britain had not been significantly changed since the reign of Elizabeth I. By the 1830s, its administration was uneven and amateur, and it was costing the Poor Rate payer too much. Hence it had to be reformed, and in February 1832 a 'Royal Commission for Enquiring into the Administration and Practical Operation of the Poor Laws' was appointed.

Through the persuasion of his friend, Nassau Senior, who had been appointed a commissioner, Chadwick became an assistant commissioner with a remit to do a field study and to report. Assistants were supposed to submit a summary of their findings; Chadwick, typically, submitted a report on his research, his recommendations and indicated the philosophy on which those recommendations were based.

> It [Chadwick's contribution] was no Selection of extract but a complete Report, very long, (one-third of the entire volume was his) brilliantly executed; and working up to six clearly formulated and practical conclusions. [3, p. 103]

The Commission was prepared to ask Chadwick to draft proposals to be incorporated in the Commission's report, but a view was taken that it would be unfair to take advantage of his work without appointing him a full commissioner. This was done, and Chadwick was launched on a long, distinguished career as a reformer.

Although Chadwick had made a name in connection with the Poor Law reform, his lasting reputation came out of what was to be his life's best work. After the initial report on the Poor Law, progress on the reform was hindered by political procrastination and personal animosity, with the result that Chadwick was virtually excluded from the continuing discussions.

Because of his painstaking methods, Chadwick had looked at the causes of poverty and, from his investigations into the living conditions of the working population in England and Wales, he could hardly have failed to understand the connection between poverty and ill health and an insanitary environment. This enquiry was initiated by the government following a resolution in the House of Lords, the Poor Law Commission being instructed to carry out that investigation.

By 1841, the report on the enquiries, and the conclusions which Chadwick was drawing were almost complete but, because of political pressures, he was instructed to drop the report. However, shortly after, political control changed and he was required to complete the report.

When it was completed, there was again political interference and, on the grounds that it would cause offence, the government refused to publish it as a government report, but Chadwick was allowed to print it under his own name as his personal view ('The sanitary conditions of the labouring population of Great Britain'). It was a brilliant success and the king's printer produced many more copies than was usual for such a publication with 10 000 being distributed free of charge.

There had been previous reports with which Chadwick had been associated, and which had centred on the improvement of houses. Before he completed the 1842 report, Chadwick had changed his views, and the report advocated a shift from the improvement of the house to the improvement of its external sanitation and drainage.

Furthermore, it proposed a system; house drainage, main drainage, paving and street cleansing were now to be considered as integral parts of a single process mechanically motivated by the constant supply of water at high pressure. [3, p. 211]

THE ROYAL COMMISSION ON THE HEALTH OF TOWNS

Following further political pressures for legislation to make sanitary reform possible, and in order to prepare the way, a 'Royal Commission on the Health of Towns' was set up.

The general principles of his [Chadwick's] Report were not to be questioned by the Royal Commission. Instead the Comission was to demonstrate the various means of applying these principles. [3, p. 123]

The Commission was instructed to follow Chadwick's plan of action and it heard reports about the sanitary conditions in 50 of England's largest towns in which lived about 18% of the total population.

The Royal Commission submitted reports to Parliament in 1844 and 1845, but when a Bill was introduced it was so heavily criticized that it was abandoned. Much of the opposition to the proposed legislation came from the Health of Towns Associations, and similar bodies.

London's Association, founded in 1844 and created by Chadwick's friend, Dr Southwood Smith, was supported by many of the day's most eminent politicians. It had as its objectives the dissemination of knowledge of the evils arising from the existing insanitary environment.

THE CLAUSES ACTS AND PRIVATE LEGISLATION

By 1847, similar Associations had been created in many of the more populous cities and towns. Many of these towns had already established the practice of promoting private legislation to enable them to carry out improvement to their areas. Because similar powers were being sought,

Parliament enacted **The Town Improvement Clauses Act 1847**. This Act set out clauses which local authorities could incorporate into their own legislation and, as such clauses had already been approved, opposition to them was unlikely when new Bills containing them were introduced into Parliament.

The City of Liverpool had pioneered environmental and public health legislation in its **1846 Liverpool Sanitary Act**. This Act took powers to abolish some local bodies, such as the Commissioners of Sewers, and gave Liverpool's council sole powers to deal with drainage, paving and cleansing, etc. It also gave the council powers to appoint an officer of health, an inspector of nuisances, and a surveyor. Dr W.H. Duncan, a distinguished local physician who knew Chadwick, Southwood Smith, and William Farr was appointed as the officer of health and Thomas Fresh was given the post of inspector of nuisances.

The duties of the Medical Officer of Health are set out . . . and they are drafted as widely as possible. Under a later section [of the Act] the duties of the Inspector of Nuisances are defined, and it is clear that he was to be an officer of the Council independent of the Medical Officer of Health but compelled, by the nature of his functions, to co-operate closely with him. [4, p. 36]

Although Chadwick was very much aware of the non-medical skills required in providing a sanitary environment, his 1842 report contained a recommendation that it would be good economy to appoint an independent medical officer to 'initiate sanitary measures and reclaim the execution of the law' [4, p. 37].

The Liverpool Act became law in late 1846, and Dr Duncan took up his appointment as officer of health on January 1847.

THE PUBLIC HEALTH ACT 1848

There were further delays in making statutory provision for sanitary reform and, by 1848, there was no positive sign of progress until a cholera epidemic intervened – Britain had experienced previous epidemics of cholera and the death toll was fresh in mind. The fear of cholera made the need for sanitary reform more urgent.

The measure placed before Parliament in 1848 was far reaching as it had to create a code of sanitary legislation and an administrative machine to carry it into effect.

As the Bill went through its parliamentary stages, it was pruned and watered down. Wide opposition was generated and on many grounds, some of which reflected a fear of losing a vested interest or the reduction of personal rights. So as to get some measure on the statute book, the government appears to have surrendered to almost all the opposition. Even Chadwick argued for dropping the Lord's smoke clauses to placate manufacturers who might, otherwise, have jeopardized the whole Act [3, pp. 324–5].

The Bill, passed against a background of fear and the turbulence of the Chartist movement, was the first major public health legislation. The Act gave mainly permissive powers for the formation of Local Boards of Health. It empowered the appointment of paid officials and there was a statutory duty requiring Local Boards of Health to appoint a surveyor, inspector of nuisances and an officer of health, this latter post, statutorily protected, was available only to qualified medical staff.

The 1848 Act vested responsibility for all sewers in the Local Boards of Health. It became illegal to build a house without drains, a sanitary convenience, and an ashpit. All streets in a Board's district had to be cleansed. Except for private streets, all streets had to be paved and drained. Slaughterhouses and common lodging houses had to be registered with the Board, and cellars less than 7 feet high were prohibited for use as dwellings. Powers were also given for cleansing filthy houses.

Because of the complex pattern of authorities existing in London, the Act, which was to last for five years, did not extend to the city or the metropolitan area of London. It established a **General Board of Health**, which was to have oversight of Local Boards of Health, but this Board suffered one particular defect in that its

President was not necessarily a Minister accountable to Parliament for its activities.

When the General Board of Health was set up, Lord Morpeth, who had been the parliamentary pilot, became its President and Chadwick the paid Commissioner. The third Commissioner was Lord Ashley who was a well-respected philanthropist. Southwood Smith, who had been a mainspring of the Healthy Towns movement, was made the chief medical inspector under the **Nuisances Removal and Diseases Prevention Act of 1848**, which was enacted to give operational powers not provided in the Public Health Act 1848 and was a response to the threat of cholera.

The 1848 Act was permissive and could be adopted by the then local authorities, which could create a local board of health. Those authorities that previously had wished to improve environmental conditions in their town had had no central authority to advise them; they now had the General Board of Health. The Board could compel the establishment of a Local Board of Health in exceptional local circumstances, such as the death rate exceeding 23 per 1000 in seven successive years or, if on a petition by 10% of the rate payers, an enquiry by a superintending inspector reported that a Local Board was desirable.

The cholera epidemic, which co-incided with the 1848 Act and the establishment of the General Board of Health and Local Boards of Health, was protracted and wide spread. It started in Scotland in October 1848 after ravaging Europe and, by June the following year, it was in full force and was very severe in London, the Midlands and parts of Wales. There were 53 293 deaths in a population of about 15 million [2, p. 68].

THE ADULTERATION OF FOOD

Mention is made above about the adulteration of food partly as a consequence of the enlargement of the cities and towns and their isolation from what had been their 'door step' sources of food. Even before 1800 there had been an increasing tendency to adulterate food. Much of this was a

fraud on people rather than a means of injuring their health but, while the adulteration of, say, bread with alum fell into this category, there were some forms of adulteration which were positively dangerous.

The analytical skills needed to detect such adulteration were scarce, although some chemists practiced in this field. One of these was Frederick Accum, a skilled and well-known scientist. He undertook analyses over a long period of time and, in 1820 published *A Treatise on Adulterations of Food and Culinary Poisons*, and this was the first time that the issue had been discussed openly and objectively [5, p. 101]. Sadly, Accum left to live abroad to avoid humiliation for a trivial offence.

Further publications of a less authorative nature appeared from time to time to keep the issue alive, but in 1848 a book by John Mitchell (quoted in [5] and see also [5], pp. 106–108) largely resumed where Accum had left off. There was little public awareness of food adulteration, and no public body had power to deal systematically with it.

ASHLEY'S HOUSING ACTS

The various enquiries carried out into environmental conditions in the first half of the nineteenth century had all shown dramatically the bad conditions under which people lived. The survey which resulted in Chadwick's 1842 report, 'The sanitary conditions of the labouring population in Great Britain' was matched by Engels' 'The condition of the working classes in England in 1844' [6]. Engels is thought to have derived much information from earlier surveys.

Housing conditions *per se* were bad, and there was much overcrowding; many people shared houses and many lived in cellars. At the time Liverpool secured its Sanitary Act 1846, 7668 cellars were inhabited by about 30 000 people [6] out of a population of 370 000,

Because of the low income of working families, many were unable to rent separate accommodation, and common lodging houses and houses in multiple occupation were common [4, p. 230]. In 1851, despite the difficulties associated with such shared dwellings, two Acts, promoted by Lord Ashley, gave powers in respect of lodging houses. The first of these, **Common Lodging Houses Act 1851**, gave controls over common lodging houses which laid foundations for later forms of control; and the second Act, **Labouring Classes Lodging Houses Act 1851**, gave powers to the then local authorities to create common lodging houses as a means of reducing homelessness. Later, having become Lord Shaftesbury, Ashley admitted that his legislation had had little practical support.

THE GENERAL BOARD OF HEALTH

Strictly, the Ashley housing Acts fell into the second time phase, and it is necessary to look again at the General Board of Health. The Board was created by the Public Health Act 1848 which, itself, had a life of only five years. Under its three members, the Board was very active in attempting to establish a public health system.

Inevitably, it created opposition as it conflicted with vested interests and under Chadwick's influence, it had centralizing tendencies. Many of the Board's alleged faults were commonly ascribed to Chadwick, who became regarded as an evil genius guiding it. Because of the Board's unpopularity, the government failed to secure its renewal at the end of its five-year life. The Public Health Act 1848, however, survived.

Chadwick and Southwood Smith both retired from paid employment in 1856, but although Chadwick continued to be an influence for many more years, he never again held public office.

A new General Board of Health was set up in 1853 under the presidency of Sir Benjamin Hall. He appointed an advisory body which included Dr Neil Arnott, John Simon and William Farr. Simon was later appointed as the Board's salaried medical officer and, when the Board was disbanded in 1858 and the duties transfered to the Privy Council, John Simon became the Privy Council's medical officer, and began a career of immense importance in the development of the public health service.

COMMUNICABLE DISEASES TO 1900

A significant feature of nineteenth century social life was the impact of communicable diseases such as cholera, diphtheria and scarlet fever. There was an interrelationship between the incidence of such diseases, poor domestic environments, and the inadequacy of the sanitary infrastructure. The incidence of communicable diseases was great, the mortality rate very high, and there was little understanding of the causes of such diseases and the mechanics by which they were spread. Indeed, the actions proposed by Chadwick and others were based on the 'miasmic' (noxious vapours) theory of the spread of disease.

The Public Health Act 1848 was followed by a massive cholera epidemic, and there was a further major visitation by the disease in 1853–4, when the first General Board of Health had fallen into disfavour.

Nevertheless, those two outbreaks saw the beginning of the better understanding of the disease and how it was spread. John Simon formed views on this but the major advances were the work of John Snow.

> It is difficult . . . to appreciate the full measure of Snow's achievement, since what he proved seems so obvious, but . . . the climate of opinion before the days of bacteriology was completely different from that of the present time. Then, and for many years afterwards, the miasmic theory of the origin of infectious diseases was the one which was most generally believed. The theory was that soil polluted with excrement or refuse of any kind gave off an atmospheric 'miasma' which was the cause of certain epidemic diseases. There was nothing specific about it, and indeed it was commonly believed that one disease could change into another; for example even after the clinical distinction between typhoid and typhus had been made, it was commonly believed that one could change into the other. The 'miasmatic' theory was that on which the early movement for sanitary reform was based. [2, p. 68]

The results of Snow's first enquiries into the transmission of cholera appeared in a pamphlet in

1849 after the second epidemic. He continued his work in the later outbreak, also making use of the statistical material prepared by William Farr of the Registrar General's Office. Out of these investigations came further publications recording his findings and conclusions, the practical importance of which he demonstrated in the celebrated *Broad Street pump*. In this 1854 incident, the cases of cholera in a population served by contaminated water drawn by that pump dramatically declined when its use was discontinued by the removal of the pump handle.

Although Snow was not able to demonstrate the causative organism (that was left to a German bacteriologist, Robert Koch, in 1883), he rightly argued that a primary source of infection was consuming water polluted by infected faeces. Snow further demonstrated that propagation through the consumption of infected water was not the only method of spread, and he described the classical methods of disseminating such diseases through bad personal and culinary hygiene.

Simon and Chadwick's belief in the miasmatic theory was understandable in the light of contemporary medical knowledge, but the reforms they promoted were appropriate in laying the foundations for the improvement of public health.

Cholera returned in 1866 as an epidemic disease, but other infectious diseases, especially those related to social conditions, were of continuing importance, especially during the last three decades of the nineteenth century. Diphtheria was important, and scarlet fever frequently left severe and permanent complications.

Records show that the two diseases were often confused in the years following the onset of industrialization, possibly because of the common symptom of sore throats. After about 1830, scarlet fever resumed its virulence having been for some years in a milder form.

Up to 1856, returns of scarlet fever and diphtheria were combined, and Simon said that the disease was unknown to the vast majority of British doctors until 1855. In 1860, Duncan writing of Liverpool experience, said that diphtheria was of minor importance, and that if it was a new disease it had only appeared about three years earlier.

In 1863, the annual death rate from scarlet fever was about 4000 per million children under the age of 15 (a note on John Simon, see [4] p. 42). After the two diseases were distinguished, scarlet fever remained the more significant until about 1885, when diphtheria became more common, and for 60 years remained a major cause of infantile deaths.

Although the mortality rate from scarlet fever, and to a lesser extent diphtheria, declined, the incidence declined at a slower rate. The virulence of haemolytic bacteria of the genus *streptococcus* seems to have declined, but other factors may also have been important. The decline antedated modern chemotherapy, but slight improvements in housing, including a reduction in overcrowding, and slightly better dietary regimes may well have been contributory factors.

The incidence of most communicable diseases was greatest in the sections of the community that were poorest in terms of housing, nutrition, wealth and leisure. Tuberculosis, was a disease that affected all classes. It was endemic but its incidence was greatest in poorer areas where housing was bad, nutrition poor because of poverty, ignorance, or social habits, and where workers laboured in damp, dusty, or hot conditions, and where the work necessitated long, excessive hours of strenuous toil.

After about 1850, the incidence of tuberculosis declined continuously. There was no useful drug to combat the disease but rest, reduced stress, improved diet and fresh air were held to be curative and, from the last quarter of the century, sanatoria providing treatment on these lines were built.

THE ADULTERATION OF FOOD TO 1900

While chemistry was more advanced in the mid-nineteenth century than medical science, little was done to follow the work of Accum in 1820 until almost the middle of the century, when John Mitchell showed that there had been a continued increase in food adulteration.

Food at that time was seriously adulterated, and it was discovered that the public had become accustomed to the flavour of such foods and liked neither the flavour nor appearance of unadulterated food. Some pioneers, such as the emerging co-operative societies, which aimed to provide a fair service (including pure food) for their members, met strong consumer opposition, and one society experienced such difficulty in selling unadulterated tea that it employed a lecturer to tell its members what good tea was really like!

Mitchell's work induced an active response, and much publicity, especially through articles published in the *Lancet*. Following public pressure, parliament appointed a select committee to enquire into food adulteration. The facts which were unearthed made parliamentary action inevitable, and resulted in the **Adulteration of Food Act 1860**.

The Act disappointed radical reformers, and evidence suggests that it was a failure. It gave no sampling powers to local authorities, but allowed the appointment of public analysts to deal with suspected food presented by private citizens prepared to pay for the analysis.

The position created by the 1860 Act was clearly unsatisfactory, and it was unlikely to achieve the reforms that were desired. In 1860 it was exceptional for there to be legislative interference in the free working of the economy, but the 1860 Act was a breach in that dyke.

In the decade that followed, there was a persistent stream of criticism and demands were made for more effective safeguards. In 1868, proposals were made to amend the 1860 Act. Those intentions met with obstruction and delay, and not until 1872 was the law amended by the **Adulteration of Food, Drink, and Drugs Act 1872**.

Progress towards a satisfactory code was being made slowly. The 1872 Act made it an offence to sell food, drink, or drugs which were not of the 'nature substance or quality' demanded by the purchaser, and this has been the basis of all later food control legislation. The Act gave limited powers to appoint public analysts, but its most important provision was to permit inspectors of nuisances, as well as private persons, to acquire samples of food for analysis. This power resulted in systematic and increased sampling of foods,

and a marked increase in the number of cases of food adulteration being detected.

Despite the improved legislation, the 1872 Act still had some deficiencies, and a select committee was appointed in 1874 to examine how the 1872 Act was working. Out of its findings, the **Sale of Food and Drugs Act 1875** was passed.

The 1875 Act, although amended and extended later, formed the basic legislation followed in later revisions of the law. Some important issues had to be decided on appeal to the High Court, including the reversal of the judgement that an inspector purchasing a sample for analysis could not be prejudiced. Much of the then adulteration, the addition of water to milk and spirits, was fraudulent rather than a danger to health – provided the water was pure!

The public analysts had a crucial role. The Society of Public Analysts was formed in 1874, and most of the practitioners were members. It published its proceedings, gave a stimulus to analytical chemistry, and developed new tests and standards of purity. In particular, the Society played an important role in establishing the limits beyond which an article of food would be regarded as being adulterated, and many of its recommended standards achieved statutory recognition.

MILK AND MEAT TO 1900

For urban populations, the supply of milk and meat has always presented problems. For many years, the main source of milk for town dwellers was cows kept in sheds within the built-up area. For the supply of meat, the practice was to buy animals at country sales, drive them into the towns and slaughter them in small, back street slaughterhouses. Back street cowsheds and slaughterhouses were conducive to the transmission of disease and the creation of serious nuisance.

Cattle, closely confined in insanitary sheds, were very susceptible to disease. Tuberculosis, in particular, could be transmitted to those who drank the milk. Furthermore, in an age when food adulteration was extensively practised, milk was adulterated by the fraudulent addition of water. For residents near to the cowsheds there were nuisances from odours, flies and the disposal of manure. The coming of the railways made possible the rapid carriage into the towns of rurally produced milk, and this was the prime cause of the decline of the town-kept cow population.

Slaughtering animals in the small, urban slaughterhouses created nuisances from noise, odours, flies and the disposal of the by-products of slaughter. For many people the trade itself was repugnant.

The recognition of the potential for nuisance and the sale of diseased meat led to the early regulation of the trade by some of the growing towns. **The Manchester Police Act 1844** gave powers to control the slaughtering of animals to prevent nuisance, for the licensing of new and the registration of existing slaughterhouses, and for the appointment of slaughterhouse inspectors who had power to inspect not only slaughterhouses, but meat and other foodstuffs.

The 1844 Act also showed that, at that time, there was no concept of an impartial and uncorrupt administration, as inspectors appointed under the Act were required to make a statutory declaration that they would act honestly.

A similar local Act in 1846 gave Manchester Borough Council powers to licence butchers or fishmongers shops.

Although the Sale of Food and Drugs Act had been passed in 1875, its provisions were augmented by **The Public Health Act 1875** which authorized medical officers of health and inspectors of nuisances to inspect food exposed or deposited for sale; it gave powers to seize unfit food; it made provision for the named officers to enter slaughterhouses and premises used for the sale of meat, so that animals slaughtered could be inspected.

HOUSING TO 1900

Reference has already been made to Lord Shaftesbury's 1851 Lodging Houses Acts. These Acts had little impact. Despite the poor conditions

under which most of the population lived, it was not until 1868 that there was further significant legislation. That Act and a subsequent housing statute in 1879 (both designated as the **Torrens Acts**) made changes which enabled local authorities to deal with individual insanitary houses. While these were useful powers, they did not permit local authorities to deal with areas of bad housing.

Some areas of bad housing were demolished under commercial pressures. With no security of tenure, possession of a tenanted house could be obtained easily by the owner, who would sell if he had a favourable offer from a developer or a railway company wanting access to a town centre. The first statutory powers to deal with areas of unfit houses were obtained by the City of Manchester in private Act legislation in 1867.

Further social pressures resulted in legislation in 1875 and 1879, which permitted local authorities to deal with areas of insanitary houses by clearing them and redeveloping the sites. Of the two Acts, collectively known as the **Cross Acts**, the first, the **Artisans and Labourers Dwelling Improvement Act 1875**, allowed councils to deal with unhealthy houses by buying the land and buildings for the purpose of improvement. Councils were allowed to build houses or let the land for building subject to schemes having special regard to providing accommodation for the working classes. Where owners refused to sell land, provision was made for compulsory purchase.

There was an interesting connection between the 1875 Cross Act and **the Public Health Act 1875**, for the latter gave powers to councils to make building bye-laws. Progressive local authorities adopted such bye-laws, and were thus able to have some control over the building standards for houses built to replace the insanitary dwellings that had been demolished.

Although some legislative provision had been made, the operation of the Torrens Acts and Cross Acts was expensive, and many local authorities showed little initiative in tackling insanitary housing conditions in their areas. Because of public pressure, Parliament appointed two select committes of the House of Commons in 1881 and

1882, and the **Artisans Dwelling Act 1882** resulted from those enquiries.

Despite this and the efforts of the Local Government Board, progress was slow, and public opinion reflected this. In 1884, a Royal Commission was appointed to enquire into the housing of the working classes. A number of very distinguished people served on that commission, and it heard evidence from such prominent public figures as Lord Shaftesbury (who conceded that his lodging house legislation of 1851 had not been a success), and Chadwick who appeared as president for the Association of Sanitary Inspectors.

Out of the work of the Royal Commission came the **Housing of the Working Classes Act 1885**. The Act required appropriate local authorities to use the powers they already had with regard to insanitary housing in order to achieve proper sanitary conditions of all dwellings in their district; it gave powers to make bye-laws to deal with houses let in lodgings, and required the supervision of tents and vans used for dwellings.

With tenure pattern for housing being heavily dominated by rented dwellings, it is important to note both that some charitable trusts provided 'working class' houses, and managed their properties with some enlightenment. In this regard, Octavia Hill (granddaughter of Southwood Smith) pioneered better housing management and, in particular, worked with the tenants of houses to improve their living standards.

In 1890, housing legislation was consolidated in the **Housing of the Working Classes Act 1890**. In terms of practical housing administration, the Act had three main parts dealing with unhealthy areas and improvement schemes, unfit dwelling houses, and powers for local authorities to provide lodging houses. This Act, both consolidating and pioneering, provided the administrative procedures and concepts which were followed in subsequent revisionary housing measures.

Although the housing legislation noted was enacted with good intentions, it was flawed to the extent that to implement it required local authorities to spend considerable sums of money which they had to raise themselves. At this time, local authorities were traditionally careful spenders of their revenue, and only in rare cases was there to

be found a zeal for improving the local housing. Some of the large northern industrial towns engaged in longer term plans, and were enterprising in finding legal authority for carrying out their plans of improvement.

AIR POLLUTION TO 1900

By the early 1850s, air pollution was still a major problem in London and the large cities. There was an increasing number of factories which burned coal, and the population continued to grow, which resulted in a rise in air pollution from coal-burning fires. The growth of mining, metal and chemical industries in the rural areas created air pollution in the countryside.

There was little effective control of air pollution in terms of both legislation and field enforcement. However, the situation was changing gradually, and failure to secure legislation focused attention on the problem.

Simon tried to secure some provision for smoke control in the City of London and eventually succeeded in 1851. While this measure applied only to the City there was strong pressure for the powers to be extended to the whole of London. In 1852, a petition to Parliament resulted in the promotion of an appropriate Bill to control smoke in London. The opposed Bill was pruned to meet the demands of critics, but it emerged as the **Smoke Nuisance (Metropolis) Act 1853**.

There was a bonus for this success in that the prime minister, Lord Palmerston, insisted that the Act should be properly enforced. Out of the defence arguments arose an interesting concept.

> . . . the danger now was whether or not the defendant had used best practicable means . . . This formula, so common it became abbreviated to b.p.m. and it persists to this day . . . it began as a great obstacle to the enforcement of clean air laws, it evolved into an indispensible prescription for their effective enforcement. [7, p. 74]

There were further improvements to smoke control in the **Local Government Act 1858**, and the **Sanitary Act 1866**, but despite the powers in the 1866 Act, local sanitary authorities were unable to reduce the smoke burden. There were three reasons for this failure. Some local Act powers were flawed by faulty procedural requirements; the fines imposed by magistrates were often derisory; and any improvement in industrial air pollution was offset by the increased pollution from the additional dwellings built to house the growing population.

THE EMERGENCE OF A CENTRAL POLLUTION INSPECTORATE

After about 1830, the alkali industry grew rapidly and large quantities of acid were discharged, despite the fact that by 1836 a remedy for this was known. Many plants in the chemical industry produced not only visible smoke, but also invisible fumes which were dangerous to health, and damaged the fabric of buildings and plants. Such emissions were fairly localized and usually came from plants situated in rural areas.

In 1862, this issue was brought before the House of Lords and a 'Select Committee was appointed to enquire into the injury resulting from noxious vapours evolved in certain manufacturing processes and into the law relating thereto'. [7, p. 21]

The prime mover in this, Lord Derby, was anxious not to make the issue one of landowners versus factory owners, but he wanted to discover whether legislative control was possible.

The select committee, advised by more skilled experts than had testified to earlier enquiries, reported very quickly and recommended that there should be legislation, and that it should be enforced by independent officers free of local control and influence.

A Central inspectorate could ensure consistency, exchange information in control technique, and acquire an expertise that would not be possible amongst officials acting for a score or more local boards of health, boards of Guardians and the like. [7, p. 22]

The Bill, introduced in 1863, fell short of the recommendations of the select committee, but it did create an inspectorate within the Board of Trade and, thus, gave victory to the centralists. The Bill was opposed but was enacted as the **Alkali Act 1863**, and this made provision for the first **Alkali Inspectorate**.

The Act was a landmark. It confirmed the view that central government should take action to protect the public from noxious vapours; it allowed, for the first time, for inspectors to enter factories to protect not the workers, but people and property outside; the inspectors were to be experts from the beginning, would serve a central department and be insulated from local interference.

The 1863 Act was to last only for five years, but was renewed and the Inspectorate became established and its role was gradually expanded. It devised methods of working which became characteristic of its operation – patience and few prosecutions.

In the 1880s attention was being focused on industrial smoke in urban areas, and on domestic smoke in London. The struggle for clean air involved combating the argument that control action was not justified, because smoke was not proved to be injurious to health. Previous work had shown a correlation between smokey fog and mortality.

In 1880, the Hon. F.A.R. Russell published a book on London fogs, in which he showed that London fogs increased mortality but, that because the effect was slow and diffused throughout the population, it received little attention.

OCCUPATIONAL HEALTH TO 1900

Much attention had been focused on the lot of the factory worker, and especially the juvenile employee; less note had been taken of the conditions under which shop workers laboured. Many shop premises were ill ventilated, overcrowded with stock, and had very limited welfare facilities. Shop assistants worked very long hours and had limited facilities for refreshment or rest. In very many larger shops, the assistants lived on the premises in attics over the shops.

In 1873, an attempt to limit hours of shop work failed but, because of pressure, a House of

Commons Committee looked at the position in 1886, and declared that the long hours worked normally were ruinous to health, especially to young women. Three hundred London doctors petitioned Parliament to support the Bill before it. The **Shop Hours Act 1886** limited the working hours of young people to 74 per week including meal times. This Act was short lived and a further Parliamentary committee examined the position and, although the 1886 Act had failed, similar provisions were made in the **Shops Act 1892**, but even that Act was flawed and it had to be amended in 1893 and 1895.

One group of workers whose practices were changed as a consequence of industrial development were the farm workers, where mechanical aids had been introduced. These increased productivity, but could be extremely hazardous, and specific legislation had to be introduced to give protection against some of the more dangerous machines.

As central government became aware of its incapacity to supervise the expanding number of premises which should be visited, intervention in industrial activities had to be increased. At first, the difficulty was met by increasing staff, but the **Workshop Regulation Act 1867** brought most manual workers under supervision and, experimentally, local authorities were involved.

The experiment lasted for four years, and was then abandoned. The reasons for the failure were that the powers given to local authorities were impracticable to work, and local authorities, on the whole, failed to administer the Act satisfactorily. In some cases, there was deliberate inaction and, in others, local influence adversely affected the local inspectorate. Thus, the **Factories Act 1871** enacted simply 'it shall cease to be the duty of the local authority to enforce the provisions of the Workshops Acts 1867–71 and it shall be the duties of the inspectors and sub inspectors of factories to enforce the provisions of these Acts' [1, p. 230].

For some years, the enforcement of occupational health law was unsatisfactory. This was partly the consequence of changes in the legislation, which failed to provide either comprehensive powers or an efficient administrative system.

Even the changes made by the **Public Health Act 1875** caused confusion.

By 1891, further factory legislation was required. Local authorities were again involved in occupational health issues and, in the **Factory Act 1891**, they were made responsible for the sanitary conveniences in factories and for cleanliness, ventilation, overcrowding and limewashing in workshops. Local authority inspectors were given the same powers for their duties as factory inspectors under the principal Act.

In making this change, central government rehearsed all the arguments for not using local authorities but decided, on balance, that they had the staff and the local knowledge that was required. Local authorities were required to notify the factory inspectorate of workshops found within their area.

From the evidence available, it seems clear that local authorities performed rather better under the new Act, but still not well enough, and an 1895 Act required them to report back to the factory inspector of action taken to deal with complaints from him. This and other changes in local government attitudes lead to a more vigorous enforcement, and the employment of specialist officers to do the work.

CONSTITUTIONAL AND INSTITUTIONAL DEVELOPMENTS

1875 was a year notable for the legislation enacted that involved environmental health issues. In many ways, the **Public Health Act 1875** was one of the most important statutes of the century, for it contained specific provisions to improve public health, and it created an administrative framework within which local government was to develop in the following century or so.

Following **The Public Health Act 1848**, the public health service experienced many difficulties in establishing itself and, in particular, it never enjoyed the political protection of a high-ranking minister. Even when John Simon was responsible to the Privy Council for the public health service, the situation was little improved despite his enthusiasm, administrative skills, and incisive reports.

After considerable pressure, agreement was reached in 1868 for the appointment of a **Royal Commission to examine the problems of sanitary administration**. There was a change in government, and the incoming Liberal administration appointed a Royal Commission in 1869. It was to examine the sanitary circumstances in England and Wales but excluded London, and it was to look at central as well as local organization.

Simon had strong views as to what was needed – a strong central administration overseen by a minister, a system of local, all-purpose sanitary/public health authorities, and comprehensive new public health legislation building on experience and responding to contemporary need. Simon was not to see all of these achieved, despite the recommendations of the Royal Commission's report in 1871. That report was accepted fully, and out of it sprang three Acts of Parliament.

In many ways, the most important of those three Acts was the **Local Government Board Act 1871**. This established the **Local Government Board**, which became responsible for Poor Law and public health functions, and other relevant ancilliary activities. Under the **Public Health Act 1872**, an attempt was made to simplify the system of local authorities by mapping out areas for which would be created a local authority to exercise within its area all the Sanitary Acts, thus creating urban and rural sanitary authorities. The Local Government Board was also empowered to create sanitary authorities for ports.

While the creation of the Local Government Board was an important step in the creation of a comprehensive local government system which would enjoy specific parliamentary support, there were other factors to note. It was significant that the proposal for the 1869 Royal Commission was acceptable to the government, and to the opposition which had initiated the proposal. Thus it was probable that future legislation would be easier to achieve because of an informal concensus of view.

Perhaps of greater significance was the change in informed public opinion towards issues which had social importance and, with the weakening of

laissez-faire influences, interventionist policies became much easier to introduce and defend. Political power was shifting from centre and rightist bases, towards a somewhat more radical stance which underpinned the desire in influential quarters to extend the franchise into the lower middle classes.

In practical terms, the third Act, the **Public Health Act 1875**, made the greatest impact. This Act provided a comprehensive range of environmental health powers dealing with local authority areas and powers, sewage, drainage, water supplies, nuisances, offensive trades, the protection of food, infectious diseases, highways, street markets, slaughterhouses and the making of bye-laws.

The Act of 1875 was drafted with some vision. Its provisions gave substance to an administrative system which was flexible and amenable to extension, and it made possible the very great progress made in the last quarter of the century in improving the sanitary circumstances of the country.

In 1876 the **Sanitary Institute of Great Britain** was founded. This organization was initiated by a distinguished group of people, including Chadwick, and was dedicated to the exchange of knowledge and to the examination of candidates for professional qualifications in surveying and as inspectors of nuisances. It later became the **Royal Sanitary Institute**, and is now the **Royal Society for the Promotion of Health**. For many years, it continued to examine sanitary inspectors, but later formed part of the examining body known as the Royal Sanitary Institute and the Sanitary Inspectors Examination Joint Board. The Royal Society of Health continues to have a diminishing interest in the overseas qualifications of environmental health officers.

In 1883, the **Sanitary Inspectors Association** was founded as an amalgamation of smaller local bodies, and the organization has continued, using various designations, to expand in membership and influence. It currently operates under a Royal Charter as the **Chartered Institute of Environmental Health**. Its first President was Chadwick and while formerly the Institution members were all qualified environmental health officers, other grades of membership are open to persons holding some approved qualification appropriate to environmental health practice.

THE NOTIFICATION OF COMMUNICABLE DISEASES

A flaw in the Public Health Act 1875 was its failure to create a system for the notification of cases of infectious diseases. This was a long perceived need and medical officers for areas where communicable diseases were most prevalent – the densely populated inner cities – had recognized the impediment to epidemiological enquiries caused by the lack of the information which notification would provide.

Some local authorities took private Act powers which enabled them to require notification of some diseases. Fourteen years were to elapse before there was attempted a general notification requirement – in 1889, the **Infectious Diseases Notification Act** was passed which allowed local authorities to adopt powers to require notification.

This was an inadequate measure, but it remained for a decade until supplemented by the **Infectious Diseases Act (Extension Act) 1889**, which required all sanitary authorities to adopt the 1889 Act. The 1889 Act listed 11 diseases which had to be notified to the sanitary authority and, furthermore, it empowered the Local Government Board to list other disease by order.

Although the notification of communicable diseases was not compulsory until near the end of the century, various powers existed which allowed local authorities to act to prevent such diseases, but the lack of knowledge of *all* cases clearly hampered satisfactory control. In this context, Frazer wrote:

> The system of notification . . . has proved to be of the greatest possible value to medical officers of health in dealing with epidemics because early notification is vital to prevent further cases arising. [4, p. 181]

The compulsory notification of specified communicable diseases was consolidated in the **Public Health Act 1936**. Subsequently further diseases were added to the list either by regulations or, notably, by the **Food and Drugs Act 1938**, which required the notification of food poisoning, and there was a further consolidation in the **Public Health (Prevention of Disease) Act 1984**.

The control of communicable disease at ports of entry was a feature of the early development of public health (see Chapters 2 and 13).

REGISTRATION OF BIRTHS AND DEATHS

Apart from the ten yearly census, public authorities had few authoritative statistics to guide them. A Select Committee of the House of Commons was appointed in 1833 to investigate the position with regard to births and deaths, and from their recommendations came the **Births and Deaths Registration Act 1836**.

The objectives of this Act were to establish the General Register office, to appoint a **Registrar General**, and to institute a system of registering all births and deaths. Before that date, the only statistics were to be culled from parish registers.

The reputation achieved by the Registrar General's Office in the next 40 years was mainly due to Dr William Farr, who was appointed the compiler of medical statistics. His work was pioneering and his reports were fundamental to the development of epidemiology and of demographic studies. Farr's appointment is believed to have been due to Chadwick, and Farr is included, with Chadwick, among the great pioneers of public health.

MINISTRY OF HEALTH

Noted above was the formation of the Local Government Board. Because of subsequent developments and extensions in the Public Health and Poor Law services, the Board was identified as being a less than satisfactory administrative machine.

The formation of a Ministry of Health had been advocated for many years by various persons for a variety of reasons. By 1918, it became obvious that changes had to be made in public health administration and, in 1919, the Ministry of Health was established to take over the functions of the Local Government Board and other duties. It was made responsible for some social services and most activities which had a health connotation, although a notable exception was the retention of the occupational health service by the Factory Inspectorate. The first Minister of Health was Dr Christopher Addison, later associated with housing legislation.

COMMUNICABLE DISEASES 1900– PRESENT

Although there were no further epidemics of cholera, other communicable diseases continued to be important in the first half of the twentieth century. The virulence of scarlet fever appeared to decline after about 1883, but it is difficult to assign a reason.

The disease with which scarlet fever was most associated, diphtheria, was, however, to remain a serious cause of infant mortality until the 1940s. There was a slow decline to around 300 deaths per annum per million children under 15 in the period 1921–5, and that remained a plateau until 1940 when immunization was available which virtually eliminated the disease.

Although anti-toxin was first used to treat the disease in 1895, and a satisfactory immunization regime was available in 1923, it was not utilized until 1940. Subsequently, a continuous immunization campaign has kept the disease under control with only an occasional case arising.

One communicable disease which was a potent cause of infant death was **summer diarrhoea**. The incidence and mortality rate had already been declining for 20 years, but in 1911 there were still 31 000 deaths of infants under 1 year due to diarrhoea, but by 1931 this was reduced to 11 705. There was medical controversy as to its cause, and the state of bacteriological science at the century's turn was such that it could throw no positive light on the causes or the mode of transmission.

The best opinion took the view that it was fly borne, and this was an opinion well supported by the fact that the disease was prevalent in summer when flies bred in back street stable middens, and that the disease declined when the horse ceased to be a major form of transport. There were other factors in reducing the disease's incidence, such as higher standards of domestic hygiene and baby care.

For **tuberculosis**, a 'social' disease, both the incidence and the mortality rate continued to fall, although there were temporary distortions in the pattern in both the time and place of cases. The environmental conditions imposed by two world wars and economic depression encouraged continued decline. Factors which have contributed to the improved circumstances include better nutritional standards, improved domestic hygiene, better occupational hygiene, reduced working hours with less physical stress, reduced overcrowding and better housing conditions.

Immunization against tuberculosis has played a part, as has the more recent (post-1945) availability of chemotherapy. Nevertheless, there have been some disturbing trends in urban communities with a high proportion of ethnic population, or where there is poverty. Immigrants may be at especial risk where they arrive from areas where there has been no chance to acquire natural immunity and where, on arrival, dietary changes and poor housing may be contributory factors.

The elimination of **smallpox** in 1980, following the WHO campaign, has been a relief to public health workers. The two varieties of smallpox have been the cause of epidemics in the UK.

Although for many years smallpox was epidemic in Britain it is probably true that since 1914 major smallpox has always been exotic though it has not always been possible to prove this as source tracing has not always been successful. [2, p. 56]

The public health control of smallpox developed because it was a serious disease with a high mortality rate. The control encompassed vaccination, notification, isolation, and effective disinfection regimes. After 1906, the incidence of Asiatic smallpox – variola major – dropped to negligible proportions, but variola minor continued to be a serious problem with 70 000 cases in the UK between 1925 and 1931.

The elimination of smallpox as a human contagious disease represents a triumph for international control and co-operation. It is perhaps an irony that probably the last cases of smallpox occurred in Britain, the home of vaccination, through the accidental release of laboratory specimen viruses.

The incidence of communicable disease does vary and illnesses have different importance at different times. In the 1980s and 1990s sexually transmitted disease was emphasized with the spread of HIV/AIDS (acquired immune deficiency syndrome) which is a socially threatening condition. Cholera became more widespread internationally and the risk of importing cases through speedy air travel was important. Domestically meningoccal meningitis became increasingly common and there was a high degree of awareness of the risk of importing rabies. Also important have been outbreaks of legionnaire's disease and food-borne disease due to *listeria*.

TREATMENT OF COMMUNICABLE DISEASES

The high incidence and mortality of communicable diseases in the nineteenth century reflects the poor domestic environment of most people, a low standard of medical and nursing care because medical science had yet to make its major advances, and the lack of drugs to treat the diseases. That the position gradually improved was due to the provision of drainage, safer water supplies, better refuse disposal, improved housing, and better diet.

Significant discoveries concerning the causative organisms of many serious diseases were not made until the last quarter of the nineteenth century.

Modern chemotherapy may be said to have started in 1910 when Ehrlich discovered salvarsan and made the treatment of syphilis possible. Perhaps the next important step was the introduction in the 1930s of the sulphonamide drugs, which were a product of the dyestuffs industry. These transformed the treatment of many diseases, as did the introduction of penicillin, the discovery of Sir Alexander Fleming, during the Second World War. In the post-1945 period, the development of new drugs and antibiotics has proceeded apace.

Perhaps beginning with vaccination against smallpox, introduced by Jenner in the late eighteenth century, there have been major advances in dealing with communicable diseases by the development of immunization regimes. Vaccination gives protection against infection, and modern thought is still that 'prevention is better than cure'.

HOUSING 1900–PRESENT

At the turn of the century, the basic housing legislation was still the **Housing of the Working Classes Act 1890**, although amending Acts were passed in 1900 and 1903. Despite this legislation, the standard of housing for poorer people left much to be desired, although there had been some slum clearance and house building in London and northern cities.

A feature of the growth of the built environment was that not until 1909 were there any provisions for town planning. The planning powers in the **Housing and Town Planning Act 1909** were permissive for local authorities which showed little enthusiasm to exploit its provisions, although some did. The provisions, permitting the control of land use, were intended to act as a brake on unrestricted development which had little regard to amenity and community interests. House construction was subject to little control because of the inadequacies of building bye-laws.

As far as housing was concerned, the 1909 Act amended the Housing of the Working Classes Act 1890, and made it mandatory in all districts. It prohibited for the first time the erection of back-to-back houses, which were still being constructed in some northern industrial cities. The Act also recognized that public utility societies, such as building societies, could be responsible for house building.

The relationship between planning and a satisfactory built environment had been recognized. In 1898 Ebenezer Howard published his seminal work, *Tomorrow, a Peaceful Path to Real Reform*, which advocated the building of new garden suburbs that were self-sufficient and isolated from other suburbs by a green belt, but with easy means of communication with them. Howard, a practical person as well as a philosophical theorist, was the driving force of the Garden Cities Association and he witnessed the successful founding of Letchworth Garden city in 1902. The 'new town' movement developed largely from Howard's initiatives.

There was a further Housing and Town Planning Act in 1919, but the housing provisions of the 1909 and 1919 Acts were repealed by and re-enacted in the **Housing Act 1925**.

Because of the shortage of houses and promises made to service men returning from the war, attempts were made to stimulate house building, and powers were taken in the **Housing Act 1919**. The shortage of houses is indicated by the fact that nationally in 1911 9.1% of the population lived at more than two per room, and by 1921 the census showed that this had risen to 9.6%. With the aid of government subsidies 176 000 houses were built under the 1919 Act by local authorities at considerable cost.

Further Housing Acts in 1923 and 1924 were designed to continue the stimulation of house building, but at a less extravagant rate of subsidy. This legislation was successful and by 1927 an annual output exceeding 270 000 dwellings was achieved.

These early 1920s Housing Acts were designed to stimulate house building, but they did little to address other housing problems, and the much amended and extended 1890 Act was no longer able to meet current needs. In view of this, the existing legislation concerning the repair, maintenance and sanitary condition of houses was consolidated by the **Housing Act 1925**.

By the late 1920s, it became apparent that much remained to be done to deal with the unsatisfactory housing situation. Building houses for sale rather than for renting was more profitable and the output of rentable houses declined.

It was estimated that there were several million insanitary houses:

> The outside estimate . . . was 4 000 000 but . . . that would depend upon the definition of a slum. In other words, a slum is what the Medical Officer of Health of the District believes to be a slum. What was beyond doubt, however, was that the slum evil in many of the industrial towns, especially London, Liverpool, and Glasgow was of vast dimensions, and that much harm to the Public Health was being caused by the delay – inexplicable to many people – in dealing with this problem as a matter of the greatest possible urgency. [8, p. 60]

The **Housing Act 1930** was the government's response. It was not a fully comprehensive measure as it omitted to deal with overcrowding, but made provision for the clearance of insanitary housing, and it prescribed procedures to be followed to make clearance and improvement areas. It required housing accommodation to be provided in advance for those to be rehoused and created the principle that compensation should not be payable in respect of unfit houses.

With regard to the proposed improvement areas, which were envisaged as being large areas of houses and other properties, local authorities were empowered to demolish or repair unfit dwellings, buy land and demolish buildings so as to leave a developable site. Local authorities had to deal with overcrowding, which Parliament failed to define.

The concept of the improvement area was directed against urban decay. While local authorities used the clearance powers widely, they were reluctant to experiment with improvement areas.

The **Housing Act 1935** made changes in the procedures for dealing with redevelopment, although this was little used. The Act did, however, tackle the problem of overcrowding by defining it. It required local authorities to survey all houses below a given rateable value and to certify the numbers of persons allowed to dwell in such houses. Local authorities were also empowered to deal with overcrowding cases of which it became aware. The **Housing Act 1936** consolidated previous practical, as opposed to financial, housing legislation, and considerable slum clearance and repair activity was stimulated.

The Second World War brought virtually all housing activity, slum clearance, and new building to a stop. What repair resources were available were diverted to dealing with war damage, so that there was little routine maintenance of houses.

At the end of the war, housing was in extreme stress. Physically, the housing stock had been depleted by air raids; many houses had drifted into unfitness because of lack of maintenance; few of the formerly unfit houses had been demolished; and very few new houses had been built. Sociologically, the position was exacerbated by the effective demand for higher housing standards; by the abandonment of houses perceived as being unfit for habitation; and the increased rate of household formation.

The housing question became important politically and sociologically, as well as from the aspect of public health. It became apparent that future action would have to encompass the removal of unfit housing, the elimination of overcrowding, and the repair and improvement of the housing stock.

In the years after 1948, there was a succession of Housing Acts designed to promote competing political programmes for house building, slum clearance and improvement. **The Housing Act 1949** made the first provision for the improvement of houses through grant aid although, in the light of subsequent developments, this was an experimental and meagre approach.

The Housing Act 1954 required local authorities to survey all the houses in their district to determine which dwellings were unfit for habitation. These surveys revealed the magnitude of the task. In the big cities, the rate of unfitness was staggering. In Birmingham, 16% of all houses were judged to be unfit, in Manchester 33%, and in Liverpool 43%.

The Housing Act 1957 was a fundamental restatement of housing law, which made significant changes to the law relating to repair and clearance of unfit properties. For the first time, England and Wales were given a statutory defini-

tion of what constituted a fit house, and that definition was wide enough to permit a liberal interpretation of what constituted unfitness. Prior to that the standard of unfitness had to be related to the general local standard of housing; the new definition applied nationally and allowed districts where housing standards were low to bring their housing gradually to the national level.

The Housing Act 1964 contained important provisions relating to the supply of water to houses and the possibility of grant aid in that regard. Attention began to focus on other aspects of housing that could affect human health, such as the improvement of houses, the universal provision of standard amenities, and the upgrading of whole areas by the repair and improvement of the houses and softening of the external environment.

The Housing Act 1969 was largely the legislative outcome of the report of the **Denington Committee** (*Our Older Homes – a call for action*). It suggested the need for a fresh approach to house improvement, and emphasized the impact a bad external environment had on housing. Out of this legislation came the concept of the general improvement area.

It was, of course, impossible to discuss housing except by understanding what constituted a satisfactory house. While the Housing Act 1957 had set out a standard of fitness, it did not address such questions as space and amenity.

In 1953, a working party under Mr Parker Morris was set up to enquire into, and make recommendations for, standards of accommodation in houses. The report from that working party was well received, and the standards it promoted were adopted widely by local authorities and better house builders. However, at a later date, in the interests of financial economy, these standards were less observed.

In the 1970s and 1980s, there were further Housing Acts. Most of these were designed to liberalize and stimulate the repair, renovation and, especially, the improvement of houses individually and in areas. With **The Housing Act 1974** came the concept of the **housing action area**, where the intention was to provide minimum repair and improvement to houses which were of poor standard and likely to be included in clearance proposals within ten years. This was an imaginative approach to the challenge to provide early improvement of living conditions in houses which were approaching the end of their useful life. Sadly, the impact of inflation on building and improvement costs made the schemes impracticable, except to a standard of repair and improvement to ensure a 30-year life.

This Act also made radical, and enhancing, changes to the improvement grants schemes, and initiated a decade of great activity in the rehabilitation of houses.

The Housing Act 1980 was designed to tidy up the provisions for house improvements, but it also made radical changes to tenure patterns, including the power of tenants of local authority owned dwellings to purchase the houses at substantial discounts. This was a right denied to tenants of rented houses in other ownership.

By the early 1980s, it was realized that the postwar housing legislation needed consolidation, and this was achieved in **The Housing Act 1985** which drew the threads together but made few changes.

The main object of the **Housing Act 1988** was to alter, again, the pattern of tenures. The main thrust of the previous decade had been towards increased owner occupation of houses, and houses sold out of the rented stock for owner occupation obviously diminished the rented sector pool, which caused difficulties. By introducing new forms of tenancy, it was hoped to induce more owners to put houses into the pool for renting, but this did not occur.

The Act also introduced a scheme to create housing action trusts in which it was hoped that large, run-down council housing estates would opt for management by such trusts, which were promised liberal support denied to local authorities to enable them to deal with their own houses.

It had also become apparent that the liberalization of the house improvement scheme had led to much grant aid being given for properties not in the greatest need of repair and improvement, and the **Local Government and Housing Act 1989** aimed to redress that balance. There was also a great need to make the improvement grant system less cumbersome to operate. The 1989 Act

addressed these problems, making radical changes in housing law including a new concept of the fitness of a house, the nature of grants available (but retaining the concept of a mandatory grant), and provided for the testing of an applicant's ability to contribute to the cost. These new provisions and procedures made most local authorities revise their private housing sector activities.

In the 1980s there was a significant shift in political opinion in respect of public involvement in housing policies, from considerations of the health and welfare of house occupiers, to financial and sociological aspects. Local authority tenants were empowered to buy their houses, thus introducing enclaves of private property into monolithic, council-owned estates. It gradually became very difficult for councils to build new houses to enable them to continue to provide rented accommodation. Increasingly, the private sector and housing associations were entrusted with the provision of rented housing, while the drive towards increased owner occupation encouraged private house building.

The statutory overcrowding provisions remained, but were largely ignored as being irrelevant in the postwar era with most local authorities working to their own, higher standards.

Throughout the industrial period, dwellings used for multiple or common occupation have been a problem. Multiple occupation continued as a serious issue in many towns and, although grant aid became available for improving such properties, many continued to be grossly unsatisfactory. There was much pressure by interested groups to secure legislation that would permit a more effective control, but the law remains to be comprehensively overhauled.

The worst housing provision has always been considered to be the **common lodging house**. In intewar years, the privately owned common lodging house run for profit virtually disappeared, and those that remained were frequently owned by charitable organizations, and developed almost on institutional lines.

In the 1970s and 1980s, the situation changed as numbers of smaller properties were adapted. This was usually done by a charitable body to provide sheltered accommodation for small groups of socially vulnerable people. In addition, former commercial premises were often adapted as night shelters for people who would otherwise sleep in the open. The common lodging house remains a social and public health hazard, but one which often needs a compassionate approach.

FOOD 1900–PRESENT

Although local authorities had had powers to inspect food for many years, it was becoming apparent that some control over the premises in which food was handled was required if clean and safe food was to be available. The **Public Health Act 1925** introduced the first powers to deal with food premises and, although the requirements were modest, they extended to water and washing facilities and cleanliness in certain food premises. A start had been made on the road to better food hygiene.

By 1920, large-scale adulteration of food had ceased, although there were foods which were easy to sophisticate, a typical example being milk. The basic law with regard to food adulteration had remained unchanged since 1875, and clearly needed to be consolidated. This was done in the **Food and Drugs (Adulteration) Act 1928** which was to remain in force for a decade. The Act neither re-enacted the food safety provisions of the 1925 Public Health Act, nor included supplementary food safety powers.

The Ministry of Health advised through Memo 36/Foods how the Act was to be operated. A similar Ministry Memo (Memo 3/Foods) laid down inspection standards with regard to meat.

Some local authorities understood that their powers to deal with food-borne diseases and insanitary conditions in food premises were inadequate and, especially in the 1930s, through private Act legislation, they took some regulatory powers of registration of some types of food premises and their occupiers.

The **Food and Drugs Act 1938** was both consolidatory and innovatory. It had three main parts: the protection of food supplies, the sampling of food and drugs, and the control of certain food premises. It made provision for the inspection of food and for the control of some premises in which food was handled. It gave the ministers powers to make regulations in respect of the registration of some food premises and some practices of food handlers. It reaffirmed sampling procedures and the provisions with regard to warranties, and it made possible the control of such premises as slaughterhouses, knacker's yards, cold stores and markets.

Regrettably, the new Act did not come into force until after the outbreak of war, but although its full implementation was delayed, especially with regard to the potential advances in food hygiene legislation, the war period was particularly active and productive in terms of food control.

Faced with food shortages, a rationing and food control system ensured that the diet of the public was better than it had ever been. To ensure that food was the most nutritious available, a considerable number of regulations were promulgated, and most of these later found a place in permanent food law.

The 1938 Act made provision for ministers to introduce regulations on a variety of topics related to food safety, and in 1955 the first regulations designed to provide a food hygiene code were introduced. These were for general application to food premises, and were followed by comparable regulations for docks and warehouses, market stalls and delivery vehicles, and slaughterhouses. These were timely because in 1954 the meat trade ceased to be subject to control. The slaughterhouses which had been closed by the policy of concentrating slaughtering facilities were able to apply for the renewal of their licences, but very many failed to achieve the standards required and remained closed.

After the 1938 Act had been passed there were numerous changes in the food industry and its practices, especially in the replacement of small factories and shops and the development of larger scale production, distribution and retail units. There was a need for the modernization of the core legislation. This was achieved in the **Food and Drugs Act 1955**. Much food control law was contained in regulations which could be easily changed but, nevertheless, that law continued to lag behind developments in food technology and retailing, areas that were perpetually responding to market forces to meet changes in taste and lifestyle.

After the 1955 Act, there were many updating amendments to existing food law and, particularly, to the regulations, as attempts were made to meet current needs. Other developments were to come.

After the experiences of the period between 1920 and 1945, there was a view that food adulteration was a solved problem. After about 1950 the industry changed to the large scale processing of food, which resulted in a lowering of compositional standards.

The post-1945 period saw major increases in the number of cases of food-borne diseases. While notified cases of food poisoning have increased significantly, much attention has been focused on unnotified incidents. Enquiries into causes and effects have suggested that changes in diet and dietary and social habits were major causes. Also implicated was poor food hygiene, which resulted in a call for more public information and training of food handlers.

The increasing importance of good food hygiene brought the realization that it was difficult to act swiftly and decisively to deal with food premises that were so insanitary as to pose a serious risk to health. In 1971 the City of Manchester took powers in the **Manchester Corporation Act 1971** to enable its environmental health officers to close insanitary food premises by direct application to the courts. The value of this power was clear and the **Food and Drugs (Amendment) Act 1976** gave similar, but less rigorous, powers to local authorities generally. The Manchester powers, slightly modified, were applied to the other nine metropolitan district councils in Greater Manchester when, countywide, local act legislation was consolidated.

There was pressure from all sides to review the food law and in 1977 the ministers asked for the views of interested bodies as to how the food law should be amended or re-cast. Many organizations, including the Institution of Environmental

Health Officers, responded. However, no action took place except to find parliamentary time to produce the **Food Act 1984**, which consolidated the existing law but made few changes of significance.

From 1973, the whole issue of food legislation was complicated by European union legislation. By the time the UK joined the EU there had been a great deal of EU legislation, including laws relating to food, that had to be accepted as they stood.

After 1973, the UK was able to participate in the discussions which preceded further food legislation, but was always at a disadvantage because Continental systems of food control were considerably different to those in the UK. There followed a considerable flow of statutory instruments converting EC directives into UK law.

From the 1970s into the 1980s, the many organizations that had an interest in food legislation continued to press for amending legislation. This was met with little success until, after a series of food safety incidents, central government conducted a survey of views and issued a white paper on food safety. In due course, the **Food Safety Act 1990** was passed.

This legislation provided some satisfaction for those who had been pressing for change. However, although the Act conceded many principles that had been urged upon the government, the actual fulfilment of those principles was to be met largely by regulations. Control through statutory intruments has important advantages as they are easier to amend or extend, but they are also normally the means of writing in the detail to clothe the principles in the legislation and, as such, may fall short of real expectations or needs.

OCCUPATIONAL HEALTH AND SAFETY 1900–PRESENT

Factory law was reviewed, extended and consolidated by the important **Factory and Workshops Act 1901** which was divided into ten parts covering many aspects of industrial employment.

For many years, the work of the Factory Inspectorate had been increasing, and it had been difficult to do enough inspections. Despite the indifferent performance of local government in assigned health and safety duties, it was considered imperative that that their role should be extended. As a result, local authorities were made responsible for sanitary accommodation in all factories, and for creating a more effective system for dealing with 'homework'.

When the Shops Bill was before Parliament, there was opposition to bad working environments and excessive hours. In 1910, Hallworth and Davies said that a large number of shop assistants in London on most days of the week worked all their waking hours [8, p. 64]. At a drapery store employing about 30 assistants, the staff worked until at least 10.00 pm on five nights of the week; 'They were herded at night into a dilapidated house in one of the neighbouring mean and dirty streets and, although they seldom left the shop before 10 o'clock at night they had to be in the dormitory by 11 o'clock' [8, p. 64].

There was an unsuccessful attempt in 1909 to give shop workers some of the health protection which factory workers had, and there was a wish that the legislation, not then usually an environmental health function, would be enforced by the Factory Inspectorate.

However, the **Shops Acts 1912** and **1913** brought consolidation of the law and some improvement. But the law was still insufficient and inadequately enforced and demonstrated that shop workers' conditions, like those of the factory workers, were being improved in piece meal fashion.

The legislative position remained unchanged until the **Shops Act 1934**, which introduced important changes. It controlled the hours of work for those under 18 years of age and, for the first time, it introduced health and welfare provisions for workers in shops, and in offices attached to shops.

Shop working hours were to be enforced by Shops Act authorities (county and county borough councils). The welfare provisions, which included sanitary and washing facilities, heating and ventilation, facilities for taking meals and the provision of seats for female workers, became the responsibility of sanitary authorities (rural and urban districts, municipal boroughs and county boroughs).

Up to this time, environmental health officers had had a declining interest in work involving workshops as such places decreased in number and became factories in which, as officers, they had much more limited responsibilities. The Shops Act 1934 changed this, and there was a renewed interest in occupational health. On the whole, the work of the local authorities under the welfare provisions of the 1934 Act was so well done that it was, later, to lead to greater involvement in occupational health and safety.

Although better provision was made for shop workers, there were still many non-industrial workers who had no occupational health protection at all, and this was to remain the case for some time.

In the immediate post-war period, the government found the opportunity in 1946 to set up an interdepartmental committee, chaired by Sir Ernest Gowers, to look at the needs of non-industrial workers. **The Gowers Committee** reported in 1949 and its report had a delayed, but important, impact on occupational health and safety legislation. The consolidating **Shops Act 1950** owed little to the influence of the Gowers Report. The **Factory Act 1951** was a consolidation of previous legislation, and it met the perceived need of the industrial worker. However, it gave little further protection to land workers or those in non-industrial employment.

Post-war developments in agricultural practices, machinery and the chemical control of weeds and pests posed a substantial threat to the health and safety of the workers involved. The first occupational health legislation which implemented recommendations of the Gowers Committee was the **Agriculture (Safety, Health and Welfare Provisions) Act 1956**. The enforcement of this Act was entrusted mainly to the Agricultural Inspectorate and not to local authorities. whose role under this Act was equated with their, then, limited duties under factory legislation.

The Offices Act 1960, a private member's Bill, followed Gowers' recommendations. The Secretary of State could make regulations, after consulting interested bodies, prescribing standards for offices. However, such regulations were never made, probably because other measures were being prepared, and the Offices Act 1960 was never put into operation.

In 1963 the **Offices Shops and Railway Premises Act** was passed. It excluded many non-industrial workers, but it did cover offices and wholesale and retail premises. Most enforcement duties were assigned to local authorities, and records of local authority activities were subsumed into national statistics. Factory Inspectors had some concurrent powers, and Superintending Inspectors of Factories had oversight over local authority work to ensure uniformity of practice and standards of enforcement.

Under this Act, regulations were made prescribing health and safety standards. Environmental health officers, to whom the local authority role was largely assigned, were experienced in the hygiene of buildings, and the administration associated with legislation, but they needed to learn new skills in ergonomics and the safe operation of powered machinery.

When the Bill was before Parliament, there was opposition to it being made a largely local authority function. In theory it is easier for a central authority to achieve common standards of performance and enforcement, and there can be little opportunity for local influence to minimize the scale of activity. But central authority is never likely to have the local knowledge of the pattern of the problem; or to be subject to the constant probing of the elected members of councils responsible for enforcement; or to have an inspectorate which should be sensitive to local cultural patterns and traditions. In contrast, centrally organized inspectorates can invest heavily in specialist skills and supporting scientific staff.

The 1963 Act was important to local authorities in respect of their involvement in the enforcement of occupational health and safety, and it gave them an opportunity to make a mark.

Although this Act was a large step forward, it still did not protect all non-industrial workers, and the law needed further extension. Legislation to protect workers had been developed on an *ad hoc* basis with separate inspectorates for different working environments, and there were gaps and

overlaps in jurisdiction. It was obvious that the system needed a radical overhaul to enable it to deal with changes in technology. patterns of trade and commerce, lifestyles and public expectations.

It was clear that conditions within the workplace could affect the public outside. Processes were often hazardous to the worker on the shop floor and to others in and outside the factory. Many thought that in order to promote safety, healthy working conditions and to avoid prosecutions for infractions of the law, improved education and training were needed. Others urged cooperative efforts to reduce hazards, improve health and replace coercion and confrontation might be profitable.

In 1970 a **Committee of Enquiry** was set up under the chairmanship of **Sir Alfred Robens** to review the system of securing health and safety at work. It reported in 1972 [9] and it recommended:

1. a more united and integrated system to increase the effectiveness of the contribution to the health and safety at work made by the state;
2. conditions for more effective self-regulation by employers and employees;
3. a Health and Safety Commission with an executive arm to be called the Health and Safety Executive;
4. a continued enforcement role for local authorities which, ultimately, would be responsible for most of the non-industrial sector.

The Committee also laid down two other principles: no self-inspections or dual inspections were to be undertaken.

The recommendations of the Committee found expression in the **Health and Safety at Work, Etc. Act 1974**, which brought six significant changes for environmental health authorities. Their role was to be expanded and the officers they appointed to administer the Act would have concurrent powers with Health and Safety Executive officers. Thirdly, the subordinate role given under the 1963 Act was removed and the local authority inspectorates were given equality of status with those of the Health and Safety Executive. Additionally, the changes required local authority inspectorates to recognize the Health and Safety Executive as the Commission's administrative machine and, fifthly, to support and co-operate with the Executive field staff.

The sixth change was in the administrative procedures. Although these brought new concepts to environmental health departments, they were readily and advantageously adopted.

The new creation was not perfect. Environmental health officers felt aggrieved at the time, because continued Crown immunity meant that they were excluded from inspecting civil service establishments (except those of the Health and Safety Executive), and they could not deal with premises occupied by other local authorities which were located in their area. It was also recognized that environmental health officers would need additional skills. Factory inspectors saw local authority officers as a challenge, an attitude later exacerbated by civil service retrenchments.

There was an unsubstantiated fear that local authority elected members would interfere with their officer's operations. The civil servants were ill informed about the local government system, its traditions, training, and capacities and the practical achievements of the environmental health service. These were matched by similar misunderstanding in local government circles of the civil service role, qualifications and training.

If the two major arms of enforcement were to work harmoniously to produce an effective national system with uniform standards of performance and enforcement there had to be introduced a system of liaison. Nationally, a liaison committee, Health and Safety Executive/Local Authority Committee (**HELA**) representing the Local Authority Associations and the Health and Safety Executive was established as a forum to discuss problems, especially in the field of common standards, information exchange, statistics and developments, and to make recommendations for changes perceived to be necessary.

The HELA set up sub-groups to have regard to training, standards of enforcement and statistics and, in 1984, a Local Authority Unit was established. This Unit, designed to give local authority views open access to the system and to harmonize practices and approaches, was staffed, in part, in technical aspects, by environmental health officers and factory inspectors. It has been responsible for developing uniform standards and raising the local authority profile in this important work.

Locally there is appointed in each Health and Safety Executive area a senior factory inspector to act as the local Enforcement Laison Officer whose remit is to assist in the solution of local demarcation and technical problems, and to call periodic meetings of local authority counterparts for discussions, and exchanges of experience.

The local authority role was defined in the **Health and Safety (Enforcing Authority) Regulations 1977**. It was always the intention to extend the local authority role and, in 1983, discussions started with the object of revising these Regulations. But despite agreement between the officers engaged in this task, there was considerable delay in new regulations (**Health and Safety (Enforcing Authority) Regulations 1989**) being promulgated, but the changes made were less extensive than originally envisaged.

AIR POLLUTION CONTROL 1900–PRESENT

This period is characterized more by the better understanding of the air pollution problems, the emergence of air pollution monitoring, and the growths of organizations committed to securing improved air quality, than by improvements in the pollution control legislation. The emergence of pressure groups arguing for powers to deal with polluted air reflects a movement which straddles the turn of the century.

By the 1880s, the relationship between air pollution, fog formation, and increased mortality had been accepted. In London and other big cities, choking winter fogs were commonplace. A **Fog and Smoke Committee**, an organization which had the practical help of many distinguished people, was established in London in 1880. However, the precise casual relationship between air pollution and ill health had still to be defined.

The political difficulty of controlling domestic smoke was also understood, and the Fog and Smoke Committee was determined to try educational means to overcome the problem.

In 1882, the Fog and Smoke Committee became the **National Smoke Abatement Institution** which developed into a powerful lobby, but was replaced in 1896 by the **Coal Smoke Abatement Society**. While this organization was primarily a London body, which for some time employed its own smoke inspectors, similar organizations were being formed in northern industrial towns.

Manchester, in many ways the cradle of the clean air movement, had a special sub-committee to research into air pollution. In 1909, it became the headquarters of the **Smoke Abatement League of Great Britain**, which was an amalgamation of a number of societies including Manchester's own **Noxious Vapour Abatement Committee**. It is important to emphasize the interest which these local societies had generated, and how they recognized that the strength of a unified organization was more likely to be an effective pressure group. Although there were now two national organizations, the League sought the co-operation of provincial local authorities leaving London to the Coal Smoke Abatement Society.

The First World War restricted the activities of the two major groups, but they resumed their campaigns after 1919. The Coal Smoke Abatement Society continued its pressure on politicians, and this led to a Ministry of Health Departmental Committee in 1926 and, later, the **Public Health (Smoke Abatement) Act 1926**. This Act was of minor importance in dealing with the smoke pollution burden, but it marked the increased interest in air pollution, and led to changes in the attitudes of central government.

There were some interesting developments in the mid-1920s. E.D. Simon, a leading industrialist, politician, and former Lord Mayor of Manchester wrote, in conjunction with a London environmental health officer, a book entitled *Smokeless City*. Apart from showing that the significance of domestic smoke was understood, the book makes clear that fuel and appliance technology were available which could have reduced air pollution from domestic fires.

The increasing interest in air pollution induced central government to consider providing local authorities with advice. When the Alkali Inspectorate declined to be involved, it was decided that the task of collecting information should be given to one of three Ministry of Health officials. Ministry minutes of the day recorded resistance to the idea of promoting further smoke control measures. It was considered that the public was not ready for measures as no causal connection had been established between polluted air and ill health. Whoever wrote that was unaware of the documented circumstantial evidence that showed a clear correlation between smoke, fog and increased mortality.

J.C. Dawes was then selected to be the advisory officer. He was a refuse disposal expert, an environmental health officer by profession who, later, was president of the Institution of Environmental Health Officers from 1938 to 1952.

In 1929 the Smoke Abatement League and the Coal Smoke Abatement Society amalgamated to form the **National Smoke Abatement Society** (NSAS). The League, based in Manchester, had appointed a full-time secretary, and the amalgamation was a positive move forward. Fortunately, the new body was able to retain the services of many of its prominent lay members who worked for the cause of clean air, and the support of environmental health professionals. It was recognized that smoke control was mainly the province of the environmental health officer and the support given by them for the movement for clean air was crucial.

It was, however, a lay member of the NSAS, who produced the seminal concept of the smokeless zone. Charles Gandy, a Manchester barrister, conceived the idea. Manchester City Council, long committed to clean air, supported the concept.

Although the positive relationship between air pollution and ill health had still to be established, in 1923 Dr James Niven drew attention to the air pollution in Manchester, the diminished sunlight and the high incidence of pulmonary and other diseases.

From about 1928, some local authorities began measuring air pollution. Although the equipment then available was relatively crude, it did at least yield measurements which could be used as evidence, and compared over different time periods and geographical areas. Despite this and other research, practical action had to be delayed until after the Second World War.

In 1946, the City of Manchester was able to secure, in a private Act of Parliament, powers to establish a smokeless zone. Other authorities, encouraged by the NSCA, took similar powers. The new powers took some time to implement, and it was not until 1954 that Manchester had its first smokeless zone.

Local authorities became more interested in air pollution control and appreciated the transboundary nature of smoke pollution. This recognition made it easier to establish local committees to co-ordinate local smoke abatement, and some of these organizations were successful and long lived.

Despite the increasing pressure, little had been done by central government to give adequate powers to local authorities to deal with smoke, especially domestic smoke.

In December 1952, London, as a consequence of persistent temperature inversion, suffered a particularly dense and persistent fog which had disastrous consequences in terms of human mortality. Later statistical analyses suggested that the mortality in excess of the normal figure was in the order of 4000.

Under pressure, the government appointed a committee under a promient industrialist. Sir Hugh Beaver, to investigate the problem and make recommendations.

The committee made rapid progress, but there was more pressure and a private member, Gerald Nabarro, approached the NSAS for a draft Bill and other assistance. That Bill failed, but the pressure on government was so great that it adopted a similar Bill and, during its passage, Mr Nabarro acted as the principal spokesman on amendments suggested by the NSAS.

The Beaver Committee was aware that much was needed to be done, but there could be no quick solution. The aim would be to secure an 80% reduction in air pollution in the heavily populated areas in 10–15 years.

The new legislation in the **Clean Air Act 1956** embodied principles which had been proposed for years by bodies pressing for clean air, and by the authorities responsible for controlling air pollution.

Air pollution from industrial coal burning plants was a lesser problem, because the economies achievable by the proper combustion of the fuel had made companies install adequate plant and operate it with skilled engineers.

The new legislation proposed to deal with domestic smoke by adapting the smokeless zone principle into **smoke control areas**, in which all premises would be subject to some control. The control over industrial premises was already available, but domestic premises would be required to be able to burn smokeless appliances and fuel. Although the grant was only to be 70% of the cost of the change, that level was chosen to reflect the fact that the new appliances would be much more efficient and burn less fuel. No grant was available for commercial premises which, nevertheless, had to comply.

The new interest in air pollution control caused a re-examination of the powers of the Alkali Inspectorate and local authorities. The Beaver Committee had urged that the central and local inspectorates should work closely together, and the subsequent closer contact brought better cooperation and improved working arrangements.

Many of the larger authorities argued that they could be responsible for all air pollution control but, finally, they were left with responsibility for a few installations while some for which they had previously been responsible were transferred to the Alkali Inspectorate. Three large local authorities were allocated control over three small-sized power stations.

One effect of the Clean Air Act 1956 was a major increase in the monitoring of air pollution by local authorities, and the development of a national survey assisted by the local authority statistics. When the UK became a member of the EU, it was required to meet the air pollution standards set down by it, and this necessitated a re-arrangement of the monitoring activities.

OTHER FORMS OF POLLUTION

Originally, the investigation into air pollution was directed against the products of combustion of coal, but after about 1970 there was increased interest in other gaseous pollutants, especially those emanating from internal combustion engines.

There began to develop a keen public interest in all forms of pollution, and this found expression in the control over the deposition of hazardous wastes. The first control was exercised in the early 1970s by the then equivalent to the district council through a licensing system (see also Chapter 43).

Pressures for more effective law persisted and arising from these pressures the **Control of Pollution Act 1974** was passed. This Act was designed to give better control over various forms of pollution, including air pollution and the pollution of land. This coincided with the reorganization of local government and the duty of dealing with hazardous wastes was given to 'waste disposal authorities' which, in England, were the county councils.

The anti-pollution movement grew increasingly strong, and there was much public pressure for protection from environmental pollution, including noise pollution. As a result, the **Water Act 1989** was passed and new measures to control water pollution.

The **Environmental Protection Act 1990** gave measures for the control of other forms of pollution. The objectives of the 1990 Act included the creation of an integrated national pollution inspectorate, which would involve local authorities in the control of certain scheduled industrial processes. The Act also strengthened the controls dealing with the disposal of waste on land.

The pressures for more comprehensive environmental control included very considerable international pressure for action to be taken to deal with pollution problems which had trans-boundary effects, such as the pollution of international water courses, and the acidification of rain by the emission of sulphur gases from the combustion of fossil fuels. There was great interest in global warming, the rising CO_2 levels and the use of chlorofluorocarbon compounds.

THE ROYAL COMMISSION ON ENVIRONMENTAL POLLUTION

Royal Commissions of Enquiry are one of the prestigious ways by which the UK government institutes a formal enquiry into a particular topic. The enquiry is carried out by a body of distinguished people who are not necessarily experts in the particular topic under review, but who are capable of mounting a sustained and penetrating enquiry by means of examining papers and listening to oral evidence from expert witnesses.

Most Royal Commissions are appointed for a single task, but the Royal Commission on Environmental Pollution is a standing Commission, which has undertaken a series of investigations into issues of pollution and on each enquiry has published an authoritative report.

THE DEVELOPMENT OF LOCAL GOVERNMENT

Environmental health control has been associated with local government for many years; indeed, it would be true to say that local authorities emerged because they were originally environmental health authorities. The history of local government is a specialist topic, and all that is noted here are the steps which created local government bodies to which reference is made in past, and some existing, environmental health legislation.

The **Public Health Act 1848** established **Local Health Boards**. The **Public Health Act 1872** created the **sanitary authorities** which would be responsible for all sanitary functions within their areas. The **Public Health Act 1875** created **Urban and Rural Sanitary Districts** with the former comprising either municipal boroughs, local government districts, or an Improvement Act district. Rural sanitary districts were the responsibility of the Board of Guardians.

The **Municipal Corporations Act 1882** created a modernized form of **municipal borough**, and the **Local Government Act 1888** set up **county councils** and **county boroughs**. This Act also created the **London County Council** and, with 32 **Metropolitan boroughs**, replaced a wide miscellany of former authorities.

Urban District and Rural District Councils emerged from the **1894 Local Government Act** to replace the urban and rural sanitary districts.

After the **Public Health Act 1872** the Local Government Board could approve the establishment of **Port Sanitary Authorities** and assign functions to them. Furthermore, under the **Public Health (Ports) Act 1896**, the Local Government Board was empowered to invest in Port Sanitary Authorities duties in respect of communicable diseases.

The **Local Government Act 1929** reformed the Poor Law system. It abolished the Boards of Guardians and vested their social and medical work in **county councils and county boroughs**.

There were major changes in the pattern of local government in London and the Midlands in the 1960s. In the Greater London area, 34 London Boroughs were set up to take over the functions of a large number of smaller authorities, and London Boroughs had powers similar to those of county boroughs except that some did not become Education Authorities.

After a long deliberation by the Redcliffe–Maude Committee, proposals to change local government to a series of single-purpose authorities was not accepted by the government, and the **Local Government Act 1972** was used to create a new system. The 1300+ councils in England and Wales were reduced to about 400 **shire districts**.

Metropolitan counties were created to cover London and six other conurbations. Additionally, 36 **Metropolitan district councils** were established by amalgamating a number of authorities. Constitutionally, these councils were very similar to the former county boroughs and, indeed, in most cases a former county borough formed the core of a new metropolitan district. The shire districts had limited functions but were responsible for housing and environmental health, but the metropolitan districts were 'all purpose' authorities. A comparable system of regional and district councils was created for Scotland.[1]

In 1986, the Greater London and the six metropolitan counties were abolished. Functions which could not be returned to district councils were assigned to 'residuary bodies'. The Greater London and the metropolitan counties had no environmental health functions other than the disposal of refuse.

PROFESSIONAL RELATIONSHIPS

The **Public Health Act 1848** required Local Boards of Health to appoint an 'officer of health' and an inspector of nuisances. Both were separate appointments and, in this the Act followed the **Liverpool Sanitary Act 1846**. The duties of neither office were prescribed, but those of the **medical officer of health** were influenced by advice from the Local Government Board.

Following the **Public Health Act 1872** the Local Government Board made a series of orders prescribing qualifications, appointment, salaries, and tenure of office of medical officers of health and **inspectors of nuisances**. In 1891 the medical officers of health in London had their duties defined.

In 1910 the **Sanitary Officers (Outside London) Order** defined the medical officer's duties and it applied also to inspectors of nuisances. The conditions of office and tenure of medical officers and sanitary inspectors were prescribed by the **Public Health (Officers) Act 1921**. That Act required that their dismissal could only be with the consent of the minister, and it also required that the term 'inspector of nuisances' be replaced with the designation **'sanitary inspector'**.

Between that date and 1974, various other orders of a similar kind were promulgated, and these had the effect of requiring public health inspectors to work under the general direction of the medical officer of health.

In 1955, the designation was changed to public health inspector by the **Sanitary Inspectors (Change of Designation) Act 1955**, and the current designation of environmental health officer began to be adopted about 1970, and became accepted as the designation after local government re-organization in 1974.

POSTSCRIPT

Although this chapter is long, it affords only a brief introduction to the way environmental health control has evolved. Most of the topics covered have, elsewhere, detailed accounts of the way progress has taken place, and the debates which have preceded all changes.

From the account given it should be apparent that, while there has been a continual stream of environmental health legislation, there have been periods in time (c. 1875, the 1930s, 1974, and the 1980s) when activities have been taking place simultaneously in several streams of activity. Experience also suggests that changes only come as a consequence of pressures on government, and such pressures are now tending to arise from public perception rather than from official sources.

Environmental health has always been in the lead in 'social' legislation and, thus, has tended to reflect contemporary political and economic thinking. Because of this environmental health law is subject to the impact of deregulation and provides good illustrations of the conflict between the need to provide adequate protection and a perceived need to reduce the burdens of compliance.

The Environmental Protection Act of 1990 is being gradually implemented with local authorities strengthening air pollution control to enable Central Government to meet EU standards.

Housing post-1990 has been in a quiet phase reflecting changes in social policy and economic fortune. Health and safety continues to be dominated by deregulation issues and compliance with approved codes of practice.

In the field of food safety there is to be witnessed a balancing act between deregulation and protection and there are likely to be changes in enforcement as the fashion changes from regulations to approved codes of practice.

[1]A review of the structure of local government in Scotland, Wales and the non-metropolitan areas of England in 1994/95 has led to proposals for single tier authorities in the whole of Scotland and Wales and in certain parts of England.

REFERENCES

1. Hutchins, B.L. and Harrison, L. (1911) *History of Factory Legislation*, P.S. King & Son, London.
2. Gale, A.H. (1955) *Epidemic Diseases*, Pelican, London.
3. Finer, S.H. (1956) *The Life and Times of Sir Edwin Chadwick*, Methuen, London.
4. Frazer, W.M. (1950) *A History of Public Health*, Ballière, Tindall and Cox, London.
5. Burnett, J. (1960) *Plenty and Want*, Pelican Books, London.
6. Engels, F. *Conditions of the Working Class in 1844*.
7. Ashby, E. and Anderson, M. (1979) *Politics of Clean Air*, Clarendon Press, Oxford.
8. Hallworth and Davies, p. 60.
9. Safety and Health at Work, Cmnd 5034 (1972), HMSO, London.

2 International aspects

Eric W. Foskett

INTRODUCTION

Chapter 1 gives an indication of the influences that have produced domestic environmental health legislation, of how a fairly comprehensive code of such legislation has developed and how, in the main, each increment has built on preceding law.

Although the end product is UK parliamentary legislation, the roots of which can often be traced to the influence of domestic pressure groups, it would be wrong to think that there is no evidence of external influences. Indeed, since about 1850 external considerations, foreign thinking and foreign practices have been working to mould British environmental health legislation.

INTERNATIONAL CONTROL OF INFECTIOUS DISEASES

International moves to control the spread of communicable disease were among the earliest influences on domestic environmental health control (see also Chapter 13). This was to be expected because the epidemics of cholera which ravaged early Victorian Britain spread in from Europe, and had, in turn, reached Europe from distant sources. The medieval 'black death', in the form of bubonic plague, was similarly an imported disease. These epidemics record the fact that the spread of infection has always been associated with man's mobility, whether that has resulted from a nomadic existence, the pursuit of war, trade, or, more recently, pleasure.

As nations became aware of illness which travellers could import, they tried defensive quarantine systems and, in so doing, created codes of legal constraints on the movement of travellers and goods. Early quarantine systems were generally enforced by the customs services, and probably the need to reduce trade constraints when world trade was expanding was a major influence in attempting to minimize the restrictions imposed by quarantine procedures.

From 1851 until the late 1930s, a series of **International Sanitary Conferences** took place in an attempt to prevent the importation of exotic diseases. The usual procedure was a conference at which a **Convention** (a form of treaty) was negotiated and signed by the attending parties. A Convention normally needed ratification by governments before it was binding, even though signed by a responsible minister. Having been ratified, it became binding and there was a duty to carry it out. The first Conferences were held with a genuine desire to make progress, but they were hampered by lack of epidemiological knowledge. Later Conferences had the advice which stemmed from medical knowledge, but this advice was largely ignored.

By the middle of the nineteenth century, mortality from endemic communicable disease was great. The disease that caused the greatest alarm in the UK was cholera. Cholera spread rapidly, and caused a high mortality. Furthermore, while the indigenous scarlet and enteric fevers affected all classes, the incidence of cholera was concentrated in the overcrowded slums. And, with an improvement in communications and the continuing expansion of foreign trade, there were considerable social, economic and medical pressures for some forms of control.

The importance of a public health system which dealt with the problems of imported disease, whether the agent was human, animal, or a commodity, was recognized by the British government and, using the powers in the **1872 and 1875 Public Health Acts**, established **Port Sanitary Authorities**.

> The Local Government Board, under these Acts assigned to the new authorities duties and powers necessary for the effective carrying out of the sanitary requirements in connection with shipping including precautions against the admission of the major infectious diseases. [1]

By this time, the old concept of quarantine was being seriously challenged. Contemporary medical authorities advocated the substitution of medical inspection for quarantine, and this view was adopted at the Vienna International Sanitary Conference in 1874. This led to the formalization of the international regulation of communicable disease and, because no international agency was available, regulation was achieved by means of a treaty.

The seventh International Sanitary Conference was held at Vienna in 1892, and from it came the 1892 International Sanitary Convention. This focused attention on the spread of cholera by westbound shipping, and it formed a useful starting point for effective international public health control.

The control of cholera was by no means complete and a further conference in Dresden in 1894 was needed to ensure that the signatories to the treaty notified each other of cholera cases.

Although by signing the treaties and conventions the UK bound itself to carry out the provisions of those agreements, statutory measures were needed to give powers of action to appropriate authorities. **The Public Health (Ports) Act 1896** enabled the Sanitary Conventions to be observed. The Local Government Board gave Port Sanitary Authorities powers under the **Infectious Diseases Prevention Act 1889**, and it made regulations dealing specifically with cholera,

yellow fever and plague: it abandoned quarantine and adopted medical inspection procedures.

In the last decade of the nineteenth century, a number of International Sanitary Conferences were held which resulted in minor modifications of the Sanitary Conventions.

At the eleventh International Sanitary Conference in Paris in 1903, two advances were made. A further International Sanitary Convention was negotiated which added plague to the diseases to be controlled; secondly, the Conference generated the concept of a permanent international health organization. Thus, in 1907, the Office International D'Hygiene Publique was established in Paris, France. This created a system of reporting the worldwide incidence of infectious disease, and the organization laid the foundations for the Paris International Sanitary Conference in 1911/12.

The main reasons for calling the 1911/12 Conference were the advances in medical knowledge that made essential the recasting of the 1903 Convention, which was concerned with only plague and cholera. Local conferences in the USA and the West Indies had discussed yellow fever and this was now considered. The Conference produced the International Sanitary Convention 1911/12, which consolidated the control procedures for cholera and plague, added yellow fever to the list, and replaced the Conventions signed in 1892, 1893, 1894, 1897 and 1903.

In 1923, the **League of Nations** set up in Geneva, Switzerland, an Office complementary to the Paris Office. This new establishment, which was advised by a health committee of medical specialists who were independent of their governments, was able, within two years, to issue weekly epidemiological reports giving the world position with regard to the five convention diseases.

Paris hosted an International Sanitary Conference in 1926, and a Convention was negotiated that year which added typhus and smallpox to the list of convention diseases. The British government ratified this Convention, and promulgated the comprehensive **Port Sanitary Regulations 1933**.

Fifty countries participated in the fourteenth and last International Health Conference in Paris in 1938. This was notable because, for the first time, serious attention was paid to the current state of medical knowledge. Also for the first time, the Conference addressed the problems of road and sea travel and, in particular, air travel, which increased the possibility of importing patients in the incubation periods of an exotic disease, and the possibility of importing insect disease vectors.

During the first 40 years of the twentieth century, international agencies began to emerge, which created initiatives that formerly had depended on the interest of a single or a few governments. The onset of the Second World War precluded any development of the ideas generated by the 1938 Conference, and that war virtually ended the health activities of the Paris and Geneva Offices.

In 1944 the emerging United Nations created the **United Nations Relief and Rehabilitiation Administration** (UNRRA), which was designed to meet the needs of those parts of Europe and Asia which fell under the control of the Western Allies, and where civil administration and public and environmental health services had broken down.

In 1946, 60 countries attended an International Health Conference in New York. This Conference assumed the functions of UNRRA and formed the **World Health Organization (WHO)** (see below).

One weakness of earlier agencies and Conventions was that their work came to fruit slowly because agreements were subject to protracted ratification procedures. The new WHO constitutional position became important because, while its decisions were binding on its members and ratification was not necessary, member states could participate in formulating proposals.

An important early step by WHO was to secure international collaboration in controlling epidemics. A new code was adopted by the WHO Assembly in 1951. **The International Sanitary Regulations 1951**, which modernized and replaced the 13 International Sanitary Conventions, came into force on 1 October 1952.

Because the International Sanitary Regulations were binding upon the WHO's members, the government's ultimate response was to revise the law relating to the domestic control and notification of disease through the **Public Health (Ships) Regulations 1979**, the **Public Health (Aircraft) Regulations 1979**, and by the **Public Health (Control of Disease) Act 1984**. This body of law prescribed measures to control communicable diseases which are to be taken at points of entry into the country.

In dealing with world health problems, WHO does not confine itself to publishing the framework of action which members are to follow, but it also embarks on practical health programmes. A significant example of this is found in the smallpox eradication scheme: WHO persuaded governments to act together to eliminate smallpox and then promoted, co-ordinated and monitored national vaccination programmes.

Communicable diseases are a prime example of trans-boundary environmental problems. In controlling them, there has to be a supra-national organization with the ability to prescribe control measures which national governments follow in order to take local action not only in their own interests but in the interests of international health.

THE EUROPEAN UNION

After 1945 serious consideration was given by European countries as to the future organization of their economic systems. Initially, a number of politicians concluded that, although the immediate challenge was to work out a successful system for economic growth and accountability, there should be some form of political unity by adopting a federal system of government.

Recent developments in the Community have shown differences of opinion on this score, but there can be little doubt that the gradual loss of some sovereign rights by states as they have sought to comply with European economic developments has raised anxieties on this issue.

Because environmental issues, whether they affect public health or not, can, and do, have a profound effect on economic policies and activity, the Community has regarded it proper to 'legislate' on many aspects of environmental control. As a result, this has changed many aspects of UK environmental health law and practice.

The history of 'pure' UK public health law has seen no real distinction between law relating public, personal and environmental health. Indeed, there have been many statutes which have encompassed all three. However, because personal and public health matters are deemed by the Community to be social issues, the view has been that in the absence of a social services remit in the Treaty of Rome and other Community constitutional legislation, the Community cannot operate in the field of public and personal health without a constitutional change.

CREATING THE EUROPEAN UNION

Adherence to the **1957 Treaty of Rome** by the UK has had a profound effect. Note is made above that the effect of signing international conventions was to create a treaty which, once signed and ratified, required full compliance by signatory powers. The **Treaty of Rome** and, later, the **Single European Act, 1986** and the **Treaty of Maastricht 1993**, were instruments of the same order – freely entered agreements but requiring compliance.

The deliberations noted above led to the formation of the **European Coal and Steel Community** in 1952. After long negotiations, the Treaty of Rome was signed in 1957 and that established the European Economic Community. In 1958 the **European Atomic Energy Community** was created and, the EU became operative with France, Italy, West Germany, Netherlands, Belgium and Luxembourg. The UK was not a member and was instrumental in establishing EFTA, the **European Free Trade Area**, as an economic counterblast.

In the 1960s, the UK made an application to join the EEC, but was not admitted. In the early 1970s, applications to join were made by Denmark, Norway, Ireland and the UK. Norway withdrew but the three others became members with effect from the beginning of 1973. Greece joined in 1981 and Spain and Portugal in 1986.

The **Treaty of Rome 1957** has been supplemented by the **Single European Act 1986** and the **Treaty of Maastricht 1993**. This Act changed the name of the organization to the European Community (EC), it extended the Community's field of action, it changed the relations between the Community's institutions and their operational roles, and it gave formal legal status to European *political* co-operation. It introduced the concept of the 'qualified majority' as a substitute for the original requirement of a unanimous decision being needed to pass new 'legislation'. The effect of this was that no single member could block the passage of a measure – that would need the votes of at least two members, and one of those would have to be one of the major members.

THE EUROPEAN COURT

Essentially, the EU operates by creating 'law' which members must obey. All legal systems need a judicial element to inflict punishment for infractions of the 'law' and, to determine what the law really means. To achieve this the EU has a **European Court of Justice**, which acts both as a judicial court and as the equivalent of a supreme court, which is an essential feature of a federal system.

The Court sits in Luxembourg and it has 13 judges each apppointed for six years. The appointments are made with the agreement of the member states, the judges being drawn from the judiciaries of member states. The Court's function is to ensure, in accordance with the rule of law, that the Treaties are implemented. The Court is assisted by six advocates general.

EUROPEAN UNION LEGISLATION

To achieve a common market, action has been directed, *inter alia*, to removing anomalies in the laws of member states, to establish common standards in units of measurement and the composition of commodities, and removing inequalities affecting citizens of member states. These wide-ranging activities are achieved through EU legislation, and this is achieved by a protracted and complex process:

> Community legislation is elaborated, discussed, adopted and interpreted by the Institutions . . . of the Community. [2, 12]

Haigh continues by discussing the different types of Community legislation thus:

> There are several types of Community legislation set out in article 189 of the treaty of Rome . . . they are: Regulations, Directives, Decisions, Recommendations, and Opinions. The last two have no legal force and should not be regarded as legislative instruments. Indeed, the Treaty does not use the word legislation. A *regulation* is directly applicable law in the Member States, and is mostly used for rather precise purposes . . . It has so far been used only rarely for environmental matters. A *directive* is binding as to the results to be achieved, but leaves the Member States the choice of form and methods. It is therefore the most appropriate instrument for general purposes particularly where flexibility is required to accommodate existing national procedures and, for this reason, is the instrument most commonly used for environmental matters. A decision is binding in its entirety upon those to whom it is addressed. It has been used in the environmental field in connection with international conventions and procedural matters. [2. p. 12]

THE EUROPEAN PARLIAMENT

Although the EU tends to resemble a giant bureaucracy, it has a democratically elected Parliament which is gradually becoming more powerful. It is directly elected, and each state is represented by a number of Members of the European Parliament (MEPs), the number approximating to the population, although the smaller countries are somewhat over represented.

Each state prescribes the method by which it will elect its representatives, and in the UK, England, Wales, and Scotland have single MEP constituencies, which are about equal to six Westminster parliamentary seats. A candidate succeeds by obtaining more votes than any other candidate. In Northern Ireland the seats are determined by proportional representation.

Italy, France, Germany and the UK each have 81 MEPs – other states have a smaller number according to the size of their populations, making a total of 518 MEPs. The number of votes is likely to be adjusted as the membership of the EU expands. MEPs do not sit as part of a national bloc, but with MEPs from other countries having the same political affiliation.

The European Parliament elects a president and it does much work through committees. Each committee has a chairperson and two deputy chairpeople. The composition of the committees reflects the parliamentary strength of a country, but every state is represented on every committee.

THE COUNCIL OF MINISTERS

This is the top level political organ of the EU. Each country is represented by a single member. This is usually either the foreign minister or prime minister but the council can consist of other ministers if there are specific policy programmes to discuss. For instance, when the Common Agricultural Policy is being discussed the Council would probably consist of the 12 agriculture ministers.

The Council is chaired by a president and the presidency rotates on a six-monthly cycle.

THE COMMITTEE OF PERMANENT REPRESENTATIVES

Because the Council could not remain in session all the time, there is a committee of Permanent Representatives composed of staff with diplomatic status. The function of this institution is to ensure that there is constant contact between the member states at appropriate diplomatic levels.

THE EUROPEAN COMMISSION

The Commission is the EU's bureaucracy – its civil service. It works through 22 directorates general, which resemble civil service departments in that each one is responsible for a particular programme area. The programme areas do not necessarily 'shadow' the functions of the UK civil departments. This means that a function which, in UK terms, would be a cohesive, single activity may well, in the EU, have sectors located in more than one directorate.

Each directorate has a director general and the process is over seen by 17 commissioners each of whom, having been nominated by his or her own government, holds a short-term political appointment. The UK appoints two such commissioners and, by convention, each of the two main parties nominates a commissioner.

The function of the commission is to initiate EU policy, to defend EU interests and to ensure that EU policy forms a consistent whole. The Commission is the EU's executive – it initiates legislation to meet its perception of need. Because of its treaty obligations, the UK government has to adjust its own domestic legislative programme to enact the law it needs to comply with EU policy as communicated in directives.

DIRECTIVES

The passage of a directive from conception to delivery is long and tortuous. This is understandable in view of the number of member states who have to be consulted. Directives, promulgated by the Council of Ministers after considering the formal written opinions of the European Parliament, are binding on all member states. They have the force of domestic law and may take precedence over it, and they can be enforced through the EU's judicial system.

While directives are created by complex procedures, each member state can participate in their drafting, and can attempt to secure exemptions or modifications applicable to it alone, or to a small group of countries. In attempting to protect their interests, member states have various opportunities for intervention:

1. at a pre-drafting stage as soon as a member state becomes aware that a directive is being projected;
2. at the drafting stage when officials of the Commission are writing a proposal for formal submission to the Council;
3. when a firm draft is published and is available for examination by the government of each member state;
4. when a proposal is being considered, as it must be, by a committee of the European Parliament;
5. when it is under consideration by the Committee of Permanent Representatives who are civil servants seconded to the EU by member states;
6. when the issue is to be considered by the Council of Ministers.

It has, however, to be remembered that whereas at one time a single state could block an issue at the Council of Ministers, that is now possible only with two or more states acting in concert.

It is clear that the most effective intervention is as early in the drafting stage as possible, and this can only be done if it is known that a directive is being drafted on a particular topic. While governments can take the initiative at any of the above stages, any individual organization has an advantage to the extent that it cannot only attempt to influence the EU organizations, but it can also bring pressure to bear to persuade its own government to act.

Although directives emanate officially from the Commission, they may be in response to deficiencies perceived by a directorate general in an existing directive: or to meet the needs of a programme of the commission; or to satisfy initiatives taken by member states or pressure groups; or as the consequence of a complaint made to the Commission.

Directives are required to be subsumed into domestic legislation by each member state in such a way that the tenor of EU policy is observed, while the state is able to preserve its own legal precedents and procedures.

Increasingly, directives enable member states to have an acceptable system which conforms to the EU requirements, but which also permits a local choice. An example of this is to be found in Directive 85/337/EEC 'on the assessment of certain public and private projects in the environment'. Popularly known as the environmental impact directive, this prescribes certain developments which must be subject to a proper environmental impact assessment. However, a further schedule lists developments which the government of a member state may choose to include in the list of mandatory assessment requirement, or deal with in another way.

ENFORCEMENT

Enforcement through the EU's judicial system made be precipitated by the apparent failure of a state to comply with a directive's requirement, and which has been detected or referred by a pressure group or an individual to a directorate general.

There are other methods of enforcement, such as a physical check on actual compliance with EU requirements, either by experts nominated by a Commission or by officers of a directorate. This already exists in the inspection of slaughterhouses and meat hygiene by veterinary officers appointed by the Commission. Such a practice is already establishing a precedent for the creation of supranational inspectorates.

CREATING A DIRECTIVE

The origin of a directive is referred to above, but it passes through a long series of stages before it emerges as EU legislation. There are certain formal steps that have to be taken in a sequence, just as there are for a UK Bill. The process involves the initiating directorate, the Commission, the European Parliament and its committees, and the Council of Ministers. Interspersed with, or preceding, these various stages there are opportunities for consultation on, and the review of, drafts. The whole process may well be started off by the ground work being carried out by a working party of extra-Commission experts.

The reason for the gestation of a directive being so protracted is that so many different interests have to be satisfied in producing legislation that harmonizes all national legal processes and technical standards.

The directives are not created in isolation. There are other international organizations that are seeking internationally agreed procedures and standards, and the EU strives to ensure that its directives are compatible with the proceedings of other organizations, such as WHO and the Food and Agriculture Organization.

As described above, the initiation of a new directive may come from a number of sources. These may include the Commission's perception of a specific need to amend existing legislation or propose a new measure, or the origin may lie in a representation made to one of the directorates general.

From the beginning, there is a long series of consultations and amendments, and it is at this stage where influence can be brought to bear on the form of the proposal by interested or involved governments or organizations.

There is another important element. At first sight the EU's organization might appear to be an inflexible bureaucracy, but in the long run it has to meet the will and the needs of the members of the EU, and for this purpose it must, as far as is possible appear to be reasonable. One of the ways it achieves this is to promulgate programmes of objectives and actions. In 1987, for example, it produced an environmental programme which supplemented two previous programmes. The 1987 programme set out the environmental targets it was hoped would be achieved in the EU by 1992. By this, member states could prepare themselves and shape their administrations to be able to cope with the drafts of directives when they appeared and be prepared to comment and discuss them, and to make budgetary provisions.

In addition to programmes of this nature, the Commission also produces yearly 'work programmes', which enable member states to plan their own measures and programmes more effectively.

PROMULGATION AND IMPLEMENTATION

When a directive has gone through all the legislative processes, it appears finally before the Council of Ministers. The Council can adopt a measure by a qualified majority, but a unanimous vote is required to send the proposal back to the Commission for re-examination.

The legislative implementation of a directive by a member state has been discussed above, but there is also the practical implementation.

The EU's approach to implementation is that the government of each member state is that state's 'competent authority'. Each state, by joining the EU, assumes duties towards it, and one of those duties is to secure compliance with directives. The state can appoint subordinate bodies to implement directives, e.g. the National Rivers Authority for the polluted water course. But the state itself remains the competent authority and, in the last resort, is the organization that must ensure that there is compliance or face enforcement proceedings before the European Court.

INFLUENCING EU POLICY

This section is devoted to showing how external events and organizations can influence UK legislation, and included are comments on how EU policies, which will affect UK legislation, may be influenced.

Two things flow from the EU's position of regarding central government as always being the competent authority. Firstly, the channel of communication is initially from the EU to central government. The appropriate ministries receive an intimation from their counterpart directorates of new developments, in the form of requests for information and comments on draft proposals.

Secondly, there grows up personal contact between UK civil servants and their EU equivalents. This personal contact is to be commended as it promotes confidence and informal discussion as a precursor to more detailed and serious negotiations – each side is better able to bring pressure on the other.

When dealing with a development, the UK ministry has to be able to frame appropriate responses. This is done out of ministry technical or professional resources, or by consultation with outside bodies. Both of these processes are suspect. There is no guarantee that the information available within the ministry is as expert as the civil service believes it to be, and an incomplete, or inaccurate, response may be generated. Furthermore, the process of consultation may be flawed by being inadequate. Ministries tend to accumulate lists of people and organizations they think must be consulted, and those lists may not represent the best sources of comment on a particular issue.

Ministries have, of course, a duty to make effective representation to directorates so as to preserve the UK's interests; every other member state is similarly occupied. This means that ministry pressures on directorates have to be effective which, in turn, demands the best sources of information.

Thus the first, and possibly the most effective, means of influencing EU policy lies with the appropriate minister and ministry. Hence, because non-civil service interests often suspect that the representations being made are inadequate, they resort to the legitimate practice of lobbying ministers, MPs, and civil servants to try to make sure that their views are heard and taken into consideration. In addition, some of the pressure is also put on MEPs (including those MEPs who do not represent a UK constituency, but may be a member of a particular European Parliament committee) and EU civil servants. For example, the Chartered Institute of Environmental Health has developed strong links with a number of European civil servants.

In attempting to put pressure on the EU's legislative process interested parties are doing no more than they do in connection with domestic legislation where lobbying to effect changes in policy is recognized as being part of the democratic process. It is fair for all views to be aired when legislation is being prepared, and not simply those that government finds convenient in supporting its case. What has to be watched is the potential for corruption and misrepresentation.

There are other ways in which directorates may be influenced. Being from an international organization, the EU's bureaucrats are usually impressed by approaches from an international organization that presents views which purport to represent a wider picture than a purely national case. Because of this, it is advantageous for an organization to be a member of a pan-European group in addition to belonging to domestic bodies.

An interested body may make representations in Brussels of its own case, although it will need to understand that probably the case will be seen as special pleading.

It is important for interested organizations to influence bodies that have similar interests so that together they can adopt a united stance on issues that affect them. Such organizations usually promote their views in print, and are prepared to promote a specific activity to secure the backing of the EU.

THE FOOD AND AGRICULTURE ORGANIZATION (FAO)

The Food and Agriculture Organization is the oldest agency of the United Nations Organisation (UNO). It arose out of the consideration of the problems of feeding the world population in postwar circumstances. Its headquarters are in Rome and this is an acknowledgment that the FAO walks a path pioneered by an Italian organization – **the International Agriculture Institute**. The FAO also had roots in the League of Nations, which in the 1930s looked at problems of nutrition and its relation to issues of health. The first director of the FAO was Lord Boyd-Orr, a British nutritionist.

The activities of the FAO are far reaching and include a scientific programme to develop better plant breeding, pest control, and the elimination of certain animal diseases.

The principal impact of the FAO on environmental health is through its interest in animal health, and through the international control and standardization of food composition through the **Codex Alimentarius**. The latter influences UK legislation directly and indirectly through the EU. As noted above the EU tries to ensure that its legislation is compatible with other international recomendations. Not all members of UNO are members of the FAO.

THE WORLD HEALTH ORGANIZATION

WHO is an agency of the UNO. It was formed in 1948 in Geneva, Switzerland, following a preliminary International Health Congress held in New York in 1946. The 1946 Conference took over the United Nations Relief and Rehabilitation Administration, which had been set up by the Allies to enable it to stabilize civil administration in areas liberated from enemy occupation.

Critics of the former international organizations were not slow to point out their imperfections, as though perfection could easily be achieved in countries medically and environmentally deprived, lacking economic resources, and an experienced and dedicated civil service.

> The World Health Organization is independent; and its decisions, unlike those of the health organizations of the League of Nations, do not need to be endorsed by a higher authority. Its constitution is wide enough to permit it to undertake any health work within the limits of its budget. [3]

One specific weakness already referred to was that earlier agencies found their work slow to be effective, because each agreement negotiated had to be subject to further ratification by each government. The new constitution of WHO overcame this by taking powers to make its decisions binding on its members. That power was conceded because provision was also made for members to be able to influence the 'legislation' which WHO produces. Member states may propose reservations which, if accepted, are incorporated into the measure. If such reservations are not accepted and not withdrawn, the measure is not then binding on the proposers.

The WHO organization operates through 11 divisions and 5 'offices' and from the environmental health aspect, 3 divisions – Communicable Diseases, Environmental Sanitation, Epidemiology and Health Statistics – are of especial significance.

As noted above, WHO secured worldwide collaboration in dealing with certain communicable diseases through the International Sanitary Regulations, and it is interesting to note the designation 'regulations' in substitution for 'convention' as an indication of the changed status of the legislation.

WHO has to operate in an area in which boundaries are unclear, and in which other agencies have an interest. For this reason, WHO works co-operatively with other UN agencies, especially the FAO in respect of nutrition and zoonoses, and the International Labour Office (ILO) with regard to occupational health issues.

THE INTERNATIONAL LABOUR OFFICE

Although the Second World War spelled the virtual end of the Paris health office, the International Labour Office was more fortunate in that, being based at Geneva, it was not subject to military occupation, although it did have to move its operational base temporarily to Montreal, Canada. After 1945 it became an agency under the aegis of the UN and, in so doing, became a major social force. Members of the UN were not automatically members of the ILO and, after 1945, there were some difficulties because within the major political blocs there were different views as to the role of trade unions.

The work of the ILO continued to develop along the inter-war years lines, and it has taken the practical step of having member countries visited by expert delegations to ascertain the scope of their labour laws, and their methods of administration and enforcement.

During the last half century, the standards evolved by the ILO have gradually become the leading external influence upon the labour law of many countries. [4, vol 9, p. 27]

The origins of the ILO can be traced to a privately organized body intended to arouse interest in international co-operation to promote better working conditions for labourers.

After the First World War, the International Labour Office was established in Geneva by the League of Nations, under Part XIII of the Treaty of Versailles. The ILO has a governing body which is unique in that it is tripartite and represents governments, and an equal number of representatives of organized labour and employers. It provides a forum for the discussion of labour and other social issues, and it has developed a consensus on appropriate policies and standards. It created an International Labour Code, which laid down minimum standards of national labour legislation and administration.

For member countries, it provides technical assistance, expert missions, and study grants, and it has developed comparative labour statistics, methods of carrying out manpower surveys, vocational training programmes, and the rehabilitation of handicapped workers.

The ILO operates by adopting conventions and recommendations. The conventions are designed as model legislation which member states are expected to ratify as soon as possible, and those states which do not are expected to report annually on their actions on matters which are the subject of conventions. Recommendations are a form of authorative guidance to members [4, Vol 9, p. 28]

A weakness of the ILO has been that it has to make conventions and recommendations to enable the least developed countries to adopt them. As a consequence, some more developed countries declined to ratify conventions or to follow recommendations which prescribed standards lower than those that they had already adopted for themselves.

Nevertheless, the ILO wishes to ensure that when local legislation is claimed to be superior to a convention, it really is. When the Health and Safety at Work, Etc Act 1974 was introduced, the ILO wished to send an inspecting delegation to the UK. This was postponed for a short while, but in due course the delegation came and saw examples of the enforcement of the legislation, both in the industrial sector and in the commercial sector, dealt with by the local authorities.

The UK is usually represented at conferences and committees by senior members of the Health and Safety Executive. While the ILO was intended to satisfy many of the aspirations of the trade union movements, which had developed strongly in the first half of the twentieth century (and were especially and increasingly interested in welfare and safety), it also caused some diminution in the movements' domestic influence because of the formal contacts between the ILO and governments.

As there is a close connection between the occupational environment and health, it is not surprising to find that the early actions of the ILO were the calling of conferences to improve the health of seamen.

A brief reference should be made to the apparent clash of activities in the field of health and safety at work between the EU and the ILO. Both of these organizations have an interest in the health, safety and welfare of workers, but in each case that interest is derived from different sources.

The ILO's interest stems from the fact that it has been specially created to promote better health, safety and welfare of people while they are at work, and has no *prima facie* concern with the competitiveness or otherwise of the employing company. On the other hand what the EU is concerned with most is that no employer is able to achieve a competitive advantage by reducing the cost of health and safety activities. The stance of the EU is thus to require the achievement of a standard minimum of health and safety provision.

THE UN ENVIRONMENTAL PROGRAMME

The UN Environmental Programme, an agency of the UN, has its headquarters in Nairobi, Kenya, and regional offices elsewhere in the world. It is much less well known than it should

be and appears in many ways to be overshadowed by WHO.

The Programme is particulary concerned with issues relates to the degradation of the environment, and especially those that affect developing countries. The resources of such countries in terms of trained technicians, finance and equipment are frequently inadequate and living standards are low and result from a low gross national product, which not only keeps the people poor, but restricts their ability to earn foreign currency with which better resources could be purchased.

In many third world countries, the need for foreign currency has lead to the exploitation of natural resources with little regard to geological, hydrological, biological or ecological consequences. Such countries have also been exploited by some industrialized countries, who have deposited hazardous waste materials that cannot be dumped at home. To make the situation worse, many developing countries are in 'harsh climate' zones and in areas where there are frequent natural disasters.

With the acknowledged trans-boundary effects of many environmental problems, difficulties, such as the reduction of tropical rain forests, have not only a local effect but also impinge on the global environment. The Programme has responded to this and is particularly concerned with the following issues:

1. protecting the atmosphere by combatting climate change and global warming, ozone layer depletion, and trans-boundary air pollution;
2. protecting the quality of fresh water sources;
3. protecting ocean and coastal area resources;
4. protecting land resources by combatting deforestation and desertification;
5. conserving biological diversity;
6. managing biotechnology in an environmentally sound way:
7. managing hazardous wastes and toxic chemicals in an environmentally sound manner;
8. protecting human health and the quality of life, especially the living and working environment of poor people from environmental degradation.

The possible short- and long-term effects of some global environmental changes have been discounted in some non-academic circles, for example, little thought appears to have been given to the effect on insect breeding by relatively modest increases in average temperature. The work of the Programme on transboundary and even global environmental issues is bound to have an effect on many countries, both developed and developing countries.

In June 1992 an international conference was held in Rio de Janeiro, Brazil at which national governments made agreements on environmental protection which are likely to have longer term influences on environmental policies.

THE INTERNATIONAL FEDERATION OF ENVIRONMENTAL HEALTH

The International Federation of Environmental Health was initiated by the then Institution of Environmental Health Officers. It was not the first attempt to create an organization linking environmental health professionals internationally. In the USA and Canada an organization, the International Federation of Sanitarians, was established in the 1960s and this continued for a number of years before being wound up.

The International Federation of Environmental Health was inaugurated in 1985, and was incorporated as a UK company in 1986. It acts as a Federation of national organizations of environmental health professionals and as such, it has no individual members. It has a colateral organization of Associated Bodies, which are mainly academic institutions that have an environmental health interest.

The Federation is a relatively new organization and is continuing to expand. It has a wide spectrum of objectives which include encouraging the co-operation of environmental health organizations; the exchange of information and experience; and the organization of contact between individual members of the constituent bodies.

The Federation endeavours to influence national environmental health policies by asking Member organizations to follow the policies adopted by

the Federation. Thus the Federation adopted a policy development suggested by the Swedish Environmental Health Officers Association relating to the assignment of wider public roles in environmental protection. It also adopted a policy suggestion made by the Californian Environmental Health Association which asked Members to ask national governments to ensure that when negotiating trade agreements under GATT [General Agreement on Tariffs and Trade] there would be no undesirable environmental consequences to either party.

The first policy statement was promulgated at the inaugural World Environmental Health Congress in Australia in 1988 and this endorsed the WHO Declaration of Alma Ata. The fourth policy statement emerged from the 3rd World Environmental Health Congress held in Malaysia in 1994 and this made the adoption an holistic approach to environmental health and the primacy on environmental health professionals formal Federation Policy.

One of the foundation concepts of the Federation is that environmental health problems are not constrained by man-made boundaries. Each Member organization is assumed to accept an awareness of international and global problems. There are, however, more localized issues and to deal with these Member organizations are being drawn together in regional groups with the object of generating local thought and action on regional issues and to keep the Federation Council aware of regional and local problems.

It aims to make effective links with such international organizations as WHO, the UN, and the EU, and to represent a global view on environmental health issues. The Federation takes the view that environmental health problems are best solved by sharing knowledge and experience, and that all the environmental health professional's organizations have much to teach others, just as they have much to learn from others.

POSTSCRIPT

It is normally assumed that the forces which impinge on law making are domestic in origin, but this is clearly not the case. Some of the external influences are indirect in nature – for example, the writings of influential people – and find expression in domestic pressures for either innovative new legislation or the revision of existing law.

Another important source of influence is to be found in international movements, and those which spring most readily to mind are the international environmental groups, such as Friends of the Earth and Greenpeace, and the international charitable agencies, such as the United Nations Childrens Fund, War on Want, and the International Red Cross. The experience and research done by such organizations are powerful influences which may, later, be reflected in changes in environmental health law.

The Treaty of Maastricht has provisions which may prove to be important for environmental health. It contains provisions relating to social benefits and the UK Government has taken a reserved position as far as mandatory compliance is concerned, but such 'social legislation' has an environmental health content and vice versa.

Basic EU treaties preclude the inclusion of public health issues but these may be seen to be within the remit of Maastricht.

REFERENCES

1. Frazer, W.M. (1950) *A History of Public Health*, Methuen, London, p. 213.
2. Haig, N. (1987) *EEC Environmental Policy in Britain*. Longmans, London.
3. Brockinton, W. Frazer (1952) *The World Health Organization*, Pelican, London, p. 210.
4. *Encyclopedia Britannica* (1980 edition), Encyclopedia Britannica Inc, Chicago.

3 The organization of environmental health in England and Wales

William H. Bassett

THE NATIONAL FRAMEWORK

The environmental health function in England and Wales is mainly operated at the local, community level through district and London borough councils, but the framework for that operation is set nationally. In non-metropolitan areas in England, county councils undertake some environmental health work, principally refuse disposal and food composition and labelling although in Wales the district councils also carry out waste disposal and regulation.

The local government structure of the metropolitan areas in England and in Wales and Scotland is being reviewed by a Local Government Commission and this may result in some areas becoming unitary authorities and being responsible for all local government functions. This will include the whole of Wales and Scotland and selected areas in England.

CENTRAL GOVERNMENT DEPARTMENTS

There is no single ministry responsible for the whole environmental health function, although the Department of Health is the focal point for the broader public health activity, and also for the health-related aspects of environmental health. Within the organization of the Department of Health is the office of the chief medical officer who, as well as having medical officers and scientists under his control, has a chief environmental health officer and several environmental health officers to advise on these issues.

Responsibility for the various facets of environmental health is divided between different central departments, and the main areas of division are:

1. Department of Health (DoH).
   (a) broad overview of health effects of environmental issues – microbiology and toxicology of the environment;
   (b) communicable disease control;
   (c) health promotion;
   (d) food safety and hygiene;
   (e) National Health Service – including food and environmental aspects.

2. Department of the Environment (DoE):
   (a) housing;
   (b) waste management;
   (c) environmental protection, including air and noise pollution;
   (d) water;
   (e) sewerage and sewage disposal;
   (f) building regulations;
   (g) bye-law approvals, e.g. dog control.

3. Ministry of Agriculture, Fisheries and Food (MAFF):
   (a) food composition, standards and labelling;
   (b) poultry and red meat inspection;
   (c) imported food controls;
   (d) pest control;

(e) animal health and welfare;

(f) food science and technological research.

4. Department of Employment:

(a) occupational health and safety.

5. Home Office:

(a) bye-law approvals, e.g. law and order including prohibition of the consumption of alcohol in specified public areas;

(b) licensing;

(c) Sunday trading.

THE WELSH OFFICE

The position in Wales is different in terms of the organization of central government departments, and the way in which the environmental health function is handled.

The Welsh Office is a separate and independent government department. It reproduces, in microcosm, all the Whitehall departments, but there are some notable variations. In line with arrangements for Scotland and Northern Ireland, the parliamentary head is the Secretary of State for Wales, who is a cabinet minister, and is assisted by two parliamentary under secretaries.

Head of the civil service in the Welsh Office is a permanent secretary, with direct responsibilities for finance and establishment. Two deputy secretaries head up the remaining operational groups. Somewhat like Whitehall, there is a separation of agriculture, particularly animal health, which is under one deputy secretary, while the housing, environmental protection and health groups are under the other. Curiously, responsibility for management of the National Health Service in Wales is a direct responsibility of the permanent secretary, although the health professional group, headed by the chief medical officer, has a direct input into its operation.

Housing, health and social services policy forms another group, headed by a permanent under secretary, who parallels the chief medical officer. There are five operational divisions within that group: housing, architects and surveyors, local authority, social services/family practitioner services, health policy and social work services. Water and environmental protection form another small division responsible directly to the deputy secretary.

The confusing management structure disguises the essence of the Welsh Office operation, which benefits from most departments being housed under one roof. While there is a Welsh Office presence in Whitehall, the bulk of the permanent staff are housed in Cathays Park, Cardiff. Unlike the London operational departments, which are separated both physically and by ministerial control. there is a day-to-day contact between the civil servants of Welsh Office across all of the divisions and groups. As a result, co-operation between those sections responsible for health, protection of the environment, agriculture, housing and finance is easier than with the UK central departments.

ENVIRONMENTAL HEALTH OFFICERS IN CENTRAL DEPARTMENTS

The effectiveness of the formulation and operation of environmental health policy within the English system depends upon the particular environmental health interests of each government department.

The environmental health officers in the Department of Health are mainly concerned with food safety. They also work closely with and advise the Ministry of Agriculture, Fisheries and Food. In other parts of Whitehall where environmental health policies are being considered and legislation formed they have less influence. Environmental health officers are currently employed at the Health and Safety Executive and Inspectorate of Pollution, and secondment from local authorities occurs from time to time at the Department of the Environment. There is an urgent need for the appointment of environmental health officers to other central departments, particularly to the Environment department, to deal with functions of those departments which fall within the remit of local authority environmental health officers.

In 1990, an environmental health officer was appointed by the Communicable Disease Surveillance Centre at Colindale (part of the Public Health Laboratory Service). This was a welcome development to co-ordinate local authority aspects of epidemiological work on communicable disease, and assist with training.

The Welsh Office presently has a chief environmental health officer with one environmental health officer assistant, based in the health profession group at Cardiff. Because of the cohesive structure, they are able to operate across the departmental boundaries to a great extent. There are, however, some limits to the Welsh Office operation. A number of services are subject to influence from Whitehall departments. For instance, the food safety element of the agriculture department is generally handled directly from London, and the Treasury has just the same pervasive influence as it has in other government departments.

THE ROLE OF THE CENTRAL GOVERNMENT DEPARTMENTS

This takes several forms:

Legislative

The drafting and processing of statutes and subordinate legislation relating to environmental health.

Once the Government has decided that there is a need for a change in the current legal provision it may well issue a **consultation paper** (sometimes called a 'green paper') which will seek the views of interested persons and agencies. Having considered the results of such consultation, the Government may issue a **command paper** commonly known as a 'white paper', which indicates the broad lines of legislation which the Government intends to introduce. It is thus a statement of intent to introduce legislation.

The issue of consultation and command papers are not required in the process of legislation, but are often used by Government as a way of gauging support for a proposed measure.

Administrative

Each central department will advise local authority environmental health departments about the implementation of legislation and on particular issues of concern to the government. This is done through the issue of ministerial circulars or through the local authority associations. There is also the very important need for each department to maintain close liaison with local authorities and their representative bodies in order to obtain information about environmental health issues generally. The arrangements will include contact on a regular basis with the local authority associations, and with the Chartered Institute of Environmental Health acting on behalf of the profession. Through these contacts local authorities at both elected member and officer levels are able to influence government policy as implemented through its legislative and advisory programmes, and to keep the government advised generally on the state of environmental health.

Monitoring

In some circumstances, central government has established direct monitoring arrangements over environmental health activity at local level. For example, MAFF acts as the 'competent authority' so far as EC law on meat hygiene is concerned, which requires it to exercise a direct surveillance role. Generally, however, the monitoring role is less direct and is undertaken through the wide network of contacts which central government has with the local authority and professional associations.

All central departments require local authorities to provide specified statistical and other information, and this includes aspects of the environmental health service. This is particularly prevalent so far as the Department of the Environment is concerned in respect of its housing function. Quarterly returns in certain aspects of local housing activity are necessary, as is the submission of an annual housing strategy review which is linked to bids for capital spending authority. Quarterly returns to DoE are also required under the Environmental Protection Act part I dealing with the authorization and control of scheduled processes. Quarterly returns to MAFF are now required in respect of activity under the Food Safety Act 1990 and returns are made to the Department of Health on fish and shellfish safety.

The regional offices of the Department of the Environment have a particular role in relation to the annual allocation of spending approvals for the housing function, and there is an annual meeting with each local authority at which its housing policies and spending bids are discussed. An annual return is also made to the Health and Safety Executive.

The trend is towards greater central monitoring and control over local authority activity and, although this has not so far affected the environmental health function to any significant degree, other than by the increased governmental control over local authority finance generally, there are indications that this may come. For example, there has been discussion about the possibility of requiring local authorities to submit annually to the Department of the Environment their plans for dealing with litter within the context of the Environmental Protection Act and recycling plans under that Act now need to be submitted to the Department of the Environment.

Direct service provision

There are some areas of environmental health activity where, as an exception to the general approach, direct services are provided at national level, either within a central department or by a quasi-autonomous body. Examples of such activities are:

1. The drinking water inspectorate: this is part of the Department of the Environment and is responsible for assisting the Secretary of State in monitoring the activities of the water undertakers with particular reference to drinking water quality.
2. Inspectorate of Pollution: again part of the Department of the Environment, this Inspectorate shares responsibility with local authorities for the enforcement of pollution legislation. There are proposals to merge the Inspectorate with the NRA and the drinking water inspec-

torate as an Environment Agency. These proposals are contained in the Environment Bill, scheduled for enactment in 1995.
3. The Health and Safety Commission is a quasi-autonomous body working under the direction of the Secretary of State for Employment, and has overall responsibility for occupational health and safety through the framework of the Health and Safety at Work, Etc. Act 1974. Within its auspices is the Health and Safety Executive, the Commission's operational arm, which shares the enforcement of legislation with local environmental health departments.
4. A National Meat Hygiene Service will take over from local authority environmental health departments' responsibilities for red and white meat slaughterhouses from 1 April 1995.

LEGISLATIVE ENFORCEMENT ON A SHARED BASIS

There are two main areas of environmental health enforcement activity where there is a shared role between central body and local authorities, i.e. air pollution and health and safety. There is a specific mechanism in place to bring the two inspectorates together in both cases to ensure the proper degree of collaboration and, through that, a consistency of approach to enforcement. While the detail differs to suit the particular circumstance, both the arrangements are based around the establishment of a collaborative body, IPLA for air pollution and HELA for health and safety, which contains representatives from both enforcement agencies. Within both the Inspectorate of Pollution and the Health and Safety Executive there is also a small local authority unit, staffed from both Inspectorates in each case, where the main technical tasks of collaboration are achieved, i.e. the production of technical guidance notes, codes of practice etc. The local authority unit within the HSE is headed by an environmental health officer.

There are arguments to support an extension of the use of structures affecting the provision of environmental health services which are based upon a highly specialized core within central government and a fieldwork, operational arm within local government, on the pattern of present health and safety structures. One obvious candidate would be the proposed Environment Agency where there is an opportunity to develop a specialized/coordinating centre supported by environmental health department fieldwork through which some activities currently undertaken by central authorities could be devolved to the local authorities.

LOCAL AUTHORITY ASSOCIATIONS

These comprise the Association of County Councils (ACC), the Association of Metropolitan Authorities (AMA), the Association of District Councils (ADC) and the Association of London Boroughs. The two with most influence over environmental health issues are the AMA and the ADC. Both comprise bodies of elected members nominated from constituent local authorities, and have a committee structure which mirrors that found generally in local authorities. This includes a committee for the debate of environmental health issues. There are proposals to merge the three main associations (ACA, AMA and ADC) to create a single representative body.

There are similar organizations in Scotland (the Convention of Scottish Local Authorities – COSLA) and in Northern Ireland (the Association of Local Authorites in Northern Ireland – ALANI).

The organizations are there to provide a national voice and to lobby and influence on behalf of local government. They are assisted by full-time officers which, in the case of the ADC, includes an environmental health officer. Both are supported by groups of chief environmental health officers, and of other local authority professions, seconded by local authorities, who advise members on the formulation of policy. These associations and their professional advisors perform a vital role in making the government aware of environmental health concerns at a local level, and in influencing the shape and content of the government's legislative programme. The roles

are also exercised through political channels (the associations are organized on party political lines), through the use of sympathetic MPs and members of the House of Lords during the legislative process; and by being consulted on government policy decisions through green and white papers and draft legislation.

Through the various organizational links which the Chartered Institute of Environmental Health and the local authority associations have, environmental health officers are represented on a wide range of national bodies. These include LACOTS, the Advisory Committee on Toxic Substances, the Royal Society for the Prevention of Accidents, the Tidy Britain Group, the Local Authority Associations Working Group on Aids and the National Drugs Forum. Similar bodies span the whole spectrum of environmental health and such 'net-working' is a very important aspect of the organization of the function and of the promotion of environmental health officers' professional objectives.

The elected members for the associations also play a full part in representing local authority interests affecting environmental health on other bodies, e.g. the Advisory Committee on Pollution of the Sea, the Central and Local Government Forum.

LACOTS

The Local Authorities Co-ordinating Body on Food and Trading Standards (LACOTS) was established by the Local Authority Associations in 1978. Its original purpose was to co-ordinate trading standards activity throughout the UK and to promote common interpretation of statutes and consistency of enforcement. In 1992, and following the Food Safety Act 1990, its remit was extended to exercise a similar role in respect of environmental health food safety. LACOTS is an unincorporated body constituted by and accountable to the ACC, AMA, ADC, COSLA and ALANI. The organization is controlled by a management committee comprising elected members nominated by the local authority associations.

LACOTS' main activities are reflected in its terms of reference:

1. To provide centralized local government machinery for the consideration of issues arising in connection with local authority trading standards, consumer protection and food law functions.
2. To co-ordinate the operational practice of local authorities at the professional/technical level for the purpose of performing the above functions.
3. To participate in consultations with Central Government and its agencies, trade and industry, European institutions and enforcement practitioners in Member States.
4. To provide a central point for the collection, dissemination and exchange of enforcement information including the maintenance of a national register of road traffic convictions and other records.

LOCAL OMBUDSMAN

Where a person considers that they have been unfairly treated by a local authority, they can ask the local ombudsman to investigate to see if there has been maladministration. The local ombudsman is independent and impartial, and has the same powers as the High Court to require the production of information and documents for investigation. Maladministration occurs if a council does something in the wrong way, does something which it should not have done, or fails to do something which it should have done. The ombudsman cannot question the decision of a council, but rather the way in which that decision was reached.

As a first stage, the ombudsman will advise the local authority that a complaint has been received and ask for it to provide information in respect of the matter complained of, and indicate whether the matter is one which can be resolved between the local authority and the complainant. The ombudsman will upon consideration decide whether further action or more detailed investigation, is needed.

The majority of complaints are resolved after an initial investigation. If further investigation is undertaken, it is likely to involve detailed examination of documents and interviews with officers involved in the matter. If, however, following a full investigation the ombudsman finds maladministration, he provides a formal report which must be considered by the council which must inform the ombudsman of the action it intends to take to remedy the grievance.

The local ombudsman does not have power to enforce a local authority to take action to remedy a grievance. However, if he is not satisfied with the response of the local authority, he may issue a further report. The ombudsman may suggest compensation be made to the complainant if loss has been suffered as a result of the maladministration. The majority of cases considered by the ombudsman relate to planning and housing issues, and relatively few to environmental health.

An example of an ombudsman enquiry in respect of environmental health related to a complaint that a local authority had not taken action to deal with nuisance caused by barking stray dogs kennelled at an RSPCA premises. The environmental health officers concerned were of the view that a statutory nuisance existed, and were in discussion with the RSPCA to achieve improvements in the management and construction of the premises. These discussions did not achieve results within a timescale acceptable to the complainant. The ombudsman found the local authority guilty of maladministration in that they did not use the powers available to them to the full extent, or as expeditiously as they could have done.

THE CHARTERED INSTITUTE OF ENVIRONMENTAL HEALTH

Aims and objectives

The organization which was in due course to become the Chartered Institute of Environmental Health (CIEH) was founded in London in 1883. Having proved an ability over the ensuing 100 years to establish and maintain professional standards, the Institution of Environmental Health Officers (IEHO) was granted a Royal Charter in 1984.

In 1994 as a mark of the profession's quality and worth Her Majesty the Queen granted the professional body a new title – the Chartered Institute of Environmental Health.

The primary objective of the CIEH is the promotion of environmental health and the dissemination of knowledge about environmental health issues for the benefit of the public. The CIEH represents the views of its members on environmental and public health issues and is independent of central and local government.

The majority of the Institute's 8500 members are employed in local government to enforce a wide range of legislation on issues such as food safety, pollution, housing standards, safety at work and infectious disease and to educate the public on matters of hygiene and safety. A significant number of members work in the private sector either for individual companies or as private environmental health consultants. There are also environmental health personnel working in central government and non-commercial organizations in addition to those teaching environmental health in universities and colleges throughout the country.

For organizational purposes the membership is divided into 17 Centres. Fifteen of these are geographical and two are functional (Port Health and Commercial & Industrial). The Centres are run by a Centre Council elected from the membership in the designated area. The Centre elects representatives to the General Council in proportion to the number of members in the Centre; the General Council is the governing body of the CIEH.

There are seven categories of membership ranging from student membership for those people pursuing an approved technical or professional course in environmental health through to corporate membership for those who are both qualified in environmental health and have passed an Assessment of Professional Competence after two years of professional practice.

Student members are encouraged to use the services provided for members, to take part in educational activities of the Institute and to attend meetings of the Centres and Branches to which they belong.

Activities

Prime among the activities of the CIEH are those which achieve the objects laid down in the Charter which emphasize the importance of education, training and the maintenance of high standards of professional practice and conduct by all its members.

The Institute undertakes the following activities in pursuit of maintaining professional standards and meeting the obligations of the Royal Charter:

1. The holding of Branch and Centre meetings for the conduct of business and the discussion and development of good practice.
2. The provision of seminars, study weekends and other opportunities for professional development at both local and national level.
3. The holding of an annual Environmental Health Congress and the Annual General Meeting of the CIEH.
4. The monitoring and approval of qualifying courses in environmental health, the assessment of professional competence and the promotion of continuing professional development among the membership.
5. The convening of technical committees and working parties at national level to develop policy and recommendations for good practice and to respond to consultation documents published by government departments and other organisations with concerns for environmental health.
6. The distribution of a weekly newspaper and a monthly journal and the publication of texts, practice notes and policy documents on environmental health issues.
7. The provision of advice to members on educational, constitutional and technical issues.
8. Liaison with officials of the UK government, the European Union and the World Health Organization on developments in environmental health.

Further details are available from: CIEH, Chadwick Court, 15 Hatfields, London SE1 8DJ. Tel: 0171 928 6006.

THE AUDIT COMMISSION

The Audit Commission for Local Authorities in England and Wales is an independent body, established under the provisions of the Local Government Finance Act 1982. Its objectives are to appoint auditors to local authorities and to help authorities to bring about improvements in efficiency, directly through the auditing process and through the 'value for money' studies which the Commission carries out. The auditors appointed may be from the publicly owned District Audit Service or from private firms of accountants.

The Commission members include senior people from industry, local government, the accounting professions and the trade unions.

Although waste collection, street cleansing and the cleansing of public conveniences were amongst the first local government activities to be studied by the Commission, it first turned its attention to the core environmental health function in June 1990 with the publication of an information paper *Environmental Health – Survey of Food Premises* [1]. This reported the results of a survey of the condition of food premises, undertaken jointly by the Commission and the CIEH, which indicated that almost one in eight food premises in England and Wales presented significant or imminent health risks, with different types of premises presenting different health risks. It was also noted that almost 46% of the food premises visited as part of the survey had not been inspected within the previous year (a quarter of these had not been visited within previous 3 years) and 5% had never been visited. This initial interest in the food safety activity was followed in December 1990 by the publication by the Commission of a broader study *Safer Food: Local Authorities and the Food Safety Act 1990* [2]. This study looked at the likely effect of the impending implementation of the Act and its regulations on environmental health departments. One of the conclusions reached was that a better structure was required to achieve common standards of Food Law enforcement (Since this report LACOTS' role has been expanded to deal with Food Safety – see p. 52).

The Commission next took an interest in the general management of environmental health, and in July 1991 published *Towards a Healthier Environment: managing environmental health services* [4]. This study considered the management and use of necessarily scarce resources in providing an efficient, effective and economic environmental health service and in particular:

(a) discussed the wide-ranging activities of the environmental health function in local authorities (Figs 3.1 and 3.2);

(b) considered the changes facing the profession including recent legislation;

(c) analysed the problems facing the service and the ways they were being tackled.

The principal findings of this study were that:

1. Each authority should develop a corporate policy for the delivery of environmental health services.
2. Each environmental health department should:
   (a) translate that policy into departmental objectives, consistent with available resources;
   (b) assemble information on local environmental health needs and target resources appropriately;
   (c) determine the style of its intervention, for example, a responsive or pro-active stance;
   (d) set out clear task allocations to staff.
3. Operational activity must be informed by accurate and detailed information systems, premises registers, risk assessment.
4. Consistency must be sustained through explicit priorities and protocols as well as cultural norms.
5. Service effectiveness must be monitored through staff management information systems and relevant output measures.
6. Authorities should assure the quality of their services through systematic evaluation of their activities including a performance cycle.

These conclusions are illustrated in Fig. 3.3.

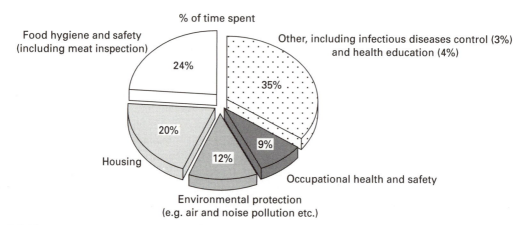

Fig. 3.1 Time spent on core activities – there are four major areas of activity. (Source: CIPFA, 1989–90. From: Audit Commission (1991) *Towards a Healthier Environment*, HMSO, London.)

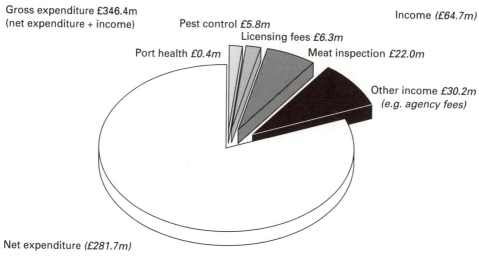

Fig. 3.2 Environmental health income and expenditure: 1989–90. Less than 20% of gross expenditure is recovered by fees and charges. (Source: CIPFA, 1989–90 (grossed up estimates). From: Audit Commission (1991) *Towards a Healthier Environment*, HMSO, London.) From 1 April 1995 income from meat inspection charges will go to the National Meat Hygiene Service and not to local authorities.

The Commission next looked at the activities of environmental health officers in the housing field and in September 1991 published *Healthy Housing: the role of Environmental Health Services* [3].

This report identified the health risk related to house condition, the condition of stock and the role of the environmental health department in enforcing the relevant legislation. The study applied the general conclusions of the earlier report on environmental health services generally [4] and again concluded that there was a lack of clear policies and strategies, inadequate information on the scale and location of housing problems in each area and a wide variation in the performance of staff. The Commission's proposal for managing the housing function is shown in Fig. 3.4.

In April 1993 and jointly with CIEH the Audit Commission published a study of the reaction of Chief Environmental Health Officers to these

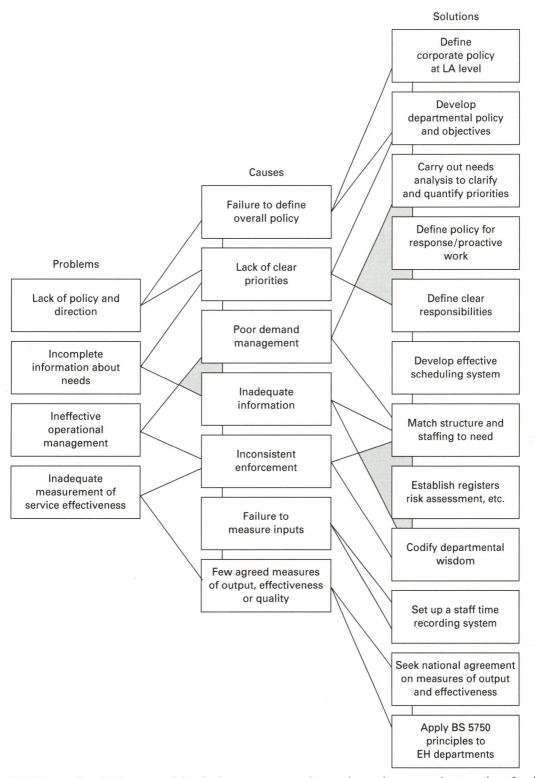

Solutions

Define corporate policy at LA level

Develop departmental policy and objectives

Carry out needs analysis to clarify and quantify priorities

Define policy for response/proactive work

Define clear responsibilities

Develop effective scheduling system

Match structure and staffing to need

Establish registers risk assessment, etc.

Codify departmental wisdom

Set up a staff time recording system

Seek national agreement on measures of output and effectiveness

Apply BS 5750 principles to EH departments

Causes

Failure to define overall policy

Lack of clear priorities

Poor demand management

Inadequate information

Inconsistent enforcement

Failure to measure inputs

Few agreed measures of output, effectiveness or quality

Problems

Lack of policy and direction

Incomplete information about needs

Ineffective operational management

Inadequate measurement of service effectiveness

Fig. 3.3 Clear policy, fresh managerial attitudes, greater team integration and more precise targeting of activity are required. (Source: Audit Commission (1991) *Towards a Healthier Environment*, HMSO, London.)

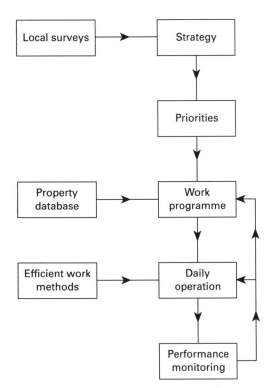

Fig. 3.4 Effective housing work by environmental health officers. Effective housing work must be based on a number of key elements. (Source: Audit Commission (1991) *Healthy Housing: the role of environmental health services*, HMSO, London.)

reports [5]. Unfortunately less than 40% of authorities responded to this survey which generally showed that the Commission's reports were appropriately timed and of high quality. This study was more in the nature of a customer survey by the Commission than an attempt to identify what effect the reports had effected on the operation of the environmental health service.

One of the more recent roles of the Commission has been to assist local authorities in the development of performance indicators which are intended to identify areas of poor performance for remedial action. Such systems are also encouraged by the Citizens Charter [6]. The system introduced so far through the Publication of Information (Standards of Performance) Direct-

ive 1992 (issued by the Commission through its powers in the Local Government Act 1992) does not deal specifically with the environmental health service although there are some general indicators which do relate to the service, e.g. responding to the public, handling of complaints about service, etc. The Commission has, however, specified environmental health indicators for use starting in 1994/95.

The Commission exercises its functions through:

1. the issue of national reports (as with those discussed above) which publish the results of surveys into particular activities and which draw attention to good practice – in effect these provide benchmarks against which to judge the performance of individual local authorities; and
2. detailed audits at individual authorities at which time the national guidelines are taken into account. These audits were undertaken at most environmental health departments following the national study on the management of the environmental health service and of environmental health aspects of housing.

THE EUROPEAN FRAMEWORK

Most UK legislation on environmental health is now resultant from EU requirements and in particular those relating to environmental protection, food safety and health and safety. More information is given about this in the appropriate chapters.

There is also an increasing trend for administrative involvement by the EU in the work of UK environmental health departments, e.g. reports on activity under the Food Safety Act have to be submitted by each department through the UK government. There is discussion about the future role of the 'EU Inspector', particularly in respect of meat hygiene.

The process involving EU Law is dealt with in Chapter 2 but it should be stated here that there is a limited opportunity to influence European policy.

THE LOCAL FRAMEWORK

With the few exceptions identified in the previous section, the environmental health function is located at district local authority (community level). There is general recognition in the UK that there are strong advantages in the core environmental health service operating at the community level where it will be in close contact with the population it serves and the environmental problems which it faces. This approach is supported by WHO [7].

The present system is, in the main, a product of the major scheme of reorganization of local government in 1974, which established a two-tiered system of district and county councils across England and Wales. This has been subsequently amended by the abolition of the Greater London Council and of the metropolitan county councils, so that the system is now single tier (district) in London and the other 36 metropolitan areas, and two-tiered in non-metropolitan areas. There are a few environmental health activities placed at county council level in non-metropolitan areas, e.g. food standards (composition and labelling) and waste disposal, although in Wales waste disposal and regulation is a district council function. Agency arrangements are sometimes used through which the district council operates the food standards function on behalf of the county council. This structure in non-metropolitan areas is currently being reviewed and it is likely that there will be an increase in single-tier (unitary) government. This will include a unitary system for all of Scotland and Wales and in selected areas in England.

THE ENVIRONMENTAL HEALTH CONTROL SYSTEM

According to Wilfried Kreisel, director of the Division of Environmental Health for WHO:

Organization has become a crucial issue in environmental management and health, especially so in the last 20 years. In many countries, actions in the environment are not coherent and many environmental health policies and programmes have become fragmented as governments have reshuffled environmental management responsibilities among public agencies and private interests. [8]

This comment is certainly applicable to the UK where the degree of 'reshuffling' has been significant, e.g. the privatization of the sewage, sewage disposal and water industry in 1989.

Kreisel sees that a key to solving this problem is the concept of moving beyond the boundaries of environmental health units, to organize environmental health as a broader system in which environmental health outcomes depend on what is done by other agencies of government and by private sector enterprises, and on the messages that reach people through the mass media and community groups. In UK terms, this means that the environmental health department (unit) must do much more than simply enforce legislation. It must be at the centre of a total system of environmental health control.

Such a concept now embraces the UK system of environmental health control based on the environmental health departments (units) located at district council level. But this was not the case at the time of the 1974 reorganization, which was mainly an allocation of specific functions. It has been developed since 1974 by the environmental health profession along the lines being promulgated by WHO and outlined in the Introduction. Its essence is the creation in each district and London borough council of an environmental health department, or separate unit within a larger department, to which all the council's environmental health functions are allocated and which is also given the specific role of taking the lead to maintain complete environmental health surveillance over the district. This latter role is performed through the establishment of a comprehensive network of liaison arrangements with other departments and organizations, both inside and outside of the council – hence the '**extended environmental health unit**'.

The production of an effective control system is essentially a team task involving all those whose efforts are critical to the environmental health

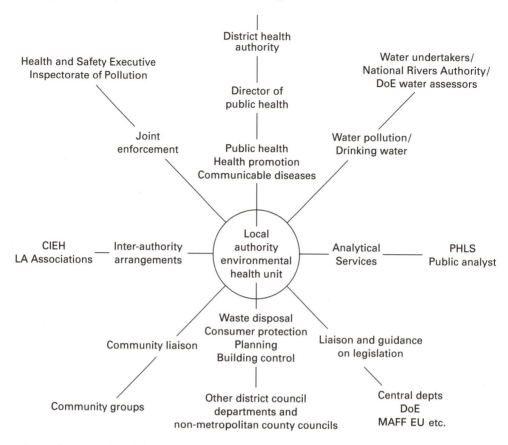

Fig. 3.5 The environmental health control system through the extended environmental health unit.

function. The breadth of this extended unit is illustrated in Fig. 3.5.

THE ENVIRONMENTAL HEALTH UNIT
Tasks

It follows that, since the environmental health unit is the focal point of a much broader system of control, the tasks to be performed within the unit will be diverse and the following groupings indicate the range of activities.

Surveillance
An essential task for the unit is to undertake an ongoing and total surveillance over those environmental issues which affect health. To successfully achieve such an objective involves both the establishment of a wide range of direct activities within

the unit, and of collaborative/monitoring arrangements with other organizations involved in environmental monitoring, both statutory and non-statutory. Direct monitoring activities carried out by staff within the unit or under contract to them may include:

1. the sampling of food and water for both microbiological and chemical assessments;
2. environmental sampling for the detection of heavy metals, asbestos, legionella, etc.;
3. detection of atmospheric pollutants;
4. assessment of contaminated land:
5. monitoring of radiation levels in air, food stuffs, land and water;
6. assessment of proposals for new development, e.g. housing, highways, industrial, etc.

Amongst the collaborative arrangements for identifying further information neccessary to form a total picture of the state of environmental health of an area will be those with the following:

1. National Rivers Authority – the pollution of water abstraction sources, rivers, streams, etc., effluent standards and consents.
2. Water undertakers and water assessors within the Department of the Environment – drinking water quality, the exchange of analytical information and the identification of potential problems.
3. Director of public health of the District Health Authority – public health statistics including mortality and morbidity figures and communicable diseases.
4. HM Inspectorate of Pollution – monitoring of pollution from scheduled processes.
5. Health and Safety Executive – enforcement and accident statistics relating to occupational health and safety and identification of priority enforcement areas.
5. Veterinary service of the Ministry of Agriculture, Fisheries and Food – notifications of zoonoses and hazards to public health arising from animal-related issues, the results of testing of feeding stuffs and meat for residues, etc. This is facilitated through the establishment of Zoonoses Groups on a county basis.

Provision of information

The Environmental Information Regulations 1992 require a wide range of bodies including local authorities to make available to the public environmental information which it holds relating to:

1. the state of any water or air, the state of any flora or fauna, the state of any soil or of any natural site or other land;
2. activities or measures (including noise or other nuisance) which adversely affect anything in (1) above, or
3. any measures (including environmental management programmes) which are designed to protect against these concerns.

There are some restrictions on these requirements, e.g. in respect of commercial confidentiality and information subject to legal proceedings. There are other statutory requirements relating to environmental information, e.g. for authorizations of processes under Part 1 of the Environmental Protection Act, 1990; where such specific requirements are not as onerous as the 1992 Regulations the latter will prevail and where they are more onerous then the more liberal regime will apply, and under the Environment and Safety Information Act 1988 under which registers of information on enforcement notices served under the Health and Safety at work Etc. Act 1974 must be kept available for public inspection.

These requirements fall on the whole range of public bodies involved in environmental issues, e.g. Health and Safety Executive, National Rivers Authority, etc., but the environmental health department should be seen as a location at which all such information is gathered together and made available to the public. Such a service enhances the central role of the department in environmental management.

Enforcement

One of the core functions of the unit is the enforcement of legislation, primarily statute law and secondary legislation, but also local legislation including bye-laws. The main areas of legislation involved are:

1. food inspection and food safety and hygiene:
2. meat hygiene and animal welfare:
3. communicable disease prevention and control:
4. health and safety at work and during recreation;
5. housing standards;
6. environmental protection including statutory nuisances:
7. licensing:
8. drinking water surveillance.

The inspection of premises in order to enforce legislation is one of the main tasks of the environmental health department and the way in which this is approached is crucial to its effectiveness. The inspection activity must be structured so as to take full account of the risks inherent in any particular premises or type of premises. Thus more attention and a greater frequency of inspection should be given to those premises whose operations and/or past record involve a greater risk to public health.

The need for such an approach has been stressed by the Audit Commission [3, 4] and by the UK Government through the Department of Health. Thus risk assessment and an inspection programme based on it are essential ingredients of the enforcement function. Enforcement is discussed in more detail in Chapter 8.

Service provision

Local authorities provide a wide range of environmental health services directly to the community, some being statutorily required and others being discretionary. These include:

1. refuse collection and street cleansing (statutory);
2. pest control;
3. dog warden (statutory);
4. food hygiene training;
5. health promotion.

These services may either be provided directly by the environmental health unit or by others on a contract from the unit. The provision of cleansing services must in any event be subject to the competitive tendering provisions of the Local Government Act 1988, and it is important that the client function in this case is performed within the environmental health unit since this involves the identification and monitoring of standards for this service.

Some services may be provided by the environmental health units as the result of an agency agreement with the body carrying the primary responsibility for that service. Examples are arrangements with a county council for the operation of the food standards function, and with the water undertakers for the sewerage function and for the control of rodents in sewers. In these cases, the primary authority retains control over the standards of the service and for resource allocation, while the district council bears responsibility for the operation of the service within those parameters.

Investigative

The unit provides a point of reference for community complaints about issues which are of concern to them, and these require investigation and determination. Many will be investigations within a legal framework which may lead to the institution of legal proceedings, e.g. statutory nuisances, while others will have no statutory remedy and will require persuasion if the problem is to be eliminated.

The number of complaints received by environmental health units from one neighbour about the activities of another are high and rising. These involve a wide range of concerns including noise, bonfires and general unacceptable behaviour. The investigation of such complaints is often lengthy and very time consuming and frequently does not have an entirely acceptable result. Some environmental health units are attempting to deal with this by encouraging the setting up of voluntary conciliation services through which these types of neighbour disputes may have an informed and negotiated solution agreed by both parties. Not only do such agencies relieve the local authority of often abortive work but they may also be more likely to produce more effective solutions in some cases.

Educative/publicity

An increasing amount of the unit's attention is being given both to the provision of environmental health information to the community on a full range of issues, e.g. food hazards, heart disease, environmental pollutants, etc., and also to the need to inform the community of services available and involve them in decisions about the content of those services and the ways in which they are made available.

The provisions of the Food Safety Act 1990 and the Health and Safety at Work, Etc. Act 1974 both provide for training to be given to staff employed in activities covered by the legislation – in effect the whole range of employment. Many employers look to the environmental health department for assistance and the Chartered Institute of Environmental Health validate such courses through those departments. Further information is given in Chapter 6.

Innovative

One of the essential tasks of the unit is to try new things, and to experiment in the solution of problems. In historic terms, it has been the efforts of individual local authorities, or groups of them, which have led to major legislative change regarding clean air, food hygiene, dog control and health promotion.

A legitimate function of the unit is to stimulate change to the approach and operation of the environmental health service through experimentation. Current examples are the creation of 'community contracts' for the street cleaning function in York, a scheme for the retrieval of supermarket trollies in Exeter (now embodied in national legislation through the Environmental Protection Act 1990), and arrangements for health promotion in Oxford. Both the Chartered Institute of Environmental Health and the Local Authority Associations have a vital role to play in promoting such innovation locally, and in pressing for national change based upon the success of local initiatives.

The Environmental Health Unit is often the lead department in a local authority's initiative to improve its environment. Environmental management strategies and the Healthy Cities initiative are examples of this.

There is a developing role of environmental health officers undertaking sponsored research as an aspect of environmental health as part of study for a higher degree and some work may often lead to new ideas for environmental health policy and practice.

Agency services

The last ten years have seen a growth of agency and advisory services to the general public, both within local authorities and by others. For example, there are numerous housing advice centres provided both by district councils and also by voluntary agencies. Some environmental health departments operate agency services for the undertaking of work related to renovation grants, and also for 'stay-put' schemes to enable elderly or disabled people to live more comfortably in their own homes (see Chapter 20). These agency services include surveys, the identification of defects, the production of specifications, the letting and supervision of contracts and the identification of funding arrangements including grant aid.

Customers for environmental health services

Over the last few years there has been increasing attention given to the identification of the customers for public services and a need to closely relate to them in terms of service standards and delivery. At Government level this has identified itself in the form of the Citizens Charter [6] which has four main aims:

1. **Quality** – A sustained new programme for improving the quality of public services.
2. **Choice** – Choice, wherever possible between competing providers, is the best spur to quality improvement.
3. **Standards** – The citizen must be told what service standards are and be able to act where service is unacceptable.
4. **Value** – The citizen is also a taxpayer, public services must give value for money within a tax bill the nation can afford.

Customer relations is now firmly placed as an issue within the environmental health service and one facet of this is the setting of performance indicators (see p. 58). There are also changes in green consumerism, i.e. a demand for greater care and protection of the environment through the identification of environmental-friendly goods and for higher standards generally in the environmental health function.

As part of the response to these changes, there is an increasing tendency to establish at local level widely based collaborative groups to consider the environmental issues relating to that area. Sometimes called the Environmental Protection Forum, these groups will include representatives of statutory and voluntary bodies. The latter, for example, may involve the Chamber of Commerce, Friends of the Earth and local consumer groups. A central, co-ordinating role by the environmental health unit in these groups is essential.

Such changes in the public perception of environmental health issues demand a much closer relationship between the environmental health unit and its community.

Policy formulation

The determination of local policies for the environmental health function is a matter for each district council individually in the light of its own problems, resources and priorities. The process of policy formulation is generally initiated informally by discussion between the chairperson of the Environmental Health Committee and the director/chief environmental health officer, at which time professional and political objectives relating to the service can be identified and structured. Proposals for new policies or changes to existing policies are then made by the chief officer to the Committee which forms resolutions in the form of recommendations to a meeting of the full council.

Many councils operate on the basis of a forward plan, in which case policy initiatives will be identified on, say, a rolling, three-year basis. Throughout this process the effectiveness of the relationship beween the chief officer and the chairperson is crucial. As part of the streamlining of management processes within local government, which has been stimulated by the 'competitive' environment created by the government in the second part of the 1980s, main committees like the Environmental Health Committee are restricting their concerns to matters of policy determination, resource allocation and monitoring, leaving the operation of services within those parameters to directors/chief environmental health officers. In some cases, authorities have seen a need to 'bridge' these two management systems by the creation of Member Working Groups. These are non-executive bodies which monitor and guide the operation of services on an informal basis working closely with operational managers.

The derivation of environmental health policies has several sources and these include the following:

1. Legislative duties: legislation may prescribe duties to be undertaken by local authorities and, in some cases, may even prescribe the standards to be achieved, e.g. each local authority is under a duty to enforce the Health and Safety at Work, Etc. Act 1974 in premises allocated to it, and many of the standards to be achieved are prescribed by legislation.

2. Legislative discretion: some legislation allows the local authority to decide for itself whether or not it wishes to use certain legislative powers, e.g. the adoption of a registration process for skin piercing.

3. Professional initiative: policies may be initiated by the director/chief environmental health officer as a result of:
   (a) personal initiative;
   (b) initiative by the professional staff of the environmental health unit;
   (c) suggestions from the Chartered Institute of Environmental Health, or other professional organization, or by the local authority associations;
   (d) discussion between colleagues at county chief environmental health officer groups or national conferences.

4. Member/political initiatives.

5. Community pressure, e.g. customer surveys, etc.

The role of elected members

It is the council as a corporate body, i.e. its elected representatives, which is responsible in law for the delivery of services. This includes the environmental health service and the relationship between the members, both individually and in formal groupings of committees, etc., and officers is crucial to the effective operation of the organization and of the environmental health unit. According to the Widdicombe Report [9], councillors, while retaining overall legal responsibility for the delivery of services, should seek to leave the day-to-day management of those services as far as possible to officers.

This relationship was further considered by the Audit Commission in its Management Paper No.1. *The Competitive Council* [10] and four main roles for elected members were identified:

1. Policy formulation: this role was identified earlier in this chapter and is seen as being the most significant role.

2. Representation: each member represents their ward and will bring to the council departments

issues affecting the community in those areas. The degree of contact between elected members and environmental health units in this regard is very significant, and ranges from the pursuit of complaints on behalf of individual constituents to the submission of petitions which may represent thousands of people. This role should not be confused with the responsibility for the operation of services which is a chief officer matter. It is a right of access to that operation on behalf of the community. Members also form a vital link between the council and the community, and this is particularly important to the environmental health service since those links with the community are so critical.

3. Performance review: having established policies and allocated resources, members should be organized in such a way as to effectively monitor the implementation of these policies and appraise their performance. In many councils, performance review committees are established to undertake this task.

4. Operational management: elected members have responsibility to ensure that an adequate management organization exists, and that clear responsibilities have been assigned to chief officers. Apart from this, the Audit Commission supports the views of the Widdicombe Committee that elected members should leave detailed operation to officers.

There is continuing debate about ways in which local authorities should manage their affairs and improve the decision-making process. Following the Widdicombe Committee studies [9], the Secretary of State published a consultative paper, The Internal Management of Local Authorities in England [11], and this has been studied by a working party composed from the local authority associations, Local Government Management Board, Audit Commission and others. It is anticipated that the Government will make proposals to further regulate the internal management of authorities in 1995.

Elected members from local authorities also have a significant part to play in the organization of local government at national level, particularly through the local authority associations. These associations also nominate elected members onto other national bodies, e.g. local authority members sit as commissioners on the Health and Safety Commission. They also have formal liaison committees with other public bodies, e.g. joint consultative committees with health authorities and county councils.

Delegation of authority

The Local Government Act 1972 allows a council to delegate decision making to committees, subcommittees and officers. The correct use of this power is also critical to the effective operation of services, and should take full account of the principles of proper member/officer relationships as outlined above. Delegation needs to be undertaken as a formal process by clear definition through resolution of the council. What is not clearly delegated in such a scheme remains a matter for the full council to determine.

Because the environmental health service contains a high level of legislative enforcement, delegation to its chief officer is usually greater than to any other chief officer, and will need to indicate each legal process delegated, e.g. service of notices, institution of proceedings, etc., under each piece of legislation.

Organization

Location

Within the district or London borough council, the environmental health unit is normally established as a separate department under a chief environmental health officer or director of environmental health, who will be a chief officer and member of the council's chief officer group or management team. Where this is not the case, the unit will be located as a separate operational group within a directorate, which will include other services.

There is a wide range of service groupings within such directorates, but it is common that the environmental health service is linked with the housing service. Such directorate posts are often held by environmental health officers but, where this is not the case, it is essential for arrangements to be made which ensure the direct provision of professional environmental health advice to the chief officer group, the council and its committees and sub-committees.

Structure
The way in which the environmental health department or unit is structured will depend upon local perceptions of problems and needs. However, it is usual for the four main functional areas, i.e. food, environmental protection, housing and health and safety, to be given particular status within the structure, either by the creation of a specialist team to deal with each or by identifying individual environmental health officers, usually at principal officer or section head level, to undertake specific responsibility for that function across the whole of the council's area. Code of Practice No.9 issued under the Food Safety Act requires that food authorities should appoint at least one environmental health officer with particular responsibility for food hygiene and safety matters.

There are often significant differences in organizational approach between rural authorities, with large geographic areas where problems are often diffused over wide areas and where travel distances for staff are great, and urban areas where the problems are often more acute and intensified.

The approach in rural areas tends to be one of a geographic allocation to environmental health officers, where responsibility is taken for all, or a wide range of, environmental health activity in that one district, with or without further technical support. In the more concentrated urban area, officers tend to specialize in one aspect of environmental health, e.g. food hygiene or health and safety, either individually or as part of a specialist team. It is possible to have an approach which involves a mixture of both in that, while the majority of activities may be dealt with on a district, generalized basis, some activities, e.g. noise control, can be the subject of a more specialized approach.

The three approaches are shown in Fig. 3.6 but only in diagrammatic form. The actual structures required to operate such systems are more complex and involve a different number of managerial levels, e.g. there may be a deputy chief environmental health officer, and the use of technical support staff.

The requirement to bring all of these separate activities together, and to link them to the liaison arrangements with the other agencies to ensure total environmental health surveillance, is achieved through the establishment of a departmental (unit) management grouping. This is often supported by the designation of particular environmental health officers to link with identified agencies. For example, a principal environmental health officer may be asked to provide structured liaison with the National Rivers Authority, and then report back through the internal management system

Staffing
Just as the establishment of an effective environmental health system relies upon a team beyond the unit, the extended environmental health unit, so the operation of the unit itself is essentially a team task. The types of staff found in the unit will include:

ENVIRONMENTAL HEALTH OFFICERS The proper use of the broad training and skills of the environmental health officer is critical to the production of an effective control system. Organizationally, structures will usually provide for such officers either to be responsible for a wide range of environmental health activity across a defined area of the district (generalized approach), or for concentrating the use of more intensive skills in a particular facet, e.g. environmental protection (specialized approach). In both cases the environmental health officer will normally be a team leader of the section dealing with this particular work, and will be supported by technical and/or scientific staff.

TECHNICIANS AND TECHNICAL OFFICERS Supporting and complementing the work of the environmental health officer in particular aspects, e.g. meat

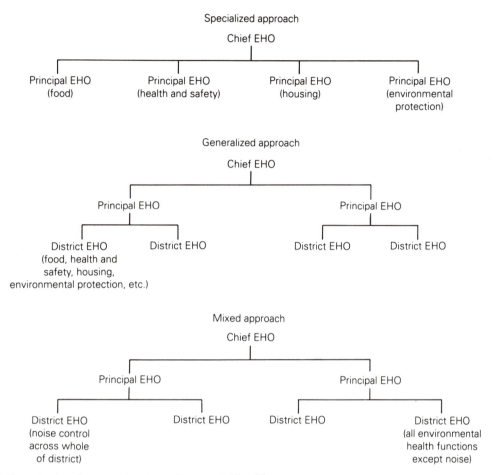

Fig. 3.6 Organizational approaches to environmental health.

inspection, food control, health and safety, and housing. This group is diverse and contains staff with a wide range of knowledge and skills.

The creation of the correct balance between the professional and technical staff is an important, and often difficult, issue for the unit to achieve. Essentially, this balance is between the broader environmental skills of the environmental health officer, and the more specialized in-depth skills of the technician. Environmental health technicians qualifying through the National B.Tec. courses are trained in all the main areas of activity, but in more detail in one or more areas, e.g. food hygiene, housing or health and safety, while technical officers will be trained only in one

particular area of the unit's work, e.g. pest control.

OTHER PROFESSIONAL STAFF It is increasingly common to find environmental health units employing professional staff other than environmental health officers. This situation is likely to increase over the next few years with the intensification of environmental health legislation, e.g. Environmental Protection and Food Safety Acts introduced in 1990; the increase in complexity of environmental issues, e.g. industrial pollution control; and the shortage of environmental health officers. Thus increasingly microbiologists, food scientists, chemical engineers and other professionals are likely to become part of the team forming the environmental health unit.

ADMINISTRATIVE AND CLERICAL STAFF Provide the necessary administrative support from within the unit to the professional and technical staff.

The unit requires a wide range of support from other departments of the council and from other agencies. The main requirements are for:

1. Personnel, accountancy, legal and computer services – usually provided in-house by the council, through the mechanism of a service level agreement with the unit which specifies the service required, how it is to be provided and the cost.
2. Engineering services – advice may be required on the engineering aspects of water supplies, waste disposal, land contamination, etc. This is either provided in-house by the relevant department, or by the appointment of private consultants on a project basis.

MEDICAL Arrangements are made between the chief environmental health officer and the director of public health of the district health authority for the provision of medical advice to the unit. In addition, the authority needs to appoint a Consultant in Communicable Disease Control to work with the environmental health department (see Chapter 16).

VETERINARY Where there is a meat inspection function, (the local authority role in meat inspection will be taken over by the national Meat Hygiene Service from 1 April 1995), the required veterinary input is provided either on a part-time or full-time basis. This is accomplished by the appointment of one or more veterinary surgeons within the environmental health unit, or by the engagement of a private veterinary practice on contract. More irregular veterinary advice, e.g. for issues relating to animal welfare, is usually provided by retaining a local practice.

ANALYTICAL The nature of environmental health control requires a wide variety of analytical and scientific services to be provided. In the larger units, this may be produced by the establishment of a scientific support team within the unit, and most units perform scientific analysis to some degree, e.g. the processing of noise recording tapes. Most units will, however, require support from outside agencies. Microbiological support is usually provided by the public health laboratory service in relation to the examination of food and water, and for the investigation and control of communicable disease. There are some areas of the country, however, that are not provided with such a service, and in these cases the unit will use other hospital facilities or private microbiological services.

Those units with responsibilities for the monitoring of the composition, etc., of food are required to appoint a public analyst who will be either employed by a council, district or county, or be in private practice. Other private analytical practices will be used on an ad hoc basis, e.g. for the identification of asbestos fibres.

The principles embodied in the organization of the unit are shown diagrammatically in Fig. 3.7. This cannot be taken as being typical of any particular type of local authority, it simply illustrates the organizational approach to establishing a structure.

Case studies of environmental health units

Clearly, there is no one model of service organization for environmental health that is appropriate to all authorities. The problems encountered in different localities and especially the variation in demographic and socio-economic characteristics which are, perhaps the most significant determinants of local service requirements, demand that each council reviews local priorities and develops structures suited to the local conditions.

In addition, in recent years, the increasingly tight constraints on local government finance and the rapidly changing conditions in which services operate, have resulted in circumstances where it is necessary to challenge preconceived ideas about the roles of environmental health departments, and how they should operate.

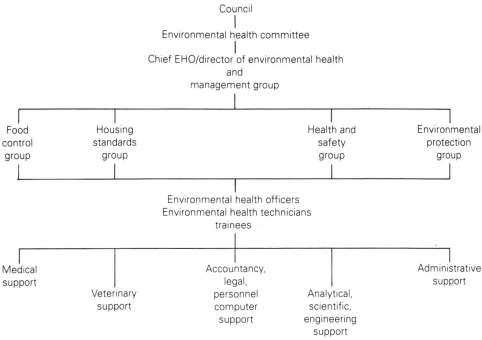

Fig. 3.7 The environmental health unit.

In order to give a feel to the range of problems and approaches to the organization of environmental health units, three case studies are included in the appendix in this chapter.

Inter-departmental organization

There is a need for an effective working relationship to be established between the chief environmental health officer and the unit, and other departments of the authority. Essentially, this is planned at two levels.

Management team
The chief environmental health officer/director of environmental health should be a member of the council's management team (or chief officer group), at which level the corporate planning of the organization takes place and major policy is formulated for presentation to members. The environmental health service, as a major district council service, must be professionally represented at this group if the significance of the service, and of other services upon it, are to be given full account.

Departmental
An effective arrangement needs to exist with most of the other departments of the council. Apart from the provision of support services, particular care needs to be taken to establish close links with the following departments:

1. Planning: access to the planning control function, assessment of proposals and recommendations on them by the environmental health department.
2. Building control: access to building regulation approval applications, assessment and comment.
3. Highways: environmental health implications of highway proposals and the implementation of noise insulation schemes.
4. Leisure: implementation of 'Health for All' targets (see Chapter 12) through leisure activities.

5. Housing: the integration of housing policies and programmes to ensure the effective use of resources and comprehensive housing strategies.
6. Waste disposal: waste disposal, recycling and waste regulation.
7. Education: hygiene control of the school meals service and the promotion of environmental health education in schools.
8. Social services: hygiene of the meals on wheels service and planning/implementation of care in the community policies.
9. Consumer protection: enforcement of the Food Safety Act 1990.
10. Fire protection: liaison on fire prevention aspects of health and safety and housing.

(The last five activities in non-metropolitan areas are functions of the county council, and should therefore be the subject of inter-authority arrangements.)

Project teams

One common feature of the organization of local authorities is the establishment of project teams or groups composed of officers with relevant qualifications and skills to work together across departmental boundaries to achieve specific objectives which the council has indentified. Environmental health departments play a full role in such groups and indeed they will lead in several areas, e.g. Environmental Strategy, Health of the Nation Groups, Area Renewal Teams, etc.

Inter-sectoral arrangements

In addition to the need to establish liaison structures with those agencies who are directly monitoring environmental health issues or who are providing direct support to the unit, it is also necessary to establish inter-sectoral links with those public bodies who are either providing significant environmental health services, or services where joint planning with environmental health is desirable and with whom it is therefore necessary to reach agreement on approaches, policies and programmes. These include the following.

District health authorities

Collaboration on health education, communicable diseases and the promotion of public health generally is achieved by arrangements between the chief environmental health officer and the director of public health and also, at member level, through the statutory Joint Consultative Committee (local authorities/health authorities).

The relationship between the chief environmental health officer and the director of public health is an important one since there are clear, effective arrangements for communicable disease control to be established and operated (see Chapter 16), joint plans to be agreed on health prevention and for non-communicable environmental hazards, and a substantial environmental health input is required into the public health function. The state of public health of an area is a fundamental factor in the setting of environmental health policies and targets, and information on this needs to be gained through these liaison arrangements. DHAs and LAs need to work together to achieve a shared undestanding of the health needs of the population. The annual report of the director of public health needs to reflect the major environmental health issues and the steps being taken by environmental health units to deal with them. The two officers will also need to agree a system for the provision of medical advice to the environmental health unit. This relationship was considered in some detail in the Acheson Report on the public health function [12] and advice on the relevant arrangements is contained in NHS Management Executive Health Service Guideline HSG (93)56 issued in November 1993.

County councils

The existence of a two-tiered system in non-metropolitan areas brings a need for a further set of relationships. Effective and close co-operation is required at both elected member and officer levels to secure the integration of policies and programmes in such a way that environmental health objectives and standards will be enhanced, or at the very least not detrimentally affected, through county council services. These arrange-

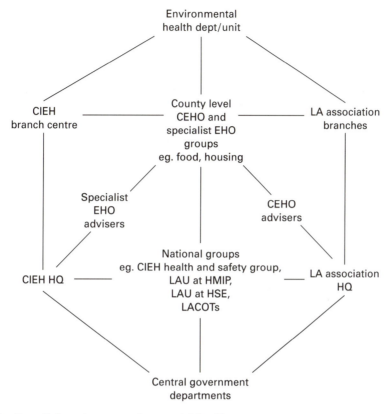

Fig. 3.8 Interauthority collaboration on environmental health.

ments should be both formal, i.e. joint consultative committees of elected members, and informal, i.e. a good relationship and regular discussion between the chief environmental health officer or his or her representative, and chief/senior officers in the various county council departments. It is the difficulty of ensuring effective arrangements between the two tiers which has, among other things, led to the current review of the system and the proposal for more single tier goverment.

Inter-authority arrangements

One of the difficulties inherent in a locally based environmental health system is that of achieving the necessary level of collaboration between the various environmental health units in order to produce the required degree of consistency in the enforcement of national legislation. Collabora-

tion is also required to combine the effort needed to react to legislative proposals, identify common problems and solutions, and generally to produce a national level picture of the environmental health function, bearing in mind the lack of a single focal point within the central government structure.

This collaboration is sought through two streams, the Chartered Institute of Environmental Health and the local authority associations, although there are 'bridges' between the two mainly by way of some environmental health officers operating in both streams. An outline of these arrangements is shown in Fig. 3.8. Central to these arrangements are the County-based specialist groups, e.g. food safety, health and safety, housing and environmental protection, under the guidance of the CEHO's Group. [13] The most recent improvement to the system is the establishment of LACOTS (see p. 52)

Concern about the general effectiveness of enforcement by local authorities does, however, continue and in January 1994 the President of the Board of Trade published the terms of reference of a scrutiny review of the organization of local authority enforcement functions[1] (see Chapter 8).

One dimension of inter-authority collaboration which has not yet been exploited to any degree is that of the provision of services one to another. Local authorities are able to provide their services to other public bodies, including other authorities. through the provisions of the Local Authorities (Goods and Services) Act 1970 and the Local Government Act 1972, and this includes all environmental health services. While a few of those services, e.g. cleansing services, must be subjected to the compulsory competitive tendering provisions of the Local Government Act 1988, the majority are only subject to local agreement.

One of the products of the 1988 Act requirements is a realization of the mutual benefits which there might be in authorities sharing the provision of services in such a way as to produce more cost effective working. There is scope for the development of this approach in the environmental health service. For example, an authority may decide that a relatively minor pest control function could be more effectively provided by a neighbouring environmental health unit with a large meat pest control; or a smaller unit may decide that, rather than attempt to recruit and retain environmental health officers with specialist knowledge, say, in environmental protection, it should purchase these services from a colleague environmental health unit which has a greater requirement for these skills. Whether it be by an extension of the competitive tendering requirements or by the implementation of cost effectiveness procedures by national government or by the Audit Commission, such arrangements are likely to be looked at with increasing regularity.

COMPULSORY COMPETITIVE TENDERING (CCT)

The principle of the compulsory exposure of local authority services to competition by tender was first put into practice by the Local Government, Planning and Land Act 1980 as a first step by the newly elected Conservative Government to improve the efficiency and effectiveness of local government. The 1980 Act requires competition with the private sector for the construction and maintenance work carried out by local authorities, e.g. highways, housing and sewerage, and also requires the establishment of separate direct labour organization (DLO) accounts together with a need to earn a rate of return prescribed by the Secretary of State.

This was followed by the Local Government Act 1988, which was based upon the government's perception of creating further opportunity for substantial savings and increased efficiency by exposing a much wider range of functions to competition. The Act defines the following activities as requiring to be subjected to a process of competition as laid down in the Act and regulations made under it:

1. refuse collection;
2. cleaning of buildings including public conveniences;
3. other cleaning including street cleaning;
4. school and welfare catering;
5. other catering;
6. grounds' maintenance;
7. repair and maintenance of vehicles;
8. management of sport and leisure facilities;
9. housing management.

The Secretary of State has the power by regulation to add to this list of defined activities and it is intended to add legal, finance, information technology, personnel and construction-related services, e.g. architecture and engineering for contract starts in the late 1990s. As indicated, the process of competition is tightly controlled both by the Act and by regulations, with particular emphasis being placed on the elimination of unfair competition, i.e. authorities unfairly favouring their in-house tenders. The process is also the subject of administrative advice from the Department of the Environment (see DoE circulars 8/88, 19/88, 1/91, 10/93 – additional advice on CCT for 'white-collar services' was issued in 1994) and close attention from the Audit Commission in their scrutiny of local authority activity. Separate accounts need to be established for each defined activity where the in-house direct service organizations (DSOs) are successful, and there are rate of return provisions. The Secretary of State is also given extensive powers to enquire into an authority's performance under the Act, and to limit or end its operation in the event of a failure to achieve the Act's requirements.

It will be seen that certain environmental health services, i.e. the cleansing services, are part of the activities which now have to be subjected to competition, and that the remainder or any part of the environmental health function could be affected in addition by the Secretary of State, although these are no current proposals in this direction.

ENVIRONMENTAL HEALTH AND THE COMPETITIVE ENVIRONMENT

The competitive environment into which local authorities have been placed arises not just from the extension of compulsory competitive tendering through the local Government Act 1988, but also from a series of other initiatives taken by the government during the second half of the 1980s, e.g. the enabling role and performance targets.

These challenges in total represent the 'competitive environment' for local authorities whose response has been of fundamental importance. This response has included:

1. Examination of the structure: organizational structures have been re-examined to ensure effectiveness in the competitive environment. A new criterion has been the need to differentiate between client and contractor for services subject to compulsory competitive tendering, i.e. separating those parts of the organization which let and control contracts from those parts (DLOs and DSOs) which undertake the contracts as operational units. This same approach is being more widely applied to other services. The provision of central services, e.g. accountancy and legal services, has also been reformed with service level agreements being introduced to establish the required levels of

service and costs for the administrative support of each service.
2. Member/officer relationships: these have been re-examined to produce greater operational efficiency.
3. Cost effectiveness: this has increased emphasis on the operation of services as they are gradually being exposed to competition.
4. Alternative providers: these are being sought for services outside the defined activities. The value of looking outside the council for provision of services, both directly to the public and in support of the authority services, is being assessed increasingly. In some local authorities, management buyouts have occurred in cleansing, leisure, legal, grounds maintenance and other services.
5. Charges for services: as a way of increasing income to the council, these are being re-assessed. Additional income is possible not only by introducing new charges or increasing existing charges, but also by extending the provision of services to other public service organizations through the Local Authorities (Goods and Services) Act 1970 and the Local Government Act 1972.

In total this response, which has been widely seen across local government, represents a revolution in local authority management and a new culture has been created in our thinking towards the way in which authorities plan and operate. The environmental health service is an integral part of the local government system and is, therefore, directly affected by the changes which have been and are still taking place.

FUTURE CHANGES TO THE ORGANIZATION OF ENVIRONMENTAL HEALTH

The changes in approach to the management of local authorities, as identified in the previous section, have created unique opportunities for environmental health officers to improve the nature and substance of the service. In particular, there are likely to be opportunities to assess the use of environmental services provided by private agencies. This has been done for many years for certain services like pest control and meat inspection, but the opportunities to do so are widening with the establishment of private environmental health consultancies and house condition surveys, food hygiene audits and health and safety inspections can, for example, be purchased by the environmental health department from such agencies.

A trend in the opposite direction may be for some environmental health departments to undertake work for other agencies, e.g. pest control for the water undertakers, and for there to be a greater level of co-operation between environmental health units and the provision of services one to another. Such changes are in their infancy but, if taken forward in a substantial way, could lead to a very different environmental health department/unit to that which exists at present. It may be possible for a small core of professional environmental health and administrative staff to act as a client organization, and to arrange for the provision of a total environmental health service on the basis of specification and contracts, some with an operational unit working within the council, some with another local authority environmental health department and some with outside agencies and consultancies.

[1] See the Report of the Interdepartmental Review Team, Department of Trade and Industry 1994, ISBN 0 85605 332 5, which indicates general satisfaction and noted that real improvemnts have been made in local authority enforcement.

REFERENCES

1. Audit Commission (June 1990) *Environmental Health Survey of Food Premises*, HMSO, London.
2. Audit Commission (December 1990) *Safer Food: Local Authorities and the Food Safety Act 1990*, HMSO, London.
3. Audit Commission (September 1991) *Healthy Housing: The Role of Environmental Health Services*, HMSO, London.
4. Audit Commission (July 1991). *Towards a Healthier Environment: Managing Environmental Health Services*, HMSO, London.
5. IEHO and Audit Commission (April 1993) *The Audit Commission Study of Environmental Health: An Assessment by Chief EHOs*, CIEH, London.
6. *The Citizen's Charter – Raising the Standard* (July 1991) HMSO, London.
7. WHO (1978) *Role, Functions and Training Requirements of Environmental Health Officers (Sanitarians) In Europe*, WHO Regional Office for Europe, Copenhagen.
8. Kreisel, Wilfried (1989) 'Affecting change – environmental health in the 1990s', address to the NEHA AEC.
9. Report of the Committee of Enquiry (1986) *The Conduct of Local Authority Business* (Cmnd 9797), HMSO, London.
10. Audit Commission (1988) *The Competitive Council*, Management Paper No. 1, HMSO, London.
11. *Local Government Review – The Internal Management of Local Authorities in England* (July 1991) DoE, London.
12. The Report of the Committee of Enquiry into the Future Development of the Public Health Function (1988) *Public Health in England* (Cmnd 289), HMSO, London.
13. Bassett W.H. (1992) Setting sail for new joint efforts. *Municipal Journal*, No. 22, 29 May–4 June.

FURTHER READING

Byrne, Tony, *Local Government in Britain*, Penguin, London.
Denis, J. (1989) *The Business of Government*, Chambers, Edinburgh.
Greenwood, J. and Wilson, D., *Public Administration in Britain*, 2nd edn, Unwin Hyman, London.

APPENDIX

CASE STUDY NO. 1: ENVIRONMENTAL HEALTH IN WARWICK

John Kirk

Introduction to Warwick District

Warwick District is situated at the heart of England bordered by the Cotswolds, Coventry and Stratford-upon-Avon. It is marketed to its several million visitors each year as England's historic heartland. Included in the District are historic Warwick with its fine castle, Kenilworth with its magnificent ruined castle and Royal Leamington Spa with all its regency elegance, surrounded by a mix of picturesque villages. In all its population is 118 000 and it covers an area of 28 253 hectares.

The industrial base of the area for a long time was manufacturing, much of which is based on parts for the automotive industry. The demise of the British motor car industry took its toll on the area with 6500 jobs being lost between 1981 and 1987. However, such is the attraction of the area with its good communications, quality of life and skilled labour force that overall in this period employment grew by 3300 jobs. The diversification of industry continues with the most notable recent recruits being Conoco Oil and EMI Music Services. Currently the unemployment level is 6.1%.

The District has considerable interaction with its neighbouring towns, particularly Coventry. This is perhaps particularly based on work opportunities and the provision of good quality, if relatively expensive, housing.

The area seeks to balance the protection of its heritage and existing quality of life with its need to change and develop.

Management philosophy

The underlying philosophy was built on four concepts, namely the need for strategic planning, the need for specialization, the increased use of technical support staff, and the need for Environmental Health Services to be involved in the wider role of health within their district.

Environmental health work combines a high level of reactive work in dealing with requests for services from members of the public, with the need to ensure that pro-active work such as food inspections is carried out to an appropriate level. The use of strategic planning techniques is a way of defining the workload to be done, quantifying this where possible, deciding what the service wants to achieve, and then prioritizing the workload against the resources available. This approach brings some degree of order to the workload presented to Environmental Health Services and enables over time the service to measure its performance.

The increasing complexity of issues presented leads to the necessity to employ persons with specialist knowledge in the key areas of environmental health. The use of EHOs to fulfil the need for specialist knowledge is an important aspect of the approach in Warwick. The knowledge and expertise of EHOs, particularly the holistic approach based on the assessment of risk and their general health background, when applied in a series of specialisms was felt to be the way to proceed. This approach does not exclude the employment of specialist knowledge outside the field of environmental health, e.g. a chemist. It does mean that EHOs will be less available for routine but important tasks faced by Environmental Health Services. This leads to the employment of technical support staff to carry out routine inspection work. In support of this concept two other developments are seen as necessary, namely the devolvement of responsibility to EHOs and the necessary training and educational support.

The devolvement of responsibility to individual EHOs requires a belief in the ability of the EHOs involved and allowing them ownership of their particular area of work. Warwick District expressed its belief in their ability and through the development of a work programme allowed ownership to be transferred to EHOs without losing control of the overall direction of the Department. Training and educational courses were supported to build on the expertise already available.

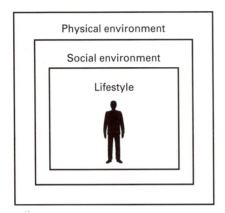

Fig. 3.9 Factors affecting health of the individual.

The Council sees itself as a major agency in the prevention of ill-health and the promotion of good health. It does however recognize that it is not the only agency concerned with health. The Council is a locally elected body involved in health, it enforces a range of public health legislation and is involved in problems with the District which affect people's health. It is therefore very aware of local needs and concerns. The Council is concerned to maintain existing standards of health protection, to improve standards of health protection, and to actively promote the health of people within its District

Fig. 3.10 Warwick District Council Health Strategy – mission statement.

The involvement in the wider preventive role within its area is based on the concept that the health of an individual is affected by that person's lifestyle, by their social environment and by their physical environment. There is also a relationship between these aspects; therefore in order to achieve real improvements in the health of individuals within an area it is necessary to consider all three. The implementation of this concept obviously involves liaison with the many other agencies involved in health.

This concept is shown diagrammatically in Fig. 3.9.

The philosophy into practice

The implementation of the philosophy outlined above involved an initial set of changes, and the evolution of these changes through time. The starting point was the organization of the Environmental Health Department of Warwick District Council prior to the adoption of the changed philosophy. The structure was based on two operational divisions and an administration division. The two operational divisions were based on the generalist principle with each being responsible for a geographic half of the district. The EHOs working within the divisions were generalists. There were no programmes of work existing.

The initial changes took two forms:

1. the development of a strategic and programmed approach to environmental health work;
2. the restructuring of the Department along more specialist lines.

Strategy and programmes

A Health Strategy was written setting out the mission statement of the Council on health and a set of primary and secondary objectives for environmental health. The mission statement, reflecting the wider role of the Department and the Council in health, is shown in Fig. 3.10.

Five primary objectives were produced, namely:

1. To ensure that food supplied, manufactured or stored in the District is fit for human consumption and of good quality so as to protect the health of people and also to promote a healthy diet.
2. To ensure that the standard of housing in the District is such as to protect and promote the health of people in the District.
3. To ensure that the levels of pollution in water, on land and in the air, including pollution by noise, are such that they do not adversely affect the health of people in the District.

4. To ensure that workplaces in the District present no health risk to, and promote the health of, people who resort to them.
5. To ensure that activities, situations or premises within the District do not pose a threat to the health of people in the District and to promote the health of people within the District.

Within each primary objective secondary objectives were set, for example the following secondary objectives were devised under the food primary objective:

1. All food businesses within the District to comply with food legislation, observe hygiene practices and have adequately trained staff.
2. All meat produced at slaughterhouses within the District to be fit for human consumption.
3. Food available within the District to be fit for human consumption.
4. To control outbreaks of food poisoning in the District.
5. To encourage the adoption of a healthy diet in the District.

An annual work programme was devised based on the secondary objectives. Each secondary objective was looked at and the work planned to be carried out to meet that objective was detailed in the work programme. The details in the programme dealt with the number of inspections to be carried out during the year, for example food premises, health and safety premises. The programme also set response times for requests for service ranging from requests for pest control services to complaints regarding noise and housing conditions. Where possible specific measured targets were set. A progress report on the achievement of the work programme was produced at the halfway mark through the year and an annual report based on the work programme was produced at the end of the year. The half-yearly report was used to assist in the writing of the work programme for the following year.

The Strategy is agreed by the Environmental Health and Control Committee, and the work programme is agreed by that committee each

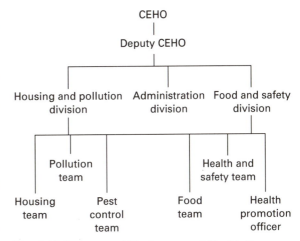

Fig. 3.11 Structure of Environmental Health Department, Warwick District Council.

year. The half-yearly progress report and the annual report are submitted to the committee.

Organization

The divisional structure was retained and the geographical split of functions was replaced by a functional split. One division took responsibility for housing and pollution, the other for food and health and safety. Other functions were allocated to the appropriate division.

The evolution of the new structure and the strategic planning enabled other developments to take place. These were an increased use of technical support staff, a strengthening of the EHO expertise in the specialist areas, and the transference of responsibility for and ownership of the targets in the work programme to the staff dealing with that particular aspect of the work. The development by the EHOs of considerable levels of expertise in their particular areas of work proceeded very quickly and was one of the factors which led to a further evolution of the departmental structure. Within the two divisions there was a demand for increased specialization basically to form two teams in each division. The structure shown in Fig. 3.11 was the result of this development and is the current departmental structure.

All increases in staffing have been in the technical support area:-

1. An additional Technical Officer in housing to deal with routine complaints.
2. Two Food Safety Inspectors were appointed following the Food Safety Act 1990 in order to undertake food hygiene inspections of food premises in order to meet Department of Health targets.
3. The appointment of a Health Promotion Officer was made to take on the work involved in the wider health role, to pick up work being undertaken on AIDS, smoking, diet, being done by EHOs.
4. A further appointment was a Consumer Advice Assistant whose task was to deal with food premises registrations, requests for information on food safety, routine food complaints and the maintenance of a computer data base on food premises. This post was office based and forms a vital part of the food team.

These appointments resulted in EHO time being freed to undertake the more exacting work in their specialisms.

The development of the wider role in health was reflected in the Health Strategy and prior to the appointment of the Health Promotion Officer specific projects were allocated to individual EHOs to pursue. Examples of the projects allocated were the development of a Smoking Policy for the Council; the development of a Food Policy; specific work on AIDS such as corporate training and the setting up of a needle exchange scheme. The appointment of the Health Promotion Officer led to such work being given to that person and also to an examination of the wider role of the Department and the Council in the health of the local population. It is interesting to note that a recent evaluation of the role of the Council which led to the production of a Corporate Strategy reflected the wider role in governance of the Council. The Council's overall mission statement was defined as follows:

The Council's purpose is to:
Provide high quality democratic government within the District, enabling its citizens to take pride in their District and to enjoy a good quality of life at a cost which they perceive to be fair.

The factors contributing to quality of life were identified as:

1. economic opportunity;
2. environment;
3. health and well being;
4. safety;
5. housing;
6. equal opportunities;
7. social/recreational;
8. law and order.

The Health Strategy and the philosophy of the wider health role fit well into the Corporate Strategy.

A further development leading from this wider role in health was the need to have liaison with other agencies involved in health. Contacts with the health authority, particularly the health promotion service, were good and a joint initiative was launched involving not just Warwick District Council and the Health Service but a county-wide strategy based on the World Health Organization targets. The Strategy called Warwickshire Health For All 2000 involved the following agencies.

1. Warwick District Council;
2. Stratford-upon-Avon District Council;
3. North Warwickshire Borough Council;
4. Nuneaton and Bedworth Borough Council;
5. Rugby Borough Council;
6. South Warwickshire Health Authority North Warwickshire Health Authority } now Warwickshire Health Authority
7. Rugby Health Authority;
8. Warwickshire County Council;
9. Warwickshire Family Practitioner Committee (now Warwickshire Family Health Services Authority).

The voluntary sector was also involved through the local offices of the Council for Voluntary Service.

Each of the agencies involved obtained the commitment of their organization to the objectives set out in the Strategy document.

Future developments

The management system is continually evolving in the Department but the basic tenets of the philosophy are still holding good.

The increase in expertise among the EHO-led teams dealing with housing, pollution, food and health and safety is opening up the possibility of removing the divisional structure and the creation of a flatter structure based on smaller teams with operational team leaders. A new structure based on four such teams was introduced in April 1995.

The development of EHO education, particularly postgraduate, is moving towards the obtaining of masters degrees in appropriate subjects. The latter structure it is hoped may provide opportunities for EHO career development which does not involve movement into management.

There is a need to develop a career structure for technical support staff, hopefully linking into the EHO structure.

CASE STUDY NO. 2: THE ENVIRONMENTAL HEALTH SERVICE IN SALFORD

Bruce Jassi

Introduction to the City of Salford

Salford is situated in the south-west of the Greater Manchester area. It has a long history; its origins go back to the eleventh century. It was part of the cradle of the Industrial Revolution in the nineteenth century and as such the urban congestion and pollution gave rise to a number of problems which are still the main source of work for the Environmental Health Service, mainly pollution and housing issues. The images of Salford in the past are renowned world-wide through the paintings of L.S. Lowry which show social, physical and environmental deprivation. At the beginning of this century, Salford was the most crowded place, in terms of population density, in the world; however, there have been significant improvements in the factors affecting the quality of life in the City since that time. The Council, through a positive working relationship with other stake-holders in the City, have replaced 60% of all the slums and overcrowded properties in the inner City since the War, Unfortunately their replacement by high-rise tower blocks is now one of the main housing problems facing the City. The City was the first in the country (and Europe) to complete a smoke control area programme for the whole of its area. Currently nearly 35% of the private sector housing stock is unfit and we have significant problems with derelict, contaminated land and air pollution from motor vehicles. Though our predecessors in Salford have made a tremendous improvement in the quality of life of every inhabitant of the City, considerable challenges remain for current and for future generations of managers.

The 1991 Census figures (as adjusted) give the population of Salford at 230 000. Ethnic minorities comprise 2.6% of the population. Like other major and industrial conurbations, Salford has suffered population decline by migrations to rural areas and since 1981 the population has declined by 11%. Interestingly there are nearly two trees for every member of the population for the City which goes some way to dispel the image of the cloth cap Northern town. The City area is 9687 hectares (about 24 000 acres). Forty per cent of this area is open green space or moorlands. There are about 100 000 domestic properties, 35 000 of which consist of Council-owned dwellings; in addition, there are over 8500 commercial properties. There are approximately 7000 privately rented properties and 1200 known houses in multiple occupation, though this figure is a gross underestimation of the real picture as the City has a major university and college of further education and is in close proximity to two universities in Manchester. Over half of the 55 000 private houses were built before 1919, and many are either unfit or in a state of substantial disrepair.

The City has seen substantial decline in regeneration in the 1980s. Unemployment, which still stands at one in eight of the working population, combined with a difficult urban environment and insufficient economic investment, has resulted at times in some social unrest. Despite these setbacks, the City Council has been visionary in its approach to its problems. The Salford Quays dockside regeneration and development is renowned throughout the world as a classical piece of inner city regeneration. Its gearing ratios of external funding of 10 : 1 are far greater than those in the docklands of London. Salford Quays provides a vision of the modern City of Salford.

There are no significant large-scale employers in the City, apart from the City Council, and the closure of primary industries like steel and coal and power stations in the City have left a need for redevelopment of major parts of the City. However, the Trafford Park Development Corporation has recently obtained permission, after appeal, to develop a Regional Shopping Centre which should be a major boost to the economy. The City is currently reviewing its economic and tourism strategies with a view to encouraging inward investment and attracting European funding.

The City Council is the largest employer with nearly 13 000 staff. There are 11 departments of which the multi-divisional Environmental and Consumer Services Department is one. Its Chief Officer is responsible for Environmental Health, Trading Standards, Markets, Client Services and 'arm's length' DSO organizations. The Department has nearly 380 staff. The Chief Officer is currently an Environmental Health Officer but the post is open to any suitably qualified and experienced manager.

Organization of the Environmental Health Service

In the past the Department consisted of several divisions which were functionally based. Environmental Control provided traditionally services like pollution control, food, and health and safety. The large Urban Renewal Division provided a complete package of renovation grants, house surveys, public health problems and houses in multiple occupation. Over the years there had been considerable stagnation in terms of development of the Department and meeting the challenges of change.

With the appointment of a new Chief Officer in 1991, a total review took place involving all staff from all levels of the Department. Unproductive rivalry and 'Chinese Walls' between sections and functional divisions were removed for the areas of Environmental Health, Trading Standards and Urban Renewal. Three new area teams were created under a general management structure. These Teams cover the City on a holistic basis for all matters relating to Urban Renewal, Trading Standards or Environmental Health. Currently the Heads of these three Teams include an Environmental Health Officer, Trading Standards Officer and a Waste Management professional. These individuals are the Area Managers and they report directly to the Chief Officer for the purpose of service delivery in their areas.

Supporting each Area Manager is a Deputy Manager. There is also a number of principal officers spread among the teams who have a lead role for a functional service, e.g. pollution, food, etc. The Department is very much moving away from a functional base hierarchy, however the service on the ground is still delivered by specialist officers. These specialist officers meet once a month in a Specialist Forum to discuss and update themselves on issues relating to their specialism. This is led by the Principal Officer who is the Lead Officer for the function. All the staff within an Area Team, regardless of their specialism, are under the direction of the Area Management Team consisting of an Area Manager and Deputy Area Manager.

Structures pre- and post-1992 are shown in Figs 3.12 and 3.13.

The Council aims to achieve a 'Community strategy' which involves core values of:

1. consultation and participation with the public and external bodies;
2. quality services and customer care;
3. corporate working and partnerships.

The Department produces an Annual Service Action Plan (Business Plan) for each service. It carries out quarterly reports using the principle of management by objectives to constantly review and refocus its resources on priorities. All these documents are sent to the main Committees and Council for approval. A system of SIMMS (Staff Information, Monitoring and Management Systems) captures the information to produce the

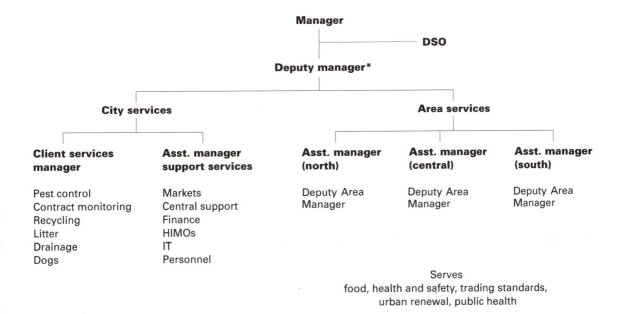

Environmental and consumer services manager

Deputy environmental and consumer services manager

Administration	**Urban renewal**	**Environmental control**	**Trading standards**	**Manual services**
Central administration	HMOs		Commercial practice	<u>Client function</u>
		Food safety		Refuse collection/
Home safety/health	Grants		Commercial standards	Street cleansing monitoring
education/training		Pollution control		
	Homecare			Dog warden service
Markets		Health and safety		
	General			Pest control and drainage
DSO				
				Vehicle maintenance
Refuse collection				monitoring
Street cleansing				
Winter weather				

Fig. 3.12 Outline structure of the Salford City Council Environmental and Consumer Services Department prior to 1992.

Manager ——————————— **DSO**

Deputy manager*

City services   **Area services**

Client services manager	**Asst. manager support services**	**Asst. manager (north)**	**Asst. manager (central)**	**Asst. manager (south)**
Pest control	Markets	Deputy Area	Deputy Area	Deputy Area
Contract monitoring	Central support	Manager	Manager	Manager
Recycling	Finance			
Litter	HIMOs			
Drainage	IT			
Dogs	Personnel			

Serves
food, health and safety, trading standards,
urban renewal, public health

Fig. 3.13 Outline structure of the Salford City Council Environmental and Consumer Services Department after 1992.
* The Deputy Manager also controls a Strategy Division which comprises a marketing manager and performance/ CCT Manager and deals with service development.

quarterly reports and the Service Plans. An extensive computerization programme carried out in 1993 will also be used in future for monitoring purposes and to improve our cost centre budgeting systems.

Team work is emphasized with regular team meetings, departmental newsletters and team development training. Nearly 2% of the staff costs of the Department are spent on training using a training strategy and an annual training plan derived from a needs assessment of each individual, carried out jointly by the individual and the line manager. The Department has a complement of eight Trainee EHOs at any one time and we are very active in training EHOs. Sixteen out of 18 managers in the Department have or are currently completing nationally recognized management qualifications, e.g. DBA and MBA.

In terms of service delivery, the Area Team is able to identify problems and be aware of developments in its patch. There is more cross-fertilization between different professions enabling holistic solutions to be developed to multi-causal problems. Specialist officers are used as the nature of the problems currently facing the Department (e.g. air pollution, contaminated land, houses in multiple occupation, consumer protection) require many inputs from different professions but these inputs need to be concentrated and in depth.

In the past 2 years the Department has moved away from predominantly EHO-based service. In 1991 there were 41 field EHOs, in 1993 there were 24. There has been a proportionate rise in the number of Technicians and the development of career paths and posts for non-professional staff, e.g. Technical and Scientific Officers posts and grades. There has also been a substantial strengthening of the support staff and the delegation of clerical and administrative duties previously done by professional staff to clerical staff. The current completion of the computerization process of the Department has enabled further administration to be delegated and to be cut. Considerable participation takes place through Specialist Project Teams known as Task Teams within the Department, e.g. IT and CCT, along with a pro-active working relationship with the Trades Unions and the adoption of an open, positive and participative management style. The Chief Officer operates through a Departmental Management Team consisting of a Deputy Manager, three Area Managers, Client Services Manager, Central Support Services Manager, performance CCT Manager and Marketing Manager. The Team meets weekly and reviews operational policies and actions of the Department on a monthly basis through team reports, quarterly reports, monthly budget reports and assessment of corporate and environmental issues. Each member of the Team, using cascade briefings, communicates the information with his line managers and the staff and there are regular Team Briefings for all staff along with the publication of a Departmental Newsletter.

Quarterly reports are sent to Committee for review and in addition each Councillor gets a half-yearly Ward Report about the work of the Department and issues of special interest in their Ward. Service Action Plans and Annual Reports regularly go to Committee and the Department is in the process of producing Annual Plans and Reports for publication.

Liaison arrangements

Regular liaison meetings take place with the Area Health Authority, mainly through the Consultant in Communicable Disease Control (who has an office within the department) and the Director of Public Health. These are mainly based on development of Infectious Disease policies and control mechanisms, however considerable planning is being undertaken to develop initiatives to manage the health of the population with regard to pollutants in the atmosphere. The Department also liaises with the Director of Social Services to develop Community Care policies and practices in line with the Care in the Community legislation and working in conjunction with the Area Health Authority.

Regular liaison also takes place with the water companies (this has been an area of considerable concern in the City and major reports have been sent to the Policy and Resources Committee of the Council with representation at Board level from the North West Water plc) and with the National Rivers Authority, Health and Safety Executive, and HMIP, on matters relating to pollution control and health and safety.

At Chief Officer level liaison takes place with senior Regional Officials in the Department of the Environment and Department of Trade and Industry on housing and development issues. The Department regularly lobbies Government over changes to legislation, e.g. in 1993 a lobby was organized and an audience was granted with the Under Secretary of State of the Department of the Environment when the difficulties of funding the demand for mandatory grants within the City were raised.

The Authority is part of the Association of Greater Manchester Authorities (AGMA). This is a residual body resulting from the abolition of the Greater Manchester County Council and it enables the ten Greater Manchester Authorities, covering a population of 2½ million, to get a strategic overview of issues in Greater Manchester, e.g. European funding, transport and other matters requiring political resolution. The AGMA has a number of Committees and Working Parties to try to resolve issues on a Greater Manchester basis, for example, there is a Trading Standards Committee which oversees work done on Trading Standards in Greater Manchester as well as the services provided by the Lead Authority on Specialist Trading Standards Service (Manchester). Other issues that are discussed include Waste Management, Waste Regulation and the Chief Officer was actively involved in the sale of the Greater Manchester Scientific Service Laboratory to a private company and has been nominated non-Executive Director of the privatized organization.

The Greater Manchester Area, since 1974, has had a liaison group of Chief Officers covering Environmental Health and since 1986 this liaison group has been expanded to include Trading Standards. The Greater Manchester Chief Officers Group for Trading Standards and Environmental Health meets once a month to discuss inter-authority issues and policy, e.g. consistency

of enforcement. The Chief Officer Group also has a number of Technical Working Parties with the aim of promoting consistency and closer working relationships between specialist EHOs in the ten different authorities. It has been successful in organizing a number of regional and national seminars as well as working with national organizations like ITSA, CIEH, LACOTS and the Audit Commission.

Problems facing the department

Externally imposed problems include both budget cuts and financial constraints. In the 4 years 1991–1995, £1.4 million (or 40%) of the non-DSO budget has been lost. This means that over 35% of the staff have left in the non-DSO side, however, the changes and cuts have not only been achieved without any compulsory redundancies but also with significant improvements to both the remuneration packages and equipment used by staff. For example, nearly £300 000 has been spent on information technology in the Department and over £40 000 a year is spent on training. More community-based services are being demanded from Departments in line with the Community Strategy and additional services are also being requested, e.g. major expenditure on anti-graffiti and litter, by the public and elected members. Therefore demands on the Department are going up but resources are being severely curtailed. The public are also now, as a result of the Citizens Charter and other developments in consumerism, more aware of their rights and as a result are complaining to the Department for redress from third parties. This further puts a strain on the reactive work of the Department and curtails the pro-active work which is increasingly being demanded by Central Government, in terms of pro-active inspections on food hygiene, health and safety and pollution control.

The City has major problems with housing disrepair and other areas. Progress has been made with the declaration of a Renewal Area and a 50% improvement in the amount paid in renovation grants between 1991 and 1994 (£2–3.1 million). New methods also need to be learned about working with the private sector and developing packages for urban regeneration. The voluntary sector also has a key role in tackling these local problems. Another major issue is the ubiquitous problems of air pollution in a congested urban area with major transport routes passing through. Recent proposals to put a 14-lane super highway through the north of the City will compound this problem in the entire City. A response is needed in terms of monitoring, in terms of abatement and in terms of lobbying for changes on this important area.

Ultimately the Authority's Environmental and Consumer Services Department may need to change from a purely public service-based approach to a public service ethos with an underlying commercial imperative approach. Satisfying the customer is fine and laudable but it must be done within existing resource constraints. There has been massive change in the way Salford manages and there is plenty of confidence within the Department to face the challenges of the future.

CASE STUDY NO. 3: ENVIRONMENTAL HEALTH IN SELBY

Nevil Parkinson

Introduction to Selby District

Selby District, the most southerly District Council area in the county of North Yorkshire, was formed in 1974. Today the District, which covers an area of 280 square miles and includes much of the fertile Vale of York, has a population of approximately 95 000 living in a network of small market towns and villages.

Just outside the north of the District lies the historic and popular tourist city of York, while to the south is Doncaster. Selby District occupies an excellent location with regard to the national communications network with junctions serving the A1 trunk road and the M62 motorway. The London Kings Cross/Edinburgh East Coast railway line traverses the District, served by principal stations at York and Doncaster.

Traditionally the District has supported a large agricultural population, but in recent years the economic base of the area has changed, with the power industries employing significant numbers of local people. The Selby Coalfield is one of the most modern coalfield areas in Europe and supplies two large power stations in the south of the District – Drax (4000 Megawatts) and Eggborough (2000 Megawatts) which burn 15 million tonnes of coal per year. Selby, the largest town in the area, lies at the heart of the District and is the administrative centre for many local government and other services. The town has a number of locally important industries, including chemical production and food processing, besides being a thriving port. Tadcaster, the second largest town in the District, is famous for its brewing and quarrying industries.

Organizational philosophy

In 1990 the Council appointed management consultants, Cooper Lybrand Deloitte, to formulate a new mechanism at Member and Officer level for monitoring and reviewing the Council's performance.

A Statement of Strategic Intent was first agreed and introduced by elected members in order that the Authority could provide the framework to plan for the future with some confidence. It was felt that what was needed at member level was a body with specific responsibility for the introduction and co-ordination of policy formulation, responsibility for monitoring achievement against pre-set plans and reviewing internal levels of performance (Fig. 3.14).

At Officer level the consultants established that there was considerable scope for re-organizing the existing structure so as to provide the opportunity for creating accountable business units to enable the new management approach to respond to the challenges ahead in the ever-changing nature of local government. For the manual services, e.g. housing repairs, refuse collection, etc., the Council clearly separated the client and contractor activities along with the establishment of a Board of Directors, the membership of which ensures no conflict of interest.

Improving customer care, service delivery and value for money were the main objectives of the new management style.

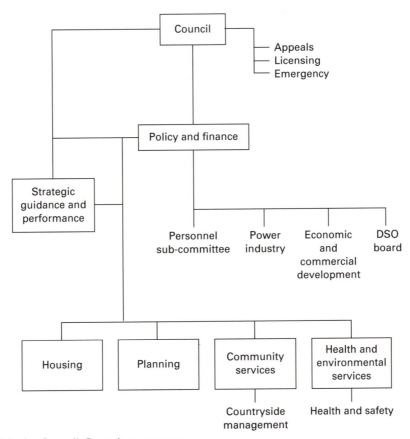

Fig. 3.14 Selby District Council Committee structure.

As part of the restructuring of the Authority's department, Public Sector Housing was divorced from the original Environmental Health & Housing Department. I did not agree with this aspect of the reorganization as I have always regarded housing as an essential part of the environmental services of the authority because of its close links with environmental health and planning.

The executive management of the Authority consist of a Chief Executive and three Directors with the following organizational responsibilities (Fig. 3.15).

Organizational structure – environmental health

This review of the establishment came at an opportune time for the reassessment of the Environmental Health functions in so much that major changes in legislation and management were being introduced in the following areas: Environmental Protection Act, Food Safety Act, Home Improvement Grants and compulsory competitive tendering in areas of refuse collection, street cleansing, pest control and public convenience cleaning.

The Section also took advantage of the review to introduce EHO specialization under a Chief Environmental Health Officer. With the exception of the Financial Services Department, deputy chief officer posts have been removed from all other department structures creating a flat management organization, each section head being responsible directly to the Director of the department with the emphasis clearly placed on performance management. A scheme of performance-related pay has not yet been adopted by the Council.

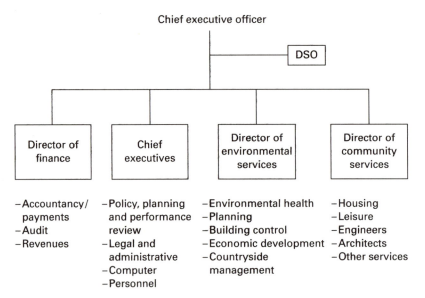

Fig. 3.15 Selby District Council management structure.

The original organization of the department was based on multi-disciplinary EHOs; the new organization substituted specialist teams arranged as shown in Fig. 3.16 with the opportunity for officers in a particular team to transfer into a new specialization after 2 years in order to maintain a wide level of experience and to promote career development. It should be noted that the administration section was also reorganized to ensure that the clerical assistants were allocated to a specific team, responsible to a Principal Environmental Health Officer.

Performance management of the Authority

Performance Management is all embracing including staff appraisal, the development of a 5-year mission statement known as the Statement of Strategic Intent, the development of strategic plans and business plans, followed by performance monitoring.

Statement of strategic intent
The Statement of Strategic Intent governs everything which the Council does. Each Committee report begins with the extract from the Statement which the recommendations in the report are designed to further. This Statement is revised annually and sets out the mission statement of the authority.

Strategic plan
The Strategic Plan contains all the new initiatives which are 'one off' projects to be completed by the Council within the financial year and which are regarded as high priority in the use of available resources. These initiatives may be as a result of changes in statute, e.g. Environmental Protection Act authorization, or new street cleansing standards. In some cases there will be items in the strategic plan which will eventually need to be incorporated into the Business Plan.

Business plan
Every section within the authority has a Business Plan setting out the actions and targets on the detailed day to day work of the section. The Business Plans are reviewed at the end of each year and are supported by a list of key indicators by which the Council committees gauge performance.

Key indicators
Key indicators are values that reflect performance within the Business Plan, e.g. total number of

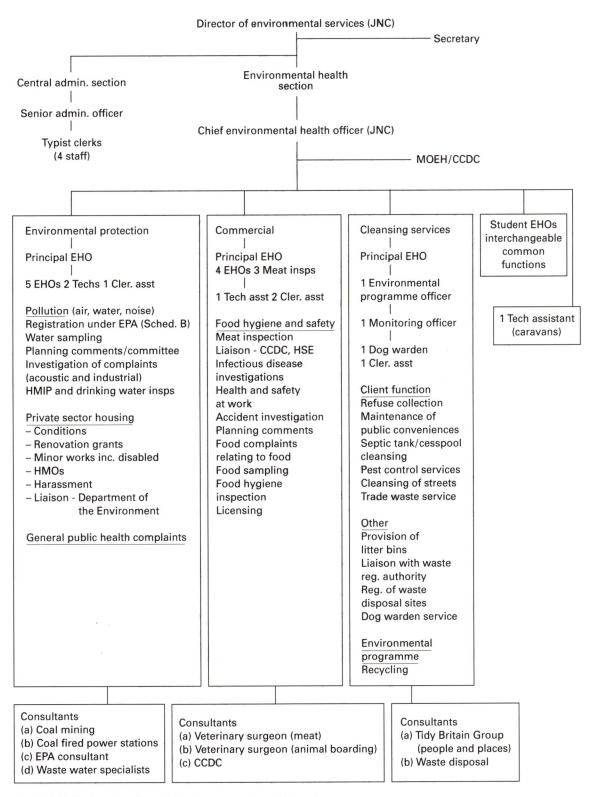

Fig. 3.16 Selby District Council Environmental Health Section.

food hygiene visits, number of private water samples, number of refuse collection default notices issued. They are reported for 2-month periods and presented in a manner that allows comparison with the previous 2 months. Finally a cumulative total is presented for the year to date.

Quality statements

The latest initiative to be introduced in order to improve still further the quality of service delivery to the customer is the preparation of Quality Statements (QS) to serve as an adjunct to each Business Plan.

The statements set out the procedures to be followed when each action of the Business Plan is carried out and include the Aims, Statement of Policy, Frequency and Standards to be applied in carrying out the action (an example is given in Fig. 3.17).

Staff appraisal

All staff are subject to annual appraisal. The process involves the setting of individual targets, identifying training needs, and assessing overall performance together with achievement of targets set for the previous year.

Performance monitoring

The annual performance of the Council is monitored by the new Strategic Guidance & Performance Committee. However, each committee of the Council has the responsibility for monitoring the Key Indicators of the Business Plans for which they are responsible. This is carried out in each committee cycle.

The day to day Business Plans are reported to the Management Team on a monthly basis to identify achievement or otherwise of targets.

The Strategic Initiatives are reported upon to both the Management Team and the Strategic & Performance Guidance Committee on a regular basis and are reviewed annually.

Use of information technology

The Environmental Health Section is now completely computerized. It has a performance mon-
itoring system which is an essential element for the retention of information on officer's visits and allows an assessment to be made in relation to compliance with response times set in the Business Plans.

In addition the computer system can act as a data base in relation to the activities of the department, and allow commercial premises to be identified for inspection on a priority basis. Details are maintained of licences, notices and registrations. The system may be used to complete national statistical returns. Information stored can also allow the automatic production of standard letters, notices, housing renovation grant schedules and grant calculations and payments can be made.

As we move towards the possibilities of compulsory competitive tendering for environmental health services and to assist in the compilation of service level agreements, a time management system has been introduced. Each officer accurately records the day to day work and the travelling time associated with that work. In addition time devoted to administration work is also recorded. Thus the section manager may monitor carefully the costs of staff time in specific areas.

More recently contract monitoring software has been installed to allow the section to carry out routine checks on the performance of contracts let by the Council.

For the future we will be evaluating new technology that allows the use of hand-held computers for carrying out inspections of commercial premises. An officer's daily work will be down loaded to the main computer after returning to the office. Such an arrangement has the potential to extend this by use of a telephone modem to allow officers to work from home. This may have benefits in becoming more competitive and the section has been given permission to pilot the system, but this has been delayed because of local government reorganization.

Use of technical support staff

The Environmental Health Section has recognized the useful contribution Technicians/ Technical Assistants make to the section's work.

SELBY DISTRICT COUNCIL
Specimen quality statement - Schedule B process – Environmental Protection Act (EPA)

Aim

To control emissions to atmosphere on processes identified in regulations made under the EPA known as Schedule B processes and to make a register available to the public on such processes.

Policy

The District Council will provide resources to process applications for authorization under the EPA Schedule B processes.

Business plan reference

E.H.B.P. 5.10

Frequency/standard

In accordance with EPA Regs and Guidance Notes – New Processes authorized within 4 months. Existing Process authorized within 12 months

Procedures

1. Some pre-discussion may take place between EHOs and the applicant.

2. On receipt of the application it shall be processed by the clerical section and immediately entered in the public register index.

3. Without delay the application shall be passed to the EHO who will assess the application to ascertain whether in his/her opinion it is duly made. In addition the officer will also consider any *claim for confidentiality of information and within 14 days* give a decision to the applicant as to whether the Council is prepared to accept a matter as confidential or not.

4. If an application is not considered to be duly made it shall be either returned to the applicant with an accompanying letter indicating the matters which are outstanding. Alternatively, letters should be sent to the applicant seeking additional information. It is also essential to ensure that the correct fee has been submitted.

5. If an application is deemed to be duly made it shall be returned to the clerical officer who will notify the Yorkshire and Humberside Pollution Advisory Council for inclusion on their data base. A copy will then be sent to the HSE and if appropriate to the Nature Conservancy body.

6. The application shall then be returned to the EHO for processing of the application within the timescale.

7. The officer may require to discuss further with the applicant matters together with a site inspection before drafting out an authorization.

8. All authorizations shall be in the name of the Chief Environmental Health Officer and shall be checked by the Principal Health Officer (Environmental Protection).

9. A letter shall accompany all authorizations setting out, in addition to other matters considered relevant by the Case Officer, the appropriate maintenance fee which is then due.

10. The authorization shall then be placed on the public register.

11. The clerical officer shall ensure that receipt of maintenance fees is kept under observation, and a reminder sent, where failure to make the appropriate payment has occurred.

12. Appeals to the Secretary of State for the Environment shall be processed in accordance with the statutory procedure laid down.

Fig. 3.17 Selby District Council Specimen Quality Statement – Schedule B Process – on the Environmental Protection Act (EPA).

Technicians are essential members of the specialist teams of officers.

Emphasis is placed on qualified technicians and opportunities are offered for qualification training such as BTec in Environmental Health. However, other qualifications are recognized depending on the area of work i.e. HND in Building for the Housing Technicians. The most recent post in the structure is to the commercial team to work in Food Hygiene and Health & Safety at Work. The holder of this post is a qualified dietician, has considerable expertise in food hygiene training and has the CIEH's advanced Health and Safety Certificate.

In order to recognize and encourage qualified technicians the Section has successfully implemented career grades linked to experience and qualifications. This also allows the section to equally benefit from the investment in people.

Liaison arrangements

Elected members and officers of the Council play a very active part in supporting the furtherance of local government and the profession at both national and local level. Staff are encouraged to write and present professionally related papers and formulate comments on draft documents from Government departments, ADC and the CIEH.

Liaison at North Yorkshire County level is primarily based on the North Yorkshire Chief EHOs Group and the specialist groups of officers set up by this body. This helps considerably in bringing about uniformity of standards and as an authority closely linked to the South and West Yorkshire conurbations, membership of the Yorkshire & Humberside Pollution Advisory Council and the Yorkshire & Humberside Clean Air Society is essential. The North Yorkshire Chief EHO's Group strongly supports the ADC with two of its group members being members of the ADC Chief EHO's Group. Liaison arrangements with the District Health Authority are maintained at Chief EHO level with certain functions allocated down to Principal EHO level.

The North Yorkshire District Control of Infection Committee is attended by the Chief EHO. Liaison committees have also been established in order to monitor the environmental problems associated with coal mining and electricity power generation. These meet at 6-monthly intervals and involve members and officers of Selby District Council, North Yorkshire County Council and, in the case of power generation, Wakefield and Leeds Metropolitan Authorities.

Representation on liaison working parties of bodies such as Water Companies and National Rivers Authorities, Public Health Laboratory/ MAFF, is shared amongst officers of the Section who are chosen for their expert knowledge and ability to represent the Council and the Section.

Use of consultants in environmental health

It will be seen from the staffing structure (Fig. 3.16) for Environmental Health that the District Council strongly believe in the use of specialist consultants particularly in relation to mining and power generation. In each of these areas consultants are retained on an annual basis plus an hourly consultancy rate after the initial 8–10 days work.

Other consultancies within the section, such as civil engineers, Warren Spring Laboratories, Universities and the Tidy Britain Group, are employed as one-off contracts.

Over the years I have found, particularly when dealing with environmental issues relating to large utility industries, that experience and expertise lies within those industries and that it is necessary to look carefully for former professional scientific and engineering staff who have worked in the industry concerned and who are now in private practice. This approach has proved extremely effective in bringing about considerable environmental improvements for local communities.

The cost of this support to the section is approximately £25 000 per year. Running alongside this professional support is the extensive Air Quality Monitoring carried out by the DC at an additional cost of £20/30 000 per year.

The Environmental Health Section is now very well placed to meet with confidence the challenges of CCT and customer demands of the next decade.

4 The organization of environmental health in Scotland

Charles Gibson

There are several differences between the system of environmental health which operates in Scotland, and that which operates in other parts of the UK. These differences embrace both the structure of the local authorities and the functions which are undertaken by environmental health departments. In this chapter, where there is no reference to a Scottish way of working, it can be assumed that the arrangements are similar to those for England and Wales.

LOCAL GOVERNMENT SYSTEM

In Scotland the system of local government is organized for the time being on a two-tier basis, with nine regional councils, 53 district councils and three multi-purpose island councils. The regional councils are responsible for large-scale services such as police, roads and education, while district councils have responsibility for services of a more local nature such as housing, parks, public cleansing and environmental health. Due to their geographical situation and the difficulty of communication with the mainland, the three island councils are multi-purpose authorities which are responsible for all services carried out by both regional and district councils.

In July 1993, the government published the white paper 'Shaping the Future – The New Councils', which gave details of the proposed single-tier struc-

ture for local government in Scotland, which will replace the existing councils in 1996.

The present structure of district, regional and islands councils is to be replaced by 28 unitary authorities which will all be responsible for providing the full range of local authority services. There is no departmental structure recommended for the new unitary authorities and it will be up to each council to make arrangements for the delivery of services in their area.

The first elections for members of the proposed new councils will be held in the spring of 1995. There will be a transitional year to enable the new councils to establish themselves and to make arrangements for the transfer of staff and property before finally taking over the full range of responsibilities from the present councils in April 1996.

CENTRAL GOVERNMENT FRAMEWORK

The central government framework in Scotland also differs from that in England and Wales, with departments set up in the Scottish Office, which are closely concerned with the work of local government. The various aspects of environmental health work are divided among the following government departments of the Scottish Office:

1. Home and Health Department
   (a) public health

(b) communicable diseases
(c) health education
(d) environmental issues
(e) licensing
(f) emergency planning.

2. Environment Department
   (a) housing
   (b) building regulations
   (c) public cleansing
   (d) waste management
   (e) water supplies
   (f) air pollution
   (g) environmental protection.

3. Agriculture and Fisheries Department
   (a) food control
   (b) meat inspection
   (c) slaughterhouses
   (d) milk and dairies
   (e) pest control.

Each government department comprises a number of sections which have different responsibilities allocated to them. They advise local authorities on their specialized function, and issue circulars and guidance on new and amended legislation. As in England and Wales, the Scottish Office departments maintain a close liaison with individual local authorities and with the Convention of Scottish Local Authorities. This is the collective body on which regional, district and islands councils are represented. There is also a line of contact between the Scottish Office departments and the Royal Environmental Health Institute of Scotland, which is the professional body which acts on behalf of the environmental health profession.

In Scotland, the central government framework is very similar to the system described for England and Wales. However, because the government departments are responsible to the Secretary of State for Scotland for local government affairs, the Scottish departments enjoy a considerable degree of autonomy. This can result in particular functions beings discharged in a different manner from England and Wales, with variations taking account of the Scottish local government structure and allocation of functions.

These functions will be gone into in some detail later, but the following are examples of the differences:

1. Food law enforcement: district council environmental health departments in Scotland deal with all aspects of food control, including composition and labelling, food hygiene and unsound food.
2. Waste disposal: this is a district council function undertaken by the vast majority of environmental health departments.
3. Milk and dairies: district council environmental health departments have responsibility for registration of dairy farms and for the hygiene standards at these premises.

THE CONVENTION OF SCOTTISH LOCAL AUTHORITIES (COSLA)

COSLA has a committee structure covering the functions of regional councils and district councils. The committee dealing with the environmental health function is the Environmental Services Committee, which also deals with waste management and general environmental issues. This Committee is assisted in its activities by a number of officer advisers, six of whom are directors of environmental health with Scottish local authorities. The main functions of the COSLA are to represent and co-ordinate the interests of the local authorities, to provide advice to government departments and agencies on proposed legislation, and to raise issues and highlight areas where it is considered that government or local government action needs to be taken.

THE ROYAL ENVIRONMENTAL HEALTH INSTITUTE OF SCOTLAND (REHIS)

REHIS is the professional body which represents the interests of the environmental health profession in Scotland. It has in its membership representatives of all officers who are engaged in the various aspects of environmental health work. By far the largest proportion of the membership comprises environmental health officers, but provided they are suitably qualified, other officers may be given full membership.

Membership includes a number of consultants in public health medicine, veterinarians and meat inspectors, and persons involved in various aspects of environmental health education. Representatives from each of these groupings may be elected to the executive council of the REHIS. Elected members of local authorities and health boards, and persons engaged in commercial activities associated with environmental health, are eligible for associate membership.

In addition to representing the professional interests of environmental health officers, the REHIS's main aims are to promote environmental health throughout Scotland and to secure the proper organization of the recruitment, training and qualifications of environmental health officers, meat inspectors and poultry inspectors. This is achieved by overseeing the professional training of, and by examining, environmental health officers and meat inspectors, by organizing regular training courses, and by holding an annual national conference and exhibition.

Regular newsletters are published covering a wide range of topics of interest to the membership. Also, an annual report on environmental health in Scotland, and a compendium of conference papers are published each year.

TRAINING AND QUALIFICATION OF ENVIRONMENTAL HEALTH OFFICERS

In Scotland, the route leading to full professional qualification in environmental health entails obtaining a BSc degree in environmental health, and undertaking a period of practical training and assessment leading to the Diploma in Environmental Health of the Royal Environmental Health Institute of Scotland.

The four-year degree course, which is held at the University of Strathclyde, follows a course syllabus approved by the REHIS. The practical training element requires students to complete 48 weeks of practical training with a local authority, following a programme prescribed by REHIS.

This is normally undertaken in four annual stages with students obtaining placements with local auhtorities who oversee the practical training during the university recess periods. An alternative is for students to undertake practical training 'end-on' by being taken on by a local authority for the required period after graduating. The final stage is a two-day assessment of competence involving interviews and practical tests, which if completed satisfactorily results in the granting of the Diploma in Environmental Health. REHIS is also responsible for the organization of courses in meat and poultry inspection. The syllabus for these courses is approved by the Agriculture and Fisheries Department. Courses and examinations, which lead to the relevant certificate being awarded, are organized by REHIS.

REHIS is consulted by government departments and the Convention of Scottish Local Authorities on proposed legislation and environmental health issues, and advises its members and individual local authorities on a wide variety of topics. The office which deals with the business and administrative affairs of REHIS is in Edinburgh at the following address:

The Royal Environmental Health Instititute
  of Scotland
3 Manor Place
Edinburgh
EH3 7DH
Tel: 0131 225 6999
Fax: 0131 225 3993

NATIONAL CO-ORDINATING GROUPS FOR ENVIRONMENTAL HEALTH

Because Scotland is a small country (the population is just over five million), it has been possible to establish national co-ordinating bodies to provide a forum at which major environmental health issues can be discussed. The two most important examples of this are described below.

The Scottish Environmental Health Group

This group was set up in 1977 by the former Scottish Home and Health Department, following the reorganization of the health boards and local authorities in 1975, to discuss important environmental health and communicable diseases issues. Its membership comprises representatives of the following: the Home and Health Department; the Agriculture and Fisheries Department, the Environment Department; The Health and Safety Executive; the area Health Boards; the Communicable Diseases Scotland Unit; the Environmental Health (Scotland) Unit; and approximately one-third of the country's 56 directors of environmental health who attend on a rotational basis. The group meets twice a year and operates most successfully as a forum for the discussion of public health issues of importance or concern.

The Scottish Food Co-ordinating Committee

This Committee was formed in 1983 in recognition of the fact that there was a need to co-ordinate and monitor the work of the 56 district and island councils in food law enforcement, in order to ensure uniform standards throughout the country. It has since developed into a highly respected body which, in addition to the role of co-ordinating enforcement of food law, has undertaken projects, surveys and studies into the safety and standards of various foods. Its membership comprises public analysts, observers from government departments, microbiologists, nutritionists and trading standards officers, plus directors of environmental health representing the network of local liaison groups, which are established in a regional basis throughout Scotland. It also acts as a consultee of, and advisor to, COSLA, government departments and the food industry, and provides a professional officers' response to issues relating to food.

There are also two specialist units set up under the Common Services Agency of the Scottish Office – Home and Health Department, namely the Environmental Health (Scotland) Unit and the Communicable Diseases (Scotland) Unit, both of which merit special mention, since they have important roles to play in the overall environmental health scene in Scotland.

The Environmental Health (Scotland) Unit

This unit was set up in 1989 under the Common Services Agency of the then Scottish Home and Health Department in order to act as an independent national advisory body on environmental health issues.

The principal functions of the Unit as described by the director of the Unit at the time of its formation are:

1. to advise and liaise with health boards, local authorities, the Scottish Office and other relevant bodies in the epidemiological and medical aspects of environmental health hazards;
2. to investigate environmental hazards to health and to undertake relevant epidemiological research;
3. to facilitate the education and training of appropriate professions;
4. to publish reports on environmental health in association with the Communicable Diseases (Scotland) Unit; and
5. to publish an annual report.

The director of the Unit is a former senior medical officer in the Scottish Home and Health Department, supported by a senior veterinarian and a former director of environmental health.

The Communicable Diseases (Scotland) Unit (CDS)

CDS is at Ruchill Hospital, Glasgow, and was established in 1969 as a consequence of the epidemic of typhoid in Aberdeen in 1964. It is part of the Common Services Agency of the Scottish Health Service, along with the Blood Transfusion Service, the Ambulance Service, the Information and Statistics Division and other national services, and has responsibility for the surveillance of communicable diseases and other infections in Scotland:

1. Surveillance of infections through the collection and analysis of microbiological and other epidemiological data from medical, veterinary and environmental sources.
2. Co-ordinating with health boards and environmental health departments in the surveillance,

investigation and control of infection, e.g. influenza, meningitis, listeriosis, AIDS, salmonellosis and other food-borne infections, hospital infections, etc. at district, area and national level.

3. Surveillance of vaccination programmes, e.g. measles, whooping cough, mumps, rubella etc.
4. Advising on immunization, malaria prophylaxis, etc. for overseas travel.
5. Advising the Scottish Office – Home and Health Department on infection problems.
6. Teaching and training medical undergraduate and postgraduate students, nurses, environmental health officers, etc.
7. Liaison with other national surveillance organizations, e.g. The Public Health Laboratory (PHLS) in England and Wales, The US Centers of Disease Control (CDC), and WHO.

Over 50 medical and veterinary laboratories in Scotland forward information weekly to the CDS relating to micro-organisms identified from man, animals or other sources, e.g. food, water, sewage, and abbatoir drains. Other data sources include the Registrar General's Weekly Returns on Notifiable Infections, family doctor 'spotter' practice and ad hoc telephone information. The data is published in the CDEH Weekly Report for distribution within Scotland, elsewhere in the UK, WHO and national surveillance centres in other countries.

During the 1970s, medical, veterinary and environmental health liaison groups were established in different health board areas of Scotland. These groups have proved invaluable in promoting closer working relationships in the investigation and control of infection. The appointment to the staff at CDS of an environmental health adviser, a nursing officer and a veterinary adviser has also ensured improved liaison with these allied professions, all of which have an important role to play in the control of infection.

In August 1993, the Communicable Diseases (Scotland) Unit and the Environmental Health (Scotland) Unit were amalgamated to form the new Communicable Diseases and Environmental Health (Scotland) Unit. In March 1994 the title of the Unit was changed to the Scottish Centre for Infection and Environmental Health (SCIEH). The functions of the two former units remain unchanged but the new management arrangement will allow for sharing of services such as information technology, data processing and administration. It is intended that the amalgamation will further enhance the cooperation that already exists between the various professions which are involved with problems which stem from environmental sources.

THE ENVIRONMENTAL HEALTH FUNCTION

As in other parts of the UK, most of the work concerned with environmental issues is carried out by the district councils through their environmental health departments. The range of functions is also similar to that in other parts of the country, and a typical structure is illustrated in Fig. 4.1.

The environmental health officers are employed as both advisers and enforcement officers. They give assistance and advice on matters concerning the surroundings in which we live and work. They also put into effect procedures which are sometimes necessary to ensure compliance with the requirements of Acts and Regulations. As well as environmental health

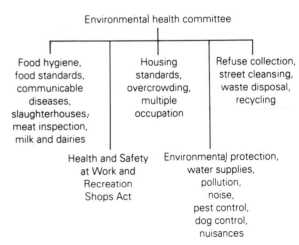

Fig. 4.1 Typical structure of an environmental health department.

officers, typical departments would have technical support staff, pest control officers, dog wardens and, where there are slaughterhouses in their area, meat inspectors and veterinary officers[1]. The environmental health team of experts have the common goal of raising standards within the environment, protecting all sections of the community from potentially harmful substances and situations.

In order to fulfil its role effectively, the environmental health team has available to it professional advice from a number of sources. These include public analysts, public health laboratories, the Health and Safety Executive, the Industrial Pollution Inspectorate, the consultants in public health medicine in the area health boards and the Scottish Centre for Infection and Environmental Health. The close links with government departments at the Scottish Office also play an important part in maintaining liaison in environmental health issues. The co-operation and liaison which has developed over the years means that the local authorities' environmental health staff could be considered to be part of an extended team, with an extensive system of professional and technical advice at their disposal. They, in turn, contribute to the work of these other agencies in as far as it related to environmental health matters. Taken in its entirety, the system provides a highly efficient and effective service to councils and communities in every kind of environmental health issue as shown in Fig. 4.2.

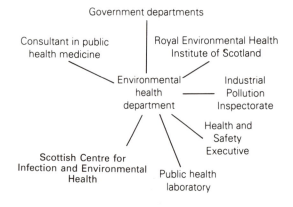

Fig. 4.2 Environmental health in structure.

THE LOCAL GOVERNMENT ENVIRONMENTAL HEALTH DEPARTMENT

At the present time, environmental health is the responsibility of the 53 district and three island councils. There is no rigid pattern which prescribes the way in which councils must discharge their environmental health functions. A number of factors are instrumental in determining the most suitable arrangement, two of the most important being population and area. The topography and remoteness of parts of the country have resulted in a very uneven population spread, and this has also played a part in areas covered by each local authority. The district council with the largest population is the City of Glasgow with over 700 000 inhabitants. At the opposite end of the scale, Badenoch and Strathspey has a population of just over 10 000. Similar extremes can be demonstrated when the areas of the districts are considered. Argyle and Bute, in the west country, extends to over 3700 sq km whereas Clydebank in the central belt of the country has an area of only 22.5 sq km.

These variances have been instrumental in determining the type of department best suited to the particular needs of each area. The tendency has been for the authorities with the largest populations, such as the four city councils, to set up departments for separate activities such as environmental health, public cleansing, building control and parks. In the less populated districts, the opposite occurs with many environmental health departments having responsibility for the wider range of functions. It follows that the degree of specialization in such fields as health and safety, food control, public cleansing or pollution control, is mainly confined to the larger authorities, with the smaller ones operating on the general practice principle. It is envisaged that the management practice will continue after the Unitary Councils take control in 1996.

The tasks of the department

The tasks undertaken in environmental health departments in Scotland are similar to those described for England and Wales. The notable exceptions to this are in the fields of food control, waste disposal (operational and regulatory) and milk and dairies.

Food control

All district councils in Scotland are responsible for all aspects of food control. This function is discharged through the environmental health departments. Each district has a public analyst to whom samples are submitted to ascertain compliance with standards for composition, labelling and fitness. Samples for bacteriological quality are submitted to the public health laboratories of the area health boards.

Waste disposal

As well as being responsible for providing and operating waste disposal facilities which are capable of dealing with waste arising from within their areas, district councils have responsibility for enforcing the general waste provisions of the Control of Pollution Act 1974, for licensing private sites and for monitoring standards. This combined operational and regulatory function is undertaken by the vast majority of environmental health departments which have public cleansing as part of their responsibilities. Where public cleansing is undertaken by a separate cleansing department, the regulatory responsibilities are normally undertaken by the environmental health department.

Milk and dairies

The registration and licensing of dairy farms, milk processing plants, dealers and retailers of milk is an environmental health function in Scotland. These responsibilities extend to monitoring hygiene standards of both the premises and the product, and to ensuring compliance with the bacteriological and compositional standards laid down for the various grades of milk.

LEGISLATION APPLYING TO SCOTLAND

A proportion of the legislation dealing with environmental health applies to the entire UK.

Examples of this are the Control of Pollution Act 1974, the Health and Safety at Work Etc. Act 1974, and the Food Safety Act 1990. The vast majority of the legislation enforced by environmental health officers does not fall into this category, however, and has been drafted specifically for Scotland. This legislation falls into two categories:

1. acts and regulations which are peculiar to Scotland, and
2. acts and regulations which are similar to those which apply in other parts of the country but which reflect the different Scottish Office, local government and court/legal systems.

An example of legislation which falls into the first category is The Civic Government (Scotland) Act 1982. This Act gives powers to district councils to deal with, *inter alia*, repairs to buildings, licensing of street traders, late catering licences, control of dogs and the making of bye-laws – all of which are used by environmental health departments in the discharge of their duties.

A second example is the Licensing (Scotland) Act 1976. Although primarily concerned with the conditions attached to the issue of liquor licences, it also contains provisions which relate to food hygiene standards in licensed premises, and can also enable the licensing authority to impose noise control standards where music or entertainment is provided in licensed premises.

The second category above is the area into which the vast majority of the legislation enforced by environmental health officers in Scotland falls. The legislation is similar to the English equivalent, and is designed to achieve the same objective, e.g. compliance with food hygiene standards and housing standards.

FINANCIAL ACCOUNTABILITY

The Commission for Local Authority Accounts in Scotland (the Accounts Commission) has responsibility for ensuring that all local authority accounts are externally audited. The Accounts Commission, through the office of Controller of Audit, exercises this function either directly using its own staff, or by the use of private firms of approved auditors. The accounts of environmental health departments are subject to this process, which · requires the Auditor to ensure that all statutory requirements have been met and proper practices observed in the preparation of the accounts.

The Accounts Commission is also empowered under the Local Government Act 1988 to undertake value for money studies in areas which include environmental health functions. These studies can lead to recommendations being made aimed at improving economy, efficiency and effectiveness, and at highlighting areas where management can be improved.

COMPETITIVE TENDERING

The principal sections of the Local Government Act 1988 require a range of local authority services to be exposed to competition, and lay down the rules under which tenders must be invited. The provisions of the Act apply to Scotland, as they do to other parts of the UK, and could in future years significantly change the traditional role of local authorities as the providers of services, including those which are currently undertaken by environmental health departments.

[1] In April 1995 the responsibility for meat inspection and slaughterhouses was transferred from district councils to the National Meat Hygiene Service.

FURTHER READING

Chartered Institute of Public Finance and Accountancy (1988) *Guide to Local Government Finance in Scotland*.

Royal Environmental Health Institute of Scotland (1988) *Environmental Health in Scotland*.

Scottish Food Co-ordinating Committee (1989) *Food Enforcement and Surveillance in Scotland*.

Scottish Home and Health Department (1989) *Health Bulletin 47/5*, Scottish Information Office.

Scottish Information Office (1975) *Local Government in Scotland*.

Scottish Office (1993) *Shaping New Councils*.

5 The organization of environmental health in Northern Ireland

Brian Hanna

The present system of local government in Northern Ireland dates from 1973. There are 26 single-tier local authorities: 2 city councils, 13 borough councils and 11 district councils. The population of these councils varies from Belfast with 296 700 to Moyle with 15 100.

LOCAL AUTHORITY FUNCTIONS

The powers and functions of local authorities are limited in that they are not responsible for health, social services, education, housing, water supply, sewerage nor planning. There is, however, a legal requirement that they be consulted on planning decisions. Responsibility for these services is shown in Table 5.1.

Table 5.1 Responsibility for services in Northern Ireland

Health and social services	– Health and Social Services Boards
Education	– Education and Library Boards
Housing	– Northern Ireland Housing Executive
Water supply and sewerage	– Department of the Environment
Planning	– Department of the Environment

ENVIRONMENTAL HEALTH FUNCTIONS

Environmental functions, with the exception of those listed above, are the responsibility of district councils and include waste collection and disposal, food (including composition and labelling) and consumer protection.

Environmental health officers are employed by Belfast City Council and by four group committees representing the 25 district councils outside Belfast. Officers are allocated to district councils to carry out the environmental health functions of the councils. They also carry out work relating to water pollution control for the Department of the Environment (NI) and to housing for the Northern Ireland Housing Executive.

These group committees are set up under powers given in the Local Government Act (Northern Ireland) 1972 and the Local Government (Employment of Environmental Health Officers) Order (Northern Ireland) 1973. Each group has an employer council which employs the environmental health officers on behalf of the group committee. The group committee is composed of two councillors from each of the councils in the group.

Belfast has a director of health and environment services, and each group has a chief administrative environmental health officer who is responsible for the supervision of all the environmental health officers within the group. There are also at group headquarters specialists in food/health education, pollution control, housing and an officer responsible for training.

Within local authorities, environmental health officers are organized in separate departments with each authority having a director of environmental health or chief environmental health officer (director of health and environmental services in Belfast), who is a chief officer and, in most cases, is a member of the council management team.

ENVIRONMENTAL HEALTH AT GOVERNMENT LEVEL

There are six environmental health officers employed by the Department of the Environment's Environment Service: one director of environmental protection; one chief environmental health officer; two senior environmental health officers and two environmental health officers. These officers not only provide services to the Department of the Environment but also advise and assist all other Northern Ireland government departments.

Environmental health matters at government level are mainly the concern of:

1. the Department of the Environment (housing, pollution, water and sewerage, planning, and licensing);
2. the Department of Health and Social Security (food, health education, and communicable disease);
3. the Department of Agriculture (food, dog control, animal diseases, and pesticides); and
4. the Department of Economic Development (health and safety, and consumer safety).

LIAISON ARRANGEMENTS

Liaison between the groups, Belfast and the Department of the Environment Inspectorate is maintained by regular meetings of the chief administrative environmental health officers, director of

health and environmental services in Belfast, and the chief environmental health officer at the Department of the Environment. Committees, composed in the main of specialist officers also meet regularly. These committees are concerned with food, housing, pollution control, general environmental health, health and safety liaison, consumer safety, training liaison, and radiation monitoring. These committees are given the opportunity to consider and comment on proposed legislation, as is the Northern Ireland Centre of the Chartered Institute of Environmental Health.

LEGISLATION

Legislation in Northern Ireland follows British legislation very closely, and the following gives some guidance in this respect.

Public health

Nuisances, drainage, sanitary conveniences, offensive trades and burial grounds are dealt with under the Public Health (Ireland) Acts 1878 to 1907. These Acts were amended regularly, and until the Environmental Protection Act 1990, corresponded fairly closely to British legislation.

Food

Food legislation is contained in the Food Safety (Northern Ireland) Order 1991, which follows the Food Safety Act 1990. Food hygiene regulations and food composition and labelling regulations follow British legislation. The enforcement of composition and labelling is the responsibility of district councils, and is carried out by environmental health officers.

Consumer protection

Consumer safety is the duty of district councils and is enforced by environmental health officers. The relevant legislation is the Consumer Protection Act 1987 and the Consumer Protection (Northern Ireland) Order 1987, and various consumer protection safety regulations which apply to the UK as a whole. District councils have responsibility for the Construction Product Regulations 1991 which are made under the European Communtites Act 1972.

Occupational health and safety

Occupational Health and Safety is covered by the Health and Safety at Work (Northern Ireland) Order 1978. There are many other relevant statutory provisions including the Factories Act (Northern Ireland) 1978, the Office and Shop Premises Act (Northern Ireland) 1966 and various regulations. The provisions in Northern Ireland closely follow the provisions in the rest of the UK particularly as the majority of legislation is now directed by the European Community.

Enforcement responsibilities are allocated in a similar way to Great Britain by using main activity criteria. However no provision has been made for the transfer of enforcement responsibility by agreement because Section 18(2)(b) of the Health and Safety at Work etc. Act 1974, and therefore Regulations 5 and 6 of the Health and Safety (Enforcing Authority) Regulations 1989, have been omitted from the equivalent Northern Ireland legislation.

The Health and Safety Division of the Department of Economic Development undertakes a similar role to that of the Health and Safety Executive, except in relation to agricultural activities where the enforcing authority is the Department of Agriculture.

The Health and Safety Liaison group made up of environmental health representatives from Belfast City Council, the four Group Committees, the Department of the Environment and a health and safety inspector from the Department of Economic Development, meets regularly to agree responsibility for enforcement, to discuss matters in relation to uniformity of enforcement and to arrange training programmes.

The Health and Safety Agency for Northern Ireland was established by the Health and Safety at Work (Northern Ireland) Order 1978 to promote health safety and welfare at work, to approve codes of practice and to issue guidance, to review enforcement strategies, to appraise proposed and existing legislation, to carry out and encourage research, to encourage training and to provide information and advice.

Waste management

Waste collection and disposal is the responsibility of district councils, who are also responsible for the licensing of waste disposal sites, street cleaning, litter and abandoned motor vehicles, and the issue of consignment notes for hazardous and special wastes. Responsibility within councils for these duties varies, but environmental health officers are involved in all to a greater or lesser degree. Legislation is found in the Pollution Control and Local Government (Northern Ireland) Order 1978, the Pollution Control (Licensing of Waste Disposal) Regulations (Northern Ireland) 1980, the Pollution Control (Special Wastes) Regulations (Northern Ireland) 1981, the Transfrontier Shipment of Hazardous Waste Regulations (Northern Ireland) 1989 and the Collection and Disposal of Waste (Northern Ireland) Regulations 1991.

Refuse collection is subject to compulsory competitive tendering from 1 April 1994 and street cleaning from 1 April 1995.

Noise control

Controls over noise nuisance, noise on construction sites, loudspeakers in the street, noise abatement zones and powers to issue and approve codes of practice for the minimization of noise are contained in the Pollution Control and Local Government (Northern Ireland) Order 1978. The legislative controls are similar to those contained in the Control of Pollution Act 1974 and are enforced by district councils in Northern Ireland. (The part dealing with noise abatement zones has not yet been implemented.)

Atmospheric pollution

The principal legislation enforced by councils is in the Clean Air (Northern Ireland) Order 1981, the

Pollution Control and Local Government (Northern Ireland) Order 1978, and the nuisance provisions of the Public Health (Ireland) Act 1878. This legislation is broadly similar to that contained in the Clean Air Acts of 1956 and 1968. Non-scheduled processes and domestic air pollution are controlled by district councils through environmental health officers.

The Health and Safety at Work (Northern Ireland) Order 1978 does not contain a similar provision to section 5 of the Health and Safety at Work Act 1974. Emission to the atmosphere regulations have not been made. The Alkali Etc. Works (Northern Ireland) Order 1991 lists both the noxious or offensive gases and the registrable (scheduled) processes or works. The Department of the Environment, Northern Ireland, may by order under Article 25 of the Clean Air (Northern Ireland) Order 1981 vary or add to the list of gases or works. The Alkali and Radio-Chemical Inspectorate of the Department of the Environment, Northern Ireland, enforces the 1906 Alkali, Etc. Works Regulation Act and the Alkali, Etc. Works (Northern Ireland) Order 1991.

A new system of industrial air pollution control is currently proposed for Northern Ireland. This will bring in controls broadly similar to those contained in Part I of the Environmental Protection Act 1990.

The Air Quality Standards Regulations (Northern Ireland) 1990 implement the EC directives requirements in relation to sulphur dioxide, suspended particulates, lead in the air and nitrogen dioxide.

The Radioactive Substances Act 1993 extends to Northern Ireland.

Water pollution

Legislation covering the management of water resources and prevention of the pollution of water in Northern Ireland is contained in the Water Act (Northern Ireland) 1972. Its provisions relating to the prevention of water pollution are broadly similar to those previously contained in the Control of Pollution Act 1974 in that a 'consent' is required to make a discharge of trade or sewage effluent, or of any polluting matter to a waterway or

underground stratum. The Food and Environment Protection Act 1985 covers dumping at sea.

The Water Act (Northern Ireland) 1972 confers functions connected with water management on the Department of the Environment for Northern Ireland and the Department of Agriculture. The issue of consents and the investigation of pollution incidents is carried out by environmental health officers (water pollution) employed by the groups and Belfast, but working and reporting directly to the Department of the Environment.

The nuisance provisions of the Public Health Acts still apply and are operated by district council environmental health officers in respect of water courses.

Housing

The statutory framework for controlling housing conditions in Northern Ireland has less in common with that of England and Wales than is to be found in other core areas of environmental health.

The principal legislation is contained in the Housing (Northern Ireland) Orders of 1981 and 1983, as amended, and the Rent (Northern Ireland) Order 1978. The Housing (Northern Ireland) Order 1992 brought a number of provisions of the aforementioned Housing Orders into line with the corresponding parts of the Housing Act 1988 and the Local Government and Housing Act 1989.

Housing Order powers concerning housing conditions, including those relating to individual unfit houses and houses in multiple occupation, are enforced by the Northern Ireland Housing Executive rather than by district councils. A considerable amount of survey and assessment work is, however, carried out on behalf of the Northern Ireland Housing Executive by district council environmental health officers.

District councils do, however, have important powers under the Rent (Northern Ireland) Order 1978 to ensure fulfilment of repairing obligations in the regulated tenancy sector through the service of certificates of disrepair and enforcement action to secure compliance with their requirements. The responsibility for controlling the conversion of restricted tenancies, for which rents are tied to pre-1978 levels, to regulated tenancies by the issue of regulated rent certificates also rests with district councils.

A further addition to district council housing powers effected by the Housing (Northern Ireland) Order 1992 was an amendment to the Rent Order which grants specific authority to district councils to prosecute offences of illegal eviction or harassment of tenants.

Communicable disease

Communicable disease is legislated for in the Public Health Act (Northern Ireland) 1967 and the Health and Personal Social Services (Northern Ireland) Order 1972. Health and social services boards, through their directors of public health and consultants in communicable disease control (CCDCs), enforce this legislation which includes notification of disease, prohibition from work of carriers, contacts, etc.

There are four health and social services boards which are co-terminus with the four group committees employing environmental health officers. Belfast forms part of the Eastern Health and Social Services Board. Some environmental health officers are authorized officers under the above legislation, and environmental health officers are involved in, for example, the investigation of an outbreak of food poisoning. Bacteriological examination of water and food is carried out for all of Northern Ireland by the Northern Ireland Public Health Laboratory at the City Hospital, Belfast.

The directors of public health liaise with the chief administrative environmental health officers in relation to communicable disease and provide medical advice when required.

Port health

Port health is also the responsibility of health and social services boards. Powers are contained in the Public Health (Aircraft) Regulations (Northern Ireland) 1971 and the Public Health (Ships) Regulations (Northern Ireland) 1971.

District councils act as agents of the boards, and environmental health officers at the ports carry out the full range of port health duties associated with infectious diseases and hygiene. The inspection of imported food is enforced by district councils under the Imported Food (Northern Ireland) Regulations 1991 as amended and the products of Animal Origin (Import and Export) Regulations (Northern Ireland) 1993. These latter Regulations are jointly enforced with the Department of Agriculture for Northern Ireland.

Drinking water

The main public water supply in Northern Ireland is the responsibility of the Department of the Environment (Northern Ireland). The Government has not yet proceeded to privatize this service but remains committed to do so at the earliest practicable date.

Provision of a sufficient wholesome supply of water to houses is required by the Water Supplies and Sewerage Act (Northern Ireland) 1945, the enforcement of which is the responsibility of district councils.

District councils, through their Environmental Health Departments, carry out systematic programmes of sampling on behalf of the four Area Health and Social Services Boards and also in relation to their duties under both food control and health and safety at work legislation.

The Government is currently finalizing arrangements to implement European requirements relating to water quality. This will be done by means of regulations made under a draft Water and Sewerage Services (Amendment) (NI) Order.

The work of monitoring water quality under these new arrangements will be carried out by the Department of the Environment's Environment Service. A public register of information will be maintained about drinking water and an annual report will be published. The Department will also be required to inform both District Councils and Area Health and Social Services Boards of any circumstances, in relation to a public water supply within their respective areas, likely to give a significant public health risk.

Dogs and other animals

An extensive range of dog control measures, enforceable by district councils, was provided in the Dogs (Northern Ireland) Order 1983. These include requirements concerning annual licensing (fee £5, with 50% discount to elderly owners who live alone and exemption for guide dogs for the blind and hearing dogs for the deaf), and the provision of penalties for allowing dogs to stray or to attack persons or livestock.

Provision is also made for the issue of Fixed Penalty notices for keeping a dog without a licence, allowing a dog to stray, failure to display identification and permitting fouling of footpaths contrary to bye-laws.

Similar powers to control dangerous dogs as apply in England and Wales were introduced in Northern Ireland by the Dangerous Dogs (Northern Ireland) Order 1991. These powers too are enforced by district councils.

Pet shops, animal boarding, riding and zoological establishments require licensing under the Welfare of Animals Act (Northern Ireland) 1972. This Act is enforced by the Department of Agriculture for Northern Ireland.

Pest control

Legal powers in Northern Ireland derived from the Rats and Mice (Destruction), Act 1919 the Prevention of Damage by Pests Act 1949 not being applicable in Northern Ireland.

Caravans and camping

The Caravans Act (Northern Ireland) 1963 is similar in its provisions to the Caravan Sites and Control of Development Act 1960.

Swimming, boating, etc.

Swimming, boating, etc. is controlled by public health and health and safety legislation with local bye-laws.

Entertainment licensing

Entertainment licensing by district councils is under the Local Government (Miscellaneous Provisions) (Northern Ireland) Order 1985, which follows the provisions of the Local Government (Miscellaneous Provisions) Act 1982.

Acupuncture, tattooing, ear-piercing and electrolysis

Acupuncture, tattooing, ear-piercing and electrolysis are required to be registered where the district council has applied the Local Government (Miscellaneous Provisions) (Northern Ireland) Order 1985, which is similar to the Local Government (Miscellaneous Provisions) Act 1982.

Powers are provided to make bye-laws.

Hairdressing

Registration of premises is required under the Hairdressers Act (Northern Ireland) 1939 and SR & O No. 86 of 1939. Powers to make bye-laws similar to the Public Health Act 1961 are provided.

THE FUTURE

Since local government reorganization in Northern Ireland in 1973, environmental health officers have been caught up in arguments for and against the group system. This system was favoured by the Institution of Environmental Health Officers, because it seemed the best way to provide specialist officers for small districts and would avoid the disintegration of the environmental health inspectorate if officers were employed by separate bodies, such as the Department of the Environment and the Northern Ireland Housing Executive.

Following a review of the group system for the administration of public health and building control by Dr R.J. Dickson in March 1985, his report was considered by the Environment Committee of the Northern Ireland Assembly. The

Department of the Environment (Northern Ireland) produced a local government consultation paper in November 1988 which stated: 'it was accepted by Dr Dickson and the Environment Committee that these services are run to a high standard and are well received by the general public.'

This consultative paper proposes that individual councils should be responsible for the appointment and employment of officers carrying out statutory building control and environmental health functions within the council area. It also proposes that new mandatory joint committees for environmental health and building control functions should be set up to serve 25 of the councils. Belfast was not included in the arrangement and the appointment and employment of specialists was to be by the new joint committee.

Responses have been made to this consultative paper including one from the Northern Ireland Centre of the Institution of Environmental Health Officers, which proposed, amongst other things, that a working party comprising all bodies with interests in the environmental health function be set up. It was proposed that the working party should take into consideration the substantial diversification of activities of environmental health departments which had taken place, the emerging changes, and the importance which the government places on a strong, impartial consumer voice which the environmental health service represents.

Unfortunately this working party never materialized and the whole matter was overtaken by events in the form of the Northern Ireland Local Government Auditor's Value-for-Money (VFM) study.

The results of this VFM study have sparked off another attempt by the Department of the Environment (NI) to change the Group environmental health system. New regulations – the Local Government (Employment of Group Environmental Health Staff) Order (NI) 1994 – have been produced and these will come into effect on 1 April 1995.

The broad thrust of the new regulations is to return the employment of district council environmental health officers to each district council and establish a Group headquarters within each of the four areas. These Groups will continue to employ EHOs and to have political representation. They will operate in a planning and monitoring role only providing direct operational services to district councils when requested. District councils would be free to seek environmental health services from other sources or provide them directly themselves.

Time will tell whether or not these changes prove beneficial. However, there is no doubt that environmental health officers will continue to work within both central and local government in Northern Ireland to ensure that environmental health services meet the needs of the people of the Province.

FURTHER READING

Dickson, Brice, *The Legal System of Northern Ireland – The Law in Action*, SLS Legal Publications, Belfast.

6 Training and professional standards

Hazel O. Carter

TRAINING OF ENVIRONMENTAL HEALTH OFFICERS (EHOs)

To become qualified as an EHO a person needs to complete an approved undergraduate or postgraduate course of study and a period of practical training. Successful completion of these elements will lead to the award of the Certificate of Registration of the Environmental Health Officers Registration Board which is the formal qualification recognized for practice as an EHO: a degree in Environmental Health is not the full professional qualification.

Accredited Environmental Health courses all cover the same basic syllabus although the emphasis may vary from course to course. Science, technology, statistics, social science, public administration and law are studied at a general level, and food, occupational health, pollution and housing issues are looked at in more depth.

Laboratory work, case studies, visits, group work and tutorials make the courses varied and interesting. Group work is encouraged in all aspects of the course, and students are also expected to do a lot of work independently. This is good preparation for a career which can involve both working alone, and as part of a team.

Some of the approved courses offer a part-time route which enables people already working in environmental health as technicians to obtain the professional qualification whilst still remaining in employment. However, practical training remains an important element of the course and a balance has to be struck between receiving 220 days' training as an EHO and carrying out day to day technical duties.

The majority of students pursue an integrated course of study where practical training occurs in the third year of 4-year degree course. In 1996 there will be some scope for flexibility enabling those students who are not able to find a 1-year practical training placement during their course to undertake training during a 2-year period at the end of their degree course.

Competition for practical training places is fierce and candidates need to be both keen and persistent to secure a place. At least 50% of the practical training has to be spent in a local authority, working and learning alongside qualified EHOs. This gives the student the opportunity to sample all aspects of the work. The remaining months can be spent in the same or a different authority or with environmental health practitioners in the private sector. A list of approved courses is provided in the appendix to this Chapter.

TRAINING OF ENVIRONMENTAL HEALTH TECHNICIANS

Environmental health technicians are drawn from a variety of backgrounds and provide technical support to the work of environmental health departments. Some technicians are drawn from a building trades background, others from nursing or the food industry or from experience in applied sciences.

There is no specific prescription for or definition of the work of a technician and it depends upon the needs of each employer. Many technicians pursue the BTec National Diploma or Higher Diploma in Environmental Health Studies and in turn these courses can be a stepping stone into the professional qualification route. Technicians are eligible for non-corporate membership of the CIEH (see Chapter 3) and those pursuing the BTec are eligible for student membership. A list of BTec courses is provided in the appendix to this Chapter.

ASSESSMENT OF PROFESSIONAL COMPETENCE

When a person qualifies to practise as an EHO he or she is eligible for Graduate Membership of the CIEH. After at least 2 years of professional practice a Graduate Member can apply to take an Assessment of Professional Competence and become a full Corporate Member of the chartered body.

The assessment requires the candidate to submit a log which summarizes the work they have undertaken during 2 years of practice. A case study is prepared which deals with a particular problem tackled during the 2 year period and the candidate attends a professional interview.

The assessors use the case study and interview to determine whether the candidate has developed seven core skills to a level which is acceptable for Corporate Membership. The core skills are:

1. investigative;
2. analytical;
3. interpretive;
4. communicative;
5. educative;
6. organizational;
7. attitudinal.

CONTINUING PROFESSIONAL DEVELOPMENT

The CIEH's scheme of Continuing Professional Development (CPD) was introduced in July 1992 on a voluntary basis. The competence of members of the CIEH is vital to the continued development and standing of the environmental health profession. Each member of the Institute has a personal responsibility to maintain his own professional competence to the collective benefit of all members. Similarly, the Institute acknowledges that it has a responsibility to invest resources in assisting members to meet their commitment.

The scheme, in principle, requires Graduate and Corporate Members to undertake and record at least 20 hours of CPD activity each year. Such activities as training courses, seminars, Branch and Centre meetings, research and the writing/presentation of papers can all be relevant to the scheme.

The headquarters of the institute is:

The Chartered Institute of Environment Health (CIEH)
Chadwick Court
15 Hatfields
London SE1 8DJ
Tel: 0171 928 6006.

APPENDIX

ACCREDITED QUALIFYING COURSES IN ENVIRONMENTAL HEALTH (PROFESSIONAL ROUTE)

BSc Degree in Environmental Health/Science (Four-year course)

Nottingham
Nottingham Trent University
Burton Street
Nottingham
NG1 4BU
Tel: 0115 9418 418
Mrs A. McCarthy – Course Leader

Cardiff
Cardiff Institute of Higher Education
Western Avenue
Cardiff
CF5 2YB
Tel: 01222 551 111
Mr A. Curnin – Course Director

Leeds
Leeds Metropolitan University*
Brunswick Terrace
Leeds
LS2 8BU
Tel: 0113 2832 600
Mr T. Moran – Course Leader

London
University of Greenwich*
Rachel MacMillan Building
Creek Road
London
SE8 3BU
Tel: 0181 316 8200
Mr S. Allan – Course Director

King's College, London*
Biosphere Sciences Division
Kensington Campus
Campden Hill Road
London
W8 7AH
Tel: 0171 836 5454
Mr N. Parkinson – Director of Studies

Middlesex University
School of Applied Sciences
Bounds Green Road
London
N11 2NQ
Tel: 0181 368 1299
Mr R. Beaumont – Course Leader

Manchester
Manchester Metropolitan University*
Department of Biological Science
Chester Street
Manchester

M1 5DG
Tel: 0161 247 2000
Ms S. Powell – Course Leader

Salford
University College Salford*
(Joint with University of Salford)
Frederick Building
Frederick Road
Salford
M6 6PU
Tel: 0161 736 6541
Ms T. Gurney – Course Contact

University of Salford
Dept of Environmental Health & Housing
  Salford
M5 4WT
Tel: 0161 745 5000
Ms D. Rennie – Course Tutor

Ulster
University of Ulster
Shore Road
Newtonabbey
Co Antrim
N Ireland
Tel: 01232 365 131
Mr H. Harvey – Subject Director

Bristol
University of West of England
Faculty of Applied Sciences
Coldharbour Lane
Frenchay
Bristol BS16 1QY
Tel: 0117 965 6261
Ms Lucy Walmsley – Course Director

Postgraduate Qualifications in Environmental Health (Two-year MSc courses for science graduates)

Bristol
University of the West of England
Department of Science

* These courses are also offered part-time for persons who wish to continue in employment.

Coldharbour Lane
Frenchay
Bristol
BS16 1QY
Tel: 0117 965 6261
Dr R. Keen – Course Director

Birmingham
University of Birmingham
School of Biological Sciences
Edgbaston
Birmingham
B15 2TT
Tel: 0121 414 3494
Mrs J. Higgit – Senior Tutor

CENTRES APPROVED TO OFFER BTEC QUALIFICATIONS IN ENVIRONMENTAL HEALTH STUDIES

National Certificate

Weston Super Mare College, Avon
01934 621 301
North East Wales Institute of HE, Clwyd
01978 290 666
Cornwall College, Cornwall
01209 712 911
Bournemouth & Poole College of FE, Dorset
01202 747 600
Peterlee College, Durham
0191 586 2225
RAMC Training Group, Hants
01252 340 251
Blackpool & The Fylde College, Lancashire
01253 52352
College of North East London, London
0181 802 3111
Norfolk College of Arts & Technology, Norfolk
01553 761 144
Basford Hall College, Nottingham
01602 704 541

Salford College of Technology, Salford
0161 736 6541
Suffolk College, Suffolk
01473 255 885
West Suffolk College, Suffolk
01284 701 301
North East Surrey College of Technology, Surrey
0181 394 1731
Matthew Bolton College of F & HE, West Midlands
0121 446 4545
Leeds College of Building, West Yorkshire
0113 2430 765

National Diploma

Bournemouth & Poole College of FE, Dorset
01202 747 600
College of North East London, London
0181 802 3111
Suffolk College, Suffolk
01473 255 885
Leeds College of Building, West Yorkshire
0113 2430 765

Higher National Certificate

College of North East London, London
0181 802 3111
North East Surrey College of Technology, Surrey
0181 394 1731
Leeds College of Building, West Yorkshire
0113 2430 765
University College, Salford
0161 736 6541
Weston-Super-Mare College of Further Education
01934 621 301

Higher National Diploma

University College, Salford
0161 736 6541

Part Two
Environmental Health Law and Administration

7 Environmental health law

Frank B. Wright

SOURCES

This book is concerned with the law of the UK. The UK comprises Great Britain and Northern Ireland, with Great Britain made up of England, Wales and Scotland. The Channel Islands and the Isle of Man are Crown dependencies and are not part of the UK. The UK constitution is not contained in any single document but has evolved over the course of time. It was formed originally by customary law and later by the common law, then by statute and convention. The UK is a constitutional monarchy. It is governed by the Sovereign who is both the Head of State and Head of Government. The organs of government are the legislature (Parliament), the executive and the judiciary. Although the powers of the monarchy are now very limited, restricted primarily to advisory and ceremonial functions, there remain important duties which are reserved for the Sovereign. These include the summoning, the proroguing and the dissolving of Parliament, the appointment of Ministers, including the Prime Minister, and the appointment of judges and certain senior officials.

International treaties, entered into on behalf of the UK, are concluded by Ministers acting under the royal prerogative. Ministers are responsible to Parliament. International treaties must be incorporated into UK law by an Act of Parliament.

The international and European dimension (see also Chapter 2)

There is a presumption of interpretation that in incorporating an international treaty the UK intends to fulfil its international obligations. However, where the words of an Act of Parliament are clear and unambiguous, they must be given effect even if the decision results in a breach of international law. The primary sources of Community law consist of the three founding Treaties (European Coal and Steel Community, European Atomic Energy Community and European Economic Community) with their Annexes and Protocols, which supplement the Treaties; the Convention on Certain Institutions Common to the European Communities (1957); the Merger Treaty (1965); certain treaties on budgetary matters; treaties on accession and their annexes; the Act of Council concerning direct elections from the European Parliament (1976); the Act of Council concerning direct elections from the European Parliament (1976); the Single European Act (1986) and the Treaty on European Union (1992). The Treaties of the European Communities and European Community law were incorporated into UK law by the European Communities Act 1972 and the European Communities (Amendment) Act 1993. The courts of the UK have not demonstrated any reticence in applying Community law and construe UK legislation so far as possible in conformity with the purpose of EC legislation. Where it appears to the courts that there is inadvertently conflicting UK legislation they will endeavour to give effect to Community law.

Common law

The earliest laws of which there is documentary evidence date from the Anglo-Saxon period of history before the Norman Conquest. These laws related to particular areas such as Kent, Wessex and Mercia. As a centralized system of law developed customary law gave way to national law. The national law came to be known as common law. Common law was developed by the King's judges and is derived entirely from case law. In addition to settling principles of law, which were to be observed nationally, the courts began to establish formal rules of procedure for those who wished to bring cases before them. Court rules established that actions had to be commenced by royal writ and set out in an accepted form. Difficulties emerged in relation to the use of writs and forms of action. Litigants who were unable to get satisfaction petitioned the monarch who in turn handed the petitions to the Lord Chancellor. The Lord Chancellor set up the Court of Chancery which was guided by principles of fairness or equity in coming to a decision. The law of equity became established in the fifteenth century. Both common law and equity came to operate as parallel systems, each bound by its own judicial precedents. The Supreme Court of Judicature Acts 1873–75 reorganized the existing court structures and brought together the common law courts and the Courts of Chancery. This legislation has now been consolidated in the Supreme Court Act 1981. Where common law and equity conflict, the law of equity prevails. All courts administer the principles of common law and equity and grant the remedies of both as the case demands.

Statute law including the Parliamentary process

An Act of Parliament which has been given royal assent and placed on the parliamentary roll is the law and must be given effect by the courts (see *British Railways Board* v. *Pickin* [1974] A.C. 765). Parliament is made up of three elements: the Sovereign, the House of Lords and the House of Commons. In order for a legislative measure to become an Act of Parliament and be recognized as such by the courts it has to undergo one of several procedures. The measure is drafted, usually by Parliamentary counsel to the Treasury, and presented to the House of Commons or House of Lords, more usually the House of Commons, as a Bill. Before a Public Bill becomes an Act of Parliament it must undergo five stages in each House. First Reading; Second Reading; Committee Stage; Report Stage, and Third Reading. The First Reading is a formality. There is no debate at this point. Nowadays this stage constitutes an order to print the Bill. At the Second Reading there is a debate on the principles of the Bill, whilst the Committee Stage sees the Bill examined in detail, clause by clause. In most cases the Committee Stage takes place in a Standing Committee, or the whole House may act as a Committee. At the Report Stage there is a detailed review of the Bill as amended in the Committee stage. On the Third Reading the Bill is finally debated. These stages can be taken quickly although the process normally takes a number of months. Much depends on the Bill's political importance. A Bill may be first considered in either House but it has to pass through both Houses to become law. Both Houses must agree the same text of a Bill, so that the amendments made by the second House are then considered in the originating House, and if not agreed, sent back or themselves amended, until agreement is reached. Under the Parliament Acts 1911 and 1949, if the House of Lords rejects any other Public Bill (except one to prolong the life of a Parliament) which has been passed by the Commons in two successive sessions, then the Bill will become law without the consent of the Lords, unless the Commons directs to the contrary. The royal assent is signified by letters patent to such Bills and Measures as have passed both Houses of Parliament (or Bills which have been passed under the Parliament Acts 1911 and 1949). The Sovereign has not given royal assent in person since 1854. The power to withhold assent resides with the Sovereign but has not been exercised in the UK since 1707, in the reign of Queen Anne. Public Bills promoted by a Member who is not a member of the Government are known as Private Members' Bills.

Delegated legislation

This is law made by subordinate authorities acting under law-making powers delegated by Parliament or the Sovereign. Many statutes empower Ministers to make delegated legislation. Such legislation includes the following:

Orders in Council

The Sovereign in Council, or Privy Council, was the chief source of executive power until Cabinet government developed in the eighteenth century. Membership of the Privy Council is automatic upon appointment to certain government and judicial positions in the UK. Membership is also accorded by the Queen to eminent people in the UK and independent countries of the Commonwealth of which Her Majesty is Queen, on the recommendation of the British Prime Minister. The Privy Council Office is headed by the Lord President of the Council, a Cabinet Minister. Orders in Council are approved by the Queen in the presence of three Privy Councillors (enough to constitute a quorum) after which it is announced that the Queen held a Privy Council. The matters considered, however, will have previously been recommended by the responsible departments of government. Orders in Council may be made by Ministers acting under the royal prerogative. See, for example, Section 84 Health and Safety at Work etc. Act 1974 which provides that Her Majesty may by Order in Council extend the provisions of the Act outside Great Britain.

Statutory Instruments

Many thousands of Statutory Instruments are issued annually by Ministers of the Crown acting under delegated powers provided by Acts of Parliament. Statutory Instruments are of considerable importance as a source of environmental health law because of the detailed technical nature of the law enforcement role. Each one published is allocated a number for the year, see for example Clean Air (Emission of Grit and Dust from Furnaces) Regulations 1971 (S.I. 1971 No.162). Statutory Instruments fall into four broad categories: **Affirmative Instruments**, which are subject to the approval of both Houses of Parliament before they can come into or remain in force; **Negative Instruments**, which are subject to annulment by resolution of either House; **General Instruments**, which include those not required to be laid before Parliament and those which are required to be so laid but are not subject to approval or annulment and **Special Procedure Orders** against which parties outside may lodge petitions.

Bye-laws

Local authorities (i.e. district and London Borough councils) have long had power, delegated by Parliament and subject to confirmation by Ministers, to make bye-laws, see for example bye-laws made for the good rule and government of local authority areas and bye-laws for the prevention and suppression of nuisances made under the Local Government Act 1972 section 235. *The Code of Practice on Noise from Model Aircraft* (1982) also refers to bye-law making powers of local authorities. Bye-laws must be consistent with the common law and statute and must not be made if provision for that purpose has already been made, or is or may be made by any other enactment.

European Community secondary legislation

The EU has policies on environmental conservation and protection, health, agriculture, fisheries and food, social policy including employment protection and health and safety at work, consumer protection, transport, energy and industry, amongst others. Many of these policies affect the work of the environmental health officer. The law-making powers of the Community institutions are to be found in Article 189 of the EEC Treaty. It is there provided that:

In order to carry out their task the Council and the Commission shall, in accordance with the provisions of this Treaty, make regulations, issue directives, take decisions, make recommendations or deliver opinions.

These measures, described as 'acts' are defined as follows:

- **A regulation** shall have general application. It shall be binding in its entirety and directly applicable in all member states.
- **A directive** shall be binding in its entirety, as to the result to be achieved, upon each member state to which it is addressed, but shall leave to the national authorities the choice of form and methods.
- **A decision** shall be binding in its entirety upon those to whom it is addressed.
- **Recommendations and opinions** shall have no binding force.

Regulations must be recognized as legal instruments and do not need national implementation – indeed it is impermissible to do so (*Commission* v. *Haly* Case 39/72 [1971] E.C.R. 1039). Most of the EU legislation affecting the work of the environmental health officer takes the form of directives. Examples of such directives are:

1. 89/391/EEC Council Directive on the introduction of measures to encourage improvements in the safety and health of workers at work, 12 June 1989.
2. 89/397/EEC Council Directive on the official control of foodstuffs, 14 June 1989.
3. 89/437/EEC Council Directive on hygiene and health problems affecting the production and the placing on the market of egg products, 20 June 1989.
3. 89/428/EEC Council Directive on procedures for harmonizing the programmes for the reduction and eventual elimination of pollution caused by waste from the titanium dioxide industry, 21 June 1989.

The Court of Justice has held that in certain circumstances, at least, directives and decisions might contain directly effective provisions (*Grad* v. *Finanzamt Traunstein* Case 9/70 [1970] E.C.R. 825). For this to occur two conditions must be fulfilled. First, there must be a clear and precise obligation and secondly it must not require the intervention of any act on the part of institutions of the Community or the Member States. Individuals may invoke before their national courts, as against the State, such provisions despite the fact that they are contained in directives or decisions rather than regulations. Governments of Member States to which directives have been addressed are obliged to implement them within the period of time specified. Failure to do so could lead to an action in the European Court of Justice by another Member State or, more likely, by the Commission. (See Articles 169 and 170 EEC Treaty.)

Actions are also possible in the domestic courts of the Member State. In two recent cases (joined), *Francovich* v. *Italian State* and *Bonifaci* v. *Italian State* [1992] I.R.L.R 84, it was held that where a Member State fails to enact the legislation required in order to achieve the objective prescribed by a directive it may be possible for an aggrieved individual to take remedial action directly against his Member State government. One possible route might lie in the context of the principles established by the European Court of Justice in Francovich.

Francovich implied that where damage is suffered through the acts or omissions of a private party which are incompatible with directly applicable provisions of a directive which has not been implemented by appropriate legislation, an action in damages will lie against the State. However, it would appear that three conditions must be fulfilled before such liability can be created. In the first place, the objective sought by the directive must include the creation of rights for individuals. The second is that the content of those rights must be ascertainable from the provisions of the directive itself. The third condition is the existence of a causal link between violation by the State of its duty to implement the directive and the loss sustained by the individual. Where these three conditions are met, Community law directly confers on individuals the right to obtain compensation as against the State. Recommendations and opinions have no binding force but may be indicative of important policy orientations and Member States may take such measures into account when enacting national legislation or when making administrative directions.

THE COURTS AND TRIBUNALS

European Court of Justice

The European Court of Justice is composed of 13 judges and 6 advocates-general appointed for renewable 6-year terms by the Governments of the Member States. The Court exists to safeguard the law in the interpretation and application of the Community Treaties, to decide on the legality of decisions made by the Council of Ministers or the Commission, and to determine violations of the Treaties. Cases may be brought before it by Member States, the Community institutions, firms or individuals. Its decisions are directly binding in all Member States. A Court of First Instance consisting of 12 judges appointed by common accord by the Governments of the Member States hears staff cases, cases involving EC competition law and certain applications under the European Coal and Steel Community Treaty. There is a right of appeal from this court, on matters of law, to the European Court of Justice.

The jurisdictions of the UK

There is one legislature for the UK but three separate legal jurisdictions: England and Wales, Scotland and Northern Ireland. These jurisdictions have separate law, judicial procedure and court structure, although there is a common distinction between civil and criminal law.

The judicature of England and Wales

The supreme judicial authority for England and Wales is the **House of Lords**. It is staffed by the Lord Chancellor and 10 Lords of Appeal in Ordinary (Law Lords) who are members of the Upper House of the legislature. Cases are normally heard by a panel of five Law Lords. Each Law Lord expresses his own opinion in the form of a speech. In recent years a number of environmental health cases have been heard in this court. (See for example *Alphacell* v. *Woodward* [1972] A.C. 824, *Salford City Council* v. *McNally* [1976] A.C. 379, and *Austin Rover Group Limited* v. *Her Majesty's Inspector of Factories* [1990] A.C. 619.) **The Supreme Court of Judicature** comprises the **Court of Appeal**, the **High Court of Justice** and the **Crown Court**. The Court of Appeal has two divisions: a Criminal Division and a Civil Division. The jurisdiction of the Court of Appeal includes civil and criminal appeals from the three Divisions of the High Court, including divisional courts, from the county courts, from the Employment Appeal Tribunal, from the Lands Tribunal and the Transport Tribunal. For civil cases the Master of the Rolls is the most senior judge. The President of the Family Division and the Vice Chancellor sit occasionally. The Criminal Division is presided over by the Lord Chief Justice. There are 28 Lords Justices to carry out the work of the two Divisions. They are assisted on occasion by High Court judges. Three Appeal Court judges will normally hear a case and a majority is sufficient for a decision. The High Court of Justice is the superior civil court. Its work is carried on by 83 High Court judges in three divisions: Queens Bench Division, the Chancery Division and the Family Division. The Queens Bench Division deals with commercial and maritime law and with civil cases not assigned to other courts. Within the Queens Bench Division there is the Divisional Court which reviews decisions of governmental and other public bodies and hears appeals from lower courts (See for example *R*.v. *Health and Safety Commission exparte Spelthorne Borough Council* (1983) The Times 18 July 1983). The Chancery Division is concerned mainly with equity, bankruptcy and contentious probate business and the Family Division deals with matters relating to family law. Sittings are held at the Royal Courts of Justice in London or at 26 Crown Court centres throughout England and Wales. High Court judges sit alone to hear cases at first instance. Appeals from lower courts are heard by two or three judges, or by a single judge of the appropriate division. Under the provisions of Section 81 Environmental Protection Act 1990, for example, a local authority may take action in the High Court for the purpose of securing the abatement, prohibition or restriction of any statutory nuisance where they are of the opinion that proceedings for an offence of contravening an abatement notice would not provide a sufficient remedy. (See for example *Hammersmith London Borough Council* v. *Magnum Automated Forecourts Ltd.* [1978] 1 W.L.R. 50).

Most minor civil cases, including most cases under the Housing Acts, are dealt with by the 300 **county courts** throughout England and Wales. These courts are staffed by county court judges (who also sit as circuit judges in criminal cases) and district judges for smaller claims. Magistrates' courts can hear certain classes of civil cases, including family matters and debt collection, whilst committes of magistrates license public houses and restaurants, clubs and betting shops. The Crown Court, brought into being by the Courts Act 1971, has an exclusively criminal jurisdiction. It sits in some 90 centres, divided into six circuits, and is presided over by High Court judges, full-time circuit judges, and part-time recorders and assistant recorders, sitting with a jury of 12 lay persons in all trials which are contested. It deals with a wide range of serious criminal offences, including those relating to environmental pollution, health and safety at work and food hygiene, the sentencing of offenders committed for sentence by magistrates' courts and appeals from lower courts. Magistrates usually sit with a circuit judge or recorder to deal with appeals and committals for sentence.

Minor criminal offences (summary offences) are dealt with by some 30 000 justices sitting in 620 **magistrates' courts**, which usually consist of three lay magistrates, sitting without a jury. The magistrates are advised on law and procedure by a fully qualified clerk to the justices. In the busier courts, a full-time, salaried and legally qualified stipendiary magistrate presides alone. There are at present around 80 stipendiary magistrates in England and Wales.

The Scottish judicature

Scotland has a legal system which differs substantially from that of England and Wales. Scotland is divided into six **Sheriffdoms**, each with a full-time Sheriff Principal. The Sheriffdoms are further divided into sheriff court districts, each of which has a legally qualified, resident sheriff or sheriffs, who are the judges of the court. The **sheriff court** has a wide civil jurisdiction. Appeals against decisions of the sheriff may be made to the Sheriff Principal and thence to the **Court of Session** or directly to the Court of Session which sits only in Edinburgh and from there to the House of Lords in London. There will normally be at least two Scottish judges hearing appeals from the Scottish courts in the House of Lords. In criminal cases sheriff's principal and sheriffs have similar powers; sitting with a jury of 15 members they may try more serious cases on indictment, or sitting alone, may try lesser cases under summary procedure. Judges in the Sheriff Court may not impose a sentence of more than 3 year's imprisonment. Cases will be committed to the **High Court of Justiciary** if the sheriff forms the view on reading the papers that on conviction a court may wish to impose a more severe sentence. The High Court of Justiciary consists of the same judges who sit in the Court of Session. It has jurisdiction over all of Scotland in respect of crimes committed unless a statute otherwise provides. It is both a trial and an appeal court. As a court of first instance it comprises a single judge sitting with a jury of 15. As a court of appeal it sits only in Edinburgh and then comprises at least three judges. In recent years a number of environmental health cases have been heard in this court. (See for example *Strathclyde Regional Council* v. *Tudhope* (1982) SCCR 286, *Docherty* v. *Stakis Hotels Ltd.* (1991) SCCR 7, *Kvaerner Govan Ltd.* v. *Her Majesty's Advocate* (1992) SCCR 10 and *Lockhart* v. *Kevin Oliphant Ltd.* (1993) SLT 179.) There is no appeal to the House of Lords in criminal cases. Minor summary offences are dealt with in **district courts** which are administered by the district and the islands local authorities and presided over by lay justices of the peace (of whom there are about 4400) and, in Glasgow only, by stipendiary magistrates. (See also Chapter 4.)

The Northern Ireland judicature

In Northern Ireland the legal system and the courts structure closely resemble those of England and Wales; there are however differences in enacted law. (See also Chapter 5.)

Industrial tribunals

Members of Industrial Tribunals in England and Wales, Scotland and Northern Ireland, amongst their other duties, hear appeals against the service of improvement and prohibition notices issued by inspectors acting under powers granted under the Health and Safety at Work etc. Act 1974. Industrial Tribunal Chairmen are legally qualified and are appointed by the Lord Chancellor. Lay members serving on tribunals in Great Britain are appointed by the Secretary of State for Employment following their nomination by the CBI and TUC. Lay members serving on tribunals in Northern Ireland are appointed by the Department of Economic Development, Northern Ireland. Appeals may be made from a tribunal on a point of law only. The appeal is to the High Court (or the Court of Session in Scotland) and must be made within 42 days of the date of the entry of the decision in the Register.

THE LAW RELATING TO STATUTORY NUISANCES

Since 1838 when Edwin Chadwick, one of the founding leaders of the public health movement, sent Poor Law medical investigators into the London slums and issued in 1842 his *Report on an Enquiry into the Sanitary Condition of the Labouring Population of Great Britain* (see Chapter 1) which led to the nineteenth century Public Health Acts, the suppression and abatement of nuisances has been an important local authority responsibility. It is true that remedies to deal with nuisances were available at the time of

the Chadwick Report but resort to the law in the nineteenth century was the prerogative of the rich. In addition strong social pressures were at work in militating against such court actions and the procedures were both unwieldy and time consuming. Consequently local authorities had, and continue today to have, an important role to play in this area of environmental protection, first because of the clear public interest in maintaining public health standards and a pollution-free environment and secondly because for an individual bringing a nuisance action can be prohibitively expensive.

The law of nuisance can be divided into public and private nuisance. **Public nuisances** are crimes, although they can be tortious in some circumstances. An act or omission which materially affects the reasonable comfort and convenience of a class of Her Majesty's subjects is a public nuisance and a criminal act. It is possible to obtain an injunction to restrain a public nuisance through the Attorney General on a relator action. Under the Local Government Act 1972 section 222 local authorities are entitled to take **injunction proceedings** in the High Court in order to prevent harm to inhabitants of their area. Aside from these two avenues the right to take action is only available if special damage has been suffered.

Private nuisances are always tortious and the principal remedies are damages and an injunction. A private nuisance is 'the unlawful interference with a persons use and enjoyment of land, or of some right over or in connection with it'. It is thus a property right. The basis for a claim in private nuisance is founded on a balancing exercise centred around the question of reasonableness, and in assessing this balance the court will take into account the locality of the nuisance, the duration of the nuisance and any hypersensitivity on the part of the plaintiff.

The law of statutory nuisance was consolidated in the Public Health Act 1936 after previous Acts in 1848, 1855, 1860 and 1875. The law was updated in a piecemeal fashion and again consolidated in Part III of the Environmental Protection Act 1990.

The control of statutory nuisances

It is the duty of every local authority to inspect its area to detect statutory nuisances and investigate complaints. If, having done so, it is satisfied that a statutory nuisance exists and is likely to recur, it should serve an abatement notice. A statutory nuisance is a nuisance at common law. This is a private nuisance of public health significance, that is one created by unlawful interference with a person's use or enjoyment of land. This can take the form not only of physical damage to land but also by causing discomfort to the owner or the occupier. An element of repetition is required because a one-off incident will rarely constitute a nuisance. It is also necessary to put the alleged nuisance in the context of the locality, for something which may be nuisance in a residential area may not be in a purely industrial location.

Statutory nuisances with which the legislation is concerned are those created by any premises in a state deemed prejudicial to health generally or which, owing to the emission of smoke, fumes, gas or noise or (in the case of industrial, trade or business premises) dust, steam and smells, are prejudicial to health or a nuisance.

Section 79 of the Environmental Protection Act 1990 places a duty on every local authority to cause its area to be inspected from time to time to detect whether a nuisance is likely to occur or recur. Thus if an individual within an area makes a complaint the local authority is obliged to investigate it and if there is a failure to do so the remedy of judicial review will lie to an aggrieved applicant. Section 80 provides that where a local authority is satisfied that a nuisance exists, or is likely to occur or recur, they must serve an abatement notice on the person by whose act, default or sufferance the nuisance is attributable or if that person cannot be found or the nuisance has not yet occurred, on the owner or occupier of the premises from which the nuisance arises or continues. The following categories of statutory nuisance are listed in the Environmental Protection Act 1990 section 79:

(a)   Any premises in such a state as to be prejudicial to health or a nuisance;

Note 'premises' includes land and, subject to subsection (12) and section 81A(9), any vessel. A vessel powered by steam reciprocating machinery is not a vessel to which this Part of this Act applies.

(b)   Smoke emitted from premises so as to be prejudicial to health or a nuisance;
Note: This provision does not apply to smoke emitted from a chimney of a private dwelling within a smoke control area, dark smoke emitted from a chimney of a building or a chimney serving the furnace of a boiler or industrial plant attached to a building or for the time being fixed to or installed on any land, smoke emitted from a railway locomotive steam engine, or dark smoke emitted otherwise than as mentioned above from industrial or trade premises. This provision also does not apply to premises occupied on behalf of the Crown for naval, military or air force purposes or for the purposes of the department of the Secretary of State having responsibility for defence, or occupied by or for the purposes of a visiting force.

(c)   Fumes or gases emitted from premises, which are private dwellings, so as to be prejudicial to health or a nuisance.

(d)   Any dust, steam, smell or other effluvia arising on industrial, trade or business premises and being prejudicial to health or a nuisance.
Note: This provision does not apply to steam emitted from a railway locomotive engine.

(e)   Any accumulation or deposit which is prejudicial to health or a nuisance.

(f)   Any animal kept in such a place or manner as to be prejudicial to health or a nuisance.

(g)   Noise, including vibration, emitted from premises so as to be prejudicial to health or a nuisance; Note: This provision does not apply to noise caused by aircraft other than model aircraft and not to premises occupied on behalf of the Crown for naval, military or air force purposes or for the purposes of the department of the Secretary of State having responsibility for defence, or occupied by or for the purposes of a visiting force.

(ga) Noise, including vibration, that is prejudicial to health or a nuisance and is emitted from or caused by a vehicle, machinery or equipment in a street; Note: This provision does not apply to noise made by traffic, by any naval, military or air force of the Crown or by a visiting force, or by a political demonstration or a demonstration supporting or opposing a cause or campaign.

(h) Any other matter declared by any enactment to be a statutory nuisance;

Other matters declared by other enactments to be a statutory nuisance are:

Public Health Act 1936, Section 141

Any well, tank, cistern, or water-butt used for the supply of water for domestic purposes which is so placed, constructed or kept as to render the water therein liable to contamination prejudicial to health.

Public Health Act 1936, Section 259

1. Any pond, pool, ditch, gutter or watercourse which is so foul or in such a state as to be prejudicial to health or a nuisance.
2. Any part of a watercourse, not being a part ordinarily navigated by vessels employed in the carriage of goods by water, which is so choked or silted up as to obstruct or impede the proper flow of water and thereby to cause a nuisance, or give rise to conditions prejudicial to health.

Public Health Act 1936, Section 268

A tent, van, shed or similar structure used for human habitation:

(a) which is in such a state, or so overcrowded, as to be prejudicial to the health of the inmates; or
(b) the use of which, by reason of the absence of proper sanitary accommodation or otherwise, gives rise, whether on the site or on other land, to a nuisance or to conditions prejudicial to health.

Mines and Quarries Act 1954, Section 151

A shaft or outlet of certain abandoned and disused mines where:

1. (a) it is not provided with a properly maintained device designed and constructed as to prevent persons from accidentally falling down the shaft or accidentally entering the outlet, or
   (b) by reason of its accessibility from a highway, or a place of public resort, it constitutes a danger to members of the public.
2. A quarry which is not provided with an efficient and properly maintained barrier so designed and constructed as to prevent persons from accidentally falling into it and which by reason of its accessibility from a highway, or a place of public resort, constitutes a danger to members of the public.

Remedies for statutory nuisances

The procedures for the remedy of statutory nuisances are set out in Part III of the Environmental Protection Act 1990. An expedited procedure is set out in Section 76 Building Act 1984 where the need for a remedy is perceived to be urgent. (See below.)

It is the duty of every local authority to cause its area to be inspected from time to time to detect any statutory nuisances and, where a complaint of a statutory nuisance is made to it by a person living within its area, to take such steps as are reasonably practicable to investigate the complaint.

Abatement notice procedure

Section 80(1) Environmental Protection Act 1990 provides that where a local authority is satisfied that a statutory nuisance exists, or is likely to occur or recur, in the area of the authority, the local authority shall serve a notice (**'an abatement notice'**) imposing all or any of the following requirements:

1. Requiring the abatement of the nuisance or prohibiting or restricting its occurrence or recurrence.

2. Requiring the execution of such works, and the taking of such other steps, as may be necessary for any of those purposes.

The abatement notice must specify the time or times within which the requirements of the notice are to be complied with.

The abatement notice must be served on the person responsible for the nuisance except where:

1. the nuisance arises from any defect of a structural character, when it must be served on the owner of the premises, or
2. where the person responsible for the nuisance cannot be found or the nuisance has not yet occurred, when it must be served on the owner or occupier of the premises.

The person served with the notice may appeal against the notice to a magistrates' court within the period of 21 days beginning with the date on which he was served with the notice. If a person on whom an abatement notice is served, without reasonable excuse, contravenes or fails to comply with any requirement or prohibition imposed by the notice, he will be guilty of an offence. The notice may also require the execution of works, and the taking of any such steps, as may be necessary for the purpose of the notice or as may be specified in the notice. The notice must specify the time or times within which the requirements of the notice are to be complied with.

Appeal procedure

A person served with an abatement notice has 21 days from the service of the notice in which to appeal against the notice to a magistrates' court. The grounds of appeal are set out in regulations made under Schedule 3, Environmental Protection Act, the Statutory Nuisance (Appeals) Regulations 1990 (SI 1990 No. 2276) and the The Statutory Nuisance (Appeals) (Amendment) Regulations 1990 (SI 1990 No. 2483). These include:

(a) that the abatement notice is not justified in terms of Section 80;
(b) that there has been a substantive or procedural error in the service of the notice;

(c) that the authority has unreasonably refused to accept compliance with alternative requirements or that their requirements are unreasonable or unnecessary;
(d) that the period for compliance is unreasonable;
(e) that the best practicable means were used to counteract the effect of nuisance from trade or business premises.

The regulations further provide for the suspension of an abatement notice pending the court's decision, unless the local authority overrides the suspension in the abatement notice with a statement to the effect that the notice is to have effect regardless, and that:

(a) the nuisance is prejudicial to health;
(b) suspension would render the notice of no practical effect; or
(c) any expenditure incurred before an appeal would be disproportionate to the public benefit.

If a person on whom a notice is served without reasonable excuse contravenes any requirements of the notice he will be guilty of an offence under Part III Environmental Protection Act 1990.

Sentencing powers for contravention of an abatement notice

A person who commits an offence on industrial, trade or business premises is liable on summary conviction to a fine not exceeding £20 000. Other persons are liable to a fine not exceeding level 5 on the standard scale (currently £2000) together with a further fine of one-tenth of that level for each day on which the offence continues after conviction. Furthermore, if the person served fails to execute all or any of the works in accordance with the abatement notice the local authority may execute those works and may recover from the person in default their costs incurred in so doing except such of the costs as that person shows was unnecessary in the circumstances. In proceedings brought by the local authority to recover such costs, the person in default cannot raise any question which he could have raised on appeal against the notice.

Expedited action for defective premises (Building Act 1984, Section 76)

Where it appears to a local authority that any premises are in such a state as to be prejudicial to health or a nuisance, and that unreasonable delay in remedying the defective state would be occasioned by following the somewhat lengthy procedure set out in Part III Environmental Protection Act 1990 the local authority may serve on the person on whom it would have been appropriate to serve an abatement notice under the Environmental Protection Act 1990, a notice stating that the local authority intends to remedy the defective state and specifying the defects that they intend to remedy. The local authority may then, after the expiration of 9 days after service of such a notice, execute the necessary works to remedy the premises' defective state, and recover their reasonable expenses from the person on whom the notice was served.

However, if, within 7 days after the service of the notice the recipient of the notice serves a counter-notice that he intends to remedy the defects specified in the first-mentioned notice, the local authority must take no action unless the person who served the counter-notice fails within what seems to the local authority to be a reasonable period of time to begin to execute works to remedy the defects, or having begun to execute such works fails to make reasonable progress towards their completion. In proceedings to recover expenses for work carried out in default and initiated by the local authority the court must inquire whether the local authority were justified in concluding that the premises were in a defective state, or that unreasonable delay in remedying the defective state would have been occasioned by following the procedure prescribed and if the defendant proves that he served a counter-notice shall inquire whether the defendant failed to begin the works to remedy the defects within a reasonable time, or failed to make reasonable progress towards their completion, and if the court determines that the local authority was not

justified in using this provision the local authority shall not recover the expenses or any part of them.

A local authority must not serve a notice under this provision or proceed with the execution of works in accordance with a notice so served, if the execution of the works would, to their knowledge, be in contravention of a building preservation order under section 29 of the Town and Country Planning Act 1947.

Proceedings in the High Court

Where a local authority considers that proceedings for an offence under Section 80 would afford an inadequate remedy in the case of any statutory nuisance they may take proceedings in the High Court to secure the abatement, prohibition or restriction of the nuisance. (Usually by way of injunction.) See further *Hammersmith London Borough Council* v. *Magnum Automated Forecourts Ltd.* [1978] 1 W.L.R. 50. In such proceedings it will be a defence to prove that noise was authorized by a construction site consent under section 61 Control of Pollution Act 1974.

Individual action by persons aggrieved by statutory nuisances

Nowadays environmental health departments of local authorities are often understaffed and may be unable to deal fully with every statutory nuisance in their district. This provision enables any person, after giving 21 days notice to the defendant (3 days in case of noise) to make a complaint to a magistrates' court on the ground that he is aggrieved by the existence of a statutory nuisance. This is a more expeditious and economic form than an action for private nuisance in the county court. If the magistrates' court is satisfied that the alleged nuisance exists, or that although abated it is likely to recur on the same premises or, in the case of a noise nuisance is caused by noise emitted from or caused by an unattended vehicle or unattended machinery or equipment and is in the same street as before, the court must make an order for either or both of the following purposes:

(a) requiring the defendant to abate the nuisance, within a time specified in the order, and to execute works necessary for that purpose;
(b) prohibiting a recurrence of the nuisance, and requiring the defendant, within a time specified in order, to execute any works necessary to prevent the recurrence.

The court may also impose on the defendant a fine not exceeding level 5 on the standard scale (currently £2000) together with a further fine of an amount equal to one-tenth of that level for each day on which the offence continues after the conviction.

If the magistrates' court is satisfied that the alleged nuisance exists and is such as, in the opinion of the court, to render premises unfit for human habitation, an order may be made to prohibit the use of the premises for human habitation until the premises are, to the satisfaction of the court, rendered fit for that purpose. Before instituting proceedings for such an order against any person, the person aggrieved by the nuisance shall give to that person such notice in writing of his intention to bring such proceedings and the notice must specify the matter complained of.

If a person is convicted of an offence a magistrates' court may, after giving the local authority in whose area the nuisance has occurred an opportunity of being heard, direct the authority to do anything which the person convicted was required to do by the order to which the conviction relates. It is most important for individual complainants to note that if they wish to make complaint to the local authority or to a magistrates' court that sufficient and proper evidence is gathered (dates, times, severity and length of nuisance if it has occurred and the numbers of people affected), or strong evidence to show that the statutory nuisance is about to occur.

Power of entry

Any person authorized by a local authority may, on production, if so required, of his authority, enter any premises at any reasonable time for the purpose of ascertaining whether or not a statutory nuisance exists; or for the purpose of taking any action, or executing any work, authorized or required by Part III Environmental Protection Act 1990. It should be noted however that admission to any premises used wholly or mainly for residential purposes shall not except in an emergency be demanded as of right unless 24 hours' notice of the intended entry has been given to the occupier. If it is shown to the satisfaction of a justice of the peace on sworn information in writing that admission to any premises has been refused, or that refusal is apprehended, or that the premises are unoccupied or the occupier is temporarily absent, or that the case is one of emergency, or that an application for admission would defeat the object of the entry; and that there is reasonable ground for entry into the premises for the purpose for which entry is required, the justice may by warrant authorize the local authority, by any authorized person, to enter the premises, if need be by force. The warrant will continue in force until the purpose for which the entry is required has been satisfied. An authorized person entering any premises has wide powers. He may take with him such other persons and such equipment as may be necessary; carry out such inspections, measurements and tests as he considers necessary for the discharge of any of the local authority's functions under Part III; and take away such samples or articles as he considers necessary for that purpose. The authorized person must secure any unoccupied premises on leaving.

For the purpose of taking any action, or executing any work, authorized by or required under Part III in relation to a statutory nuisance within section 79(1)(ga) Environmental Protection Act 1990 caused by noise emitted from or caused by the vehicle, machinery or equipment any person authorized by a local authority may after notifying the police and on production (if so required) of his authority enter or open a vehicle, machinery or equipment, if necessary by force, or remove a vehicle, machinery or equipment from a street to a secure place.

If entry has been gained to any unattended vehicle, machinery or equipment the authorized person shall leave it secured against interference or theft in such manner and as effectually as he found it. If the unattended vehicle, machinery or equipment cannot be left secured the authorized person must immobilize it by such means as he considers expedient, or remove it from the street to a secure place taking care not to cause more damage than is necessary. The local authority must then notify the police of its removal and current location.

A local authority may recover its reasonable expenses in executing the powers set out above.

A person who wilfully obstructs any person acting in the exercise of any powers set out above will be liable, on summary conviction, to a fine not exceeding level 3 on the standard scale.

If a person discloses any information relating to any trade secret obtained in the exercise of any powers set out above he shall, unless the disclosure was made in the performance of his duty or with the consent of the person having the right to disclose the information, be liable, on summary conviction, to a fine not exceeding level 5 on the standard scale.

FURTHER READING

Bailey, S.H. and Gunn, M.J. (1991) *Smith and Bailey on the Modern English Legal System*, 2nd edn., Sweet and Maxwell, London.

Bassett, W.H. (1995) *Environmental Health Procedures*, 4th edn., Chapman and Hall, London.

Haigh, N. (1989) *EEC Environmental Policy and Britain*, 2nd rev. edn. Longman, Harlow, Essex.

Lasok, D. and Bridge, J.W. (1994) *Law & Institutions of the European Communities*, 6th edn. Butterworths, London.

Neal, A.C. and Wright, F.B. (1992) *The European Communities' Health and Safety Legislation*, Chapman and Hall, London.

Rogers, W.H.V. (1989) *Winfield and Jolowicz on Tort*, 13th edn., Sweet and Maxwell, London.

Spencer, J.R. (1989) *Jackson's Machinery of Justice*, Cambridge University Press, Cambridge.

Tolley's Environmental Handbook: A Management Guide (1994) Tolley Publishing Co., Croydon, Surrey.

8 Enforcement of environmental health law

Peter E. Beeching

BACKGROUND

The body of law relating to environmental health does not exist within one faculty but can be found in many different areas of activity which relate to the general concept of environmental health. Not all law relating to environmental health will be enforced by the environmental health officer; much of it falls to other enforcement agencies such as Her Majesty's Inspectorate of Pollution, the National Rivers Authority, the Health and Safety Executive, county councils and other departments of district councils.

This chapter deals with the practical aspects of the enforcement of environmental health law by local authorities, although the general principles and considerations do have a wider application.

Self enforcement

Since the 1970s there has been a trend in environmental health law towards the concept of self enforcement, most noticeably within the Health and Safety at Work, etc. Act 1974 and the Food Safety Act 1990. The concept of 'self enforcement' places responsibility for complying with legislation squarely upon the person running a business or undertaking an activity. There can be no reliance upon the enforcing authority to inspect and draw attention to failures to comply with the law. The Control of Pollution Act 1974 also pursued this idea but in a different format.

This included the introduction of codes of practice produced as statutory instruments to provide guidance on the standards to be achieved to limit noise in respect of certain activities, e.g. the flying of model aircraft, audible intruder alarms, construction sites and ice-cream van chimes.

Deregulation

During the early 1990s there has been an increasing concern at the amount of legislation and regulation affecting business and environmental health legislation has been identified as being particularly burdensome. Concern was expressed about the extent of, and need for legislative requirements. The way in which the law was being enforced in respect to its application to situations, the consistency of enforcement, both between and within enforcing authorities and the spirit in which it was being applied were also questioned.

This concern led to the establishment of seven 'Deregulation Task Forces' within the Department of Trade and Industry with the following terms of reference:

To advise Ministers on priorities for the repeal or simplification of existing regulations and enforcement methods so as to minimise the costs to business; to advise Ministers on the best way of developing and maintaining consultation on the introduction and enforcement of new regulations including those arising from EU measures; bearing in mind the considerations of public health, safety and security which underlie the regulatory system [1].

In January 1994 the Task Forces put forward some 605 proposals for deregulation resulting in the Deregulation and Contracting Out Act 1994 which includes a power to 'abolish and reform outdated and burdensome regulations without sacrificing necessary protection'.

Further to this two 'scrutiny reviews' were set up in January 1994 to consider:

1. the organization of local authority enforcement functions;
2. fire legislation and fire safety enforcement;

The terms of reference of these reviews were: to investigate the organizational arrangements for the enforcement functions of local authorities and to report on the scope for minimizing business compliance costs and enforcement costs, as well as reducing inconsistences in enforcement by removing any duplication and improving co-ordination within and between enforcement functions. The study:*

1. reviewed experience of co-ordination of enforcement, particularly within existing unitary authorities and also within and between other authorities;
2. assessed the scope for wider co-ordination of regulatory functions by all authorities; and
3. made recommendations on the means available to central and local government to promote good practice.

There is therefore a move to reduce the 'burdens on business' to provide more guidance and quasi-control over the way in which legislation is enforced to ensure a more acceptable and consistent approach based on professional judgement and assessment of risk.

Attitude towards enforcement

In order to effectively undertake the enforcement of legislation the enforcing officer must be aware of the background to that legislation, the thinking behind it and what it is designed to achieve. Legislation should not be enforced because it exists but because it will achieve something either in terms of positive improvement or in terms of reduction of risk, e.g. of food poisoning or of accidents. When challenged an enforcing officer must always be able to defend actions/requirements on the basis of what they will achieve and not on the basis of the blind enforcement of the letter of the law.

Enforcement officers should have an awareness of the commercial effect of their requirements on the business or individual charged with meeting those requirements. Thus the seriousness of the effect of non-compliance must be balanced against the cost of compliance in monetary and other resource terms and in practical application. This approach is embodied in legislation dealing with pollution from industry in the concept of 'BATNEEC' – Best Available Technology Not Entailing Excessive Cost – but the principle applies to all dealings with businesses and individuals upon whom requirements are made.

Consistency

The need for consistency of approach both between officers within a local authority and between officers employed by different authorities across the country is also self evident. Such consistency however becomes more difficult to achieve as the emphasis of enforcement moves away from the application of the letter of the law to professional judgement and risk assessment. The use of national codes of guidance as issued in respect of the Food Safety Act 1990 [2] for example becomes more important, as does the adoption of the '**Home Authority**' principle whereby the local authority with the headquarters of a national or regional company in its area takes responsibility for agreeing standards which are to be applied nationally to that company. Before taking action against such a company an individual local authority liaises with the home auth-

---

* See 'Local Government Enforcement – Report of the Interdepartmental Review Team (1994), HMSO, London.

ority as to the problem experienced and the agreed national standard.

The emphasis of enforcement has thus moved during the last decade away from strict application of the letter of the legislation to enforcement based on professional judgement, risk assessment, working with business to achieve reasonable and cost-effective programmes of compliance and consistency of approach both locally and nationally. In enforcing environmental health legislation the environmental health officer must be aware of the context of the enforcement activity and those other matters indicated above.

INSPECTIONS

Any inspection must be undertaken with a clear view of the purpose of the inspection and the context in which the inspection is to be made. It is necessary to make adequate preparations before embarking upon an inspection, such as researching the records, contacting appropriate people, ensuring that adequate and proper protective clothing and equipment required is available, ensuring that the timing of the inspection is appropriate to the purpose and having a clear view of the available courses of action to deal with the conditions that may be discovered.

There needs to be some method of targeting inspection resources to best effect to ensure that the potentially greatest risks are addressed as a priority. This is achieved by the **programming** of inspections.

Inspection programming

Programming of inspections is carried out using existing information from whatever source is available. The main source of information will of course be from previous inspections undertaken on a particular premises. The information contained on various registers, both statutory and informal, will also give an overview of the numbers and types of property and businesses to

be assessed. Information gained from complainants and from officers' individual knowledge of the area will also be of use.

The Audit Commission for Local Authorities and the National Health Service in England and Wales have published papers on '*Environmental Health Survey of Food Premises*' and '*Safer Food: local authorities and the Food Safety Act 1990*', both of which give guidance on the effective use of resources [3,4]. There is similar guidance available to local authorities in respect of the enforcement of health and safety at work legislation through HELA (Health and Safety Executive Local Authority joint committee [5]).

Risk assessment*

The Food Safety Act 1990 Code of Practice No.9 [2], revised 1994, deals with food hygiene, inspections and sets out guidance on the 'Priority Planning and Programme of Inspections'. It states that each authority should draw up a programme for food hygiene inspections and ensure that inspections are undertaken within that programme. Those premises posing a greater risk should be inspected more frequently than those with a lesser risk.

The Code of Guidance contains a model risk assessment scheme for the priority classification of food premises. The scheme is based on 'pointing' set criteria to consider:

1. the potential hazard to human health from the business by assessing the method of processing of food, the number of consumers likely to be put at risk if there is a breakdown in food hygiene and safety procedures;
2. the level of current compliance (i.e. at the latest inspection) with the food hygiene legislation;
3. confidence in existing management control systems.

Assessment of these matters will, through a set pointing scheme laid out in the code of practice, indicate a degree of risk and thus a priority within

---

* In January 1995 LACOTS issued a draft guidance note on Risk Assessment. This contains advice on the application of risk assessment principles to food hygiene inspections.

the system and a required minimum frequency of inspection.

Although the Code of Practice relates specifically to food hygiene inspections and the risk assessment scheme is specific, the principles contained within the scheme can be applied to all premises and types of business to be inspected by environmental health officers and others.

The three main questions to be asked in assessing likely risk are:

1. What is the potential hazard from the business activity at the premises?
2. What is the level of compliance with current legislation?
3. What is the level of competence of the existing management control system?

As an example, if these questions are applied to houses in multiple occupation the areas which would be considered in assessing risk are:

1. In respect of the potential hazard: the size layout, height and type of letting of the house.
2. In respect of compliance with legislation: the existence of adequate means of escape in case of fire, the number of people living in the house, the provision of amenities and the extent of disrepair.
3. In respect of the existing management: the type of manager (e.g. managing company, absent landlord, resident landlord), the effectiveness of the current management of the property, history of harassment, illegal eviction, past level of complaint.

These factors and others which may be considered relevant can then be rated using an appropriate scheme and the risk assessment and priority for inspection established. This approach can be applied to all types of business and premises.

Recording of information

Having assessed the degree of risk and programmed inspections accordingly there is a need to consider the process and type of system to be used for recording information. There are a number of information technology systems which

have been developed specifically for recording and manipulating environmental health information. These systems have been developed in collaboration with environmental health officers and meet general needs. It is however likely that every environmental health organization will require some specific or different way of dealing with some information in order to meet a special need and most information technology companies will be able to provide bespoke additions to meet such requirements (see Chapter 15).

In assessing the way in which information is to be recorded and stored, whether by using paper or information technology, it is vital to consider what information is to be stored, what use is to be made of it, and how it is to be collected. Information should only be collected if there is a positive use for it. Information should not be collected simply because the system can handle it and it may come in useful some time but it is currently difficult to imagine how.

Information collected from inspections will be by questioning and observation by the inspector. The inspector must be able to record the information collected in a clear and accurate manner and in an easily retrievable form.

The use of inspection forms for all types of inspection is now almost universal. Such forms are helpful in ensuring that information is recorded in a standard way and can be easily retrieved for central record and statistical purposes. The inspector must however take care to ensure that the completion of the form does not govern the inspection. The inspection should be undertaken using the form as an *aide mémoire* with additional notes being made as necessary.

Whatever recording systems are used it is important to remember that they are a tool to be used by the inspector. In order for the maximum benefit to be derived from this tool accurate and full information must be provided but the requirements of the information system are not the purpose for the inspection. The use of information technology and audiorecording of inspection notes either during the inspection or immediately afterwards is becoming a more common practice. Such systems enable the production and storage of records and the production of documentation to implement required action following an inspection to be undertaken directly from the 'inspection' notes without an intermediate stage involving the inspector in non-productive administration.

Preparation for inspections

Before undertaking an inspection the inspector must be clear as to the **purpose** of the inspection.

Code of Practice No.9 Food Safety Act 1990 [2] states that:

> Food hygiene inspections have two main purposes. First, the authorized officer should seek to identify potential risk arising from the activities carried on such as processing, cooking, handling and storage of food. Second they should identify contraventions of the Food Safety Act 1990 and food hygiene and processing regulations and seek to have them corrected. Authorized officers should be prepared to offer advice where it is appropriate or requested to encourage the adoption of good food hygiene practice.

Every inspection has a purpose which can be set out in these terms; unless the inspector is clear as to the purpose of the inspection it is unlikely to achieve its full potential and ultimately the improvements which are potentially necessary may not be achieved in full.

Preparation for the inspection also includes ensuring that the necessary **protective clothing** is available, this clearly applies to food hygiene inspections, but also inspections of building sites, warehouses and other potentially dangerous areas require adequate protective clothing to be worn. Such clothing must be worn to protect the inspector and also to set an example to the workforce, particularly where there is a lack of understanding of the value of protective clothing and a consequential reluctance to wear it.

Equipment to be used during the inspection must be in good working order, properly calibrated where appropriate, clean and well presented.

The inspector must be aware of the **history of the premises/business** to be inspected and of any

particular issues relating to it by researching records and past inspection information.

Consideration must be given to the **timing of the inspection**. This will to some extent depend upon the purpose of the inspection; however, where it is not essential to undertake the inspection at a particular time or to witness a particular event or activity, regard should be had to the needs and wishes of the owner and occupiers of the premises or the owner and staff of the business.

Unless it would defeat the purpose of the inspection **prior notice** should be given and where possible a mutually agreed time set. Where a house is to be inspected it is important to make arrangements with both the owner and tenants and if a tenant is not present to ensure that they have no objection to the necessary inspection being undertaken. In such circumstances the tenant should be offered the opportunity to speak to the inspector individually and not in the presence of the owner if they so wish. A similar opportunity should be given to members of a workforce where appropriate, for example where inspections are made under the Health and Safety at Work Etc. Act 1974.

Undertaking an inspection

Having decided the purpose of the inspection and made the necessary arrangements the **technique of inspection** to be employed will depend on the circumstances and purpose of the inspection. Traditionally inspection techniques have concentrated on a visual and physical examination of premises and equipment – the 'walls floors and ceilings' approach. This approach provides only limited information.

Where handling practices are observed these are only an indication of what is happening at the time. This approach is thus clearly inadequate for most purposes and must be supplemented by information gathered in other ways.

In most cases an inspection of a premises of whatever type will be undertaken in the company of the owner or a manager who will be able to provide further information. Discussion with this person and the inspection of appropriate documents where available can help in identifying particular areas for attention.

Where a large premises is being inspected it may be appropriate to adopt the concept of '**unit inspection**' whereby the premises is divided into sub-areas or units and each unit is given its own priority within the risk assessment scheme and dealt with on its own merits. Such an approach is particularly useful in respect of premises such as department stores where there is a wide range of risk between the various activities being undertaken.

Having undertaken a **general inspection** in many cases it will be necessary to concentrate attention on the **critical control points**. These are the points which will show whether a **risk** exists and whether the action being taken to control a **hazard** is effective in keeping the risk within acceptable limits.

The difference between hazard and risk can be illustrated by the following example. Asbestos fibres are a hazard and hazard analysis shows that the ingestion of asbestos fibres causes lung damage. However following the identification of the hazard in the early 1980s a risk analysis was undertaken which showed that in respect of asbestos used in dwellings, as long as the asbestos used was undamaged then the risk to the occupants was so small as not to be measurable. Thus although the hazard remains the risk is infinitesimal and thus no action was required.

Hazard assessment at critical control points is an inspection technique which looks at hazards and risk throughout a process and identifies particular points of control required to deal with the risk. This approach must be underpinned by full inspection at appropriate intervals.

Having undertaken an inspection which, where appropriate, will have included discussions with the owner, manager, tenants of a house, union representatives, individual staff members and others able to provide information it is necessary to relate the *conclusions* to those affected.

Notification following inspection

In most cases the immediate conclusions of the inspection should be related to the responsible person upon the completion of the inspection and before leaving the premises. They should be advised of the general findings, of any particular areas requiring attention, the inspector's intended course of action in respect of those matters and when, if further action is to be taken, it can be expected. If there are areas which require further consideration by the inspector and upon which an immediate comment cannot be made the responsible person should be advised and told when advice will be given on those issues.

It is important to advise all those people involved in providing information of the outcome of the inspection where they have a direct interest. For example tenants of a house in multiple occupation should be advised of the service of notice on the owner and copies of the notices made available to them should they so wish. Union or other worker representatives should be made aware of action taken under the provisions of the Health and Safety at Work Etc. Act 1974.

Quality of inspections

The quality of inspections is important and management procedures must be in place to **monitor** the quality of inspections undertaken to ensure that as far as possible they are carried out to a uniform and adequate standard and that the interpretation and action taken by officers following an inspection is consistent within the authority and in line with national guidelines. Quality assurance systems to ensure that this occurs should be introduced, they should be clear and defined. Guidance on the requirements for such a system can be found in BS5750. Whether a system is to be approved under that British Standard or not, the requirements of the system are the same.

COMPLAINTS AGAINST A THIRD PARTY

All complaints must be taken seriously because however trivial they may seem initially the matter is important enough to the complainant for him to have made the complaint. It is essential that the complainant is kept fully informed of the progress and outcome of the investigation and, if no action is to be taken, advised that is the case and told of any alternative course of action which may be available.

The effective investigation of a complaint requires a process to be followed which ensures that all relevant facts are taken into account and explained, that the complainant is aware of what is happening and what is required of them, that any legislative procedures used are followed and that all information is accurately and fully recorded.

Receipt of complaints

The person receiving the complaint should ensure that they accurately record the nature of the complaint, the name, address and availability of the complainant including a telephone contact where possible, note any constraints as to contact, e.g. the complainant does not wish to be contacted at work or does not want anyone to call at their home. The use of a proforma for the recording of this initial information is helpful and most environmental health departments will have such proforma.

The recipient of the complaint must then decide on the most appropriate person to deal with the complaint. It may be that the complaint is not one to be dealt with by the environmental health department, in which case it should be referred to the appropriate one. In all cases the complainant should be advised of how the complaint will be dealt with, advised of the name, where possible, and contact number of the investigating officer and given a timescale within which to expect an initial response.

Response

The **response** to the complaint will vary having regard to the nature of the complaint and the constraints placed upon the investigating officer by the complaint. In many environmental health departments it is not considered a good use of valuable resources to fully investigate every complaint at the initial stage. This approach is particularly taken when complaints relate to domestic noise where experience has shown that an initial

letter to the person complained of advising that there has been a complaint and asking for co-operation in reducing the offending activity results in a majority of cases being resolved. This approach places the onus on the complainant to come back if the problem continues or recurs.

It is vital for the complainant to be aware of how the complaint is being pursued and the expectation of them. It is good practice to produce an advice leaflet for those types of cases where a policy decision has been made not to investigate upon initial complaint.

Where a complaint is to be investigated the investigating officer should contact the complainant within the timescale indicated to them in order to discuss the complaint, obtain more details and explore the implications of the appropriate investigation. In a limited number of cases such contact will not be possible due to constraints imposed by the complainant. Such cases should however be the exception.

This initial response should again identify what is expected of the complainant. Their wishes as to the nature and extent of the investigation should be taken into account as far as possible. A complainant's identity should not be revealed unless their express consent has been obtained.

The investigation

The **investigation** of the complaint will vary in detail depending upon the type and nature of the complaint. The following general principles will however apply to all investigations:

1. The investigation must be thorough, looking at all relevant facts.
2. The investigating officer must act with integrity and keep confidences; where information to be given cannot be kept in confidence the person giving that information must be advised.
3. All people involved in the investigation must be kept advised of progress, any decisions made, and of outcomes.
4. The investigation and the facts revealed must be recorded accurately and fully, either at the time or immediately after the investigating officer has received the information.

5. A sequential record of the investigation should be kept.
6. Where statutory action is a possible outcome of the investigation all actions which are part of the investigation should be undertaken having regard to statutory requirements and the rules of evidence.

Where the investigation is into a complaint of nuisance there are a number of specific areas which the investigating officer will need to address. In many cases where there is only one complainant, the investigation should consider why there is only one complainant. Is it because that person is the only one affected or is he being unreasonable, or are others affected but do not know how to complain, or are afraid of complaining?

Where possible, the alleged nuisance should be witnessed by the investigating officer. This will not always be possible in cases where the problem is transient and occurs at irregular intervals. If action is to be taken without the problem being witnessed, the investigating officer must be sure that the complainants are prepared to give evidence in court to support their allegations.

In deciding whether a nuisance exists, regard must be had to its severity, frequency, length of time over which it occurs, the number of people affected and the defences which are available within the legislation.

Action following investigation

Having completed the investigation the investigating officer must make a judgement as to the most appropriate course of action to deal with the problem complained of, having regard not only to the legal situation but to the direct effect of the action on the problem being experienced.

The action to be taken should be appropriate to the matter being investigated. The purpose of the action is also relevant; is there a need to punish someone for their actions or is there a need to remedy the problem or both and which is the priority.

It is not for the investigating officer to make moral judgements nor to determine the extent of punishment but to use professional judgement to ensure that the investigation is brought to the most appropriate and effective conclusion.

Conciliation services

The use of conciliation services may be effective in respect of domestic complaints. These are generally provided by voluntary organizations within local areas. They bring together people who have a disagreement with the aim of enabling those people to resolve their differences through discussion and agreement on a way forward and where appropriate agreeing compromises and changes to lifestyle. The conciliation approach can only be effective where there is a willingness on both sides to address the problem with a chance of resolving it between themselves. Such services have proved effective and a number of local authorities are actively supporting either the creation or extension of such services.

REMEDIES

Upon completion of an inspection, or upon completion of investigation of a complaint, a decision has to be made on the action appropriate to remedy the situation that exists. The range of action available varies from no action at one extreme to prosecution and/or closure of a business or dwelling at the other.

In deciding upon the action to be taken the following criteria should be applied:

1. seriousness of situation;
2. effect on others;
3. degree of risk to others and numbers of people likely to be affected;
4. previous record of person responsible;
5. knowledge and ability of person responsible;
6. effect of action on likelihood of recurrence;
7. range of options available;
8. guidance, i.e. codes of practice;
9. statutory duty of local authority;
10. appropriateness of available courses of action.

These criteria should be considered as a whole, although clearly the weighting given to each will vary dependent upon the individual circumstances. The courses of action open to achieve a remedy will vary with the legislation available to address the issue. Individual pieces of legislation and remedies available for individual breaches of legislative requirements are covered in the other chapters of this book dealing with specific areas of work. In general terms however the following courses of action are available to local authorities and their authorized officers to deal with situations which require remedy.

No action is a course which may be taken either where there is no proven problem or where the breach of legislation is so minor as to have no effect. No action may be taken but a note must be made on file to the effect that a breach has been noted, such information would then be available to be taken into account in future.

Informal action is probably the most common course of action taken by environmental health officers to remedy situations which come to notice. The majority of people and businesses wish to comply with the law and live in peace with their neighbours. They will therefore positively respond to informal requests to either do something or refrain from doing something to overcome the problem which exists.

Informal action is generally appropriate where there is no great risk to human health, where the person responsible has a good record of responding to previous requests or has had no previous contact with the department, and generally in situations where the inspector considers that the appropriate remedy will be achieved within a reasonable time without recourse to formal action.

Informal action can be either written or verbal, if verbal it must be recorded in writing for record purposes. Informal action must make it clear to the recipient what is required, by when, and what the consequences of non-response will be. The consequences of non-compliance will of course vary from no further action to formal action of some kind. It must be remembered that judgements to use informal action are subject to review by the local government ombudsman (see Chapter 3).

Formal action to afford a remedy can take a number of forms depending upon the nature of the provisions of the legislation which apply. The

forms of action available are service of notices, closure of businesses or premises, prosecutions, formal warnings, all of which can either be taken immediately or following non-compliance with some previous form of requirement.

Notices

Various legislation enforced by environmental health officers includes provision for the service of notice either requiring action to do something, to stop something or to undertake works. Examples are a notice under the Housing (Management of Houses in Multiple Occupation) Regulations 1990 to clean the common parts of a house in multiple occupation; a notice under the provisions of the Environmental Protection Act 1990 requiring the abatement of a noise nuisance by ceasing the noisy activity between certain times; and a notice under the provisions of section 352 of the Housing Act 1985 requiring the provision of adequate means of escape in case of fire from a house in multiple occupation.

All notices have to be prepared carefully in order to ensure that they are accurate, are making requirements which are within the scope of the statutory provisions being used, and are served on the correct person or persons.

There are appeal provisions in relation to all notices and grounds of appeal are set out in the legislation. If a notice is inaccurate or wrongly served, a subsequent successful appeal will not only prove to be embarrassing, but may also be costly to the local authority in terms of court costs and lead to difficulty in dealing with the problem addressed by the notice in subsequent future action.

The notice must be accurate and based on information obtained by a full and properly recorded inspection (where appropriate) and other research. All inspection and other notes used in the preparation of the notice should be retained for use if necessary in any subsequent court hearing. Normally only notes made at the time of an inspection or immediately after are admissible as evidence, and it is thus important that the original notes are in a form that can be used for this purpose.

The notice must be **in the correct form**. In the case of notices served under the provisions of the Housing Acts, there are prescribed forms regulations which set out the detailed form which the notice must take. Where no 'prescribed forms' exist, the notice should be written and in such a form as to clearly state the powers under which the notice is served, the requirements of the notice and any appeal which there may be against it.

In all cases, however, a notice must be **addressed fully and accurately** to the person upon whom it is to be served and served correctly. Where notice is served on more than one person, it must be served on each separately. The details of how a notice should be **served** and upon whom varies in detail from Act to Act but in general the requirements are that service is achieved by giving the notice to the person to whom it is addressed or sending it to him at his last known address or in the case of a registered company to the registered office. Service by post should be by recorded delivery. If the owner of a property is not known a notice may be served by addressing it to 'the owner' and leaving it at the property to which it relates.

The local authority can require any person with an interest in the premises to provide information as to all persons having an interest by service of a requisition for information under the provisions of the Local Government (Miscellaneous Provisions) Act 1976 section 16.

A notice must **specify what is required in clear terms.** In some cases, it is necessary to specify the work to be undertaken to meet the requirements of the notice and in such cases actual works must be specified. In the case of a notice served under the provisions of section 352 of the Housing Act 1985 for the provision of adequate means of escape in the case of fire, it is not sufficient to specify 'carry out such works as are necessary to provide an adequate means of escape in case of fire'. The detailed works required to each door, floor and staircase along with other works must be specified.

A period of time must be given for the works to be carried out, or the nuisance remedied, or the action undertaken. In the case of notices served under the provisions of the Housing Act 1985 requiring works to be carried out, the notice must specify a date by which works must commence and a period of time in which they must be completed. The time given for compliance with the notice must be reasonable. This will vary according to the type and extent of the action required to comply with the notice.

The notice must be **authenticated** by the signature of the proper officer (a facsimile signature can be used). A proper officer of the local authority is an officer who has been appointed to undertake the functions of the local authority in a specific area of responsibility. The officer will also require specific delegated authority to serve notices under each section of legislation used if the decision to serve the notice is to be made by that officer.

Appeals

In almost all cases, there is a **right of appeal** against a notice. The grounds of appeal are specified in the relevant legislation: they vary in detail but in general terms relate to the following:

1. the notice is not justified;
2. there is a material informality, defect or error in, or in connection with, the notice.
3. the local authority has refused unreasonably to approve alternative works;
4. the works required are unreasonable in character or extent or are unnecessary;
5. the time allowed for compliance is not reasonable;
6. the notice should have been served on someone else instead of, or in addition to, the recipient.

The period allowed for appeal is normally 21 days, and if an appeal is lodged the notice is normally held in abeyance until such time as the appeal has been determined.

Enforcement of notices

The formal procedure for the enforcement of notices will vary from notice to notice, but there are two general methods of enforcement:

1. prosecution; and

2. the undertaking of works in default

but these are not mutually exclusive.

It is an offence not to comply with the terms of a notice, served under the provision of the legislation enforced by environmental health officers. Prosecution is normally taken in the magistrates' court where penalties involving fines and/or imprisonment may be imposed.

There are **statutory defences** for noncompliance in a number of circumstances. For example, where a notice is served under the Environmental Protection Act 1990 requiring the abatement of a noise nuisance in respect of a construction site, it is a defence to show that the alleged contravention amounted to the carrying out of the works in accordance with a consent under section 61 of the Control of Pollution Act 1974 (which is a consent to undertake works within set conditions laid down by the local authority prior to the commencement of work). Also, under the provisions of the Environmental Protection Act 1990 relating to the disposal of special waste, it is a defence to show that all reasonable precautions were taken and that due diligence was exercised.

In addition to, or instead of, undertaking prosecution for non-compliance, the local authority may in many cases where works have been required undertake those **works in default** of the responsible person and recover the costs of so doing. The works undertaken have to be those specified in the notice, and only those. Any other works found to be necessary either have to be undertaken with the prior agreement of the persons responsible, or have to be the subject of an additional notice served and enforced in the normal way.

The cost of the works has to be reasonable, and in subsequent action to recover costs the local authority may well be required to show that the costs incurred are reasonable. It is therefore necessary to have sufficient documentation to show this is the case, which may well, in all but the smallest of jobs, involve obtaining estimates from a number of contractors, or using a schedule of rates which has been the subject of competitive tender.

Expenses are recoverable from the person upon whom the notice was served, can be recovered in instalments, and are made as a charge on the property in cases where the works undertaken are on a specific property. There is an appeal against the service of a demand for the repayment of expenses incurred within 21 days of service, but no matter which could have been raised in appeal against the service of the notice can be raised at this stage.

The closure of a business or premises is available to a local authority in particular circumstances defined within specific legislation. There are specific powers contained within the Food Safety Act 1990 which permit an authorized officer where he believes that there is an imminent risk of injury to health in respect of a premises to serve an emergency prohibition notice. This ensures the immediate closure of the premises or the immediate prevention of the use of a piece of equipment or a particular process. An emergency prohibition order must be applied for within 3 days. The magistrates court (in England and Wales) has power to issue such an order and may also issue a prohibition order following a successful prosecution by a local authority for a breach of hygiene or processing regulations.

The Housing Act 1985 contains provisions enabling a local authority to require the closure or demolition of a dwelling which is unfit for human habitation and where the cost of remedying the defects is such that repair or improvement would not be the most appropriate course of action. This procedure is somewhat different from the other examples cited in that it is not designed to be a punishment for some wrong doing by the owner but rather the result of an exercise to find the most appropriate course of action to deal with a particular circumstance but having no regard to the history of the case or why the circumstances exist.

There are powers within the Housing Act 1985 for a local authority to **take over the management** of a house in multiple occupation by means of a control order where the living conditions in the house are such that an order is necessary to protect the safety, health or welfare of the residents. (See Chapter 20.)

A further example is to be found in the Health and Safety at Work Etc., Act 1974 in respect of **prohibition notices** which are available to an authorized officer where he is of the view that there is an activity being undertaken, or about to be undertaken, which will involve the risk of serious personal injury.

Clearly the use of any of these powers has a major effect upon the person against whom the action is being taken and the inspector must therefore be very sure that such action is warranted and necessary. There are appeals against such action in all cases generally, with the availability of compensation should the appeal prove successful.

Prosecution for non-compliance with any legislation should not be pursued unless there is a clear reason and the prosecution will achieve either an improvement in the situation, provide a suitable punishment or act as a warning to others of the consequences of non-compliance with legislation in terms of action to be taken.

The Food Safety Act 1990 Code of Practice No. 2 [2] sets out factors which should be taken into account when considering whether to prosecute. The factors are:

1. the seriousness of the alleged offence;
2. the previous history of the party concerned;
3. the likelihood of the defendant being able to establish a due diligence defence;
4. the ability of any important witnesses and their willingness to co-operate;
5. the willingness of the party to prevent the recurrence of the problem;
6. the probable public benefit of a prosecution and the importance of the case e.g. whether it might establish legal precedent in other companies or other geographical areas;
7. whether other actions such as issuing a formal caution or an improvement notice or imposing a prohibition, would be more appropriate or effective;
8. any explanation offered by the affected company.

Although these criteria are written in respect of prosecution relating to matters covered by the Food Safety Act 1990 they can, with the exception of the matter relating to due diligence which is specific, be used in the consideration of any prosecution and form a useful checklist of matters to be considered prior to taking a decision as to whether or not to prosecute.

Prosecutions should be brought without unnecessary delay. It is in the interests of all parties to deal with them as quickly as possible.

All legal proceedings are subject to be requirements of the **Police and Criminal Evidence Act 1984** and the codes of practice made under that Act. The requirements should be taken into account throughout the whole process which brings a case to prosecution, as failure to comply with the requirements is likely to lead to a prosecution being lost on a procedural issue rather than being considered on its merits under environmental health legislation.

The use of **formal cautions** in accordance with Home Office circular 59/1990 is available to enforcing officers within a local authority. It is important that formal cautions are used in a uniform and consistent way and therefore the circular sets out the principles of the use of formal cautioning.

The purpose of a formal caution is:

1. to deal quickly and simply with the less serious offender;
2. to divert them from the criminal courts;
3. to reduce the chance of them reoffending.

The following conditions must be met before a caution can be administered: –

1. There must be evidence of the offender's guilt sufficient to give a realistic prospect of conviction.
2. The offender must admit the offence.
3. The offender must understand the significance of a caution and give informed consent to being cautioned.
4. The administration of a caution must be in the public interest; in order to decide whether this is the case the following factors should be taken into account:
   (a) the nature of the offence;
   (b) the likely penalty if the offender was convicted by a court;
   (c) the offender's age and state of health;

(d) previous history;

(e) attitude towards the offence.

In view of the seriousness and possible subsequent effects on the offender the use of formal cautions should not be entered into lightly and a set procedure should be established. Such a procedure could, following the decision that a formal caution would be appropriate, involve the following steps:

1. The offender is offered the formal caution procedure as a way of dealing with the offence in writing, he is advised of the consequences and his agreement to this course of action and formal admission of the offence is requested.

2. If the offender is in agreement with the procedure he is requested to provide a declaration to that effect, failure to provide the declaration (which can be provided by the local authority for the offender's signature) within a given time leaves the option of prosecution open.

3. The formal caution must be delivered in person by a senior officer, probably the chief officer in most cases.

4. A record of the formal caution is kept by the authority with a copy being given to the offender. The formal caution can then be taken into account in deciding action in the case of further offences and can be cited in court if prosecution is taken within 3 years of the caution.

Cautioning of suspected offenders

Although the provisions of the Police and Criminal Evidence Act 1984 relate only to police officers, codes of practice are issued to guide others with a duty to investigate and charge offenders. The appropriate Code of Practice is Code C (Code for the Detention, Treatment and Questioning of Persons) which sets out the following guidance.

A person who there are grounds to suspect of an offence must be cautioned before any questions about it (or further questions if it is his answers to previous questions that provide grounds for suspicion) are put to him for the purpose of obtaining evidence which may be given to a court in a prosecution. He need not therefore be cautioned if questions are put for other purposes, for example, to establish his identity, his ownership of, or responsibility for, any vehicle or the need to search him in the exercise of powers of stop search.

When a person who is not under arrest is initially cautioned before or during an interview he must at the same time be told that he is not under arrest, is not obliged to remain with the officer but if he does, may obtain legal advice if he wishes.

The caution shall be in the following terms:

'You do not have to say anything unless you wish to do so, but what you say may be given in evidence'. Minor deviations do not constitute a breach of this requirement provided that the sense of the caution is preserved.*

When there is a break in questioning under caution, the interviewing officer must ensure that the person being questioned is aware that he remains under caution.

A record shall be made when a caution is given. As soon as the interviewing officer believes that a prosecution should be brought and there is sufficient evidence for it to succeed he shall cease questioning.

An accurate record must be made of each interview with a person suspected of an offence. The record must state the place of the interview, the time it begins and ends and must be made during the course of the interview unless it is the investigating officer's view that this would not be practicable or would interfere with the conduct of the interview. The record must constitute either a verbatim record of what has been said or an account of the interview which adequately and accurately summarizes it.

If the interview record is not made during the course of the interview it must be made as soon as practicable after its completion and the reason for not completing it during the interview recorded.

---

* The wording of the caution is under review by the Home Office in the light of provisions of the Criminal Justice and Public Order Act 1994, which removes the right of silence.

Powers of entry

Power of right of entry into private property is an important statutory power conferred upon authorized officers for the purpose of enabling them to carry out their duties and responsibilities. The environmental health officer is vested with extensive powers of entry, which should always be used judiciously, tactfully, and strictly for the purpose for which it is given.

On appointment an environmental health officer should be issued with an instrument of authorization, normally signed by the chief executive, which will set out the legislation under which he is authorized to act. This authorization should be carried when it is intended to use formally the statutory powers of entry, at other times a suitable identity card should be carried as a minimum.

There are a number of general principles contained within the various legislation giving right of entry to authorized officers in respect of environmental health, although the detail varies from Act to Act:

1. The officer seeking entry must be duly authorized in writing by the local authority and must, if so requested, produce an authenticated document showing that authority.
2. Entry must be required for a specific purpose, e.g. ascertaining whether there is, or has been, any contravention of the legislation under which entry is made; whether circumstances exist which would require the local authority to take action or execute works, or to undertake such action or works that may be necessary. Action can only be taken in respect of the specific purpose for which entry was obtained.
3. Entry may be obtained at all reasonable hours; however entry may not be demanded as of a right unless 24 hours' notice of entry has been given in respect of any premises other than a factory, workshop or workplace. In respect of entry under the provisions of the Housing Acts, the notice of intention to enter is normally 7 days to both the occupier and the owner (if known), unless entry is required to a house in multiple occupation in which case 24 hours' notice is required.

4. If admission is refused, or it is expected that it will be refused, or the premises is unoccupied or the occupier is absent, or to give notice of intended entry would defeat the object of the entry, application can be made to a justice of the peace for a warrant authorizing entry onto the premises, if need be by force. Notice of intention to apply for a warrant must be given to the occupier unless either the premises is unoccupied, or to do so would defeat the object of entry.

An authorized officer entering any premises by virtue of these powers may take with him such other persons as may be necessary, and on leaving an unoccupied premises shall leave them as effectively secured against trespass as he found them.

A warrant shall remain in force until the purpose for which entry was required has been resolved. In the case of the Food Safety Act 1990, the warrant remains in force for 1 month.

Any person entering a premises who in so doing gains access to a trade secret shall not divulge that information, other than if required to do so as part of his official duties. **Obstruction** by any person to willfully prevent the execution of a warrant shall render them liable to a fine and a continuing daily fine for each day in which the obstruction to entry continues. If an occupier obstructs the owner of a premises from undertaking work which he is required to do by action taken, the owner may obtain a court order requiring the occupier to permit the execution of the work.

Delegation of powers

Many of the powers contained within environmental health legislation are powers of the local authority, although some legislation, e.g. Health and Safety at Work, Etc., Act 1974 gives powers direct to an authorized officer appointed by the local authority.

In order to use the law in a practical way to achieve its aims, it is obviously not possible for the local authority itself to serve notices, take enforcement action, or arrange for works in default to be undertaken in every individual case where such action is required. There is thus provision within the Local Government Act 1972 for a local authority to delegate any of its powers to an officer of the council, authorized for that specific purpose, or to any group of members of the council, i.e. a committee or sub-committee of the council.

For the purposes of the day-to-day running of environmental health, and for the purpose of providing a response to circumstances within a realistic timescale, the chief environmental health officer (or equivalent) is normally appointed the proper officer, and given delegated powers to undertake an extensive range of duties and actions on behalf of the local authority. The extent of delegation will vary from authority to authority, but in general terms should include those matters which require a professional as opposed to a political decision, e.g. the service of notices requiring compliance with the law. There needs to be a clear resolution in respect of each delegation, as it may be challenged and be required to be produced in court.

REFERENCES

1. *Deregulation Task Forces Proposals for Reform* (1994) HMSO, London.
2. Food Safety Act 1990, Codes of Practice – HMSO, London.
3. *Environmental Health Survey of Food Premises*, Audit Commission for Local Authorities in England and Wales (1990) HMSO, London.
4. *Safer Food: local authorities and the Food Safety Act 1990*, Audit Commission for Local Authorities in England and Wales (1990) HMSO, London.
5. *Priority Planning of Health and Safety Inspections in the Local Authority Sector* (1987) HELA, London.

FURTHER READING

Department of Trade and Industry (1994) *Deregulation, Cutting the Red Tape*, HMSO, London.

Fisk, D.J. Chief Scientist, Department of the Environment (1993) *Risk Assessment and Environmental Health Resource Management* Paper presented to Institution of Environmental Health Officers Congress, 1993.

Hutter, B.M. (1988) *The Reasonable Arm of the Law?; The Law Enforcement Procedures of Environmental Health Officers*, Clarendon Press, Oxford.

Blake, L., Malcolm, R. and, Pointing, J.W. (1993) *Prosecuting Food Safety Act Offences* Institution of Environmental Health Officers, London.

9 Pest control

Veronica Habgood

INTRODUCTION

The control of pests is a long-established public health function of local authorities. A pest may be defined as a creature which in a particular situation is seen as undesirable whether for health and hygiene purposes, or for aesthetic or economic reasons. Pest control is the term applied to activities designed to identify, reduce or eliminate pest populations in any given situation.

Control of pests through local authority intervention is primarily concerned with preventing a risk to public health in whatever situation they may be encountered. Diseases caused by bacteria, viruses, protozoa and fungi may be transmitted actively through a bite or a sting; or passively via contaminated food or from contaminated food preparation surfaces and equipment. Insects and rodents are the most common pests associated with risks to public health. Rats and mice have been shown to transmit salmonellosis and leptospirosis (Weil's disease) to humans; cockroaches and pharaoh's ants can transmit pathogenic bacteria; fleas and bedbugs may cause infection at the site of a bite, in addition to transmitting pathogenic organisms to a host's blood. Feral pigeons and seagulls may be carriers of *Salmonella* and their presence, particularly close to food premises, is undesirable.

Within local authorities, the function of pest control, because of the intrinsic link to health and hygiene, is most often the responsibility of the environmental health service. The execution of the pest control function however will vary considerably between local authorities. For many local authorities, the pest control function amounts solely to the provision of advice, together with the enforcement of the provisions of the Prevention of Damage by Pests Act 1949, Public Health Act 1936 and the Food Safety Act 1990, and an assortment of minor legislation. Many local authorities have now contracted out their pest control function, although the service is not yet the subject of compulsory competitive tendering. Others still provide a full advisory and treatment service. The policy with regard to charging for treatments varies between local authorities and with the type of pest infestation.

LEGAL PROVISIONS

A miscellany of legislation of direct and indirect relevance to pest control has been produced. Generally, from a public health stance, the legal provisions provide for:

1. the duties of local authorities;
2. the prevention of risk to health, and nuisance;
3. health and safety in the use and storage of pesticides;
4. applications of relevance to particular pests.

The following is a summary of the most relevant provisions in respect of pest control.

Prevention of Damage by Pests Act 1949

The Prevention of Damage by Pests Act 1949 is primarily concerned with the control of rats and mice, and the prevention of loss of food through infestation. Infestation is defined as the presence of rats, mice, insects or mites in such numbers or under such conditions, that there is a potential risk of substantial loss or damage to food.

A duty is placed on local authorities under section 2, Prevention of Damage by Pests Act 1949 to ensure that their district is kept free from rats and mice. To this end, local authorities are required to:

1. carry out inspections from time to time;
2. destroy rats and mice on any land which the local authority occupies, and keep that land free, so far as practicable, from rats and mice;
3. enforce the provisions of the Prevention of Damage by Pests Act 1949 in respect of the duties of the owners and occupiers of land.

A duty is also placed on the owner or occupier of land to notify the local authority in writing where substantial numbers of rats and mice are living on their land, excluding agricultural land. The expression 'substantial numbers' is not defined. The law essentially places the responsibility for maintaining land free from rats and mice on owners and occupiers.

Where local authorities are aware of circumstances where action should be taken to destroy rats or mice on land, or where there is a need to keep the land free from rats or mice, they may serve a notice on the owner or occupier of the land, requiring steps to be taken within a reasonable period of time to effect specified treatment, structural repair or other work. The local authority can carry out the work in default of the person(s) on whom the notice was served, and recover the costs.

Other provisions of the Prevention of Damage by Pests Act 1949 are concerned with infestations in connection with the business of manufacture, storage, transportation or sale of food. These provisions are administered by the Ministry of Agriculture, Fisheries and Food, who may delegate powers to the local authority. Further provision in respect of the infestation of food can be found in the Prevention of Damage by Pests (Infestation of Food) Regulations 1950.

Public Health Act 1936: sections 83–85

The provisions of sections 83–85, Public Health Act 1936, deal with action available to local authorities in the case of filthy and verminous premises, articles or individuals. The expression 'verminous' includes reference to the eggs, larvae and pupae of insects and parasites. In the case of premises which are considered to be verminous, or in such a filthy or unwholesome condition as to be prejudicial to health, the local authority has the power to serve a notice on the owner or occupier of the premises specifying works that are to be effected to remedy the condition of premises, or to remove and destroy the vermin. Works may be carried out in default of the owner or occupier, and the costs recovered from them. Similarly, in the case of filthy or verminous articles, the local authority must require that those articles be cleaned, purified, disinfected or destroyed, or, if appropriate, removed from the premises to prevent injury or danger of injury to the health of any person.

In the case of verminous persons and their clothing, either the local authority or the county council may remove that person with their consent, to a cleansing station. A Court Order may be obtained from a magistrate's court requiring the person's removal to a cleansing station, if that person refuses to consent to their removal. County councils or local authorities may provide cleansing stations for the purpose of exercising these functions, although many local authorities no longer have access within their area to such facilities.

Public Health Act 1961: section 37

Section 37, Public Health Act 1961 prohibits any person who trades or deals in household articles (a 'dealer') from preparing for sale, selling, offering or exposing for sale, or depositing with any person for sale or preparation for sale, any household article known to be verminous. Any household article being prepared for sale, offered or exposed for sale or deposited for sale in any premises, can be disinfected or destroyed on or off those premises under the authorization of the proper officer of the local authority.

Food Safety Act 1990

The provisions of the Food Safety Act 1990 are not directly concerned with pests and pest control. However, under section 8, Food Safety Act 1990, it is an offence to sell food that is unfit for human consumption or so contaminated that it would not be reasonable to expect it to be used for human consumption. Food contaminated as a result of a pest infestation may therefore be construed as being unfit for human consumption, although each case should be considered individually.

Under Regulation 6, Food Hygiene (General) Regulations 1970 it is an offence to carry on a food business on or at an insanitary premises or place, the condition, situation or construction of which is such that food is exposed to risk of contamination. Again, evidence of an infestation of rodents or insects is indicative that food may be exposed to the risk of contamination, and the proprietor of the food business may be liable to prosecution.

Regulation 25, Food Hygiene (General) Regulations 1970 (as amended) requires that the walls, floors, doors, windows, ceiling, woodwork and other parts of the structure of every food room be kept clean and in such good order, repair and condition as to prevent, so far as reasonably practicable, the entry of birds and any risk of infestation by rats, mice, insects or other pests. Remedial work can be effected through the service of an Improvement Notice issued under section 10, Food Safety Act 1990.

Other legal provisions

Powers are given to local authorities under section 74, Public Health Act 1936 to deal with nuisance or damage caused in built-up areas through the congregation of house doves, pigeons, sparrows or starlings. No bird which has an owner can be seized or destroyed. All reasonable precautions must be taken to ensure that birds are destroyed humanely, and nothing may

be done which is contrary to Part 1, Wildlife and Countryside Act 1981.

Provisions exist to deal with the presence of rodents, insects and vermin on ships and aircraft, where their presence may be a threat to public health. The Public Health (Aircraft) Regulations 1979 and the Public Health (Ships) Regulations 1979 are applicable in these circumstances. Powers are exercisable by the Director of Public Health, not the local authority environmental health function.

The Rag Flock and Other Filling Materials Regulations 1981 require that in addition to the standards of cleanliness specified in respect of each kind of filling material, all filling materials must be free from vermin. In this context, vermin includes the eggs, larvae and pupae of insects and parasites.

Where rats are threatened by or infected with plague, or are dying in unusual numbers, the Public Health (Infectious Diseases) Regulations 1988 require the local authority to report the situation to the Chief Medical Officer for England (or Wales) and to take all necessary measures for destroying rats in their area, and for preventing rats from gaining entry to buildings.

The Public Health (International Trains) Regulations 1994 will make provision for the 'deratting' of international trains leaving the UK in the unlikely event that rats from a plague control area are or are suspected of being on board.

A wide range of other legislation exists, dealing largely with the control of particular species. These requirements are concerned with ensuring the humane destruction of wild animals, health and safety for pest control operatives and the public, protection of the environment and limitations on the control of certain species.

PLANNED PEST CONTROL

Pest control can be expensive, whether it takes the form of the eradication of pests, the provision and maintenance of measures to prevent an infestation or the implementation of legal controls.

Where pests are to be controlled through the application of chemical, physical or biological measures, a planned, co-ordinated approach is essential to maintain health and safety, reduce poor results and prevent the ill-considered choice of pesticide and its associated undesirable effects. Planned pest control can be considered in five stages:

Recognition that an infestation exists, its extent, nature and identification of the species present.

Appreciation of all the factors which may influence the effectiveness of the treatment.

Prescription of the exact measures that need to be taken, whether proofing, hygiene control or the application of pesticides, together with the relevant health and safety measures.

Implementation of the prescribed measures by trained personnel.

Determination of the effectiveness of control, and follow-up where appropriate.

Health and safety considerations

All pesticides are inherently dangerous, not just to their target organism, but to man, domestic animals, non-target groups and the environment. Safe use in their storage, handling and application is therefore necessary.

The advertisement, sale, supply, storage and use of any pesticide is only permitted where approval has been given by the relevant Minister under the Control of Pesticides Regulations 1986. These Regulations were made under Part III, Food and Environment Protection Act 1985. Approvals are normally granted for individual products and specified uses. A pesticide may only be used where an approval has been granted, and the manner specified in the approval. Approvals are reviewed annually by the Advisory Committee on Pesticides, under the auspices of the Ministry of Agriculture, Fisheries and Food. The Food and Environment Protection Act 1985 also makes provision for information about pesticides to be available to the public and for the publication of Approved Codes of Practice for the purpose of providing sound practical guidance. The Approved Code of Practice has no legal status, but failure to have due regard to the advice is admissible in any proceedings against a person

under the Food and Environment Protection Act 1985. The Control of Pesticides Regulations 1986 additionally require that employers have a responsibility to ensure that employees are trained in the safe, efficient and humane use of pesticides.

Persons handling pesticides must also have due regard to the provisions of the Health and Safety at Work Etc. Act 1974, and in particular to the Control of Substances Hazardous to Health Regulations 1994.

Training for those handling pesticides should include not only the preparation of formulations for application, but also relevant health and safety legislation, first aid and emergency arrangements, handling of pesticide containers within and outside the store, records of stock, its movement and usage.

Guidance has been produced by the Health and Safety Commission on the correct use and storage of pesticides for non-agricultural use [1]. The document sets out the criteria for the proper storage of pesticides having regard to the quality and type of pesticides being stored. The criteria relate to the siting of the store; the adequacy of its capacity; the construction using fire and corrosion-resistant materials; the provision of suitable means of entrance and exit; the capability to contain spillage and leakages; freedom from damp and frost; lighting and ventilation; precautions against theft or vandalism; organization and provision of suitable facilities to accommodate the intended products. Where handling of pesticides takes place, provision should be made for personal protective equipment, personal washing facilities, protective clothing accommodation, storage of empty containers and waste and suitably designed and equipped preparation areas. Attention must be paid to stock rotation, maintenance and an awareness of potential hazards.

PEST CONTROL THROUGH DESIGN AND CONSTRUCTION

The eradication of infestation is an established function of local authorities. Of equal importance is the provision of advice in regard to the design and construction of buildings. This can be an effective proactive tool. Consideration must be given to the risk of infestation according to the use to which a building may be put, the effect of building location and the acceptability of infestation. Any form of infestation in health care premises would pose an unacceptable risk; food premises would be considered high risk, and domestic, detached or semi-detached buildings, low risk.

In general, buildings should be designed to prevent access and harbourage, and building materials should be such that they are unsuitable for nesting purposes. Intervention at the planning approval stage, or during the early design stage of renovation work, will enable good practice in design and construction to be adopted.

External walls should be designed and constructed to ensure there are no holes greater than 5 mm, and that access to any wall cavity which may offer harbourage is prevented. Airbricks should be protected by wire mesh or possess openings less than 5 mm. Smooth-faced finishes deter climbing. Internal walls, partitions and ceiling cavities should prevent access to other parts of the building, and be designed to prevent harbourage. Hollow spaces behind skirting boards, architraves, decorative moulding and panels are to be avoided. The use of silica aerogel within stud partitions will eliminate insect pests through desiccation. Insulation materials may be used for nesting by rodents; rigid foams have shown less susceptibility to damage than semi-flexible foams.

When closed, doors should not permit access or a gnawing edge. Doors closing onto a level threshold will ensure this. Self-closing doors are recommended, to reduce access by rodents when doors are accidentally left open.

Birds, particularly feral pigeons, can be discouraged from alighting and roosting by ensuring that the number of ledges is reduced to a minimum, and any remaining surfaces are inclined at least 45° from the horizontal. Access to roof spaces can be denied through careful attention to design and construction detail.

Ductwork, trunking and service pipes can offer easy access to all parts of a building, unless closely built in, or the openings sealed. Widespread infestation of many system-built buildings by cockroaches or pharaoh's ants may arise through the migration of insects via communal building components and fittings. Of particular concern are district heating systems, where an ideal warm environment conducive to the survival of insects is present. Cables, pipes, sanitaryware and ducting passing into or out of a building should also be tightly fitted to prevent access or egress of insects. A diverse range of pipe and wire rat guards are available to prevent ingress via soil and rainwater pipework.

In multi-occupied buildings, communal facilities such as refuse chutes and lifts can provide access to all levels of a building. Rodents may damage the service components through gnawing. In refuse collection bin rooms, food scraps may encourage infestation. A self-closing, tight-fitting metal door, or a timber door with metal kick plates will act as a deterrent.

Food premises

Design and construction considerations beyond those described may be applicable in food premises and other high risk buildings. The elimination of voids and the creation of space around fittings, and the coving or splaying of junctions at walls, floors and ceilings, will reduce the potential for harbourage and facilitate effective cleaning. Whilst fly screens at windows are effective in preventing the entry of flying insects, their design is not always conducive to effective cleaning and their use should be judiciously considered. Advice from LACOTS (see page 52) sanctions the use of fly screens where there is a positive risk of contamination of food, and it is reasonably necessary to protect food from that risk.

RODENTS

Rodents are mammals with a characteristic gap between their front and back teeth known as the diastema. The rodents most commonly encountered by environmental health departments are *Rattus norvegicus* (the brown, common or sewer rat) and *Mus domesticus* (the house mouse). *Rattus rattus* (the black, or ship rat) is less common in the UK and its presence may be confined to port areas. Grey squirrels (*Sciurus carolinensis*) may be of significance in certain areas of the UK.

Public health significance

Rats and mice will readily infest both domestic and commercial premises, particularly where there is stored food. Entry may be gained through poor design, construction and maintenance of the building fabric, or via containers of food, where few precautions are taken during transport and movement of goods. Stored food may be eaten or contaminated; packaging, the building fabric, fixtures and fittings may be damaged or soiled through gnawing and defaecation, causing economic loss and nuisance. An infestation may be indicative of poor standards of hygiene and housekeeping, particularly in food premises, coupled with a lack of awareness of suitable preventive measures.

Rodents may also be involved in the transmission of disease. Organisms giving rise to Weil's disease (leptospirosis), plague, trichinosis, salmonellosis, tapeworm and rabies may be carried by rats and mice. Once established, with shelter and a supply of food, both rats and mice will readily breed, giving rise to significant populations within a relatively short space of time.

Characteristics

The **brown rat** (*Rattus norvegicus*) (Fig. 9.1) is generally brownish-grey in colour, with a paler greyish belly. The tail is thick and shorter than the head and body and is nearly always pale below and dark above. An adult may weigh on average 340 g. The snout is blunt and the ears small and furry. Droppings may be grouped or scattered and are ellipsoidal or spindle shaped.

The brown rat is a burrowing animal, and will live indoors, outdoors or in sewers and enjoys both rural and urban environments. It may frequently be found at landfill sites and railway embankments and possesses climbing and swimming skills. The diet of a brown rat is that of an omnivore but with a preference for cereals and a need for water. It will rarely venture far from a nest site in search of food – up to 660 m in the case of adult males. Foraging for food takes place mainly at night. All brown rats exhibit a cautious reaction to new objects.

By contrast, the **black rat** (*Rattus rattus*) (Fig. 9.1) has a black or dark brown body with a pale, sometimes white belly. The tail is thin and longer than the head and body. An adult weighs up to 300 g. The snout is pointed, and the ears large, translucent and furless. Droppings are scattered and banana or sausage shaped.

The black rat is non-burrowing and is rarely found in sewers. It has superior climbing skills. The diet is omnivorous, with a preference for fruit and vegetables. In common with brown rats, a cautious reaction is extended to new objects.

The **house mouse** (*Mus domesticus*) (Fig. 9.1) is brownish-grey with a thin tail which is much longer than the head and body. Adults weigh up 25 g. The snout is pointed and the ears small, with fine hairs. Droppings are scattered and thin spindle shapes.

The house mouse rarely burrows but has good climbing skills. It may be found both indoors and outdoors and is ubiquitous. The diet is omnivorous, with a preference for cereals. Behaviour is erratic, and there is a transient reaction to new objects.

Identifying an infestation

Evidence of the presence of rats or mice can be established without necessarily sighting an animal. Typical signs, both inside and outside premises, include damage to building materials, packaging and food from gnawing. Tooth marks may be evident, and will help to indicate if the rodent is a rat or mouse; mice tend to nibble from the centre of a grain, rats often leave half grains or small pieces of debris. Holes, which may be the entrance to a nest, will typically be about 80 mm in diameter in the case of rats, and 20 mm in the case of mice. These holes may appear in the ground or in floors, walls and the base of doors. Footprints may be evident in dusty environments. Rats are creatures of habit and will regularly use

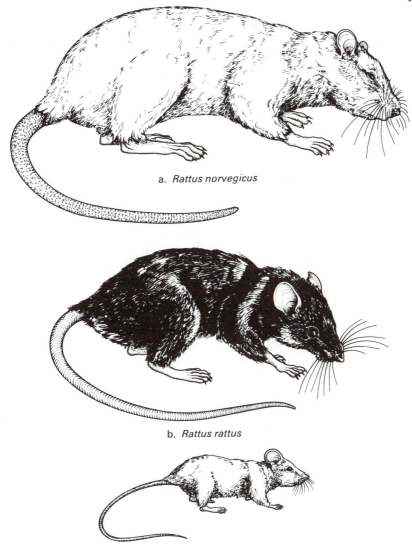

a. *Rattus norvegicus*

b. *Rattus rattus*

c. *Mus domesticus*

Fig. 9.1 The brown rat (*Rattus norvegicus*); the black rat (*Rattus rattus*), and the house mouse (*Mus domesticus*). (Source: Burgess, N.R.H. (1990), *Public Health Pests*, Chapman & Hall, London, p.139, fig. 16.1.)

the same run from one place to another. The run will exhibit characteristic 'smear' marks, as the grease and dirt from the rat's fur makes contact with surfaces. Outside, soil and vegetation will become flattened. Droppings will aid identification of the types of infestation, and whether or not the infestation is current. A soft, wet appearance is indicative of fresh droppings, becoming dry and hard after a few days. Old droppings have a dull appearance.

Control principles

Rodents require food, water and shelter to survive. Preventive measures to repel an infestation in the first instance can be achieved through attention to design, construction and maintenance of buildings, in addition to good housekeeping. The latter is especially important in food and other high risk premises. Effective cleaning of all parts of premises and equipment is essential, together with storage of food in rodent-proof containers, maintenance of refuse storage and collection points in a clean condition and regular inspection of premises for anything that may encourage rodents or offer harbourage.

Where an infestation has been established, the use of a rodenticide will be required until control of the infestation has been achieved. Remedial work in the form of repair and proofing, coupled with a revision of hygienic practices will help to prevent reinfestation.

Rodenticides are poisons used to kill rodents following a single or multi-dose of poisoned bait. The chemicals most commonly used are anticoagulants. Anti-coagulants interfere with the production of prothrombin, which clots blood quickly when blood vessels are damaged. The animals therefore die from internal or external haemorrhaging. Over time, sub-lethal ingestion of anti-coagulants has given rise to resistance to some of the more common formulations, in particular warfarin. Multi-dose anticoagulants include difenacoum, diphacinone, coumatetralyl, bromadiolone and warfarin; single-dose anticoagulants include brodifacoum and flocoumafen. Other rodenticides interfere with the rodent's metabolism: alpha-chloralose, effective against mice where temperatures do not exceed 16°C, reduces the body temperature, resulting in death from hypothermia; calciferol causes a fatal disruption of calcium metabolism; norbormide interferes with the blood supplying the vital organs.

Rodenticides will only be effective if ingested and therefore tend to be combined with a food that is appealing to the rodent. Foods commonly used are cereals and grains. Pellets, pastes and sachets containing poisoned bait may also be employed. Rodenticidal dusts spread along runs will be picked up on the feet and fur of passing animals, and ingested during preening. The behavioural characteristics of rodents must be taken into account when laying poisoned bait. Locations should be selected carefully, having regard to the evidence of infestation. Laying unpoisoned bait until the rodents are feeding readily will help to overcome a cautious reaction and 'bait shyness'. Once feeding is established, poisoned bait can be laid. Care should be taken to ensure that humans and other animals cannot gain access to the poisoned bait, and that foodstuffs will not be contaminated. Use may be made of bait trays or boxes. The bait should be checked every 2–3 days, and topped up according to manufacturer's instructions. Untouched bait should be removed. The infestation may take a few days to 3–4 weeks to be eradicated, particularly where multi-dose rodenticides are in use.

Where no further 'takes' have been recorded for a week, it is likely that the infestation has been eradicated, and all bait should be removed. It may be expedient to maintain permanent baiting sites on farmland, or where effective proofing measures are impracticable.

Other treatments that may be applied in particular circumstances include:

1. **Trapping** can be used to eliminate small infestations or as a temporary means of preventing re-infestation. Approved 'break-back' traps are recommended, which should be placed on runs or at the entrance to harbourage. Traps have limited application.
2. **Gassing** is used outdoors to kill rats in burrows. Extreme care must be exercised when using this technique. Tablets are placed in burrows and exit holes sealed. On contact with moisture, a gas is liberated which kills the rats in the sealed burrow. Hydrogen cyanide in the form of a calcium and magnesium cyanide mixture and phosphine are approved for use in the UK.

Control of rats in sewers

The practice of sewer baiting to control rat populations in the sewerage system has decreased in recent years. The responsibility for sewer baiting rests with the Sewerage Undertakers, created by the Water Act 1989. Sewerage Undertakers make their own arrangements for sewer baiting; work may be contracted out to local authorities or undertaken by the Sewerage Undertaker or their subsidiary company. Within the Thames Water area, all but nine local authorities carry out sewer baiting on behalf of Thames Water Utilities plc.

Test baiting may be used to assess the extent of populations and to target treatment. Access to the sewers is gained via manholes. Test bait or poisoned bait is deposited on the benching alongside the invert. Alternatively, where no benching is present, or the angle too steep, a bait tray can be fixed to the side of the manhole. A rope leading from the bait tray to the benching enables rats to reach the bait easily. Usually, one manhole in each direction from an affected area is baited. In many systems, however, infestations are such that all manhole points are baited.

Grey squirrels

Grey squirrels (*Sciurus carolinensis*) are common residents in urban areas and will give rise to complaints from time to time. The body is about 250 mm long with a 220 mm bushy tail. The winter coat is grey with a white underside; the summer coat shorter and brownish-grey above. Grey squirrels have no public health significance, but may be a nuisance due to the damage caused to trees, fruits and the fabric of a building. The animals are determined and ingenious, and any proofing measures must take this into account. Destruction of squirrels may only be a temporary measure, since the area is likely to be recolonized.

Approved cage and spring traps can be used throughout the year. Poison baiting can be employed both indoors and outdoors, subject to the statutory provisions of the Control of Pesticides Regulations 1986 and the Grey Squirrels Warfarin Order 1973. The traditional method of squirrel control is shooting and drey poking, which is usually carried out during the winter months.

COCKROACHES

There are a large number of species of cockroach throughout the world but only two are commonly found in the UK *Blatta orientalis* (the **oriental cockroach**) is found throughout the UK, usually in warm indoor environments such as restaurants, hospitals, prisons and other institutional premises. *Blattella germanica* (the **german cockroach**) favours similar environments, particularly kitchens, bakeries, district heating systems and other warm, moist areas. It is sometimes known as the 'steamfly'.

The lifecycle of the cockroach is one of incomplete metamorphosis. Females produce egg cases (oothecae) which contain eggs. The eggs hatch into nymphs, which resemble small versions of the adult. The lifecycle progresses through a number of nymphal stages, depending on the species, before becoming fully grown and sexually mature.

Public health significance

Both adults and nymphal stages will feed on a variety of organic foods, including food intended for human consumption, refuse and material in drains. Regurgitation of gastric fluids onto food and indiscriminate defaecation contaminate fresh foods and surfaces. Scavenging occurs over wide areas, and tends to take place at night. Cockroaches are unable to survive more than a few weeks without a supply of water or high water-content foods. Both the oriental and german cockroach are known to carry pathogenic organisms such as Salmonellae and Staphylococci, although evidence to suggest transmission of disease is scant. Their presence in premises will frequently give rise to feelings of revulsion, particularly where large numbers are exposed.

Characteristics

Blatta orientalis is dark brown to black in colour and 20–25 mm in length. Males and females differ in appearance, the females possessing small, vestigial wings (Fig. 9.2). Males pass through seven nymphal stages, the females, ten. Between five and ten dark brown oothecae are produced during adult life, each containing about 15 eggs. Adults can live for up to 300 days. The preferred temperature range is 20–29°C.

The climbing ability of oriental cockroaches is not particularly effective, and the species is most likely to be found on horizontal surfaces or rough vertical surfaces.

By contrast, *Blattella germanica* is mid-brown in colour with two distinctive dark longitudinal

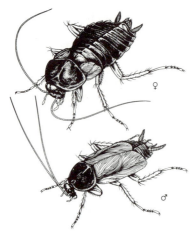

Fig 9.2 Oriental cockroach (*Blatta orientalis*). (Source: Burgess, N.R.H. (1990), *Public Health Pests*, Chapman & Hall, London, p.41, fig. 6.3.)

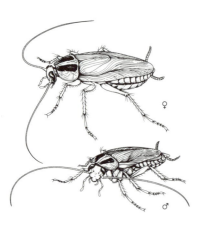

Fig. 9.3 German cockroach (*Blattella germanica*). (Source: Burgess, N.R.H. (1990), *Public Health Pests*, Chapman & Hall, London, p.36, fig. 6.2.)

bands in front of the wings (Fig. 9.3) and a length of up to 15 mm. Males pass through five nymphal stages; the females, seven. Between four and eight oothecae are produced during adult life, each containing about 35 eggs. The female carries the ootheca until just before the eggs hatch. Adult males can live for 120 days; the female life is much shorter. German cockroaches prefer temperatures within the range 15–35°C, and a relative humidity of around 80%.

German cockroaches move quickly and are adept climbers. During the daytime they will seek harbourage on both horizontal and vertical surfaces.

Identifying an infestation

Since both species of cockroach will not readily emerge during daytime, and night inspection may be impractical, careful observation is necessary to establish the extent of any infestation. Visual evidence will include the presence of egg cases and faecal spotting. A strong sour smell is frequently noticeable. Pyrethrum sprays can be used to 'flush out' cockroaches from less accessible areas such as behind equipment, pipework and voids and crevices within the structure. Cockroach traps with a sticky surface can be left out overnight to determine the extent of infestation, and, additionally, can be used to monitor the effectiveness of treatment.

Control principles

Preventive measures should be employed to reduce the likelihood of an infestation in the first instance. Consideration should be given to the design, construction and maintenance of the building fabric, paying particular attention to the avoidance of voids and crevices. The adoption of good hygienic practices in food premises will discourage infestation. Thorough cleaning and removal of food debris should be undertaken.

Where an infestation has arisen, successful control will only be achieved through a planned programme of treatment, coupled with the adoption of preventive measures. The favoured method of treatment is through use of a residual insecticide, applied as a spray. The active ingredient may be fenitrothion, carbamates such as bendiocarb and propoxur, and pyrethrins. Boric acid and hydramethylnon may be incorporated in scatter baits or pastes for use in less accessible areas.

Residual sprayed insecticides should be applied to wall and floor surfaces and around places likely to offer harbourage, using a suitable spray nozzle configuration. Cockroaches will be readily 'flushed' into other areas of a building or adjoining building. Treatment should therefore commence at the most distant point of the infestation, working towards the centre of the infestation. Dust injection of inaccessible voids may be used additionally. Follow-up treatment is necessary in the case of the oriental cockroach because the oothecae are resistant to the effects of insecticides. A residual effect should be maintained for up to 3 months after the initial treatment, to control emerging nymphs. Treatment for german cockroaches should consider harbourage areas at height, because of their superior climbing ability. Residual insecticides have the disadvantage of dead and dying insects in evidence. These should be removed and suitably disposed of on a daily basis.

In some situations, the use of insecticides is undesirable. Insect growth inhibitors have been recently introduced with some success, particularly in block treatments in system-built premises. Juvenile hormones applied to the nymphal stages in the cockroach's lifecycle inhibit metamorphosis into the sexually mature adult, thus preventing reproduction. The treatment may take a number of weeks to be effective.

FLEAS

Adult fleas are ectoparasites of warm-blooded animals. They tend to be host specific, but will readily feed on other species in the absence of their primary host. The number of local authority treatments for fleas has increased greatly in the past 10 years. Most treatments are carried out in respect of the **cat flea** (*Ctenocephalides felis*). The **human flea** (*Pulex irritans*) is present throughout the UK but with improved standards of personal and domestic hygiene is becoming an increasingly rare occurrence. The **rat flea** (*Xenopsylla cheopis*) will infest the black rat (*Rattus rattus*) acting as the vector for plague. Bird fleas (*Ceratophyllus* spp.) are generally host specific and feed rarely on human blood.

Public health significance

Fleas are known to act as vectors of human disease such as plague and typhus and may transmit the dog tapeworm (*Dipylidium caninum*). Human and cat fleas however, are more likely to give rise to an irritant reaction, where bites are scratched and become swollen and infected. The irritation is thought to be due a reaction to the anti-blood clotting agent contained in the insect's saliva.

Characteristics

All fleas are laterally compressed, which allows them to move easily through their host's hair. The hind legs are long and well developed for jumping and the eye is black and prominent. A row of stiff, backward-facing spines run along the back. Both human and cat fleas are about 2 mm long and dark brown or mahogany in colour. The cat flea can be distinguished from the human flea by the presence of a prothoracic comb (spines) (Fig. 9.4). The lifecycle is a complete metamorphosis.

The cat flea lays oval, white, translucent eggs, about 1 mm long on the hair of the host. These readily fall off onto bedding, carpets or upholstery. After 2–3 days, the eggs hatch, and white larvae, up to 5 mm long, emerge. The larvae feed off animal debris, and the excreta of adults. After three larval stages, lasting up to 4 weeks, the larvae spin a cocoon and pupate. The adult flea is ready to emerge within a week, but may not do so until the vibration of a passing blood meal is sensed. In this way, fleas can remain dormant in the cocoon for up to 12 months. This explains how heavy infestations of fleas arise in premises which have been vacant for a period of time. The fleas feed on blood from the host. Cat fleas will also feed from dogs, small rodents and humans.

In common with the cat flea, the human flea will lay pearly white, oval eggs, about 0.5 mm in length, in the clothing or bedding of its host. The larvae which emerge 2 or 3 days later are white and bristly, and feed on dust, fluff, shed skin, hair, dandruff and faecal pellets of adults. Pupa-

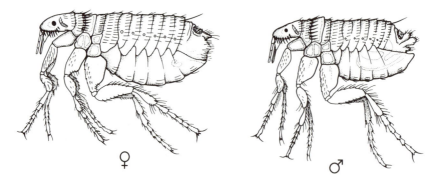

Fig. 9.4 Cat flea (*Ctenocephalides felis*). (Source: Burgess, N.R.H. (1990), *Public Health Pests*, Chapman & Hall, London, p.80, fig. 9.3.)

tion follows in the same manner as that of the cat flea. The adult flea will remain dormant in the cocoon until a suitable host passes nearby. Human fleas will live on blood from the host, but spend more time on the host's bedding or clothing than on the host itself.

Identifying an infestation

The fleas may be seen on the host animal or on bedding or clothing. More commonly, humans will be alerted to the presence of fleas as a result of being bitten. The bites of cat fleas tend to be confined to the lower legs and ankles, whereas bites of human fleas tend to be concentrated around the waist and abdomen.

Control principles

Both adults and larvae can be readily controlled provided that both the host and its environment are treated. This generally involves the concurrent use of a contact insecticide (e.g. pyrethrin) and an insect growth regulator (e.g. methoprene), together with efficient vacuuming of carpets and upholstery, and replacement or thorough washing of the host's bedding or clothing. Aerosols containing both a contact insecticide and an insect growth inhibitor are readily available for public use, although many people prefer the infestation to be dealt with by a trained pest control operator.

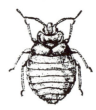

Fig. 9.5 Bedbug (*Cimex lectularius*).

BEDBUGS

Bedbugs (*Cimex lectularius*) are ectoparasites of humans, feeding largely during night time on human blood. During the hours of daylight, they inhabit cracks and crevices in furniture, pictures and wallpaper seams.

Characteristics

Adults are about 6 mm in length, with flattened bodies and red-brown coloration when unfed (Fig. 9.5). Their bodies show a rich mahogany colour as they become engorged with blood up to six times their original size following a blood meal. Adults can survive for 6 months between feeds. A characteristic almond smell and the presence of faecal spotting is evident during an infestation. Eggs are yellowish-white and laid in crevices. A minimum room temperature of 14°C is required before the eggs will hatch; the optimum being about 25°C. The nymphs pass through five developmental stages, each requiring one or more blood meals. The lifecycle is 6–7 weeks, but

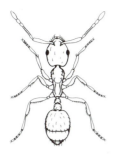

Fig. 9.6 Pharaoh's ant (*Monomorium pharaonis*). (Source: Burgess, N.R.H. (1990), *Public Health Pests*, Chapman & Hall, London, p.99, fig. 12.3.)

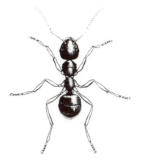

Fig. 9.7 Common black ant (*Lasius niger*). (Source: Burgess, N.R.H. (1990), *Public Health Pests*, Chapman & Hall, London, p.98, fig. 12.2.)

may be considerably longer under adverse conditions.

Identifying an infestation

Infestations are generally associated with areas of social deprivation and poor standards of personal hygiene. Bedbugs however can easily be introduced into any home where infested second-hand furniture and other effects are purchased. Much stigma is still attached to the presence of bedbugs in a home, although they have not been implicated in the transmission of disease. Bites will tend to be evident on parts of the body exposed at night, and produce swelling, unpleasant irritation and possible secondary infection.

Control principles

Treatment with a residual insecticide containing pyrethrins will control an infestation. The insecticide should be applied to all surfaces and furniture over which the bedbugs will crawl. Bedding and clothing can be washed and tumble dried, which will kill bedbugs and eggs; mattresses may be steam treated at a cleansing station or disposed of.

ANTS

Pharaoh's ants (*Monomorium pharaonis*) are a yellow-brown colour and approximately 2 mm in length (Fig. 9.6). They are associated with indoor

environments, particularly hospitals, prisons, housing estates with district heating systems and other warm institutional premises. Under optimum temperatures (30°C), the ants will breed prolifically and readily form new colonies when the original one is under threat. Workers will scavenge widely in search of food, and may be found in refuse rooms, the vicinity of drains, food rooms, sterile rooms and in hospital wards. Their mandibles are strong enough to chew through packaging and plastics.

Control principles

Control is difficult, and colonies may persist for years in some premises. Conventional treatment involves the use of residual insecticidal sprays containing bendiocarb and poisoned baits containing hydramethylnon. Use of such treatments may not affect the queen, who will continue to produce eggs. Juvenile hormone baits containing methoprene are very effective, since the growth regulating hormone will be introduced to the nest, sterilizing the queen and suppressing the development of larvae into adults. Treatment must be thorough, ensuring that all colonies are subject to control. Effective control may not be achieved for up to 20 weeks.

The **common black ant** (*Lasius niger*) may be dark brown or black in colour and 3–5 mm in length (Fig. 9.7). It generally lives outside, but may invade buildings in search of food. Although omnivorous, ants have a predilection for sweet

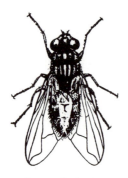

Fig. 9.8 Common house fly (*Musca domestica*).

foods. Nests may be found by observing the trail of ants. Common nesting sites are around foundations, under paving slabs, the edges of flower beds and lawns, often where there is sandy soil. To control ants, an insecticidal spray or dust containing bendiocarb will be effective. Proprietary insecticidal sprays available to the public will only provide temporary relief in heavier infestations.

FLIES

The habits and lifestyles of many flies lead to contamination of food and implicates them as carriers of enteric disease. Flies will indiscriminately feed on faeces, rotting food and refuse and fresh foods. Material from these sources will adhere to leg and body surfaces, and may be deposited during a subsequent feeding stop. During feeding, flies regurgitate the contents of their gut over the food, releasing organisms from an earlier meal. Defaecation occurs randomly both during a meal and at rest. A number of flies are of public health significance in the UK.

House flies

The **common house fly** (*Musca domestica*) has a well-differentiated head, thorax and abdomen and two broad wings. Adult flies are 6–9 mm in length with a 13–15 mm wingspan (Fig. 9.8). The abdomen is grey and black in the male, but more yellowish and black in the female. The female lays 120–150 eggs at a time on organic matter. These are white and about 1 mm long. Within 8–48 hours the eggs hatch into tiny larvae. These

maggots feed voraciously and pass through the three larval stages in a minimum of 4–5 days. The larvae then pupate, the pupa hardening and changing in colour from yellow through red, brown and finally, black. This stage takes 3–5 days under optimum conditions, but may take several weeks in cold or adverse conditions.

The adult fly will be attracted to breeding sites which will provide food and warmth for larvae. Decaying animal and vegetable matter, human and animal faeces and even fresh foods are favoured sites.

The **lesser house fly** (*Fannia canicularis*) is similar in appearance and lifestyle to the common house fly, breeding mainly in refuse and the soil of chicken runs, but not usually travelling between waste matter and human food.

Bluebottles or **blow flies** (*Calliphora* spp.) are widely distributed. Their lifecycle is similar to the common house fly, preferring decaying animal matter, kitchen refuse containing meat or fish, or fresh meat on which to deposit or 'blow' eggs. The adult fly is 10–15 mm long, with a 25 mm wingspan, and has a distinctive dark blue shiny body, large compound eyes and a loud buzzing flight.

Greenbottles (*Lucilia sericata*) have a similar life cycle and habits to bluebottles, but are smaller in size, being about 10 mm long, with coppery metallic green colouration.

Flesh flies (*Sarcophaga* spp.) are larger than bluebottles and have a grey chequered colouring. They feed on carrion and decaying animal matter, and may be found in the vicinity of dustbins during the summer months, but rarely venture indoors.

Fruit flies (*Drosophila* spp.) are small flies about 2 mm long, with a wingspan of 3–4 mm and a greyish-yellow body. They are associated with fermenting matter such as decaying fruit and vegetables, yeasts and vinegar. Large numbers in food premises are a nuisance and may give rise to contamination of food.

Cluster flies

Cluster flies can give rise to a nuisance where large numbers congregate around buildings prior to hibernation in the autumn, or on leaving their hibernation in the spring. They will use roof spaces or cavity walls for shelter. Common species include the cluster fly (*Pollenia rudis*), the autumn fly (*Musca autumnalis*), the green cluster fly (*Dasyphora cyanella*), the yellow swarming fly (*Thaumatomya notata*) and the window fly (*Anisopus fenestralis*).

Principles of control

Control is most easily effected through the removal of organic matter and the maintenance of refuse areas in a clean and tidy condition. Drains and gullies should be free from organic debris. Where appropriate, fly screens can be installed at opening windows. Self-closing doors or the use of heavy duty plastic door strips can prevent flies from entering food rooms. Electronic flying insect killers attract flying insects to an electrified grid with ultraviolet light. The dead insects are caught in a catch-tray, which must be emptied regularly. These devices should not be sited over open food or food equipment. Sticky fly papers have some application in storage and refuse areas, although they may be considered aesthetically unpleasant, and should be changed frequently.

Both 'knock-down' and residual chemical treatments containing pyrethroids can be applied, although some resistance has been noted. Fly baits based on sugar and incorporating a housefly pheromone and an active ingredient such as methomyl can be successful. To break the lifecycle, a larvicide, diflubenyuron, has been approved for use in fly control. The application of any insecticide in food premises should be used only as a back-up to physical controls. Where treatment is carried out, all food and equipment coming into contact with food should be removed or protected from the insecticide and dead insects.

INSECTS OF STORED PRODUCTS

This is a large group of insects comprising beetles, weevils and moths, which readily attack food during manufacture, processing, storage or trans-

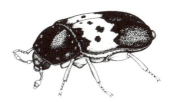

Fig. 9.9 Larder beetle (*Dermestes lardarius*). (Source: Burgess, N.R.H. (1990), *Public Health Pests*, Chapman & Hall, London, p.107, fig. 13.6.)

portation. All have a four-stage lifecycle, and most damage is done by the larvae who live in the food, contaminating it with waste products and secretions. Adults further contaminate food through excrement, empty pupae and dead bodies. These pests are not vectors of disease.

Beetles

The **larder** or **bacon beetle** (*Dermestes lardarius*) is a member of the hide beetle species. It can be a serious pest in food premises. The adult is about 12 mm in length with a dark body and a distinctive light band across the body (Fig. 9.9). Larvae are dark brown and covered with tufts of hair. The larvae will eat any material of animal origin, including meat, bone, hide, fur and wool. Their presence in food premises is indicative of poor hygiene.

The **flour beetle** (*Tribolium confusum*) and **rust-red flour beetle** (*Tribolium castaneum*) are commonly found in flour mills and animal feed mills, but will also feed on other stored foods such as nuts, dried fruit and spices. The larvae of these species are almost identical; adults differ in the shape of their antennae. Both beetles may reach 4 mm in length and under favourable conditions can live for 18 months. Adults produce bitter secretions which taint foods.

The **saw-toothed grain beetle** (*Oryzaephilus surinamensis*) is commonly found in bulk grain stores, but will also attack rice, dried fruits and nuts. The adult is about 3 mm in length and a dull brown colour with distinctive serrated ridges on the thorax (Fig. 9.10). Larvae are about 5 mm long and pale yellow. Established infestations can be widespread and difficult to control.

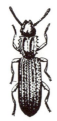

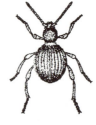

Fig. 9.10 Saw-toothed grain beetle (*Oryzaephilus suri-namensis*).

Fig. 9.12 Spider beetle (*Ptinus tectus*).

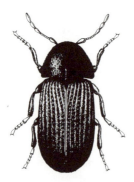

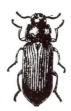

Fig. 9.13 Yellow mealworm beetle (*Tenebrio molitor*).

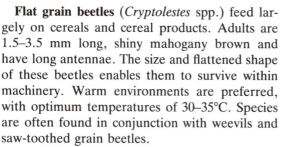

Fig. 9.11 Biscuit beetle (*Stegobium paniceum*). (Source: Burgess, N.R.H. (1990), *Public Health Pests*, Chapman & Hall, London, p.102, fig. 13.1.)

Flat grain beetles (*Cryptolestes* spp.) feed largely on cereals and cereal products. Adults are 1.5–3.5 mm long, shiny mahogany brown and have long antennae. The size and flattened shape of these beetles enables them to survive within machinery. Warm environments are preferred, with optimum temperatures of 30–35°C. Species are often found in conjunction with weevils and saw-toothed grain beetles.

The **biscuit beetle** (*Stegobium paniceum*) is a pest found in both commercial and domestic food stores. Adults are 2–3 mm in length and mid to dark brown in colour (Fig. 9.11). Infestation can be widespread because of the ability of adults to fly. The preferred food of larvae is cereal products and dried vegetable material such as that found in packeted soup. Larvae have the ability to chew through most packaging.

A related species is the **cigarette** or **tobacco beetle** (*Lasioderma serricorne*). This beetle will survive in a similar habitat to the biscuit beetle,

but is less common in the UK. In tropical regions, extensive damage may be caused to tobacco and cigars.

The **spider beetle** (*Ptinus tectus*) is common in the food industry, infesting grain, flour, spices, dog biscuits, nuts and dried fruits. In the domestic situation it is associated with old birds' nests and may cause damage to clothing and fabrics. The adult is 2–4 mm in length, mid brown in colour and the rounded body is covered in fine hairs (Fig. 9.12).

Yellow mealworm beetles (*Tenebrio molitor*) are usually associated with birds' nests and when found in food premises are indicative of neglected hygiene practices. Adults may reach 15 mm, and are a shiny dark brown (Fig. 9.13). The lifecycle may take a year to complete. Preference is for cereals or cereal products, but the beetles will scavenge on dead insects, birds or rodents. The **dark mealworm beetle** (*Tenebrio obscurus*) is a similar beetle, but less common in the UK. The **lesser mealworm beetle** (*Alphitobius diaperinus*) may be found on imported products such as oilseed, rice, bran and cereals. It requires warmth and is more frequently found in piggery and poultry units.

The **grain weevil** (*Sitophilus granarius*) can be recognized by the presence of a prominent snout

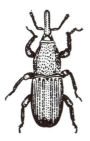

Fig. 9.14 Grain weevil (*Sitophilus granarius*).

at the front of the head (Fig. 9.14). Adults are 3–4 mm in length and dark brown to black. Eggs are laid inside grains of cereal and the larva remains in the grain, feeding and pupating, before the adult emerges through a small exit hole. This activity produces large quantities of dust and faecal material known as 'frass' and may cause significant economic loss. Infestation can go undetected for a period of time, and can be introduced into new areas where grain is moved. The **rice weevil** (*Sitophilus oryzae*) and the **maize weevil** (*Sitophilus zeamais*) are similar to each other, but can be distinguished from the grain weevil by being less shiny and having four distinct orange patches on the wing cases. They are imported in grain and cereals.

Moths

The larvae of a number of species of moth will readily feed on cereals, dried fruits, spices, chocolates and nuts. The **warehouse** or **cocoa moth** (*Ephestia elutella*) is the foremost moth pest of stored food in the UK. A wide range of foods are attacked, including cocoa beans and chocolate products. The larvae will contaminate food through faecal pellets and from trailing strands of silk produced as they move through the food. The silken threads are difficult to remove and in heavy infestations may hang in festoons from packaging. The larvae are creamy white with dark spots on each segment, and up to 12 mm long. The moths are 14–16 mm long with pale buff or grey wings (Fig. 9.15).

The **tropical warehouse moth** (*Ephestia cautella*), also known as the almond or dried currant moth, is frequently imported into the UK. The

mill moth or **mediterranean flour moth** (*Ephestia kuehniella*) prefers cereals and may be found in flour mills and bakeries. The larval silk may block chutes and choke sieves and milling machinery. The **indian meal moth** (*Plodia interpunctella*) is imported in foods such as peanuts, cocoa beans and dried fruit. The larvae may be yellowish and do not have dark spots on the segments. Adult moths have reddish-brown wing tips.

Mites

Mites that infest stored products are pale fawn to brown in colour and not usually visible as individuals without magnification. They enjoy humid conditions and feed on moulds which form on food products. The **flour mite** (*Tyroglyphus farinae*) and the **cheese mite** (*Tyrophagus casei*) are the most common species. Heavy infestations may give rise to an allergic dermatitis in persons handling infested products.

Controlling insects of stored products

To reduce the spread of an infestation where insects may be inadvertently introduced into premises, good housekeeping practices are essential:

1. inspection of incoming goods and separation of new stock from old;
2. effective stock rotation;
3. regular inspection of goods stored for extended periods;
4. frequent cleaning of storage areas and removal of any spillages;
5. maintenance of the building fabric and suitable ventilation, where appropriate.

Where an infestation has arisen, insecticides are usually employed. Badly damaged or heavily infested products may have to be destroyed. A sprayed residual insecticide or an insecticidal dust containing an appropriate active ingredient such as pirimiphos-methyl or fenitrothion can deal with an infestation. However, fumigation by trained operators using methyl bromide may be the only satisfactory treatment for some infestations.

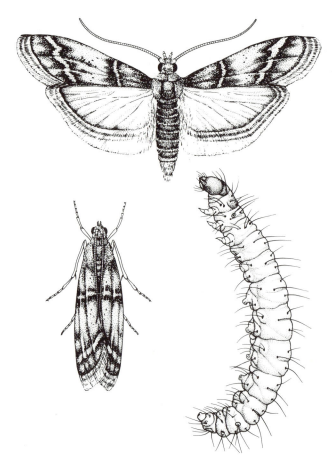

Fig. 9.15 Warehouse or cocoa moth (*Ephestia elutella*). (Source: Burgess, N.R.H. (1990), *Public Health Pests*, Chapman & Hall, London, p.118 fig. 14.4.)

WOOD-BORING INSECTS

The term 'woodworm' is used generally, to describe any beetle whose larval stage attacks timber. In all cases, eggs are laid in cracks and crevices of dead wood, fence posts, seasoned wood, door and window frames, structural timbers and furniture. The larvae hatch and burrow into the wood, tunnelling randomly, excreting a 'bore dust' or 'frass' characteristic of the species. In the final larval stage, a pupation chamber is constructed close to the surface, where the larva pupates. Adult beetles emerge some weeks later and leave the timber through an exit hole. The size and shape of the exit holes and the presence of 'bore dust' close to the infested timber, will help to determine the species of beetle. The lifecycle can take between 2 and 10 years, depending on the species.

The **common furniture beetle** (*Anobium punctatum*) is 3–5 mm in length with a dull medium brown coloration and a 'humped' thorax (Fig. 9.16). It leaves exit holes of about 2 mm diameter. This beetle is widespread in the UK and may cause extensive damage, seriously threaten-

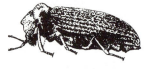

Fig. 9.16 Common furniture beetle (*Anobium punctatum*).

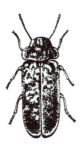

Fig. 9.17 Death watch beetle (*Xestobium rufovillosum*).

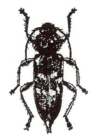

Fig. 9.19 House longhorn beetle (*Hylotrupes bajalus*).

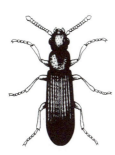

Fig. 9.18 Powder post beetle (*Lyctus brunneus*). (Source: Burgess, N.R.H. (1990), *Public Health Pests*, Chapman & Hall, London, p.112, fig. 13.11.)

ing the structural integrity of floors and roof timbers and ruining the appearance of furniture.

The **death watch beetle** (*Xestobium rufovillosum*) is 5–9 mm long and has a dark brown mottled appearance (Fig. 9.17). The lifecycle may take up to 10 years to complete and the emerging adult leaves exit holes about 4 mm diameter. This beetle is found in the Southern two-thirds of Britain and favours hardwoods such as oak and willow. Serious structural weakening can occur over a period of time.

The **powder post beetle** (*Lyctus brunneus*) (Fig. 9.18) is about 6 mm long and leaves exit holes about 1 mm diameter. It commonly feeds on the sapwood of felled hardwoods and produces large quantities of powder from the timber. The **house longhorn beetle** (*Hylotrupes bajalus*) (Fig. 9.19) is about 16 mm long and leaves oval-shaped exit holes about 3 mm by 6 mm. It will infest seasoned softwoods and can cause extensive

structural damage during its four to five year life cycle.

Two **wood-boring weevils** (*Pentarthrum huttoni* and *Euphyrum confine*) will also attack timber, particularly that which has been damaged through fungal action. Adult weevils are 2.5–4.5 mm long and dark brown in appearance with a typical weevil 'snout'. Exit holes are similar in size and shape to those of *Anobium punctatum*. The lifecycle can take 8 months to complete. The adult weevils are commonly found in basements, cellars and other sub-ground floor areas of buildings.

Control principles

Infestation can be prevented through the use of timbers which have been impregnated under pressure with a residual insecticide. Surface treatments will discourage females from laying eggs but will have no effect on larvae in the timber. Frequent examination of older, stored furniture will enable early recognition of an infestation and permit remedial and preventive action to be taken.

In all cases of infestation by wood-boring insects, treatment should be carried out by specialist personnel. Unsound structural timbers may need to be removed and destroyed, and replaced with sound, seasoned timbers treated with a residual insecticide. Treatment of timber or furniture *in situ* generally involves the application of a residual insecticide by brushing, spraying or injection. Lindane has routinely been used in the past, but there has been a move towards photostable pyrethroids such as permethrin and cypermethrin. Small infested items can be fumigated using methyl bromide.

OTHER PESTS OF PUBLIC HEALTH SIGNIFICANCE

Feral Birds

The presence of large numbers of **pigeons** (*Columba livia var*) or **starlings** (*Sturnus vulgaris*) in urban areas frequently gives rise to complaints of nuisance. Fouling of pavements and buildings where the birds roost and nest, noise and the blockage of gutters and rainwater pipes with feathers, nests and dead birds are common complaints. There is little evidence to substantiate the claim that these birds transmit disease to man, although pigeons have been shown to be infected with ornithosis and salmonellosis. Pigeons in particular may gain access to food premises, contaminating food and machinery.

Control principles
Pigeons are attracted to urban areas by the presence of food dropped deliberately or accidentally by the public. Limiting the availability of food through a prohibition on feeding of pigeons and strict regulation over the storage and collection of refuse containing food waste will go some way towards discouraging these birds. Under the Wildlife and Countryside Act 1981, both pigeons and starlings may be taken or killed by authorized persons, provided that approved methods are used.

Trapping is effective for pigeons, but less so in the case of starlings. A number of suitable designs are available; all permit birds to enter the trap freely, but deny exit. The traps may be placed on the ground but more commonly in urban areas on the flat roof of low rise buildings. Bait, usually a mixture of maize and wheat or a proprietary mix, is placed inside and outside the trap. Water should also be provided inside the trap. The trap should be left open for a period of about a week to allow the birds to become accustomed to its presence. When the birds are feeding freely, the trap is closed. The trap should be checked daily

and all unringed birds humanely destroyed, usually by cervical dislocation. Ringed birds should be returned to their owners.

Stupefying or narcotic baits, approved for use under the Food and Environment Protection Act 1985, can be used in urban areas, but may present a public reaction if unconscious or dying birds are evident. Pre-baiting is carried out for up to 28 days, after which alpha-chloralose is added. Narcotized bait is usually laid before dawn and left for a few hours before being cleared away. A search must then be made for all affected birds. Ringed birds and non-target species should be allowed to recover; pigeons should be destroyed humanely. Repellents and scaring devices can be employed to prevent roosting and perching on buildings. Netting can be applied to buildings, but will only be viable if the mesh size is suited to the size of the bird. Gels can be applied to ledges and windowsills. Over time, however, their performance is impaired by birds attempting to land and flattening the gel or covering it with droppings. Spring-tensioned wire positioned around ledges is really only suitable for pigeons. Acoustic methods of scaring include sirens, ultrasound and recordings of the distress calls of the target species. Some success has been claimed using birds of prey.

Shooting can be used effectively for small numbers of birds, but is likely to give rise to an adverse public reaction.

Brown-tail moth

The **brown-tail moth** (*Euproctis chrysorrhoea*) may give rise to localized concern amongst the public. The adult is of no public health significance; the larvae, however, are covered in fine hairs which can cause severe irritation and skin rash. The caterpillars emerge from a silky tent in which they have hibernated in April/May, and feed on fruit trees, blackthorn, hawthorn and oak. The larvae are covered in thick tufts of brown hair with two white lines of hair tufts on their backs and two orange warts. The hairs are easily detached and can make contact with human skin. Many of the hairs are barbed and resist washing and brushing off. Hairs in the eyes can

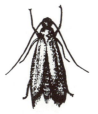

Fig. 9.21 Common clothes moth (*Tineola bisselliella*).

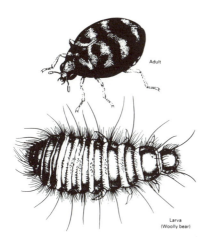

Fig. 9.20 Carpet beetle (*Anthrenus verbasci*). (Source: Burgess, N.R.H. (1990), *Public Health Pests*, Chapman & Hall, London, p.103 fig. 13.2.)

cause serious discomfort. The larval stage is usually completed by June.

Control principles
Control may be exercised through the cutting out and burning of the overwintering tents of the larvae between November and March. Alternatively, insecticidal sprays can be applied in mid September or mid May. Sprays based on permethrin, trichlorophon or diflubenzuron may be approved for control of these moths.

Carpet beetle

The **carpet beetle** (*Anthrenus verbasci*) is found in domestic premises in carpets, clothing, stuffed specimens, animal furs and skins and may be associated with birds' nests. The adult beetles are 1.5–4 mm long, with dark bodies, mottled with patches of lighter coloration, giving rise to distinctive wavy patterns (Fig. 9.20). The larvae are segmented and dark in colour, with tufts of bristles which give them the common name 'woolly bear'. The larvae cause extensive damage to non-synthetic fabrics and animal fur and skins. Adults feed on pollen and nectar.

Control principles
Control involves the removal and destruction of heavily infested materials, together with thorough

vacuuming. A residual insecticide containing fenitrothion, bendiocarb or permethrin may be applied.

Clothes moths

The term 'clothes moth' is applied generally to species of moth which commonly damage natural products of animal origin such as wool, fur and feathers. The three common species are the **common clothes moth** (*Tineola bisselliella*) (Fig. 9.21), the **brown house moth** (*Hofmannophila pseudospretella*) and the **white-shouldered house moth** (*Endrosis sarcitrella*). All adult moths are 8–10 mm long, shun light and are not strong flyers. The larvae are white, and through feeding, cause holes and damage to blankets, clothing and carpets.

Control principles
Control is achieved through careful storage of articles with naphthalene crystals or mothballs. Dichlorvos strips can be used in enclosed situations. A residual insecticide can be applied to the structure of premises, or to packaging, where approved for use. Where an infestation has occurred, heavily infested articles should be removed and destroyed.

Fur beetle

The **fur beetle** (*Attagenus pellio*) lives in birds' nests and is frequently found in the domestic situation. The lifecycle and habits of this beetle are similar to the carpet beetle. In appearance, however, there are differences. The adult beetle is about 5 mm long, and black, with distinctive white spots: one on each of the wing cases, and

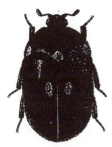

Fig. 9.22 Fur beetle (*Attagenus pellio*). (Source: LGMB/ADAS, *Pest Control: a reference manual for pest control staff; invertebrates*, LGMB, Luton, p.68.)

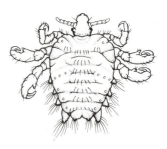

Fig. 9.24 Crab louse (*Phthirus pubis*). (Source: Burgess, N.R.H. (1990), *Public Health Pests*, Chapman & Hall, London, p.92, fig. 11.2.)

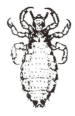

Fig. 9.23 Head louse (*Pediculus humanus capitis*).

three at the base of the prothorax (Fig. 9.22). The larvae may be up to 12 mm long with a long 'tail' of silky hairs. Control is the same as that for carpet beetles.

Lice

All lice have well-developed mandibles for biting and piercing skin, enabling them to suck the blood of their host. Three lice are of public health significance: the **head louse** (*Pediculus humanus capitis*), the **body louse** (*Pediculus humanus corporis*) and the **crab** or **pubic louse** (*Phthirus pubis*).

Characteristics
Head and body lice are 2–4 mm in length and pale grey to light brown in colour. The crab louse is about 2 mm in length and greyish. All lice are darker in colour following a feed.

Head lice (Fig. 9.23) are widely found in the UK and primarily affect children. Despite their prevalence, there is still much embarrassment associated with an infestation. Eggs are laid at the base of the hair and hatch leaving the pale-

coloured egg casing, known as a 'nit' on the hair. The nymphs feed on blood until sexual maturity. Transmission is through physical contact.

Body lice live in the clothing of the host, moving to the host to feed. Survival is reliant on the same clothing being worn at no more than 3-day intervals. Transmission is via infested clothing or physical contact.

Crab lice (Fig. 9.24) favour the coarser body hair found in the pubic areas and underarms and spread through intimate contact. All lice will cause irritation and scratching may give rise to secondary infection. Body lice may transmit typhus, trench fever and relapsing fever.

Control principles
Control of head and crab lice can be achieved through application of insecticidal shampoos or lotions containing malathion or carbaryl. In the case of body lice, infested clothing should be destroyed or disinfested at a cleansing station.

Mosquitoes

About 30 species of mosquito are present in the UK, occupying different aquatic habitats such as coastal salt waters, brackish inland waters, stagnant ponds and water-filled hollows in trees and logs. The two main mosquito groups in the UK are the **anophelines** and the **culicines**. In general, all have slender bodies, long legs and a well-developed proboscis. The length of the body is dependent on the species, but will range from 7 to 15 mm (Figs 9.25 and 9.26).

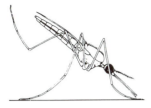

Fig. 9.25 Anopheline mosquito. (Source: Burgess, N.R.H. (1990), *Public Health Pests*, Chapman & Hall, London, p.71, fig. 8.4.)

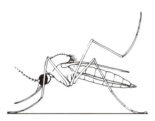

Fig. 9.26 Culicine mosquito. (Source: Burgess, N.R.H. (1990), *Public Health Pests*, Chapman & Hall, London, p.71, fig. 8.4.)

Characteristics

Eggs are laid on water, and hatch within a few hours. The larvae will breathe oxygen by moving to the surface of the water. The larvae feed on organic matter and micro-organisms in the water or on the surface. After four larval stages, the larvae pupate, forming a comma-shaped pupa which can propel itself using paddles at the bottom of the abdomen. The adult mosquito emerges from the pupa onto the surface of the water. Females alone will bite and suck blood; the males feed on the nectar of flowering plants. Females are attracted to a host by heat and exhaled carbon dioxide. A blood meal is required before viable eggs can be laid. During feeding, a small amount of anticoagulant saliva will be injected into the host to prevent the blood from clotting. The irritation, swelling and erythema associated with a mosquito bite is an antibody reaction to this anticoagulant.

Public health significance

The mosquito has significant public health importance in tropical and sub-tropical regions; the female being the vector of malaria, yellow

fever, filariasis, dengue fever and forms of viral encephalitis. In temperate regions the effect of a mosquito bite causes discomfort and possible secondary infection as a consequence of scratching. No link has been established between the transmission of the human immunodeficiency virus (HIV) and a mosquito bite.

Control principles

Effective mosquito control relies on knowledge of the species involved. However, in general, mosquito control should be aimed at both the larval and adult stages of the lifecycle. Breeding sites can be removed through emptying natural or man-made containers of water, draining puddles, ditches and small pools, and channelling water to increase the flow.

The larval stages can be eliminated in a number of ways. The application of an agent such as light oil or lecithin will reduce the surface tension of the water, preventing the larvae from obtaining oxygen. These agents spread readily over a large area, and can be applied aerially. Consideration must be given to the ecological effect. Larvicides containing permethrin, pirimiphos-methyl or chlorpyrifos which are applied to breeding sites do not have approval for use in the UK. The use of methoprene, the insect growth regulator and a biological control agent, the bacterium *Bacillus thuringiensis israelensis*, have been used for larval control in developed countries.

Adult mosquitoes can be eliminated using 'knock-down' agents or residual insecticides. Hand-held aerosols can be used in a domestic environment. Individual protection can be achieved through the application of suitable insect repellents to exposed parts of the body or the use of mosquito coils or candles containing citronella to deter the insects. In tropical areas, sleeping accommodation can be protected by a mosquito net impregnated with a suitable insecticide. Windows and doors can be fitted with mosquito proofing.

Plaster beetles

Plaster beetles (*Lathridiidae* spp.) are small dark brown beetles, 1.5–2.5 mm long, that have a

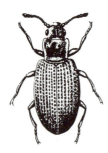

Fig. 9.27 Plaster beetle (*Lathridiidae* spp.).

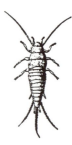

Fig. 9.28 Silverfish (*Lepisma saccharina*).

predilection for damp and humid conditions (Fig. 9.27). They can be significant where infestation occurs in food premises. Control over humidity or removal of damp conditions will remove any problems, although a residual insecticide can be applied.

Psocids

Psocids or **booklice** (*Psocoptera* spp.) are generally found in high humidity situations where they feed on moulds. Damp wallpaper, book bindings and food packets are favoured, and damage may occur where significant numbers are present. These insects are 1–1.5 mm long, wingless and greyish in colour, although the colour may reflect their food. Infestations spread readily through the movement of infested books or foodstuffs. Their presence in domestic situations frequently gives rise to complaints.

Control principles
Control can be achieved through improving hygiene and environmental conditions. Infested food packets should be destroyed and storage areas treated with a residual insecticide.

Silverfish

Silverfish (*Lepisma saccharina*) are commonly found in damp situations such as bathrooms, kitchens and pantries. They may be up to 20 mm long, with carrot-shaped wingless bodies and three bristly tails (Fig. 9.28). The colour is a silvery-grey. They feed on protein-rich gums and binding pastes in books and packeted foods,

wallpaper paste and fine textiles. The lifecycle may take up to a year to complete. Silverfish are of no public health significance, although severe infestations may be a nuisance.

Firebrats (*Thermobia domestica*) are similar to silverfish, but require a warm, dry environment and a preference for starchy foods.

Control principles
Control of silverfish and firebrats can be achieved through attention to hygiene or the application of residual insecticides based on synthetic pyrethroids, carbamates or organophosphates.

Wasps

The **common wasp** (*Vespula vulgaris*) is frequently found nesting in roof spaces, cavity walls, trees or in the ground. Nests are constructed each year from chewed wood pulp, which is converted into a paper-like substance and formed into many cells within an outer layer. The nest will be expanded during the season to accommodate the growing colony, which may reach many thousands. The wasps seen outside the nest are workers, 10–20 mm in length, with a distinctive

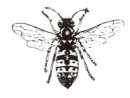

Fig. 9.29 Common wasp (*Vespula vulgaris*).

yellow and black banding and a 'wasp-waist' (Fig. 9.29). As cold weather approaches, the new queens find a suitable place for overwintering and the rest of the colony dies. The queens emerge from hibernation in spring and form new colonies. Wasps are usually a nuisance in late summer when the workers forage in search of sweet substances, and, if provoked, will sting.

Control principles

Control is effected through the application of insecticidal dust at the entrance to the nest. Workers will then carry the insecticide into the nest, spreading it to other wasps in the colony. Pyrethroids tend to excite wasps, and active ingredients such as carbaryl, bendiocarb and iodofenphos are generally used. Operatives should be protected against aggressive behaviour by wasps, should the nest be disturbed. Care must be taken to avoid treatment having an effect on beneficial wasp and bee species. General application of residual insecticides to loft spaces may present a risk to bats.

ACKNOWLEDGEMENTS

Many thanks to Dr Burgess and Helen Hadjidimitriadon, the artist, for their kind permission to reproduce some of the drawings from Burgess, N.R.H. (1990) *Public Health Pests*, Chapman & Hall, London.

REFERENCES

1. Health and Safety Commission (1991) *The Safe Use of Pesticides for Non-Agricultural Use: Approved Code of Practice*. HMSO, London.

FURTHER READING

Bassett, W.H. (1995) *Environmental Health Procedures*, 4th edn, Chapman & Hall, London.

British Standards Institute (1992) *BS 5502: 1992, Buildings and Structures for Agriculture Part 30: Code of Practice for Control of Infestation*.

Building Research Establishment (1980) *Reducing the Risk of Pest Infestations: design recommendations and literature review*, BRE, Aylesbury, Bucks.

Burgess, N.R.H. (1990) *Public Health Pests* Chapman & Hall, London

Cornwell, P.B. (1979) *Pest Control in Buildings: a guide to the meaning of terms*, 2nd edn. Hutchinson, London.

Kettle, D.S. (1990) *Medical and Veterinary Entomology*. CAB International, Wallingford, Oxon.

Local Government Management Board/ADAS (1992) *Pest Control: a reference manual for pest control staff*, LGMB, Luton.

Munro, J.W. (1966) *Pests of Stored Products*, Hutchinson, London.

Sprenger, R.A. (1991) *Hygiene for Management*, 5th edn, Highfield Publications, Doncaster.

Various Information Papers and Monographs produced by the Building Research Establishment and the Ministry of Agriculture, Fisheries and Food.

10 The control of dogs

Veronica Habgood

INTRODUCTION

The UK may be considered to be a nation of animal lovers, but the increased number of dogs, particularly in urban areas, and the heightened public awareness of the health and aesthetic issues arising from the lack of control by owners over their animals has led to an increasing number of complaints to the Police and local authorities. The major issues relate to stray animals, dangerous dogs, fouling in public places and noise nuisance from barking dogs. In recent years, therefore, the Government has been put under pressure to strengthen the legislative measures in respect of dogs. The resulting law has introduced new powers and responsibilities for local authorities and a need for close co-operation between local authorities, the Police and organizations such as the RSPCA and Wood Green Animal Shelters. Within local authorities, it is frequently the environmental health service which has responsibility for matters concerning dogs.

CONTROL OF STRAY DOGS

It is estimated that on any day in the UK there can be up to 500 000 uncontrolled dogs on the streets and at least 200 000 are registered each year as strays [1]. These dogs can cause road accidents, kill or maim livestock, bite or attack members of the public and deposit tonnes of excrement, daily.

These problems associated with stray dogs have been recognized in statute law since 1906, when the Dogs Act 1906 placed a duty on the Police to accept and detain any stray dog taken to a police station by a member of the public. Additionally, both the Police and local authorities have exercised their discretionary powers in rounding up and dealing with strays. The Local Government Act 1988, offered local authorities discretionary powers to seize and destroy stray dogs. Following this, many local authorities established a dog warden service. The provision of such a service was however discretionary and complementary to that provided by the local Police. Arrangements for kennelling, and charges for kennelling and, where necessary, destruction varied between local authorities and their relationship with the Police, voluntary organizations and private kennels.*

Increasing public concern about issues relating to dogs, together with the perceived success of local authorities operating a discretionary scheme, culminated in new statutory duties for local authorities in respect of stray dogs under the Environmental Protection Act 1990. These provisions have been exercisable from 1 April 1992, since when, the Police have no longer exercised their discretionary powers in rounding up strays. The public, however, will still be able to take

---

* The police functions relating to stray dogs are under review – see 'Review of Police Core and Ancillary Tasks – Interim Report', Home Office, October 1994.

stray dog to a police station, pursuant to the Dogs Act 1906.

Environmental Protection Act 1990: sections 149–151

Every local authority is required to appoint an officer whose function is to administer the duties required under the Environmental Protection Act 1990. These duties can be discharged through the appointment of dog wardens, who will be responsible for day to day activities in connection with the seizure and detention of stray dogs. Dog wardens may be local authority employees or contractors.

Where a dog, which is believed to be a stray, is found in a public place, the officer has a duty to seize and detain the animal. If the dog is on private land, the officer must receive the consent of the owner or occupier of the land before seizing the dog. 'Stray dog' is not defined, but implies that there is no person in charge of the dog for the time being. A duty is placed on any person who finds a stray dog, to either return it to the owner, or take it to the Police or local authority, where particulars of the dog and the name and address of the finder will be taken. The person finding the dog may keep it for at least 1 month, or hand it over to the local authority or Police to be dealt with.

Where the owner of the dog can be identified through a collar tag, the officer must notify that person by notice, that the dog has been seized and where it is being held. The notice must give the person 7 days to collect the dog and pay the necessary charges, otherwise the dog is liable to be disposed of or destroyed. A public register containing prescribed particulars of seized dogs is required to be kept by the officer. Such particulars, prescribed in the Environmental Protection (Stray Dogs) Regulations 1992, include a brief description of the dog, including any distinguishing characteristics; information recorded on the collar and tag; the date, time and place of seizure; date and service of any notice; the name and address of any person claiming to be the owner, to whom the dog was returned, and the date of return. Where the dog is disposed of, the date

of disposal; method of disposal (destruction, gift or sale); the price, where sold and the name and address of the person effecting the destruction, receiving or purchasing the dog.

Seized dogs may be detained in kennels provided by the local authority, or a voluntary organization or private kennels with an arrangement with the local authority. Arrangements must be made for receiving and dealing with dogs found or reported outside usual working hours. The charge to the owner on collection of a stray dog is based on the cost per day of kennelling the dog, together with a sum of £25, prescribed by the Environmental Protection (Stray Dogs) Regulations 1992. There is no automatic entitlement to the return of a dog unless the full amount is paid; however local authorities do have the discretion to determine that a dog be returned to the owner without full payment of the costs.

Dogs must be kept for a minimum of 7 days following seizure or service of a notice on the owner, whichever is the longer. Dogs which are injured, or in poor health, can be destroyed before the end of 7 days to avoid suffering. In this instance, the advice of a veterinary surgeon should be sought. Following the 7-day detention period, where a stray has not been reclaimed, the officer must determine the most appropriate means of disposal. The local authority may make their own arrangements for selling or giving the dog to a person who in the officer's opinion will care for the dog properly, or may have an arrangement with a voluntary organization, who will attempt to find a suitable owner. Any person who has purchased or received a dog in good faith, has the ownership of that dog vested in them, such that the original owner has no rights to reclaim the dog. Alternatively, the dog may be destroyed in a humane manner.

The cost to local authorities in exercising their duties in respect of the control of stray dogs will vary, depending on the arrangements made for the appointment of dog wardens and kennelling. Estimates of the direct cost of these function were made in a Department of the Environment survey in 1991 [2], and ranged from £23 000 p.a. in a mixed urban-rural district council, to £205 000 in a city council area.

Control of Dogs Order 1992

This Order, made under the Animal Health Act 1981, requires every dog on a public highway or in a place of public resort, to wear a collar, with the name and address of the owner inscribed on the collar or on a plate or badge. A number of exceptions are provided for: these include dogs registered with the Guide Dogs for the Blind Association, dogs used in emergency rescue work, dogs being used by the Armed Forces, Police or Customs and Excise and dogs used for sporting purposes. Any dog found on a highway or in a public place without a collar may be seized and treated as a stray pursuant to the provisions of section 3, Dogs Act 1906 or sections 149–151, Environmental Protection Act 1990.

DANGEROUS DOGS

A number of well-publicized incidents involving attacks by certain breeds of dog has led in recent years to a tightening in the legal controls in respect of 'dangerous' or 'vicious' dogs.

Until 1991, the law concerned with controlling attacks on the public existed within the Dogs Act 1871 which was concerned with dogs which were dangerous and not kept under proper control, and the Town Police Clauses Act 1847, which made it an offence for a ferocious dog to be at large. In 1989, these provisions were extended by the Dangerous Dogs Act 1989. This provided for the making of a Court Order requiring that a dog be handed over for destruction and the owner disqualified from keeping a dog in the future, where a dog was deemed to be dangerous and not kept under proper control. The Dangerous Dogs Act 1991 provides for even more stringent control.

Dangerous Dogs Act 1991

Section 1, Dangerous Dogs Act 1991 applies to certain prescribed breeds of dog bred for fighting or possessing the characteristics of a type of dog bred for fighting. To date, the breeds prescribed are:

1. pit bull terrier;
2. Japanese Tosa;
3. Dogo Argentino;
4. Fila Braziliero.

The provisions of the Dangerous Dogs Act 1991 are enforced by the Police or an authorized officer of the local authority. Additionally, the local authority role in controlling stray dogs will inevitably bring them into contact with prescribed breeds.

The Dangerous Dogs Act 1991 prohibits the breeding of prescribed dogs, their sale or exchange; the offering of such dogs as gifts or their importation. Furthermore, after 30 November 1991, no person is permitted to have one of these breeds in their possession, unless it has been exempted. Arrangements have been made for compensation to be paid to owners whose dogs are not exempt and have to be destroyed. The provisions in relation to compensation and exemption are contained in the Dangerous Dogs Compensation and Exemption Schemes Order 1991 (as amended). Such exempted dogs are registered and the owners issued with a certificate of exemption. To gain a certificate of exemption, an owner must arrange for the dog to be neutered, permanently implanted with a transponder, tattooed with the dog's exemption reference number, covered by third party insurance, kept in secure conditions at home and when in a public place, muzzled and held on a lead by someone aged at least 16. Additionally, the owner must provide the Police with the name, age and gender of the dog, together with the address at which the dog is kept.

The transponder is implanted in the scruff of the dog's neck and an electronic reading device passed within 100–1300 mm of the transponder will produce a digital display which will uniquely identify the dog on the Index of Exempted Dogs. The tattoo is the most simple means of determining whether or not a dog has been exempted, but in circumstances when this is difficult to read, the transponder comes into its own. The Index of Exempted Dogs is administered by a contracted private company which can be contacted by the Police or local authority.

Identification of prescribed breeds

One of the major difficulties encountered by those concerned with the legislation is the identification of the prescribed breeds, in particular the pit bull terrier and dogs with pit bull terrier characteristics. In 1992, the Department of the Environment estimated there were between 5000 and 10 000 pit bull terrier types in the UK [3]. Guidance has been provided by the Department of the Environment [3], and the RSPCA have a small number of qualified expert witnesses. Standards laid down by the American Dog Breeders Association include reference to behavioural characteristics in the identification of dangerous dogs [4]. A High Court Ruling in 1993 [5] determined that these behavioural characteristics could be taken into account during any proceedings to confirm whether a dog fell within the prescribed description.

The onus of proving a dog is not a prescribed breed or exhibits characteristics of a prescribed breed rests with the plaintiff. The difficulty in positively identifying a prescribed breed has lead to a series of appeals and dogs being kept kennelled at Police or local authority expense in excess of 15 months.

'Specially dangerous dogs'

Provisions also exist by virtue of the Dangerous Dogs Act 1991, for the Secretary of State to make an Order in respect of other 'specially dangerous dogs'. The Order will apply certain requirements in respect of the need for such dogs to be kept on a lead and muzzled in a public place, and prohibiting such dogs from being abandoned and being allowed to stray. No Orders have yet been made. The Secretary of State can also prescribe the kind of muzzle to be used. In all events it must be sufficient to prevent a dog biting a person. To date, no such muzzles have been prescribed, although reference can be made to British Standard 7659:1993 – Dog Muzzles.

Dogs dangerously out of control

Any breed of dog which is dangerously out of control in a public place is dealt with under section 4, Dangerous Dogs Act 1991. Proceedings may be taken against the owner or person for the time being in charge of the dog. 'Dangerously out of control' means that there are grounds for reasonable apprehension that the dog will injure a person, whether or not it actually does so; and 'public place' means any street, road or other place (whether or not enclosed) to which the public have or are permitted to have, access for payment or otherwise. An aggravated offence is deemed to have been committed where the dog injures any person.

In the case of a dog which is allowed to enter a place which is not a public place and where it is not permitted to be, for example, a private garden, the owner or person in charge of the dog is guilty of an offence in the case where there are reasonable grounds to suspect that the dog will injure someone or guilty of an aggravated offence in the event that the dog causes actual injury. An aggravated offence may be dealt with summarily or on indictment, and carries a more severe penalty than a non-injury offence.

Seizure of dangerous dogs

Powers are available under sections 4–5, Dangerous Dogs Act 1991, enabling the Police or local authority to seize a prescribed breed which is in a public place and which is not exempt, or if exempt, is not muzzled and kept on a lead, or is a prescribed 'specially dangerous dog' or is a dog which is dangerously out of control.

In general, the Dangerous Dogs Act 1991 provides for the destruction of a seized dog. Where no proceedings are to be brought and a dog has been seized, a Justice of the Peace may order the immediate destruction of the dog. In the case of a prescribed dangerous dog, or where an aggravated offence has been committed, the court is obliged, following a successful conviction, to order the dog's destruction. It is suggested that where there is any doubt as to the positive identification of a prescribed dangerous dog, an order for the dog's destruction is not sought until after a successful conviction. The court may also disqualify the offender for whatever period it thinks fit, from having custody of a dog.

In cases where an owner is convicted of an offence under the Dangerous Dogs Act 1991, the Court may not order the dog's destruction until the end of the Appeal period, and in the event of an Appeal, once the Appeal has been withdrawn or determined.

DOG WARDENS

To fulfil the statutory duties under the Environmental Protection Act 1990 and the Dangerous Dogs Act 1991, local authorities have generally provided a dog warden service through the direct employment of dog wardens or through a contractual arrangement. In most cases, the duties of a dog warden will comprise both statutory and non-statutory functions. These functions include:

1. The seizure and detention of stray dogs, dangerous dogs and associated duties under the Environmental Protection Act 1990 and the Dangerous Dogs Act 1991.
2. The enforcement of bye-laws and orders relating to the fouling of public areas, including 'Poop-Scoop' schemes; identification of dogs under the Control of Dogs Order 1992; the control of dogs on highways.
3. The investigation of complaints relating to the keeping of dogs, particularly in relation to general welfare and nuisance from barking or the accumulation of faeces.
4. The provision of advice in respect of the licensing of pet shops, animal boarding establishments and dog breeding premises.
5. Health education, through the provision of information to the public promoting the dog warden service; the production and distribution of publicity material concerned with the keeping of dogs; education of the public through talks and presentations.

The emotive nature of dog-related issues necessitates the appointment of someone who is sensitive to the sentiments of dog-lovers, but nonetheless, is capable of acting in a enforcement capacity. The job relies on fostering good public relations and building up a close working relationship with the Police and animal welfare agencies.

Dog warden equipment

To carry out the duty of seizing stray and dangerous dogs, dog wardens must be properly equipped, not only to protect themselves, but also to ensure that dogs are seized and transported with due regard to their welfare. Generally, a suitably equipped 'transit-type' van is adequate for most Local Authority use. Desirable features include:

1. driver separation, with vision panel to rear compartment;
2. aluminium or imperviously lined rear compartment, with drainage;
3. wash hand basin with hot and cold water supply;
4. active ventilation from rear compartment and good interior lighting;
5. side and rear door entry;
6. two to four steel-mesh kennels with opaque dividers;
7. a separate puppy box/kennel;
8. low-loading sill;
9. storage space for dog warden equipment and paperwork;
10. blankets, rubber mats, bowls, food and water for dogs.

The dog warden must be provided with protective equipment. This will generally include a helmet with a heavy duty visor; chest, forearm, groin, leg and foot guards together with heavy duty leather gloves. For seizing dogs, slip/rope leads; short and long catch-poles; a throw net and metal guard muzzles. A first aid kit should be readily accessible, and a camera can be useful for identification purposes. Radio contact with the local authority offices will facilitate a quick response to complaints concerning stray dogs and enable the dog warden to call for assistance, where necessary.

DOG CONTROL

A miscellany of legal controls is available to local authorities to provide for control in matters such as canine defecation and noise.

Fouling in public places*

Complaints concerning dog fouling in public places are commonplace in most local authorities. Although unpleasant aesthetically, the major issue associated with dog fouling is the potential risk to human health. All dogs may carry parasitic worms in their intestines, including the roundworm *Toxocara canis*. The worms are most commonly found in young dogs. Eggs from the roundworm are disseminated into the environment via the faeces of the dog. These eggs may remain viable for a period of years. Humans become infected through ingestion of viable eggs. Children are most at risk because of the nature of play, which may bring them into contact with contaminated ground. Much attention is therefore focused on the maintenance of dog-free children's play areas in public parks and beaches. Each year, a number of children exhibiting the clinical symptoms of toxocariasis are identified. These symptoms are a form of blindness or eye disease and physical damage to the viscera caused by migrating larvae, which hatch from the eggs. Surveys have shown that asymptomatic infection with *Toxocara canis* is common, indicating that up to one million people in the UK have been infected at some time [6]. *Toxocara canis* cannot develop into an adult roundworm in the human.

The control of *Toxocara canis* and other worm infestations in dogs can be readily controlled through the administration of anthelmintic ('worming') preparations, together with the control of canine defaecation. Individuals can reduce the risk of infection by maintaining good standards of hygiene in the home. Such measures include discouraging dogs from licking people; maintaining separate food bowls, utensils, toys and blankets for pets; not allowing dogs to sleep on beds and washing hands after handling the dog.

Public Health Act 1875: section 164 and Open Spaces Act 1906: sections 12 and 15

Bye-laws can be made under these provisions to control the entry of dogs into prescribed areas of parks, recreation grounds, beaches and promenades and to maintain dogs on leashes in prescribed areas at prescribed days and hours. There is also provision to require owners to clear up faeces within prescribed dog exercise areas. Model bye-laws have been produced which can be adopted by local authorities, subject to confirmation by the Home Office.

Litter (Animal Droppings) Order 1991

The Litter (Animal Droppings) Order 1991 applies the provisions of Part IV, Environmental Protection Act 1990 in respect of litter and refuse, to dog faeces on land which is not heath or woodland or used for grazing animals. The Environmental Protection Act 1990 requires local authorities, certain Crown authorities, designated statutory transport undertakers and occupiers of certain other land, to keep their land clear of litter and refuse. The effect of the Order is not to create an offence in respect of dog fouling, merely to ensure that any faeces are removed.

Local Government Act 1972: section 235

The provisions of section 235, Local Government Act 1972, enable local authorities to make bye-laws for the purposes of 'good rule and government'. Model bye-laws were reviewed in 1990, and have been produced in respect of dog fouling in certain public places. Local authorities wishing to adopt the bye-laws must seek the approval of the Home Office. There is no statutory requirement for local authorities to adopt the bye-laws.

Removal of canine faeces byelaws

To assist local authorities in fulfilling the duty under Part IV, Environmental Protection Act 1990, the removal of canine faeces ('poop-scoop') bye-laws made under section 235, Local Government Act 1972, have been enthusiastically adopted by many councils. The bye-laws apply in respect of designated footways, footpaths, grass

* For a review of the legal provisions see the Summary Report of the Advisory Group on Litter – Review of the Litter Provisions of the Environmental Protection Act 1990. DoE, July 1994.

verges, parks and other open spaces and pedestrianized areas within local authority areas. The effect of the bye-laws, is to require persons in charge of a dog within the designated areas to remove any faeces deposited by their dog.

The adoption of these byelaws requires effective publicity, together with capital expenditure for the provision of suitable receptacles, education of the public geared towards toilet training of dogs and high profile enforcement action. Guidance is available to local authorities on introducing a 'poop-scoop' scheme [7], and a number of contractors can supply suitable equipment and publicity material.

Whilst many local authorities favour the provision of a dedicated receptacle and suitable cardboard 'scoops' or bags for the removal and disposal of dog faeces by owners, some have introduced specially designed 'dog toilets' in parks and other open spaces.

The design of 'dog toilets' varies, but most essentially comprise a distinguishable area, normally of sharp sand, which may or may not be partially enclosed by low-level fencing. The sand offers an attractive surface for dogs and encourages defaecation. Additionally, one or more vertical timber posts encourage dogs to urinate in the area. The success of 'dog toilets' relies on a high level of maintenance. First, the sand must be regularly cleaned to remove faecal matter (twice weekly, or more often where there is heavy usage); secondly, the sand must be periodically disinfected, perhaps on a monthly basis; and finally, the sand should be replaced at least annually.

'Poop-scoop' bye-laws can also be applied to the gutters of a carriageway subject to a 30 mph speed limit, and additional bye-laws provide for an offence where a dog is permitted to foul prescribed carriageways.

Nuisance

The noise from barking dogs is a frequent complaint to environmental health departments, and one which is often difficult to resolve. Dogs which are not properly trained or controlled, or are kept in unsuitable environments may cause noise by barking. Dog breeding premises and animal boarding establishments have been the focus of well-publicized allegations of noise nuisance, some of which have been the subject of enquiry by the Local Government Ombudsman. Prolonged and persistent barking may constitute a statutory noise nuisance, which can be dealt with under Part III, Environmental Protection Act 1990 (see Chapter 7). Advice concerning training to reduce the incidence of barking and the use of proprietary 'anti-barking' devices can often be provided by the dog warden.

Accumulations of dog faeces on premises may also give rise to a statutory nuisance or risk to public health and can be dealt with similarly under Part III, Environmental Protection Act 1990.

Welfare

The welfare of dogs is not of direct concern to environmental health departments, although conditions which give rise to concern may be encountered. In these circumstances, referral should be made to one of the animal welfare agencies such as the RSPCA.

CONTROL OF RABIES

Rabies, or hydrophobia, is a viral zoonosis transmitted via the saliva of a rabid animal. The saliva is introduced by a bite, or more rarely through a scratch or break in the skin. Rabies occurs worldwide and is spreading across Europe to northern France. No cases of indigenous rabies have been reported in England and Wales since 1902, the only reported cases having been contracted abroad. Canine and feline animals are the main vectors in Europe, particularly the fox and dog. There is much concern at the risk of rabies being introduced into the UK through the accidental or intentional importation of rabid animals aboard ships, aircraft and more recently, via the Channel Tunnel link. The occupations at most risk are animal handlers at quarantine kennels and zoos, port health inspectors, veterinary surgeons, animal health inspectors and dog wardens.

Rabies (Importation of Dogs, Cats and Other Mammals) Order 1974

Statutory powers provide both a pro-active and reactive approach to dealing with rabies. The Rabies (Importation of Dogs, Cats and Other Mammals) Order 1974 [as amended], prohibits the landing in Great Britain of any animal brought from outside Great Britain, except in accordance with the terms of a licence which has been issued in advance. Animals landed within the terms of the order are subject to a quarantine period of 6 months, at the owners' expense.*

Rabies (Control) Order 1974

The Rabies (Control) Order 1974 provides for measures to be taken in the event of an outbreak of rabies. Such measures include the declaration of an infected area; the seizure and destruction of the suspect animal; restriction on the movement of animals in and out of an infected area; action to control dogs, cats and other animals through leashing or muzzling; seizure, detention or destruction of animals not kept under proper control; compulsory vaccination of animals; prohibition on events and activities where animals are brought together and the destruction of foxes within the infected area.

Rabies outbreak contingency plans have been produced by animal health authorities; i.e. London boroughs, metropolitan authorities and county councils. These plans set out the action to be taken in the event of an outbreak of rabies in their area, including publicity, liaison with other statutory bodies, manpower, equipment and similar considerations.

Public Health (International Trains) Regulations 1994

In regard to the Channel Tunnel link, the operators have introduced various measures during the design and construction of the tunnel, to minimize the likelihood of foxes, dogs and rodents gaining access to the tunnel. However, there is always the possibility of 'stowaway animals' on trains, and the Public Health (International Trains) Regulations 1994 will address this situation. A 'stowaway animal' is defined as 'any animal on board an international train, except one which is being lawfully transported through the tunnel, or smuggled through the tunnel'. The effect of this Statutory Instrument is to require any member of the train crew to report the presence of a stowaway animal to the train manager. The train manager then has a duty to report that sighting to the local authority environmental health service at the next designated stopping place for that service. Where the animal is a rabies suspect, either the train manager or the local authority, will advise the Ministry of Agriculture, Fisheries and Food who will be responsible for any necessary rabies control measures. Where the stowaway animal is not a rabies suspect, the local authority is able to require the deratting, decontamination or disinfestation of the train.

REFERENCES

1. Moore, S.R. and Dhaliwal, P. (1992) Campaign on dogs. *Environmental Health*, **100**(6), 152–154.
2. Price Waterhouse (1991) *Resource Implications of s. 149–151 Environmental Protection Act 1990 (Dog Control) for the Department of the Environment*, Price Waterhouse, London.
3. Department of the Environment/Welsh Office/Home Office, Environmental Protection Act 1990, Part IV. Control of Stray Dogs. Circular 6/1991 DoE.
4. *R.* v. *Knightsbridge Crown Court*, ex. p. *Dunne* [1993] *Q.B.D.* and *Brock* v. *Director of Public Prosecutions* [1993] Q.B.D. *The Times Law Reports*, 23 July 1993.
5. UK looks set to adopt US standards on Pit Bull Terriers (1992) *Environmental Health News*, **8**(28), 4.
6. Gillespie, S.H. (1993) Human toxicariasis. *CDR Review*, **3**(10), R140–R143.

---

* Qualified exceptions apply to dogs originating in the EU States which are offered for sale in the UK. See the Rabies (Importation of Dogs, Cats and Other Mammals) (Amendment) Order 1994.

7. Home Office (1990) Review of Dog Byelaws. Circular 93/1990.

FURTHER READING

Department of the Environment/Welsh Office (1989) Action on Dogs: The Government's proposals for legislation. A Consultation Paper.

Department of the Environment/Welsh Office/ Home Office, Environmental Protection Act 1990, Part IV. Control of Stray Dogs. Circular 6/1992 DoE.

Department of Health and Social Security/Welsh Office (1977) Memorandum on Rabies.

Health and Safety Executive (1990) *The Occupational Zoonoses*, HSE, London.

Home Office/Department of the Environment/ Welsh Office/Scottish Office (1990) The Control of Dogs: a Consultation Paper.

Home Office (1990) Review of Dog Byelaws. Circular 93/1990.

Institution of Environmental Health Officers (1991) *Dogs – Control by Local Authorities: Report of Dogs Survey 1991*. CIEH, London.

Price Waterhouse (1991) *Resource Implications of s. 149–151 Environmental Protection Act 1990 (Dog Control) for the Department of the Environment*, Price Waterhouse, London.

Tidy Britain Group (1993) *Local Authority Survey – Control of Dog Fouling*.

11 Public safety and health

Richard J. Palfrey

INTRODUCTION

There is something that is curiously beguiling about most of the attractions which make up the present day leisure industry. They have elements of surprise, excitement and mystery together with their often unique transient nature to be sampled today, or gone tomorrow. They are intended to transport their participants from the familiar to new sensations and excitement. Ensuring the safety of these events are a whole range of Environmental Health Controls which go unnoticed in the main until some serious mishap occurs.

FAIRGROUNDS

Fairground apparatus has become increasingly sophisticated in recent years, and the potential for serious personal injury is high if safe working practices are not established and rigidly followed.

Fairgrounds have features which are difficult and complex, ensuing from the wide variety of largely non-standard devices, the diversity of sites and method of operation. In the travelling section of the industry, there are problems of repeated 'build up' and 'pull down'.

There continues to be a high level of public and media concern about fairground safety. Between 1986 and 1993 there were 11 fatal accidents at fairgrounds, three to employees and eight to members of the public. In the same period there were 645 major accidents involving the public.

Accidents continue to occur, the latest fatalities being at a pleasure park at Coney Island, Porthcawl at Easter 1994.

Code of Safe Practice

Useful advice can be found in Fairgrounds and Amusement Parks: A Code of Safe Practice (1992) (HS(G) 81 [1]) prepared by the HSE through the Advisory Committee for Health and Safety in the Amusement Industry. The Code deals with:

1. designing, manufacturing, supplying and modifying amusement devices;
2. assembling and dismantling passenger-carrying devices, and general passenger safety;
3. testing, examining, maintaining and safely operating devices;
4. training ride operators and attendants;
5. installing, using and maintaining electrical equipment;
6. gas safety and fire precautions.

Each ride is required to have a log book recording operating particulars, together with a record of any alterations or repairs which could affect structural safety. This must be kept for 5 years. The Code requires an initial test, before first use, of all new fairground rides and thorough examination by an independent, competent, trained person of every ride at least once in every 14 months. Any defects must be notified in writing and copied to HSE where there are implications for similar devices elsewhere. In addition a daily inspection of each ride is required before the commencement of operation and a record made in a register to be kept for at least 1 month.

All passenger carrying amusement devices should have arrangements for the support and retention of passengers either incorporated in the basic design or, where appropriate, additionally provided on the ride. Such devices (seat belts, lap bars, enclosing harnesses, etc.) are required by the Code to be capable of being positioned or fastened so that they do not inadvertently open during the course of the ride. Where a ride is to be unsuitable for certain categories of passenger, e.g. small children, clear notices or other devices should be displayed prominently to indicate the extent of the exclusion.

Detailed objectives are set for operators building up or pulling down rides, a situation which arises more frequently in the travelling sector of the industry. Precautions such as numbering parts, the order or sequence of assembly and dismantling, and the careful handling of components to reduce risk of damage, are included.

Special emphasis is paid to the stability of the ride, consideration being given to the varying ground conditions and the behaviour characteristics of particular rides. Regular checking to ensure that original standards are maintained is also required.

Obligations are placed upon ride operators and attendants to ensure that passengers are correctly positioned, that safety equipment is being used and is properly in position and fastened, before the ride cycle is commenced. Cautionary notices are required to be prominently displayed, indicating clearly reasonable passenger conduct.

The ride operators should be alert in observing passengers during the ride cycle wherever practicable, and should be prepared to slow down and bring to rest any ride, should the onset of an emergency become apparent.

There are, additionally, age and training requirements for operators and attendants. The safe use of electricity, emergency fire arrangements, the safe use of flammable liquids, gas, ammunition and explosives and other matters are also dealt with.

Definition and enforcement

Fairgrounds are defined in the Health and Safety (Enforcing Authority) Regulations 1989 as meaning any part of premises which is, for the time being, used wholly or mainly for the operation of any fairground equipment, other than a coin-operated ride, non-powered children's playground equipment or a swimming pool slide.

This definition is narrow when compared with the definition of fairground equipment, and was drafted in this way to exclude certain types of lower risk equipment to ensure, for example, that coin-operated children's rides outside of shops do not constitute a 'fairground'. (Similar equipment, however, in a fairground site will be the responsibility of the HSE.) Fairgrounds at premises otherwise allocated to local authorities, e.g. in holiday camps, will fall to the HSE for inspection.

Enforcement of the provisions of the Health and Safety at Work, Etc. Act 1974 is the responsibility of the Health and Safety Executive (HSE) by virtue of schedule 2 of the Regulations.

Fairground equipment

The definition of fairground equipment is not included in the Regulations, but it is to be found in the Health and Safety at Work, Etc. Act 1974 as amended by the Consumer Protection Act 1987. Fairground equipment is here defined as any fairground ride, any similar plant which is designed to be in motion for entertainment purposes with members of the public on or inside it, or any plant which is designed to be used by members of the public for entertainment purposes, either as a slide or for bouncing upon. In this definition, the reference to plant which is designed to be in motion with members of the public on or inside it includes a reference to swings, dodgems and other plant which is designed to be in motion wholly or partly under the control of, or to be put in motion by, a member of the public.

Although playground equipment is excluded, the Code does cover the use of amusement devices in other premises, making it of use to local authority inspectors who come across equipment, the use of which may constitute only a minor activity on the premises.

The Code is not an 'approved' code, but it has been agreed by the Advisory Committee on Health and Safety in the Entertainments Industry and by the fairground associations – the Association of Amusement Parks and Piers of Great Britain, the Showman's Guide of Great Britain and the British Amusement Catering Trades Association – it is expected that their members will meet its requirements.

A series of guidance notes has also been produced by the Health and Safety Executive in the Plant and Machinery Series. These describe various factors that contribute to accidents on fairground apparatus. The guidelines are based on HSE reports of incidents, visits to fairgrounds by inspectors and the considerable experience of fairground operators. The range of passenger-carrying amusement devices so far covered by these guidance notes include the waltzer (PM47), the octopus (PM48), the cyclone twist (PM49), the big wheel (PM57), the paratrooper (PM59), the chair-o-plane (PM61), roller coasters (PM68) ark/speedway devices (PM70), water chutes (PM71) and the trabant (PM72). Another source of information is 'Fairground User's Safety Guide' published by ROSPA.

Playground equipment

Playground equipment and rides may now also be found in hotels and restaurants where section 3 of the Health and Safety at Work, Etc. Act 1974 will apply. While the Code of Safe Practice is principally aimed at fairground activities, it contains useful guidance on standards which could be required for children's rides. A useful guide on playground equipment standards is the booklet, *Playground Management for Local Councils*, issued by the National Playing Fields Association [2].

The Entertainment Services National Industry group (NIG) of the HSE is also prepared to give advice on standards through the HSE Area Enforcement Liaison Officer Service.

HAIRDRESSING

Hazards

The occupational hazards are numerous. The industry is made up of very small units, usually employing a high proportion of young people and there are always large numbers of trainees and others waiting to enter the industry.

The most frequent occupational problems encountered are those of dermatitis of the hands and the ergonomic problems resulting from long periods of standing in tiring postures. Recently, there has been a growing awareness of the possible long-term hazards associated with the chemical dyes and sprays that are frequently found in these premises, and the risks from customers infected with transmissible blood diseases.

However, although there has been concern about the occupational hazards of hairdressing, it is not generally held to be a high-risk activity in respect of the transmission of serious infections. But some of the hairdressing practices employed may result in infection passing from customer to customer, if hairdressing implements are not sterilized. Therefore the promotion of hygiene in the salon is important.

The two major infections about which there has been most concern, AIDS and hepatitis B, are both capable of transfer by small amounts of blood and serum (from an infected hairdresser or customer) to breaks in the skin. Although there is no danger if these diseases are not present (it is unlikely that the AIDS virus can survive for long periods on equipment anyway), it is poor practise to rely on this being the situation and so high standards of hygiene and positive methods to ensure the destruction of likely organisms must be employed.

Less serious infections, including spots, boils, abcesses, impetigo (both streptococcal and staphylococcal), herpes, ringworm, headlice and warts may also be passed from person to person if hygienic practices are not employed.

Legislation

There is specific legislation covering hairdressing salons. Local authorities may make bye-laws which relate to hairdressers and barbers under section 77 of the Public Health Act 1961 for the purpose of ensuring the cleanliness of the premises, equipment and staff.

All hairdressing businesses must also comply with the requirements of the Health and Safety at Work Etc. Act 1974, and local authorities are the enforcing authorities for these premises.

Under the Control of Substances Hazardous to Health Regulations 1994 (COSHH), there is an obligation to carry out an assessment of risks in the use of substances used at work. Exposure must then be adequately controlled (see Chapter 28). These provisions are important in the hairdressing trade.

Hygiene

The main vehicles of bacterial transmission are razors, scissors, clippers and styptic, with brushes, combs, massagers, rollers, towels and hands presenting only an occasional risk. To eliminate risk, it is wise to avoid the use of open razors, replacing them with disposable razors or disposable blade razors, which can be discarded after use. Electric razors can be difficult to sterilize and should also be avoided.

The use of scissors cannot be avoided, but if skin is punctured, wounds should be immediately treated, (e.g. with a prepacked spirit swab,) and left to dry. The scissors should not be used again until they have been sterilized by autoclaving, boiling or soaking them in 70% alcohol chlorhexidine in alcohol for 30 minutes. Because of the time required for treatment, hairdressers often find it helpful to keep two or more pairs available for use. Scissors should be washed regularly in hot water containing detergent, and then dried or wiped with an alcohol wipe before allowing to dry.

Manual clippers with non-detachable blades should not be used, and care should be taken to ensure that the blades of electrical clippers are correctly aligned to avoid cuts to the skin. When this happens, the blades should be removed and treated as above. Properly adjusted clippers only need a regular wipe over with an alcohol wipe.

Styptic, used to stop bleeding, should not be applied directly onto broken skin. It should either be applied on gauze or cotton wool or applied in aerosol form. It is recommended that it is not used and that bleeding is controlled by wiping with a gauze, cotton wool or by waiting for the bleeding to stop naturally.

Combs, brushes, massagers, etc, may be cleaned by washing with hot water and detergent after each customer, drying and using an alcohol and chlorhexidine wipe.

Towels, capes and gowns require no special precautions but should be laundered regularly. Disposable paper items are more hygienic and are especially recommended for customers with skin problems. Apart from alcoholic disinfectants and bleach for blood spills, chemical disinfectants are not generally recommended in hairdressing salons, as they may regularly become contaminated and their concentration may vary. They are also often toxic and corrosive.

Automatic autoclaves are recommended as being the most effective means of sterilizing hairdressing equipment, and these should be used wherever possible. Glass bead sterilizers use the dry heat method of sterilization. These instruments need time to heat up and may be difficult to use for some items as they can only sterilize the parts in contact with the hot beads. It is also often argued that these instruments may also blunt pieces of equipment with sharp cutting edges.

If sterilization is not possible by either of the above methods, disinfection may be accepted by boiling or steaming for at least 10 minutes in equipment specially designed for hairdressing instruments. Ultra-violet light apparatus often found in hairdressing salons does not sterilize equipment and is, therefore, not as efficient as the use of autoclaves, etc.

Useful guidelines on satisfactory methods of sterilization and disinfection have been produced by the Public Health Laboratory Service entitled Guidelines for hygienic hairdressing [3]. The Department of Health has also produced an AIDS information leaflet for hairdressers.

Premises and equipment should be kept clean and staff should follow good standards of personal hygiene. The salon should be kept clean using proprietary cleaners but, specifically, alcohol-based disinfectant is recommended for surfaces which need to be wiped three or four times a day. Staff should wash their hands before and after each customer. If staff suffer from dermatitis, disposable gloves should be worn.

Product safety

Considerable advice is now available on the composition and safety of products supplied to hairdressing businesses. These products will not present a risk to health and safety if they are used sensibly and in accordance with instructions supplied by manufacturers. A useful source of information in this respect is the HSE publication, *How to Use Hair Preparations Safely in the Salon* [4]. This booklet gives advice on the storage and sensible use of hair preparations. Hair preparations are governed by the Cosmetic Products Regulations 1978 which, among other things, requires that cosmetic products shall not be liable to cause damage to human health when applied under normal conditions of use. These Regulations lay down safety standards for all cosmetic products, including appropriate labelling requirements.

ACUPUNCTURE, TATTOOING, EAR PIERCING AND ELECTROLYSIS

During the 1970s, considerable concern was expressed at the possible transmission of blood diseases as a result of skin piercing activities. Although this concern was initially associated with the spread of the hepatitis virus, the growing awareness of the dangers of AIDS and HIV made the control of these potentially dangerous activities essential.

Health and safety aspects

General duties are placed on operators of these businesses by the Health and Safety at Work, Etc. Act 1974 to conduct their operations in ways which are, as far as reasonably practicable, safe

and healthy, and do not put staff or customers at risk. Cosmetic and therapeutic skin piercing when not carried out under medical control and supervision, is allocated to local authorities for enforcement of the Act. Where a peripatetic practioner carries out work in a client's private home, this is the responsibility of the Health and Safety Executive.

Adoptive powers

Many local authorities, however, feel that the detailed duties in the codes of practice and byelaws made under Part VIII of the Local Government (Miscellaneous Provisions) Act 1982 are more beneficial, and use these specific powers.

The powers are adoptive, and district and London borough councils are able to choose the provisions they wish to apply within their areas.

Acupuncture and tattooing, ear piercing and electrolysis are treated separately for the purpose of making a resolution to adopt the powers, and local authorities may resolve that any of these activities be controlled, or that different ones be controlled, from different dates. Provision is made for adequate publicity before a resolution takes effect. Acupuncture is not defined in the Act but is generally taken as meaning 'the insertion of needles into living tissue for remedial purposes'. Tattooing is referred to in the Tattooing of Minors Act 1969 as 'the insertion into the skin of any colouring material designed to leave a permanent mark'.

Registration

The effect of passing a resolution is to require the registration of persons undertaking skin piercing activities, unless the activities are undertaken by a registered medical practitioner or a dentist. Premises must also be registered. Where a person travels offering skin piercing services, the person's home must be registered.

There are no transitional periods for the benefit of existing traders. Existing traders, therefore, must ensure that they register early, and local authorities must ensure that they are able to process these applications before their resolution takes effect.

Registration cannot be refused, but where a previous registration has been cancelled by a magistrates' court as a result of a conviction for an offence under the local authority's bye-laws, the court's consent must be obtained before a person can be re-registered. The registration certificate issued and a copy of the bye-laws must be displayed prominently on the premises, and a reasonable fee is payable to the local authority for registration. Failure to display the registration certificate or bye-laws is an offence.

Offences

It is an offence punishable by a fine to level 3 to carry on any of the skin piercing activities unregistered. A similar fine is possible for a contravention of bye-laws. A court can also suspend or cancel a registration by order instead of, or in addition to, levying a fine.

Bye-laws

Model bye-laws have been produced by the Department of the Environment and the Welsh Office and are used as a basis for councils to adopt. They contain provisions to secure the cleanliness of premises, sterilization of instruments and hygiene of the practitioners. Codes of practice are also drawn up by most councils to assist practitioners in complying with their bye-laws. Most codes are derived from *A Guide to Hygienic Skin Piercing* by Norman D. Noah MB MRCP MFCM and published in 1983 by the PHLS Communicable Disease Surveillance Centre, Colindale (ISBN 0-901144-10-X).

The British Acupuncture Association, the Traditional Acupuncture Society and the Register of Oriental Medicine have also produced codes of practice.

Guidance has been given to local authorities on the risk of infection from skin piercing activities by the Health and Safety Executive in an advisory circular, LAC(T) 5.6.1 *Risk of Infection from Skin Piercing Activities*.

PUBLIC ENTERTAINMENT LICENCES

Purpose of licensing

The objective of this regime is to ensure that such events are adequately controlled, that there is proper hygiene and safety and that nuisance is avoided.

Licences for music and dancing

The Local Government (Miscellaneous Provisions) Act 1982 provides that public dancing, music or other public entertainment of a like kind can only be provided under the terms of a licence. Any person providing such an entertainment without a licence is liable to a fine of £20 000 and/or imprisonment for up to 6 months, and there are punitive measures for breaches in the terms, conditions and restrictions of a licence of a fine of up to level 5 and/or imprisonment of up to 3 months (The Entertainments (Increased Penalties) Act 1990).

There are exceptions to the licensing requirement in respect of music in places of worship, at religious meetings, at pleasure fairs and at entertainments held in the open air, unless the local authority has adopted the provisions relating to outdoor entertainments.

Licences can be granted for one or more occasions and relate to the entertainment, rather than the premises. Licences are required for either live or recorded music (although in the latter case there is no requirement for a licence in premises licensed for the sale of intoxicating liquor), or whether the entertainment is by the public or by a performer.

Private entertainment

Care must be made to distinguish between public entertainment, which requires a licence, and private entertainment which does not under these provisions. It will be a matter of fact and degree in each case as to whether entertainments are private or public, and this is not always an easy decision to make. There is, however, guidance in Home Office Circular 95/84 and from a number of decided cases. The test set out in the case of *Allen v. Emerson* [1944] KB 362 [1944] 1 A11 ER 344 DC gives guidance 'where public entertainment will be provided in a place open to members of the public without discrimination who desire to be entertained and where means of entertainment are provided'. There is no reference to payment, as payment for admission is immaterial to a person's status as a member of the public. Where a charge is made, the above judgement can be considered in the light of the test in *Gardner v. Morris*: 'it is not whether one or two (or any particular number) members of the public are present but whether on the evidence, any reputable member of the public, on paying for admission could come in'. (1961 59 LGR 1987 and *Frailing* v. *Messenger* 1867 31 JP 423.)

Bona fide guests of members of clubs are not regarded as members of the public. (*Severn View Social Club and Institute Ltd* v. *Chepstow Licensing JJ* (1968) 1 WLR 1512.)

However, the device of becoming a member of a 'club' merely on the immediate payment of a fee and completion of an application form has been discredited (see *Panama (Picadilly) Ltd.*, v. *Newberry* (1962) 1.WLR. 610)

The Home Office view is that it is likely that events will be required to be licensed if large numbers of people are able to gain admission simply upon payment of the required fee. This view was upheld in the High Court in the case of *Lunn* v. *Colston-Hayter* (Times Law Reports 28 Feb. 91).

Premises available to the general public, such as a function room in a public house, when used for a private purpose, e.g. a wedding reception, would not fall to be licensed on that occasion.

For information on the licensing of private places of entertainment see the note on page 183.

Licenses for sporting events

The second category of entertainment for which a licence is required consists of, or includes, any public contest, exhibition or display of boxing wrestling, judo, karate or similar sport. There are exceptions to this requirement for these entertainments when held at pleasure fairs, and when taking place wholly or mainly in the open air. The Fire Safety and Safety at Places of Sport Act 1987 requires a licence for indoor sporting events which the public attends. Sports entertainment at sports complexes also requires a licence.

Musical entertainment in the open air

The third category applies to any public musical entertainment held wholly, or mainly, in the open air and on private land. There are exemptions for events such as fetes etc. This requirement relates to open-air pop festivals (see below) and other open air entertainments in which music is a substantial ingredient. This control is adoptive and the procedure requires publicity following the appropriate resolution with the provisions becoming effective from the date specified in the council resolution.

Application for licences

Schedule 1 of the 1982 Act contains detailed provisions as to the procedure for applying for licences and the powers of local authorities to impose conditions.

The procedure for making an application is found in paragraph 6 of Schedule 1 of the Act. Applications for the grant, renewal or transfer require the applicant to give 28 days' notice to the local authority, chief police officer and fire authority. Where the required notice has not been given, the local authority has some discretion to consider it, but a pre-requisite to this is that consultation takes place with the fire authority and chief officer of police. Applicants must furnish such particulars and give notice as the local authority may prescribe by regulations.

Subject to limited exceptions, a reasonable fee must be paid and the amount is at the discretion of the local authority. However, the fee must not be arbitrary, unreasonable and improper and should not exceed the cost of administration of the licensing system. The exceptions relate to licences for buildings occupied in connection with places of worship and for village, parish or community halls and similar buildings. The local authority may also remit the fee where the entertainment is of an educational, charitable or similar purpose.

Licence conditions

Licences are issued subject to standard conditions prescribed by regulations made by the licensing authority. Every licence then granted, renewed or transferred is presumed to have been issued subject to these conditions unless they have been expressly excluded or varied. It is open to the holder of a licence to apply for conditions to be varied. When attaching conditions, it should be borne in mind that these must relate to safety, health and the prevention of nuisance.

The hours of opening are best controlled by special conditions as hours of opening are linked closely with liquor laws.

There is a limit on the conditions that may be attached to a licence for an outdoor entertainment. These relate to the safety of those present, provision of access for emergency vehicles, the provision of adequate sanitary appliances and the prevention of noise nuisance. (HSE Guidance Notes GS50 and IND(G)102L.)

Provisional licences

A good feature of the 1982 Act is that it permits the issue of provisional licences, subject to confirmation, for premises about to be constructed, or under construction or alteration. This is useful for those engaged in elaborate or costly proposals, as it gives an early indication of whether or not the project is likely to receive a licence.

Consultation

When considering an application, the licensing authority is required to consider the observations submitted by the chief officer of police and the fire authority. Conditions adopted by many local authorities also require public notices of application to be given. It appears, however, that no other person has a right of objection, although any observations made would be considered.

Although no guidance is given in the 1982 Act as to the hearing of objections when they are made, the applicant should be informed of the nature of the objections so that he or she can respond. In these situations, procedures for dealing with applications must be considered carefully or they will lead to appeals against licensing authority decisions. All applications must be dealt with in accordance with terms of natural justice, though in many cases an oral hearing will not be necessary and can be dealt with by written representation only. If an oral hearing is arranged it is wise for objectors to state their case first.

Offences

Where entertainments are provided without the necessary licence or in contravention to the terms, conditions or restrictions of a licence an offence is committed. The only statutory defences are to prove that due diligence had been exercised, that all reasonable precautions had been taken or that a special order of exemption is in force under section 74(4) of the Licensing Act 1964. These orders automatically override any conditions as to permitted hours. An investigation of a breach of hours in licensed premises should therefore include a check on whether a special order of exemption is in force.

Public conveniences at places of entertainment

Certain local authorities are empowered to require sanitary facilities to be made available for public use in 'relevant' places (see below) by S20 Local Government (Miscellaneous Provisions) Act 1976. The requirement by written notice can be occasional – for such occasion specified in the notice – or provided for continuing use. There is only a right of appeal against the latter, although unreasonable requirements under the former may be challenged in any prosecution for non-compliance.

Relevant place means any of the following places:–

1. A place which is normally used or is proposed to be normally used for any of the following purposes, namely:–
   (a) the holding of any entertainment, exhibition or sporting event to which members of the public are admitted, either as spectators or otherwise;

(b) the sale of food or drink to members of the public for consumption at the place:–
2. A place which is used on some occasion or occasions or proposed to be used on some occasion or occasions for any of the purposes aforesaid.
3. A betting office.

A duty is imposed to have regard to the needs of disabled persons when complying with a notice. There may be some overlap with the requirements of some licensing procedures.

Pay parties*

In view of the dangers to the public and the nuisance caused by so called 'pay parties', the Entertainments (Increased Penalties) Act 1990 raised the penalties for the use of premises for which no licence was in force, or for contravention of the terms and conditions of a licence imposing a limit on the number of people who may be present at the entertainment to a £20 000 fine or 6 months' imprisonment. The Criminal Justices Act 1988 (Confiscation Orders) Order 1990 gives magistrates the power to order the confiscation of the proceeds, where these exceed £10 000, made by people convicted of these offences.

'Pay Parties' is the most commonly used generic name given to these events, the different names given to the various types of pay party reflecting both the size and venue of the event:

1. Acid House Party, Dance Parties, Raves and Warehouse Parties.
2. The smallest pay parties often held in domestic premises are called 'Blues Parties' or 'Shebeens'.

(See Joint Home Office and Department of the Environment Guidance booklet 'Control of Noisy Parties' September 1992.)

Powers of entry

There is a provision in the 1982 Act for the entry of places of entertainment by the police, or by authorized officers of the licensing authority and the fire authority, for enforcement of the licence. Proceedings for alleged breaches of the Schedule may be instituted by any person and there is no limitation in the Act.

Revocation

If convicted of an offence under the Act, the licence may be revoked. The principles of natural justice apply, and the holder of a licence should, even though convicted of an offence, have an opportunity to state his or her case. There is a right of appeal against any adverse decision of a licensing authority, but the holder of a licence is not bound to implement the decision until either the 21 day appeal period has passed or the appeal has been determined. The appeal period cannot be extended. The procedure for an appeal is given in section 34 of the Magistrates' Courts Rules of 1981. Appeals are by way of re-hearing and the appellate court is entitled to substitute its own opinion as to the fact or merits of the case. (It would no doubt give some consideration to the fact that the original decision has been made by an elected representative body.) As the magistrates' court can only summons those against whom it can make an order, only the licensing authority can be summoned to appear. If observations or objections were considered in arriving at a decision, it would be for the licensing authority to bring evidence of these before the magistrates' court.

An appeal against the decision of the magistrates' court may be brought to the crown court with 21 days, but in this case there is provision to extend this time for giving notice of appeal.

The Private Places of Entertainment (Licensing) Act 1967

In areas where this Act has been adopted, private dancing, music or other entertainments of a like kind, which are promoted for private gain, must also be licensed. A definition of 'private gain' is found in the London Local Authorities Act 1991.

---

* Sections 63–67 of the Criminal Justice and Public Order Act 1994 give the police new powers to deal with 'raves' (a gathering of 100 or more people at which amplified music is played at night and which is likely to cause serious distress to inhabitants). These powers include the removal of people attending and seizure of sound equipment.

The Act is an adoptive one and therefore only applies if the appropriate authority – district councils, the London boroughs or the council for the Isles of Scilly – so resolve. The procedure for adopting the Act, together with the requirements as to publicity, etc., are laid down in Part II of the Schedule to the Act, and the powers available enable control of events involving music and dancing including 'pay parties'.

When licences are granted, they can be made subject to terms, conditions or restrictions imposed by the licensing authority. This may include conditions providing power of entry to private premises for which generally there is no right of entry. Those also applicable to public entertainments will usually be equally relevant.

Enforcement provisions are identical to the provisions found in the Local Government (Miscellaneous Provisions) Act 1982, in respect of public entertainment and, as with that Act, any person may prosecute for the breaches defined in section 4 of the Act.

Investigations into alleged contraventions of this Act need care and the procedures of the Police and Criminal Evidence Act 1984 must be followed.

When licences are refused, appeals to a magistrates' court are available and the appeal is in the form of a re-hearing of the application.

Private parties not for gain

In the case of private parties which are not held for gain and do not come within the scope of licensing legislation, the powers available to local authorities are restricted solely to the noise nuisance abatement powers of Part III of the Environmental Protection Act 1990. This includes the power under section 81[5] to seek a High Court injunction if the Authority considers that summoning proceedings would provide an inadequate remedy (see Chapter 7).

POP FESTIVALS

Background

These often accommodate in excess of 100 000 people and employ many hundreds of staff and comprise a major sector of the leisure industry.

Guide to Health, Safety and Welfare at Pop Festivals and Similar Events [5]

This 1993 guide indicates the key points in the planning and arrangement of a pop concert. Advice is given on health and safety, fire and emergency planning and venue facilities.

Legislative controls

Under the Local Government (Miscellaneous Provisions) Act 1982a local authorities may adopt the controls for public musical entertainments taking place wholly, or mainly, in the open air and on private land. These were included specifically to control pop festivals. Whether the particular festival has the requisite degree of music, giving rise to a need for a licence, and whether it is a public or private entertainment, must be determined for these controls to be relevant.

Licence conditions can be imposed in the interest of the health and safety limited to securing:

1. the safety of performers and other persons present;
2. adequate access for emergency vehicles;
3. the provision of adequate sanitary accommodation;
4. preventing neighbourhood disturbance by noise.

The law of nuisance (see Chapter 8) also provides a broad and powerful restriction on any kind of potentially intrusive activity. With the approval of the attorney general, local authorities or individuals who have reason to feel unhappy at the prospect of a pop festival (or indeed of any large gathering) can take the matter to the High Court and, if they can prove a likelihood of substantial and unreasonable interference to the community, they will obtain an injunction. This will effectively put the promoter at risk of proceedings for contempt of court if a nuisance is caused as a result of the pop festival. (Such action has been taken successfully by Windsor and Maidenhead BC and Newbury DC in relation to 'pay parties').

Although the law of nuisance is not a very flexible means of control, it can give local authorities a very effective negotiating weapon.

The essence of a nuisance is a condition or activity which unduly interferes with the use or enjoyment of land. This has been applied to a number of cases involving the congregation of crowds and in the case of *A.G.* v. *Great Western Festivals Ltd.* (unreported) to pop festivals in particular. The features of a pop festivals which might amount to a nuisance include noise, trespass and damage to adjoining property, traffic congestion and pollution by litter. The normal remedy for a nuisance is an action for an injunction. For temporary events, such as pop festivals, it will usually have to be a *quia timet* injunction – one granted before an event on the basis of evidence showing a strong possibility that a nuisance will occur.

The Noise at Work Regulations 1989 will also apply to persons at work at the pop festival.

The general duties of the Health and Safety at Work, Etc. Act 1974 will also apply, including the management of Health and Safety at Work Regulations 1992 (see Chapter 25) and these powers may prove useful in dealing with the many other hazards, such as laser equipment, disco lighting and pyrotechnics encountered on the site.

Other legislation such as the Theatres Act, the Cinemas Act and the Building Regulations may also be relevant.

Forward planning

To ensure the success of any large pop festival, it is essential that planning starts at least 6 months before the event, that sufficient funds are available to invest in the event, and that an efficient back-up organization and management policy is established. It will, therefore, be necessary to set up a working party composed of the promoters, local authority, police and fire officers and representatives of voluntary organizations at an early stage.

Many of the faults and failures of festivals in relation to matters which are the concern of the local authorities have arisen, not only through a lack of co-operation between promoters and local authorities, but also through not allowing the time for such co-operation to be really effective. The prime responsibility rests with the promoters. It remains, however, a major responsibility of a local authority to create conditions under which such co-operation is possible.

In the initial stages, the local authority should be concerned with the location and suitability of the site, estimated attendance figures, legal and financial implications, and all of the possible public health problems. Standards must be identified and met and the necessary safeguards observed.

If local legislation requires an application to be made for a public entertainment licence, this should be made clear to the promoters, who may then take the appropriate action in good time.

Sites vary from fields to theatres to sports stadia – and even on occasions lakes and rivers. The choice of site, therefore, has a direct bearing on the standards which will need to be applied.

Prediction of numbers

It is not possible to plan for a pop festival without a reasonable idea as to the numbers expected to attend. Prediction of numbers is undeniably a difficult task, particularly for those with little experience of pop festivals.

Standards

Attention needs to be paid to the following issues all of which are dealt with in the Guide:

1. crowd safety;
2. structural stability of stages, etc.;
3. protection of water sources;
4. refuse and litter;
5. food safety;
6. washing facilities (one for every five sanitary conveniences);
7. drainage;
8. pest control;
9. noise;
10. sanitary accommodation (one closet per 100 females and three closets for every 500 males plus 1.5 m run of urinal per 500 males);
11. access and signs for disabled people;

12. fire prevention and fighting (also see *Guide to Fire Precautions in Existing Places of Entertainment and Live Premises* (1990) HMSO, ISBN 0.11.340907.9);
13. power supply;
14. medical services;
15. security;
16. management of site and stage.

Other outdoor events

A Code of Practice for Outdoor Events [6] provides guidance on safety management at outdoor shows and meetings. It indicates standards for crowd control and site operations at events ranging from national atheletic meetings to agricultural festivals and car boot sales.

Managing Crowd Safety (IND(6)1426) published by HSE gives guidance on management responsibilites for such events.

SAFETY AT SPORTS GROUNDS

A sports ground is any place where sports or other competitive activities take place in the open air, and where accommodation has been provided for spectators, consisting of artificial structures or of natural structures artificially modified for the purpose (Safety at Sports Grounds Act 1975).

The Wheatly Report, commissioned in 1972 as a result of the Ibrox Park disaster, resulted in the passing of the Safety at Sports Ground Act 1975. The Act requires all designated sports grounds (those in respect of which a designation order is in operation) with a capacity of over 10 000 people to be issued with safety certificates issued by the local authority. This capacity may be changed by order, and can be different for different classes of sports grounds. The Act was considerably extended by provisions contained in the Fire Safety and Safety of Places of Sports Act 1987 giving certifying authorities similar powers in respect of regulated stands, i.e. covered stands with a capacity of 500 or more spectators.

The 1975 and 1987 Acts are administered in London and conurbations by the London borough councils and metropolitan authorities, respectively, and in the rest of England and Wales by county councils. In Scotland, the work is carried out by regional or island councils.

It is the duty of every local authority to enforce the Act and its regulations, and arrange for periodic inspections of designated sports grounds. Powers of entry to, and inspections of, any sports ground for this purpose are provided by section 11 of the 1975 Act.

The Football Spectators Act 1989 was introduced to control admission to designated matches by a membership scheme. It also provides for the safety of spectators by means of licences and safety certificates.

Safety certificates

Safety certificates may only contain conditions to secure safety at the sports ground, and may include a requirement to keep records of attendance and maintenance of safety measures. Before a certificate is issued, the local authority is required to consult the building authority and the chief officer of police.

When determining an application for a safety certificate, it is their duty to determine whether the applicant is a qualified person, that is, one who is likely to be in a position to prevent contravention of the terms and conditions of any certificate issued. The form of application is contained in the Safety of Sports Grounds Regulations 1987 which, among other things, lay down the procedure for making an application under the Act. Safety certificates may be amended either with or without the application of the holder, but amendments must be limited to safety measures. Transfers of certificates are provided for, but the local authority's duty to determine whether the person is a qualified person remains. In both cases, consultation must take place between the chief officer of police, the fire authority and building authority before the local authority amends or transfers the certificate. Any alteration to a sports ground which may affect safety must be notified to the local authority in advance.

If a person is judged by a local authority not to be a qualified person, there is a right of appeal to the magistrates' court as there is against the inclusion or omission of anything from a certificate or a refusal to amend it.

Where a general safety certificate is in force, its provisions take precedence over certain other pieces of legislation which may impose terms and conditions. This may well effect the licence conditions issued in respect of any public entertainments licence.

Prohibition notices

A special procedure is detailed in the Act for dealing with situations where serious risk is posed to spectators, and in that situation local authorities have power to serve prohibition notices which specify the matters giving rise for concern, and restrict or prohibit admission to, or to parts of, a sports ground until matters have been remedied. These notices take effect immediately. A person aggrieved by a prohibition notice may appeal to the magistrates' court against the notice, but in view of the overriding requirement for safety, the bringing of an appeal does not have the effect of suspending it.

Offences

Various offences are detailed in the Act, including contravention of the certificates, and its terms or conditions, etc. These are punishable by fine or summary conviction, or fine and/or imprisonment for not more that 2 years on indictment.

Guidance

Useful guidance on sports ground safety is included in the voluntary code, *Guide to Safety at Sports Grounds* which was issued jointly by the Home Office and the Scottish Home Office and Health Department [7]. Advice is given in this document (which is known as the 'Green Guide') on the construction and layout of grounds, including details of access and egress and ground capacity estimation, terracing, barriers, stands, etc., as well as for other matters covered by a certificate. The third edition in 1990 incorporated lessons from the Hillsborough, Sheffield tragedy in

1989 and the Bradford City fire in 1985. Its recommendations may be put into statutory form by inclusion in Safety Certificates. The information contained in the guide is especially applicable to football grounds, but the advice is also of use in dealing with a variety of sporting events at grounds where the gathering of crowds may present a safety problem.

Toilet facilities at stadia

Published by the Sports Council in association with the Football Trust in 1994 this guide offers advice on evaluating existing toilet facilities, improving standards, and choice of equipment for new installations. It applies to rugby and hockey stadia, as well as to football grounds.

Specific guidance is given on planning, location and access, design of toilet areas, fittings and materials, and provision of toilets for family areas, disabled spectators, non-spectator use, and portable toilets. The section on design recommends that before finalizing any designs which omit doors or lobbies to toilet areas, the local environmental health officers should be consulted.

A chapter is devoted to the subject of the ratio of toilets to the number of male and female spectators – the guide makes the following minimum recommendations for newly constructed or refurbished stadia and stands, per accessible area:

	Urinals:	WCs:	Wash hand basins:
Male	1 per 70 males	1 per 600 males, but minimum of 2 per toilet area	1 per 300 males, but minimum of 2 per toilet area
Female	—	1 per 35 females, but minimum of 2 per toilet area	1 per 70 females, but minimum of 2 per toilet area

Copies of the guide are available, price £12.50, from: Publications Department, The Sports Council, 16 Upper Woburn Place, London WC1H 0QP, ISBN 1 873831 40 4.

Indoor sporting events

Safety at indoor sporting events is controlled by the public entertainments licence procedure detailed in Schedule 1 of the Local Government (Miscellaneous Provisions) Act 1982 (see page 181). These are not covered by the Safety at Sports Ground Act 1975.

Health and safety enforcement

Responsibility for enforcing the Health and Safety at Work, Etc. Act 1974 in sports grounds falls to local authorities (unless they are sports grounds under the control of local authorities). However, because there are overlapping responsibilities relating to safety of sporting events at sports grounds, there is a need for liaison between the various authorities involved. It is the Health and Safety Commission's policy that the provisions of the 1974 Act should not generally be enforced if public safety is adequately covered by enforcement of the specific legislation in the 1975 Act. In cases of an urgent threat to life or injury, however, the use of the Act's powers would not be precluded if they could eliminate the risk or reduce it.

CINEMAS

Legislation

The main piece of legislation concerning the exhibition of films is the Cinemas Act 1985, which consolidates the Cinematograph Acts of 1905 and 1952, the Cinematographic (Amendment) Act 1982 and related enactments. This Act made no change to the previous law except that, on the recommendation of the law Commission, it amended provisions derived from the Sunday Entertainments Act 1937 so as to extend the exemption from the Sunday Observance Act 1780 to cover exhibitions produced by means of videos.

Licences

Subject to certain exemptions film exhibitions may only be given in premises which have been licensed by the local authority in which they are situated. Before the consolidating legislation was passed, licensing control related to exhibitions of 'moving pictures' produced on a screen by means which include the projection of light. This definition was not flexible enough to encompass changes in modern technology, and did not include video exhibitions which are transmitted by signal. While control now extends to videos shown in clubs and pubs, it does not extend to exhibitions of moving pictures arising out of the playing of video games and, therefore, places such as amusement arcades and public houses do not require to be licensed under this legislation.

Licence conditions

The granting of a licence is discretionary and, subject to regulations made under the Act, licensing authorities may impose terms and conditions on the licence. The terms and conditions which may be imposed are not limited to those for securing safety but, when imposed, the test to be applied is that they should be reasonable and in the public interest. Subject to these restrictions, there is no fetter upon the power of the licensing authority. Model licensing conditions are detailed in Home Office Circulars No. 150/1955 and 63/1990.

The London Inter-borough Entertainments Working Party has also produced their own set of rules relating to the showing of films for inclusion in licences issued under the Cinemas Act.

Film exhibitions for children

When granting a licence, the licensing authority has a duty to impose conditions or restrictions prohibiting the admission of children to film exhibitions involving the showing of works designated unsuitable for them. The familiar classification of films is not based on statute, but is undertaken by a body known as the British Board of Film Classification. Their system of classification, the object of which is principally to indicate which films are considered suitable for the viewing by children, has been adopted by local authorities. For the classification of films by the Board see Home Office Circular No. 98/1982 and 63/1990.

Any film exhibition organized wholly or mainly for children requires the consent of the licensing authority and in these circumstances they can impose special conditions or restrictions. A statutory obligation to provide for the safety of children's entertainments is contained in the Children and Young Person's Act 1933.

Applications for licences

When applying for a licence, or for its renewal or transfer the applicant must give 28 days' clear notice of intention to the licensing authority, the fire authority, and the chief officer of police. When the requisite notice has not been given, the licensing authority can still grant a licence, but only after consultation with the other two authorities. (The mere sending of a letter does not constitute consultation). Licences are granted for periods of up to 12 months. Fees for licences may be fixed by the licensing authority, but they must not exceed the sum stipulated in the Fees for Cinema Licences (Variation) Order 1986. These are currently set at £173 in the case of a grant or renewal for 1 year, and in the case of a grant or renewal for any less period £58 for each month for which a licence is granted or renewed, but in this case the aggregate of the fees paid in any year is not permitted to exceed £173. The maximum fee for a transfer of licence is £35. These figures can be amended by order of the Secretary of State. (Useful advice on fees is contained in Association of District Council's Circular 1986/119.)

Regulations

Section 4 of the Act requires film exhibitions to comply with regulations made by the Secretary of State. To date no regulations have been made but, by virtue of the Interpretation Act 1978, the Cinematograph (Safety) Regulations 1955 as amended, and the Cinematograph (Children) No. 2 Regulations 1955 have effect.

Exemptions

Certain exhibitions are exempted from the requirement to obtain a licence. These include exhibitions in private dwellinghouses where the public are not admitted and where there is no private gain, or where the sole or main purpose is to demonstrate or advertise products, goods or services or to provide information, education or instruction.

Where the public are not admitted, or admitted without payment, or the exhibitions are given by an exempted organization and conditions regarding private gain etc., as above, are fulfilled, no licence is required. Exempted organizations are defined in relation to a certificate given by the Secretary of State. This exemption does not apply to certain exhibitions for children as members of a club, the principal object of which is attendance at film exhibitions, unless in a private house or as part of the activities of an educational or religious institution, or to exempted organizations in cases where the premises are used for an exhibition for more than 3 days out of the last 7 days.

It is not necessary to obtain a licence when premises are not used for more than 6 days in a year, and where film exhibitions are held occasionally and exceptionally, and the occupier has given at least 7 days' notice in writing to the fire authority and the chief officer of police, and he or she complies with any regulations of conditions imposed by the licensing authority and notified to him or her in writing. Strictly speaking, licences are required where film exhibitions take place in premises on a regular basis, even if less than six times per year, as the use would not be exceptional, but many authorities do not require a licence in these circumstances.

Film exhibitions which take place in buildings or structures of a movable character only need to be licensed (by the licensing authority where the owner normally resides) where he or she has given at least two days notice to the fire authority and the chief officer or police, and he or she complies with any conditions imposed by the authority in writing.

Sunday opening

The Sunday Observance Act 1780 is not contravened by staging film exhibitions on a Sunday, but a licensing authority is entitled to impose conditions, including those aimed at preventing employment, where a person has been employed for the previous 6 days. There are exceptions to this restriction in cases of emergency notified to the licensing authority where a rest day is given in lieu and where an employer has, on making due enquiry, reasonable grounds for believing that a person has not been employed for the earlier 6 days.

Offences

Where premises are used without a licence or consent (in respect of children) or where terms, conditions or restrictions are contravened, those responsible for the organization or management, as well as the licence holder, are guilty of an offence. A maximum fine of £20 000 is stipulated for operating without a licence, and in other cases level 5 on the standard scale. In addition, a court can order the forfeiture of anything produced to the court relating to the offence, as long as the owner has been given an opportunity of appearing to show cause why it should not.

If the owner of a licence is convicted of an offence as stipulated in section 10 of the Act, or failed to provide for the safety of children, the licensing authority may revoke his or her licence.

Power of entry

Right of entry to inspect premises to see whether the relevant provisions are being complied with is given to constables and authorized officers of licensing and fire authorities. Inspections by the fire authority to check on fire precautions, however, require 24 hours' notice. When authorized by warrant, constables or authorized officers of the licensing authority can enter and search premises when they have cause to believe that an offence has been, is being, or is about to be committed. This power is subject to the restrictions of section 9 of the Police and Criminal Evidence Act 1984, and authorized officers must produce authority when requested. Any person who intentionally obstructs an officer is liable on summary conviction to a fine not exceeding level 3 of the standard scale.

A constable or authorized officer who enters and searches any premises under the authority of a warrant issued under section 13 above, may seize and remove apparatus or equipment, etc. which her or she believes may be forfeited under section 11.

Appeals

A person may appeal to the crown court against a refusal or revocation of a licence or terms, conditions or restrictions subject to which a licence is granted as he or she may against the refusal to renew or transfer a licence. Appeals in Scotland are to the sheriff's court. Refusals in England and Wales in relation to Sunday opening and any conditions in that respect are to the crown court. Where a licence has been revoked, it remains in force until the determination or the abandonment of the appeal or, if successful, it is renewed or transferred.

Local authorities in Greater London have powers to vary licences and grant provisional licences, but other authorities have no power to grant a licence except in respect of premises actually in existence.

Where introductory music is played at any premises, or is featured in an interval or at the conclusion of a show, it is considered part of the exhibition provided the total time taken amounts to less than one-quarter of the time taken by the film exhibition. A Public Entertainment Licence is therefore not required.

Video juke boxes

Commercial premises which promote cinematographic exhibitions (video juke boxes) as a means of attracting custom come within the Act's control. It is not necessary for a charge to be made for admission for a licence to be required if the exhibitions were advertised and the sums paid for the facilities or services are for private gain. Additional requirements in respect of television exhibitions in Part 4 of the Cinematographic (Safety) Regulations 1955 have to be complied with.

Health and safety enforcement

Responsibility for enforcement of the provision of the Health and Safety at Work, Etc. Act 1974 in cinemas lies with local authorities. However, where the main purpose of a cinema premises is for educational or vocational training, similar to that provided in the mainstream education system, such premises will be the responsibility of the Health and Safety Executive.

THEATRES

Generally speaking, any premises used for the public performance of plays is required to be licensed. The only exceptions to this arise in respect of buildings under the control of the armed forces or in buildings known as 'patent theatres' where the performance may take place by virtue of 'letters patent'. Licence authorities are the London boroughs and district councils elsewhere.

The law relating to theatres was formerly embodied in the Theatres Act 1843 and, at this time, this piece of legislation gave the Lord Chamberlain powers of absolute censorship over the presentation of any stage play. To assist in this measure, copies of every new stage play were required to be submitted to him. In these early days, theatre going was something of a hazardous affair and the records show that in 1884 alone it was calculated that, worldwide, 41 theatres were burned down involving the death of over 1200 people. From these tragedies, lessons were learned and there followed important decisions and action regarding public safety, fire precautions and fire-fighting. The Public Health (Amendment) Act of 1890 enforced stricter fire regulations, but within a few years there followed demands that all theatre planning should be subject to municipal or state control. It was not until the Theatres Act 1968, however, that this legislation was repealed and the role of the Lord Chamberlain in respect of censorship was abolished. Copies of scripts of all new plays are now sent to the British Museum. The censorship measures were replaced by provisions for the prevention of obscene performances vested in the courts, rather than by adminstrative or executive action.

Licences

When considering the need for a licence, the term 'play' is usually taken to mean any dramatic piece – whether improvized or not – by one or more persons who are actually present and performing. What the performers do, whether it consists of speech, singing or action, must constitute the whole or a major part of a performance and involve the playing of a role. For example, a dialogue between persons in costume or action without words may constitute a dramatic piece. Ballets, whether they fall within the above definitions or not, do require a theatre licence, but theatre licences do not cover public music or dancing events. Where, however, the music is incidental to a play, or it takes place in the interval, or the music and dancing forms part of a musical comedy, a public entertainment licence is not required. It is not unusual for a building to hold both licences.

Full licences are granted for periods of up to 1 year, but there is also provision to grant a licence in respect of one or more occasions (an occasional stage play licence).

When a full licence is applied for, the licensing authority and chief officer of police in whose area the premises are situated, must be given at least 21 days' notice of intention to make application. The information to be given with an application must be in accordance with regulations prescribed by a licensing authority. An application for a renewal of a licence must give at least 28 days' notice of intention. Where, however, the application is for one or more particular occasions, only 14 days' notice is required to be given, and there is, in this instance, no obligation to inform the chief officer of police.

Appeals

Where a licensing authority refuses a licence, there is a right of appeal to a magistrates' court by way of complaint for an order, and the licensing authority will be a defendant. Although the chief officer of police has to be notified of an application, he or she is not party to appeal proceedings, even if the decision to refuse a licence was made after considering his or her recommendations to do so. There is no right of appeal against a licensing authority decision to issue a licence. Persons aggrieved by a decision of a magistrates' court may appeal to the crown court. When granting a licence, a licensing authority may impose conditions and restrictions, but they must act judicially in doing so, and the restrictions which the licensing authority are empowered to make are strictly controlled. They relate in the main to matters of health and safety, and do not extend to restrictions on the nature of plays or the manner of the performance.

Licence conditions

It is worth emphasizing that conditions which can be imposed by a licensing authority when granting, renewing or transferring a licence are strictly limited to protecting physical safety and health. This is usually achieved by adopting local conditions which are principally aimed at providing a safe means of escape. This is achieved by providing an escape route which allows normal people to get out from a theatre after an outbreak of fire to a place of safety by their own efforts, without being placed in jeopardy while doing so. In addition, the conditions will require a sufficient number of well located exits with adequate lighting and direction signs throughout. Equipment and areas of potential hazard are required to be protected and an efficient exit drill procedure to ensure orderly exit is essential.

In addition to these physical requirements, control of psychological factors conducive to panic need to be addressed and alarm procedures should reflect this. Fire escape drills are helpful, but it should be borne in mind that in a building whose occupants are transient may be of limited value unless permanent staff are trained to help the temporary occupants. This is usually reflected in a requirement for the provision of adequate stewards or attendants. These requirements are even more vital in situations when an audience consists mainly of children, and it is not unusual

for theatrical performances to which section 12 of the Children and Young Persons Act 1937 applies to provide increased numbers of stewards. It is essential to liaise with the fire and rescue services when considering these aspects of a theatre licence. As to the provisions of exits, entrances, etc., see also the Public Health Act 1936, section 59 for further powers.

Conditions related to health include the provision of adequate ventilation, the prevention of overcrowding and the provision of adequate sanitary accommodation and washing facilities, including facilities for the use of disabled persons. Guidance on this may be found in the British Standard 6465: Part 1: 1984 Sanitary Installations, and powers for requiring it are contained in section 20 of the Local Government (Miscellaneous Provisions) Act 1976.

In older, purpose-built theatres, it is not unusual to find large spans of unsupported ceilings, often decorated with ornate plaster mouldings. In these circumstances, conditions often require the regular inspection of these features and the provision of certificates of safety. For further advice on the safety of ceilings and the responsibility of licensing authorities, see Home Office Circular No. 264/1947.

Relationship to liquor licences

When a theatre licence is granted, the licensee acquires the right to sell intoxicating liquor if he or she notifies the clerk to the licensing justices of his or her intention to do so, unless the licensing authority has issued the licence subject to restrictions prohibiting the sale of liquor. When imposing such restrictions, it is important that the local authority considers each application on its merits, for it is not permitted to attach a restriction in pursuance of a general rule.

Where liquor is permitted to be sold by virtue of a theatre licence, the provisions of the Licensing Act 1964 apply, and it is therefore only permitted to be sold during the ordinary permitted hours applicable to licensed premises. A condition can be imposed by the licensing authority, however, limiting the sale of liquor to the times when the premises are used as a theatre. If such a condition is not imposed, the theatre can also sell liquor when it is not in use as a theatre, including days such as Sundays, Christmas Day and Good Friday, when no performances take place. Extensions of the permitted hours as in other licensed premises is not permitted.

Fees

The person applying for the grant, renewal or transfer of a licence must pay the licensing authority a reasonable fee. This requirement is waived in respect of occasional licences if the performance is of an educational or like character, or is to be performed for a charitable or other like purpose.

Provisional licences

As with many other forms of licensing, it is possible to grant a provisional licence where premises are under construction or alteration. In such circumstances, a provisional licence may be issued if the licensing authority is satisfied that the completed premises would be in accordance with its requirements. A licence will be granted subject to conditions that it would be of no effect until confirmed.

Sunday performances

By virtue of section 1 of the Sunday Theatre Act 1972 licensed theatres are permitted to open on Sundays, despite the prohibition contained in the Sunday Observance Act 1780. Theatres are, however, required to be closed by 2 am (3 am in Inner London) after Saturday night performances and must remain closed until 2 pm.

Offences

It is an offence to use unlicensed premises and any person concerned in the organization or management of a performance is liable, on summary conviction, to a fine of up to level 4 on the standard scale, or imprisonment for 3 months, or both. A similar penalty is available for the breach of the licence conditions, and in this instance a licence can be revoked. Fines of up to £1000 and up to 6 months' imprisonment can be imposed for presenting or directing obscene plays, and those that incite racial hatred or provoke a breach of the peace by the use of threatening, abusive or insulting words. In the case of the latter offence, proceedings can only be authorized with the consent of the attorney general.

Authorized officers of licensing authorities have certain powers of entry, and wilful obstruction of an officer is an offence.

It should be noted that, in many instances, the law concerning the licensing of theatres is also contained in local Acts which may supplement, modify or supersede the general law.

Health and safety enforcement

Enforcement of the provisions of the Health and Safety at Work, Etc. Act 1974 in theatre premises is reserved to the Health and Safety Executive but may be transferred to the local authority by local agreement.

DEALING WITH LICENSING APPLICATIONS

Although most routine matters relating to licensing administration are delegated to officers of a council, decisions on whether or not to grant licences are usually dealt with by a committee. It is important that sound administrative procedures in accordance with the rules of 'natural justice' are followed to avoid procedural difficulties at later stages.

Committee hearings of licensing application are generally more informal than court hearings as the rules as to evidence do not apply and it is not given under oath. Nonetheless, the committee must endeavour to ensure that fair and orderly hearings take place and that applicants are given the opportunity of being heard before applications are refused, even if not expressly required by the law. An applicant should be permitted to be accompanied by a legal or other representative if desired and as much notice of the hearing as is practicable should be given, in order to enable him to prepare his case adequately.

Similarly, any body or person wishing to make representations in respect of an application should also be given the opportunity of appearing before the committee.

It is important that committee members are given copies of every document. It is also desirable for the applicant to be informed of the nature of any objections to the application so that he can respond to them.

Whilst local variations to procedure will exist there are certain elements which should be followed:

1. Those present should identify themselves and the chairman of the meeting should ascertain whether the applicant, if unaccompanied, was aware that he could be represented.
2. The chairman or appropriate officer of the council should open the hearing with an outline of the relevant details of the application.
3. The applicant be invited to present his case, following which he may be questioned by members of the committee. Persons who have made representations may also be afforded this opportunity.
4. Comments are then invited from the technical officers including the Police and fire authority where present, following which the applicant should be permitted to ask questions of the officers.
5. The applicant should then to allowed to make a final statement. It is vital that the case of any party is prosecuted in the presence of the other and it is essential that all the committee members remain present throughout the hearing.
6. Committee members should confine themselves to asking questions and must not indulge in any discussion of the merits of the case.
7. Any request for adjournment should be granted if refusal would prejudice a fair hearing and deny the applicant natural justice.
8. The applicant, third parties and officers of the council may be asked to withdraw at the end of the hearing to allow the committee to consider the matter. The committee's legal adviser and minutes secretary will remain and if it is

necessary to seek clarification and further advice parties may be recalled.
9. When a decision is reached the parties will be recalled and the decision announced to the applicant, together with an explanation of any conditions which are to be attached or reasons for a refusal. The information is then given in writing as soon as practicable together with details of any rights of appeal.

LIAISON WITH THE LICENSING JUSTICES

Although the administration of Liquor Licensing Legislation in England and Wales is undertaken by the licensing justices this does not preclude environmental health departments from playing a significant part in the process.

The formal system of notification of applications includes the requirement for the proper officer of the district council to be notified. The proper officer is responsible for returning comment on behalf of the council and directors of environmental health, when designated as proper officers, are in an excellent position to coordinate the response and achieve improvements relating to food hygiene and health and safety.

A procedure must be set up to consult each relevant department of the council and coordinate the replies directly to the licensing justices. Where matters are raised it is often the case that an applicant will deal promptly with any deficiencies, or at least give a written undertaking to deal with them within a reasonable timescale, in order to ensure that a liquor licence is granted. If facilities are lacking or substandard and no informal agreement can be obtained it is open to the proper officer to object to the issue of the licence. This will entail a personal appearance at the hearing and so a system of early notification of this course of action to the council's legal representatives should be in place in the internal administrative procedures.

In order to keep the licensing justices informed of environmental health officers' continuing interest in premises which they licence it is useful to send copies to them of any notices of requirements served. It is also useful to keep the licensing justices informed of Public Entertainment Licence decisions as these often also relate to premises having liquor licences in some shape or form.

SWIMMING AND LEISURE POOLS

To obtain the benefits and pleasure which swimming can give, the water of a swimming pool must be fresh and crystal clear, attractive in appearance, and free from harmful and unpleasant bacteria. To achieve these characteristics, the water must be in a state of chemical balance. Only minimum amounts of chemicals should be used if they are not to cause discomfort to the delicate membranes of the bathers' eyes, nose, throat and skin.

The water supplied to pools will often be of varying quality, and therefore it can be seen that, apart from knowledge of the delicate adjustments necessary to maintain the correct balance, some knowledge of the quality of water making up each pool is necessary.

Pool pollution may arise from a variety of sources – dust, hair, body grease and excretions from the nose and throat, for example, collect on the surface of the water (the top 16 cm of water contains 75% of bacterial pollution). Many of the insoluble pollutants, such as dirt, sand from filters and precipitated chemicals, may find their way to the bottom of the pool. In addition, there may be forms of dissolved pollution, such as urine, perspiration and cosmetics, and chemical pollution produced by reaction in the water treatment. While many of these factors are unpleasant and a nuisance, rather than a risk to health, they must all be considered when designing a pool and selecting a water treatment plant. However, the most serious pollution comes from the living organisms introduced by the bathers themselves, and it is this form of pollution that gives rise to a number of unpleasant conditions and diseases, and poses the most serious risk unless the pool is properly controlled and facilities, such as showers and footbaths, are provided to reduce pollution loads. (See Fig. 11.1.)

Standards of operation

Primary responsibility for pool water quality obviously lies with the pool operator, although environmental health officers have a key role, through their enforcement of public health and safety legislation, to ensure pools are maintained in a clean and safe condition. It is therefore essential that operators receive adequate training and knowledge to ensure the correct balance between treatment and pool usage.

Sampling techniques

The use of correct sampling techniques is essential to provide reliable information to determine whether disinfection is being carried out properly or not:

1. Although many pools will now have automatic monitoring equipment these are not a substitute for routine testing by the operator, although they may allow a reduced programme of tests.
2. Training of pool operators should include advice on how to act effectively on the results and, as many of the tests require matching of colours, operators should be examined to ensure that they have no difficulty in reading results correctly.
3. Whilst almost any sample of water from the distribution system may be typical of the whole this is not the case with swimming pools where pollution and disinfectant levels vary. The bottom at the deep end may receive little or no pollution over a period of time whilst continuing to be disinfected whilst the shallow end could contain pollution added only a short time before the sample was taken. The state of the water therefore depends a great deal on the concentration of disinfectant and its speed of action.
4. Normally sampling is done at the shallow end of a pool when bathers are present and active, but instructions as to the proper place and time of sampling cannot be rigidly stipulated.
5. Frequent residual determinations of deep end samples should be taken but samples for

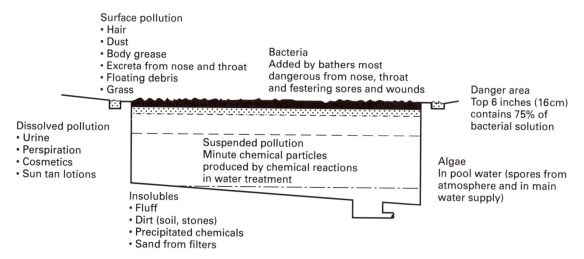

Fig. 11.1 Physical, chemical and biological pollution of swimming pools.

bacteriological analysis at the deep end need not be done so frequently. For special pools (paddling, diving and remedial pools) variations on sampling technique are a matter of common sense.

6. A record should always be kept of the place, time, and use of the pool, the pH and the amount of chlorine (residual and free) in the water. These do not need to be kept permanently but are useful evidence of the state of a pool over the previous few weeks.

7. The frequency of tests depends upon the use of the pool, its equipment and past performance and heavy use, changes in disinfectant and recent failures will require more frequent bacteriological checks. No pool however should go without its occasional bacteriological check with the samples being taken unannounced on a day and time when the pool is in use.

8. Particular care must be taken to avoid contamination of samples and to neutralize the disinfectant in samples taken for bacteriological examination.

9. When samples are taken for bacteriological analysis a chlorine determination should be made on another sample at the same time and place as the first.

10. As results of bacteriological examinations are not immediately available, regular and frequent determinations of free residual (of chlorine is used) are an important check on the condition of the water and a guide to any action required. For no pool should this be less frequent than two to three times a day.

11. Pool attendants should be trained to do the tests, but officers should also do a test when they visit. Test kits must be properly maintained and kept clean at all times with any glassware being thoroughly washed in clean water to remove test reagents before making subsequent tests.

12. Reagents have a 'shelf life' and require replacing at regular intervals and should be properly stored when not in use.

Purification

All swimming pools should be equipped with adequate purification plants to remove sources of pollution. The most usual method is to recirculate pool water after chlorination, filtration and aeration. By maintaining sufficient levels of a chosen disinfectant, usually chlorine, in the water, the rapid and immediate destruction of bacteria is assured. In any pool, water is also constantly being discharged, as part of the filtration process, and being replaced with fresh water. Pollution can also be progressively diluted. However, although a significant amount of pollution may be removed at the first turnover, the proportion falls with successive turnovers, and even after the water has been through the filter system several times, a small proportion of pollution remains.

The **turnover rate** of a pool is determined by the number of hours it takes to pass the total pool water volume through the filter. This influences the choice of filter and its operation during each 24-hour period. However, when choosing a filter it should be borne in mind that not all pool water will actually pass through a filter in a single turnover due to remixing of the filtered water when it is returned to the pool. It has been estimated that even in a pool with good circulation, something like seven 'turnovers' are required in order to filter 99% of the pool water.

The following rates of turnover are suggested as being minimum requirements:

1. **Private outdoor pools** with a small bathing load, would normally need a filter with an 8-hour turnover period.
2. **Private indoor heated pools** would require a 6-hour turnover period.
3. **School pools** which are often heavily used, require a turnover of less than 2 hours. (These figures will only be relevant if plant is well maintained and operated in good condition.)

Filtration

From the foregoing, it will be seen that the selection of a filter should be undertaken with great care as it has an important bearing on the ultimate clarity, appearance and safety of the pool water. The filter is the heart of any pool installation, and without an effective one problems will arise in maintaining pool water in an acceptable condition for bathing. It is the correct use of a filter, in association with correct chemical disinfection, that maintains pool water bright and clear.

Filters are generally of the pressure type using sand, diatomaceous earth, or cartridges as the filtering medium.

Sand filters

These are basically of three categories, depending on the rate of flow of water through the sand bed. The system employed by each type is similar. Water, under pressure, flows through a bed of graded sand enclosed in a container. These filters ultimately reach a point when they are unable to deal with further particulate matter, and they are cleaned by 'back washing'. The reversal of the water flow disturbing the sand particles and allowing the filtered-out debris to be backwashed to waste. Such filters, although expensive to install, are simple to operate and can be inexpensive in use, as the filter medium is reused time and time again.

Diatomaceous earth filters

Although of varying designs, these filters tend to work on the same filtration principle as sand filters. This involves the use of a fine fabric supported within the filter vessel through which the water flows. Diatomaceous earth is introduced to the vessel as a filter powder, and forms a fine coating over the fabric. This layer removes the dirt from the water until, when fully loaded as shown by a rise in pressure, the water flow is reversed, and the filter powder and dirt are discharged to waste. These filters can be very efficient and give good quality water when operated correctly. They do tend to be more expensive to use as the diatomaceous earth has to be discharged to waste.

Cartridge filters

These filters are normally used in small pools, and rely on the passage of water through pads of bonded fibre and/or foam. The dirt-coated pads are removed and replaced at intervals because it is uneconomic to try to clean dirty pads.

This system can be relatively inexpensive to purchase and operate, but the efficiency of filtration, while adequate, may not be as high as those types described above.

Sterilization

Whilst filters are an essential part of the water treatment process, a sterilant or disinfecting chemical has to be used to ensure that water is kept free from harmful bacteria and other organisms. While many disinfectants, such as ozone, brominel and iodine are available, to date only chlorine has satisfied all the major requirements. Its effectiveness, low cost, speed of kill, and relative ease of control, makes it the most likely disinfectant to be encountered.

Chlorine

In many pools, chlorine is injected automatically in controlled quantities. In most large pools, this method of sterilization is very sophisticated, and samples of water are tested and dosed to maintain continuous control of the levels of free and combined chlorine. As a result, many of the problems associated with high combined chlorine levels, chlorinous odours, stinging eyes and skin irritation can be eliminated. Usually, the dose of chlorine is maintained at a sufficiently high level to produce a free residual of 1.5–3 ppm, but where there is heavy use, levels of up to 5 ppm free chlorine should not give rise to complaint, provided the pH is carefully controlled (7.4–7.6 pH being considered ideal).

There are, at present, four main chlorine donors used for swimming pool water treatment, and the chlorine content varies according to the donors chosen.

Sodium hypochloride
This form of chlorine liquid is widely used, and is an accepted method of chlorination. It is marketed commercially under a number of different names, and contains 10–15% chlorine. Because this product is very caustic and has a very high pH (pH12) great care must be taken in its handling. In use it can cause the pH of the pool water to increase, will tend to increase total dissolved solids, and can cause scale and corrosion of metal pipes and valves. As this material can decompose quickly if stored incorrectly – in heat, light or in metal containers – it is inadvisable to order more than one month's supply at a time. Fig. 11.2 shows a full sodium hypochlorite treatment system.

Isocyanurates
These materials offer the advantage of being stable in sunlight, making them suitable for use in outdoor pools. They are available in powder or granule form, are safe to handle and have a long shelf life. The granules are added directly to the pool water or in solution through a feeder. They dissolve to leave no sedimentation and, being slightly acid, have little effect on pH levels. Depending upon their form, they have relatively high levels of available chlorine – sodium dichloroisocyanurate 56% and trichloroisocyanuric acid 91%. When using these materials, cyanuric acid levels should be maintained at between 25–50 ppm – if it rises above 150 ppm, 'chlorine-lock' can occur.

Calcium hypochlorite
This is available in tablet or granular form, and is usually made into a 6% solution to be pumped into the circulation. The material contains 65% minimum of available chlorine which is stable if stored in cool, dark conditions prior to dilution. In use, this material has the advantage over sodium hypochlorite of not causing the pH level to rise by as much, and it does not add nearly as much total dissolved solids (TDS). A disadvantage is that a much larger dosing pump is required, and it needs constant agitation to keep it soluble when made up in solution.

Determination of residual chlorine
For low concentrations of chlorine in pool waters, use is made of the Palin-DPD (diethyl-p-phenylenediamine) test for chlorine and phenol red tablets (containing a reagent to counter chlorine bleaching) for the pH test. Reliable and simple to use, these kits use tablets and comparator discs to monitor chlorine and pH levels.

Chemistry of chlorine in pool water
When chlorine and water are mixed, the free chlorine killing agent hypochlorous acid, is formed, together with hypochlorite ion and hydrochloric acid. The hypochlorous acid combines with organic pollutants (body fluids, dead skin and ammonium compounds) to form chloramines

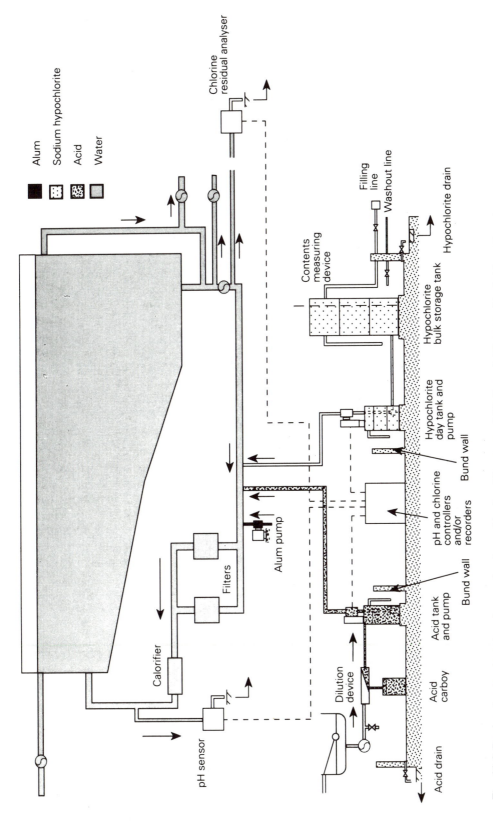

Fig. 11.2 Pool water treatment systems using hypochlorite. (Courtesy of Wallace & Tiernan, Tonbridge, Kent.)

Alum

Sodium hypochlorite

Acid

Water

Chlorine residual analyser

Contents measuring device

Filling line

Washout line

Hypochlorite bulk storage tank

Hypochlorite drain

Hypochlorite day tank and pump

Bund wall

pH and chlorine controllers and/or recorders

Bund wall

Acid tank and pump

Acid carboy

Dilution device

Acid drain

Alum pump

Filters

Calorifier

pH sensor

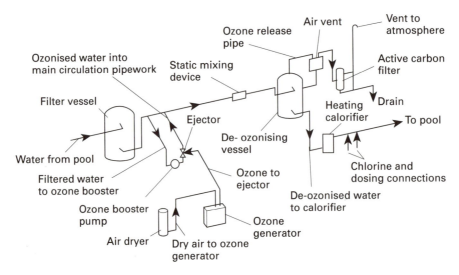

Fig. 11.3 Ozonization of swimming pool water.

– combined chlorine. The hypochlorous acid (free chlorine) is rapid acting, whereas hypochlorite ion is slow acting, and the percentage of these constituents is influenced by the pH, e.g. the efficiency of free chlorine is approximately 100% higher at pH 7.5 than it is at pH 8.0, and the former figure should be aimed for. However, in addition to adding bacteria to a pool, bathers constantly add nitrogenous matter, and chlorine is also needed to deal with these pollutants and remove chloramines in the pool water. Both hydrochloric acid, which reduces the pH of the water, and nitrogen trichloride can be formed unless adequate hypochlorous acid is added. Control of the amount of chlorine added is therefore essential to ensure a satisfactory free chlorine level, and that the proportion of combined chlorine is maintained at about one-third of the total chlorine present.

Breakpoint chlorination

If insufficient chlorine is available in a pool, the combined chlorine level will rise, the water may lose colour and clarity, and nitrogen trichloride may be produced resulting in complaints of smarting eyes and skin irritation among bathers. If sufficient chlorine is added, it will combine with the pollutants and break them down to harmless substances. Further additions of chlorine will then

be present in the water as **free chlorine**, available to deal with further pollution as it arises. A 'breakpoint' occurs and the residual falls, and from this point free chlorine can exist together with combined chlorine. This is the system adopted in most pools in this country.

Ozone

The use of ozone in the purification of swimming pool waters is practised extensively throughout Europe, and appears to be finding some favour in the UK. The initial cost of an ozone installation is high, but it is claimed that if used in a new pool complex, the cost difference may be largely offset by capital savings in heating and ventilation plant.

It is also claimed that ozone has several advantages over chlorine in that it is an effective bactericide, and is also effective against viruses. It oxidizes organic matter and the resultant pool water has excellent clarity. It has, however, a short life in solution, and is toxic and aggressive. As ozone does not remain in water as 'residual' ozone, it is necessary to chlorinate to provide residual protection in the water. The amount of chlorine necessary is, however, greatly reduced, and the process still results in an improved atmosphere in the pool hall with a noticeable lack of characteristic monochloramine odour. Fig. 11.3

shows a diagrammatic layout of an ozonization plant. The dose of ozone should be about 2 mg/l.

'Slipstream' ozonation is now available. This treats only 10% of the water with ozone, the rest being treated by a normal filter and chlorine dosing system.

Bromide

Treatment of swimming pool water with bromide is sometimes encountered, as it is claimed to counteract some of the disadvantages of using chlorine as a disinfectant. It has been widely used in the USA since the 1940s, and is commonly used in its solid form under the name of Dihalo, which combines bromine (66%) and chlorine (28%). It has been predicted that the use of this disinfectant may increase in coming years, although its relatively high cost may restrict its use.

In France, liquid bromine has been used in swimming pool water treatment, and its innocuousness to bathers has been confirmed in a number of toxicological studies. Its bactericidal, viricidal and algicidal properties are comparable with chlorine, and it is claimed that because the connection between its bactericidal activity and the pH is slight, this factor can be kept at a level where the risk of irritation is minimal.

The bromine content of water can be readily measured by chemical methods using colorimetry or by electrochemical methods. Reagents used are orthotolidine or DPD – the former being most sensitive.

Other disinfectants

Iodine chlorine dioxide, ultra-violet light and metal ions (electro katadyn system) have been used, mainly outside the UK, but their use is rare as all have disadvantages.

The determination of pH values

pH is the expression used to indicate the degree of acidity or alkalinity of water. Pure neutral distilled water has a pH of 7.0; and a figure below 7.0 will indicate that the water is acidic, above 7.0 that the water is alkaline. Normal waters contain a variety of substances in solution. Calcium and magnesium salts give the water its characteristic hardness, for example, and traces of many other compounds are naturally present, and are affected by changes in pH.

Alkaline conditions can give rise to irritation if the pH rises much in excess of pH 8.0, and the effectiveness of chlorine as a sterilant is also greatly reduced.

In 'hard' water areas, another problem can arise with a high pH: the precipitation of calcium salts, which results in a cloudy pool and blocked filters. Should this occur, the filter must be thoroughly backwashed as the accumulation of the deposit may set hard and possibly ruin the filter.

If the pool water is allowed to go acidic, even very slightly, two major difficulties arise. Firstly, corrosive conditions will exist, and any metal parts of filter systems etc. in the pool will be attacked, and any alkaline floor and wall finishes, such as the proprietory 'marbelite', may also suffer. Secondly, in acidic conditions, unpleasant compounds are formed by the interaction of chlorine and polluting substances, which cause irritation to mucous membranes and eyes, and give rise to the so-called 'pungent odour of chlorine'.

This is the reason for most of the complaints of 'over chlorination', and the cause is not an excess of chlorine, but the formation of these irritant and smelly compounds, due to the presence of too little chlorine in an acid water.

This is the reason for maintaining pool water at around pH 7.4 to 7.6, i.e. slightly alkaline. It will give some protection against the accidental production of acid conditions, while still allowing effective performance by the chlorine.

In measuring pH values, advantage is taken of the fact that certain dyes, known as indicators, change their colour in a definite and reproducible manner and degree, according to the pH value of the solution with which they are mixed. Phenol red or diphenol purple are the most suitable for pool water, their ranges being pH 6.8 to 8.4 and 7.0 to 8.6 respectively. Both are available in tablet form. For very accurate measurement of pH, a meter should be used.

Algal control

Algae are tiny aquatic plants which often first appear in pools as brown or green slimes on steps, walls and floors. If they are allowed to establish themselves, they can be a considerable nuisance. They grow rapidly, increase chlorine demand, block filters and are the main cause of discoloured water. In correctly maintained pools, algal problems are rare. Weekly additions of algicide will establish a buffer against temporary or inadvertent loss of chlorine, which may create the conditions which favour rapid algal growth.

Care must be taken when using algicides of the quaternary type, as over dosing may lead to excessive foaming or the formation of a foam layer on the surface of the pool.

Total dissolved solids (TDS)

The addition of water treatment chemicals to pool water results in an increase in the amount of solids dissolved in the pool water. When these increase to undesirable levels the colour, clarity and appearance and taste of the water can be adversely affected, to the discomfort of bathers. A maximum of 1500 ppm should not be exceeded. The choice of disinfectant can have a significant affect on the TDS content of pool water, and control can be obtained by accurate control of pH value (7.3–7.5), the use of minimum quantities of chemicals, regular backwashing of filters and dilution of pool water with fresh water.

Alkalinity

Alkalinity is the quantitative analysis of the amount of alkali present in the water a bicarbonate, which will act as a 'buffer' and be readily available to react with fluctuating pH conditions and maintain the clarity and comfort conditions in the pool. A level of around 100 mg/l is desirable. It must not be allowed to rise above 220 mg/l, otherwise corrosion can result. High levels of alkalinity can be lowered by the addition of hydrochloric acid to the pool water.

Water quality guidelines

It is recommended that where water quality values are set, they are seen as objectives for operators to follow, rather than as rigid or inflexible standards.

Colony counts and the test for *Escherichia coli* and other coliform organisms provide simple tests for checking the bacteriological quality of swimming pool water.

If coliform organisms are absent and pH and disinfectant residual levels maintained at correct levels, the risk to bathers will be minimal. Colony count tests, which determine the number of organisms capable of living in the pool water, although regularly carried out, are not essential for assessing bacteriological safety. They are, however, useful as indicating the general quality of the water and that filtration and disinfection processes are operating correctly. A range of values can be established for each pool, depending on the local circumstances and disinfectant used. These will, after a time, establish a norm for the pool, and this can be used to identify significant changes in water quality. This is more useful to the enforcement officer than the actual numerical results themselves.

Guidelines on appropriate bacteriological standards are to be found in the Department of Environment booklet, *The Treatment and Quality of Swimming Pool Water* [8]. The absence of coliform organisms with colony counts not greater than 10 (and always less than 100 organisms per ml) at 24 hours gives a good indication that the quality of the pool water is satisfactory. Counts above 100 organisms per ml require investigation. Occasional counts of up to 10 coliform organisms, in the absence of *E. coli*, are acceptable provided they do not occur in consecutive samples, pH and disinfectant levels are satisfactory, and the colony count levels are within the established norm for the pool.

Where there are persistently poor results which may indicate disinfection and filtration failures, a full investigation and sampling programme must be implemented. In these circumstances, it may also be necessary to look for the presence of *Pseudomonas aeruginosa* and possibly *Staphylo-*

coccus aureus, as extra indicators of water quality.

Procedures for taking samples are described in detail in Report 71 on *The Bacteriological Examination of Drinking Water Supplies* [9].

Whirlpool spas*

These have become very popular forms of water recreation, and are now to be found in many hotels, clubs and leisure centres etc. In theory, their disinfection should be relatively simple, but their very popularity and the heavy loading they are subjected to make this a difficult task unless a strict regime is utilized.

Spa pools are commonly disinfected with Dihalo (bromine), although more are changing to hypochlorite disinfection for easier and more efficient control.

Most pools run at a temperature around body heat (37°C), and this may induce bathers to sweat heavily. In leisure and fitness centres, pools are often used after heavy exercise often without showering before immersion, and because the pool volume is small pollution levels will be high. The combination of pollution, temperature and bathers being close together in a confined space, coupled with inadequate surface water removal, insufficient filtration and unbalanced water can lead to discomfort and danger. The water temperature is ideal for skin rash inducement and respiratory infection, unless disinfection is efficient.

Pseudomonas aeruginosa folliculitis has been the most commonly identified infection associated with whirlpool spas, with the characteristic rash developing anywhere between 8 hours and 5 days after bathing (mean incubation period 48 hours). When investigating complaints, it is important to differentiate this rash from others of an eczematous nature, sometimes associated with solid bromine treated pools. The folliculitis may, on occasions, be associated with mastitis and otitis externa in the bathers. Circumstantial evidence has also linked whirlpool spas to occasional urinary tract infections, and they may serve as sources

of other infections including legionellosis and Pontiac fever. Defective maintenance or operation are usually common in reports of outbreaks.

The Swimming Pools and Allied Traders Association (SPATA) has produced standards for the installation and operation of commercial spa pools, and there is mention of SPATA in the Department of Environment booklet, *The Treatment and Quality of Swimming Pool Water* [8]. These guidelines should be followed to ensure trouble-free operation. It is also recommended that, in addition to emptying and refilling pools at least weekly, the pH value, disinfectant concentration and temperature be tested regularly during the day, and records be kept in a log book. From time to time, tests for alkalinity, total dissolved solids and surface and calcium hardness should be undertaken. Control of bathing load and enforced intervals between bathing sessions can assist in maintaining water quality.

Biological standards may be found in SPATA's *Standards for Spa Pools* [10], which states that the biological conditions of the water shall be at the judgement of the environmental health officer for the area. Notwithstanding this, the standard recommended for spa water are:

1. Total plate count at 37°C should not exceed 100 colonies for 1 ml of sample water.
2. No *E. coli* in 100 ml of sample water.

The suggested health and safety guidelines for public spas and hot tubs issued by the US Department of Health and Human Services suggests that, 'The presence of organisms of the coliform group, or a standard plate count of more than 200 bacteria per millilitre or both in two consecutive samples or in more than 10% of the samples in a series shall be deemed as unacceptable water quality.'

The health and safety aspects of pools

Guidance on safety in swimming pools, the risks associated with their operation, and the precautions to be taken to achieve a safe environment for the public who use them and the

*Also see 'Hygiene for Spa Pools' 1994. PHLS Press and Publications, 61 Colindale Avenue, London NW9 5DF. £6.50. ISBN 0 901144 371.

employees who work in them, is to be found in the Health and Safety Executive/Sports Council Publication *Safety in Swimming Pools* [11]. This booklet outlines standards of good practice as a basis for decision making by managers on what arrangements are best for their pools.

The risk of drowning in a swimming pool, compared with the overall national drowning problem, is not high with only 3–5% of drownings occurring in pools. Compared with the estimated 150 million visits to swimming pools each year, the figures are small. However, any death which can be avoided, especially in such a controlled environment, where all risk should be removed, is inexcusable. The problem is therefore primarily one of management.

Existing legislation, which controls safety in swimming pools, is to be found in the Health and Safety at Work, Etc. Act 1974 and the Public Health Act 1936.

The Health and Safety at Work. Etc. Act 1974 places certain general obligations on all pool operators, and these responsibilities extend to protecting the public who may use the pool and any contractor working at pool premises. The Health and Safety Executive is the enforcing authority at local authority run pools, including school pools. At pools which form part of residential accommodation (hotels, holiday camps, etc.) and leisure complexes, enforcement is the responsibility of the local authority.

The Public Health Act 1936 contains powers for local authorities to make bye-laws for the regulation of swimming pools under their management. Model bye-laws are available from the Department of the Environment, and cover aspects such as water purity, hygiene, behaviour and the prevention of accidents.

Even though the above legislation exists, effective safety relies on the general acceptance and adoption of recognized standards, such as the following.

Safe design of the pool structure, systems and equipment
Good design is essential for a safe pool environment, and safety is one of the important factors considered by the Sports Council when consider-

ing schemes submitted for grant aid. Designers and sponsoring authorities are encouraged to meet the standards recommended in the booklet [11].

Details on the structure and finishes of the pools and buildings are outlined to avoid dangerous situations, such as abrupt changes in floor level in wet areas being built into a pool. Precautions to prevent persons, particularly young children, having accidents or falling through open ledges of stairways and landings are included. Good planning and circulation layout ease management problems and enhance safety. Floor and wall surfaces and features next to wet circulation areas should not present a hazard to bathers, and slip-resistant flooring and well-designed walls, which avoid sharp edges, projections or abrasive finishes, are recommended to minimize these hazards. Suitably toughened glazing – as specified in BS6206 – should be used in areas adjacent to wet circulation routes to reduce the risk of injury and damage.

Entry to and exit from a pool should not only be safe but easy, and the design and sighting of these facilities must be suitable for the pool.

Pool edges should be clearly visible – colour contrasted – so that bathers can avoid hitting the edges when diving or jumping in. This may not be feasible where the pool takes the form of a gently sloping 'beach', but in such leisure pools this is not so critical.

The profile of the pool bottom should not be a hazard to swimmers in the pool or those jumping in, and for rectangular pools the Sports Council have recommended a number of possible pool profiles, with water depths ranging from 2 m deep water to 90 cm shallow water with gradients of not more than 1 in 15. In irregular-shaped leisure pools, profiles will depend on pool layout and any features present.

Wave machine openings, sumps, or inlets or outlets of the pool water circulation system should have suitable protective grilles or covers, designed to prevent trapping. Undue suction should not be created at openings which could result in a body being held against the grilles.

Any safety signs used should comply with the Safety Signs Regulations 1980, and the content and location of signs needs careful consideration as part of the overall safe pool environment. Clear signs, showing depths of water, areas where it is safe to swim or dive, and those giving instruction on the safe use of diving or other equipment are particularly important. Examples are given in *Safety in Swimming Pools* [11].

The installation of heating, ventilation and air conditioning systems in pools needs careful consideration, as these factors can indirectly affect pool safety. They also promote rapid corrosion of pool-side structures if out of balance by permitting excess humidity.

A comfortable temperature should be maintained in the swimming pool hall and changing areas, and a maximum temperature of around 27°C of water with the air temperature about 1°C higher, to avoid excess condensation, is suitable.

Effective, draught free ventilation should be provided, and humidity and air movement should be balanced to achieve comfortable conditions.

Adequate lighting, either natural or artificial, should be provided to avoid excessive glare or reflections from the pool water, to avoid solar gain, and to ensure that the whole of the pool and its base are easily visible to lifeguards and bathers.

Wet and corrosive conditions in pools can compound the risks from electricity. Designers should be aware of the various risks of shock, burns, fire or explosion, and take these dangers into account.

Maintenance requirements and safe working practices

The correct planned maintenance of buildings and plant is essential in ensuring the health and safety of pool users and employees. Arrangements should therefore be made for their thorough inspection and examination, either by utilizing manufacturers' instructions or by pool operators devising them as part of the pool operating procedure. Maintenance should take place at the specified intervals and records kept of any remedial work carried out.

Buildings should generally be inspected annually, but where high humidity levels increase the risk of corrosion, and chemicals in the atmos-

phere may increase the risk, some structures may require more frequent inspection, e.g. every 6 months.

Any steam boilers and plant should be maintained to the standards required by sections 32–35 of the Factories Act 1961, including a regular, thorough examination by a competent person. After each examination, a certificate should be obtained and kept available for inspection.

Staff should be adequately trained for their pool duties and useful courses to provide this training are organized by the Institute of Baths and Recreation Management (IBRM). These include courses for supervisors, attendants and plant operators. Courses designed for the latter include technical aspects of pool water treatment.

Asbestos may be found in swimming pool premises, since at one time it was widely used for insulation and fire protection. All work with asbestos is now subject to the Control of Asbestos at Work Regulations 1987, and its associated codes of practice. Generally speaking, only persons licensed by the Health and Safety Executive under the Asbestos (Licensing) Regulations 1983 may work on asbestos.

Access to exterior windows for cleaning can pose special problems in swimming pools. Suitable guidance on this aspect of maintenance can be found in *Prevention of Falls to Window Cleaners* [12].

Fixed electrical installations should be inspected and tested to the standards in the current edition of *Regulations for Electrical Installations* published by the Institution of Electrical Engineers [13]. Because of the adverse conditions of a pool environment, tests should be done at least annually.

The pool water treatment system

Whatever system of disinfection, filtration and circulation is used it must be operated safely. The main risks associated with treatment systems include risks to bathers from unclear water, and risks to bathers and employees from chemicals used in disinfection systems. There is the added danger to employees who often have to work on these items of plant in confined spaces. Written health and safety policy statements should include an assessment of all of the hazards associated with all aspects of the plant and the precautions to control the risks. Adequate staff training should be provided.

Advice on delivery, storage and handling of chemicals is given in a series of Department of the Environment booklets (see reading list) giving guidelines for the design and operation of plant using different disinfectants. All chemical containers should be clearly labelled with their contents, and the packaging and labelling should comply with the Chemicals (Hazard Information and Packaging) Regulations 1993.

Storage facilities should be secure, dry, well ventilated, clearly marked and sited well away from public entrances and ventilation intakes. Safe systems of work should always be followed to safeguard employees from harmful materials; these may include the provision of protective clothing and, in some cases, respiratory protection. First-aid provision should be adequate to deal with the consequences of chemical splashes, etc.

Where any major, uncontrolled release of toxic gas is possible, written emergency procedure for dealing with such an incident should be prepared, and should include evacuation procedures and the notification and co-ordination of emergency services.

While the Department of the Environment booklets give good advice on the safe design and operation of the common disinfection systems, the more important hazards associated with these systems are:

SODIUM HYPOCHLORITE AND ACID SYSTEMS Used with automatic dosing systems these have been known to release chlorine gas when water pumps have failed. Correct siting of pumps to avoid them losing their prime and the provision of interlocks to prevent incorrect dosing, as well as additional sampling points and correct maintenance procedures are measures to be adopted to eliminate this hazard.

ELECTROLYTIC GENERATION OF SODIUM HYPO-CHLORITE This can sometimes produce hydrogen and, occasionally, chlorine gas. In view of the flammable nature of hydrogen the selection, siting and maintenance of electrical equipment is likely to be a specialist job.

OZONE SYSTEMS These present hazards from the chemicals used and from the electrical ozone generating process. Guidance on the health hazards associated with ozone is to be found in *Ozone Health Hazards and Precautionary Measures* [14]. Ozonators should be provided with automatic shut down devices to cope with any abnormal operation.

Where ozone devices are installed to remove ambient odours in changing rooms, ozone levels must not be allowed to exceed the recommended occupation health limits set out in the HSE Guidance Note *Occupational Exposure Limits* [15].

CHLORINE GAS SYSTEMS Chlorine gas is particularly hazardous and, in view of the advice contained in the statement on the use of chlorine gas in the treatment of water of swimming pools issued by Department of the Environment Circular 72/78 recommending that this use should cease by 1985, it will only be rarely found. Where it is found, the advice contained in the HSE Guidance Booklet *Chlorine from Drums and Cylinders* [16], and the Department of the Environment booklet, *Swimming Pool Disinfection Systems Using Chlorine Gas – Guidelines for Design and Operation* [17] should be followed.

ELEMENTAL LIQUID BROMINE SYSTEMS Being less hazardous than other pressurized gas systems, the main problems of these systems relate to spillage. Adequate supplies of neutralizing material should be provided to deal with such emergencies.

CALCIUM HYPOCHLORITE, CHLOROISOCYANURATE, HALOGENATED DIMETHYLHYDANTOIN AND SOLID ANCILLARY SYSTEMS The main risks relate to general chemical handling and the generation of chlorine gas if chemicals are mixed or stored incorrectly.

PH ADJUSTMENT BY THE USE OF CARBON DIOXIDE The system of metering carbon dioxide gas into the water circulation system is becoming more popular as it eliminates the risk of chlorine gas generation – unlike acid and hypochlorite systems. However, because of the risk of asphyxiation, carbon dioxide should be stored outside of buildings.

SAND FILTERS When it is necessary to enter filter vessels the advice published by the HSE in *Entry into Confined Spaces* [18], should be followed.

Supervision arrangements to safeguard pool users

All pools require supervision if they are to be operated safely. Pool operators should therefore consider carefully the main hazards associated with their pool, and make detailed arrangements to deal with them. The precautions taken by the pool operator must include a written operating procedure, which sets out the organization and arrangements for user safety, including details of staff training requirements. This is particularly important when a pool may be used without constant poolside supervision. These should be constantly reviewed and updated so take account of incidents experienced at the pool, thus keeping the procedures relevant.

By displaying suitable signs and posters such as those based on the *Swimming pool user's Safety Code* published by RoSPA [19], bathers can be made aware of potential hazards and encouraged to act responsibly.

Generally, the Department of the Environment has recommended that a minimum water area of 2 m^2 per bather be allowed for physical safety, but this is only a guideline and operators must assess the maximum number that can be safely admitted to their pool, taking account of bathers' behaviour and also the capacity of the pool water treatment system.

Where it is deemed necessary to provide constant poolside supervision, sufficient adequately trained lifeguards should be provided and effectively organized and supervised. Because of the variety of pool facilities and users, it is not feasible to make specific recommendations for lifeguard numbers. These must be arrived at by taking account of all relevant local factors, although as a starting point some advice on minimum numbers is set out in the publication.

REFERENCES

1. Health and Safety Executive (1992) HS (G) 81 *A Code of Safe Practice at Fairs*, HMSO, London.
2. National Playing Fields Association (1983) *Playground Management for Local Councils*, London.
3. Noah Norman, D. (1987) *Guidelines for Hygienic Hairdressing*, Public Health Laboratory Service, Colindale.
4. Health and Safety Executive, *How to Use Hair Preparations Safely in the Salon*, HMSO, London.
5. Health and Safety Executive, Home Office and Scottish Office (1993) *Guide to Health, Safety and Welfare at Pop Festivals and Similar Events*, HMSO, London.
6. Code of Practice for Outdoor Events, National Outdoor Events Association, 7 Hamilton Way, Wallington, Surrey SM6 9NJ.
7. Home Office and Scottish Home Office and Health Department (1990) *Guide to Safety at Sports Grounds*, HMSO, London.
8. Department of the Environment (1984) *The Treatment of Swimming Pool Water*, HMSO, London.
9. Department of the Environment, Department of Health and Public Health Laboratory Service (1983) *The Bacteriological Examination of Drinking Water Supplies*, Report 71, HMSO, London.
10. Swimming Pools and Allied Traders Association (1983) *Standards for Spa Pools*.
11. Health and Safety Executive and Sports Council (1988) *Safety in Swimming Pools*. Sports Council, London.
12. Health and Safety Executive, *Prevention of Falls to Window Cleaners*, Guidance Note GS25, HMSO, London.
13. Institution of Electrical Engineers, *Regulations for Electrical Installations* (current edition).

14. Health and Safety Executive, *Ozone Health Hazards and Precautionary Measures*, Guidance Note EH38, HMSO, London.

15. Health and Safety Executive, *Occupational Exposure Limits*, Guidance Note EH40, HMSO, London.

16. Health and Safety Executive, *Chlorine from Drums and Cylinders*, Guidance Booklet HS(G)40, HMSO, London.

17. Department of the Environment (1980) *Swimming Pool Disinfection Systems Using Chlorine Gas – Guidelines for Design and Operation*, HMSO, London.

18. Health and Safety Executive, *Entry into Confined Spaces*, Guidance Note GS5, HMSO, London.

19. RoSPA, *Swimming Pool User's Safety Code*, RoSPA, Birmingham.

FURTHER READING

Department of the Environment (1975) *The Purification of Swimming Pool Water*, reprinted 1980, HMSO, London.

Department of the Environment (1982) *Swimming Pool Disinfection Systems Using Sodium Hypochlorite and Calcium Hypochlorite – A Survey of the Efficacy of Disinfection*, HMSO, London.

Department of the Environment (1982) *Swimming Pool Disinfection Systems Using Ozone with Residual Chlorination – Monitoring the Efficacy of Disinfection*, HMSO, London.

Department of the Environment (1982) *Swimming Pool Disinfection Systems Using Chloroisocyanurates – A Survey of the Efficacy of Disinfection*, HMSO, London.

Department of the Environment (1983) *Swimming Pool Disinfection Systems Using Electrolytically Generated Sodium Hypochlorite – Monitoring the Efficacy of Disinfection*, HMSO, London.

Department of the Environment (1982) *Swimming Pool Disinfection Systems Using Sodium Hypochlorite – Guidelines for Design and Operation*, HMSO, London.

Department of the Environment (1982) *Swimming Pool Disinfection Systems Using Ozone with Residual Free Chlorine and Electrolytic Generation of Hypochlorite – Guidelines for Design and Operation*, HMSO, London.

Department of the Environment (1981) *Swimming Pool Disinfection Systems Using Calcium Hypochlorite, Chloroisocyanurates, Halogenated Dimethylhydantoins and Solid Ancillary Chemicals – Guidelines for Design and Operation*, HMSO, London.

Swimming Pools and Allied Trades Association (1980) *Standards for Swimming Pools – Water and Chemical*.

British Effluent and Water Association, *Code of Practice for Ozone Plant for Swimming Pool Water Treatment*.

Pool Manager's Handbook, Olin HtH.

Towards a Perfect Pool, R. Bartlett & Sons Ltd, Bristol.

Chamberlain, Malcolm, (1985) Swimming pools – established safety standards. *The Safety Practitioner*, March.

12   Health promotion

Peter F. Allen

DEFINITION OF HEALTH PROMOTION

In *The Politics of Health Education* [1], Jennie Naido gives an inclusive definition of health promotion: 'Health promotion includes a range of methods from personal education, mass media, advertising, preventative health services and community development, to organizational developments and economic and regulatory activities.' Health promotion is not the same as health education. Health promotion is broader and wider. It includes personal education and it also includes regulatory activities. This latter point is important because there is still misunderstanding concerning it and a tendency amongst some to see the regulatory or enforcement duties as the environmental health officer's 'proper' job and health promotion as something that can be done if time and resources are available. In terms of the Naido definition enforcement and education are both important parts of health promotion. Put another way it would be foolish to pursue a vigorous inspection and prosecution programme and ignore the fact that much food poisoning stems from poor understanding of food hygiene principles. Advancing food hygiene and safety, needs to take both elements into account. Enforcement and education complement each other.

Health education

Environmental health officers are generally clear about what the regulatory element has to offer but less so about the contribution that health education can make. As Ewles and Simnett say in their *Promoting Health – A Practical Guide to Health Education* [2], 'Without education for health knowledge and understanding, there can be no informed decisions and actions to promote health . . . Knowledge is power and without health knowledge, people are powerless to change their health themselves because they do not have the knowledge of alternatives and therefore cannot make informed health choices.' Therefore health education is individualist by nature and this is both a strength and a weakness. It is a strength when it provides decision makers and individual members of the public with health knowledge and understanding. However it can become a weakness if it is seen as health promotion per se. Then the individualism of health education discounts the structural factors Naido mentions such as the socio-economic or structural aspects and health promotion becomes individualistic. Thus if a person drinks heavily, then the focus is on the individual and the habit, rather than the power of the drinks industry and other structural factors such as poverty, stress or even poor housing. This is often referred to as the 'blame of the victim' approach.

The fact that we still have designated health education officers, health education units and a central body called the Health Education Authority blurs the reality of the situation, for an analysis of their work shows it to be wider than a simple individualistic approach. The designations are more a fact of history and political expediency than logic and practice.

Health promotion then is about health advancement and includes a wide range of methods to achieve that end. These methods include both individualistic and structuralist approaches; the merits of neither should be discounted.

THE HEALTH OF THE NATION

Health promotion was put firmly on the national agenda with the publication by the Department of Health in June 1991 of a green paper entitled 'The Health of the Nation' [3].

The green paper's approach was to focus debate on a number of alternative objectives and targets. It put forward three criteria for identifying key areas. Sixteen areas were considered and four were immediately rejected. Consultation was proposed on targets for the remaining 12 areas, although it was emphasized that the Government expected to proceed initially with only about half of them

The white paper

In July 1992 Virginia Bottomley, the new Secretary of State for Health, published the related white paper [4] of the same name. The white paper set out the Government's strategy for health. It:

1. selected five key areas for action;
2. set national objectives and targets in the key areas;
3. indicate the action needed to achieve the targets;
4. outlined initiatives to help implement the strategy;
5. set the framework for monitoring, development and review.

The key areas for action and national targets are:

1. coronary heart disease and stroke;
2. cancers;
3. mental illness;
4. HIV/AIDS and sexual health;
5. accidents.

In the main, the targets relate to the year 2000, but some look further to the future. Within the key areas, emphasis is placed on risk factors, such as smoking and dietary imbalances. The white paper stressed the fact that 'everyone has a part to play if the strategy is to be successful'. At national level the Government has set up a Ministerial Cabinet Committee to co-ordinate Government action and oversee implementation of the Health Strategy. A wider Health Working Group under Ministerial chairmanship was set up and brought together Government departments, statutory and voluntary bodies, industry, education, sports, trade unions, the media and others. Another aspect of the white paper was the recognition that health promotion needs to take place in a variety of 'settings' such as healthy cities, healthy schools or healthy hospitals and that specific action needed to take place in the workplace and the environment

Healthy alliances

The importance of active partnerships between the many organizations and individuals who can come together to help improve health was also highlighted with the new term 'Healthy Alliances'. The white paper saw the main 'stakeholders' as:

1. **The Government itself** – taking a range of practical measures to support the strategy as well as setting up the Ministerial cabinet Committee on Health Strategy to co-ordinate Government action and oversee implementation and development of the strategy in England.
2. **Local authorities** – responsible for a wide range of public services, many of which are linked with the strategy set out in the white paper. These responsibilities include 'education, environmental control, environmental health and food safety, transport, housing and social services'.
3. **Voluntary organizations** – 'between them they cover the whole range of health-related activity from the highly specialized to the general'.
4. **The media** – 'has a crucial role to play in providing individuals with the information necessary to make healthy choices'.

5. **The Health Education Authority (HEA)** which carries out national programmes of public education and provides a national stimulus for local activity in a variety of settings. The HEA was 'tasked' with reviewing its strategic aims and objectives in the light of the strategy for health. (Interestingly enough the HEA was founded in 1927 by officers from local government and funded to a large extent by local authorities. It passed to an independent body, following the Cohen Committee's Report in 1964 [5] when Government assumed responsibility for full funding. In 1986 it was changed from a relatively free standing, independent organization to a special health authority and became an integral part of the National Health Service, directly responsible to the Secretary of State.)

6. **Employers** – who 'have long been required to provide safe working conditions. Increasingly they are also recognizing the benefits of a healthy workforce'.

7. **Health professionals** – 'crucial to the success of the strategy'.

8. **The National Health Service** – was recorded as having a 'central role'. Regional Health Authorities 'will lead in ensuring that objectives are achieved regionally' . . . 'Hospital and Community Units, and primary and community health care services, will need to be involved in working towards these objectives'. (Neither changes in the National Health Service structure, which have resulted in the reduction in the number of regional health authorities and the merging of some District and Family Health Service Authorities, nor the creation of the internal market within the health service have essentially changed this brief.)

Neither the green nor white paper was without its critics. Linda Ewles writing in the *Health Education Journal* [6], summed up the main criticism as 'its failure to acknowledge the socio-economic determinants of health, and its emphasis on the now-familiar government style of health promotion: individual lifestyle change'. A further disappointment, Linda Ewles records, was that no money was attached to the strategy:

'once again, the David of prevention would have to fight the Goliath of treatment and care services for resources – but without a divinely-inspired catapult.

Nevertheless, what the Health of the Nation initiative has done is to provide a national strategy for health. The first time a national strategy for **health** as opposed to health services has ever been produced. It has also put health promotion firmly on the agenda nationally. Moreover in encouraging healthy alliances it empowers organizations such as local authorities and local health authorities to get together on health promotion.

Another important aspect of the initiative is that in a series of well-presented coloured graphs it laid bare the state of the national health. See for example Fig. 12.1 which sets out the death rates for accidents for all persons aged 65 and over between 1970 and 1990 and the associated target.

As the Secretary of State put it in her 'One Year On Review' [7], 'every day in England, heart disease and stroke kill nearly 550 people; every day 370 die from cancer; every day 26 perish in accidents, many of them on our roads. We all have to die some time, but the real tragedy is that many of these deaths are premature and preventable.'

HEALTH PROMOTION IN PERSPECTIVE

In order to make sense of the Health of the Nation initiative, we need to see it in historical perspective. Health promotion is not just a phenomenon of the 1990s; it has a long history. A reading of the mosaic health laws in the Old Testament book of Leviticus confirms this. That aside, the promotion of health since the mid-nineteenth century can be seen to fall into four discernible periods [8,9]. Each period is characterized by a special emphasis given to a particular type of intervention, as shown in Table 12.1.

From the 1830s to the 1880s we had, prompted by the ravages of infectious disease and popular outcry, **sanitary intervention**, when the thrust was at the very basic level of providing clean water and an adequate sewerage system, plus occasional forays into bad housing and bad food.

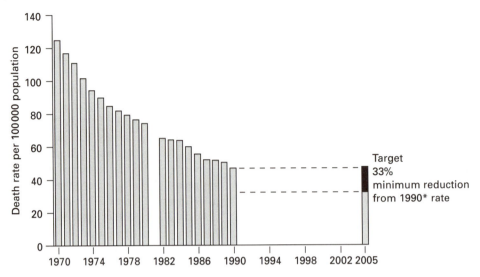

Fig. 12.1 Death rates for accidents: England 1970–90 and target for the year 2005 (all persons aged 65 and over). Rates are calculated using a 3-year average plotted against the middle year of the average. Data for 1981 were affected by industrial action by registrars and are excluded, thus rates for 1980 and 1982 are based on 2-year averages. Rates are calculated using the European Standard Population to take into account differences in age structure. (Source: Department of Health (1992) *The Health of the Nation in England. A Strategy for Health*, HMSO, London.)

Table 12.1 The discernible periods of health promotion

Period	Type of intervention
1830–1880	Sanitary
1880–1930	Personal and social
1930–1970	Therapeutic
1970–today	Holistic

From 1880 to 1930 there was **intervention at the personal and social level**, fueled by the horrendous health study of recruits for the Boer War, many of whom had to be turned down as unfit for service. The development of the school meals service, school medical service, the health and district nursing and midwifery services are all features of this period.

From 1930 to 1970, following the discovery of antibiotics and 'other drug' breakthroughs of this time, came the therapeutic intervention period, with vaccines, vitamins and contraceptives making a profound effect on health as well as on forming the view that there was 'a pill for every ill'.

However, since the late 1970s the evolution of health in the UK has been characterized by a new **holistic intervention**. This recognizes that if we are to have positive health all factors need to be taken into consideration, including such matters as poverty, inequalities associated with social class, gender, ethnicity and geographical location. These health determinants were brought starkly to life by the Black Report [10]. The corollary of this is that no one organization or profession has all the answers – that if health is to advance there is a need to welcome and encourage inputs from all directions, not least from the community itself.

WHO'S HEALTH FOR ALL/HEALTHY CITY PROJECT

The WHO 'Health for All by the year 2000' Alma-Ata declaration in 1978 [11], which has been brought to life by the Healthy City Project, is a movement born out of this new phase. In its strategy for attaining the goal of health for all by the year 2000, the WHO's European regional office is arranging its activities in three main areas:

1. promotion of lifestyles conducive to health;
2. reduction of preventable conditions;
3. provision of care that is adequate, accessible and acceptable to all

The regional office has identified 38 targets, eight of which concern the provision of a healthy environment. These relate to:

1. multisectoral policies (target 18);
2. monitoring and control mechanisms (target 19);
3. control of water pollution (target 20);
4. control of air pollution (target 21);
5. food safety (target 22);
6. control of hazardous wastes (target 23);
7. human settlements and housing (target 24);
8. working environment (target 25).

A number of organizations, including the Institution of Environmental Health officers and the then Faculty of Public Health Medicine, endorsed the 'Health for All' concept. The great strength of this initiative was that it has put health promotion on the international agenda for awareness and action. Its weakness was that, on its own, it tended to be a top down approach and therefore had the inherent danger of becoming merely a paper exercise. Not surprisingly, therefore, the 'Health for All' initiative did not really kindle enthusiasm at community level until the emergence of the WHO's Healthy City project in such places as Toronto and Adelaide. The Healthy City project focused on the local community and their health needs within the broad umbrella of the 'Health for All' objectives. The weakness of the Healthy City approach was that the early emphasis on the City did for a time preclude the notion that the project should include not only cities, but towns and villages as well.

The Government's Health of the Nation initiative of 1991 can therefore be seen as a response to the holistic period stimulated by international and local pressures. The criticisms that have accompanied the initiative especially those concerning its failure to address inequality and socio-economic differences in health can also be seen as

a response to its failure to fully take on board the new concepts in health promotion. To be fair, the Secretary of State has stated that the 'White Paper is not the last word. It is only the start of a continuing process of identifying priority objectives, setting targets and monitoring and reviewing progress.' Time will tell.

Sustaining change

It is useful to review a model of change [12] to get an objective view of how change takes place in health issues. It will be seen that change for the better is by no means automatic but is determined by a number of factors. Any health issue could be used to illustrate the model but since reduction in smoking is a key target in the Health of the Nation, this will be used. The societal model of change is set out in Table 12.2.

As can be seen from Table 12.2, for a societal change to take place there must be a gain that can be perceived and it must be at a cost worth paying. In terms of smoking, this element is certainly satisfied. Then there must be the capacity for change. A powerful group in society has few problems in making changes, but, what happens if you wish for change yet the pressure group you belong to lacks muscle? This happened in the campaign to remove lead from petrol and Des Wilson in his book '*The Lead Scandal*' [13] set out the strategy. It was done by building up a broad-based coalition built up among all sorts of organizations and across political parties. Because the same is happening at present on the smoking issue it is highly probable that before too long smoking advertisements will be banned in this country.

However we then enter the most challenging element in change. How is change to be sustained when the original campaign has run out of steam

Table 12.2 Model of societal change

Elements of change	Determining factors
Gain	Perceived – cost
Capacity	Powerful – coalition
Sustainability	Opposition – counter opposition

and it is no longer smart to campaign? Again looking at the model in Table 12.2 gives us the answer. We need to recognize that if one group in society gains through change it is likely that another group will lose and bide its time until the fires burn low under the initial campaign. That is why we are now seeing, under the guise of 'deregulation', an attempt to roll back the environmental and food safety law made in the 1970's. The 'losers' in the initial stages of change are pushing back. Similarly with smoking we should expect the initial 'losers', i.e. the tobacco industry, to counter attack.

The tobacco industry is rich and powerful. It is an illusion to think the industry as a whole will sit back and see home markets dwindle. More likely it will keep a low profile until the non-smoking campaign has run out of steam or it is no longer smart to campaign and then . . .

The above model does however highlight the factor that can sustain change, i.e. the counter opposition. In the case of smoking there is good news for the healthy alliances now being built up on the non-smoking issues between local authorities, business generally, Government and the health authorities are becoming 'structural' and will form a tough counter opposition.

Nevertheless as can be seen from the above model, change for the better is by no means automatic.

LOCAL AUTHORITY HEALTH PROMOTION

Health of the Nation saw local authorities as a major stakeholder in health promotion and went on to say 'Environmental Health Departments have a particularly important part to play and the Department of Health is developing even closer links with them and the environmental health profession'.

The nature of the services that local authorities provide and the close democratic relationship with the local communities does mean that the local authority should be a major stakeholder in health promotion. Much will depend on the vision and priorities of members and officers.

Since 1974, when the medical officer was relocated to the health authority, the environmental health officer has been the officer most readily identifiable with health. That is not to say other officers such as personnel officers do not have health functions, it is simply that the environmental health officer is clearly seen as most closely identified with health. Therefore where local authorities have been developing their potential in this field of health promotion, with one or two notable exceptions, it has been the environmental health officer who has been the lead officer:

1. **Enforcement of mandatory legislation** – local authorities' environmental health officers enforce a wide range of mandatory health legislation covering air, ground and traffic pollution, food hygiene and safety, housing standards, health and safety at work etc. Enforcing mandatory standards is an important form of health promotion which should not be ignored. Sometimes in order to get health advanced, legal enforcement is necessary.

2. **Work in connection with discretionary powers** – district councils already exercise a wide range of discretionary powers. Fairly wide ones are given in section 54 of the Public Health Act 1964 and the Home Safety Act 1961. Activities cover HIV/AIDS, alcohol and drug addiction, nutrition, women's health, men's health, heating and energy advice, home safety, occupational health and health aspects of poverty.

3. **Health promotion work in connection with health and safety and food hygiene** – faced with the critical need to stem the rising tide of food poisoning, there has been a massive demand for training. This has largely been met by environmental health officers, most of them from within the local government setting.

4. **Role model** – in England and Wales there are over 400 local authorities with 2 405 569 employees. In terms of the employment market this is a substantial segment. If local authorities take action to introduce effective health policies they can not only provide their

internal community with an opportunity for better health but they also provide a role model for local commerce and industry. Many have followed this approach on specific health promotion issues.

5. In 1993 the Institution of Environmental Health Officers (IEHO) carried out a survey [14] to establish the situation as regards smoking. They found that 85% of local authorities that responded had in fact established non-smoking policies.

6. To help local authorities the IEHO with the Health Education Authority have published 'Guidelines for Smoking Policies in Local Authorities' [14]. This excellent booklet contains a step by step guide as well as much other useful information.

7. **Campaigns and projects** – local authorities and their environmental health officers can also take action by way of campaigns and health promotion projects.

8. Restaurants, cafes and hotels are regularly inspected by environmental health officers under the Food Safety Act and therefore these officers are in a strong position to encourage above the statutory minimum standards. The Health Education Authority's 'Heartbeat Award' scheme introduced jointly by the Health Education Authority and individual local authorities has provided a means for promoting and establishing healthy eating options and no smoking areas in catering premises.

9. Some local authorities have gone further and established their own food awards for the catering industry which enhance the 'Heartbeat' standards and encourage additional health facilities such as baby changing accommodation.

10. Commercial premises, other than catering premises, can also be encouraged in a similar fashion. Three years ago Oxford City Council introduced jointly with the health authority a 'Health Award'. In order to attain the award a company must comply completely with the Health and Safety at Work Act and in addition commit itself to three approved 'green'

policies and three approved healthy lifestyle policies

11. **Participation in national campaigns** – local campaigns and projects are good but they are even better when interacting with a national campaign. Such central organizations as the Health Education Authority or the Department of Health can set the national agenda by getting national media coverage. They can also provide expertise to give a campaign direction and flair. Nevertheless, good as it can be, a central campaign on its own can sometimes alienate the very groups who are targeted. For instance some teenagers may not necessarily want to be associated with society as a whole and may take it as a symbol of their independence to act contrary to the message of a national campaign. It is here that local authorities with their amazing local networks can adapt and earth a central campaign.

12. **Provision of local health promotion accountability** – the Secretary of State for Health is responsible for all the key appointments to the Regional and District Health Service structures and is responsible to Parliament for the Health Service's effectiveness. Therefore accountability is essentially upwards. In contrast local council's accountability is to the local people who elect them. Therefore accountability is essentially downward to the local community.

13. Given this the local council is in the best position to provide local people with access to comment and participate in national health promotion initiatives. Local people through their local councils and their council's national organizations like the Association of District Councils can bring a local voice to Government discussions. Significantly many responses to the Government's Health of the Nation green paper came from local councils and perhaps more significantly the Government has made a particular point in using the Local Government Associations to progress their Health of the Nation initiative. See for example the Health of the Nation guidance [15] published jointly by all

the local councils national bodies and sent to local authorities.

14. **Local health promotion strategies** – To bring it all together, local councils through their environmental health officers can also develop local health promotion strategies. An increasing number of local authorities are already doing this. The best strategies have the following characteristics:
   (a) they provide a local health data base;
   (b) they activate other local authority departments into seeing their health contribution;
   (c) they seek healthy alliance with other local organizations;
   (d) they involve the internal community (staff) and the external community in the development of the strategy.

15. An increase in unitary authorities, which bring at local level services such as social services and education together with environmental health, housing and recreation, will enhance the impact of such local health strategies.

So local authorities through their environmental health officers can make a major contribution to health promotion and this is likely to increase with the impending changes in local government.

In 'The Health of the Nation for Environmental Health', [16] the then IEHO highlighted the work which environmental health departments are contributing towards the priorities of Health of the Nation. This document emphasizes the links between the environment and health agendas including Government strategies, and at Annex 3 gives examples of structures for corporate action for interagency working.

MANAGEMENT OF LOCAL HEALTH PROMOTION

Plan and strategy

Health promotion like any other function in environmental health needs to be properly managed. Following the Audit Commission survey [17] into the management of environmental health, there has been a considerable tightening up of the management systems within departments including the production of business of health plans. The department's health promotion policy and strategy should find its place within those departmental plans.

Organization

In one sense all members of the environmental health department should be health promotion activists but experience is now showing a need for specialists. Surveys by the CIEH indicate that it is now not uncommon for departments to employ officers specializing in such matters as HIV/AIDS, drug and alcohol abuse, home safety, food and safety education, heating and energy as well as health promotion generally. The trend has also been for these officers to be formed into a specialist unit and this trend is likely to be increased with the advent of larger unitary authorities.

In a few local authorities, these units have been placed in the chief executive's department. There are some advantages in this approach, especially initially when the local authority is seeking to develop a corporate approach to health promotion. However such units can become isolated and lose touch with the operational services. On balance health promotion units are best located within the central support services of the environmental health department where the unit's expertise can be readily accessed.

Training and education

A further implication for environmental health departments of the practice of health promotion is in terms of training and education. The Acheson Report [18] said, 'We believe that the most significant changes which need to be made to basic post graduate training in public health medicine are those relating to epidemiology, **behavioural science** and control of communicable disease and infection.' In highlighting the need for public health medicine consultants to draw on the behavioural sciences, the Acheson Report highlights the need for all natural science based-professionals involved in health promotion to do likewise. This includes environmental health officers.

In relation to student environmental health officers, the Health Education Authority's Environmental Health Consultative group in the mid 1980s sponsored a research project to determine the approach the various colleges and universities were taking in relation to teaching health education to student environmental health officers. From this and similar initiatives, some useful shifts in attitude and behaviour have occurred, both among teaching staff and students and among those members of the Chartered Institute of Environmental Health who sit on the regulating Education Committee.

At the post-graduate level recent years have also seen some signal advances in the provision of health promotion training. In 1986, the Health Education Authority (then called the Health Education Council) produced through their Environmental Health Consultative Group a 'communication skills package for environmental health practice' [19]. This package is still used and continues to 'open' minds on the pay off of using skills derived from the social sciences. In addition recent years have seen local authority personnel departments develop in-house training in a variety of communication skills, including working with the media which can be readily adapted to health promotion.

For those staff who need to develop their behavioural skills to a greater degree than can be provided by short courses, there is now a wide range of post-graduate degrees, diplomas and certificates. For example, the Diploma in Management Studies, which has a strong social science input, or the Certificate in Health Education. The new universities are offering a variety of masters degrees which include health promotion, e.g. the MSc Sociology of Health and Welfare at the University of Greenwich which has a specific health promotion module. Most offer their courses on a part-time or distance-learning basis.

Support

Environmental health staff should be able to look for health promotion support to the specialists in health promotion.

Apart from local networks, there are now two professional officer networks that give a great deal of support and advice on health promotion matters. First there is the Society of Health Education and Health Promotion Specialists. This represents the 1000 or so health promotion officers mainly in the National Health Service; some on the purchasing side and some on the provider side. Then there is the CIEH's National Health Promotion Network, which is specifically for officers working in health promotion in environmental health departments. In October 1993, their policy *Promoting Public Health* [20] was published. This covers:

1. aim and rationale;
2. environmental health promotion;
3. an environmental health approach to enhancing public health;
4. indicators of good practice within environmental health promotion;
5. document review;
6. further information and contacts.

CONCLUSION

The Department of Health's Chief Medical Officer, Kenneth Calman, commenting on the Health of the Nation initiative and looking to the future said: 'It is important to have commitment from everyone to achieve the major health gains aimed for in this strategy' [21]. Promoting health is everybody's business. The implications are illustrated in the Oxford Health Wheel [9].

THE OXFORD HEALTH WHEEL (Fig. 11.2)

In the centre is the community, showing clearly that the community has a central role in health promotion. Around the rim are the various health and non-health professionals, and organizations that have a contribution to make. Holding the

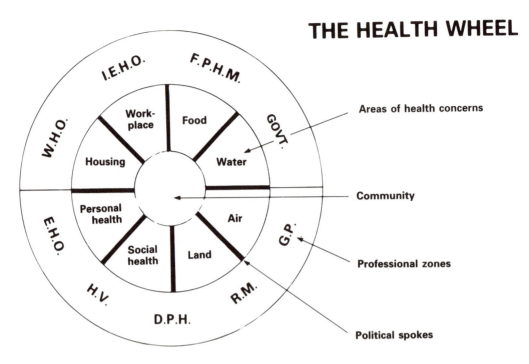

Fig. 12.2 Oxford Health Wheel.

wheel together are the 'spokes' or politicians, locally and nationally. Again we should note the key position politicians occupy. They provide the environment for health promotion to take place; they can provide encouragement or discouragement; they can provide or withhold essential resources and they can provide constitutional direction and thrust.

Between the spokes are the different areas of health concern. These will differ from place to place and from time to time. Once the health wheel starts moving, we then find that different groups who hitherto felt they had no health contribution to make in a particular area suddenly find they do indeed have something very valuable which they can contribute.

It is when this recognition dawns that health is indeed everybody's business that the wheel of health starts moving. Environmental health officers are in a unique position to share this particular gospel.

REFERENCES

1. Naido, J. *The Politics of Health Education – the limits of individualism*, Routledge & Kegan, London.
2. Ewles and Simnett (1992) *Promoting Health – a practical guide to health education*, John Wiley, Chichester, Sussex.
3. Department of Health (1991) *The Health of the Nation: a consultative document for health in England*, HMSO, London.
4. Department of Health (1992) *The Health of the Nation: a strategy for health in England*, HMSO, London.
5. Report of a Joint Committee of the Central and Scottish Health Services Council (1964) *Health Education*, HMSO, London.
6. Ewles, L. (1993) Paddling upstream for 50 years. *Health Education Journal*, **52**, (3).
7. Department of Health (1993) *The Health of the Nation – one year on*, HMSO, London

8. Kickbusch, I. Health promotion strategies for action. *Canadian Journal of Public Health*, **77**, (5).

9. Allen, P. (1991) *Off the Rocking Horse*, Greenprint, London.

10. Black, D. (1981) Inequalities in health. *British Medical Journal*, 2 May.

11. World Health Organization (1977) *Health For All by the year* 2000, WHO, Geneva.

12. Allen, P. (1994) Local authority action. Royal Society of Health Journal,

13. Wilson, D. (1983), *The Lead Scandal*, Education Books, London.

14. IEHO (1993) *Guidance to Local Authorities on Smoking Policies*, CIEH, London.

15. AMA, ADS, ACC (1993) *Health of the Nation – guidance*, London.

16. IEHO (1993) *The Health of the Nation for Environmental Health*, CIEH, London.

17. *Towards a Healthier Environment: Managing Environmental Health Series.* 1991. HMSO London.

18. Report of the Committee of Inquiry into the future development of the public health function (1988) *Public Health in England*, HMSO, London.

19. Benn, M. (1986) *EHO Communications Package*, Wetherby, M. Benn Associates.

20. IEHO & NHPN (1993) *Promoting Public Health*, CIEH, London.

21. Department of Health, (1993) *On the State of the Public Health*, HMSO, London.

22. Buzan, T. (1982) *Use Year Head*, BBC Publications, London.

23. Mehrabian, A., *Silent Messages*, Wadsworth Publishing Company, California.

24. Cockerill, M., *Live from No.10*, Faber and Faber, London.

FURTHER READING

O'Neil, P.D. (1990) *Health Crisis 2000*, WHO, Geneva.

Harrison, L. (1993) *Alcohol Problems: a resource directory and bibliography*, Central Council for Education and Training in Social Work.

Mackay, J. (1993) *The State of Health Atlas*, Simon and Schuster, London.

Foster M. (1993) *Camden and Islington HIV Prevention Strategy*, London.

Tones, B. K. and Tilford, S. *Health Education: effectiveness and efficiency*, (2nd ed, forthcoming), Chapman & Hall, London.

APPENDIX

IMPROVING COMMUNICATION SKILLS

Effective communication is one of the most important skills for environmental health staff to possess and not least in relation to health promotion where it will not happen unless we effectively communicate our health message. The following points should be considered in giving a talk.

Preparation

Questions to ask the organizer
1. What is the nature of the group?
2. How long is the session and for how long do you wish me to speak?
3. What is it they are hoping to hear from me?
4. Where will it be held and what visual aid equipment is available?
5. Plus a question for yourself: do I really have something valuable to contribute to this gathering?

Give yourself time to think over the invitation. It may be to everyone's benefit if you graciously refuse! If you decide to do the talk, then you enter what should be a very pleasurable phase of the talk – the preparation proper.

Researching the subject thoroughly
You may already know a great deal about the issue, but giving a talk is an opportunity to develop your own thoughts and your own knowledge, and look for ways to share them with your audience. The danger here is overload, getting lost in a welter of information – so much so that joy goes out of the window. Most experienced

speakers tend to clear their own mind first before looking further afield. I find Tony Buzan's 'mind mapping' approach extremely helpful [22]. This consists of getting one sheet of blank paper, writing the central topic in the middle, and then building up with the other topics around it. The advantages of this approach is that the relative importance of the various ideas fall into place, and links between different key concepts are immediately recognizable. It also stops you getting bogged down in detail and frees your mind to be creative. The added bonus is that when using this approach a good structure to the talk often emerges naturally.

Structure

The structure of presentation has three parts: the beginning, the body and the end. A common failing among speakers is to fail to get the first and last bits close enough together! There are many textbooks which will give students a way of opening and closing a presentation and it is well worth experimenting. Keeping to time is also vitally important.

Making a presentation is not unlike selling a product. A well-known formula that is used in the selling world goes under the mnemonic AIDA: Attention, Interest, Desire, Action. This method can be used with great benefit in structuring a presentation:

1. Attention: in the opening seek to secure identification with the audience.
2. Interest and Desire: build these into the main body to develop the audience's interest and commitment to the subject. And then go for,
3. Action: whether you are lecturing to a basic food hygiene course or a group of medical students, it is worth building in the action points. It gives the audience something to bite on and gives you something to aim at.

Should you write it out?

Reading out a prepared text is the death knell to communication. It is much more enjoyable and rewarding to use 'confidence' cards or a sheet with the main points listed. This enables you to be free to pick up on the audience's reactions and signs of interest, or disinterest as the case may be. Similarly, memorizing a text is equally disastrous and anchors you in the past rather than freeing you to share with the audience in the present. Experienced speakers put their main points, essential facts and phrases, on to a card or sheet. They live with these, adding or subtracting as new ideas and new insights come to them. Then, when the time comes to stand on their feet, they do not have a written barrier standing between themselves and the audience, yet at the same time they know exactly where they are coming from.

Presentation

Having invested a great deal of time in preparing a talk it would be sad to see that investment wasted at the point of delivery. So what can psychological research tell us about delivery?

Research by Albert Mehrabian [23] suggests a 55/38/7% principle: in our communications one with another, 55% of what is communicated is communicated visually, 38% what it sounds like and only 7% the words being used. Even with the latter we tend to focus on 'buzz' words or phrases. So how we present ourselves and our material visually does matter. Should we be formal or informal? We need to think in terms of the group and the occasion. What might be absolutely right for one occasion could be quite wrong with another group or another occasion. But above all we should be ourselves. Audiences can soon spot a 'poseur'. Similarly we need to give special attention to visual aids. Will they help or will they hinder? Will they assist your communication with the group or will they act as a barrier? These days every environmental health department should be developing its own slide library and these can be drawn upon. Key messages superimposed on slides can be a powerful aid to communication, but care needs to be taken that they are bullet messages rather than a 'splodge' of air gun pellets. The strength of having a slide collection is that they can be quickly turned into transparencies for the overhead projector. On the subject of overhead transparencies, it is worth noting that speakers still persist, even at major conferences, in using handwritten transparencies when, for a few pounds a professional set will enhance the visual presentation.

Since 38% of the communication is determined by the sound of the communication, it certainly helps to sound confident. The evidence will transmit itself to the group and encourage them to want to communicate with you. On the other hand, fear of failure not only makes you, the speaker, feel very uncomfortable with such symptoms as a dry mouth or heaving stomach, but it also quickly transmits itself to your audience. The topic gets lost as the audience gets nervous wondering if you are going to make it to the end. If you have that problem, take heart. A lot of famous communicators have had it too. Howard Keel was so dry mouthed before going on a Royal Command Show they even vaselined his lips; Angela Rippon, before compering the Eurovision Song Contest, said she was so nervous that she felt sick. Barbara Castle records that when she first stood up in Parliament she was lost for words. Afterwards a kind friend said to her, 'Don't worry, the last person who did that went on to become Prime Minister.' And that gives us the clue to tackling our nerves. Psychologists tell us nerves come from our fear of failure. That somehow when we stand up on our feet we will not be able to communicate and our personal world will come tumbling down round our ears for all to see. The best antidote to this is not a spot of salt in your pocket to keep your mouth moist, although that can help, but good preparation and practice. The more you do of both the more confident you will become. Then you will find that you will really enjoy the experience and so will the audience.

Communicating apart from on your feet

I have deliberately dwelt upon environmental health staff communicating on their feet, because not only is it an important area if we are to promote health, but it also brings out the two main principles which underline effective communication, be it communication with large groups, small groups, on a one-to-one basis, with the media or communicating by letter or committee report.

The first principle which should undergird all our communication is the 55/38/7% principle. I have already mentioned it in terms of giving a presentation, but it is equally important in other settings – even radio. True, the 55% visual element is lost, but that means we have to pay special, or greater attention, to the remaining 45%, especially the tone and manner of our verbal communication. With the advent of local radio, BBC and commercial, in most places and the topicality of our work, environmental health officers are continually presented with opportunities to go 'live'. Therefore, it is useful to bear this in mind if we are to maximize these useful opportunities for health promotion.

The second and the most crucial point of all is that communication is not just a one-way business. A question of getting a message across. Communication is a two-way process. It follows from this that we need to constantly think in terms of the other person or persons – to be open to their reactions and their needs. Harold Macmillan, one of the first prime ministers to appear on television just before a general election, was told as he sat down before the camera; 'There will be 12 million people watching tonight', but as he wrote later, 'I just had the sense to say to myself, no, no, no, two people, at the most three.' His presentation therefore, instead of adopting a grand public speaking style to 12 million, which would have seemed odd to the small groups watching at home, was quietly conversational. The positive response by the public to this approach, showed the master of communication certainly knew how to be an outstanding success. For this and similar insights into how prime ministers have faced the media, Michael Cockerill's book *Live from No. 10* is warmly recommended [24].

13 Port health

Peter Rotheram

DEVELOPMENT OF PORT HEALTH
(see also Chapter 2)

Systematic shipping quarantine of ships arriving from Levantine Turkey was adopted by Venice in the aftermath of the Black Death, when it became apparent that the Levant had become a permanent reservoir of plague. The Venetian ships collected valuable cargoes of silk and spices which had been transported overland to the Levant, they were isolated in quarantine for 40 days on returning to Venice to establish that they were not infected. When plague spread to the Baltic and the Low Countries, ships arriving in England from infected areas were detained by an Order of Council, but it became increasingly difficult to restrict the illicit landing of people [1]. English common law did not oblige townspeople to maintain the watch between sunrise and sunset or to detain people unless they had committed a felony. The first Quarantine Act of 1710 removed these impediments to enforcing quarantine, but it was only after the Levant Company lost its monopoly of trade with Turkey in 1753 that legislation was introduced – an Act for Enlarging and Regulating Trade into the Levant Sea 1753 and an Act to Oblige Ships to Perform Quarantine [1] 1753 – requiring all ships loading in the Levant to undergo quarantine in the Mediterranean. But the Dutch did not apply such rigorous quarantine [2] and with more than half the cotton used in England transhipped through Holland, British shipping was at a disadvantage. As a consequence the law was subsequently amended by an Act to Encourage Trade into the Levant Sea 1799 by

providing a more convenient mode of performing quarantine. Ships from the Levant were permitted to perform their quarantine in the Medway at Stangate Creek, hulks were provided for cargoes to be aired, and Parliament voted funds for the building of a lazaret at Chetney Hill.

The relaxation of quarantine was achieved amid controversy as to whether plague was 'epidemic' or 'contagious'. Charles Maclean, a ship's surgeon who had served with the East India Company, propounded an elegant hypothesis suggesting that diseases which were seasonal and could infect people more than once were 'epidemic', while those which occurred independently of season or the state of air and only infected a person once were 'contagious'. His hypothesis [3] was based on the observations of ships' surgeons that fevers, such as typhus and yellow fever, were dependent on the season and the state of the air. The experience of Southwood Smith at the London Fever Hospitals brought him to the same conclusions as Maclean, and he developed his theme on the high economic costs of disease which was adopted by Edwin Chadwick [4]. The spread of cholera to Britain prompted the Board of Health to produce a Report on Quarantine [5]; largely the work of Southwood Smith. It was decidedly anti-contagionist and led to the first International Sanitary Conference in 1851, but the resulting convention was only ratified by France and Sardinia.

The British view was that the enforced detention of ships in quarantine was only necessary when the disease was actually on board, and if the ship was in a foul condition it should be cleansed and disinfected before pratique was granted. Orders assigning to the Poor Law Authorities at endangered ports power to deal with shipping arrivals suspected of having cholera on board were issued by the General Board of Health in 1849. Section 32 of the Sanitary Act 1866 subsequently made ships subject to the jurisdiction of the Nuisance Authority in whose district they moored; regulations were introduced requiring ships to be inspected and dealt with as if they were a house. This arrangement was not entirely satisfactory when there was more than one Nuisance Authority in a port, and section 20 of the Public Health Act 1872 empowered the Local Government Board to constitute one Port Sanitary Authority with jurisdiction over the district on any port established by the commissioner of customs.

These statutory powers were consolidated in 1875 and re-enacted in the Public Health Act 1936, which changed the designation Port Sanitary Authorities to Port Health Authorities. The statutory provisions relating to port health were subsequently incorporated in the Public Health (Control of Disease) Act 1984. In Scotland, port health functions are exercised by port local authorities, designated under the Public Health (Scotland) Act 1897. A Joint Board constituted as a port health authority, precepts the constituent local authorities for its expenditure.

JURISDICTION

The functions of a port health authority are assigned directly by statute or in a statutory instrument. The area of jurisdiction of a port health authority is specified in a statutory order. It may comprise the whole or part of a customs port, including the whole of any wharf and the area within the dock gates. A port health authority may, within its district, exercise any of the functions of a local authority relating to public health, waste disposal or the control of pollution assigned to them in the order. The Prevention of Damage by Pests Act 1949 provides that the local authority for any port health district is the port health authority. They are also designated as local authorities under Parts I and III of the Environmental Protection Act 1990 and as food authorities under the Food Safety Act 1990, and may be assigned the functions of a local authority under Part I of the Slaughterhouses Act 1974. Any local authority having jurisdiction in any part of a port health district is excluded from exercising any functions assigned to the port health authority.

ORGANIZATION

Most of the work of a port health authority is undertaken by environmental health officers; where a district council is the port health authority the work may devolve on a few specialists. The whole environmental health department may be involved, particularly where the port or airport is handling traffic outside normal business hours. When the port health authority is constituted as a joint board, it will employ its own environmental health officers and administration staff and precept the constituent local authorities for any expenditure incurred. In either case, the port health authority will appoint one or more port medical officers; district health authorities have a statutory obligation to provide these services free of charge to the port health authorities. The port medical officer may also be appointed as a medical inspector of aliens, to undertake medical examinations on behalf of the immigration service. Where a port or airport is approved by the EU for the importation of produce of animal origin from third countries, an official veterinarian will have to be appointed by the competent authority.

At any port or airport the port health officers will liaise with custom officers and traffic controllers to maintain surveillance of shipping and aircraft arrivals. Customs officers will alert the port health officer whenever they become aware of any apparent contravention of the Public Health (Ships) Regulations 1979 and Public Health (Aircraft) Regulations 1979, or the Imported Food Regulations 1984. When the port health authority is not an enforcing authority under the Animal Health Act 1981, the port health officer will advise the responsible authority of any animals which are imported contrary to the rabies control legislation. Details of the cargo imported on a ship or aircraft can be cleared from a manifest which can be obtained from the carrier. This information may be computerized using direct trader input (DTI), which involves the importer entering details of each consignment on the computer system to obtain clearance from customs and port health.

INTERNATIONAL HEALTH CONTROL

Successive International Sanitary Conferences eventually led to the elimination of quarantine [6], and under the auspices of the World Health Organization (WHO) the International Health Regulations 1969 specified the maximum restrictions that could be applied to ships and aircraft involved in international commerce. They are based on the assumption that the only effective protection against the spread of epidemics is the provision of wholesome supplies of food and water, the effective disposal of waste and the elimination of vectors of disease on ships and aircraft.

Following the increasing emphasis on epidemiological surveillance for communicable disease recognition and control, the WHO agreed to strengthen the use of epidemiological principals as applied internationally, to detect, reduce or eliminate the sources from which infection spreads, to improve sanitation in and around ports and airports, to prevent the dissemination of vectors and, in general, to encourage epidemiological activities on the national level so that there is little risk of outside infection establishing itself. Following the change in the approach to dealing with cholera and the elimination of smallpox, the International Health Regulations were amended in 1973 and 1981. The diseases subject to the International Health Regulations are plague, yellow fever and cholera and provision is made in the UK for implementing the government's obligations under these Regulations in the Public Health (Ships) Regulations 1979 and Public Health (Aircraft) Regula-

tions 1979. As a result of a world-wide campaign by the WHO, smallpox was eradicated and vaccination against the disease is no longer required. Efforts to control cholera by vaccination failed to prevent the spread of the disease, and people arriving from infected areas are no longer required to have cholera vaccinations. Yellow fever and plague are controlled by measures to control the vectors of the disease. A yellow fever vaccination is required for people arriving in countries where the mosquito vector of the disease is prevalent, but this does not include the UK.

THE PUBLIC HEALTH (SHIPS) AND (AIRCRAFT) REGULATIONS 1979

These provide for people arriving on infected or suspected ships or aircraft to be placed under surveillance; the periods are calculated from the time of leaving the infected area. Measures to control the spread of lassa fever, rabies, viral haemorrhagic fever and marburg disease are also specified. Requirements for the notification and preventing the spread of other infectious diseases from arrivals at ports and airports are included in the Public Health (Infectious Disease) Regulations 1984 and 1988.

An infected ship or aircraft is:

1. A ship or aircraft which has on board on arrival a case of a disease subject to the International Health Regulations, or a case of lassa fever, rabies, viral haemorrhagic fever or marburg disease.
2. A ship or aircraft on which a plague infected rodent is found on arrival.
3. A ship or aircraft which has had on board during its voyage:
   (a) a case of human plague developed by the person more than 6 days after his or her embarkation; or
   (b) a case of cholera within 5 days before arrival;
       or
   (c) a case of yellow fever or smallpox.

A suspected ship or aircraft is:

1. A ship or aircraft which, not having on arrival a case of human plague, has had on board during the voyage a case of that disease developed by a person within 6 days of his or her embarkation; or
2. a ship or aircraft on which there is evidence of abnormal mortality among rodents, the cause of which is unknown on arrival; or
3. a ship or aircraft which has had on board during its voyage a case of cholera more than 5 days before arrival; or
4. a ship which left within 6 days before arrival an area infected with yellow fever; or
5. a ship which has on board on arrival a person who the medical officer considers may have been exposed to infection from lassa fever, rabies, viral haemorrhagic fever or marburg disease.

HEALTH CLEARANCE OF ARRIVALS

The master of a ship or the commander of an aircraft arriving from a foreign country must report to the port health authority, not more than 12 hours and not less than 4 hours before arrival:

1. the occurrence on board during the passage (or the last 4 weeks if longer) of:
   (a) death other than by accident;
   (b) illness where the person concerned has or had a temperature of 38°C or greater which was accompanied by a rash, glandular swelling or jaundice, or persisted for more than 48 hours; or has or had diarrhoea severe enough to interfere with work or normal activities.
2. The presence on board of:
   (a) a person suffering from an infectious disease or who has symptoms which may indicate the presence of infectious disease;
   (b) any animal or captive bird of any species including rodents and poultry, or mortality or illness among such animals or birds.
3. any other circumstances which are likely to cause the spread of infectious disease.

If none of these circumstances prevail, the ship or aircraft does not require health clearance (**free pratique**) unless otherwise directed by an author-

Table 13.1 International code of signals health clearance messages

Q	My vessel is 'healthy' and I request free pratique.
QQ	*I require health clearance
ZU	My Maritime Declaration of Health has a positive answer to question(s) (indicated by appropriate number(s)).
ZW	I require a port medical officer.
ZY	You have health clearance.

*By night, a red light over a white light may be shown, where it can best be seen, by ships requiring health clearance. These lights should only be about 2 m (6 ft) apart, should be exhibited within the precincts of a port, and should be visible all round the horizon as nearly as possible.

ized officer of the port or airport health authority. Otherwise the specified signals (Table 13.1) should be shown on arrival and no person may board or leave the ship or aircraft other than a customs officer, immigration officer, the pilot of a ship or an authorized officer until health clearance has been granted. These restrictions on boarding or disembarking do not apply when only the presence on board of any animal or captive bird requires reporting, unless plague has occurred or is suspected among rats and mice or there has been abnormal mortality among them. When health clearance is required, a **maritime or aircraft declaration of health** has to be completed by the master or commander, except in the case of arrivals from Belgium, France, Greece, Italy, Netherlands, Spain or the Irish Republic. Control measures to prevent the spread of infectious disease from ships and aircraft that are 'suspected' or 'infected', or which have arrived from an infected area may include medical examination, or the disinfecting of any person suffering from or exposed to infectious disease, disinfection or disinsectation of ships, aircraft or clothing, measures to prevent the escape of plague infected rodents and the removal of any contaminated food or water other than the cargo.

AIRCRAFT DISINFESTATION

In order to minimize the risk of aircraft spreading vectors of disease, the commander of an aircraft which has landed in a risk area may be required to produce details of the application of residual insecticides or in flight disinsection. The WHO has recommended [7] an initial treatment with permethrin to produce an even deposit of 0.5 g/m^2 on carpets and 0.2 g/m^2 on other surfaces (these rates may be halved for subsequent treatments). For the purpose of in flight disinsection, an approved aerosol formulation is required to be dispensed uniformly in the enclosed space at the rate of 35 g/100 m^3. The serial numbers of the aerosol dispensers used in the treatment should be entered on the aircraft's declaration of health. In no circumstances should insecticide be used on an aircraft, unless it has been specifically approved for that purpose.

SHIP DISINFESTATION

A ship arriving from a foreign port must have a **deratting certificate** issued in a designated approved port showing that the ship has been deratted within the previous 6 months, or a **deratting exemption certificate** issued in either an approved port or a designated approved port showing that the ship was inspected and found free from rodents and the plague vector. The list of approved and designated approved ports is published by the WHO, and amendments are notified in the Weekly Epidemiological Record [8]. If the certificate was issued more than 6 months previously, the ship must be inspected at an approved port and if necessary deratted at a designated approved port. Where the ship is proceeding immediately to a designated/approved port, the validity of the certificate may be extended by 1 month. This provision would be applied where the amount of cargo remaining on board prevents the inspection of all the spaces for the issue of a deratting exemption certificate. If evidence of rodents is found during the inspection of a ship, the port health officer is authorized to require the master to apply the appropriate control measures. These may be either trapping, poisoning or fumigation of the infested spaces, together with the elimination of any harbourage.

Disinfestation methods on ships

The construction of various ship types (Fig. 13.1) together with the limited time available to disinfest ships, limit the options for treatment. Consequently, acute poisons such as sodium fluoracetate or fumigation with hydrogen cyanide or methyl bromide may be required. These will usually be undertaken by a contractor, but it is the responsibility of the port health officer in charge to specify the treatment required and to have regard to the safety aspects. Acute rodenticides should only be used in spaces which can be secured to prevent access, while fumigation is taking place the crew will have to be accommodated ashore. Care will be required if it is intended to fumigate food with hydrogen cyanide or leave food exposed to hydrogen cyanide during fumigation.

If a ship, aircraft or cargo infested with rats arrives from an area in which plague is present, or if there is undue mortality among them, then fumigation should always be required. As methyl bromide is three times heavier than air, its use is particularly appropriate for the fumigation of foodstuffs, or a fully laden ship. Methyl bromide and hydrogen phosphide are also used for the elimination of arthropod infestations of cereals, nuts, dried fruit and herbs and spices, such fumigation may take place prior to shipment or after loading on board the ship.

With regard to in-transit fumigation, the International Maritime Organization recommends that the ship's master should obtain approval from his national administration. At least two members of the crew, including one officer, should be trained with particular reference to the behaviour and hazardous properties of the fumigant in air, the symptoms of poisoning and emergency medical treatment. They should brief the crew before the fumigation takes place and the ship should carry gas detection equipment, at least four sets of protective breathing apparatus, together with the appropriate medicine and first-aid equipment. It is the responsibility of the fumigator to ensure that all spaces treated are gas tight and that warning notices have been posted at the entrances to any spaces considered unsafe. Adjacent

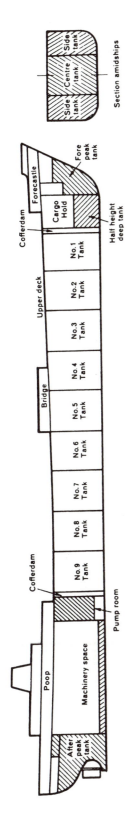

Tanker 15BH WB20500T incl. 14500T in clean ballast tanks DTf3300T

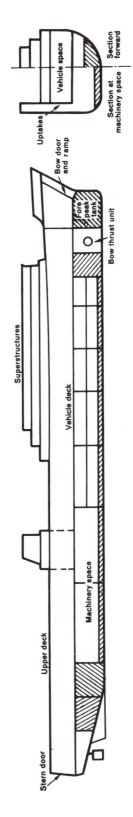

Ro Ro Cargo Coll BH to U dk 10 to 2nd dk WB350T incl. DTf90T

Fig. 13.1 Profiles illustrating decks, superstructures, spaces and tanks. (Reproduced by kind permission of Lloyds Register of Shipping, London.)

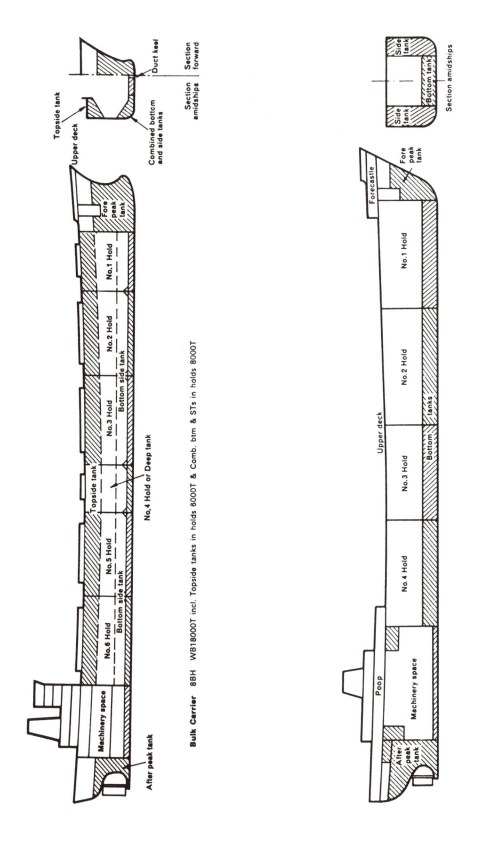

Bulk Carrier 8BH WB18000T incl. Topside tanks in holds 6000T & Comb. btm & STs in holds 8000T

Ore Carrier 6BH WB10000T

Figure 13.1 continued

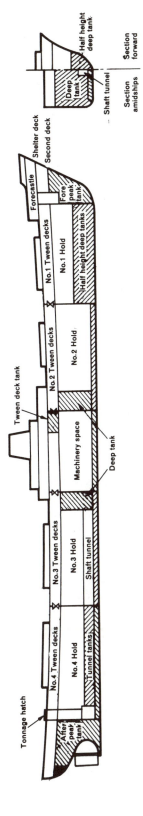

General Cargo Ship Coll BH & APBH to S dk 7 to 2nd dk WB4200T incl. DTma890T DTmf890T Tunnel tanks 400T UnDk a20T f20T

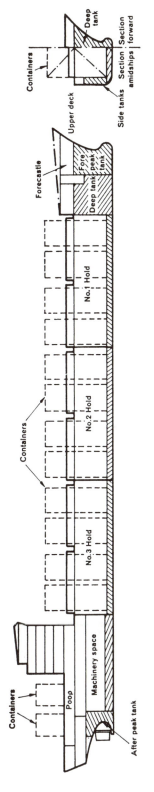

Container Ship 6BH WB2400T incl. DTf300T STs in Nos. 1 & 2 holds 1350T

Figure 13.1 concluded

spaces, accommodation and working spaces should be checked for the level of gas concentration at least at 8 hour intervals and the readings recorded in the ship's log book [7].

SHIPBOARD SANITATION

The provisions of the Public Health Acts relating to filthy, unwholesome and verminous premises or articles and verminous persons (see Chapter 16) apply to ships as if the vessel were a house, building or premises within the district, and the master or other officer in charge the occupier. In regard to statutory nuisances (see Chapter 7) the Environmental Protection Act 1990 defines 'premises' to include any vessel. An abatement notice may be served on the master of a vessel, as if he or she were the occupier of premises on which a statutory nuisance exists or is likely to occur. Except for a ship belonging to Her Majesty or visiting forces, the person in charge of a ship may be ordered to remedy any conditions on board which are prejudicial to health, and statutory nuisances may be dealt with summarily.

The standardization of sanitary measures to be taken on ships is specified by the WHO in the *Guide to Ship Sanitation* [9]. It provides practical recommendations for protecting food and potable water, the disposal of waste and elimination of pests, which are necessary to prevent the spread of disease.

International trains

An international train is a shuttle train or through train operating through the Channel Tunnel, and the person designated as the **train manager** on a journey terminating in the UK is responsible for advising the enforcement authority of the presence of any animal or sick person aboard the train. The Public Health (International Trains) Regulations 1994 define the enforcing authority as the port health or local authority at any place designated as a control area, freight depot or terminal control point. In relation to the records to be kept by an international train operator and

in the event of a health alert, the Secretary of State is designated as the enforcing authority.

Where a stowaway animal which is or was at the time of its death capable of carrying rabies, plague or viral haemorrhagic fever is suspected aboard an international train, the enforcement authority at a stopping place may require the train and its contents to be deratted, disinfected or decontaminated. There are also powers for the disinfection of decontamination of any rolling stock or any article on board where a sick person has been identified on the train.

Sick traveller means a person who has a serious epidemic, endemic or infectious disease, or whom there are reasonable grounds to suspect has such a disease, it does not mean venereal disease or infection with human immunodeficiency virus (See Chapter 16).

WATER SUPPLIES

Every port and airport is required by the international health regulations to have a supply of pure drinking water. Potable water for ships and water boats must be obtained only from those water points approved by the port health authority. Water boats should have independent tanks and pumping systems for potable water. Hydrants for the supply of water from ashore should be located so as to prevent contamination. Supply pipes should be above the high water level of the port, and drainage openings for pipes need to be above any water surge from passing ships. Water supply hoses require a smooth, impervious lining and should be used exclusively for the delivery of potable water, when not in use the ends should be capped.

Ships' storage tanks for potable water should be independent of the hull (Fig. 13.2), unless the tank bottom is at least 60 cm above the deepest load line. The bottom of the tank should not be in contact with the top of any double bottom tank, pipe lines carrying non-potable liquids should be routed so they cannot contaminate the potable water supply. A manhole on the tank top should have a coaming to keep the opening clear of the deck, and overflow pipes should have the open

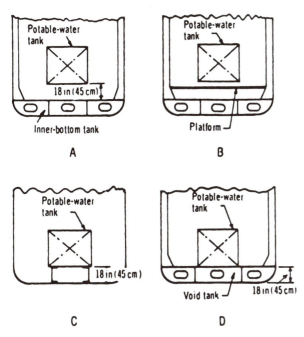

A

B

C

D

Fig. 13.2 Acceptable location of potable water in relation to bilge space of inner-bottom tank. (Source: Lamoureux, V.B. (1967) *Guide to Ship Sanitation*, World Health Organization, Geneva (Reprinted with amendments, 1987.))

end pointing downwards. Where tanks do not meet these recommendations, the water may be used for domestic purposes aboard ship, or should be chlorinated before its use as potable water.

Chlorine should preferably be applied as a hypochlorite solution, with equipment which will produce a free chlorine residue of 0.2 mg/l. Whenever any potable water tanks or any part of the supply system has been contaminated, serviced or repaired they should be cleansed, disinfected and flushed before being put back into operation. The chlorine solution for disinfection should be 50 mg/l for 24 hours, or in an emergency 100 mg/l for 1 hour. The heavily chlorinated water should be discharged and the system flushed with potable water before the system is used to supply potable water. Automatic chlorinators on an ultra-violet sterilization system should be fitted where low pressure evaporators are used for desalination. Sea water obtained when within 32 km of the land should never be used to produce potable water.

IMPORTED FOOD CONTROL

Enlargement of the European Union took effect on 1st January 1995, with the accession of Austria, Finland and Sweden. The European Economic Area (EEA) comprises the States of the EU together with Norway and at a date to be agreed Liechtenstein. Iceland is a member of the EEA for limited areas of trade, in particular fishery products.

For veterinary and phytosanitary purposes trade within the EEA (other than live shellfish and fishery products) is undertaken under the same harmonized conditions as apply to trade within the EU. Live shellfish and fishery products entering the EU from within the EEA are to be treated in the same way as products originating in the EU for health certificate purposes, but they are treated as third country imports for veterinary checks purposes.

The Products of Animal Origin (Import and Export) Regulations 1992 and The Products of Animal Origin (Third Country Imports) (Charges) Regulations 1992 implement Council Directives concerning veterinary checks on trade within the EEA and the organization of veterinary checks on products imported from third countries. [10,11]

With regard to trade within the EEA veterinary checks may be made on imports from another member State and the place of destination to ensure that all animal and public health conditions relating to imports have been complied with. Checks of such products during transport to their destination shall only be made, if an infringement of the Regulations on any animal or public health conditions relating to the importation or transport is suspected.

Products of animal origin may only be imported into the EEA through ports and airports which have been designated as Border Inspection Posts (BIPs) for specified products. A product of animal origin includes any product containing meat, raw and rendered animal fat, products obtained from eggs other than finished foods, recognizable milk products, and fishery products other than processed foods which contain less than 10% of a fishery product.

The importers of a product subject to veterinary checks are required to give prior notice of the arrival of consignments at a BIP and submit a Certificate for Veterinary Checks form, together with the veterinary certificate accompanying the product. Every consignment from a third country is subject to a documentary and identity check to verify the origin of the product and establish the requisite health marks and stamps are present, and that no indiction of rejection of the consignments has been given. Unless a reduced checking regime has been agreed for a specified product, or products arriving from a particular country, physical checks must be undertaken on all consignments. In particular, each consignment must be inspected to check that the conditions of transport have maintained the products in the required state, and that any temperature specifications have been complied with. An organoleptic examination to check for abnormalities rendering the product unfit for the use given on the veterinary certificate must be carried on 1% of the items in the consignment (with a minimum of 2 and a maximum of 10). For loose products the examination has to be made of at least five separate samples distributed throughout the consignment.

Addition physical and laboratory examination are carried out in the event of doubt, or when either information from another member state or when a result from the examination of a previous consignment has been unfavourable. If all the checks are satisfactory the consignment can be released for free movement in the territory of the EAA, provided the importer has paid the prescribed charges and received back a completed copy of the Certificate of Veterinary Checks signed and sealed from the BIP.

When physical checks on food entering the EAA show that the product may not be cleared for human consumption, the consignment must be re-dispatched outside EAA territory, destroyed or used for purposes other than human consumption where specific EC rules permit. Any costs of re-dispatching, destruction or using the product for purposes other than human consumption are to be charged to the importer or his representative. Where checks at the point of marketing indicated that the required checks at an inspection post at the point of arrival in another member state have not been complied with, the competent authority in that member state should be notified and the Commission informed in cases of repeated non-compliance.

It is proposed to introduce regulations covering both animal and public health aspects of products of animal origin, with a single regulation for each group of products. The Food Safety (Fishery Products) and (Live Bivalve Molluscs and Other Shellfish) Regulations 1994 stipulate that the specified import conditions should be enforced through the Products of Animal Origin (Import and Export) Regulations 1992. They also specify the requirements for establishment numbers, health mark and health certificates, the Fresh Meat (Import Conditions) Regulations 1995 are intended to replace the Importation of Animal Products and Poultry Products Order 1980 and the requirements of the Imported Food Regulations relating to fresh meat. These will be followed by further regulations dealing with poultry meat, game meat and meat products etc., for which animal and public health conditions have been established by the EU.

Health marks and certificates

A health mark is required on any fresh meat, meat product or bulk lard imported for sale for human consumption other than:

1. vitamin concentrates containing meat;
2. pharmaceutical products containing meat;
3. gelatine;
4. rennet;
5. meat products, of which meat is not a principal ingredient and which does not contain fragments of meat.

A meat product means any product prepared wholly or partly from fresh meat (which has undergone treatment to ensure a degree of preservation), but excludes fresh meat and those products specified above (Imported Food Regulations (IFR) 12(2) and 13(1) and Schedule 1).

Fresh meat means the offal or other edible parts of a mammal or bird which has not been subject to any treatment or process other than chilling, freezing, vacuum packing or packing in a controlled atmosphere and includes minced, chopped or mechanically recovered meat and meat treated by the addition of seasonings (IFR 2).

A health mark is defined as a label, mark, seal, brand, stamp or other voucher and they must be so placed as to be legible and clearly visible (IFR 12(1) and 13(1) (a) (b)).

Where a health mark is applied to packaging or is printed on packaging, it must be applied or printed in such a manner that the health mark is destroyed when the package is opened, unless the package is not capable of being used again as packaging (IFR Schedule 3(6)).

Recognized health marks are required to be published in the London and Edinburgh Gazettes and indicate that the ministers are satisfied that the fresh meat or the meat from which the meat product was prepared, was derived from mammals or birds inspected before and immediately after death and passed in accordance with criteria satisfactory to the minister. They also indicate that the dressing, packing and preparation of the fresh meat or meat product was carried out with all necessary precautions for the prevention of danger to health. The recognition of health marks may include fresh meat or meat products derived from mammals or birds killed when wild, which were not inspected immediately before death (IFR 13(3)).

Unless the notice requiring a health mark specifies that it extends to the following description of meat or poultry meat, they are prohibited:

1. Fresh meat comprising, or forming part of, the head of any animal or bird.
2. Any part of a carcass which has been chopped or minced, with or without the addition of any spices, cereal products, salt, flavouring, vegetables or other ingredients.

3. Scraps or trimmings, viz: small pieces and trimmings being muscular or other tissues or fats weighing less than 100 g which have been removed from an animal during the preparation of wholesale cuts, the boning, cutting or trimming of fresh meat or the preparation of fresh meat for the retail trade. (IFR 12(1) and 13(4) and Schedule 5)

The health mark must be applied before importation to all livers of bovine animals, swine and solipeds by hot branding; and to the meat of all solipeds, ruminating animals, swine and venison by either hot branding or stamping with marking ink.

Health marks must be applied in the following manner:

1. Carcasses weighing more than 65 kg to the external surfaces of the thighs, loins, back, breast or shoulder (IFR Schedule 3(1)(a)).
2. Carcasses weighing 65 kg or less to the external surfaces of the thighs and shoulders (IFR Schedule 3(1)(a)).
3. Cuts of meat and offal shall each bear a health mark unless wrapped or packed, in which case both the wrapping and packaging must have a health mark. Pieces of meat, including those weighing under 100 g, must be wrapped and packaged with a health mark on both the wrapping and packaging (IFR Schedule 3(1)(b)(d)(e)(f)).
4. Large packages consigned to a poultry cutting plant for cutting, or from a cutting plant to a meat products plant for treatment, or to restaurants or canteens for direct supply to the final consumer after cooking, are required to have a health mark on the package together with a label giving the intended use and address of destination (IFR Schedule 3(2)(a)(c) and Schedule 11).
5. Either on the wrapping of poultry carcasses or on the carcass but so that it is clearly visible under the wrapping, and also on any packaging (IFR Schedule 3(2)(b)).
6. On both the wrapping and packing of poultry meat and individual cuts of offal (IFR Schedule 3(2)(c)(d)).

7. Either on the meat or the wrapping and also on any packaging of any other fresh meat (IFR Schedule 3(3)).
8. Either on the meat or the wrapping and also on any packaging of meat products (IFR Schedule 3(4)).
9. A health mark shall accompany any bulk lard (including any other rendered mammal or poultry fat), transported in any ship, aircraft, hovercraft or road vehicle. It shall state the quantity and indicate the position of the tank in which the bulk lard is carried. Additionally, it must contain a certificate to indicate that any tank, pipes or pumps, used for the loading had been inspected and found clean (IFR Schedule 3(5)).

Wrapping and packaging

In relation to any fresh meat or meat product, 'wrapping' means any material or container in direct contact with the product, while a 'package' is the outer container into which the wrapped product is placed, other than any bulk container attached to a road vehicle or trailer (IFR 12(1)).

The wrapping of fresh meat or meat products:

1. Shall be transparent and colourless, unless it provides for the protective requirements of packaging.
2. Must not alter the organoleptic characteristics of the meat.
3. Must not be capable of transmitting substances harmful to human health.
4. Except for earthenware containers for meat products, it shall not have been used previously for wrapping meat, unless the wrapping provides the protective requirements of packaging when it may be used again after cleaning and disinfection.
5. Packaging of fresh meat or meat products shall be strong enough to ensure effective protection during transportation and handling, it shall not contain fresh meat of more than one species of animal, and must not have been used previously for a similar purpose unless it is made of impervious and corrosive resistant materials, which have been cleansed and disinfected.

Temperature requirements

Fresh meat and meat products must be transported so that the following temperatures can be maintained:

1. Carcasses and cuts: +7°C (chilled), −12°C (frozen).
2. For offals: +3°C.
3. Rabbit meat, poultry meat, rabbit offals and poultry offal; +4°C.
4. Meat products as specified on the label when prepared.

Health certificate

A health certificate is required for any fresh meat (which includes chilled or frozen meat) imported for sale for human consumption, which is derived from any domestic bovine animals (including buffalo), swine, sheep, goats, solipeds or poultry, or any meat product other than:

1. Meat extract, meat consommé, meat sauces and similar products not containing any fragments of meat.
2. Whole, broken or crushed bones, meat peptones, meat powder, pork-rind powder, blood plasma, dried blood plasma, cellular proteins, bone extracts and similar products.
3. Fats melted down from animal tissue.
4. Stomachs, bladders and intestines, cleaned and bleached, salted or dried.
5. Products containing fragments of meat, but which contain a quantity of meat or meat product not exceeding 10% of the total weight of the final product ready for use, after preparation in accordance with the instructions for use issued by the manufacturer. (IFR 14(1) and Schedule 2)

The health certificate must be in the form prescribed in the regulations, expressed in the English language and issued by an official veterinarian, or in the case of meat products by any other designated person.

The designated person must certify that the meat or meat product described was obtained in accordance with the requirements of community directives. In the case of imports from third countries, the meat or meat product must be certified that it comes wholly from animals slaughtered at establishments approved for export to the country of destination, that the health mark has been affixed to the packages and that hygiene requirements have been complied with.

Rejection and re-export

Meat contravening the provisions relating to health marks and certification may be detained and must not be removed for any purpose other than exportation without the permission of the authorized officer.

The detention notice must specify grounds upon which it is based and notify the importer that the meat must be destroyed or disposed of so that it cannot be used for human consumption, unless the importer gives a written undertaking to export the food within 14 days or to prove in proceedings before a justice that the importation complies with the requirements for health marking and certification, or the importer serves a counter notice on the authorized officer.

If the importer does not satisfy the justice that the product complies with the requirements for health marks and certification, he shall condemn the fresh meat or meat product. When satisfied that importation is not contrary to these provisions, the justice shall rescind the notice prohibiting its removal.

If the fresh meat or meat product is subject to either fresh meat, poultry meat or meat product directives, the authorized officer shall provide the minister with full details of the reason for its rejection. The importer shall be notified of his right to serve on the authorized officer the counter notice within 7 days, requiring him to obtain the opinion of an independent veterinary expert on the validity of any matter specified in the notice. On receipt of the counter notice, the authorized officer shall inform the minister and request him to nominate an independent veterinary expert. The minister shall consult with the Commission on the nomination of such an expert, who must be a national of an EU state other than

the importing or exporting country. The independent veterinary expert nominated by the minister shall examine the food and shall give his written opinion to the authorized officer, who shall make it available to the person who served the counter notice. If within seven days the authorized officer does not rescind the detention notice, the food shall be dealt with by a justice of the peace (IFR 16).

Defective health marks and certificates

Where any fresh meat or meat product is not permitted due to the absence of a recognized health mark or certificate for the product, the authorized officer shall furnish the minister with all relevant information in his or her possession. The minister shall make such enquiries as he or she considers appropriate, and communicate the results to the authorized officer. If, after consultation with the minister, the officer is satisfied that the fresh meat or meat product satisfied the criteria for having a health mark or certificate, the importation may be permitted provided the authorized officer notifies the minister (IFR 15).

Inspection charges

Where an importer specifically requests a portal authority for sound reasons, to carry out the examination of any food outside business hours, the enforcing authority shall arrange such examination and may charge the importer making this request for that service (IFR 22).

Prohibited food

In addition to the provisions of the Imported Food Regulations and the Importation of Milk Regulations which prohibit the import of certain classes of food, compositional and hygiene regulations also specify foodstuffs and wrapping materials whose importation is prohibited. The port health authority is the food authority responsible for preventing the import and, in some cases, the export of food which contravenes the statutory standards contained in:

Aflatoxin in Nuts, Nut Products, Dried Figs and Dried Fig Products Regulations 1992

Antioxidants in Food Regulations 1987*

Arsenic in Food Regulations 1959*

Bread and Flour Regulations 1984*

Caseins and Caseinates Regulations 1985

Chloroform in Food Regulations 1980*

Colouring Matter in Food Regulations 1973*

Egg Products Regulations 1993

Emulsifiers and Stabilisers in Food Regulations 1989*

Extraction Solvent in Food Regulations 1993

Flavourings in Food Regulations 1992

Food Additives Labelling Regulations 1992

Food (Control of Irradiation) Regulation 1967*

Food (Control of Irradiation) Regulations 1990

Food Protection (Emergency Provisions) (Paralytic Shellfish Poisoning) Order 1991

Ice Cream (Heat Treatment, Etc) Regulation 1959*

Ice Cream Regulations 1967*

Importation of Milk Regulations 1988

Imported Food (Bivalve Molluscs and Marine Gastropods from Japan) Regulations 1992

Imported Food and Feedingstuffs (Safeguards against Cholera Regulations) 1991*

Imported Food (Safeguards against Paralytic Toxin) (Pectinidae from Japan) Regulations 1992

Lead in Food Regulations 1979*

Mastic Materials and Articles in Contact with Food Regulations 1992

Materials and Articles in Contact with Food Regulations 1987

Meat Products and Spreadable Fish Products Regulations 1984*

Mineral Hydrocarbons in Food Regulations 1966*

Miscellaneous Additives in Food Regulations 1980*

Olive oil (Marketing Standards) Regulations 1987

Potassium Bromate (Prohibition as a Flour Improver) Regulations 1990

Poultrymeat (Water Content) Regulations 1984

Preservatives in Food Regulations 1979*

Product of Animal Origin (Import & Export Regulations) 1992

Solvents in Food Regulations 1967*

Spirit Drink Regulations 1990

Sweeteners in Food Regulations 1983*

Tetrachloroethylene in Olive Oil Regulations 1989

Tin in Food Regulations 1992

* As amended.

Food Labelling Regulations 1984 (as amended)

Imported food, except for fresh fruit and vegetables, cheese, butter, fermented milk and cream products and carbonated water, vinegar, etc., must be labelled with:

1. The name of the food and an indication of its physical condition and treatment.
2. A list of ingredients (in descending order of weight at the time of preparation of the food), water not exceeding 5% of the finished product, or water which is added for the purpose of reconstitution need not be declared.
3. Subject to specified exceptions an indication of the minimum durability.
4. Any special storage conditions or conditions of use for food to retain its specific properties.
5. The name or business name and address or registered offices of the manufacturer or packer or of a seller establishment within the EU.
6. Particulars of the place of origin if its omission might mislead purchasers as to the true origin of the food.
7. Instructions for use if necessary to make proper use of the food.

When food is sold otherwise than to the ultimate consumer, the particulars may be marked on the trade documents furnished on or before delivery of the food instead of on the package or label.

Meat Staining and Sterilization

The proposed Animal By-Products (Identification) Regulations 1995 are intended to replace the system of movement permits required by the Meat (Sterilization and Staining) Regulations 1982. The import of high risk animal by-products is prohibited by EU requirements, low risk by-products are subject to the requirements for a licence under the Importation of Animal Products and Poultry Products Order 1980 as amended.

FOOD HYGIENE AND SAFETY

The Food Safety Act 1990 defines 'premises' as including any ship or aircraft as may be specified in an Order made by Ministers. Until the commencement of such an Order only a home going ship plying exclusively in inland waters, or engaged exclusively in coastal excursions, lasting not more than one day starting and ending in Great Britain and not calling at a place outside Great Britain is subject to the food safety legislation that applies to 'premises'. Powers of entry conferred by the Act include the right to enter any ship or aircraft for the purpose of ascertaining whether there is any imported food present as part of the cargo. Provision is also made in the Act (section 58) for treating any offshore installation in the United Kingdom's territorial water as if it were situated in the adjacent part of Great Britain for the purposes of food safety legislation.

Fishing vessels, including fish processing factories are subject to hygiene requirements of the Food Safety (Fishery Products on Fishing Vessels) Regulations 1992, which are intended to ensure that fish is handled and stored under hygienic conditions and protected from risk of contamination. Fish caught by a fishing vessel flying a third country flag landed in a UK port is subject to the veterinary checks regimen; such direct landings do not have to be accompanied by a health certificate.

AIR POLLUTION

The prohibition of dark smoke from chimneys (see Chapter 41) applies to vessels, as references to a furnace included reference to an engine of the vessel, and so long as the vessel is in navigable waters contained within any port, river estuary etc., for which charges other than light dues can be made in respect of vessels entering or using facilities therein.

The permitted periods in which vessels are allowed to emit dark smoke without committing an offence are contained in the Dark Smoke (Permitted Periods) (Vessels) Regulations 1958. But the provisions of Part III of the Environmental Protection Act 1990 relating to nuisances arising from smoke, fumes or gas emissions, do not apply to a vessel powered by steam reciprocating machinery. In relation to the release of other pollutants into the air, the Act can be used to abate or prevent nuisances arising from the handling of bulk cargoes [12]. The area of a port health authority includes the territorial waters to seaward of the district, in respect of any nuisance to which Part III of the Act applies.

REFERENCES

1. Salisbury Manuscripts 1602/1603, Calender State Papers Domestic 1635/1636, Calender Treasury Papers 1708 and 1714.
2. Howard, J. (1789) Lord Liverpools Papers 1786. (Account of the Lazarettos Privy Council: Levant Company to Pitt 1792).
3. Maclean C. (1796) *The Source of Epidemic and Pestilential Diseases*. Calcutta.
4. Southwood Smith, T. (1866) *The Common Nature of Epidemics*. London.
5. General Board of Health (1849) *First Report on Quarantine*.
6. Howard-Jones, N. (1975) *The Scientific Background of the International Sanitary Conference 1851–1938*. WHO Geneva.
7. International Maritime Organization (1984) *Supplement to the Recommendation on The Safe Use of Pesticides in Ships*, London.
8. WHO (1985) *Weekly Epidemiological Record*, Vol. 60, World Health Organization, Geneva.
9. Lamoureux, V.B. (1967) *Guide to Ship Sanitation*, World Health Organization, Geneva.
10. Products of Animal Origin (Import & Export) Regulations 1992.
11. The Products of Animal Origin (Third Country Imports) (Charges) Regulations 1992.
12. Schofield, C. and Shillito, D. (1990) *Guide to the Handling of Dusty Materials in Ports*, 2nd edn, British Materials Handling Board, Ascot.

14 Statistical method

Frank Oliver

Statistics as a subject can be defined as the science of the collection and analysis of numerical information. For many purposes, in environmental health and elsewhere, it is necessary to get more than a subjective impression; measurement is essential to assess the nature and scale of problems and to assess the efficacy of different possible ways of treating them. Abundant experience shows that training and experience are vital to the use of statistics. Nevertheless, people working in many fields can benefit from an understanding of basic statistics; even if they are not themselves professional statisticians they can perform some of the simpler techniques but, more important, they can understand and appreciate the results obtained by professional statisticians, together with their limitations, and can recognize problems for which professional statistical advice is necessary.

A single chapter can do no more than introduce statistics as a subject. Serious students will need to study specialist textbooks and to gain experience by tackling a variety of problems and exercises. The explanations and discussion of the various methods outlined in this chapter do no more than give an introduction to them; there is a great deal more to say about most of them and reference should be made to the works cited in the reading list accordingly. The descriptions of the techniques included in this chapter should be sufficient to enable lay people to be able to read and to understand much of the statistical analysis performed and published by others, and to cope with routine situations where such analysis is necessary themselves, but the advice of professional statisticians should be sought whenever necessary. Such help will certainly be far more useful if given at an early stage rather than after the data have been collected.

Modern developments in calculation have transformed the application of statistics. Pocket calculators, costing perhaps £15, do many of the calculations which formerly had to be performed – laboriously and inaccurately – by hand. All users of statistical methods need such calculators. Furthermore, most computer installations provide access to packages, e.g. Minitab, which enable users to do many statistical calculations without acquiring any knowledge of computer programming; it may reasonably be expected that local authority environmental health departments have appropriate numbers of terminals giving access to such packages on central computers. It is now easy to do most calculations; the difficulties arise in deciding which calculations to undertake and in interpreting the results.

COLLECTION OF DATA

The first thought of many people faced with a problem is to conduct a survey. This should be one's last thought. An enormous quantity of information is collected by the Government Statistical Service and by other bodies. Many of the results are published and available in libraries and elsewhere, and many further compilations and analyses of government-collected data can be obtained on request, although perhaps at a charge. Other information is already available in the records of institutions and can be extracted much more satisfactorily than by seeking to collect it by means of surveys.

The range of available published information varies continually, and it is not possible to present a full account which will remain useful for any appreciable length of time. Much the most comprehensive account is published by the Central Statistical Office, which brings out a new edition of the invaluable *Guide to Official Statistics* [1] from time to time. The most recent edition at the time of writing appeared in 1990. This *Guide* covers not only official statistics, it includes some statistics published by local authority associations and relevant professional bodies. Every 10 years a Census of Population is held which yields a great mass of information relating to the country as a whole, as well as to separate local authority areas; housing conditions have, historically, been a particular subject of enquiry. The reports on each census run to hundreds of volumes, which now appear rather more quickly than formerly as a result of the use of computers in the census offices. The **Annual Abstract of Statistics** [2] contains a large number of statistical series, some covering the previous several years, others a somewhat longer period, and guidance is given as to where to look for further information regarding the topics covered. **Social Trends** [3] and **Regional Trends** [4] appear annually and contain a great deal more interpretation and analysis (though fewer hard facts) than the *Annual Abstract*. The annual **General Household Survey** [5] obtains information on a variety of topics including health and housing. The Office of Population Censuses and Surveys publishes a wide range of volumes, including some in microfiche, on a variey of topics; much of the information is available for separate local authority areas. Government departments are most helpful to would-be users of the statistics which they publish in clarifying any obscurities regarding them. Many official statistics are available in computer readable form, which facilitates their analysis. The Chartered Institute of Public Finance and Accountancy (CIPFA) also publishes numerous reports on a local authority basis.

If it is really impossible to get the information from these or other existing sources, or by extracting it from existing records, it may be necessary as a last resort to collect it oneself. This will invariably be slow and expensive, will probably introduce sampling and other errors, will require great practical skills and experience, and should often be best left to professional firms who will certainly work closely with the would-be users of the results. If one decides to collect the information personally, one has to choose between a **complete census** and a **sample survey**. The former is more attractive, but will often be impossible (testing products for possible contamination may involve destroying the particular items tested, so a sample of the total is necessary), or impracticable (perhaps because the numbers involved are too large). A properly selected sample survey enables much greater attention to be paid to persons or items chosen in the sample, and greatly reduces the cost and time involved in processing the results.

If practicable, it is greatly preferable for the fieldwork to be done by **observation** rather than by interview or postal questionnaire. Investigators can assess whether freezers are at excessive temperatures, are overfilled, or are in need of defrosting and will do so more accurately than by asking their owners or users. Membership of ethnic minority groups is easier to establish by inspection than by questioning. In some cases, observation can be advantageously combined with other methods of enquiry.

Questionnaires can be filled in by interviewers or may be posted or handed to respondents. **Interviewer surveys** are preferable in that they reduce opportunities of misunderstanding questions, enable the interviewers to observe as well as question, and usually lead to higher response rates. However, there is often a case for conducting a **survey by post**. Doing so is always cheaper and often quicker, it avoids the results of unfortunate interactions between interviewers and subjects, and it enables respondents to consider their replies, consult records, etc. There are many other reasons for preferring each method to the other. The decennial censuses of population adopt a compromise arrangement whereby census enumerators visit households and leave forms with them for later collection, helping respondents to fill them in as necessary; a consequence of using this method is that the census questionnaires have to be sufficiently simple for most households to fill in unaided.

Designing a questionnaire is not something to be undertaken lightly. Questions should be readily intelligible, not only to the experts conducting the survey, but to those answering them. They should be unambiguous ('Do you prefer lined or unlined curtains?' might refer to the presence or absence of a lining, or the design of a pattern), and unbiased (during the course of a lengthy interview respondents to one survey were asked two almost identical questions, with many more agreeing that 'more public ownership would be good for the country' than agreeing, rather later in the interview, that 'more nationalization would be good for the country'). Closed-ended questions ask for one answer out of a number of possibilities, e.g. they ask respondents to say which of a number of age ranges they fall in, or whether they agree strongly, agree mildly, neither agree nor disagree, disagree mildly, or disagree strongly with some opinion, such as that much more public money should be spent on reducing pollution. Open-ended questions do not restrict possible responses in this way. Thus, they may ask respondents their ages or for their views on spending money to reduce pollution. Responses to open-ended questions must be classified by the interviewer or, usually more appropriately, by the survey organization, and this introduces possible errors of judgement; closed-ended questions are usually to be preferred.

Draft questionnaires should be tried out in pilot surveys and amended in the light of experience. Pilot surveys have many other practical advantages.

The annual reports of the *General Household Survey* invariably include the questionnaires used in the survey and filled in by interviewers during interviews; they are examples of well-designed, but extremely lengthy and complex, questionnaires which it would be impossible to use in postal surveys. It is always good practice in reporting the results of a survey to include the

actual words of the questions asked – among other advantages, this allows readers to assess possible biases in their wording. This is standard practice in newspaper reports of public opinion polls commissioned by them.

CLASSIFICATION AND TABULATION

Statistical information, however obtained, is usually presented in the form of **tables of results**. They vary from case to case, but there are certain common features of all good tables. They should have clear headings. The source of the figures should be given (so that readers can assess the reliability of the results, check them for accuracy, clear up problems of definition, coverage, etc., and know where to look for further information). Two short tables are shown (Tables 14.1 and 14.2).

Table 14.1 Cars per household, UK, Family Expenditure Survey, 1988

Number of cars/vans	*Number of households*	
0	2467	(34%)
1	3266	(45%)
2	1272	(18%)
3 or more	260	(4%)
Total	7265	(100%)

Source: Central Statistical Office (1988) *Family Expenditure Survey*, HMSO, London, Table 1.
Note: percentages do not add to 100 because of rounding.

It should be seen at a glance that the two tables relate to different years and to different geographical entities (Northern Ireland being included in the first and not the second). Table 14.1 is directly quoted from the source, although the percentages are not given there, whereas Table 14.2 is the result of analysis of the data published in the *General Household Survey*. A particular point to notice about the second table is that the lengths of time do not overlap, so that for any household it is entirely clear which category or **class interval** it falls in. (A system of intervals of the form 0 to 1 year, 1 to 3 years, 3 to 5 years, etc., would leave it ambiguous as to which inter-

Table 14.2 Length of residence of head of household by tenure, GB, %, 1986

Length of residence	Owner occupied		Rented		Total
	Owned outright (%)	With mortgage (%)	Local authority/New town (%)	Other (%)	(%)
Less than 1 year	4	12	9	23	10
1 but under 3 years	6	19	13	20	14
3 but under 5 years	6	16	11	10	12
5 but under 11 years	15	28	23	16	22
11 but under 16 years	11	12	12	6	11
16 but under 21 years	13	8	10	6	10
21 but under 31 years	23	5	11	5	11
31 or more years	22	1	11	13	10
100% equals	2510	3838	2684	1134	10166

Source: Derived from Office of Population, Censuses and Surveys (1986) *General Household Survey*, HMSO, London, Table 6.32.
Note: percentages may not add to 100 because of rounding.

val a reading of exactly 3 years should go into.) Table 14.1 is a simple or **one way table**, the only question relating to each household is which row it features in. Table 14.2 is a **two way table**, where each of the households behind the quoted percentages is classified both by row and by column.

Table 14.2 presents its results in percentage form to enable comparisons between lengths of residence among different tenure patterns to be drawn most easily. Thus it will be seen that households with mortgages have not usually lived in their homes for a long time, that households in council-owned property accord closely with the overall average length of residence pattern, that other renters are often short-term occupants, and that most owner occupiers without mortgages have been at their addresses for many years. The percentage signs at the heads of the columns emphasize that households within tenure category are broken down into length of residence.

Table 14.1 shows a distribution of discontinous or **discrete data**, in that the number of cars each household has is necessarily 0, 1, 2, etc.; Table 14.2 shows five distributions of **continuous data**, in that the head of household can have resided for any length of time, e.g. 4.7151 years, possibly within specified limits. Continous data have always to be grouped in drawing up a table, whereas discrete data need not be, as here.

DIAGRAMS

Diagrams, charts, graphs, etc., can be a good way of presenting statistics so that they make a strong impression on readers, particularly non-statistical readers. The more 'popular' the presentation required, the more likely it is that diagrams will be helpful. The annual official publication *Social Trends* (see page 239) makes extensive use of them, and can be referred to for examples of good practice. Different colours can often be used with advantage. The powerful impact made by diagrams means that extra care needs to be taken in drawing them, and there are many common fallacies which can mislead the unwary reader.

It is just as necessary to give clear headings and data sources to diagrams as to tables, for the same reasons. In drawing **graphs**, etc., axes should be clearly labelled. Axes normally intersect at zero on both scales, but it is frequently desirable to start at some other value below which there are no observations, say in graphing a time series, so that fluctuations are more easily perceived; if so, the axis should be clearly scaled accordingly and a break inserted between the bottom scale point and the origin – this break can usefully be emphasized by a zig-zag line. ('Official' practice is regrettably lax in this.)

One kind of diagram which causes many problems is where one single object is shown in

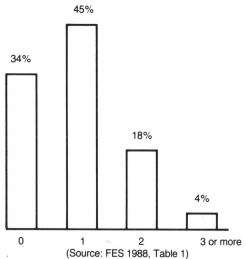

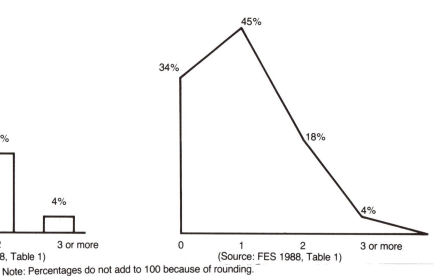

Fig. 14.1 a Bar chart of cars per household, UK Family Expenditure Survey 1988. b Frequency polygon of cars per household, UK Family Expenditure Survey 1988. Note: in a and b percentages do not add to 100 because of rounding. (Source: FES 1988, Table 1.)

different sizes to indicate different quantities. Suppose that it is estimated that the rat population of an area of waste ground was 100, 200 and 250 in successive years. A report on this might properly feature three rows each marked with the relevant year, containing 10, 20 and 25 identical pictures of a rat with a clearly marked scale, showing one picture of a rat equalling ten rats in the waste ground. On the other hand, it would be improper to draw a single rat for the first year, double its size for the second year, and increase it again for the third. The problem is that, if one doubles the length, height and thickness of the rat, one increases its volume by a factor of eight. If each dimension is multiplied by 2.5 the volume is multiplied by 15.625 (i.e 2.5 × 2.5 × 2.5). The result would be both misleading and alarmist. In order to get a rat of double the volume, each dimension should be multiplied by the cube root of 2, that is by 1.26. At best, the result would be unclear. Such diagrams are best avoided. When faced with them in other people's writings, one should be especially careful in interpreting them.

The statistics in Table 14.1 can well be illustrated by means of a **bar chart** or a **frequency polygon**, both methods being shown here (Fig. 14.1). Bar charts are commoner and are to be preferred.

Observations of different sizes are often grouped into class intervals. This is always necessary for continuous data and may be required for discrete data also. Thus, in compiling Table 14.2, households whose heads had been resident for any length of time as great as or greater than 1 year, but not as great as 3 years, were put into the second interval, and 14% of all households fell into this category. In illustrating any of the columns of such a table, the most suitable form of diagram is a **histogram**.

Where the class intervals are of equal breadth these are essentially bar charts where the bars adjoin each other. Problems arise where, as in Table 14.2, the intervals are unequal. Consider the 'Total' column, for example. Fewer households had been in place for less than 1 year than had been for 1 but less than 3 years, but a moment's thought reveals that this is because, and only because, the first interval covers a span of 1 year only while the second interval covers 2 years. One corrects for different breadths of class interval by dividing the frequency being displayed by the breadth of the interval and drawing the histogram with a height proportional to the result. (If all the breadths are equal the height is simply proportional to the frequency, as in a bar chart.) The effect of this correction is to make equal

Table 14.3 Length of residence of head of household, % GB, 1986

Length of residence	Percentage of households	Breadth of interval	Height of histogram
Less than 1 year	10	1	10.0
1 but under 3 years	14	2	7.0
3 but under 5 years	12	2	6.0
5 but under 11 years	22	6	3.7
11 but under 16 years	11	5	2.2
16 but under 21 years	10	5	2.0
21 but under 31 years	11	10	1.1
31 or more years	10	10 (say)	1.0
Total	100		

Source: Derived from Office of Populations, Censuses and Surveys (1986) *General Household Survey*, HMSO, London, Table 6.32.

Note: 100% = 10 166 households; percentages to not add to 100 because of rounding.

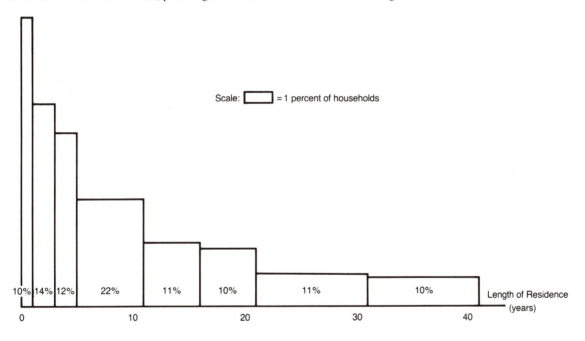

(Source: Derived from *General Household Survey*, 1986, Table 6.32)

Fig. 14.2 Length of residence of head of household, % GB, 1986. (Source: derived from General Household Survey, 1986, Table 6.32.)

areas of the histogram represent equal frequencies. Here the breadths of successive intervals are 1, 2, 2, 6, 5, 5, and 10 years, with the last interval being of indeterminate breadth. For present purposes take it as 10 years: where it is not possible to make an intelligent approximation it is

better to omit the interval from the histogram and explain the situation in a footnote to it. The histogram is calculated in Table 14.3 and the resultant graph is shown in Fig. 14.2.

Note that there is no vertical scale on the left of the diagram – any such scale would be either incorrect or confusing – but an area scale is given, obtained by calculating it for two or three different sections of the histogram

POPULATIONS AND SAMPLES

In statistics, the word **population** has a broader meaning than its non-technical meaning. It signifies the total number of units, whether human or otherwise, it is wished to make statements about, often on the basis of a **sample**. Thus as well as the population of people resident in the UK or in a particular area at any particular time, one can have the population of households, the population of dwellings, the population of cafés, etc. A cake manufacturer receiving a consignment of eggs will regard it as constituting a population of eggs, and may draw a sample for destructive testing. On the basis of the sample, the manufacturer may conclude that the rest of the population, i.e. of the consignment, is of unacceptable quality.

A listing of the members (human or otherwise) of the population is called a **sampling frame**, and such a sampling frame is usually necessary in drawing proper samples.

In any serious sampling investigation, it is necessary to choose the sample by random means. It is not satisfactory for the investigator to pick a few apparently typical members of the population, or to reach into a crate and pull out some of its contents haphazardly. A **random** sample, in the technical sense, is one in which each member of the population has a calculable and non-zero (not necessarily equal) chance of selection. A special kind of random sample, known as a **simple random sample**, is where the chances of selection are all equal and the selection of one member does not affect the relative chances of selecting others.

In principle, one can draw such a simple random sample by numbering each member of the population, writing the numbers onto small, identical cards, putting the cards into a hat or urn, stirring them up thoroughly, and drawing out the required number of cards to give the sample. If after drawing each member of the sample one returns its card to the urn before drawing the next member, so that any member can be drawn two or more times, the result is a simple random sample **with replacement**; if one does not return each drawn card so that no member of the population can be drawn more than once, it is a simple random sample **without replacement**.

In practice it is not necessary to use cards, urns, etc. Provided that the members of the population have been numbered, tables of random numbers enable one to select the numbers to constitute the sample, with or without replacement as desired. Such tables are widely available. Computer packages usually have facilities for generating random numbers which can be used for drawing samples as described above, and many packages will actually draw simple random samples of the required size directly, sparing one the trouble of using random numbers.

It is often possible to achieve greater accuracy by drawing a **stratified sample**. If one can divide the population into a number of groups or strata, so that each member falls into one and only one stratum, one can take separate random samples within each stratum and pool the results. In nation-wide samples, it is common to stratify by standard region, so that the proportions of families in Scotland and in East Anglia, for example, in the sample correspond to those in the population. Expenditure per family on tobacco in Scotland is much higher than in East Anglia, so in the Family Expenditure Survey this stratification gives a national average which cannot be too high because the sample happened to choose a rather larger proportion of Scottish households than of households from East Anglia. The pooling of the separate samples from each stratum is particularly simple if the same sampling fraction is used throughout, as is usual, but it is sometimes preferable to sample some strata more intensively than others and to take account of this in analysing the results.

In order to be useful, the system of stratification must be related to the subject of the enquiry – the closer the better.

It is sometimes overlooked that it is necessary

to have, or to construct, separate sampling frames for each stratum. This requires that the classification into strata is practicable in advance of drawing the sample. One cannot stratify individuals by their (unknown) voting behaviour at the last general election, for example.

The costs of interviewing a simple random or stratified sample of families in the UK would be very high, consisting partly or largely of interviewers' travelling costs. Such costs can be greatly reduced by confining interviewing to a suitable number of locations by taking a **multi-stage sample**. Here the population is divided into a number of first-stage units – for national surveys these are often constituencies or local authority areas. A random sample of first-stage units is drawn (perhaps using stratified sampling) and the individuals to be interviewed are chosen only from the selected first-stage units. (The choice may be done by any suitable random process; if the first stage is of constituencies, a second stage of wards or polling districts might or might not be introduced.)

Multi-stage samples are **less** accurate than simple random samples of the same size (and hence less accurate still than stratified samples of the same size), but economies in administration may allow so much larger samples to be drawn as to outweigh this loss of accuracy. National surveys usually combine multi-stage and stratification methods. It might be hoped that the gain in accuracy from the latter would outweigh the inaccuracy of the former, giving an overall sample as accurate as a simple random sample of the same size, but detailed analysis usually suggests that this is over optimistic.

Stratified and multi-stage samples are both random, in the technical sense, although not simple random. There is one commonly-used method of sampling individuals which is non-random, called **quota sampling**. Here each interviewer is instructed to go to a particular area and to interview a predetermined number of people whom she happens to meet, subject to quota controls (most interviewers are women). These quota controls, typically of age, sex and social class (as indicated by occupation), ensure that her interviewees are representative of the population

of her area in these respects. Quota samples thereby achieve the advantages of stratifying by age, sex and class, none of which are normally possible stratification criteria in random samples. By confining the interviewing to a number of preselected areas, the cost reduction advantage of multi-stage sampling is derived.

Since it is not possible to say what the probability is of most individuals meeting an interviewer and being interviewed in a quota sample, quota samples are, in the technical sense, non-random. Formal methods of analysing random samples cannot be applied to them. Nevertheless, quota samples are often used by commercial organizations and give excellent results; voting figures at general elections are predicted with reasonable accuracy by the various public opinion organizations.

Quota sampling is cheap per interview and has the advantage of the quota controls. But perhaps its greatest advantage in many contexts is speed, since interviewers do not have to spend time trying to find named individuals. At election times there are, or may be, swings of opinion which should be measured as rapidly as possible, and clearly it is necessary for public opinion polls to be published before, rather than after, the election has been held. Speed is also essential in measuring radio audiences and in assessing listeners' reactions, since people forget the programmes they heard as time passes.

The Government Office of Population Censuses and Surveys never uses quota sampling, and it is unlikely to be desirable in environmental health work. Since quota sampling is non-random, it is impossible to apply the wide variety of methods available for the analysis of random samples. Quota samples are subject to major sources of bias. Thus, some interviewers might avoid speaking to people who appear to be in a hurry, or to members of ethnic minority groups. The infirm are less likely to be out in the street. In practice, the principal bias is found to relate to occupation. Non-working housewives are much more likely to be chosen than those with jobs. Students, messengers and delivery people will be over represented at the expense of factory workers, train drivers and coalminers.

MEASURES OF CENTRAL TENDENCY

One often wants to give a single statistic which typifies a number, usually a large number, of different statistics. This single value is in some sense their 'average'. Thus, one can think of the average income in an area and compare it with the average in another area or in the same area at a different time. Looking at Table 14.1, one may ask the average number of cars per household, and at Table 14.2 the average lengths of time heads of households with different tenures have resided at their addresses. Several different measures of average are used – so it is bad practice to refer to any of them specifically as **the** average – and these measures are known collectively as **measures of central tendency**.

Consider the statistics shown in Table 14.4. The figures fluctuate considerably from month to month, but as one studies the table two features of it suggest themselves. There appears to be a tendency for deaths to be higher in the winter than in the summer, and each year there appear to be fewer deaths than in the previous year. These suggestions can be examined by use of the **mean**. In 1989 there were 1329 deaths altogether in the 12 months, and so the mean number of deaths per month was 1329/12 = 110.75. Similar calculations for 1990 and 1991 give means of 100.08 and 82.92 deaths respectively. This confirms the suggestion of a year-to-year decrease, and the further information that the decrease was much larger between 1990 and 1991 than between 1989 and 1990 emerges. In the same way, the means for successive months of the year can be found to be 137.3 (i.e. (161 + 148 + 103)/3, 129.7, 130.7, 99.3, 90.7, 74.3, 62.0, 58.7, 82.0, 85.0, 105.0, 120.3). Averaging over the 3 years in this way reveals a smooth seasonal pattern, with

the December mean over twice as great as the August mean.

If there are n observations written $x_1, x_2 \ldots x_n$, their mean is defined as $x = (x_1 + x_2 + \ldots + x_n)/n$. (The mean of values of x is usually denoted as $\bar{x}$, m or m_x, or if the values constitute a population rather than a sample as μ or μ_x.)

(Mathematicians refer to this as the **arithmetic mean** to distinguish it from the **geometric mean**, the n th root of the product of $x_1, x_2 \ldots x_n$. The geometric mean is rarely useful in statistical work.)

What is the mean number of cars per household, using the data of Table 14.1? Obviously, no cars were owned by the 2467 households which had no cars. Households with 1 car each had 3266 cars in total. Households with 2 cars each had $1272 \times 2 = 2544$ cars. Households with 3 or more cars had at least $260 \times 3 = 780$ cars, so the 7265 households had $0 + 3266 + 2544 + 780 = 6590$ cars, a mean of $6590/7265 = 0.9071$ cars per household. (This ignores fourth, fifth, etc., cars and is thus a slight underestimate.)

This extension of the basic formula for the mean may be expressed as follows. If f_1 units each have x_1 of the characteristic, f_2 each have x_2, and so on up to f_n units each having x_n, the total number of units is $f_1 + f_2 + \ldots + f_n$, and the total amount of the characteristic is $f_1x_1 + f_2x_2 + \ldots + f_nx_n$, giving a mean of

$$\bar{x} = (f_1x_1 + f_2x_2 + \ldots + f_nx_n)/(f_1 + f_2 + \ldots + f_n),$$

that is, with obvious notation,

$$\bar{x} = \Sigma f_i x_i / \Sigma f_i.$$

It is not possible to **find** the means of the five distributions in Table 14.2 because the lengths of residence of each head of household are not given

Table 14.4 Sudden infant deaths by month of death England and Wales, 1989–91

	Jan	Feb	Mar	Apr	May	Jun	Jul	Aug	Sep	Oct	Nov	Dec
1989	161	131	156	92	103	68	59	71	88	114	147	139
1990	148	121	121	110	79	81	69	60	93	77	97	145
1991	103	137	115	96	90	74	58	45	65	64	71	77

Source: Office of Population Censuses and Surveys, *OPCS Monitor DH3*, 91/1 and 92/2, HMSO, London, Table 4.

exactly, but it is possible to **estimate** them. One has to assume a value for each of the class intervals, and in default of anything better one generally takes the midpoint of each interval as its typical value. Thus 'less than 1 year' is taken as 0.5 years, '1 but under 3 years' as 2 years, and the next five as 4, 8, 13.5, 18.5 and 26 years. Some guess is needed to cope with the top, open-ended, interval – say 36 years. (In well-constructed tables, only small numbers of cases will be in any open-ended class intervals, so the exact values chosen will not greatly affect the results.) This gives the mean length of residence of heads owning their dwelling outright as $(4 \times 0.5 + 6 \times 2 + 6 \times 4 + 15 \times 8 + 11 \times 13.5 + 13 \times 18.5 + 23 \times 26 + 22 \times 36)/100 = 19.37$ years, which in view of the questionable assumptions which have had to be made should be rounded to 19.4 years (or perhaps to 19 years). That mean, together with the means for the other four distributions which can usefully be checked as an exercise dividing by the totals of the percentages given, which are not always 100 because of rounding), are given in Table 14.5 below.

Table 14.5 Mean length of residence of head of household, by tenure, GB, 1986

Tenure	Mean length of residence
Owner occupied (owned outright)	19.4 years
Owner occupied (with mortgage)	8.0 years
Rented (local authority/new town)	12.9 years
Rented (other)	10.2 years
All households	12.4 years

Source: Derived from Office of Population Censuses and Surveys (1986) *General Household Survey*, HMSO, London, Table 6.32.

The results, although not unexpected, are illuminating, but there are three sources of error in their compilation which should be kept in mind in interpreting them: they are based on a possibly unrepresentative sample rather than a complete census; they assume that the midpoints of the intervals are typical of the households in them; and they use the assumption that the typical length of residence of the '31 years or more' households is 36 years.

Although probably the most commonly used measure of central tendency, the mean has features which may be disadvantageous in particular applications. It is dependent upon just how extreme the extreme values are (so that the mean of 1, 2, 3, 4 and 30 is 8 and the mean of 1, 2, 3, 4 and 70 is 16). A small number of freakish values can produce a mean which is scarcely typical of the values to which it relates. It is necessary to make assumptions regarding typical values of open ended class intervals. And the result may well be a value which it is impossible actually to observe, e.g. 108.4 deaths or 0.907 cars.

These features can usually be avoided by the use of the **median**, the other average in common use in statistics. The median is that value which is greater than or equal to half the observations, and is less than or equal to half the observations. Referring to Table 13.4, the 12 statistics for 1989 can be arranged in increasing order as 59, 68, 71, 88, 92, 103, 114, 131, 139, 147, 156 and 161. So in 6 months there were fewer than 108.5 deaths and in 6 months there were more; the median is thus 108.5 deaths. (One takes the value midway between the two relevant observations, here 103 and 114, in cases such as this.) Similarly, in 1990 the median was 95 deaths per month and in 1991 it was 75.5 deaths – by this measure too, successive years showed an improvement. Over the 36 months as a whole, the median was 92.5 deaths, which is not the median of the three annual medians.

Analysis of Table 14.1 shows that the median number of cars per household was 1; at least half the households (actually 79%) had 1 car or less, and at least half (actually 66%) had 1 car or more. Alternatively the 3633rd household in increasing number of cars owned had 1 car (3633 = (7265 + 1)/2).

Given the original data or a table in which they are presented ungrouped, one can find the median exactly. For continuous data such as ages which have been arranged in a grouped table, one has to make an estimate of the median. If one is prepared to assume that the observations are evenly spread throughout the interval containing the median, the following simple formula gives the resultant approximation:

$$\text{approx median} = 1_m + \frac{\frac{n}{2} - f_b}{f_m} \cdot h$$

where 1_m is the lower limit of the interval which contains the median, n is the number of observations, f_b is the total number of observations below the lower limit of the median interval, f_m is the number of observations in the median interval, and h is its breadth. Thus, consider the statistics in Table 14.6, noting carefully the wording in the 'age' columns. In published statistics, ages are usually given to the nearest whole number below, so that '16 to 19' includes those aged 19 years and 11 months.

The left-hand half of Table 14.6 gives the information as published. The right-hand half is easily compiled from it for the present purpose. Since there were 110 874 single women one seeks to estimate the age of the 55 437th and 55 438th in increasing order of age. It is seen that they must have been between 20 and 25, but it is not certain just where.

h   The median estimation formula gives:

$$\text{approx median} = 20 + \frac{55\,437 - 33\,271}{44\,277}.5 = 22.50 \text{ years}$$

probably best quoted as 22.5 years in view of the assumptions necessary to obtain it. For ever married women, the formula estimates the median as 31.13 or 31.1 years, understandably somewhat larger.

It will be seen that it is not necessary to make any assumptions about the top, open ended, class interval of 40 and over. This is a minor advantage of the median over the mean; to estimate the mean some assumption about the top interval would be necessary.

It is worthwhile noting two points which sometimes confuse students. The formula correctly uses n/2, that is 55 437, rather than, 55 437.5, and the breadth of the interval '20–24' is indeed 5 years rather than 4 as might be thought (since it includes women aged between 20.0000 and 24.9999).

When statistics are presented in percentage form, as in Table 14.2, the percentages can be used directly to estimate medians. Provided that they actually do add to 100, n/2 equals 50. (If as a result of rounding they add to some other value, say 99, one should use this and say n/2 = 49.5.) For all households, the median length of resi-

Table 14.6 Legal abortions to resident women, England and Wales, 1991

Age	Single	Ever married	Age	Single	Ever married
Under 15	886	–	Under 15	886	–
15	2270	2	Under 16	3156	2
16–19	30 115	564	Under 20	33 271	566
20–24	44 277	7367	Under 25	77 548	7933
25–29	22 470	15 203	Under 30	100 018	23 136
30–34	7841	15 019	Under 35	107 859	38 155
35–39	2416	10 308	Under 40	110 275	48 463
40 and over	599	4590	Total	110 874	53 053
	110 874	53 053			

Source: Office of Population Censuses and Surveys (1993) *Abortion Statistics* HMSO, London, Table 3; OPCS series AB no 18.
Notes: 3449 women are omitted from the above table because their age and/or marital status was not recorded. The 'ever married' include the married, widowed, divorced and separated.

dence of the head can be approximated at 8.8 years, a notable contrast from owner-occupying households without mortgages where the equivalent statistic is 19.1 years.

Another statistic which is sometimes used as a measure of central tendency is the **mode**. This is a value which occurs more frequently than the values immediately smaller and larger than it. Thus Table 14.1 shows that the mode of the number of cars per household was 1 – more households had 1 car than had no cars or 2 cars. The data in Table 14.1 are said to be unimodal, in that they have only one mode. It is possible for data to have two or more modes. Surveys of household size usually discover modes of two persons and four persons; there are more two-person households than one-person or three-person households, and more four-person households than three-person or five-person households. In bimodal distributions there is no implication that the two modes should be observed equally frequently.

The concept of a mode is too useful to be confined to discrete data. For grouped distributions with intervals of equal breadth one can identify **modal intervals** or **modal ranges** as intervals which are observed more frequently for their size than their neighbouring intervals. For distributions with unequal intervals, one has to allow for this by dividing each frequency by the breadth of the interval, i.e. by finding the height of the histogram, and looking for local maxima in the results. For the ages of single women who had abortions in 1991, one finds 2270/1 = 2270, 30 115/4 7529, 44 277/5 = 8855, 22 470/5 = 4494 etc., so the modal interval was 20 to 24. For ever married women, the modal interval was 25 to 29.

Distributions of households by income usually show two modal intervals, one corresponding to retired households and the other to working households.

The mode can still be usefully found and cited even in cases where it is not satisfactory as an average. Thus, Table 14.5 shows that the modal length of residence of heads of household is under 1 year, at the extreme of the distribution.

The median is but one of a family of similar statistics which describe features of the data. The quartiles divide the observations into four equal groups, so that the first quartile is the value which at least one-quarter of the observations are less than and at least three-quarters greater than, and the third quartile cuts off the top quarter of the observations in the same way. The second quartile is identically equal to the median. With the exception of the median, such statistics as these order statistics are seldom useful unless there are a great many observations.

As with the median, exact quartiles can be read off given actual observations or an ungrouped frequency distribution. For grouped distributions, formulas analogous to that for the median give approximate values. Thus, for the single women of Table 14.6, since $n/4 = 27\,718.5$,

$$\text{approx first quartile} = 16 + \frac{27\,718.5 - 3156}{30\,115}.4$$
$$= 19.26 \text{ years}$$

and

$$\text{approx third quartile} = 25 + \frac{83\,155.5 - 77\,548}{22\,470}.5$$
$$= 26.25 \text{ years}$$

For the ever married women, the approximate quartiles are 26.75 and 35.79 years, rather larger figures.

One can define and obtain similarly four quintiles (which divide the observations into five equal slices) nine deciles (dividing them into ten equal slices), and various other measures including 99 percentiles. Decisions as to which to use depend on the data and on the problem being investigated.

MEASURES OF DISPERSION

It is often necessary to measure the unequalness of members of sets of observations. The average or mean income might be adequate to meet a household's needs, but if some households are very rich while many are extremely poor this would not be satisfactory. Again, the average bacterial content of samples of ice cream might be satisfactory, but this might conceal a number of unacceptably high readings. If a population is fairly homogeneous, a moderate sample should be sufficient to pick out its salient features, whereas a much larger sample might be needed if the characteristic being investigated varies greatly from one member of the population to another.

Various measures of dispersion exist. Perhaps the simplest is the **range**, the difference between the highest and the lowest value. This is easily found and understood, but seldom has any other merits in the context of environmental health. All too often, the range merely reflects the largest single value, the smallest being zero or nearly zero. If one is willing to accept the maximum as a measure of dispersion, it is better to use it directly.

The over-sensitivity of the range to extreme values, usually extremely large values, can often be avoided by excluding, say, the top and bottom 25%. Doing so gives the range between the first and third quartiles, called the **inter-quartile range**. Conventionally, this is often divided by two to get the **semi-inter-quartile range,** or **quartile deviation**. The inter-quartile range, of the age distribution of single women in Table 14.6 is $26.25 - 19.26 = 6.99$ years, and the quartile deviation therefore 3.50 years, considerably smaller figures than 9.04 years and 4.52 years respectively for the ever married women, a notable feature of the data of Table 14.6 which may not be evident at first glance.

However, the most generally useful measures of dispersion are based on the differences of individual values from the mean value. Some of these differences are positive and some are negative and their total will always be found to be zero, so the crude mean of the differences is itself bound to be zero. This is avoided by squaring each difference and taking the mean square deviation about the mean; this is known as the **variance**.

Suppose that during a five day week, 15 carcasses were found with a certain disease. Regardless of how many were found on each day, the mean number per day is $15 \div 5 = 3$ carcasses. If the numbers on consecutive days were 0,2,7,2 and

4, the variance would have been $\{(0 - 3)^2 + (2 - 3)^2 + (7 - 3)^2 + (2 - 3)^2 + (4 - 3)^2\}/5 = \{9 + 1 + 16 + 1 + 1\}/5 = 28/5 = 5.6$ carcasses squared.

Denoting the individual values by $x_1, x_2 \ldots x_n$, the variance may be defined as:

$$\text{var}(x) = \frac{\Sigma(x_i - \bar{x})^2}{n}$$

and this may be most easily calculated as:

$$\text{var}(x) = \frac{\Sigma x_i^2}{n} - \bar{x}^2$$

This formula always gives the same answer, thus $(0^2 + 2^2 + 7^2 + 2^2 + 4^2)/5 - 3^2 = 73/5 - 9 = 5.6$ carcasses squared.

The variance is always given in squares of the units of measurement of the original data, and this often leads to difficulties of interpretation which can be avoided by taking the square root. Doing so gives the **standard deviation**, often abbreviated to SD and denoted by σ if the data refer to a population or s if they come from a sample.

In this case, the standard deviation is the square root of 5.6, i.e. 2.4 carcasses.

Many calculators have facilities for obtaining standard deviations directly, without using the formula for the variance and taking the square root of the result. They often have two keys, one marked σ_n and the other σ_{n-1}. The first gives the standard deviation as the square root of the variance as calculated from the formulas given above, while the second gives a larger value got by dividing $\Sigma(x_i - \bar{x})^2$ by $(n-1)$ rather than by n. In the particular numerical case considered here, $28/4 = 7$ whose square root is 2.6 carcasses.

$\Sigma(x_i - \bar{x})^2/n$ is sometimes called the **population variance** and $\Sigma(x_i - \bar{x})^2/(n-1)$ the **sample variance**, with the **population standard deviation** and the **sample standard deviation** being defined accordingly. The population variance, as the mean square deviation, is more readily understood. In using samples to estimate features of populations, it is found that the sample variance gives unbiased estimates of the variance in the population, whereas dividing by n on average gives estimates which are too small. Clearly, if n is a large number the difference will be negligible, but for small numbers of observations it may be appreciable.

Given an ungrouped frequency distribution, such as that in Table 14.1, the variance and standard deviation can be found as follows:

x	f	fx	fx^2
0	2467	0	0
1	3266	3266	3266
2	1272	2544	5088
3	260	780	2340
	7265	6590	10 694

giving $\bar{x} = 6590/7265 = 0.9071$ cars as before, and

$$\text{var}(x) = \frac{\Sigma fx^2}{\Sigma f} - \bar{x}^2 = \frac{10\ 694}{7265} - 0.9071^2$$
$$= 1.4720 - 0.8288$$
$$= 0.6492 \text{ cars squared}$$

and

$$\text{SD(x)}_n = \sqrt{0.6492} = 0.8057 \text{ cars.}$$

The sample size is here so large that the two standard deviations give effectively the same answer.

Since the mean number of cars per household was 0.9071, households with three cars had 2.0929 more cars than the mean; 2.0929/0.8057 = 2.5976. so the difference is 2.60 standard deviations. Households with two cars had a difference of 1.0929/0.8057 = 1.36 standard deviations. It is usually found that most, but not all, members of a population or sample have a difference of less than two standard deviations. In this case all but 4% of the 7265 households did. This is a typical figure, all but 5% being a common result.

Just as with the mean, if the data are grouped one cannot get an exact standard deviation, but a satisfactory approximation can usually be obtained by supposing that each observation came from the midpoint of its class interval. The standard deviation, being based on the squares of differences from the mean, is heavily dependent on just how large the largest values are, and this makes it impossible to get adequate approximations faced with some distributions where the top (or bottom) class interval is open ended. If there is an appreciable number of observations in the top interval and there is no natural upper limit, the problem is essentially insoluble. Such cases are uncommon in the context of environmental health, where the original observations are likely to be available and their standard deviation, like their mean, can be calculated from them directly. In contexts where the great sensitivity of the standard deviation to extreme values would be disadvantageous, the problem can often be avoided by the use of quartile deviations instead.

It is sometimes found useful to express the standard deviation as a fraction of, or as a percentage of, the mean. The result is the **coefficient of variation**, and measures how variable the observations are in relation to their average size. Since the mean and standard deviation are both measured in the same units, the coefficient of variation is an absolute number, and this makes it possible to compare the inequality of two or more distributions measured in different units.

STATISTICAL INFERENCE

It often happens that statistics are available which relate to a sample from a much larger population. The actual members of the sample are not themselves of any or much interest, but one wants to use them to make inferences about the population from which the sample was drawn. Suppose one chooses 100 eggs from a large consignment and examines each of them for salmonella; one's impression of the consignment would be different if one knew that none, or two, or 20 of the sample were infected. One would not be interested in the eggs actually chosen for their own sake, but because of what they suggested about the consignment as a whole. In the same way, the *General Household Survey* collects detailed information about some 10 000 households each year, not because the particular households are of interest, but because they may be typical of the population of all households. The last ten years provide guidance about conditions about the end of the twentieth century, and this may well be more interesting than treating statistics relating to them as of purely historical importance.

Consider for the sake of definiteness the 7265 households of the *Family Expenditure Survey* of 1988 [6]. It was found that the mean number of cars per household in that sample was 0.9072. This result is only of interest because it suggests that in 1988 among households in general, the mean number of cars per household was 0.9072, but it is evident that, had the *Survey* happened to choose a different set of households to interview, it would virtually certainly have produced a mean other than 0.9072. It seems reasonable to suppose that if another sample would very probably have got a mean fairly close to 0.9072 this would be a better estimate of the mean in the population as a whole, than if another sample might well have produced a completely different result. Informally, one looks to the sample itself to provide a margin of error associated with each figure, so that 0.9072 ± 0.0190 would indicate a fairly exact estimate, whereas 0.9072 ± 0.1900 would give little more than an order of magnitude.

There are two wholly different techniques of statistical inference. Some of the calculations are the same in both of them and they are quite frequently confused, but a real understanding of them depends upon recognizing their differences.

In the first case, the sample is used to **estimate** characteristics of the population and to yield margins of error associated with the estimates, as with the cars per household example above.

Usually, one takes a statistic calculated for the sample to be the estimator of the equivalent statistic in the population, e.g. the mean number of cars per household is estimated as 0.9072 because this is the mean in the sample. Provided that the sample is simple random, this gives an **unbiased** estimate of the population statistic, in the sense that, even though the sample estimate may differ considerably from the population statistic as a result of having taken an unlucky sample, if one repeated the sample over and again the errors would cancel out. (The *Family Expenditure Survey* is, though random, not simple random, but an elaborate combination of two-

stage and stratified sampling designed to give unbiased estimates in this technical sense.) Furthermore, the sample mean is taken as the estimator of the population mean to accord with the **principle of maximum likelihood**, which tells one to assume that the population has the characteristics that make the sample as plausible as possible; if the population mean is 0.9072, the sample mean is more likely to be 0.9072 than if the population mean is 0.9172, although a population with that mean could certainly have given rise to the data in Table 14.1.

The Family Expenditure Survey was only taken once in 1988, but it is possible, in theory, to think of it being taken over and over again, each replication giving a mean cars per household figure. Each of the multitude of possible samples of size 7265 would have its own mean, and the actual mean of 0.9072 can be thought of as a sample of size one from the population of all such possible sample means.

It is a remarkable fact that, regardless of the pattern of the original population, the distribution of all possible sample means for random samples of any particular large size must belong to a family of distributions known as **Normal** distributions. If one draws the histogram of Normally distributed data it looks like a bell with a very large mouth, in that it rises from zero to a flat peak in the middle from which it declines symmetrically. Normal distributions are completely determined by their means and standard deviations, in the sense that any other statistic (e.g. the ninth decile) can be calculated using only the mean and standard deviation. In particular, 2.5% of all observations from a Normal distribution are larger than the mean plus 1.96 standard deviations, and, by symmetry, 2.5% are smaller than the mean minus 1.96 standard deviations. Hence exactly 95% of all observations lie within 1.96 standard deviations of the mean and 5% do not.

Consider the Normal distribution consisting of the means of all possible samples of the particular size that could have been drawn. If the mean of this distribution equals the mean in the population (μ) of the characteristic being studied, as it will for simple random samples, the sample mean is an unbiased estimator of the population mean. The standard deviation of the distribution of possible sample means is called the **standard error**; write standard error ($\hat{\mu}$) or SE ($\hat{\mu}$) to indicate the standard error of the estimate of the population mean. Denote the size of the population by N and the size of the sample by n; then provided the sample is simple random with replacement,

$$SE(\hat{\mu}) = \sigma/\sqrt{(n)}$$

where σ is the standard deviation in the population. This formula also applies to simple random samples without replacement when N is so much bigger than n that there is very little chance of drawing an appreciable number of the population more than once in a sample with replacement (so that there is little benefit to be obtained by avoiding doing so).

If σ is not known and $s = \sqrt{(\Sigma (x - \bar{x})^2/n)}$ is used as an estimate of it, the resultant estimate of the standard error is:

$$est. \ SE(\hat{\mu}) = s/\sqrt{(n - 1)} = \sqrt{(\Sigma(x - \bar{x})^2/n(n - 1))}.$$

It will be seen that the standard error does **not** depend on the size of the population or upon the sampling fraction n/N, provided that the sample is with replacement or the sampling fraction is small. That is, a sample of 100 carcasses will be just as accurate if it is taken from a population of 1000 or a population of 100 000 carcasses. This surprises some people, but if it were not so, efficiently designed samples of a thousand voters could not give fairly accurate forecasts of results of elections among 30 million voters.

For large samples, this provides a way of giving a margin of error to an estimate from a sample. Since 95% of values in a Normal distribution lie within 1.96 standard deviations from the mean, and since the distribution of sample means is Normal for large samples, there is a 95% chance that the sample mean $\bar{x}$ lies within 1.96 standard errors of the population mean, i.e. that:

$$\mu - 1.96 \ SE < \bar{x} < \mu + 1.96 \ SE.$$

This statement about x can be rewritten into an apparently synonymous statement, with apparently the same chance of being correct, about μ:

$$\bar{x} - 1.96 \ SE < \mu < \bar{x} + 1.96 \ SE.$$

It is possible to compute the entries in such statements. Thus, for the cars per household data, $\bar{x} = 0.9071$. $SD(x)_n = 0.8057$, so SE $= 0.8057/\sqrt{(7264)} = 0.009453$. Multiply by 1.96 to get 0.0185. The interval is $0.9071 - 0.0185$ to 0.9071 to $+ 0.0185$, that is:

$$0.8886 < \mu < 0.9256.$$

This statement, however, is no longer about one particular sample mean out of the distribution of all possible sample means, but about the true, though unknown, population mean. As such, it is certainly either true or false, so one cannot say that there is a 95% chance of it being true. It is a 95% **confidence interval** in the sense that 95% of intervals constructed in this way for estimates of a variety of population statistics using different samples will include the true values of the population statistics and 5% of them will not; one does not usually know whether a particular interval does or does not do so.

For greater levels of confidence than 95%, one needs wider intervals. For 99% confidence replace 1.96 by 2.58 (or more precisely by 2.576) and for 99.9% confidence replace it by 3.29 or 3.291, since 99 and 99.9% of observations from a Normal distribution lie within 2.576 and 3.291 standard deviations of its mean respectively. On the other hand, if a 95% interval looks too wide, one can lower the degree of confidence. Tables of the Normal distribution are widely published and multiples appropriate to any required level of confidence can readily be found by consulting them; alternatively, statistics computer packages can be used to obtain intervals corresponding to various levels of confidence.

The other basic method of statistical inference is known as **hypothesis testing**. Here one sets up a **null hypothesis** and asks whether the observations are reasonable on the basis that the null hypothesis is correct. If so, one accepts (or fails to reject) it; if not, one rejects the null hypothesis in favour of the **alternative hypothesis**. Accepting the null hypothesis does not mean that the sample proves it to be correct, or even the most plausible, merely that the sample is the sort of sample that would be reasonable if the null hypothesis actually were correct. In practice, there is often a variety of null hypotheses which, if they were tested individually, would each be accepted but no more than one of which could be true. The selection of the hypothesis to test is thus arbitrary, and in accepting it one must bear in mind that it has not been proved to be correct.

Thus, suppose one set up the null hypothesis that the mean number of cars per household was 0.9, the alternative hypothesis being that it was some other value. The mean in the sample was 0.9071, a difference of 0.0071 cars. Since, as before, the standard error is 0.0185 cars, the difference is $0.0071/0.0185 = 0.384$ standard errors. This is the sort of difference which arises 95% of the time, being less than 1.960 standard errors, and so the sample would be entirely reasonable given the truth of the null hypothesis, which there is thus no reason to reject. There is, however, just as little reason to reject the different null hypothesis that the mean number is 0.91, with which the sample is quite as compatible, but clearly both means cannot be correct.

On the other hand, consider the null hypothesis that the mean was 1 car per household. The difference between the (hypothesized) true mean and the sample mean was 0.0929 cars, that is $0.0929/0.0185 = 5.022$ standard errors. This is a larger difference than 3.291 standard errors, so fewer than 1 sample in 1000 would have a sample mean so different from 1 if that were indeed the true mean. Hence if the null hypothesis were correct, a 1 in 1000 fluke would be required to account for so remarkable a sample. The result is said to be **statistically significant** and the null hypothesis is rejected in favour of the alternative hypothesis that the mean is not 1 car.

Conventionally, one rejects null hypotheses if the sample would require a 1 in 20 chance to account for it. It is good practice to indicate the highest level at which the sample statistic is statistically significant – at the 5% level (1 in 20), 1% level (1 in 100), or 0.1% level (1 in 1000), corresponding in the case of large samples to 1.960, 2.576 and 3.291 standard errors respectively.

If the null hypothesis is really true and one accepts it, or is really false and one rejects it, one makes the correct decision. If the null hypothesis is true, but one rejects it as a result of an unlucky sample one is said to make an error of the first kind, or a **type I error**; if one erroneously accepts a false null hypothesis one makes a **type II error**. Faced with a given sample, one can only reduce the chance of making one type of error at the expense of increasing the chance of making the other type; to reduce both implies decreasing the standard error, which involves a larger, or more skilfully designed, sample. One's final decision may well depend on the different costs that would be incurred by making each kind of error.

SMALL SAMPLES

As stated, the means of simple random samples of fixed large size are themselves Normally distributed in repeated sampling, with mean equal to the mean in the population and standard deviation equal to the standard deviation in the original population divided by the square root of the sample size. This is true regardless of whether or not the original population is Normally distributed.

In small samples this is not true. However, it is possible to assign confidence intervals or to test hypotheses regarding the mean of data from small samples that are approximately Normally distributed, as follows. Firstly, care must be taken to divide the standard deviation by the square root of the correct number, since n and $n - 1$ will be appreciably different if n is small; if the standard deviation is estimated from the sample, the standard error is still $s/\sqrt{(n - 1)}$ as above. However, the distribution of repeated sample means is not Normal, but follows a distribution known as Student's t distribution. Tables of this are widely available. Their use involves knowing the number of **degrees of freedom**; in the present context this is n − 1, one less than the sample size. One consults the tables to obtain the values corresponding to 1.960, 2.576 and 3.291 for the Normal distribution; they are invariably somewhat larger. (As the sample size gets larger so the number of degrees of freedom increases, the t distribution becomes more and more similar to the Normal distribution and the corresponding values become nearer to those of that distribution.)

Suppose that a simple random sample of 14 restaurants is visited and checked for the presence or absence of each of a dozen possible lapses from good hygiene practice, with the following results:

Number of lapses	*Number of restaurants*
0	2
1	2
2	5
3	3
4	1
5	1
6 or more	0
Total	14

What does this tell, not about the 14 restaurants which happened to have been drawn in the sample, but about the population from which the sample was drawn? (If the 14 were not a properly chosen sample, but were those about which complaints had been received, the generality of restaurants would presumably be rather better but one could not make any satisfactory inferences about them.)

The sample looks reasonably Normal, in that it is unimodal and symmetrical, so the t distribution is appropriate. Denoting the number of lapses at each restaurant by x, it is readily found that Σx, the total number of lapses, is 30 and $\Sigma x^2 = 90$. The mean in the sample, $\bar{x}$, is found as 30/14 = 2.143 lapses per restaurant, and the standard deviation as $\sqrt{\{90/14 - (30/14)^2\}} = 1.355$.

The principle of maximum likelihood gives the estimate of the mean number of lapses per restaurant in the population as 2.143. The standard error is $1.355/\sqrt{(14 - 1)} = 0.376$ lapses. The 95% point of the t distribution with 13 degrees of freedom is found from published tables to be

2.160 (as compared with 1.960 in the Normal distribution), and 2.160 × 0.376 is 0.812. The 95% confidence interval is therefore 2.143 + 0.812, i.e. 1.331 to 2.955 lapses. (This fairly broad interval is a warning against drawing over firm inferences from very small samples.)

Alternatively, one can test the null hypothesis that in the population of restaurants the mean number of lapses is three. Since 3 − 2.143 equals 0.857, this is 0.857/0.376 = 2.279 standard errors. The 95 and 99% points of t with 13 degrees of freedom are 2.160 and 3.012 respectively, and 2.160 < 2.279 < 3.012. Hence the result is significant at the 1 in 20 level (although not at the 1 in 100 level) so one rejects the null hypothesis that the mean number of lapses in the population of restaurants is 3.

The question sometimes arises as to whether a sample is a large sample or a small sample – that is, whether the Normal distribution is applicable or whether the t distribution should be used. Some statisticians recommend a cutoff sample size of 30, but the safest policy is to treat the sample as a small sample if there is any doubt.

Note that if the sample indicates that the data are extremely non-Normal, these small sample methods are inapplicable, though, if the sample is large, large sample methods can still be used.

BINOMIAL SAMPLING

An important special case is where the sampling is **binomial**, that is where each member of the population either has or has not a certain characteristic, and one wants to make inferences about the proportion or percentage in the population with the characteristic. Examples are the proportion of carcasses showing traces of disease and the proportion of garages which failed to service a test car to a reasonable standard. Provided that the samples are large, they can be treated by the methods of the previous section; inferences from small binomial samples are outside the scope of this chapter.

Thus, 876 out of a sample of 1358 families with children under five in the 1991 General Household Survey had formal arrangements for care of their children and 482 had not. The proportion who had arrangements was 876/1358 = 0.6451, i.e. 64.51%. This proportion is the mean of 482 zeros and 876 ones, so suppose that the sample, of size 1358, was 482 zeros and 876 ones out of a large population consisting only of zeros and ones. The ones correspond to having arrangements, and the means of the zeros and ones in the population is the proportion of families with arrangements. Denote the proportion in the sample by p and in the population by π. Then, as before, the maximum likelihood estimator of π is p. The standard error is:

$$\sqrt{\frac{\pi(1 - \pi)}{n}}$$

and if π is not known this is estimated as:

$$\sqrt{\frac{p(1 - p)}{n - 1}}$$

(Since n must be large, it scarcely matters whether n or n − 1 is used.)

To assign a 95% confidence interval to the population proportion, calculate that $\sqrt{\{p(1 - p)/(n - 1)\}} = \sqrt{\{0.6451 \times 0.3549/1357\}} = 0.0130$. Multiply by 1.96 to get 0.0255. Hence the limits of the interval are 0.6451 ± 0.0255, so it can be given as:

$$0.6196 < \pi < 0.6706$$

One is 95% confident that between 62% and 67% of such families had such arrangements in 1991.

On the other hand, suppose one wanted to test the null hypothesis that two-thirds of such families had such arrangements. The sample shows a deficiency 0.0216; could this reasonably be attributed to chance? Under the null hypothesis the standard error is $\{0.6667 \times 0.3333/1358\} = 0.0128$, so the difference is $0.0216/0.0128 = 1.689$ standard errors. This is less than 1.960 and so is not significant at the 1 in 20 level, so the null hypothesis is accepted; one could reasonably attribute the shortfall to an unlucky sample and can conclude that the proportion of families with such arrangements was 2/3.

This method is only valid for large samples of, perhaps, 40 or more. Since it is applicable only to large samples, in carrying it out one always uses the Normal distribution rather than Student's t distribution.

ASSOCIATION IN TWO-WAY TABLES

Suppose that each member of a population can be classified in two different ways. A simple method of testing a sample is available to examine whether there is any connection between the two systems of classification. Thus, suppose samples of supermarkets, large food retailers and corner shops are taken, and classified as being hygienic, borderline, or unhygienic, with the following results. Do they provide any real evidence that standards vary from one kind of shop to another in the population from which the samples were drawn?

	Hygienic	Border-line	Un-hygienic	Total
Supermarkets	35	10	15	60
Large retailers	28	10	12	50
Corner shops	41	14	35	90
Total	104	34	62	200

Barely more corner shops were hygienic than unhygienic, whereas more than twice as many supermarkets were. But can one reject the null hypothesis of no association, attributing the apparent connection in the sample to chance? It will be seen that 52% of all shops were classified as hygienic; 52% of 60, 50 and 90 is 31.2, 26.0 and 46.8, and 'expected' numbers of borderline and unhygienic shops of the various kinds can be found similarly, giving the following 'expected' table:

31.2	10.2	18.6
26.0	8.5	15.5
46.8	15.3	27.9

(The elements in this table are most easily found by multiplying the two marginal totals in the table of actual observations and dividing by the overall total; thus $31.2 = (104 \times 60)/200$, etc.)

The test statistic is usually denoted by $\chi^2_{(v)}$ (where v, the number of degrees of freedom, is the product of one less than the number of rows in the table and one less than the number of columns, here $2 \times 2 = 4$). It is calculated by finding the square of the difference between the observed number in each position in the table and the expected number, and dividing by the expected number, and adding all the results. Here $(35 - 31.2)^2/31.2 = 0.463$. The complete set of results is:

0.463	0.004	0.697
0.154	0.265	0.790
0.719	0.110	1.807

which add to 5.009. This test statistic is referred to tables of the χ^2 distribution, from which one finds that it is not statistically significant. The connections found in this sample are not so strong as to rule out the theory that they were produced by chance alone. (As usual when one accepts a null hypothesis, one may be making a type II error; there may be a difference but the sample has not shown it up strongly enough.)

This test is an approximate test only, and is not applicable to very small numbers. A rule sometimes quoted is that, in the table of 'expected' frequencies, all entries must be at least of size 5, and all but one of size 10 or more, a rule satisfied here. If these conditions are not met, it may be possible to make progress by grouping similar criteria, e.g. here one could have divided shops into hygienic on the one hand and borderline or unhygienic on the other; this achieves statistical correctness but loses information.

This test of association can be used to test the difference between two sample proportions or percentages. For example, an extended survey on the prevalence of *Listeria monocytogenes* in cooked chilled food was undertaken by nine local authorities in 1989 and 1990. Among the results of the survey was the following (Table 14.7).

In 1989 the percentage with positive results was 16.9, which fell to 11.0 in the first half of 1990. Is this difference real, or could it be attributed to

Table 14.7 Listeria species in samples of commercial chilled food West and North Yorkshire Survey

	1989	Jan–Jun 1990
Listeria sp. +ve	360	150
Listeria sp. −ve	1773	1218
Total	2133	1368

Source: Report of the West and North Yorkshire Survey January 1989 to June 1990.

chance unrepresentative samples? Altogether there were 510 positive samples out of 3501, i.e. 14.6%. Had this percentage applied exactly to the 2133 samples in 1989, 310.7 would have been positive. Note that $(2133 \times 510/3501 = 310.7)$. $(360 - 310.7)^2/310.7 = 7.82$, and the remaining three places in the table give similar answers. The total of all four is 23.41. Comparing this with the entries in a statistical table of the $\chi^2_{(v)}$ distribution, it is found to be very highly significant at the 1 in a 1000 level, so the null hypothesis that there was no real change is rejected. The number of observations was so large that the decline of 5.9% could not reasonably be attributed to chance.

This test of association in two-way tables is easy to carry out using ordinary calculators, and most computer installations are programmed to do it.

CORRELATION

One often wishes to analyse the relationship, if any, between pairs of readings, where two different features of each member of the sample or population are measured. This is in contrast to cases considered up to now where only one feature of each member of the sample or population was considered, e.g. number of cars or length of residence. For example, one may collect statistics of mean temperature and of numbers of cases of reported food poisoning, in order to examine the possibility that higher temperatures are associated, for whatever reason, with larger numbers of cases. Here each observation consists of two figures – the temperature and the number of cases. Statistics of population density in a number of different areas (from the most recent census) can be compared with the number of complaints of noise per thousand residents, with a view to examining whether higher densities are associated with higher complaint rates. Having collected a number of such pairs of observations, it may well be useful to plot them on a **scatter diagram**, where, for example, each observation is shown by a point, with the temperature being shown on the horizontal axis and the number of reported cases of food poisoning on the vertical axis. One then gets a visual impression of the nature of both sets of readings and of the relationship, if any between them, for example, whether they tend to increase together or to move in opposite directions, whether they lie closely on a line, straight or curved, and so on.

Like all statistical diagrams, scatter diagrams should have clear headings, the source of the data displayed should be indicated and the axes should be labelled. If, as will often be the case, one or both of the axes do not start at zero, this should be shown by a clear break or breaks to avoid misleading the casual viewer. The only real difficulties with scatter diagrams arise in displaying freak readings, and if the number of points is too great for them to be separately distinguished. (On the other hand if the number of points is quite small, they can sometimes be labelled in order to convey useful information.)

Time charts are a special case of scatter diagrams, where time is shown along the horizontal axis and the values of a series along the vertical axis. In this case, successive points are often joined by straight lines to make the picture displayed clearer.

For example, consider the statistics in Table 14.8.

A scatter diagram, in which each point has been labelled, is shown in Fig. 14.3.

There is clearly a definite tendency for high values for smoke to be associated with high values of sulphur dioxide, but the relationship is far from exact. A measure of the direction and strength of the relationship is provided by the **correlation coefficient**, usually denoted by the Greek letter ρ if calculated from a population or by *r* if from a sample.

Table 14.8 Atmospheric pollution – micrograms per cubic metre, regions of Great Britain, 1987–8

	Smoke	Sulphur dioxide
North	13	37
Yorkshire and Humberside	23	45
North West	17	45
East Midlands	16	43
West Midlands	16	40
East Anglia	12	24
Greater London	14	42
Rest of South East	11	39
South West	8	21
Wales	11	28
Scotland	17	34

Source: Central Statistical Office (1990) *Regional Trends*, HMSO, London, Table 6.15.

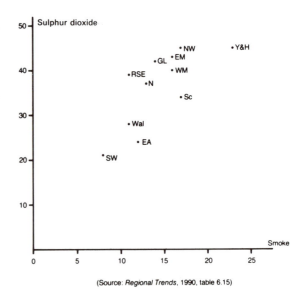

(Source: *Regional Trends*, 1990, table 6.15)

Fig. 14.3 Atmospheric pollution in micrograms per cubic metre by regions of Great Britain, 1987–88. (Source: Regional Trends, 1990, Table 6.15.)

In order to calculate the correlation coefficient, one should first find the **covariance**, a statistic of little use in itself, but which is used as an important ingredient in other calculations. If the pairs of statistics being correlated are denoted by (x_1, y_1), $(x_2, y_2) \ldots (x_n, y_n)$, the covariance is defined as:

$$\text{cov(x, y)} = \frac{\Sigma(x - \bar{x})(y - \bar{y})}{n}$$

which however is not convenient for manual calculation. The equivalent formula:

$$\text{cov(x, y)} = \frac{\Sigma xy}{n} - \bar{x}\bar{y}$$

gives the same answer more simply.

As explained above, some statisticians distinguish between the population and sample variances or standard deviations, depending on whether they divide by n or by $n - 1$; if they divide by $n - 1$ they have to modify the covariance similarly.

Denote the smoke readings by x_i and the sulphur dioxide readings by y_i. It may be found that $\Sigma x_i = 158$, so $\bar{x} = 158/11 = 14.3636$ and that $\Sigma y_i = 398$, so $\bar{y} = 398/11 = 36.1818$. $\Sigma x_i y_i = (13 \times 37) + (23 \times 45) + \ldots + (17 \times 34) = 5968$. Hence:

$$\begin{aligned} \text{cov(x,y)} &= \frac{5968}{11} - 14.3636 \times 36.1818 \\ &= 542.5455 - 519.7009 \\ &= 22.8446. \end{aligned}$$

The covariance, unlike the variance which must be positive, can be either positive or negative; the positive sign of this particular covariance indicates a positive relationship between smoke and sulphur dioxide, but the covariance in itself gives no indication of how strong that relationship is.

In order to find the correlation coefficient, in addition to the covariance one needs the variances of the two variables taken separately. The three statistics are then used in the following formula:

$$r(x,y) = \frac{\text{cov(x,y)}}{\sqrt{\{\text{var(x).var(y)}\}}}$$

In this case, since $\Sigma x^2 = 2434$, $\text{var(x)} = 2434/11 - 14.3636^2 = 14.9597$ and $\Sigma y^2 = 15110$, $\text{var(y)} = 15110/11 - 36.1818^2 = 64.5137$, so the correlation coefficient is calculated as:

$$\frac{22.8446}{\sqrt{(14.9597 \times 64.5137)}} = 0.735$$

The correlation coefficient must lie between -1 and $+1$. This particular coefficient is positive and substantial but considerably less than 1. Thus like the scatter diagram it indicates a definite but imperfect relationship. With experience, one learns to infer from correlation coefficients of different sizes what the corresponding scatter diagrams would show.

The connection measured by the correlation coefficient is a **linear** one, i.e. how closely the points on the scatter diagram lie to a straight line. It is possible for the points to lie closely on a curve, in which case the correlation coefficient would fail to bring out the strength of the relationship; again, if the points show a close upward connection on one half of the diagram, and a downward connection on the other, the correlation coefficient may be near zero.

The correlation coefficient is independent of the origin and units of measurement of x and y. In this case, if the data had been expressed in terms of thousandths of ounces per cubic yard the result would have been just the same.

It cannot be stressed too strongly that a correlation coefficient, however large, cannot in itself prove that either variable causes the other. Either may affect the other or some third factor may influence them both independently. Over the years, the number of telephones has been closely correlated with the number of reported cases of AIDS, but solely because both have risen over time – there is no suggestion of any causal relation. Alternatively, a real connection between two variables may be obscured by a third factor influencing them differently; numbers of deaths in road accidents have been negatively related to the number of vehicles on the road.

In some contexts it is usual to give r^2, called the **coefficient of determination**, rather than r, but doing so conceals whether the relationship is positive or negative.

If a correlation coefficient r has been calculated using a sample of size n, it is possible to test the null hypothesis that in the population from which the sample was drawn the correlation coefficient is zero against the alternative hypothesis that it has some other value. Under fairly general conditions one can calculate $r/\sqrt{\{(1 - r^2)/(n - 2)\}}$ and, ignoring its sign, compare the result with the critical values of the t distribution with $n - 2$ degrees of freedom. Suppose that a sample of 12 mobile ice cream vans is drawn and for each the storage temperature and the bacterial count are obtained and found to be correlated with $r = 0.65$. Using the formula given above gives a test statistic of $0.65/\sqrt{\{(1 - 0.65^2)/10\}} = 2.705$. Reference to tables of the t distribution indicates that the 5% point with 10 degrees of freedom is 2.228 and the 1% point is 3.169. Hence the sample value would, under the null hypothesis, require a rather unlikely chance to account for it and the result is said to be significant at the 1 in 20 level (although not at the 1 in 100 level), the null hypothesis is rejected, and one concludes that there is a definite association between temperature and bacterial content among the entire population of ice cream vans.

The correlation coefficient as defined above is the coefficient much the most commonly used in practice. It is sometimes called the Pearson product moment coefficient, to distinguish it from Spearman's **rank correlation coefficient**. The rank correlation coefficient is the ordinary correlation coefficient calculated using two different rankings of members of the sample or population. A principal use of Spearman's coefficient is in dealing with non-quantitative data. A panel might assess the attractiveness and quality of life in each ward of a city, ranking them from the most attractive down to the least but without calculating an index of attractiveness. The ranks themselves could then be correlated with other rankings, e.g. a ranking by reported crime rate. Although particularly useful in dealing with non-quantitative data, the rank correlation coefficient can also be used with quantitative data. Thus, the ranks of the various standard regions in terms of smoke and sulphur dioxide pollution can be found and correlated. Table 14.9 also gives the differences between the ranks and the squares of the differences.

The Yorkshire and Humberside region had the highest smoke pollution statistic and ranked first

Table 14.9 Ranking of regions by smoke and sulphur dioxide pollution, 1987–8

	Smoke	Sulphur dioxide	Difference	Difference squared
North	7	7	0	0
Yorkshire and Humberside	1	1.5	−0.5	0.25
North West	2.5	1.5	1	1
East Midlands	4.5	3	1.5	2.25
West Midlands	4.5	5	−0.5	0.25
East Anglia	8	10	−2	4
Greater London	6	4	2	4
Rest of South East	9.5	6	3.5	12.25
South West	11	11	0	0
Wales	9.5	9	0.5	0.25
Scotland	2.5	8	−5.5	30.25
			0	54.50

and second equal in terms of sulphur dioxide. The South West ranked bottom by both criteria. Scotland was among the worst for smoke, but ranked fairly low down by sulphur dioxide. The differences between the rankings are given in the column headed 'difference': these must necessarily add to zero. The squares of the differences are given in the last column. It is possible to calculate Spearman's coefficient by calculating the ordinary correlation coefficient between the ranks as usual, but a simple formula gives almost the same answer (and exactly the same answer in the absence of ties):

$$\text{rank correlation coefficient} = 1 - \frac{6\Sigma d^2}{n(n^2 - 1)}$$

Here this is $1 - (6 \times 54.50)/\{11(121 - 1)\} = 0.752$. This is an approximation to the true answer of 0.750, the difference arising from the tied ranks.

Although the rank correlation coefficient is most useful in dealing with non-quantitative data, it does have other advantages. It is robust in cases where there are small errors of measurement which do not affect the rankings, it is not liable to be distorted by a freak reading, and it does not presuppose that any relation between the criteria is necessarily linear. Nevertheless, the ordinary

Pearson coefficient is much the more commonly used.

The null hypothesis that the rankings in the population from which the sample data were drawn are independent can be tested for samples of at least moderate size by using the sample rank correlation coefficient in the same formula given above for the sample product moment coefficient and comparing the result with values in tables of the t distribution. This is an approximate test only, and does not apply to small samples of size ten or less. In such cases reference should be made to special tables.

REGRESSION

The correlation coefficient indicates whether two variables are linearly related. Perhaps as a result of finding an encouraging coefficient, one may want to calculate the best linear relation between two variables. If the variable y is linearly related to the variable x, but is also subject to other influences and, perhaps, errors of observation, the relationship can be expressed as $y = \alpha + \beta x + u$, where α and β are constants and u represents the effect of all other influences in such a manner that values of u average out to zero; these influences stop the relationship being exact. The value of β shows the expected change in y associated with a change of one unit in x. Three possible reasons for fitting such a function by estimating numerical values of α and β are

1. Data reduction. A single equation may summarize a great mass of indigestible statistical material.
2. Forecasting. Having fitted a relationship, one may be able to use it to forecast one variable on the basis of a known or expected value of the other.
3. Model estimation. It may be believed that x, in conjunction with other influences, does actually determine the values of y in accordance with a law of the form $y = \alpha + \beta x + u$, where u is the result of the other influences. One may wish to estimate the parameters α and β.

The standard procedure is known as **regression analysis**, and the resultant equation as the **regression** of y on x. In each case, one normally quotes r or r^2 together with the fitted equation, since high values are an indication of the success of the exercise. Fortunately, if one has already found the correlation coefficient little further arithmetic is needed to get the regression.

The regression of y on x is calculated as:

$$y - \bar{y} = \frac{\text{cov(x,y)}}{\text{var(x)}} \cdot (x - \bar{x})$$

This is the equation of a straight line, and by finding two points on it and plotting them on the scatter diagram, one can draw the line on it by joining them up with a ruler. The line must go through $(\bar{x}, \bar{y})$, the midpoint of the observations. The line can be rewritten in the form $y = a + bx$. The unknown parameters α and β are estimated by a and b respectively. For each value of x the fitted line gives a 'predicted' value of y, say $\hat{y}$. The errors $e = y - \hat{y}$ have the properties that (i) they sum to zero, the positive errors exactly balancing the negative errors, i.e. $\Sigma e = 0$, and (ii) the sum of the squares of the errors, Σe^2, is the smallest possible using a straight line, that is, that replacing a and b by any other values increases Σe^2. It is for this reason that the regression is often called the **least squares line**. (The values of e, the differences of actual values of y from the **fitted** regression, i.e. $y - a - bx$, should be distinguished from the unknown values of u, the differences of actual values of y from the underlying function, i.e. $y - \alpha - \beta x$.)

Consider the statistics in Table 14.10.

A glance suggests a downward trend. Denote the expenditure series by y, and write $t = -4.5$, $-3.5, \ldots 4.5$ for the 10 years. Then Σy, the sum of the ten values of capital expenditure, is 1824, $\Sigma y^2 = 336\,504$, $\Sigma t = 0$, $\Sigma t^2 = 82.5$ and $\Sigma ty = (-4.5 \times 195) + (-3.5 \times 221) + \ldots + (4.5 \times 147) = -420.0$. Hence $\bar{y} = 182.4$, $\bar{t} = 0$, var(y) = 380.64, var(t) = 8.25 and cov(t,y) = -42.0. These values enable the correlation coefficient and the regression to be calculated using the above formulas. The correlation coefficient equals -0.75, and the regression of y on t is:

Table 14.10 Capital expenditure by local authorities on sanitary services, 1983–92 £m, January 1987 prices

1983	1984	1985	1986	1987	1988	1989	1990	1991	1992
195	221	181	177	183	199	181	182	158	147

Source: Derived from Central Statistical office (1993) *United Kingdom National Accounts*, HMSO, London, Table 8.3, and Central Statistical Office *Economic Trends*, HMSO, London.

$$y - 182.4 = -\frac{42.0}{8.25} \cdot (t - 0)$$

which can be written as:

$$y = 182.4 - 5.091\ t$$

Substituting the value of the correlation coefficient into the formula for its test statistic given above gives -3.21, and reference to a book of tables of Student's t distribution indicates that this is statistically significant at the 5% level since there are $10-2=8$ degrees of freedom. Hence, over the years 1983 to 1992 there was a definite downward trend in local authority capital expenditure on sanitary services which cannot reasonably be attributed to coincidence. The regression indicates that it amounted to £5.09m (at January 1987 prices) per year.

The variable t was defined in such a manner that $t = 5.5$ corresponds to 1993. Substituting this in the calculated regression gives a prediction of $182.4 - (5.5 \times 5.091) = £154.4$ m for that year, when inflation is corrected for. Looking at the data in Table 14.10 confirms that this is a reasonable prediction, but the comparatively low value of the correlation coefficient indicates that any such prediction may be considerably in error. In any case, one should avoid using regressions to make predictions too far in advance. In this case, a prediction for the year 2024 would be negative – an impossibility for such gross data even if current influences on the series continued. Furthermore, in practice, there is almost certain to be some at present unforeseen influence which will affect the trend long before then.

It is possible to find regressions which use more than one explanatory variable; a case which often arises is when y is, or may be, related both to x and to time t, and the function $y = a + bx + ct$ can be fitted. This is called **multiple regression**,

and the goodness of fit of such a function is measured by the **multiple correlation coefficient R** or its square, the **coefficient of multiple determination R^2**. As the number of explanatory variables increases, the arithmetic soon becomes impracticable except on computers, which, however, will almost certainly have programs for performing such calculations rapidly and accurately.

MOVING AVERAGES AND SEASONAL CORRECTIONS

A plot of a regression line on a time chart, as for the local authority capital expenditure data used above, often indicates (even if the correlation coefficient is fairly large) that a straight line is not satisfactory as a form of trend. In most practical situations, the trend is complex and does not allow of simple mathematical description. The technique of moving averages enables smooth curves to be calculated, which on plotting will be found to follow the original observations reasonably closely. A common case where moving averages are particularly effective is of monthly or quarterly data where there is a strong and regular seasonal pattern.

Suppose one wants to fit a 3-year moving average to the local authority data given above. To get the average for 1984 one takes the total of the 3 years' data centred on 1984, i.e. $195 + 221 + 181 = 597$, and divides by 3 to get 199. For 1985 the moving average is $(221 + 181 + 177)/3 = 579/3 = 193$, but this could also have been found as $(597 + 177 - 195)/3$. Then for 1986, $(579 + 183 - 221)/3 = 180.3$ and so on until for 1991 $(521 + 147 - 181)/3 = 487/3 = 162.3$ and one can check the accuracy of the complete calculation by verifying that $487 = 182 + 158 + 147$.

The 5-year moving average would be found as (195 + 221 + 181 + 177 + 183)/5 = 957/5 = 191.4 for 1985, as (957 + 199 − 195)/5 = 192.2 for 1986 etc.

In many cases, the length of the moving average is arbitrary. The longer the average, the smoother the trend but the less closely it tracks the original statistics. It will be seen that the average is not available for the first and last year(s), and the longer the average the more years it is unavailable for. Unlike regression trends, the moving average cannot be projected into the future (which may well be no bad thing). It is found that moving averages may sometimes show cycles which do not exist in the original statistics. The arbitrary length of the average means that different trends sometimes show different features; thus in this example, the three year moving average shows an increase from 1986 to 1987 whereas the 5-year average shows a decline.

If there is a natural cycle of fixed length in the original statistics the moving average should be of that same length. Thus, in dealing with monthly or quarterly data, a 12 month or a four-quarter moving average should be used. (If the statistics refer to the volume of letters posted, for example, this ensures that one and only one Christmas features in each value calculated for the trend, so that it does not fluctuate according to the number of seasonal peaks included in each of its various values.) This is one reason, but not the only reason, for wanting to fit a moving average of even length. Adding four (say) consecutive values and dividing by four gives an average which is centred between two of the original observations. To get an average which can be compared directly to an original observation, it is usual to take the mean of the averages calculated in that way which fall just before and just after each observation.

Consider the statistics in Table 14.11. There has been a tendency for employment to grow over the period, but in each year there was a fall between December and March. To ensure that each value of the moving average trend gives equal weight to each season of the year, a four-quarter average is required. (245 + 265 + 266 + 270)/4 = 1046/4 = 261.5, but this centres midway between June and September of 1988. Similarly,

Table 14.11 Employees in restaurants, cafés, etc., thousands, Great Britain, 1988–92

1986	Mar	245	1991	Mar	291
	Jun	265		Jun	301
	Sep	266		Sep	288
	Dec	270		Dec	288
1989	Mar	268	1992	Mar	283
	Jun	290		Jun	306
	Sep	295		Sep	298
	Dec	297		Dec	295
1990	Mar	296			
	Jun	308			
	Sep	314			
	Dec	306			

Source: *Employment Gazette*, October 1993, Table 8.1.

(265 + 266 + 270 + 268)/4 = 1069/4 = 267.25 centres midway between September and December of that year. The mean of these, 264.375 can be taken as the centred four-quarter moving average at September 1988. This is more easily found as (1046 + 1069)/8 = 2115/8 = 264.375, and the calculation as a whole is displayed in the left-hand half of Table 14.12.

As always with moving average trends, values are necessarily missing at the beginning and end of the period. This trend is given here to three decimal places so that it can be used in subsequent calculations; otherwise it would be rounded off.

It will be seen that the actual figure for March always falls below the trend, whereas in June the actual figure is always above the trend. It is often desired to correct out the seasonal pattern to get a **seasonally adjusted** series showing what the values would have been but for these regularly recurring seasonal effects, i.e. embodying the trend together with the one-off random influences. (Perhaps the best-known context where this is done is with statistics of the unemployed claiming benefit which are published monthly, which are given in their raw form and also corrected for seasonal influences. The latter are found more useful for most purposes). Thus it is supposed that the original observations are the additive combination of the trend, the seasonal effects, and random influences. A trend can be

Table 14.12 Moving average trend re: Table 14.11

			Sum of 4	Sum of 8	Trend	Diff	Seas.	Seas. corr.
1986	Mar	245					−9	254
	Jun	265					6	259
	Sep	266	1046	2115	264.375	1.625	3	263
	Dec	270	1069	2163	270.375	−0.375	0	270
1989	Mar	268	1094	2217	277.125	−9.125	−9	277
	Jun	290	1123	2273	284.125	5.875	6	284
	Sep	295	1150	2328	291.000	4.000	3	292
	Dec	297	1178	2374	296.750	0.250	0	297
1990	Mar	296	1196	2411	301.375	−5.375	−9	305
	Jun	308	1215	2439	304.875	3.125	6	302
	Sep	314	1224	2443	305.375	8.625	3	311
	Dec	306	1219	2431	303.875	2.125	0	306
1991	Mar	291	1212	2398	299.750	−8.750	−9	300
	Jun	301	1186	2354	294.250	6.750	6	295
	Sep	288	1168	2328	291.000	−3.000	3	285
	Dec	288	1160	2325	290.625	−2.625	0	288
1992	Mar	283	1165	2340	292.500	−9.500	−9	292
	Jun	306	1175	2357	294.625	11.375	6	300
	Sep	298	1182				3	295
	Dec	295					0	295

estimated by the method of moving averages as shown. The differences between the actual values and the trend are a combination of seasonal and random effects, and are shown in the right hand half of the above calculation. These differences are collected in the auxiliary Table 14.13.

Table 14.13 Seasonal corrections re: Table 14.11

	March	June	Sept	Dec	
			1.625	−0.375	
	−9.125	5.875	4.000	0.250	
	−5.375	3.125	8.625	2.125	
	−8.750	6.750	−3.000	−2.625	
	−9.500	11.375			
Total	−32.750	27.125	11.250	−0.625	
Mean	−8.188	6.781	2.813	−0.156	1.250
	−0.313	−0.313	−0.313	−0.313	1.252
Adj. mean	−8.501	6.468	2.500	−0.469	−0.002
Seasonal	−9	6	3	0	0

The mean difference in each of the four months is found; if the random influences balanced out over the period, these mean differences would be the seasonal pattern and, by definition, add to zero. However, they usually need minor adjustment by adding or subtracting the same small amount to each of them (any need for a major adjustment is an indication of an arithmetical error). The adjusted means are as shown above, and are the best available estimates of the seasonal pattern. However, since the original data are given to the nearest integer, the seasonal pattern should also be, and the adjusted means are rounded off accordingly. (It is occasionally necessary to round one or more of them the 'wrong way' to ensure that they continue to add to zero.)

In this case, it is estimated that in March employment in restaurants, cafés, etc. is reduced by 9000 by seasonal influences, increased by 6000 and 3000 in June and September respectively, and unaffected in December. Hence the seasonally adjusted statistics are obtained by subtracting these amounts and this is done in the table above; thus for March 1988 it is estimated that employment would have been 245 − (−9) = 254 (thousands) but for the seasonal effect, and the rest of the seasonally corrected series is calculated similarly. The trend shows a much smoother increase than the seasonally adjusted series; since this latter also incorporates random influences this is not surprising.

Common mistakes in carrying out this calculation include using too many or too few decimal places. As usual, the best strategy is to keep as many as reasonably practicable during the calculation and to round off at the end, here to as many decimal places as in the original statistics. To get seasonally corrected figures, the seasonal pattern must be subtracted from the data rather than added; adding it would produce a series with twice as great a seasonal pattern as the original. The seasonal corrections can be, and should be, applied to the first two and the last two readings, even though the trend cannot be obtained for them. Indeed, one could use them for the following year or two without serious error to correct data for 1993 and 1994 as they become available without necessarily going through the entire calculation again.

This method proved satisfactory in this instance because the values of the original series were of much the same magnitude at the end of the period as at the beginning. In many cases this is not so. The seasonal pattern is usually expected to be multiplicative. Thus it might be found that there are an extra 10% or so of cases of food poisoning each August, and if the general level of food poisoning rises or falls substantially, the seasonal pattern would be expected to get larger or smaller in terms of actual numbers of cases, although not in terms of percentages. This case can be dealt with by the method explained above, first, by taking logarithms of the original data, secondly, by applying this method to the logarithms and, thirdly, by taking antilogarithms of the result. (This relies on the property that the logarithm of a product is the sum of the logarithms.) Official UK government statistics are often published in both a raw and a seasonally corrected form. The process of correction used by the Government Statistical Service uses an elaborate computer program which incorporates various sophistications not explained here but which embodies the same principles as the calculation shown above.

CONCLUSION

The various statistical methods explained in this chapter constitute a basic minimum for dealing with most frequently recurring needs. There is much more to say about their proper use, and there is no substitute for practical experience. Even so, the account given here should enable non-statisticians to apply these techniques in routine situations and to understand their use by other people. They can all be performed fairly easily using calculators, and most computer installations can do the arithmetic with minimal programming by taking advantage of standard statistical packages.

REFERENCES

1. Central Statistical Office, *Guide to Official Statistics*, HMSO, London.
2. Central Statistical Office, *Annual Abstract of Statistics*, HMSO, London.
3. Central Statistical Office, *Social Trends*, HMSO, London.
4. Central Statistical Office, *Regional Trends*, HMSO, London.
5. Office of Population Censuses and Surveys, *General Household Survey*, HMSO, London.
6. Central Statistical Office (1988) *Family Expenditure Survey*, HMSO, London.

FURTHER READING

Much the fullest and most useful guide to the availability of published statistical material, including some from non-official bodies, is the Central Statistical Office's *Guide to Official Statistics*, HMSO, London. One should always consult the most recent edition, which at the time of writing is No. 5 of 1990 (ISBN: 011 620 394 3). A new edition is planned for publication in late 1994. The Central Statistical Office also publishes a short annual booklet entitled 'Government Statistics: a brief guide to sources', which may be obtained without charge on application to the Central Statistical Office Press, Publication and Publicity, Great George Street, London SW1P 3AQ.

An account of many fallacies which over hasty use of statistics can lead one into is the classic book by Huff, D. (1975) *How to Lie with Statistics*, Penguin, London.

A brief account of the statistical methods most commonly used in the context of environmental health is Pearson, J.C.G. and Turton, A. (1993) *Statistical Methods in Environmental Health*, Chapman & Hall, London.

A full account, suitable for the layman, of the statistical methods explained in this chapter and a great many others is Anderson, D.R., Sweeney, D.J. and Williams, T.A. (1993) *Statistics for Business and Economics*, 5th edn, West Publishing Company, St Paul, Minnesota. This contains tables of the Normal, t and chi squared distributions.

A proper understanding of the basis behind statistical methods can only be obtained by a study of the mathematical principles which underly them, for which 'A' level mathematics at least is necessary. A suitable text at this level is Clarke, G.M. and Cooke, D. (1992) *A Basic Course in Statistics*, 3rd edn, Edward Arnold, London. This too contains tables of the Normal, t and chi squared distributions, and also a table of significance levels of Spearman's rank correlation coefficient for small numbers of observations.

Those proposing to make substantial use of information from social surveys, or to conduct or commission such surveys themselves, will need to make a special study of them. For this purpose Moser, C.A. and Kalton, G. (1985) *Survey Methods in Social Investigation*, 2nd edn, Gower Publishing Company. Aldershot, is particularly suitable.

15 Fundamentals of information technology and its application in environmental health

Paul B. Paddock

INTRODUCTION

For some 30 years organizations have been developing computer-based information systems. Throughout the 1960s, 1970s and early 1980s the vast majority of issues were associated with how to 'supply' information systems to organizations. As these issues have become better understood, and with many of the basic organizational systems having been automated, attention has turned to more imaginative and fruitful applications for information technology and the ascertaining of the 'demand' for information systems in organizations. What we have witnessed has been a revolution in the way people do their jobs and in the development of new systems. The computer keyboard and screen are familiar desk-top tools in many offices. This may be a computer terminal used to access a remote mainframe computer or a personal computer used for word-processing and spreadsheet calculations or, increasingly these days, a combination of both.

With this 'explosion' in information technology has come a plethora of technical terms, many of which are unknown to, or poorly understood by, **end-users** – the people receiving the printouts, manning the computer workstations, as well as those who order and pay for the technology. A basic understanding of the fundamentals and terminology of information technology will assist end-users to utilize the power of the computerized information systems introduced into an organization. In general terms, the objectives of information technology in any organization are to make the organization more efficient, to make managers more effective and to achieve a competitive advantage.

Before discussing the hardware and software components of information technology, it is appropriate to differentiate between the terms 'data' and 'information', as they are used interchangeably in everyday speech as meaning the same thing. **Data** are facts, events and transactions which have been recorded and they are the raw input materials from which information is produced. **Information** is data that have been processed in such a way as to be understood by and useful to the recipient. The mere act of processing data does not itself produce information. Fig. 15.1 describes, in outline, a model which is applicable to all information systems, whether manual or computerized, and which illustrates the important distinction between these two terms. The characteristics of good information are identified in Table 15.1

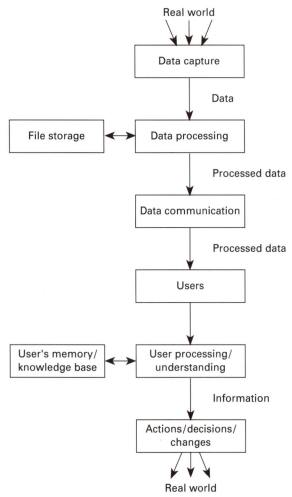

Fig. 15.1 An informations systems model.

FUNDAMENTALS OF INFORMATION TECHNOLOGY

What exactly is a computer? A **computer** is a machine which, under the control of a stored program, automatically accepts and processes data, and supplies the results of that processing. A computer can be viewed very simply using a 'systems' model (Fig. 15.2) – inputs are processed and transformed into outputs. The inputs can be provided using a keyboard or a mouse for example, whilst the outputs can be displayed on a monitor or printed out on a printer or plotter. Traditionally, there have been three types of computers – mainframe, mini- and personal or microcomputers. However, this distinction is becoming increasingly blurred due to the increasing power of personal computers (PCs). The majority of computers used in environmental health departments are of the microcomputer variety based on the IBM PC, and it is this type of machine that forms the basis of the discussion in this chapter.

Computer systems are made up of both hardware and software – either one of these elements is useless on its own. The hardware is the physical component – the bits you can touch – whilst the software is a list of coded instructions which convert the hardware from a box of electronic bits into an accounting machine or a word-processor or a drafting system, for example.

Table 15.1 The qualities of good information

1. Relevant for its purpose
2. Sufficiently accurate for its purpose
3. Complete enough for the problem
4. From a source in which the user has confidence
5. Communicated to the right person
6. Communicated in time for its purpose
7. Contains the right level of detail
8. Communicated by an appropriate channel of communication
9. Understandable by the user

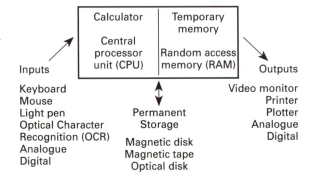

Fig. 15.2 Systems model of a computer.

Hardware components

These can be grouped into the following categories:

Central processing unit (CPU)

This is the brains of the system. Its circuitry controls the activity of the other components. Instructions are retrieved from memory by the CPU, decoded, then carried out. The CPU is typically a cabinet on a mainframe, a printed circuit board on a mini-computer or a single chip on a personal computer. A major reason for the widespread use of PCs is their relatively low cost. There are several different types of microprocessor used in PCs, of which the most popular ones are Intel's® 8086, 80286, 80386 and 80486 (80xxx) used in IBM® AT and compatible computers, and the Motorola® 68000 which forms the basis of the Apple® Mac family of computers.

Random access memory (RAM)

This is the electronic circuitry used as a temporary storage area for programs and data which are in active use. Data can be transferred from RAM to the CPU (or other components) at very high speeds because there is no physical component involved, only electronic signals. RAM is cleared when a computer is switched off or reset and, therefore, it is always necessary to transfer any changed data back to a permanent storage location (disk or tape) as part of any computer process.

The amount of RAM present in a machine is very important. Computer memory is measured in **kilobytes** (K) or **megabytes** (MB) of information. The building blocks of memory are defined in Table 15.2. Software requires a minimum amount of RAM to work properly. Unfortunately, it gets more complicated as RAM is divided into a number of blocks. The first 640 K of a PC's memory is called **conventional memory**. Any RAM present in a machine above 640 K is addressed by the CPU as either **extended memory** or **expanded memory** (Table 15.2). Many software programs now require at least 2 MB of memory in order to function adequately. As a

Table 15.2 Memory

Definitions of memory building blocks:

Bit	the smallest unit of storage in a computer; each bit can hold a single binary digit (0 or 1)
Byte	the amount of storage needed to hold one character and consists of eight bits
Kilobyte	equals 1024 bytes
Megabyte	equals 1 048 576 bytes
Gigabyte	equals 107 341 824 bytes

Different types of RAM configuration:

Conventional memory	this comprises 640 K which is available for the disk operating system (DOS) and user programmes
Expanded memory	the expanded memory specification developed by Lotus, Intel and Microsoft (LIM) allows additional RAM to be made available to user programs which have been specially written to take advantage of it; such memory is installed on an expanded memory board and comes with an expanded memory manager
Extended memory	this is general purpose memory beyond 1MB on 80286 machines (or higher) and requires an extended memory manager to co-ordinate the use of such memory

general rule, the more RAM available inside a computer, the better!

Bus

This is the electronic pathway along which all of the other components communicate with each other. The 'width' of the bus – the number of circuits – determines the size of the units of data which are transferred. A typical mainframe will have a 64-bit bus whereas popular PCs have a 16- or 32-bit bus.

Keyboard

This is the device most commonly used to communicate with a computer. For PCs there are two commonly used keyboard styles – the original PC keyboard and the 102-key (enhanced) keyboard (Fig. 15.3). Both keyboard styles possess keys

Original PC keyboard

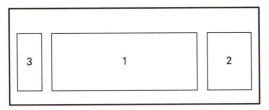

102 key keyboard

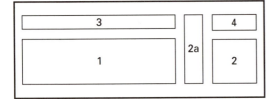

1 – QWERTY keys; same as a typewriter
2 – numeric keypad
2a – cursor control keys, insert and delete keys, etc.
3 – function keys
4 – num lock, caps lock and scroll lock lights

Fig. 15.3 Computer keyboard styles.

known as **function keys**. The effect of pressing any of these keys is entirely dependent on the program in use at the time. Function key 1 (**F1**) is used by many programmes as a **Help** key.

Screen (monitor)
A typical screen will display 25 rows of information with 80 characters on each row. Some programs are capable of using a screen's graphical capabilities to display more than 80×25 characters and to display pictures and charts. Different screens have different graphical capabilities, with the most obvious difference being monochrome and colour. Computer monitors are also available in a number of different sizes. Screens possess different resolutions which are dependent on the number of dots per inch (dpi) that can be displayed – the higher the resolution the clearer the image. There are a number of different types of PC monitor and display adaptor, the characteristics of which are summarized in Table 15.3. Further developments in monitor design centre around the radiation output from the device and

Table 15.3 Common PC adaptor types

Adaptor	Characteristics
Monochrome Display Adaptor (MDA)	Monochrome, no graphics
Colour Graphics Adaptor (CGA)	Colour, low resolution graphics
Hercules Graphics Controller	Monochrome, medium/high resolution graphics
Enhanced Graphics Adaptor (EGA)	Colour, medium/high resolution graphics
Video Graphics Array (VGA)	Monochrome or colour, medium/high resolution graphics
SuperVGA	The current standard, colour, very high resolution graphics

Table 15.4 Capacities of floppy disks

Disk size (inches)	Disk density	Storage capacity	Equivalent A4 pages
3.5	Double density	720 kb	400
3.5	High density	1.44 Mb	800
5.25	Double density	360 kb	200
5.25	High density	1.2 Mb	650

whether the monitor is interlaced or non-interlaced (this refers to the way in which the display is maintained on the screen) with the latter providing a 'flicker-free' display at high resolutions.

Disk storage
Disk capacities, like RAM, are measured in thousands or millions of bytes – kilobytes (K) and megabytes (MB) respectively. There are two basic types of computer disks called **hard (fixed or winchester) disks** and **floppy disks**. Floppy disks come in different sizes and densities (Table 15.4). Hard disks have a much higher capacity than floppy disks, with most new PCs having fixed disks with a capacity of 100–400 MB or even greater. Hard disks are also faster than floppy disks by a substantial factor. Several new developments in disk technology include optical and floptical storage as well as removable hard drives. To make things even more complicated there are two common

but different interfacing/controller systems for hard drives, IDE and SCSI, which are not interchangeable.

Printers

Printers vary in capability from adapted electronic typewriters capable of printing 20 characters per second to page printers capable of more than 100 pages per minute. The most widely used types of printer are **dot matrix** and **laser** printers, although **inkjet/bubblejet** printers are beginning to have a major impact on the market. A dot matrix printer forms characters by firing small needles (known as pins) at an inked ribbon in front of the paper. If more pins are used, a clearer image is formed. Low cost printers use nine pins whilst higher quality ones use 24. Laser printers are more expensive than dot matrix (in terms of capital cost and consumables) but they print at higher speeds and at the highest quality (usually 300 dpi, although more recent lasers have 600 dpi capability). Typical speeds are between 6 and 12 pages per minute. Some laser printers use a common language called **Postscript** which provides a range of scaleable typefaces (i.e. how the characters are drawn to convey different moods and messages, e.g. Gothic and Courier) and graphical facilities which are particularly useful when using desk-top-publishing systems. Bubblejet/inkjet printers fire ink droplets at the paper from thin nozzles, giving near-laser quality and a typical speed of two to three pages per minute. The last few years have also seen the development of colour printers, particularly in dot matrix and bubblejet/inkjet formats.

Pointing devices

Although keyboards are the preferred device in most instances for the input of new text, this is only one type of task involved in, for example, word processing operations. **Mice** and **tracker-balls** facilitate direct manipulation of a pointer/cursor allowing other, more complex, tasks to be carried out quickly and with the minimum of mental effort. Such devices contain roller-balls and movement of the ball is translated and used to move a pointer around on the screen. Other pointing devices include light pens and digitizers.

Scanners and optical character recognition (OCR)

Such devices provide a quick way of 'capturing' pictures and line art for incorporation into documents as well as inputting text into a computer by the use of OCR software. However, it should be borne in mind that such software can have difficulties in recognizing certain typefaces and styles.

CD-Roms (compact disk-read only memory)

This is a method of data storage which utilizes optical compact disk technology. Very large amounts of information can be stored in this way, but once laid on to the disk, cannot be removed. **WORM (write once read many) disks**, although similar to CD disks, allow you to save data on the disk yourself, but once this has been done, it cannot be erased. WORM disks, as with CD disks, can be removed and replaced at will. Such media provide a wealth of information.

Software components

Operating system software

The operating system controls nearly every aspect of the basic operation of the computer and provides two major interfaces:

1. between the user and the computer; and
2. between the application program being executed and the various pieces of hardware available.

There are a number of basic tasks which are carried out by most application program:

(a) transferring data to and from disks;
(b) transferring data to the printer;
(c) detecting when a key has been pressed;
(d) loading program from disk into RAM;
(e) detecting disk errors;
(f) displaying messages on the screen.

The operating system is a collection of ready-written software which is supplied with the computer which application program can use for common tasks rather than having to re-invent the wheel. The operating system is loaded into the computer when it is switched on – a process often referred to as **booting up**. Closely associated with the operating system are the utilities which provide a range of facilities associated with general housekeeping, such as taking copies of data and deleting redundant data.

Graphical user interfaces (GUIs)

This is a recent and important software development affecting the way people interact with computers. Such programs use drawings (often referred to as **icons**), boxes and characters to represent objects on the screen. A mouse is used to select the object required and so allow the user to issue instructions, e.g. to launch a particular piece of software. The most well-known example of this type of interface is Microsoft Windows®.

Programming languages

Computer programming languages have evolved through a number of levels – what are termed generations:

1. **Machine code (1st generation)** – originally used to program early computers and consisted purely of a series of 1s and 0s.
2. **Assembly language (2nd generation)** – comprised a vocabulary of short mnemonic codes each of which represented an operation to be performed by the computer.
3. **3rd generation languages** – examples include COBOL, Fortran and Algol.
4. **4th generation (4GL) languages** – developed along with a number of related tools consisting of dedicated programming and query languages, such as SQL, application generators such as those included with products like dBase III Plus® and dBase IV®, and macro languages in products such as Lotus 123® and SuperCalc 5®.

Application software

The last few years have seen substantial developments in the range of application software programs available. Originally, systems revolved around transaction processing characterized by the simple processing of highly structured data; payroll, accounts receivable, stock control to give just a few examples. Such applications enabled the inherent benefits of computer-based systems to be achieved; speed and accuracy applied to large quantities of data. Nowadays, application software covers a wide range of activities – word processing, spreadsheet and statistical analysis, database management, data communications, desk-top publishing and graphics/drawing to name but a few. More specialized software applications include project management, computer-aided design (CAD), survey analysis, questionnaire design and analysis systems (such as satisfaction and customer care surveys) and simulation software.

Networking of computers

The power and flexibility of information technology (IT) in many organizations derives from a combination of the capabilities of the individual machine and from the ways in which machines are linked and combined. Many computer systems installed in environmental health departments form parts of networks and are involved extensively in data communication.

Networks

Networks are communication systems which link together computers, storage devices, word processors, printers and even the telephone system. There are a number of different types of network with names which describe the geographical area over which their different components are spread:

1. **Wide area networks** (WANs) span separate locations which may be many miles apart and use the general telecommunications network.
2. **Metropolitan area networks** (MANs) span a single city – these require special cables which are currently being laid in some cities to provide high speed communications in order to cope with the increasing graphical content of IT and the expected growth in the transmission of video and voice data.
3. **Local area networks** (LANs) are usually restricted to a single or a few buildings and are linked by direct cables rather than by general telecommunication lines.

Each type of network may be composed of one or more types of computer system (Figs 15.4 and 15.5) with geographical links through circuits provided by the national postal, telegraph and telephone authority (PTT). These circuits could be ordinary dial-up telephone lines or dedicated circuits (leased lines) used exclusively for computer communications. Several standards apply to data transmission which are summarized in Table 15.5.

Within organizations, the simplest type of network is one where it is possible to share disks and printers between several computers. **Peer-to-peer networks** allow any computer to make its disks and printers available to any other computer on the network. The advantage of this type of network is its simplicity and its low cost. However, as performance is likely to suffer many organizations have installed networks using **dedicated servers** which supply the requested services. Each computer on the LAN needs to be connected to the network through an appropriate interfacing card, which is dependent on the type of network installed – typically Ethernet® and Token Ring® networks.

For LANs to work efficiently, network management programs are required, with examples of these being Novell NetWare®, LAN Server® and LAN Manager®. Critical to network operation is an effective server-based backup strategy, usually provided by tape drives, and it is essential to institute daily backups in order to avoid disasters!

INFORMATION TECHNOLOGY AND INFORMATION SYSTEMS

Although the boundaries between them are blurred, it is possible to distinguish three major areas of application of IT in information systems:

1. Office support systems – text handling, data storage and reference, computing, telecommunications.
2. End-user systems – decision support systems, expert systems, executive information systems, search and retrieval of information, text handling, etc.

3. Data/transaction processing

These categories overlap and interrelate. Micro-electronics and telecommunications are transforming office work which is, in turn, influencing the availability and type of information that managers use. This is especially true in environmental health departments and the remainder of this chapter will consider the uses and application of IT in the work of environmental health officers and their departments.

Computers have played an important role in local government for many years and have helped determine the way local government operates. Over the last decade the level of investment in IT has greatly increased, with the Audit Commission estimating a 700% increase in expenditure on IT equipment (excluding salaries) when compared to similar expenditure over the previous decade [1]. The Commission calculated that local government expenditure on information technology exceeded £600 million. These figures are impressive when it is realized that during the same decade local government was under severe pressure from central government to reduce costs. In order to meet the challenges they now face, many local authorities have looked to information technology for answers. In fact, without the use of such technology, changes such as the rapid introduction of the Council Tax would have been impossible. The effective use of IT has now become essential to local authorities. However, as highlighted by the Audit Commission 'IT changes often imply major organisational change' [1].

THE USE AND APPLICATION OF INFORMATION TECHNOLOGY IN ENVIRONMENTAL HEALTH DEPARTMENTS

Office support systems

Text handling

Word processors are now a common feature in most offices and can either be a stand-alone or dedicated word processor or a general purpose

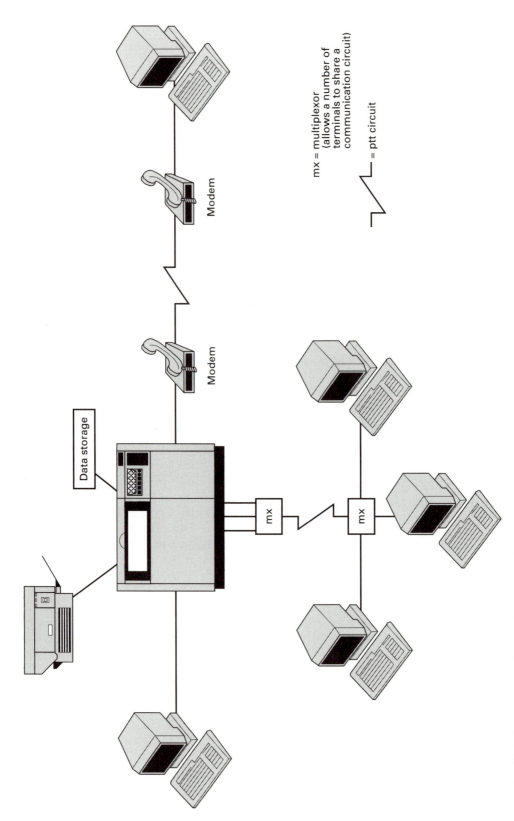

Data storage

Modem

Modem

mx

mx

mx = multiplexor
(allows a number of
terminals to share a
communication circuit)

= ptt circuit

Fig. 15.4 Components of a mainframe WAN.

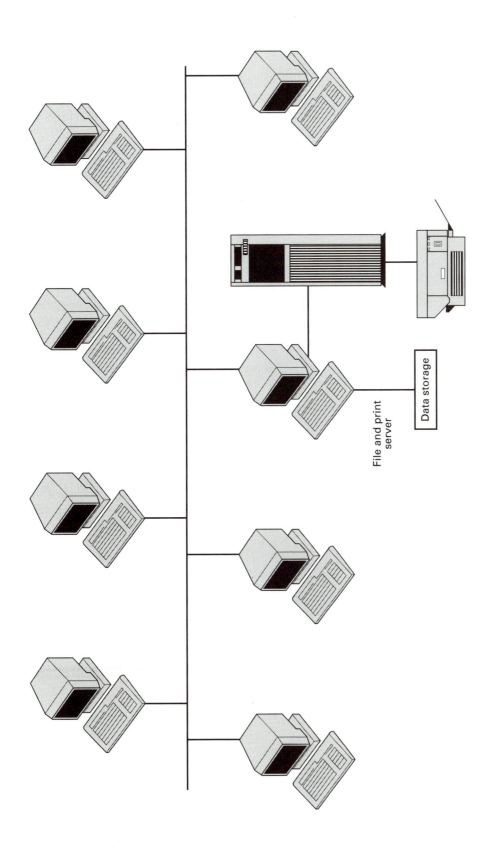

Fig. 15.5 Components of a PC LAN.

Table 15.5 Main CCITT* standards for data communications over telephone lines

Standard	Transmit	Receive
V21	300 bps†	300 bps
V22	1200 bps	1200 bps
V22 bis	2400 bps	2400 bps
V23	75 bps	1200 bps
V32	9600 bps	9600 bps
V32 bis	14400 bps	14400 bps

*Comité Consultatif International Telegraphique et Telephonique

† bps = bits per second.

micro-computer utilizing a word-processing program. Such programs allow documents to be typed, and then altered or manipulated at will without having to retype the entire document. The document is usually stored on disk so that it can be recalled for use at a later date. Word processors are invaluable for producing 'individualized' standard letters or for lengthy reports which require extensive editing and revision. They can improve productivity dramatically whilst at the same time improving quality. Facilities found in most word processors are insertion and deletion of text, automatic re-formatting when margins are altered, tabulations and columns, type styles, moving blocks of text, pagination, standard paragraphs and spelling checks. The various letters with predominantly standard paragraphs, and committee and management reports, that abound in environmental health departments, can easily be produced using such software.

Developments in software and laser printers have enabled the growth of desk-top publishing (DTP) which allows more extensive layout and graphics facilities to be incorporated into documents. This has allowed more professional quality reports and other documentation to be produced 'in-house' by departments with the elimination of traditional type setting.

Data storage, referencing and manipulation

The ability to store and access vast volumes of data is an undoubted benefit of IT in all organizations, not just environmental health departments.

All local authority departments need to maintain records for all their activities and to produce management and statistical information as required, not just by their own authorities but by various government agencies and professional institutions as well.

In the past, many departments designed their own databases, initially on paper, and subsequently using software such as dBase III Plus®. However, there are now a number of specifically designed integrated modular systems which provide useful management tools for the effective and efficient management of environmental health departments. Such systems allow properties within the authority's area to be assigned with a unique code, thereby allowing the collation of all data associated with that property. Data can also be collated with regard to specific types of property, such as commercial or houses in multiple occupation. Once stored, the database of the property and action related information is available as and when required, subject to user-defined levels of individual access, i.e. passwords. Departmental activities such as complaints received, surveys, inspections, correspondence, enforcements, prosecutions and, in some cases, time monitoring, are also maintained through modular systems. Various modules, such as those for food and health and safety, incorporate risk assessment procedures whereby it is possible to prioritize inspections on the basis of certain criteria. Modular systems also cater for the import/export of data not just between the various modules but also other application software such as word processors. By allowing the flow of data in such a manner, a computer system should render all but the initial entry redundant, as once entered onto the system it could be merged to a diary, or visit record automatically. It should be borne in mind that the collection and use of such electronic data is subject to the provisions of the **Data Protection Act 1984**. Consideration should be given to the users of any system and proprietary systems should be evaluated in relation to the data that needs to be input and the queries to be handled. This will then assist in ensuring that the system is workable in relation to the day-to-day workload. The ability of a good software solution to deal with the automatic generation of, for example, complaint- or visit-related correspondence, will in itself mean that staff may more effectively create and print their own letters directly. However, computers and software, no matter how powerful, will not run themselves; goodwill and commitment are a necessary ingredient. Therefore, it is imperative that end-users are involved in the selection of any computer system to be installed.

Telecommunications

Database interrogation

The information requirements demanded by environmental health departments cannot always be provided internally. Frequently, information must be sought from external sources such as **online databases**. For environmental health departments to search online databases the necessary connections will need to be made through a WAN, with appropriate hardware in the department, and with access being controlled by a hierarchy of passwords.

Over the last few years there has been substantial growth in the offering of online databases by many organizations (Table 15.6). The costs of searching such databases vary from host to host and are made up of telecommunication charges, time spent searching and charges for displaying and printing records. The advantages of online searching are considerable due to the extensive range of databases and resources available. However, the search needs to be comprehensively structured as the costs can quickly mount up.

Further sources of information pursued by many departments are provided by specialized CD-ROMs (Table 15.7). The range of titles is rapidly growing and they have the advantage of being straightforward and easy to use after a little tuition. These services are also regularly updated so as to incorporate new legislation, approved codes of practice and guidance for example. Many of the titles will allow 'downloading' – the transference of some of the text from the CD-ROM into a word processor or saved on a disk for use at a future date.

Table 15.6 Online databases

ABI/Inform	FSTA
Acompline/Urbaline	Foods Adlibra
AIDS Database	Geobase
AIDS Knowledgebase	Health Periodicals
Aqualine	Database
Architecture Database	Her Majesty's Stationary
ASSIA	Office
Biological and	Hseline
Agricultural Index	Ibsedex
Biosis	Iconda
British Medical	Life Sciences Collection
Association	Medline
Presscuttings	Nioshtic
British Official	PHTM
Publications	Planex
Brix	Polis
BSI Standardsline	Pollution
CA Search	Resline
CAB Abstracts	Safety
Celex	Scimp
Chemical Safety	Scisearch
Newsbase	Sigle
Cisdoc	Social Scisearch
Scad	Toxline
Compendex and	Urbaline
Compendex-Plus	Waste Info
Conference Proceedings	Water Resources
Index	Abstracts
Current Technology	
Index	
DHSS-data	
Embase	
Emhealth	
Enrep	
Enviroline	
Environmental	
Bibliography	

Source: Ford, N., Page, G. and Rennie, D. (1992) *Environmental Health Information Sources: how to use them*, CIEH, London.

Further detailed information about the online databases and CD-ROMs listed in Tables 15.6 and 15.7 can be found in the CIEH publication *Environmental Health Information Sources: how to use them* [2]. This book also provides substantial information about literature searching and

Table 15.7 Databases available on CD-ROM

ABI/Inform	Iconda
Justis	Life Sciences Collection
Aslib Index to Theses	Medline
Biological and	Metropolitan
Agricultural Index	OCLC Environment
Biosis	Library
CAB Abstracts	OSH-UK
Compact Library – AIDS	OSH-ROM/Mhidas
Compendex-Plus	PolTox
Enviro/Energyline	Science Citation Index
Abstracts	Social Sciences Citation
Environmental	Index
Periodicals	Toxline
Bibliography	UKOP
Excerpta Medica Library	Water Resources
Service	Abstracts
FSTA	
Helecon	

Source: Ford, N., Page, G. and Rennie, D. (1992) *Environmental Health Information Sources: how to use them*, CIEH, London.

highlights a varied selection of environmental health information sources.

Groupware

This is a term used to cover software aimed at supporting groups of people and includes electronic mail, diaries, scheduling, conferencing and bulletin boards.

Some environmental health departments have now instituted electronic mail systems across their LAN where messages are communicated by electronic means rather than by paper-based communication. Messages are displayed on a desk-top terminal and incoming and outgoing messages are filed electronically, if required.

The facilities of a WAN are required in order to gain access to the **Telecom Gold** service. This is an electronic mail network widely used by public authorities and private businesses alike. Within the local government sector major users include trading standards departments, social services departments and environmental health departments. Most users of Telecom Gold are organized in private networks so that information distrib-

uted between them can be controlled and managed – it also ensures confidentiality. Within environmental health, Telecom Gold is regularly used for exchanging technical information and for more urgent matters such as food hazard warnings. It can also be used as a research tool to access technical reference libraries or to request information from colleagues. Examples of databases accessible direct via Telecom gold are **Profile** (which includes the full text of most major newspapers), **Justis** (which contains the complete text of UK and European Union law reports and other related legal information) and **HSELine** (the HSE's abstract database of information on occupational health and safety). A further database accessible through Telecom Gold on a subscription basis is **Environmental Health Briefing**. This offers subscribers the chance to set up their own in-house environmental health database which is updated each week. It also offers ready prepared reports on topical issues and an awareness service on current legal and technical topics.

A further example of an electronic mail network is **Epinet** (Epidemiological Network) controlled by the Public Health Laboratory Service (PHLS) at Colindale in London. The network provides links for various bodies involved in communicable disease control including hospitals, PHLS, environmental health departments, and others.

Facsimile transmission (fax)

Substantial use is made of this technology by environmental health departments. Fax allows the transmission of an exact copy of an original document including diagrams, pictures and text. New systems on the market allow faster transmission and do not need to use special thermal paper which fades over time. Increasingly, fax cards are installed in computers and the transmission can be brought directly into a machine where it can then be incorporated into a word processor or another application program.

End-user systems

End-user computing is a large and growing field. This situation is true of many environmental health departments where managers, professional and office staff have adopted a direct, hands-on approach to computers. Such usage can assist people to develop systems which help them to perform their functions more effectively. Staff are using IT to support their provision of what is, after all, a people-centred service – one in which experience, local knowledge and professional judgement is supported and not replaced by technology.

Management, in particular senior management, has an important part to play in encouraging a positive attitude towards technology, especially as the value of informal learning is often underestimated. One of the most effective methods for individuals to gain confidence and to overcome any feelings of anxiety is to allow them to 'play' on the computer. Although this may involve investing extra time in such people, this investment often pays off as these individuals may bring fresh ideas and new ways of looking at problems. The allocation of time for training is also an important issue to be borne in mind by managers. Both informal learning and training will increase technical awareness and will promote the tendency for staff to use the information systems and technology.

When implementing any computer system in a department, it will be necessary to consider the implications and impact of computer hardware. Who is to be given a terminal? Where should terminals be positioned? The current trend is to attempt to give everyone a terminal on their desk, as this enables the system to be used more efficiently.

Hand-held technology

A new development currently on trial in some local authority departments concerns the introduction of hand-held technology in order to maximize the use of IT. Hand-held computers, coupled with portable printers, could, in the future, enable officers to automate letter and notice production on site, improving the quality, quantity and speed of service achieved.

CONCLUSIONS

The Audit Commission report *Towards a Healthier Environment: managing environmental health services* [5] identified the need for the computerization of environmental health records and the creation of property registers relating to the main function areas. The problems of implementing such a process were also highlighted in the report:

> The introduction of a computerised record system to environmental health departments is a substantial undertaking. Successful implementation demands clear commitment, the allocation of significant resources to bring it about and a fundamental review of information flows. [3, p. 32]

The present use of computers in environmental health departments can be viewed on two levels:

1. **Operational systems** – the management of departments can be assisted by the computerization of certain operational functions such as registers of commercial premises and records of inspections for example.
2. **Strategic systems** – where the use of computers can assist in the setting of or achievement of the department's strategic objectives making a direct impact on the service delivered to customers.

The development of strategic IT systems needs to relate to and support the department's objectives, as detailed in service plans, and should identify several subsystems – the core systems (finance, payroll), office systems (word processing, electronic mail, etc.) and strategic systems (complaints registers, staff monitoring, etc). A properly designed computer system should assist departments to operate at increased efficiency levels, while effectively reducing the workload on staff, by removing a vast amount of work which is duplicated with manual systems. However, a suitably designed system will require all users to be trained as appropriate if its capabilities are to be realized and exploited.

Some of the ways in which departments are using IT have been briefly discussed in this chapter, with IT being used for a multitude of purposes at both operational and strategic levels. Increasingly, the monitoring and control of costs is vital when operating in a competitive environment. With the current and future changes in the environment faced by departments, such as competitive tendering and privatization, it is important that systems are in place to cope with, control and anticipate future developments. The increasing need to provide services that are value for money, the requirement for performance indicators, increased legislative provisions, the pressure for statistical returns, the continuing need to work towards quality service provision – all these are issues to be considered in a climate of diminishing resources. IT and computerization can assist environmental health departments in facing up to these challenges . . . and beyond!!

REFERENCES

1. Audit Commission (1990) *Preparing an IT Strategy: making IT happen*, Management Paper No.7, February 1990, HMSO, London.
2. Ford, N., Page, G. and Rennie, D. (1992) *Environmental Health Information Sources: how to use them*, IEHO, London.
3. Audit Commission (1991) *Towards a Healthier Environment: managing environmental health services*, HMSO, London.

FURTHER READING

Gunton, T. (1988) *End User Focus*, Prentice Hall International (UK) Ltd, Hemel Hempstead, Herts.
Lucy, T. (1991) *Management Information Systems*, 6th edn, DP Publications Ltd, London.

Part Three
Epidemiology

16 Communicable disease – administration and law

William H. Bassett

BACKGROUND

In the reorganization of local government in 1974, responsibility for the control of infectious diseases was divided between the local authority (London boroughs, metropolitan boroughs and district councils) and the National Health Service. In broad terms, local authorities were responsible for the investigation and control of outbreaks of infectious disease and, through its appointed 'proper officer' (usually a specialist in community medicine employed by the health authority), for the enforcement of the various legislative provisions which exist for this purpose. Health authorities were responsible for a range of services contributing to the prevention, control and treatment of communicable disease and infection including health education, health visiting, immunization, hospital treatment and other relevant health services. They were also required to provide medical advice and assistance necessary in controlling infectious disease.

THE ACHESON REPORT

These somewhat vague roles led to a number of difficulties in interpretation and identification of the extent of the responsibilities of the two agencies and their officers, particularly that of the proper officer. The relationship and extent of involvement in infectious disease control between the two bodies also varied in different areas of the country. This lack of clarity led to calls for reform of the situation, and in January 1986 the Secretary of State for Social Services established an inquiry under the chairmanship of Sir Donald Acheson, the chief medical officer, with the following terms of reference:

> To consider the future development of the public health function, **including the control of communicable diseases** and the speciality of community medicine, following the introduction of general management into the hospital and community health services, and recognizing a continued need for improvements in effectiveness and efficiency; and to make recommendations as soon as possible and no later than December 1986.

The Committee reported the results of their deliberations in January 1988 [1]. The report drew attention to the fact that, 'The microbes which give rise to communicable disease and infection do not work within statutory limits and responsibilities', and the Committee therefore saw no simple solutions to the problem but suggested three ways in which an improvement could be effected:

1. Better and continuing collaboration between health and local authorities.

2. Those responsible should be able to react quickly and decisively to problems.
3. Clear recognition of the responsibilities of health authorities for the treatment, prevention and control of most communicable disease and infection, while still recognizing a continuing role for local authorities in the prevention and control of notifiable disease, particularly those which are food and water borne.

The report went on to identify a number of particular actions which could be taken to improve matters on these three issues, and these included the need for one officer in each area to be made responsible for communicable disease and infection, the establishment of District Control of Infection Committees and a review of the Public Health (Control of Disease) Act 1984.

These recommendations were generally accepted by the government and were implemented, with the exception of the review of legislation, through administrative action by the issue by the Minister of Health of Circular 88/64 (now incorporated in NHS circular HSG(93)56). This required health authorities to review the arrangement for the discharge of their responsibilities to improve the health of the population, including the control of communicable disease, and set out the framework for new administrative arrangements which are:

1. Regional health authorities should ensure that proper arrangements have been made between district health authorities and local authorities for the prevention of infection and communicable disease and the control of outbreaks.
2. District health authorities, either individually or on a joint basis where this is appropriate, should appoint a consultant in communicable disease control (CCDC) with responsibility for those arrangements and for the taking of necessary action and arranging the appropriate co-ordination. This appointee should also be designated as the proper officer of the local authority for the exercise of their control functions.
3. One of the ways in which effective collaboration is ensured is through the establishment of the District Control of Infection Committee,

which has an advisory role and one of its purposes is to assist the CCDC in producing a written policy relating to monitoring and surveillance, outbreak investigation and collaborative arrangements including channels of liaison. The membership of the Committee should comprise a cross-section of those involved and include environmental health officers from the local authorities within the health district.

The essence of these arrangements is that the legal responsibilities of both health and local authorities were left undisturbed while the appointment of the CCDC by the health authority and the addition of proper officer duties to that post by the local authorities brought together full responsibilities into one post.

The present arrangements

A further review of the recommendations was undertaken by a joint DoE/DoH Committee led by Dr Michael Abrams as part of a wider study of the operation of the public health function following changes in the organization and management of the National Health Service, i.e. the establishment of NHS Trusts and the implementation of a purchaser/provider relationship.

Revised guidance on communicable disease control has been issued in EL(91)123 which is included as Annex B to NHS Management Executive Guideline HSG(93)56. (Circ. 88/64 is now withdrawn.)

The broad framework of arrangements proposed by Circ. 88/64 and set out in the previous section still apply but greater attention has been given to some aspects:

1. The Communicable Disease Control Plan – the written policy relating to monitoring and surveillance, outbreak investigation and collaborative arrangements should be in the form of a joint plan between the health authority (HA) and the relevant local authorities (LA), through consultation between the CCDC, CEHOs, FHSA, PHLS, provider units, GP fundholders, water undertakers, port health authorities and other agencies involved.

The plan should include:

(a) a clear description of the role and the extent of the responsibilities of each of the organizations and individuals who are involved on a day to day basis or may be involved when an outbreak occurs;

(b) the arrangements for informing and consulting the PHLS Communicable Disease Surveillance Centre (CDSC), the regional health authority (RHA) and Department of Health;

(c) the arrangements which have been agreed with neighbouring LAs and HAs both for managing individual cases of infectious disease which may have implications for those authorities and for dealing with outbreaks of infection which cross boundaries;

(d) the arrangements which have been agreed amongst all the LAs and HAs involved in areas where the boundaries between these authorities overlap.

(e) arrangements for creating a control team to manage a significant outbreak of disease or other incident, the support which will be available to the team and what its duties will be. The plans for dealings with outbreaks should be sufficiently detailed and flexible to allow them to be implemented rapidly by all concerned in a situation requiring urgent action;

(f) the arrangements which have been made to provide the necessary staff and facilities outside normal working hours should this be required to manage an outbreak of disease;

(g) arrangements for dealing with district immunization programmes, both on a day to day basis and in the event of an outbreak of disease.

These joint plans are to be reviewed annually, copied to all involved and to the Regional Director of Public Health and tested from time to time by audit and simulation exercises.

2. Regional Directors of Public Health have a responsibility for ensuring that the plans are satisfactory, that there is satisfactory communication between RHAs, playing a co-ordinating role in more widespread outbreaks and undertaking regional surveillance of disease.

3. LAs should provide professional and other staff to support the CCDC and ensure that satisfactory arrangements are made for the receipt of notification of disease.

4. The CCDC should be formally appointed by each local authority as the proper officer under the Public Health (Control of Disease) Act 1984 and the appropriate control powers should be delegated formally to that person. Advisory Appointment Committees for CCDC posts should include a local authority representative.

THE PUBLIC HEALTH (CONTROL OF DISEASE) ACT 1984*

One of the Acheson Committee's recommendations was that the Public Health (Control of Disease) Act 1984 should be revised to produce a more up-to-date and relevant legislative backing to control communicable disease and infection. A review of this legislation was undertaken by the Department of Health, and a consultation document was issued in 1989 [2] outlining options for change which would better reflect both the changed perceptions of the respective responsibilities of health and local authorities and the different control requirements of current communicable disease problems. So far, however, no legislative change has taken place and the following is an outline of the present control provisions.

The Public Health (Control of Disease) Act 1984 contains most of the provisions related to the control of infectious disease.

The notifiable diseases

The diseases notifiable under the provisions of the Public Health (Control of Disease) Act 1984 are:

1. cholera

*See also 'Communicable Disease Control: A Practical Guide to the Law for Health and Local Authorities'. James Button, Public Health Information Unit, Manchester.

2. plague
3. relapsing fever
4. smallpox
5. typhus
6. food poisoning

There are also 24 diseases notifiable under the provisions of the Public Health (Infectious Diseases) Regulations 1988. These are:

1. acute encephalitis
2. acute poliomyelitis
3. meningitis
4. meningococcal septicaemia
5. anthrax
6. diphtheria
7. dysentery (amoebic or bacillary)
8. paratyphoid fever
9. typhoid fever
10. viral hepatitis
11. leprosy
12. leptospirosis
13. measles
14. mumps
15. rubella
16. whooping cough
17. malaria
18. tetanus
19. yellow fever
20. ophthalmia neonatorum
21. rabies
22. scarlet fever
23. tuberculosis
24. viral haemorrhagic fever.

Acquired Immune Deficiency Syndrome (AIDS) is not notifiable, although certain regulations relating to disease control are applied to it.

A local authority may make any disease notifiable within its area subject to an order approved by the Secretary of State for Health. An order must state the public health powers being adopted in respect of the disease and must be advertised with a copy of the order being sent to every registered medical practitioner within the district. In an emergency the local authority may make an order without the prior approval of the Secretary of State, however the Secretary of State may subsequently approve or revoke the order. If he does not respond the order ceases to have effect after one month.

The notification system

A registered medical practitioner who becomes aware, or suspects, that a patient is suffering from a notifiable disease or food poisoning, must notify the proper officer of the local authority in writing. He must provide the following information:

1. The name, age, sex and address of the patient.
2. The disease or particulars of the poisoning from which the patient is, or is suspected to be suffering, and the date, as nearly as can be determined, of its onset.
3. If the premises are a hospital, the day on which the patient was admitted, the address from which he came, and whether or not the disease or poisoning leading to the notification was contracted in hospital.

There is a standard form for notification and the medical practitioner receives a fee from the district health authority for each notification made.

Upon receipt of a notification the 'proper officer' of the local authority must, within 48 hours, send a copy to:

1. The district health authority within which the medical practice submitting the notification is situated.
2. If the certificate is for a patient in hospital who came from outside the local authority or health authority in which the hospital is situated, and that patient did not contract the disease in hospital, he must copy the certificate to the proper officer of the local authority from which the patient came, the district health authority from which the patient came and, if relevant, the appropriate port health authority.

The proper officer is also required to make weekly and quarterly returns of notifications received to the Registrar General and to notify the chief medical officer of the Department of Health by telephone of any serious outbreak of disease, or food poisoning.

The chief medical officer must also be notified if a notification of any of the following diseases is received:

1. a disease subject to the international health regulations, i.e. cholera, plague, smallpox and yellow fever;
2. leprosy;
3. malaria or rabies contracted in Great Britain;
4. viral haemorrhagic fever.

Where a local authority or port health authority have reason to believe that rats in their district are infected with plague or are dying in unusual numbers they are required to notify the chief medical officer.

DISEASE CONTROL MEASURES

Among the range of measures available to the proper officer under the Public Health (Control of Disease) Act 1984 are:

1. Control of infectious persons.
   (a) Any person who knows he is suffering from a notifiable disease or has care of a child so affected must avoid exposing other people to the risk of infection, either directly from his presence in a public place, or at school, or indirectly by exposing others to the risk of handling infected bedding, personal clothing or articles that could carry infection.
   (b) In order to prevent the spread of infection restrictions may be put on the movement and disposal of bodies of persons who have died while suffering from a notifiable disease.
   (c) A person suffering from a notifiable disease must not carry out any trade, business or occupation when there is a risk of spreading the infection. It may be necessary for the proper officer to require patients or carriers of notifiable disease not to attend work where there is a risk of their spreading infection, this is particularly appliable to food workers who are carrying organisms associated with enteritis. In such cases, the local authority is required to compensate them for loss of earnings.
   (d) If there is a reason to believe that a person is, or has been, suffering from a notifiable disease, or is suspected of carrying an organism that may infect others, an application for a warrant to examine him or her may be made to a justice of the peace.
   (e) If it is considered that a person suffering from a notifiable disease should be admitted to a hospital to prevent the spread of infection and the person refuses, a warrant may be obtained from a justice of the peace requiring him to enter hospital and be detained.

2. Control of infected premises, articles, etc.
   (a) When required, the local authority may cleanse and disinfect any premises or, when necessary, destroy any articles inside. The local authority may pay compensation for any damage resulting from its action and provide temporary accommodation while the disinfection is carried out.
   (b) The local authority may provide a disinfecting station and may remove or disinfect articles free of charge.
   (c) A person may not let any accommodation, whether it is a house or hotel, which has been occupied by persons who are known to have suffered from a notifiable disease unless the accommodation has been satisfactorily disinfected.
   (d) A local authority may prohibit home work on a premises where there has been a case of notifiable disease until such time as satisfactory disinfection has been undertaken.

3. Food control.
   The range of controls over food and food premises in order to prevent and control outbreaks of food-borne disease are dealt with in Chapter 33. Of particular relevance are the powers given in section 9 of the Food Safety Act 1990 whereby an authorized officer of the food authority may inspect, seize and remove to present to a justice of the peace food which is likely to cause food poisoning or any disease

communicable to human beings, and the powers in sections 10 and 12 to serve improvement and emergency prohibition notices.

PORT HEALTH

In districts which have been consolidated as port health districts, communicable disease control is the responsibility of the port health authority. The powers of port health authorities in respect of the control of infectious disease are contained in the Public Health (Aircraft) Regulations 1979 and the Public Health (Ships) Regulations 1979 and are dealt with in Chapter 13.

Channel Tunnel

The Public Health (International Trains) Regulations 1994 were brought in to safeguard public health in relation to the opening of the Tunnel and were made under the Public Health (Control of Disease) Act 1984. The regulations are broadly constructed so as to ensure the effective safeguarding of public health whilst minimizing the burden on the operation which would ensue from any avoidable disruption of this international service.

So far as communicable disease is concerned, the regulations provide for:

1. Notification by the train manager to the enforcement authority where there is on board a train terminating in the UK a sick traveller (i.e. one who has a serious epidemic, endemic or infectious disease or where there are reasonable grounds for suspecting such disease).
2. The enforcement authority may question train passengers where they believe there is a significant danger to public health, because they are either a sick passenger or may have been exposed to similar infections, in order to ascertain their current state of health, contact with infection and previous and intended destinations.
3. The enforcement authority to require the disinfection of rolling stock or articles on board the train.

The regulations apply not only to the Tunnel system but also to control areas designated by the Secretary of State, e.g. terminal control points for passenger services.

The enforcement authority is the local authority in whose district the control area is situated and, for situations on board train, the Secretary of State.

The diseases which are generally defined as being subject to the controls are those which are serious epidemic, endemic or infectious diseases. These are not specified but venereal disease and HIV infection are specifically excluded. All the notifiable diseases will be included in these definitions including tuberculosis. The inclusion of tuberculosis in these notifications and control provisions is interesting in that it is excluded from controls available to deal with similar concerns on ships and aircraft. There is concern, however, about the increasing prevalence of tuberculosis, hence its inclusion in respect of the Channel Tunnel controls.

There will still remain in relation to the use of the Tunnel some wider legislation controls. Of particular note are those dealing with:

1. the disinfestation of verminous persons, articles etc. (Public Health Act 1936);
2. the carriage of persons suffering from notifiable diseases on public conveyances, which includes trains, (Public Health (Infectious Diseases) Regs 1988);
3. the powers of detention and removal to hospital of infectious persons, who may also be sick travellers (Public Health (Control of Disease) Act 1984).

Reference should also be made to a 'Report Concerning Frontier Controls and Policing, Co-operation in Criminal Justice, Public Safety and Mutual Assistance Relating to the Channel Fixed Line' (Cm 2366 HMSO 2 August 1993). This sets out arrangements between the British and French Governments on these issues.

PUBLIC HEALTH LABORATORY SERVICE

The Public Health Laboratory Service (PHLS) was set up as an emergency service in 1939 at the outbreak of the Second World War to improve the microbiological and epidemiological services to deal with outbreaks of infectious disease during wartime. It became a permanent part of the public health organization of England and Wales under the National Health Service Act 1946. In 1988, the service comprised 52 public health laboratories undertaking both public health and hospital microbiology. There are also reference and research laboratories at the Central Public Health Laboratory, Colindale, London and the Centre for Applied Microbiology and Research at Porton. Since its inception, the service has monitored infections in the population including hospital infection, provided microbiological reference services, has supported local and health authorities in the investigation of disease, and has undertaken a wide range of research. In Scotland an informal network of laboratories exists and there is a national epidemiological centre, the Communicable Diseases (Scotland) Unit (CDSU), which is administered by Common Services Agency of the Scottish Office Home and Health Department.

In February 1994 a Strategic Review of all aspects of the PHLS was initiated in the light of the reforms of the NHS and other changes in relation to its work. Amongst the matters to be examined are the extent of the epidemiological role, the level of support the service should provide to local authorities and others on communicable disease work and the enhancement of the epidemiological surveillance network.*

COMMUNICABLE DISEASE SURVEILLANCE CENTRE

Established in 1977 and located at Colindale, the functions of the Centre include: national surveillance of communicable disease; advice, assistance and coordination of disease investigation and control nationally; surveillance of immunization; production of the weekly Communicable Disease Report (received by all environmental health departments); and research.

LIAISON BETWEEN AGENCIES

There are a number of authorities and bodies involved in the control of infectious disease, each with its own area of responsibility, some of which overlap and are ill-defined. In order for the system to work effectively, it is essential for there to be close liaison and co-ordination of effort between the authorities, agencies and individuals involved at all levels, both in respect of specific outbreaks and more generally.

Liaison arrangements as outlined earlier need to be established having regard to local circumstances, but in general terms a good working relationship between those involved must exist involving regular contact, the sharing of information and the appreciation of the area of expertise of the other members of the team. It is the responsibility of the chief environmental health officer and of the director of public health of the health authority to ensure that these arrangements exist and work effectively, and this should be ensured through their more general liaison on public health (see Chapter 3).

REFERENCES

1. The Report of the Committee of Inquiry into the Future Development of the Public Health Function, *Public Health in England* Cmnd 289, HMSO, London.
2. Department of Health (1989) *Review of the Law of Infectious Disease Control*, Consultation Paper, October, HMSO, London.

*A report was made to the PHLS Board in September 1994. This made several recommendations, including the promotion of a corporate image and purpose, a strategy for service development, and an organizational vision based on a network of groups of laboratories, each managed by a Group Director, a national marketing strategy and further measures to achieve economy and efficiency.

17 Food-borne disease

John Cruickshank

INTRODUCTION

The ingestion of food may give rise to disease under a variety of circumstances. Some substances are inherently unsafe, e.g. certain fungi; food may be contaminated with chemical materials such as organophosphate; food stuffs may be handled or stored incorrectly such that toxic substances may form; and food may become contaminated by infectious pathogenic micro-organisms such as *Salmonella* spp. or *Campylobacter* spp. Diseases resulting from such events are collectively known as food poisoning or food-borne disease.

Other infections acquired by mouth are due generally to direct ingestion of micro-organisms without the intervention of food as a vehicle of transmission. Such infections are called faecal-oral in type and include hepatitis A and poliomyelitis. The distinction is not absolute as some conditions, such as dysentery, though usually spreading by the faecal–oral route may occasionally be transmitted in food.

While the commonest clinical presentation of food-borne disease is gastro-enteritis, a wide range of clinical manifestations from confusion and paralysis due to central nervous system (CNS) involvement, to renal and hepatic failure may occur though usually from the less common causes of food poisoning.

Cases of food poisoning occur singly (sporadic cases) or in outbreaks where two or more cases are epidemiologically related. Tracing the origin of sporadic cases is often very difficult, but where larger numbers are involved, evidence of common factors will often lead to a particular source for the offending organisms.

NON-MICROBIAL FOOD-BORNE DISEASE

Fungi

Mushroom poisoning

The collection and consumption of wild mushrooms is enthusiastically practised in many rural parts of the UK. Some varieties are harmless and edible, others produce gastric irritation of varying degrees of severity, and a few are associated with severe disease with multi-organ involvement. There is no simple or rule of thumb method of distinguishing toxic from safe species. Fortunately, clinical mushroom poisoning is rarely seen.

The great majority of severe and of fatal cases in Europe are caused by the *Amanita* genus of fungi. They cause one of two clinical syndromes depending upon the toxins they produce. *A. pantherina* (false blusher) and *A. muscaria* (fly agaric) ingestion results in the rapid onset of gastro-intestinal symptoms followed by inco-ordination and other signs of neurological disorder due to the muscarine that they harbour. Recovery is usual within 24 hours. In contrast *A. phalloides* (death cap) and *A. virosa* (destroying angel) toxins, amanitine and phalloidin, cause an initial enteritis followed a few days later by renal and hepatic failure carrying a mortality rate of up to 90%.

Mycotoxicosis

Foods affected by toxin-producing moulds may cause illness in man or animals, sometimes on an epidemic scale. Manifestations are as diverse as gangrene and convulsions (ergotism), renal disease (Balkan nephropathy) and liver cancer (aflatoxicosis). Low levels of aflatoxins are frequently found in peanuts and may play a part in the development of liver diseases in places where food storage is conducive to fungal growth.

'Special' foods

A number of 'health foods' such as ginseng and liquorice may, if taken in quantity over long periods, cause hallucinations, nausea, vertigo and other CNS effects.

Red Whelks

The salivary glands of this shellfish, which is readily distinguishable from the edible whelk, secrete tetramine. This toxin produces alarming symptoms, including muscle weakness and vertigo, which however disappear within a few hours.

Red kidney beans

Though recognized as a cause of severe gastroenteritis since a large outbreak in 1948 was attributed to 'flaked beans', food poisoning from the consumption of raw or undercooked red kidney beans only came into prominence during the late 1970s and early 1980s, when a series of incidents were reported. A number of toxic substances can be extracted from the beans, but current evidence suggests that the haemagglutinin component is probably responsible for the diarrhoea and vomiting. Much of this substance is leached out by soaking the beans for several hours and thorough cooking will render them safe. The onset of symptoms is usually within an hour or two of ingestion and rapid recovery is the rule.

Food contaminated with chemical substances and toxins

Pesticides

These substances are used to control pests of various kinds on wheat seed, fruit trees and vegetables. If ingested they are absorbed and affect particularly the CNS. A mortality of around 8% was recorded in a large outbreak in Iraq caused by bread made from seed treated with organomercurial compounds.

Metals

Mercurials discharged into the sea may be taken up by fish and have caused nephritis and incapacitating CNS damage to persons who ate them. Minamata disease in Japan, resulting from wholesale discharges of industrial pollutants containing mercury into a bay from which the local population caught fish which formed the major part of their diet, left many persons with severe neurological damage.

Zinc leached from galvanized pans when acid materials, such as fruit, are boiled in them is toxic and causes acute abdominal symptoms. A variety of foods including apples, rhubarb, chicken, spinach and alcoholic punch have caused outbreaks. Symptoms, vomiting and/or diarrhoea, appear rapidly after ingestion, often within a few minutes. Recovery is generally quick. The presence of zinc levels in suspected foods will confirm the diagnosis.

Dinoflagellates

'Blooms' or 'red tides' of proliferating dinoflagellate organisms (*Gonyaulax* spp.) periodically infest coastal waters where they are ingested by bivalve molluscs, in particular mussels. The toxin produced by the organism is concentrated in the flesh of shellfish, but causes no harm to them. In man the toxin affects the CNS causing parasthesia of the mouth, lips, face and limbs, which may progress to a paralytic state depending upon the species of *Gonyaulax* involved. Regular monitoring of toxin concentrations in shellfish is carried out on susceptible coasts and public warnings are given when potentially dangerous levels are found.

Additives

Monosodium glutamate used extensively in Chinese cookery may induce temporary burning sensations over the trunk, face and arms, headaches, tightness in the chest and, occasionally, abdominal pain and nausea.

Ciguatera

Small tropical fish may feed on the dinoflagellate, *Gambierdiscus*, which will render their flesh toxic. They in turn are eaten by large edible fish, e.g. groupers, in which the toxin accumulates in high concentration. Rare cases occur in the UK when fish brought or sent back from tropical waters are consumed. The symptoms which develop within a few hours of ingestion are similar to those with dinoflagellates.

Food stored incorrectly

Scombrotoxic fish poisoning

Scombroid fish, tuna, skipjack and mackerel and, occasionally, herring and sardine, may become contaminated with spoilage organisms, which can convert the amino acid, histidine, in the tissue to histamine. This substance, together with other as yet poorly characterized toxins, causes acute facial flushing, rapid pulse, headaches and mild gastro-enteritis. The symptoms are alarming but short lived. Proper refrigeration of fish will prevent the proliferation of the organisms responsible. Histamine levels of 20 mg or more per 100 g or more of fish are diagnostic, but it should be noted that suspect fish must be kept refrigerated during transport to the laboratory for testing.

Solanine

Potatoes which are left to sprout or which are exposed to sunlight, such that the skin surface becomes green, will accumulate the alkaloid, solanine, in the skin and just below the surface. Peeling and washing will render them safe, but jacket potatoes have caused some cases of poisoning. A large outbreak at a school in London was associated with potatoes stored in sacks over a holiday period. Symptoms are those of gastro-

enteritis together with varying degrees of confusion and other neurological signs. Recovery within 24 hours is usual, although prolonged indisposition may occur and the occasional fatality has been recorded. It is surprising that the condition, relating to one of our commonest foods, is so uncommon.

FOOD-BORNE DISEASE CAUSED BY PATHOGENIC MICRO-ORGANISMS OR THEIR TOXINS

Incidence

While there is no doubt that the incidence of microbial food-borne disease is rising, it is not possible to make any real estimate of the true number of cases for the reason that most cases are not notified, although it is required by law. Many patients do not seek medical advice, and a large proportion of those who do consult their doctors are not able to provide histories which clearly point to food origins for their illness. Statutory notification is required of any cases of cholera, dysentery, food poisoning, typhoid fever and viral hepatitis, in England to the proper officer for the district and in Scotland and Northern Ireland to the chief administrative medical officer or director of public health. Details are contained in Supplement 1 of the Communicable Disease Report, 1990 [1]. (See Chapter 16 for the administrative and legal framework for the notification and control of food poisoning and other communicable diseases.)

Salmonellas and certain other enteric pathogenic organisms isolated by laboratories in England and Wales are referred to the Laboratory of Enteric Pathogens (LEP) in the Central Public Health Laboratory of the Public Health Laboratory Service for confirmation of identity. Information from the LEP is combined and correlated with that obtained by the Communicable Disease Surveillance Centre (CDSC), and from notifications to the Office of Populations, Censuses and Surveys. Parallel systems operate in Scotland [2] and in Northern Ireland [3]. The figures are published at regular intervals and can be regarded

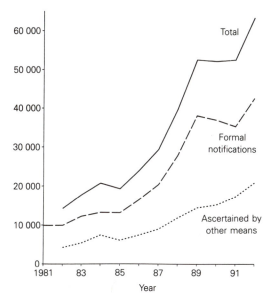

Fig. 17.1 Notifications of food poisoning, England and Wales 1981–92. (Source: OPCS. Prepared by CDSC.)

as a reasonably reliable guide to the trends in incidence of the various forms of microbial food-borne disease. Other organizations likewise compile statistics in other parts of the world, and WHO publishes a regular newsletter on the situation in Europe. In developed countries, trends seem to be similar both in numbers and in the organisms primarily responsible for food-borne disease.

Trends in the incidence of food poisoning in England and Wales are illustrated in Fig. 17.1. While the reported numbers of incidents have been rising steadily since the mid-1960s, the unprecedented increase from 1985 onwards has become the cause of grave concern. While part of the increase will be due to better surveillance and more efficient reporting, there is no doubt that the figures represent a true increase in food-borne disease in the past few years.

The situation stimulated the production of two reports: one by the Agriculture Committee of the House of Commons on salmonella in eggs [4] and the other by the committee on the Microbiological Safety of Food (The Richmond Committee) [5]. Both groups recognized the need for further research into the sources and causes of food-

borne disease and for tighter controls in the production, processing and distribution of food stuffs. To this end the Steering Group for the Microbiological Safety of Food (SGMSF) was established to provide surveillance through a number of working groups, on aspects of the food industry ranging from farm animals and abattoirs to matters concerning retailing and catering. Where potential problems are identified they are referred to the Advisory Committee for the Microbiological Safety of Food (ACMSF) whose function is to make assessments of risk and to provide advice on appropriate action. Reports from these bodies are presented to the Minister of State whose ultimate responsibility it is to consider the need for government intervention.

Organisms responsible – microbial characteristics

Six groups of organisms are responsible for the great majority of cases and outbreaks of food-borne disease. These are *Salmonella* spp., *Campylobacter* spp., *Clostridium perfringens*, *Staphylococcus aureus*, *Bacillus* spp. and small round viruses. Of these the campylobacters and salmonellas far outnumber all the others. Others, while capable of causing serious disease and from time to time outbreaks, are less often encountered. Table 17.1 summarizes the organisms according to whether their common reservoirs are human, animal or environmental.

Pathogenesis

The effects of food poisoning bacteria on the gastro-intestinal tract are either mediated through the presence of the organisms themselves or through the production of powerful exotoxins which may exert their influence in the absence of the organisms. The former are known as the infection type, and the latter the toxic (Table 17.2). Generally, the incubation period of the toxic type illnesses is shorter than the infective, as the toxins may be preformed in the food. Proliferation in the intestinal tract is necessary with the infective type before a sufficiently large number of organisms has accumulated to cause

Table 17.1 Food poisoning organisms by origin

	Human only	Animal	Environment
Common	*Staphylococcus aureus** Viruses	Salmonella spp. (non-typhoid) *Campylobacter* spp.	*Clostridium perfringens* *Bacillus* spp.
Uncommon	*Salmonella typhi* *Salmonella paratyphi B* *Escherichia coli* (enteropathogenic, enteroinvasive, enterotoxigenic) *Shigella* spp.	*Listeria monocytogenes* *Yersinia enterocolitica* *Escherichia coli* (enterohaemorrhagic)	*Clostridium botulinum* *Vibrio parahaemolyticus* *Aeromonas* spp. *Pleisomonas* spp.

*Rare phage type 42D is of bovine origin

Table 17.2 Organisms causing food poisoning – infectious and toxic

Infectious	Incubation period (hours)	Toxic	Incubation period (hours)
Salmonella spp.	17–72	*Clostridium perfringens*	8–12
Campylobacter spp.	48–120	*Clostridium botulinum*	12–36
Escherichia coli	12–72	*Staphylococcus aureus*	2–6
Vibrio parahaemolyticus	12–24	*Bacillus* spp.	2–16
Yersinia enterocolitica	Variable	*Escherichia coli*	12–60
Listeria monocytogenes	Variable	(enterohaemorrhagic)	
Aeromonas spp.	Variable		
Pleisomonas spp.	Variable		

damage and initiate symptoms. The toxin of *Clostridium botulinum* is one of the most toxic substances known to man. There may be difficulties in the detection of organisms of the toxic type in foods. Tests may be required to demonstrate the toxin which will remain after the organisms which produced it have died out. Some of the organisms causing food-borne disease may have both toxic and invasive potential.

Technical details on the biological and cultural characteristics of the organisms can be found in standard microbiology texts. The following accounts provide the information relevant particularly to their ability to cause food poisoning.

Salmonella spp.

The two major groups are those causing enteric fevers (typhoid and paratyphoid), and those causing food poisoning (the non-typhoid salmonellas). The enteric fever group consists of *S. typhi* and *S.*

paratyphi A and B. With rare exceptions these organisms infect man only. The non-typhoid group consists of over 2000 species, all of which have their primary reservoirs in animals – both wild and domestic. The classifications into serotypes are made on the basis of antigens on their surfaces (O antigens) and on their flagellae (H antigens). Kaufman and White developed a scheme using these antigens in combination to enable identifications to be made. Certain more common species can be more precisely characterized using special techniques such as phage typing and plasmid analysis and finger-printing. The organisms can grow in many foods at a wide range of temperatures from 10°C to over 40°C. They are destroyed by pasteurization temperatures and are killed in 20 minutes at 60°C. Salmonellas survive well outside a person or an animal in faeces, on vegetables, in animal feeds and in many foods for long periods. While 10 serotypes account for 90%

of all human isolates, two serotypes, *S. enteritidis* and *S. typhimurium*, constitute 80% of the total in the UK.

Campylobacter spp.

The species causing food-borne disease are *C. jejuni* and *C. coli*. They are found as part of the normal gut flora of many animals including mammals, birds and reptiles. Their growth requirements are more exacting than those for salmonellas and the organisms do not grow on food under normal circumstances. Sub-typing can be undertaken but is less precise than with salmonellas. Growth occurs up to 42°C and the organism survives well in water and raw milk.

Clostridium perfringens

This organism is found in soil, dust, vegetation and elsewhere in the environment. It will only grow anaerobically, and produces a variety of exotoxins some of which act upon the gastro-intestinal tract. Spores may be formed in adverse conditions which enable the organisms to survive circumstances which would normally kill vegetative bacteria. Five types are recognized on the basis of toxins and enzymes produced. Type A strains are responsible for most food poisoning outbreaks.

Staphylococcus aureus

Up to 40% of persons carry *Staph. aureus* in their noses and a proportion of these on their skin as well. Many strains produce enterotoxins of which there are at least five: A, B, C, D and E. Growth occurs on many foods particularly those with a high protein content and the toxin is readily produced at ambient temperatures. The organisms are killed at 60°C in 30 minutes, but the toxin will survive boiling for the same period of time. More precise identification of staphylococci is achieved by phage typing. Because of the commonness and ubiquity of this organism, such methods must be used when attempting to identify the sources of outbreaks.

Small round viruses

These agents were first identified in the faeces of patients in the town of Norwalk in the USA during an outbreak of gastro-enteritis. The organisms are detectable only by electron microscopy. Other strains are named either by their appearance, eg: Calicivirus, Astrovirus, Norwalk-like or by their geographical location of origin, i.e. Snow River agent. They appear to be entirely human in distribution and are found in sewage effluent and, consequently, in shellfish. Because it has not so far been possible to grow these organisms in culture, little is known of their biological characteristics.

Bacillus cereus

This free-living organism is widespread in the environment and is particularly, but not exclusively, associated with foods involving grains and cereals. Strains produce two distinct exotoxins, one of which causes vomiting and the other diarrhoea. Spores are formed which resist boiling and frying for short periods. There are numerous serotypes, some of which are more commonly found as pathogens than others. There is good evidence that other *Bacillus* species, e.g. *B. subtilis* and *B. licheniformis*, may also be responsible for cases and outbreaks of food poisoning.

Organisms less commonly responsible for outbreaks of food poisoning

Escherichia coli

Strains characterized by certain biological properties and known as enteropathogenic (EPEC), enteroinvasive (EIEC) and enterotoxigenic *E. coli* (ETEC) can cause gastro-enteritis, and may be defined serologically according to their somatic (O) and flagellar (H) antigens.

Another group of increasing importance consists of around 50 serotypes which are known as enterohaemorrhagic *E. coli* (EHEC) and which are now definitely associated with the conditions haemorrhagic colitis and the haemolytic uraemic syndrome. All produce a characteristic toxin known as Verotoxin (VT) and strains may be referred to as VTEC in some texts. (In the USA and Canada the same toxin is referred to as Shiga-like toxin – SLT.) *Escherichia coli* type 0157 is by far the most frequently reported strain and appears to be largely of beef or milk origin. Further typing systems have been developed and can be used for epidemiological tracing.

Shigella sp.

The dysentery group of organisms are pathogens of man only and are usually transmitted by the faecal-oral route in circumstances of poor general hygiene. Food contamination readily occurs, however, though in the UK *Shigella* spp. are rarely associated with food poisoning. There are four major species, *S. sonnei*, *S. flexneri*, *S. boydii* and *S. dysenteriae*, and numerous subtypes.

Vibrio parahaemolyticus

This marine organism is found in coastal and brackish waters. It is halophilic (salt loving) and grows best in media with high salt content. Infection is associated with seafoods and is particularly prevalent where raw fish is eaten, e.g. Japan. There are many antigenic subtypes.

Clostridium botulinum

This anaerobic, spore-bearing organism is extensively distributed in the environment and produces a powerful exotoxin affecting the CNS. The organism will grow particularly well on low acid (pH >4.5) foods such as fish, fruit and vegetables. There are seven antigenic types, A–G, each with their own distinct toxin. Human intoxications are usually with types A, B and E, though a recent Swiss outbreak was caused by type G. The toxins, powerful as they are, are readily destroyed by heat. The spores, if type A, resist boiling for several hours; those of other types are slightly less resistant.

Listeria monocytogenes

Because these organisms are very widely distributed in the gastro-intestinal tracts of wild and domestic animals, they contaminate the environment generally. They can grow over a wide range of temperatures from as low as +4°C, are comparatively resistant to disinfectants and changes in pH, and can survive extreme environmental conditions. Strains can be distinguished by serotyp-

ing, types 1/2a and 4b being most commonly found in strains isolated from pathological sources.

Yersinia enterocolitica

Like *L. monocytogenes*, these organisms are widely distributed in animals, including mammals, birds, flies and fish, and in the environment, particularly water, soil and vegetation. They may grow at refrigeration temperatures, and at pHs from 5.0 to 9.0. Many antigenic types occur of which 0:3, 0:8 and 0:9 are most frequently associated with human disease. Most clinically significant strains produce an enterotoxin, but only at temperatures up to 30°C. The part played by this toxin in mediating disease is not yet clear.

Other organisms

Evidence that *Aeromonas* and *Plesiomonas* spp. can cause food poisoning comes largely from studies in countries in the East where seafoods, raw and cooked, form a large part of the diets of the population. *A. sobria* are the most commonly isolated strains in the UK.

Cases caused by *Brucella* species are reported from time to time due mainly to the consumption of imported dairy products, usually cheese. Indigenous cases are now very rare.

The association between the protozoal parasites, *G. lamblia* and *Cryptosporidium* spp., and food-borne disease is tenuous, though one school party is thought to have been infected by the latter through tasting silage.

'HIGH-RISK' FOODS

While food-borne disease has been linked to almost every kind of food from peppercorns to chocolate bars, certain foods are far more prone to significant contamination than others. The great majority of outbreaks are associated with the following foods.

Foods of animal origin

Meats

Salmonellas and campylobacters are found in the gastro-intestinal tracts of cattle and poultry and less often in other farm animals. Contamination of meats during slaughter and processing is common, particularly so with poultry. Raw carcasses are, therefore, potentially hazardous and up to 60 to 80% of 'oven ready' chickens may yield one or other of the organisms on culture. Undercooking of red meat and poultry may therefore leave residual pathogens. Salmonellas but not campylobacters are liable to proliferate if cooked meat storage conditions are inadequate.

Dairy products
Milk always contains organisms which are derived in the main from the gastro-intestinal tract of the cow, and pathogens may be part of their flora. Raw and imperfectly pasteurized milk may be contaminated with salmonellas, campylobacters, listerias, yersinias or enterotoxigenic *E. coli*. Dairy products like creams and soft cheeses (rarely hard cheese) may, consequently also be infected.

Eggs
Salmonellas may contaminate eggs through cracks in their surfaces or, with certain strains, may infect the eggs within the oviduct. Where such eggs are lightly cooked, temperatures within the albumen of the yolk may well not be sufficient to destroy the organisms. Mayonnaise and other dishes in which raw eggs are used may also transmit salmonellas.

Shellfish

Bivalve molluscs, e.g. mussels, oysters, and, to a lesser extent, gastropods e.g. cockles, whelks are grown commercially in river estuaries, many of which are chronically and heavily polluted with human sewage. Purification processes can reliably remove bacteria but viruses become fixed in their flesh where their concentration may reach five times that in the water from which they are derived. Decontamination procedures are often ineffective and raw or undercooked shellfish are frequently the source of viral gastro-enteritis outbreaks.

CLINICAL AND EPIDEMIOLOGICAL FEATURES

The great majority of notified cases are sporadic. Since most households carry several 'high risk' foods, and since most such food is used within a short time after purchase, it is not generally possible to trace with any certainty the foods responsible for these cases.

Outbreaks may occur within families, in institutions, particularly hospitals, or within the community, usually at functions such as receptions, weddings, barbeques and dinners. Sometimes clusters of cases, in which no connection in time or place is readily apparent, are linked only in that an organism of an unusual type has been isolated from diverse sources and imaginative and assiduous investigation may be needed to establish relationships.

Salmonellosis

Enteric fever
Though not generally considered as 'food poisoning' typhoid and paratyphoid can be transmitted from a patient or carrier to further patients on food or in water soiled by urine or faeces. The disease presents after an incubation period of 10 to 14 days with fever, malaise, anorexia, aches and pains and constipation. Diarrhoea is uncommon before the tenth day after onset. The organisms are hardy and the source, always a case or a carrier, may be remote from the vehicle of transmission. In the Aberdeen outbreak of 1963 the vehicle was corned beef which had been infected in the Argentine.

Outbreaks are rare in the UK but a number have been recorded from Europe, USA and Canada within the past 20 years in which such vehicles as water, shellfish and dairy products were implicated. Carriers in domestic situations with good hygiene seem to pose little risk. Proven cases, however, working in the commercial food industry, must undergo complex clearance procedures before returning to work. Details are provided in the Public Health Laboratory Service document (CDR Supplement 1, 1990) [1].

Non-typhoid salmonellosis

PRESENTATION AND COURSE The incubation period is between 12 and 48 hours extending sometimes to 72 hours. Onset is rapid with abdominal pain, diarrhoea and often vomiting in the early stages. The stool is liquid and commonly contains little or no blood or mucus. Spontaneous uncomplicated recovery over 5 to 7 days is the usual course, supportive treatment only being needed. In the very young, frail and elderly, significant dehydration can develop within a few hours and hospital treatment with intravenous fluids may be required. Rarely the organisms become invasive and a serious septicaemic illness ensues for which appropriate treatment must be given. Mortality in outbreaks is in the region of 1 to 4%, almost entirely in the particularly susceptible individuals mentioned above.

EPIDEMIOLOGY Transmission of salmonellosis follows two basic patterns. In the first, food or, more rarely, water contaminated with the organisms is the vehicle; in the second, the organism is passed from person to person by way of direct contact with infected excreta or indirectly through handling objects, e.g. clothes, bedding or toys, contaminated with infected excreta. In effect, spread is by the faecal-oral route. Cases can, therefore, occur in an outbreak initially through the consumption of an infected food, and subsequently further persons may be infected through contact with one of the original cases having themselves no connection with the original causative circumstances. The former are known as primary cases, the latter as secondary ones. The propensity for secondary cases to occur is a characteristic of salmonellosis and is not shared with other food poisoning bacteria, except on rare occasions.

Because of the wide distribution of salmonellas in animals and the environment, a great variety of food stuffs has been associated with outbreaks from the exotic, e.g. bean sprouts and peppercorns, to the more mundane, e.g. eggs. The organisms grow well in meats, milk, eggs and dairy products, and the majority of cases and outbreaks, where traced, ultimately lead back to one or other of these sources. Currently, poultry meat, eggs and egg products are of particular importance in the UK, and are responsible for the unprecedented rise in cases in the past few years (Fig. 17.2). Strains of *Salmonellae enteritidis* are the cause of a high proportion of cases and outbreaks in the present epidemic which extends to many countries throughout the world. Fresh milk, raw or imperfectly pasteurized, and dried milks are also responsible for numerous outbreaks while red meats, whole and processed as causes of salmonellosis are rather less common than they were. The way in which these foods become contaminated in the first place takes in modern systems of feeding of commercial animals, husbandry methods and the techniques employed in food processing from slaughter to distribution. Infection may be acquired directly by eating contaminated raw foods such as milk, or undercooked meats and poultry, or eggs or egg products in which temperatures reached in cooking are insufficient to destroy the organisms. Thus raw eggs used in home-made products such as mayonnaise, meringue and glaze are regularly shown to be the source of outbreaks, and the use of pasteurized liquid egg is recommended instead where possible. The Chief Medical Officer issued guidelines to the public advising on simple procedures to prevent egg-borne salmonellosis [6].

Other cases arise from contamination or recontamination of foods during home or institutional catering procedures and are caused by failure to observe basic food hygiene rules. Food incorrectly prepared may allow the survival of contaminating pathogens, and food incorrectly stored may allow proliferation of pathogens originally present in insignificant numbers. Contamination of food at source is, however, the initial event in any food-borne salmonella incident, and control of the initial contamination is as important as food hygiene is in the long term.

A further source of salmonellas is imported food and, in recent years, the organisms have been isolated from foods as various as frogs' legs, pasta, cuttlefish, pâté and herbal tea.

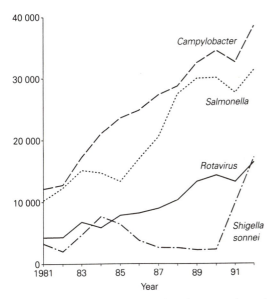

Fig. 17.2 Laboratory reports of major gastrointestinal pathogens: England and Wales 1981–92. (Source: Salmonella – LEP (formerly DEP), 1981–91; PHLS Salmonella Data Set, 1992. *Campylobacter*, *Shigella sonnei*, rotavirus – identifications from faeces reported by laboratories to CDSC.)

Uniquely, among patients with food-borne disease, those convalescent from salmonellosis may continue to excrete the organisms in faeces asymptomatically for substantial periods. Only about 50% of patients will have ceased to excrete the organism after 5 weeks and 90% by 9 weeks. This may pose problems with those involved in catering and food production.

Inasmuch as person-to-person spread is well recognized in salmonellosis, the significance of the commercial food handler excreter deserves consideration. A food handler is defined for this purpose as 'one who handles food which is either to be eaten raw or which is not to be further cooked before consumption' on the basis that adequate cooking will destroy any organisms allowed to contaminate food. No commercial food handler with diarrhoea should be permitted to handle any food at all. Clearance by serial stool examination after recovery and before returning to work is only necessary if salmonella organisms were recovered from the stool specimens in the acute phase. Persons in the food industry whose work falls outside the definition above need not be excluded from work after recovery provided they are known to practise good personal hygiene. It is, however, recognized that commercial food processing firms may not unreasonably choose to clear all food handlers as a means to encourage public confidence. Details of exclusions of personnel with salmonellosis and with other food-borne diseases are given in the PHLS (1990) [1] and WHO (1989) [7] documents. The introduction of quinolone antibiotics has provided the means for eradicating the organism in convalescent excreters.

The prospect of all food becoming free from salmonellas is remote. Because of their distribution, resistance to unfavourable environments, ability to grow in many foods at a wide range of temperatures, propensity to give rise to secondary cases and prolonged asymptomatic convalescent excretion, they are unique in the problems posed in investigation and both short and long term control.

Gamma irradiation of foodstuffs can eliminate pathogenic organisms including salmonellas from the high-risk foods. Problems still remain in the general acceptance of safety of such techniques in the perceptions of the public.

Illustrative outbreaks of salmonellosis
Outbreaks of food-borne salmonellosis generally present either as point source incidents, or extended common source incidents. In the former, most of the patients involved are infected at roughly the same time and usually at the same place or event, e.g. a wedding reception. In the latter, the organism may continue to infect people over a period of time, either because the vehicle of transmission is widely distributed both in time and place, or because it is not identified for weeks or months and cases present apparently sporadically rather than in epidemic form.

An example of the first type was an outbreak at a large psycho-geriatric hospital in which 358 patients and 50 staff developed salmonella gastroenteritis mostly over a period of 3–4 days. Nineteen patients died. Studies suggested that cold roast beef, probably contaminated while in a refrigerator, was the cause. Over 80% of the patients became ill within the usual limits of the incubation period, and the inference was that they were infected at the same meal. A small number of secondary cases occurred later.

In contrast, imported chocolate bars contaminated with *S. napoli* were distributed to many parts of the country, and cases were reported with no clear relationship either in time or place, until, careful epidemiology suggested the likely means of transmission. Similar outbreaks have occurred with processed sausage (*S. typhimurium*), with cochineal used to measure intestinal transit times in a hospital in the USA (*S. cubana*) and with contaminated baby foods in the UK (*S. ealing*). In all these incidents, the cases seemed to be sporadic and unrelated to each other, but continued to occur in spite of measures taken to prevent spread. The appearance of numbers of unusual strains however scattered they may be in distribution should raise suspicion that they may be related epidemiologically. Where common strains, e.g. *S. enteritidis*, are the cause of widespread infection, suspicion of relatedness can be slow to develop.

Campylobacter spp.

Presentation
The incubation period is between 3 and 7 days, rarely longer. Abdominal pain and cramps may be quite severe. Diarrhoea and vomiting is of acute onset, and lasts from 4 to 7 days without specific therapy. The stool frequently contains both blood and mucus. Arthritis occurs in 1 to 2% of cases, but invasive disease and other complications are rare. Erythromycin is effective in severe cases and will also reduce the duration of carriage.

Epidemiology
Though *Campylobacter spp.* can be found in the intestines of most animals, only in sheep do they cause any ill effect. Otherwise they behave as part of the normal flora. Transmission to man, however, occurs readily either through food or from contamination of the environment.

The infection in man is common world wide, and now accounts for more reported cases of gastro-enteritis than does salmonellosis (Fig. 17.2). All age groups in all climates are affected, though the incidence in temperate areas is seasonal with a rise in the numbers of cases in the summer months. As in salmonellosis, the sources of sporadic cases are usually impossible to define. Large outbreaks have been traced to the contamination of water or milk with animal excreta. An unusual form of contamination is the transfer of campylobacter from the beaks of birds, mainly magpies, to bottled milk left on the doorstep when they peck through the top to gain access to the contents. Undercooked or cross contaminated poultry is also a source, and is the only food regularly associated with the disease. In families, especially where there are young children, kittens and puppies with diarrhoea have been responsible. Secondary cases are, in contrast to salmonellosis, uncommon, although infants with liquid stools may disseminate the organism widely within a household. Carriage may occur over some weeks, but its significance is much less than in salmonellosis and exclusion of food handlers after clinical recovery is not needed, and neither is stool follow up necessary.

Illustrative outbreak
Three to 4 days after an extended family gathered for a reunion dinner cooked at the home of the matriarch, 7 of the 10 persons present developed severe abdominal cramps and diarrhoea. One child was admitted to hospital for observation with suspected appendicitis. *Campylobacter jejuni* was grown from all five stool samples submitted. Food history analysis suggested that turkey, which formed the major part of the main course, was responsible. Two of the three guests who did not become ill were vegetarian. No food from the meal was available for analysis, but a number of the patients had noticed that the meat near the bone was pink and seemed undercooked. The turkey had been cooked on the morning of the dinner after overnight thawing at room temperature. Campylobacters were isolated from other birds from the same farm as had supplied the

family. All strains were of the same biotype; serotyping was not done. Recovery took up to 9 days. In spite of there being close contact between cases and children, no secondary cases occurred.

The outbreak illustrates the severe clinical symptoms, the long incubation period and the lack of person-to-person spread characteristic of campylobacter infection. It is likely that the thawing time was insufficient and that parts of the turkey did not reach temperatures adequate to destroy the organisms.

Clostridium perfringens (welchii)

Presentation

After an incubation period of 12 to 24 hours, nausea and colicky abdominal pain is followed by diarrhoea and, less often, vomiting. The course is characteristically milder and shorter (1 to 2 days) than with salmonella or campylobacter infections, and complications rarely occur.

Epidemiology

This ubiquitous organism, which is found in human and animal excreta and in soil and dust, can readily contaminate food. Transmission through flies and other insects may also occur. The ability to cause disease, however, is dose dependent, and fairly exacting conditions for growth must be satisfied if the number of organisms sufficient to cause disease is to be reached. Cooked meats, both red and white, stews and gravies provide suitable anaerobic environments. Spores of the organism survive cooking heat, and unrefrigerated storage will provide optimum temperatures for germination of the spores at some stage during the slow period of cooling. Proliferation will occur with the subsequent production of the toxin. Toxin is only formed by actively sporulating organisms, and thus the temperature conditions allowing the spores to develop into vegetative forms are critical. The toxin is heat resistant and is not generally destroyed when the food is reheated.

Outbreaks are associated with relatively large catering concerns – where bulk cooking of sizeable cuts of meats will result in slower cooling than with the usual, much smaller, domestic sized joints and poultry. Classically, meat dishes are prepared well in advance, set out to cook for some hours or overnight at ambient temperatures, and then reheated for a short time before serving. Stock pots can provide excellent conditions for the sporulation of *Cl. perfringens* and should be discouraged. Cooling in a refrigerator will reduce temperatures sufficiently quickly so that the foods will pass rapidly enough through the critical range to prevent germination taking place.

Illustrative outbreak

Fifty-seven patients and 12 staff members from all 8 wards of a small, 200-bed mental institution developed diarrhoea over an 8 hour period. Preliminary enquiries suggested that all the patients had shared a meal at lunch time the previous day, about 12 hours before the onset of the first cases. Food histories strongly pointed to a chicken broth as the most likely source. *Cl. perfringens* type 71 was isolated from the faeces of 24 of the cases and the remnants of the broth. In the latter the same organisms were at present at a concentration of over 10^4 per ml. Enquiries into the food preparation revealed that the broth had been prepared the evening before, transferred to a number of large bowls and placed in a refrigerator overnight. In the morning, the bowls were noticed to be warmer than they should have been, and it was suspected that the refrigerator had not been working properly. The broth was put back into a vat, brought to the boil and served over the following 2 hours. The patients and staff all recovered within 3 days.

The failure to recognize that both the nature of the food and the conditions of storage provided near perfect conditions for clostridial sporulation and germination was the prime cause of this outbreak. Refrigeration temperatures should be checked and recorded at least daily, and the widely held notion that heating will render any food safe must be dispelled.

Staphylococcus aureus

Presentation

The onset is usually about 1 to 6 hours after ingestion of food containing enterotoxin, and may be dramatically severe, particularly when large numbers of people are involved in an outbreak. Abdominal pain, nausea and violent vomiting may cause rapid exhaustion, prostration and collapse. Diarrhoea may follow some hours later. Dehydration requiring intravenous fluid and electrolyte restoration is not uncommon. Recovery, however, generally follows quickly after the acute phase.

Epidemiology

Food is almost always contaminated through contact with a staphylococcal lesion on the skin of a food handler. The hand is most often the source, but other exposed parts such as the eye, ear and nose may be the infected sites. Some outbreaks in the USA have been attributed to nasal carriers without overt lesions, but such are thought to be very unusual as large concentrations of organisms, 10^6 per gram of food and 10^7 per ml of milk, are probably required to produce enough enterotoxin to cause symptoms.

Protein-rich foods provide particularly good conditions for growth of the organisms. Most frequently implicated are meats, sliced and processed, pies, cured hams and dairy products such as cream, mayonnaise, pastries and custards. Staphylococci can grow in the presence of high concentrations of salt and other food preservatives and, thus, in cured and pickled meats. Once inoculated, the bacteria multiply rapidly at ambient temperatures and within 2 to 6 hours, depending on temperature and initial contaminating 'dose', sufficient toxin is produced to initiate illness. The toxin is moderately heat stable and mild reheating or cooking, i.e. boiling for 30 minutes, may not render affected food safe.

The bovine strain of *Staph. aureus* phage type 42D may be found in raw milk from cows with mastitis and, before pasteurization was almost universally adopted, caused outbreaks from time to time. However, temperatures above 20 to 25°C

are necessary for growth and toxin production to occur.

Illustrative outbreak

Seventy-two out of 123 persons who attended a wedding reception fell ill with acute, persistent and severe vomiting between the time of the reception and when the evening's celebrations were due to begin. Many were temporarily prostrated, including the bride and groom, and a few elderly cases required hospital admission for parenteral treatment. The reception was held in a marquee on a very warm, dry day in mid-summer. The caterers prepared the food over the previous 24 hours and it was laid out in the tent at about 10 a.m. The buffet, which began at 3 p.m. consisted of meats, poultry, salads, mayonnaise, sweets with cream, salmon and pastries. Staphylococci of the same phage type were isolated from patients and from a number of the foods. Food analysis did not clearly implicate one food, but it was thought that the mayonnaise which had been used on many items may have been the major source. The catering establishment was found to be in breach of some basic food hygiene regulations, and one food handler had an eye infection from which the same phage type of staphylococcus was isolated. This person presumably transferred the organism from his eye to the food, which subsequently was kept at a high ambient temperature in the tent during which time bacterial proliferation and toxin production occurred. The two major errors were permitting an employee with an obviously infected lesion to handle food, and failure to recognize the hazard of leaving foods at high ambient temperatures for prolonged periods.

Viral food-borne disease

Presentation

The incubation period is between 12 and 48 hours and the disease presents as a mild gastroenteritis of sudden onset. Resolution is rapid, generally within 24 to 48 hours. Complications are rare but secondary cases occur frequently.

Epidemiology

Many, possibly most, cases of viral gastroenteritis, whether sporadic or epidemic, are of a person-to-person type and are of unknown origin without any demonstrable link to food.

Food-borne outbreaks, which are far less common, are particularly associated with sea-foods which are normally eaten raw, e.g. oysters, or are lightly cooked, e.g. mussels. The molluscs become contaminated during cultivation in sewage polluted waters, and depuration techniques, which can be relied upon to clear the shellfish of bacteria, are not yet shown to be reliable for viral clearance.

Outbreaks have been reported with other foods – salads and cold meats – which are not to be reheated before consumption. In some, food handlers have had an illness compatible with viral gastroenteritis at the time the food was prepared. There is evidence from a number of outbreaks that excretion of the virus may continue for some time after apparent clinical recovery in sufficient quantity to transmit the infection and convalescent catering staff should avoid handling raw or not to be reheated foods for 48 hours after symptoms have resolved.

The inability to confirm cases other than by electron microscopy, which requires very high concentrations of organisms in specimens, renders the study of outbreaks other than by epidemiological methods difficult. The viruses are no longer detectable in faecal specimens 24 to 48 hours after the onset of illness, and are not detectable yet in foodstuffs. It is anticipated that modern technology such as the use of DNA techniques will be applied to these problems in the foreseeable future.

Illustrative outbreak

A reception was held at a well-known institution to provide an opportunity for the producers of unusual and exotic foods to display their wares to invited guests representing a wide range of interests in the food trade and its regulation. The following day a number of the guests reported sudden attacks of vomiting and diarrhoea with mild abdominal pain. Investigations revealed that about 40 of the 200 persons attending had been

unwell. Electron microscopy of stool specimens of eight of the cases revealed small, round virus particles. Analysis of questionnaires completed by all those attending, whether ill or not, demonstrated a striking relationship between the eating of raw oysters and lightly cooked mussels, and the development of symptoms. The shellfish, which had been satisfactorily depurated of bacteria, had been grown in an estuary known to be heavily polluted with human sewage.

Bacillus cereus

Presentation

There are two clinical forms of the disease depending on which of two toxins is produced by the strain involved in the incident. One causes vomiting 1 to 6 hours after ingestion, and the other diarrhoea after 6 to 16 hours. Symptoms are generally short-lived and person-to-person spread does not occur.

Epidemiology

The organism is widely distributed in the environment and faecal carriage among the clinically normal population in one study was 14%. It is not surprising, therefore, that isolations have been made from many foods. Small numbers of organisms clearly are of no concern, and it is only under circumstances when spore germination can take place that sufficient organisms and toxins are produced to cause disease. The spores of different strains vary in their resistance to heat, but most will withstand boiling and quick frying.

Meat, vegetable and cereal dishes are most often implicated. The toxins are produced when contaminated food is kept warm over prolonged periods, but at temperatures insufficient to kill vegetative forms of the bacteria or to prevent the germination of the spore forms. Dishes where rice has been pre-cooked in quantity, and then kept at ambient temperature until being mildly reheated just before consumption, have been responsible for a number of outbreaks.

Cereal-based outbreaks are usually of the short incubation vomiting type, while the diarrhoeal syndrome is associated more often with other foods, but this is by no means always the case.

Illustrative case

Three groups of people complained to an environmental health department in the course of one evening that they had felt unwell and had moderately severe vomiting some 4 hours after eating takeaway chinese meals from one particular outlet. Though the main dishes varied considerably, all had had portions of fried rice. The rice had been prepared the previous day by boiling and allowed to cool overnight. When customers ordered fried rice, portions were dipped in simmering deep fat for about a minute and then placed in containers. *Bacillus cereus* was isolated from the uncooked rice in small quantities, and from the boiled rice and fried rice in large numbers. As in the case of *Cl. perfringens*, the *B. cereus*, which can grow either aerobically or anaerobically, was able to sporulate and germinate as the slow cooling process passed through optimal temperatures for these processes to occur.

Uncommon food-borne diseases

Escherichia coli

EPEC, EIEC and ETEC are particularly associated with infantile diarrhoea in developing countries, and with diarrhoea in travellers to countries with poor hygiene standards. Human carriers are the reservoir for the organisms, and sewage contamination of food and water is responsible for most cases. Outbreaks in developed countries caused by water pollution have been reported, but are rare events.

Infections associated with enterohaemorrhagic *E.coli* (EHEC, VTEC), most commonly *E.coli* 0157, are generally sporadic but clusters of cases and outbreaks are reported from time to time. Clinical presentation is of diarrhoea with heavily blood-stained stools and abdominal cramps. Between 5 and 10% of cases subsequently develop the haemolytic uraemic syndrome and renal failure may occur in a few patients. The incubation period is around 1–3 days and the very young

are the most frequently and severely affected. In the few recorded UK outbreaks beefburgers, yoghurt, turkey rolls and quiches, and polony and garlic sausages have been the likely vehicles of infection. Person-to-person spread is reported occasionally. Nearly 500 cases were recorded in 1992 – a significant increase over recent years – due in part to more widespread recognition and in part to technical diagnostic developments.

Illustrative outbreak

Over a 2 month period a cluster of over 20 cases of *E. coli* 0157 were identified in one region, 16 of which were all of one phage type. The onset of most of the latter cases clustered over a 2-week period. There was considerable geographical scatter but eight cases were from a single town. A food questionnaire was administered to all the cases and to 39 others in a case control study. A strong association with a locally produced yoghurt became apparent. Inspection of the production unit showed a basically good hygiene practice, but there were areas where cross-contamination of the milk might have occurred after pasteurization, though no direct microbiological evidence was obtained. Modifications were recommended and no further cases have occurred.

Clostridium botulinum

Presentation

A few cases may present with gastroenteritis. Most, however, show CNS involvement from the outset. Symptoms such as dizziness, double vision and inability to open the eyes fully, may progress alarmingly quickly to rapidly developing paralysis. The incubation period is 12 to 36 hours, but may be longer. Mortality varies from 15% to over 90%, in part depending on available facilities for treatment.

Epidemiology

The organism is extensively distributed in soil and mud and is, therefore, also found in animals and fish which tend to forage in or around water. In societies where raw fish or seal meats are allowed to ferment, the disease is relatively commoner because such conditions will encourage the growth and toxin production of *Cl. botulinum*. Elsewhere, home preservation by canning of many types of food and, in particular, vegetables, which are quite likely to be contaminated with spores, has been responsible for outbreaks. Boiling will not destroy the spores, though the use of a pressure cooker may enable lethal temperatures to be reached. The toxin is thermolabile, and is destroyed by cooking. Thus it is only food not subject to further heating just before consumption that constitutes a risk.

Botulism is rare in the UK – only 52 cases having been reported since the first in 1922. Twenty-seven cases were from a single outbreak in 1989 in which commercially produced hazelnut yoghurt was the vehicle of transmission. Other incidents were associated with duck, rabbit, hare, pigeon, nut brawn, meat pie, macaroni cheese and fish.

Illustrative outbreak

Four patients were admitted in quick succession to hospital with CNS symptoms suggestive of botulism. The diagnosis was rapidly confirmed by mouse inoculation. All had eaten tinned salmon from a single tin which had come from a canning factory in the north west of Canada. *Cl. botulinum* was isolated from the can opener and from the tin, and was shown to produce type E toxin, the same as that in the serum of the patients, two of whom died. Investigations showed a small defect in the can sealing which probably occurred at the factory, allowing access of the organism at a late stage in the processing.

Listeriosis

Presentation

As many cases present only a mild, 'flu'-like illness, it is likely that very few are diagnosed clinically, and that even fewer are confirmed bacteriologically. Severe disease is generally confined to the pregnant, the neonate and the immuno-compromised. Infection in pregnancy may result in abortion or in overwhelming sepsis with brain involvement in the foetus and newborn. Meningitis is the usual manifestation in the compromised. Since so many foods contain *Listeria monocytogenes*, the incubation period is difficult to estimate. Published figures vary from 1 to 70 days. Overall mortality is about 30% in the UK for severe disease.

Epidemiology

The disease, at least in its severe form, remains rare in this country. Outbreaks presenting as clusters of abortions or neonatal infection in North America and Switzerland were traced to contaminated coleslaw, milk and soft or Mexican cheeses. The only cluster of cases so far reported in the UK was epidemiologically associated with cream. *L. monocytogenes* is present in varying quantities in many foodstuffs with a particularly high incidence in chicken. soft cheeses and certain processed meats such as pâtés. However, the factors determining whether or not clinical disease will result from ingesting contaminated food remain obstinately obscure.

Yersinia enterocolitica

While most cases in the UK are probably acquired by the faecal-oral route and are not food-borne, in Scandinavia and other continental and transatlantic countries, epidemics with patterns suggesting food origin occur regularly. Ground or raw pork has been identified as an important source in Belgium, and in the USA large outbreaks involving milk or milk products have been recorded.

Vibrio parahaemolyticus

The majority of cases seen in this country have been acquired abroad, particularly in South East Asia and Japan. Cross-contamination between cooked and uncooked seafood or the use of sea water rinse have been responsible for a number of outbreaks. Imported, frozen, cooked shellfish, particularly prawns, are another fairly common source of infection. Sporadic cases of presumed local origin are occasionally seen. Other members of the *Vibrio* group of organisms, *Aeromonas spp.* and *Plesiomonas spp.* are also linked to seafood and water.

Shigellosis

The organisms (*Shigella*) are classically transmitted person to person by the faecal–oral route, and epidemics are associated with institutions where personal hygiene may be unreliable. In the past, outbreaks in which contaminated foods of many kinds were implicated, were commonplace, Nowadays, food-borne shigellosis is very rare in the UK.

THE PRINCIPLES OF INVESTIGATION AND CONTROL OF FOOD-BORNE DISEASES

Detailed consideration of the investigation, analysis and control of outbreaks of communicable diseases in general is presented in Chapter 18. This section provides a brief account of the application of the principles and practices described therein to food-borne disease.

Outbreaks may come to the attention of health authorities through a variety of sources. Notification as required by law may be received from one or more general practitioners or from hospital control of infection officers. Patients may present at accident and emergency departments. Complaints may be made directly to environmental health departments. Most outbreaks of food-borne disease declare themselves by virtue of the numbers involved over a short period of time among a well-defined group of people, e.g. coach party, wedding reception or works outing. However, in circumstances where the victims may be widely dispersed as in an outbreak caused by *S. ealing* in baby milk powder, where symptoms other than gastroenteritis prevail (botulism and listeriosis), or where other forms of transmission (person to person) might have occurred, only careful investigation will provide the basis for control.

The purpose of investigation is to stop any further spread of the outbreak as quickly as possible, and to provide information to prevent recurrences. To achieve this, the organism responsible must be identified, the food concerned defined and the means whereby contamination took place discovered. All persons who are ill and those at risk, but not ill, need to be identified, as do the contacts of these persons. The steps to be taken are, firstly, the collection of data and, secondly, the analysis of that data.

Recommendations on the investigation and control of food poisoning are issued by the Department of Health and the Welsh Office [8], the Scottish Home and Health Department [2] and the Departments of Health and Social Services in Northern Ireland [3].

Investigations

General
A history taken quickly from a number of the cases may reveal one or more possible sources common to them all. Investigations designed around a theory of the cause of an outbreak are often more fruitful than a wide approach with no clear target in mind. Unfortunately, this is not always possible.

Laboratory
Laboratory studies to determine the microbiological cause of the outbreak should be initiated at the same time as the epidemiological data are collected. Early identification of the organism responsible will influence the depth and extent of the investigation required.

Faecal samples
These should be obtained from the clinically ill, others exposed to the same possible sources and, if relevant, any food handlers involved. Suspect food should be submitted as soon as possible with proper documentation of its source, handling and storage.

Inspections
Where premises from which suspect food may have come are identified, inspection for the state

of hygiene of the kitchens and for the food handlings practices must be carried out. Environmental swabs may be taken to determine the extent and nature of any contamination of both fixed and movable fittings.

Epidemiology

In any outbreak in which there is uncertainty as to the source and/or the pattern of transmission, further investigations will need to be carried out. The purpose is to define:

1. the timing of the outbreak,
2. the place or geographical situation of persons affected at or around the time they were infected, and
3. certain personal characteristics of those involved.

This information should be obtained through questionnaires designed according to the principles given in Chapter 18.

Timing

By plotting the dates and time of the onset of symptoms against the numbers of cases, an epidemic curve can be constructed of the outbreak. The shape of such a curve will provide information as to the type of outbreak. A curve with a single high peak is characteristic of a point source outbreak, e.g. a company dinner party, when all cases are infected within a short time of each other (Fig. 17.3). A broad, lower curve suggests person-to-person spread (Fig. 17.4).

Place

Details of geographical locations of individuals at or around the times of the onset of symptoms may, in circumstances where there is no obvious occasion linking them, be useful. Apparently randomly distributed cases may be related by such things as delivery rounds, supplies of unusual foods, water sources, movement of personnel, or the attendance at particular institutions or functions.

Persons

Personal characteristics which may be relevant include age, sex, occupation, travel, medical

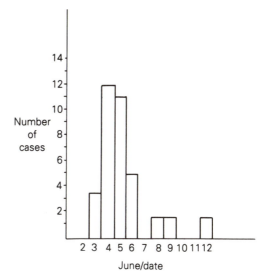

Fig. 17.3 Epidemic curve from a point source hospital outbreak caused by *Salmonella* bacteria in a chicken dish. Note the small number of secondary cases.

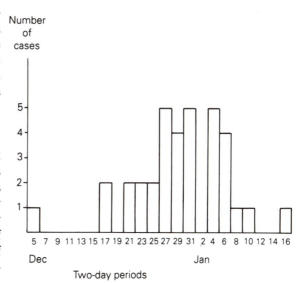

Source: CDSC.

Fig. 17.4 Epidemic curve from an extended common food source caused by commercially produced and widely distributed spiced sausage.

history, eating habits and relationships to other sufferers. The extent of food histories that are required will depend upon whether or not a particular occasion can, with reasonable confidence, be identified. Details of food eaten and not eaten from a defined menu can often be obtained without difficulty. It may be necessary, however, to ask patients to recall food eaten 3 or more days before becoming ill.

Analysis

On the basis of the information obtained it may be reasonably clear what the likely food source was. It is, however, only too easy to arrive at doubtful or even incorrect conclusions unless great care is taken in the assessment of the data. For example, asymptomatic food handlers are often found to be excreting the same organism as the victims of a food poisoning episode, and come under suspicion as the sources of the organism. This they rarely, if ever, are. Food handlers handle, and not infrequently nibble at, food they are dealing with and thus become victims themselves.

The two statistical methods used in the analysis of outbreak data are the case-control study and cohort study. Both essentially compare data from infected persons with that on uninfected persons (controls). The principles and applications of the methods are given in Chapter 19.

Control

Personnel
Patients with skin lesions or in the acute diarrhoeal phase of gastro-enteritis will be excreting large numbers of organisms and must be regarded as potentially infectious. Secondary spread is, however, unlikely with organisms other than *Salmonella* and to a lesser extent *Campylobacter*.

Patients involved in catering and food handling should be excluded from work during this phase. Patients with good personal hygiene need not be restricted after clinical recovery, and will only require clearance at follow up if involved in commercial food handling activities. Details of recommended exclusions for all food-borne infections which should be applied to patients, their contacts and food handlers are given in PHLS document (Supplement 1 CDR 1990) [1].

Food and food hygiene
Once suspect foods have been identified, the most appropriate action will depend upon the way in which contamination has taken place. Some foods, red and white meats in the raw state in particular, must be assumed to harbour pathogens. Where milk or tinned foods are suspect, failures in pasteurization or manufacturing may require investigation. Food which is adequately cooked and, if not eaten immediately, stored correctly, e.g. cooked and raw foods kept separately, at appropriate temperatures, is safe. Breaches in food hygiene standards may take many forms (Table 17.3) [9].

Veterinary aspects
Meat, poultry and other foods derived from animals may be contaminated with organisms known to cause food poisoning in man. Frequently, those organisms may neither cause any illness in the animal nor interfere with growth or weight gain. Thus those involved in the husbandry of domestic animals are more often than not unaware that any particular animal is carrying a pathogen. Moreover, so extensive is the contamination of the environment with both human and animal excreta that many vehicles from flies to feed are available whereby organisms can be transferred to and between animals. During the lairage, slaughter and processing of cattle and poultry, further opportunities for cross-contamination arise. Control at this level is clearly difficult and is the province largely of the Ministry of Agriculture, Fisheries and Food, and of the State Veterinary Service. The major problems have recently been reviewed [10]. At present, the major actions to control food-borne disease of animal origin must lie in handling practices at the level of the manufacturers, merchants and caterers.

Table 17.3 Factors contributing to 1479 outbreaks of food poisoning, England and Wales, 1970–82

Contributing factors	Number of outbreaks in which factors recorded (%)					
	Salmonella	C.perfringens	Staph.aureus	B.cereus	Other	Total
(i) Preparation too far in advance	240 (42)	464 (88)	80 (48)	54 (86)	6 (4)	844 (57)
(ii) Storage at ambient temperature	172 (30)	276 (53)	75 (45)	39 (62)	4 (3)	566 (38)
(iii) Inadequate cooling	125 (22)	313 (60)	12 (7)	17 (27)	1 (<1)	468 (30)
(iv) Inadequate reheating	76 (13)	275 (52)	5 (3)	33 (52)	2 (1)	391 (26)
(v) Contaminated processed food	100 (19)	19 (4)	27 (16)	4 (6)	86 (54)	246 (17)
(vi) Undercooking	139 (25)	74 (14)	2 (1)	1 (2)	7 (4)	223 (15)
(vii) Contaminated canned food	2 (<1)	4 (<1)	42 (25)	1 (2)	55 (35)	104 (7)
(viii) Inadequate thawing	61 (11)	34 (6)				95 (6)
(ix) Cross-contamination	84 (15)	8 (2)	2 (1)			94 (6)
(x) Raw food consumed	84 (15)		1 (<1)		8 (5)	93 (6)
(xi) Improper warm holding	15 (3)	52 (10)		8 (13)	2 (1)	77 (5)
(xii) Infected food handlers	13 (2)		50 (30)		2 (1)	65 (4)
(xiii) Use of leftovers	25 (4)	25 (5)	11 (7)	1 (2)		62 (4)
(xiv) Extra large quantities prepared	29 (5)	17 (3)	2 (1)			48 (3)
Total	566	525	166	63	159	1479

Source: Reproduced with the permission of Hodder and Stoughton Ltd and the author.

CONCLUSION

Clearly, the education of workers in the food industry provides the key to the prevention of almost all the common forms of food-borne disease. This view is endorsed by a publication of the WHO which emphasizes the role of management in this respect and presents a series of recommendations aimed at reducing the human factors in the causation of a common, but preventable, problem [7].

The reports of the Richmond Committee and the Steering Group and Advisory Committee for the Microbiological Safety of Food contain series of recommendations designed to ensure that the public can have confidence that food available to it in whatever form is, or can be, rendered safe by standard processing or catering procedures. The recommendations will form the framework upon which future legislation in this field will be developed.

REFERENCES

1. Public Health Laboratory Service (1990) *Notes on the Control of Human Sources of Gastro-intestinal Infections, Infestations and Bacterial Intoxications in the United Kingdom*, Communicable Disease Report, Supplement 1. (Undergoing revision 1995.)
2. Scottish Home and Health Department (1991) The Investigation and Control of Food Borne and Water Borne Diseases in Scotland, HMSO, Edinburgh. (Undergoing revision 1995.)
3. Department of Health and Social Services (1993) *Investigation and Control of Food Poisoning and Gastro-enteritis in the Community*, DHSS, Northern Ireland.
4. Report and Proceedings of an Inquiry of the Agriculture Committee of the House of Commons (Session 1988–9), *Salmonella in Eggs*, 108–1, 108–11, HMSO London.

5. Report of the Committee on the Microbiological Safety of Food (1990) *The Microbiological Safety of Food, Part 1 and Recommendations* Richmond, Report), HMSO, London.
6. Department of Health, Chief Medical Officer Report, Advice on Raw Eggs Consumption. Press Release 88/445.5 December 1988.
7. WHO (1989) *Health Surveillance and Management Procedures for Food Handling Personnel*, Technical Report Series 785, World Health Organization, Geneva.
8. Department of Health (1994) *Management of Outbreaks of Foodborne Illness. Guidance produced by a Department of Health Working Group*. HMSO, London.
9. Roberts, D. (1993) Factors contributing to outbreaks of food poisoning, in *Food Poisoning and Food Hygiene* (eds C.B. Hobbs and D. Roberts), 6th edn, Edward Arnold, London.
10. Johnson, A.M. (1990) Veterinary sources of food-borne illness. *Lancet*, **ii**, 856–8.

FURTHER READING

Consultants in Public Health Medicine (Communicable Disease and Environmental Health Working Group) Scottish Centre for Environmental Health (1994). Guidelines for bacteriological clearance following gastrointestinal infection. *Communicable Diseases (Scotland) Weekly Report*, **28**(26), 8–13.

Department of Health and Social Security (1986) *Report of the Committee of Inquiry into an Outbreak of Food Poisoning at Stanley Royd Hospital*, HMSO, London.

Hobbs, B.C. and Roberts, D. (1993) *Food Poisoning and Food Hygiene*, 6th edn, Edward Arnold, London.

Jacob, M. (1989) Safe food handling *A Training Guide for Managers of Food Service Establishments* World Health Organization, Geneva.

Palmer, S.R. (1989) Epidemiological methods in the investigation of acute bacterial infections, in *Medical Bacteriology, A Practical Approach*, (eds P.M. Hawkey and D.A. Lewis), IRL Press (OUP), Oxford, pp. 271–85.

Clinical Microbiology, Stokes, E.J., Ridgway, G.L. and Wren, M.W.D. (1993) 7th edn, Edward Arnold, London. (One of a number of texts providing detailed accounts of the biological and cultural characteristics of the organisms referred to in this chapter.)

18 Communicable disease control

Stephen R. Palmer

INTRODUCTION

Improvements in sanitation, housing, nutrition, and other social conditions of the British population over the last century have resulted in a dramatic decline in such epidemic diseases as cholera, typhoid, typhus, dysentery, tuberculosis and diphtheria. Medical advances in antibiotic therapy and vaccine production after the Second World War brought communicable disease further under control. Consequently, a body of opinion gained ground which saw communicable disease as a rapidly diminishing area of concern.

In the last 20 years or so, however, communicable diseases have re-emerged as a major public health issue [1]. The growth in international travel has brought significant problem from imported infections, such as typhoid and malaria, and the fear that newly discovered infections, such as Lassa fever, may become epidemic in the UK has led to the development of national policies for control. Discoveries of new diseases such as Legionnaires' disease have revealed new hazards from modern living conditions. Changes in the food industry with mass production and national and international distribution of foods have provided for widespread outbreaks of food-borne disease. Diseases such as hepatitis B and AIDS have highlighted the influence of personal behaviour and lifestyles on the risk of infection. The AIDS pandemic has ensured that communicable diseases now have a very high priority in public health. In addition to these factors, increased public awareness and expectations have ensured a high profile for infectious diseases in the political arena.

As the disease pattern has changed, so the need has grown for public health professionals to re-examine the methods of control appropriate to new circumstances. Modern public health now has to focus much more on national and international surveillance to identify and assess communicable disease problems and, increasingly, epidemiological methods are being applied to their investigation and control.

A communicable disease is the result of an interaction of an infecting agent, a host and environmental factors. Consequently, successful investigation of infectious disease incidents and their control depends upon understanding not only the microbiology of the organism, but also the environmental and host factors which result in exposure to the agent and the development of disease. The study of the interaction of these factors in a population is the basis of epidemiology, which may be defined as, 'the study of the distribution and determinants of disease in populations and its application to control'. Accurate laboratory diagnosis is usually a major factor in successful control, but epidemiological methods alone may be sufficient to introduce interim control measures. For example, the methods of spread of AIDS were identified by epidemiological methods 2 years before the infecting agent, human immunodeficiency virus (HIV), was discovered.

ORGANISMS THAT CAUSE DISEASE

Agents vary in their ability to cause disease (pathogenicity) and different strains of the same agent may cause more or less severe disease (virulence). Some agents cause disease only in certain animals. *Salmonella typhi* is a pathogen of man, whereas other agents can cause disease in several species, e.g. *Salmonella enteritidis*. The following is a classification of the infective agents.

Viruses

These consist of a single nucleic acid, RNA or DNA, surrounded by a protein envelope and measuring less than 300 nm. They cannot multiply outside of living cells.

Changes may take place in the molecular structure of the DNA or RNA during passage of the virus through a host to another, allowing it to by-pass the immunity which has been acquired by past exposure to the virus. A slow alteration in the make-up of the virus is called antigenic drift, and a sudden change is called antigenic shift. Hosts previously exposed to new strains have little or no acquired immunity, and large-scale epidemics can result.

Viruses can be identified by:

1. Electron microscopy (EM). This is used for pox viruses, e.g. chickenpox and orf, and for gastro-enteritis viruses, e.g. rotavirus and small round-structured viruses (Norwalk-like).
2. Culture. A virus may be grown from body fluids, skin, throat swabs, etc., on culture media such as cell cultures, in embryonated eggs, and in suckling mice. Most viruses can be cultured, although highly specialized techniques may be required and the yield is not usually good. Dangerous viruses should only be cultured in high containment reference laboratories.
3. Serology. Virus particles (antigens) may be detected by mixing the sample of blood or faeces (e.g. hepatitis B surface antigen in blood and the rotavirus in faeces) with antibodies against the virus. Alternatively, specific antibodies against the virus can be detected.

Following infection, the patient produces antibodies in the blood. Two blood samples are taken, the first as soon as possible after onset of illness, and the second after about 2 to 3 weeks. An increase in antibody level may be detected by a variety of techniques including complement fixation tests, immunofluorescence, radioimmunoassay, and enzyme-linked immunosorbent assays. These serological methods can be applied to population surveys for epidemiological purposes. Newer techniques are being developed in which saliva and urine are used instead of blood.

Bacteria

These are unicellular organisms without nuclei that are classified by shape (e.g. spherical cocci, cylindrical bacilli, helical spirochaetes) by their ability to stain with different chemicals, (e.g. Gram's staining (Gram-positive or Gram-negative bacteria); by culture characteristic, e.g. their dependence on O_2 for growth and their appearance on culture plates; by biochemical reactions (particularly their ability to ferment different sugars); and by antigenic structure. Some bacteria produce spores which resist heat and humidity, allowing the organism to survive for prolonged periods in the environment (e.g. *Bacillus anthracis*). Other organisms are delicate and survive for a very short time outside the body, e.g. gonococcus.

The differences between bacteria in growth requirements are used to culture selectively pathogens for diagnostic purposes. All bacteria require water for growth, but they differ in oxygen requirements. Some organisms, e.g. *Campylobacter*, require additional carbon dioxide. Most bacterial pathogens prefer a temperature of about 37°C for growth, but some will grow at refrigeration temperatures, e.g. *Yersinia* and *Listeria*, and this can be used to culture them selectively (cold enrichment). Differences in nutritional requirements of bacteria are used to make culture media, which suppress some organisms and encourage the growth of others.

Bacteria contain a single chromosome but may have additional genetic material within the cell (e.g. plasmids). Plasmids may contain genetic information coding for resistance to antibiotics. The pattern of plasmids within a bacteria can be used to type organisms. Mutation of genetic material takes place and strains with altered antibiotic resistance may emerge. These may be distinguished by their resistance pattern to a range of antibiotics.

Bacteria cause disease by two means: invasion of tissues and production of toxins. Toxins may be liberated outside of the bacteria (exotoxins), which can then circulate via the blood stream to cause tissue damage away from the site of infection (e.g. diphtheria). These toxins may be preformed in food (e.g. botulism). Toxins which are part of the structure of the bacteria (endotoxins) cause damage at the site of the infection or, when the cell dies, they can circulate around the body. Detection of toxins in blood or faeces is used to confirm certain infections, e.g. botulism.

Pathogenic bacteria may be detected by:

1. Microscopy. Light microscopy of body fluids, faeces etc., using staining techniques.
2. Culture. Bacteria may be cultured from tissues or the environment. The material is put onto plates of culture media containing nutrients, e.g. meat extract, blood or agar, and incubated at 37°C, usually for 24–48 hours.
3. Serology. As with viruses, antibody detection can sometimes be used to confirm infection, e.g. legionnaires' disease, but this is not useful for most enteric infections.

Chlamydias, *Coxiellae* and rickettsiae

These organisms, like viruses, will only multiply in living cells but are considered to be bacteria. They cause a variety of diseases. *Chlamydias* cause psittacosis and *Coxiellae* cause Q fever. Rickettsiae cause a wide range of serious illnesses, such as typhus and Rocky Mountain spotted fever, which are very rare in the UK.

Yeasts and fungi

These are forms of plant life which obtain energy by parasitism. They may live in the environment or they may be normal inhabitants of animals and man, in which case they cause disease only when the host defences are depleted, as in AIDS patients. Environmental fungi may be widespread such as *Aspergillus*, which can cause lung disease when inhaled by immunosuppressed patients; or have a limited geographical distribution and cause disease in unusual circumstances, like *Histoplasma*.

Dermatophytoses, such as athlete's foot, and nail infections are transmitted by direct and indirect person-to-person contact. Zoonotic fungi such as ringworm, are transmitted from animals to man by direct contact. Other fungi are not communicable from person to person. Diagnosis is by microscopy of lesions and sometimes culture.

Protozoa

These are single-celled nucleated organisms which may have complex life cycles involving sexual and asexual reproduction. Examples include organisms of the genera *Plasmodium* (which cause malaria), *Toxoplasma, Cryptosporidium* and *Giardia*. The latter three occur commonly in the UK.

Helminths

Tapeworms (cestodes), flukes (trematodes), and roundworms (nematodes) are all helminths (worms). They have complex life cycles which must be understood before the diseases they cause can be controlled. Most are rare causes of disease in the UK.

THE HOST

Host defences

The body has a general resistance to the invasion and multiplication of organisms. The skin and mucus membranes are natural barriers to infection, though allowing organisms to live as commensals in their surface without causing disease. The acidity of the stomach kills most organisms that are ingested. If an organism does penetrate these barriers, circulating cells called macrophages may attack and kill them.

In addition to this general protection, the immune system provides more specific defences. Foreign material such as the surface of an infecting organism is recognized by the immune system as 'foreign' (antigen). As a result, proteins called antibodies are produced by the cells of the immune system, which bind with the antigen to inactivate it and bring about its destruction. The first time the immune system meets a particular antigen, the response may be relatively inefficient. If the immune response overcomes the infection, bringing about recovery from the infection, the immune system remembers the encounter and the next occasion the antigen is encountered a more rapid response is mounted, which usually prevents the disease from developing at all. This explains why second bouts of measles or chickenpox do not occur. However, if the organism changes (like influenza) through antigenic drift (see above) it can evade the immune response and cause another episode of illness.

Host factors and disease

Certain factors may reduce immunity and place a person at greater risk of developing an infection. The elderly are at greater risk because of declining natural resistance and waning immunity; the very young are also at increased risk because of the immaturity of the immune system. Poor nutrition also increases susceptibility leading to, for example, a high mortality from measles in developing countries and a high tuberculosis rate in alcoholics and vagrants. Natural barriers may be compromised. Thus smokers are at greater risk of respiratory infections including legionnaires' disease; those taking anti-acid medication are at greater risk from gastro-intestinal pathogens.

THE ENVIRONMENT

Particular occupations may place workers at increased risk from certain diseases (e.g. psittacosis in poultry processors). Poor housing with overcrowding and lack of hygienic facilities increases the risk of disease such as tuberculosis and dysentery. Climatic conditions also influence the incidence of disease. Food poisoning is commoner in the summer, partly because many organisms multiply faster in food at higher ambient temperatures. Respiratory infection is commoner in the winter probably because of colder temperatures and more time spent indoors with poorer ventilation. Air pollution and smoking may increase susceptibility to respiratory infections. Disruption of populations because of war or famine or migration results in epidemics from poor sanitation, contamination of water supplies, increase in vermin and lack of personal hygiene.

BASIC CONCEPTS IN INFECTIOUS DISEASE EPIDEMIOLOGY

Reservoir of infection

This is where the agent normally lives and multiplies and where it depends mainly for survival. This may be man, e.g. chickenpox; animals, e.g. brucellosis; or the environment, e.g. tetanus. It is not necessarily the same as the source of infection in a particular incident.

Source of infections

Infection may arise from the organisms normally living in the person, or from another human being, an animal (zoonoses) or the environment. The source of an infection may sometimes be different from its reservoir. For example, in an outbreak of listeriosis in Canada in 1981, the reservoir of infection was a flock of sheep, from which manure was used as fertilizer on a cabbage field. Contaminated cabbages from the field were used to make coleslaw which became the source of infection for humans. When the source of infection is inanimate, e.g. food, water or fomites, it is termed the **vehicle** of infection.

Methods of spread

The routes by which an infectious agent passes from source to host can be classified as follows:

1. Food-, drink- or water-borne infection (e.g. typhoid and cholera). The term 'food poison-

ing' is often used of incidents of acute disease in which the agent has multiplied in the food vehicle before ingestion (e.g. salmonella food poisoning), and where it may have formed toxins, e.g. botulism. Other agents such as viral gastroenteritis agents may be carried on the food but do not multiply in it. This subject is dealt with fully in Chapter 17.

2. Direct or indirect contact. This includes spread from cases or carriers, animals or the environment to other persons who are 'contacts'. (A carrier is someone who is excreting the organism but who is not ill.) Within this category possible routes include:
   (a) faeces to hand to mouth spread (e.g. shigellosis);
   (b) sexual transmission (e.g. syphilis);
   (c) skin contact (e.g. wound infection and cutaneous anthrax).

3. Percutaneous infection. This includes:
   (a) insect-borne transmission via the bite of an infected insect, either directly from saliva (e.g. malaria), or indirectly from insect faeces contaminating the bite wound (e.g. typhus).
   (b) inoculation of contaminated blood or a blood product, either by transfusion, by sharing intravenous needles, by contaminated tattoo needles or acupuncture needles (e.g. hepatitis B).
   (c) the agent may pass directly through intact skin (e.g. schistosomiasis) or through broken skin (e.g. leptospirosis).

4. Air-borne: infectious organisms may be inhaled as:
   (a) droplets and droplet nuclei (e.g. tuberculosis);
   (b) aerosols (e.g. legionnaires' disease);
   (c) dust (e.g. ornithosis).

5. Mother to baby. Organisms may pass from the mother across the placenta to the baby before birth, e.g. rubella, or via blood at the time of birth (e.g. hepatitis B).

Occurrence

An infection which is always present in a population is said to be **endemic**. An increase in incidence above the endemic level is decribed as an **epidemic**, or **pandemic** when the epidemic is worldwide. Cases may be **sporadic** when they are not known to be linked to other cases, or clustered in **outbreaks** when two or more linked cases or infections occur, suggesting that there was a common source or there has been spread from person to person. Two commonly used measures of occurence of disease or infection are the **incidence** rate, the number of new cases occurring in a defined population over a specific time period expressed as a proportion of the total population, e.g. 10 cases per 100 000 persons per year; and **prevalence**, the proportion of a defined population with the disease at a point in time.

In infectious diseases propagated from person to person, e.g. measles, an epidemic occurs only when there is a sufficiently large proportion of the population which is susceptible to infection. The resistance of a population to the epidemic, because a sufficient proportion of the population is immune, is called **herd immunity**.

The **attack rate** during an outbreak is the proportion of the population at risk who were ill during the period of the outbreak. The **secondary attack rate** is the attack rate in the contacts of primary cases due to person-to-person spread.

Incubation period

This is the time from infection to the onset of symptoms. For each organism there is a characteristic range within which **the infecting dose** and the **portal of entry**, as well as other **host factors**, (e.g. age and other illness), give rise to individual variability. For example, in rabies the incubation period is shorter the closer the bite wound is to the head. The virus travels up the nerves to the brain and has less far to go the closer the bite to the head.

Communicability

The infectious agent may be present in the host and passed to others over a long period of time, **the period of communicability**. Some infections can be passed on even when the host is well. These people are then known as temporary or chronic **carriers** e.g. typhoid carriers. In some diseases, transmission from person to person occurs before symptoms develop. For example, a person with hepatitis A is most infectious to others just before they become ill.

Variables

Epidemiology involves measuring attributes or factors which vary in character or quantity. Some variables are fixed, i.e. they are either present or absent (e.g. sex, occupation and nationality), or they may be discrete (e.g. the number of people in a household); or they may be continuous, being possessed in different amounts (e.g. age, height and weight). Analysis of the distribution of fixed variables in a population will usually be by calculating the proportion of people who fall within certain categories, or the rates of occurrence of disease within sub-groups of the population (e.g. death rates by residence or occupational group). Analysis of continuous variables is more complicated since values obtained from a population will lie along a range, and these values are usually summarized by an average.

DETECTING PROBLEMS

The process of detecting trends in occurrence of disease and infection in a population and reporting information to those responsible for public health action is called **epidemiological** or **population surveillance**. Langmuir defines it as: 'the continued watchfulness over the distribution and trends of incidence through the systematic collection, consolidation and evaluation of morbidity and mortality reports and other relevant data' [2]. Epidemiological surveillance has become increasingly important in identifying outbreaks due to nationally and internationally distributed contaminated foodstuffs, and it may be the only way to detect outbreaks when the victims have travelled during the incubation period to many different destinations.

The stages of surveillance are:

1. systematic collection of data;
2. analysis of the data to produce statistics;
3. interpretation of the statistics to provide information;
4. distribution of this information to all those who require it so that action can be taken; and
5. continuing surveillance to evaluate the action.

Data may be collected especially for surveillance purposes (**active systems**) or use may be made of routine data (**passive systems**). Most active data collecting systems are based on a carefully designed standard case definition, such as the clinical reporting system set up in 1982 to monitor the AIDS epidemic. An internationally agreed case definition was essential if data from different countries were to be compared.

Passive data collection systems are usually based upon a microbiological or clinical diagnosis which is not precisely defined, and this may lead to problems of interpretation. For example, for the notifiable diseases a doctor only has to suspect the diagnosis in order to report a case. If all these were followed up, not all would be true cases. Nevertheless, such data are invaluable for monitoring trends and for detecting episodes or cases for further investigation.

The main sources of surveillance data for communicable diseases in the UK are outlined below. Possible weaknesses in the accuracy and completeness of the data should always be borne in mind.

Death certification and registration

Each week copies of death entries in the local death register for the preceding week are sent to the Office of Population Censuses and Surveys (OPCS) by all registrars in England and Wales. The underlying cause of death is coded in accordance with WHO manuals, and statistics are published weekly, monthly, quarterly and annually in varying detail.

Death certification and registration is virtually 100% complete, but errors in the data can occur at any stage from diagnosis through certification and coding, to processing and analysis. The death entry is a public document and this may sometimes deter the doctor from entering the correct diagnosis (e.g. in cases of syphilis and AIDS), although it is possible for the doctor to provide further information about the death which is not entered on the public record.

The present system depends upon identifying a single cause of death for analysis. This may be unrealistic, particularly in the elderly, and limits the usefulness of published statistics.

Infection contributing to death, but not considered to be the underlying cause of death (e.g. pneumonia complicating chronic bronchitis), will not be coded under the present routine system and, therefore, much important data on infectious diseases will not appear in published statistics. Furthermore, most infectious diseases in England and Wales do not result in death, so that in these cases mortality data are not useful in monitoring trends.

Mortality data are analysed weekly and published within 7 days of collection, and so can be used to identify increases in mortality rate quickly at the beginning of influenza epidemics.

Statutory notifications of infectious disease

The clinician making or suspecting the diagnosis is required to notify the proper office appointed by the local authority for the control of infectious disease who, in turn, sends a weekly return and these are published weekly in the OPCS Monitor. These data are corrected quarterly and analyses published quarterly and annually in the OPCS Infectious Disease Series. Similar systems operate in Scotland and Northern Ireland. The data are available quickly and are related to defined populations so that rates by age and sex can be calculated. For some diseases which are not often confirmed in the laboratory (e.g. measles and whooping cough) notifications provide an invaluable means of monitoring trends and are available over many decades. However, the clinical diagnosis may not always be correct, and most infections are considerably undernotified. (See also Chapter 16.)

Laboratory reporting and microbiological data

Laboratory reporting of infections forms the core of communicable disease surveillance in the UK.

Medical microbiologists report specified infections each week to the directors of the Communicable Disease Surveillance Centre (CDSC) and the Scottish Centre for Infection and Environmental Health (SCIEH) on specially designed forms or via new electronic reporting systems. These data are analysed and information provided within a week of receipt of the report in the weekly Communicable Disease Report (CDR) and SCIEH Report. Information is also made available via electronic systems such as EPINET.

The data are limited to infections in which there is a suitable laboratory test, and those which are easy to diagnose clinically are poorly covered. Not all microbiology laboratories report. However, the laboratory based data have proved invaluable in national and international surveillance of communicable diseases (Figs 18.1 and 18.2).

General practice reporting of clinical data

The Royal College of General Practitioners (RCGP) set up a clinical data collecting system in 1966 in a small number of volunteer practices. The data are published in the weekly OPCS Monitor. Similar systems exist in Wales, Scotland and the Oxford Region, and district based systems also have been established. The data cover diseases not usually needing hospital admissions or laboratory investigations, and can be related to a defined population. The GP surveillance data have been especially useful in influenza surveillance.

INVESTIGATING PROBLEMS

There are three complementary approaches, the epidemiological, microbiological and environmental measurement and inspection methods. In an outbreak of food poisoning, for example, the **microbiological approach** relies upon culturing the causative organism from food sources. The **environmental approach** would be to document how the food was prepared, identify faults in kitchen practices, and measure cooking and refrigeration temperatures. The additional need

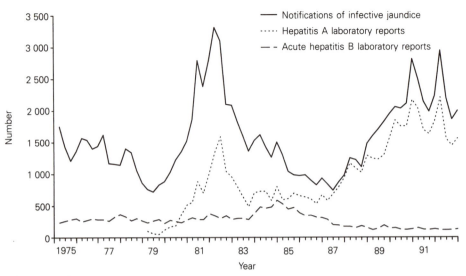

Fig. 18.1 Viral hepatitis, quarterly notifications and laboratory reports England and Wales 1975–92. (Source: OPCS, PHLS. Prepared by CDSC (data collected 31 December 1992.))

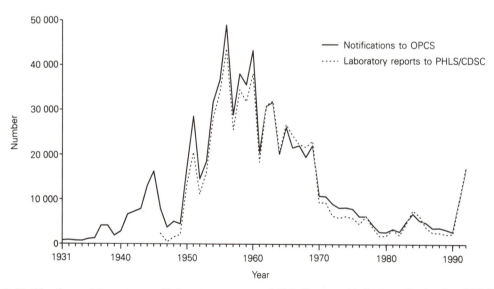

Fig. 18.2 Notifications of dysentery and laboratory reports of *Shigella sonnei* infection: England and Wales 1931–92. (Source: OPCS, PHLS. Prepared by CDSC.)

for the **epidemiological approach** is not always appreciated but can be shown as follows.

In an outbreak of salmonella food poisoning, the reservoir of infection may be commercially reared chickens, but utensils and surfaces may have been cross contaminated and bacteria transferred to other foods which, when eaten, become the source of infection. Isolation of the causative organism from food, or surfaces, cannot alone distinguish the order of events leading to the outbreak. Very often an outbreak investigation begins after all foods served have been consumed or discarded. Foods which remain may have been contaminated after the event. Sometimes the significance of the isolation of organisms from food is unknown, e.g. listeria from sandwiches bought in a shop, and only by showing an association between being ill and eating the food can the risk be clarified. The epidemiological approach looks for evidence of association between eating the food and illness.

Stages in the investigation of an outbreak

Preliminary enquiry
The purpose of the preliminary enquiry is to confirm the outbreak is genuine; confirm the diagnosis; agree a case definition; formulate ideas about the source and spread of the disease; start immediate control measures if necessary; and decide on the management of the incident.

Confirming the outbreak
An increase in the reported number of cases of a disease may be due to misinterpretation of data. There may be increased recognition of the disease because a new or more sensitive diagnostic technique has been introduced. If doctors have a special interest in a disease, it may lead to increased investigation and more frequent recognition of the disease in a locality. Occasionally, a laboratory error causes a 'pseudo-outbreak'.

Confirming the diagnosis and case definition
The clinical diagnosis is usually established by a study of the case histories of a few affected persons. Laboratory tests are essential to confirm the diagnosis in most infections, but epidemiological investigation should begin immediately and should not usually await laboratory results. A clear case definition is essential for case searching to be carried out. This case definition should be agreed by all involved in the investigation and used consistently throughout the investigation by all investigators; this is especially important in a previously unrecognized disease, or one in which there are no satisfactory confirmatory laboratory tests.

Tentative hypothesis and immediate control
The preliminary enquiry should include detailed interviews with a few affected persons, so that common features may be identified, such as an attendance at a function. Symptoms, dates of onset and possible exposures should be documented. Ideas can then be developed about the source and spread of infection, and a questionnaire designed to test these hypotheses in subsequent analytical studies. However, it may be necessary to take immediate control measures before confirmation so that further cases may be prevented. When a common vehicle or source of infection is suspected, appropriate action should be taken to interrupt the spread and control the source.

Management of an incident
If the preliminary enquiry confirms that the incident is real, a decision should be taken on its management. Small outbreaks will usually be managed informally. In serious outbreaks, an outbreak control team should be set up. This should include in addition to the environmental health officer, the consultant for communicable disease control, the local microbiologist, a Public Health Laboratory Service consultant microbiologist and a consultant epidemiologist possibly from the CDSC or SCIEH. The control team may require an administrator or non-medical epidemiologist to manage an 'incident room' where information on the outbreak should be collated and made available to those who require it. Each local authority must have an incident management plan which details the responsibilities and duties of each member of the team (see Chapter 16).

Identification of cases, collection and analysis of data
The cases first reported in an outbreak are usually only a small proportion of all the cases and may not be representative. Focusing only on these cases can be misleading. The exposed population should be identified so that thorough case finding can be carried out.

School or hotel registers, lists of institutional residents, pay-rolls and other occupational records and lists of persons attending functions associated with the disease are useful ways of identifying cases.

The aim of the enquiry will be to collect data from those affected, and those who were at risk but were not affected. The data routinely sought from cases include name, date of birth or age, sex, address, occupation, recent travel, immunization history, date of onset of symptoms, description of the illness and the names and addresses of the medical attendants. Other details will depend on the nature of the infection and possible methods of spread.

To ensure accurate and comparable records of all persons included in the enquiry and to help analysis, the data should be collected on a carefully designed standard form or questionnaire. Administration of the questionnaire will often be by face-to-face interview by a single investigator or group of investigators trained to administer the questionnaire. Interview by telephone may be useful in obtaining data quickly. When numbers are large and the enquiry is straightforward, a self-administered postal questionnaire is cheaper and quicker to administer, but the response rate and accuracy may be worse. Errors in recall can be reduced by providing background details of events, and making use of other sources to check data such as diaries, menus, discussion with relatives, etc.

The data from the cases should be analysed by time, place and person to determine the mode of spread, source of infection and persons who may have been exposed.

Time

The time of importance is the time of onset of the disease, since from this and a knowledge of the incubation period of the infection, the period of possible exposure can be determined. These data are presented graphically, usually in the form of a histogram (Fig. 18.3). In point-source outbreaks, all cases are exposed at a given time, and the onsets of symptoms of all primary cases cluster within the range of the incubation period. An epidemic which extends beyond a single incubation period range suggests either a continuing or recurring source of infection, or the possibility of secondary transmission. In outbreaks spread from person to person, cases will be spread over a longer period with peaks at intervals of the incubation period.

Place

Addresses of cases should be plotted on a map to show the geographical spread of the outbreak. Cases which do not follow the general time or geographic distribution may provide valuable evidence of the source of infection.

Cases clustering in a particular place of work or neighbourhood may indicate the existence of a point source of infection or of person-to-person spread.

Testing hypotheses

The data analysed so far may indicate that most cases ate a particular food or worked near a particular cooling tower. Great care, however, should be taken when interpreting such data. It is almost always necessary to have a control group to find out if, say, all the population are fond of a particular food or visit premises near the cooling tower. This is where analytical epidemiology is necessary [3].

Cohort and case control studies

The analytical cohort study attempts to investigate causes of disease by using a natural experiment in which only a proportion of a population are exposed to a factor such as a food, and compares attack rates in exposed and unexposed. For example, when investigating a food poisoning outbreak in an institution or hotel, it is usually possible to identify retrospectively all those exposed and to calculate attack rates in people who did and did not eat particular foods.

A case control study approaches the question from the opposite direction and begins by identifying people with and without the infection, and then tries to identify factors associated with disease. A group of cases is compared with a group of people who were not ill but had equal access to the likely source of infection. Controls can be taken from electoral registers, hospital admis-

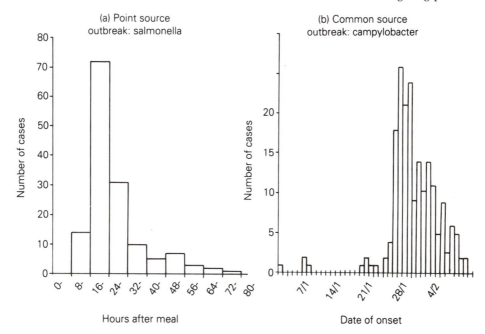

Fig. 18.3 Epidemic curves of two outbreaks. (a) An outbreak of salmonella food poisoning in people eating a buffet meal. Almost all cases occurred within the usual range of the incubation period (8–72 hours). (b) A community outbreak of campylobacter from raw milk. The contaminated milk was delivered over a period of several days so that the dates of onset cover a period greater than the incubation period for campylobacter (2–10 days); a diminishing level of contamination of milk during the week was likely.

sions lists, the telephone directory, GP age/sex registers, hotel and reception guest lists, family members of cases, neighbours of cases, acquaintances nominated by cases, and persons investigated by the laboratory but who were negative for the disease in question. The statistical power of the study can be increased by increasing the number of controls per case.

There are many possible pitfalls in conducting analytical studies and careful design is essential to minimize bias. An important possible bias may arise from the loss of cases or controls from the study because of refusal to be interviewed or failure to trace patients. Patients' recall may be biased by their own preconceptions or by press and media speculations. Cases will often have been interviewed on many occasions before an analytical study is carried out, and this may have introduced bias from suggestions made by interviewers, as well as prompting a more detailed recall. Bias may result from the interviewer knowing the disease status of the person and

Table 18.1 Contingency table

	Ill	*Well*	*Total*
Exposed	a	b	a+b
Not exposed	c	d	c+d
Total	a+c	b+d	a+b+c+d

having his or her own suspicion or prejudice about the source.

Incomplete histories may be taken in which, for example, the patient with salmonella poisoning is only asked in detail about one food. Training and experience in the technique of interviewing, and use of a structured questionnaire are safeguards.

In both cohort and case control studies, the basic analysis is by a comparison of proportions. The date can be presented in a contingency table as follows (Table 18.1):

In cohort studies, the ratio of a to a+b is the attack rate in exposed. The ratio (a to a+b) to (c to c+d), the ratio of the attack rates in exposed

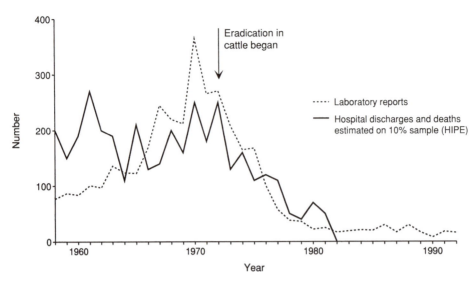

Fig. 18.4 Human brucellosis in England and Wales 1958–92. (Source: OPCS, PHLS. Prepared by CDSC.)

and unexposed, is called the **relative risk**. The size of the relative risk is an indication of the causative role of the factor concerned. In case control studies, the ratio a to a+b is not meaningful, since b is usually an unknown fraction of the total well population who were exposed. However, a statistic called the odds ratio or cross product ratio, ad to bc, approximates to the relative risk.

CONTROL

Control measures may be directed towards the source, the method of spread, or the persons at risk, or a combination of these.

Control of source

Some infections which are spread from a human source can be controlled by putting the case or carrier in isolation (e.g. diphtheria and typhoid fever). When animals are the source of an infection, it is sometimes possible to control an outbreak by eradication (e.g. rodent control for leptospirosis). Rabies may be controlled by the destruction of rabid animals and wild or stray animals, and by the muzzling of domestic dogs.

Outbreaks of food-borne zoonoses are usually controlled by removing the vehicle of infection. Eradication has played a major part in the long-term control of these zoonoses, for example, bovine tuberculosis and brucellosis (Fig. 18.4).

Environmental sources for diseases like legionnaires' disease (water cooling systems of air-conditioning plants, domestic hot water systems in large buildings or whirlpool spas) may be controlled by cleansing and disinfection. Other pathogens, which contaminate worksurfaces, utensils and equipment in kitchens, and clothing can also be controlled by the cleansing, disinfection or sterilization of these environmental sources.

Sterilization is defined as a process used to render an object free from viable microorganisms, including bacterial spores and viruses. **Disinfection** is a process which reduces the number of viable microorganisms but does not necessarily inactivate some viruses and bacterial spores.

Steam sterilization
Steam under pressure can be heated above 100°C and direct contact will kill vegetative microorganisms and their heat-resistant spores and viruses. The temperature and contact time must be precisely controlled for guaranteed results.

Hot-air sterilization

Dry heat at 160°C for 2 hours, 170°C for 1 hour or 180°C for 30 minutes will kill all microorganisms. Hot-air ovens are used for materials which will not damage at high temperatures.

Ethylene oxide sterilization

This will kill most bacteria, spores and viruses, and is usually used at sub-atmospheric pressures with an inert diluent gas. It is toxic, potentially carcinogenic and flammable. It is used for heat sensitive equipment.

Low-temperature steam and formaldehyde

This combination of dry saturated steam and formaldehyde kills vegetative bacteria, spores and most viruses.

Objects are exposed to dry saturated steam at 73°C at sub-atmospheric pressure into which formaldehyde is introduced. It is used for items not damaged by this process but unsuitable for steam or dry heat sterilization.

Sterilization by irradiation

Irradiation by gamma rays or accelerated electrons in excess of 25k Gray (Gy) provides adequate sterility. This method is used widely for single-use medical devices.

Low-temperature steam disinfection

This is a disinfection or pasteurization process which kills most vegetative micro-organisms and viruses. The process usually involves exposure to dry saturated steam at 73°C for more than 10 minutes at below atmospheric pressures.

Disinfection with washers

Washer disinfectors use physical cleaning and heat to disinfect contaminated re-usable items. Items have to be able to withstand wet heat at 80°C.

Decontamination by manual cleaning

Physical removal of contamination itself is important. It reduces the initial load for disinfection and is a necessary preparatory step before sterilization or disinfection is carried out.

Chemical disinfection

There must be good contact between the item and the disinfectant for a pre-determined minimum time period. The precise choice of disinfectant will be determined by the particular task at hand.

Boiling water disinfection

Water at 100°C for more than 5 minutes will kill most micro-organisms. Items have to be cleansed before immersion. This is a commonly used method for disinfecting small items of medical equipment.

Disposal by incineration

This is applicable to all micro-organisms where temperatures are in excess of 850°C, or 1000°C if cytotoxic drugs are in the waste stream.

Control of spread of infection

Disease spread by food, milk and water is prevented by the withdrawal or treatment of the contaminated product. Diseases spread by direct contact may be controlled by avoiding contact. Those spread by indirect contact may be prevented by hand washing. Spread by the faecal–oral route, e.g. dysentery, is prevented by hand-washing and the disinfection of surfaces in lavatories.

Diseases due to insect bites, such as malaria, typhus and yellow fever, are controlled by vector destruction, protective clothing and insect repellents. Hepatitis B and HIV infections, which can be spread by blood, are controlled by preventing accidental inoculation and the contamination of broken skin or mucous membranes by infected blood or tissue fluids. The spread of air-borne infections may be limited by ventilation in buildings. In special circumstances, physical isolation of infectious cases (e.g. Lassa fever) is required, and highly susceptible people, e.g. children with leukaemia, may be placed in protected isolation.

Control of persons at risk

Some diseases can be controlled by immunization or by giving antibiotics to persons at risk. Human immunoglobulins are commonly used for passive protection (e.g. when immunoglobulin is given to travellers to prevent hepatitis A). Rabies immunoglobulin and vaccine is given to people following the bite of a rabid, or possibly rabid animal. Antibiotics are given to contacts of cases of meningococcal infection to eradicate carriage of the organism in the nose and throat of contacts, thereby preventing them passing on the infection to others.

THE CONTROL OF IMPORTANT DISEASES IN THE UK

Acute poliomyelitis

Polio occurs worldwide, especially in children in developing countries. The virus infection is often asymptomatic, but it can cause paralysis and death or permanent disability. The virus enters the body orally, and invades the central nervous system. Diagnosis is by clinical presentation and isolation of the polio virus from faeces.

Source and spread
Man is the reservoir and the virus is present in pharyngeal secretions and is excreted in faeces. Transmission occurs by faecal–oral spread and by direct contact.

Incubation period
3–5 days.

Control
Routine immunization of all infants. Cases should be nursed with enteric precautions. Contacts should be immunized. Outbreaks can be controlled by emergency mass vaccination. Travellers to endemic areas should be immunized.

Acute encephalitis

Infection of the brain can be caused by several organisms, the commonest being viruses such as mumps. The incubation period varies with the

agent. Specific treatment may be available for certain agents.

AIDS

AIDS is the result of infection with HIV, which attacks the body's white blood cells thereby reducing resistance to other infectious agents. The pandemic of AIDS began in the 1970s, and almost all countries of the world have cases. The highest incidence at present is in Central Africa and North America. Cases present with a variety of unusual opportunist infections. Diagnosis is based on fulfilling strict clinical/microbiological criteria. At present, there is no curative treatment and most cases die within 3 years of diagnosis of AIDS.

Source and spread

The origin of HIV is uncertain, but man is the reservoir, and the virus is present in blood and body fluids. Transmission occurs by sharing blood and body fluids in three main ways:

1. anal and vaginal sexual intercourse;
2. perinatal transmission from mother to baby;
3. blood transfusions, blood products such as factor VIII, and re-use of contaminated needles by intravenous drug users.

Health workers exposed to inoculation accidents with blood have contracted HIV infection, but no risk from intimate, but non-sexual, contact has been shown.

Incubation period

Several months to many years. A median of 10 years has been suggested.

Control

All blood donations must be tested for HIV antibodies and contaminated blood removed. Only sterile needles should be used. IV drug users should not share needles. Health education should alert people to the risks from unprotected sexual intercourse with multiple partners and sharing needles, and to the lack of risk from casual contact. Confidential HIV counselling and testing should be promoted.

Treatment of other sexually transmitted infections may reduce risk.

Anthrax

An acute bacterial infection of humans and animals caused by *Bacillus anthracis*, which may be fatal. Infection is usually of the skin with an ulcer and scab formed. It may be followed within a few days by septicaemia and meningitis.

The disease is enzootic in certain African and Asian countries, but is very rare in the UK. It is an occupational hazard of persons such as wool-sorters, fellmongers, knackermen, farm workers and veterinarians in contact with infected animals or their products, e.g. blood, wool, hides and bones. Diagnosis is by culture of wounds, and treatment is with penicillin.

Source and spread
All domestic, zoo and wild animals are potentially at risk of infection. Anthrax bacilli are released from infected carcasses and form resistant spores on exposure to air. These spores contaminate soil for many years. Humans are usually infected by inoculation into cuts and abrasions from direct contact with infected animals, carcasses or animal products and contaminated soil. Inhalation or ingestion of spores may occur. Animals are infected from contaminated feed, forage, water or carcasses.

Incubation period
3–10 days.

Control
Prohibit contact with infected animals and their products. Establish environmental and personal hygiene, e.g. ventilation and protective clothing, where a special risk exists. Disinfect imports of hairs and wool. Vaccination may protect those occupationally exposed to risk. Carcasses suspected of infection should not be opened, but should be disposed of safely.

Campylobacteriosis

This occurs worldwide and is the commonest diagnosed diarrhoeal disease in the UK. It is usually caused by *Campylobacter jejuni*. Diagnosis is by isolation of the organism from faeces. Treatment is usually confined to fluid replacement.

Source and spread
There is widespread intestinal carriage in most mammals and birds. Poultry and cattle are the main reservoirs for human infection, which may be acquired by ingesting contaminated raw milk, undercooked chicken or other food contaminated in the kitchen. Direct faecal–oral spread from animals may occur, especially from puppies and, exceptionally, there is person-to-person spread. Large water-borne outbreaks have occured.

Milk from bottles pecked by magpies has been shown to cause a significant number of cases in the UK.

Incubation period
1–10 days.

Control
Pasteurize milk, chlorinate drinking water supplies, thoroughly cook meat (especially poultry), and practice good kitchen hygiene, protect doorstep-delivered milk from bird attack.

Cholera

A bacterial infection endemic in many developing countries with recent epidemics in South America. It may cause epidemics of profuse watery diarrhoea particularly among refugees and people living in overcrowded and poor sanitary conditions. Diagnosis is by faecal culture. Death due to dehydration occurs, but can be prevented by prompt fluid replacement.

Source and spread
Man is the reservoir and transmission occurs when water and food contaminated by infected faeces is consumed. Sewage contamination of

water supplies causes epidemic disease. Outbreaks due to raw or undercooked seafood have occurred.

Incubation period
A few hours to 5 days.

Control
The separation of water supply from sewage disposal effectively eradicates the disease. Infected persons should not handle food. Unchlorinated drinking water should be boiled.

Cryptosporidiosis

A recently recognized, but common, protozoal cause of gastro-enteritis, especially in children worldwide. It can cause life-threatening disease in immunosuppressed patients. Diagnosis is by identification of oocysts in faeces under light microscopy. There is no specific therapy.

Source and spread
Cryptosporidia have been identified in the faeces of most animal species. Human infection results from person-to-person faecal–oral spread, especially in children, and from raw milk or direct contact with farm animals, especially calves. Water-borne outbreaks have been reported.

Incubation period
1–10 days.

Control
Ensure personal hygiene. Pasteurize milk and ensure adequate filtration of drinking water and maintenance of swimming pools.

Diphtheria

Caused by the bacterium *Corynebacterium diphtheriae*, which produces a toxin leading to sloughing of epithelial tissue in the throat and the formation of a membrane, sometimes with cardiac and nerve involvement. The fatality rate is high if not treated early. Mass immunization has made this a rare disease in temperate climates where it was once common. In tropical countries, skin and wound infections are more common. Diagnosis is by culture of the organism from the throat or nose or wound swabs. Treatment is with antibiotics and, possibly, specific antitoxin.

Source and spread
Man is the reservoir, and transmission occurs via droplets and nasal and skin discharges to close contacts of cases or carriers. Rarely transmission occurs via contaminated food such as milk.

Incubation period
2–5 days.

Control
Routine immunization of all infants. Isolate infected cases. Search for carriers in close contacts and eradicate carriage with antibiotics. Contacts should be quarantined, put under daily surveillance for a week and given antibiotics if not previously immunized. All previously immunized contacts should be given a booster dose.

Escherichia coli – enterohaemorrhagic strains

This is a newly recognized (1982) cause of bloody diarrhoea (haemorrhagic colitis) and kidney disease (haemolytic uraemic syndrome) which has a significant mortality. It is caused by strains of *E. coli* which produce verocytotoxin (VTEC strains) most commonly in the 0157 group. Diagnosis is by isolation of the organism from faeces. The value of antibiotic treatment is unclear.

Source and spread
Cattle are the probable reservoir. Food-borne outbreaks particularly associated with undercooked hamburgers, and raw milk have occurred. Person-to-person faecal–oral spread, especially in nurseries has been documented. Water-borne outbreaks have been reported.

Incubation period
12–60 hours.

Control
Thorough cooking of raw meat, pasteurize milk, chlorinate water supplies, good kitchen and personal hygiene.

Giardiasis

This is a common cause of diarrhoea due to infection with the protozoa *Giardia lamblia*. Symptoms tend to be prolonged or intermittent abdominal pain, and loose stools. Diagnosis is by identification of the organism in faeces by light microscopy. Treatment is with metronidazole.

Source and spread
Man is the usual reservoir, with person-to-person faecal–oral spread, especially between young children in nurseries. Zoonotic infection in North America is relatively common with beaver and muskrats contaminating water supplies.

Incubation period
5–25 days

Control
Good personal hygiene. Exclude children with diarrhoea from nursery or school. Filter and chlorinate water supplies.

Legionnaires' disease (see also Chapter 27)

A relatively uncommon form of pneumonia caused by the bacterium *Legionella pneumophila*, which has a fatality rate of about 20 per cent. The immunosuppressed, aged, heavy smokers and those with pre-existing heart and lung disease are at greatest risk. Point source outbreaks associated with hotels and hospitals are reported. Diagnosis is by isolation of the organism from sputum or biopsy, and by serological identification of antibodies. Treatment is with antibiotics.

Source and spread
Legionella are free living organisms which are ubiquitous in standing waters and soil, and colonize plumbing systems, cooling towers, etc.

Most environmental isolations are not related to cases of infection. Human infection occurs when aerosols of contaminated water are created and inhaled. The risk of infection will depend upon the dose of the organism present in the aerosol, and the susceptibility of the person exposed. Aerosols can be created by air conditioning cooling towers, domestic showers and taps. Person-to-person spread does not occur.

Incubation period
2–10 days.

Control
Domestic water should be routinely chlorinated. All buildings with wet cooling tower systems should be identified, and cooling towers regularly cleaned and disinfected. Where possible, dry cooling systems should replace them. Domestic water supplies should be maintained at a temperature for hot water of more than 50°C and for cold water of less than 20°C. In an outbreak, higher temperatures and hyperchlorination may be necessary to render water systems safe.

Leprosy

A chronic bacterial infection caused by *Mycobacterium leprae*, which causes skin and nerve damage, and may lead to traumatic injury and deformation. Several forms are recognized, some of which may heal spontaneously. It is still common in the tropics and sub-tropics. Diagnosis is by clinical presentation and identification of the organism in skin scraping or biopsy material. Treatment is with long-term antibiotics. Physiotherapy and surgery may help deformities.

Source and spread
Man is the reservoir. Transmission does not occur very readily, and usually only in household settings, probably from contact with nasal discharges.

Incubation period
Several years.

Control

Early identification and treatment of cases. Infectious cases should be isolated until treatment established. Examine all household contacts. Treatment may need to be given to children in the household to prevent illness.

Leptospirosis

A sporadic bacterial disease of varying severity transmitted by contact with infected animal urine. The causative agent is the spirochaete *Leptospira*, with over 170 serotypes. It occurs worldwide, with areas in which host-adapted serotypes predominate, e.g. *L. hardjo* in cattle in the UK. Weil's disease, a particularly severe form with liver and kidney involvement, is caused by infection with *L. icterohaemorrhagiae*. Diagnosis is by serology. Treatment is with antibiotics.

Source and spread

Most animal species may be hosts of leptospires, but the main natural reservoirs for human infection vary with the serotype: *L. canicola* in dogs, *L. hardjo* in cattle and *L. icterohaemorrhagiae* in rats. Leptospires are excreted in urine which contaminates the environment, especially watercourses. Humans are infected by direct contact with the animal or contaminated environment, and leptospires enter the body through abrasions, wounds or mucous membranes. Person-to-person spread does not occur.

Incubation period

3–20 days.

Control

Control rodents. Avoid swimming in, or drinking from contaminated waters. Protective clothing is needed for workers at special risk.

Listeriosis

A relatively uncommon, but increasingly recognized, bacterial disease in humans caused by *Listeria monocytogenes*. It occurs worldwide.

Cases are almost exclusively in pregnant women, neonates, immunosuppressed patients and the elderly. It can cause fatal meningoencephalitis and abortion. Diagnosis is by culture of the organism. Treatment is with antibiotics.

Source and spread

The agent is widely distributed in animals, birds, humans and soil. The main reservoir for human infection is not clear. The organism is excreted in animals faeces. Outbreaks of food- and milk-borne infection have occurred in humans. Soft cheeses and paté have been identified as high-risk foods. Listeria grow slowly at normal refrigeration temperatures. Cross-infection in hospitals has been reported.

Incubation period

Uncertain, but probably a few days.

Control

Ensure good personal hygiene and care in the storage and preparation of food. Heat-treat dairy products. Ensure safe handling of infected animals, and avoid contact with possibly infected materials during pregnancy.

Lyme disease

This infection, with the spirochaete *Borrelia burgdorferi*, causes a characteristic skin rash, erythema migrans, followed by variable cardiac, nerve and joint manifestations. In certain parts of North America and in Scandinavia, it appears to be a common disease, but it is still rare in the UK. Diagnosis is based on clinical features. Laboratory confirmation is difficult: reliable serological tests are still to be developed and isolation of the organism is not a routine procedure. Early treatment with antibiotics may prevent the more serious sequelae.

Incubation period

Days to several weeks.

Source and spread

Deer and mice are known to be reservoirs in the USA. Transmission to humans is via the *Ixodes* tick, which feeds on infected animals, but many patients do not remember being bitten. Person-to-person spread does not occur.

Control

Avoid tick infested areas. Remove ticks from the skin quickly. Cover exposed parts of the body when in tick infested areas. Early treatment with antibiotics.

Malaria

Worldwide, malaria is one of the most important infections and a common cause of death. Malaria is caused by one of the four species of the protozoan parasite *Plasmodium falciparum, P. ovale, P. malariae* and *P. vivax*. It occurs in the tropics and sub-tropics. Diagnosis is by clinical presentation and identification of organisms in the blood. Treatment is with chloroquine, quinine and other antimalarials. Chloroquine resistance of the parasite is a major problem throughout the world.

Source and spread

Man is the reservoir and transmission occurs via the bite of the *Anopheles* mosquito.

Incubation period

Usually 10–15 days. May be much longer with *P. vivax*.

Control

Protect against mosquito bites by staying inside after dark and covering arms and legs and using a repellant spray. Eradicate mosquito breeding sites. Insecticide spraying of dwellings. Prompt treatment of cases. Travellers to endemic areas require chemoprophylaxis for which medical advice must be sought. (For mosquito control generally, see Chapter 9.)

Meningococcal meningitis and septicaemia

Meningitis is an infection of the brain lining by various bacteria or viruses, causing severe illness;

it has a high mortality if untreated. Viral meningitis is usually less severe than bacterial meningitis. The latter may be associated with a generalized (blood) infection (septicaemia), which has a worse prognosis.

Infection caused by the meningococcus receives the greatest public health attention in the UK, where it is endemic with cyclical epidemic waves.

Diagnosis of bacterial meningitis is by the isolation of the organism from blood or cerebro-spinal fluid. Viral meningitis is more usually diagnosed serologically. Treatment is by appropriate antibiotics.

Source and spread

The natural reservoir of the meningococcus is the human nasopharynx. The carriage rate for all meningococci in the normal healthy population is about 10%. Transmission occurs by droplet spread between people who are close contacts. Only a small proportion of people who acquire the organism ever develop the disease.

Incubation period

2–10 days.

Control

All cases of meningococcal meningitis and septicaemia should be notified promptly to public health authorities. Household and kissing contacts should be traced and offered antibiotics to clear pharyngeal carriage in an attempt to prevent transmission to other susceptible contacts. A vaccine against groups A and C is available and trials of group B vaccine are underway. Group B is the commonest form of the disease in the UK. In Africa and Asia, group A disease is more common and a vaccine is offered to travellers going to highly endemic areas.

Plague

A highly dangerous bacterial infection with *Yersinia pestis*, which historically caused plague in large epidemics. Its main geographical distribution today is in Asia. Diagnosis is by direct microscopy of lesions and culture of the organism. Treatment is with antibiotics.

Source and spread
The natural source of bubonic plague is the brown rat and rat flea. The flea ingests infected blood, and Y. *pestis* multiplies in the flea's stomach, and is excreted in its faeces or is regurgitated. Rats are infected by flea bites. Humans are infected by rat flea bites, or by handling infected rats, or by person-to-person droplet spread (pneumonic plague). The death of infected rats causes fleas to seek other hosts, such as the black rat which carry fleas into close contact with humans.

Incubation period
2–6 days.

Control
Isolated cases. Travellers to endemic areas can be immunized. Antibiotics may be given to contacts to prevent disease. Control rodents.

Psittacosis, ornithosis

A febrile bacterial infection with *Chlamydia psittaci* causing fever and pneumonia. It occurs worldwide. Diagnosis is by serology and treatment is with tetracyclines and erythromycin.

Source and spread
Psittacine and other birds, including ducks, turkeys and pigeons, are the usually identified source of human infections. Sheep strains may infect pregnant women. Infection is via inhalation of aerosols or of infected dust contaminated by bird faeces, nasal discharges, or sheep products of gestation or abortion. *C. psittaci* may survive in dust for many months. Person-to-person transmission of avian or ovine strains is rare. Outbreaks occur among aviary and quarantine station workers, and poultry processing workers.

Incubation period
Usually 4–15 days.

Control
Quarantine infected birds. Provide good ventilation of poultry processing plants and heat-treat feathers. Pregnant women should avoid contact with flocks during lambing in enzootic areas.

Q fever

A disease caused by *Coxiella burnetti*, which presents with fever, pneumonia and sometimes endocarditis. It occurs worldwide. Diagnosis is by serology and treatment is with antibiotics.

Source and spread
Many animals, as well as ticks, are natural hosts. The reservoir for human infection is usually sheep and cattle. The organisms are abundant in placentae and birth fluids, and remain viable in dust and litter for months. Infection results from inhalation of contaminated dust, handling infected carcasses, or by consumption of contaminated milk, or possibly, tick bites.

Incubation period
2–4 weeks.

Control
Pasteurize milk. Take hygienic precautions in abattoirs. Prevent contamination of urban areas with infected straw, etc.

Rabies

A viral infection of the central nervous system which is invariably fatal in the non-immunized. Rabies occurs in all continents except Australia and Antarctica. The British Isles are rabies free. Diagnosis is by visualization of the virus in brains of animals, and by serology in humans. There is no definitive treatment available.

Source and spread
The virus can infect all warm-blooded animals and birds. Two cycles of transmission are recognized: urban dog rabies, which is now largely confined to the less developed countries; and sylvatic or wildlife rabies, which is the main type

in the USA and much of Europe with various reservoir hosts, e.g. skunks, raccoons and foxes in the USA and Canada; Arctic foxes in the Arctic; mongooses and jackals in Africa; foxes in Europe; blood-feeding bats in South America; and other bats in the Americas and Europe. Rabies is fatal in carnivores, and it is the population density which determines the maintenance and spread of infection by biting. Transmission among bats by contrast is by aerosol inhalation. Most human infections are from bites of domestic carnivores or, in South America, vampire bats. Person-to-person transmission has resulted from infected corneal transplant grafts.

Incubation period
This can be from 10 days to a year or longer. The incubation period is shorter the nearer the bite is to the head.

Control
In enzootic areas, avoid contact with wild animals and promptly cleanse any bite wounds. Specific immunoglobulin is vital as soon as possible after exposure. Pre- and post-exposure vaccination can be given. In enzootic areas, vaccinate dogs, cats and cattle. Quarantine all carnivores on importation (6 months in Britain for carnivores). Some countries require vaccination of dogs and cats before importation. Vaccinate dogs at frontiers between enzootic and rabies-free areas. (For the control of dogs generally see Chapter 10.)

Relapsing fever

A widely distributed bacterial infection caused by *Borrelia* species with high fatality. The endemic form is tick-borne and occurs in Africa, the Americas, Asia and, possibly, parts of Europe. Epidemic relapsing fever is louse-borne, and is limited to parts of Asia, Africa and South America. Diagnosis is by microscopy of blood or culture of the organism. Treatment is with tetracycline.

Source and spread
Man is the reservoir of epidemic louse-borne infection. Infection occurs when the louse is crushed on the bite wound by scratching. Endemic tick-borne relapsing fever is transmitted from the natural wild rodent reservoir by tick bites to humans.

Incubation period
5–15 days.

Control
Treat cases, clothing, and bedding with insecticide. Control ticks.

Shigella dysentery

Of the three main types, *Shigella sonnei* is the commonest in the UK, usually causing transient mild diarrhoea in children. *S. flexneri* and *S. dysenteriae* are usually imported infections, and more often cause severe bloody diarrhoea. Diagnosis is by isolation of the organism from the faeces. Treatment is fluid replacement, and antibiotic therapy in severe cases.

Source and spread
Humans are the reservoir and the organism is excreted in faeces. Prolonged carriage is possible. Transmission is usually by the direct faecal–oral route, especially within families with small children, and in nurseries and schools. Food-borne outbreaks have occurred, and in developing countries water-borne outbreaks occur due to sewage contamination of drinking water.

Incubation period
1–7 days.

Control
Strict personal hygiene. Sanitary disposal of faeces and protection of water supplies. Infected persons should not handle food. Children with diarrhoea should be excluded from school until symptom free and stools are formed. In school outbreaks, supervision by staff of handwashing in young children and adequate provision of hot water and clean towels in toilets is imperative.

Tetanus

This occurs worldwide, but is rare in the UK. Painful contraction of muscles is caused by a toxin produced by *Clostridium tetani*. Diagnosis is usually based on clinical presentation. Treatment is with specific immunoglobulin and penicillin.

Source and spread
Clostridia are normal intestinal flora, and also survive as spores in the soil. Infection may be by contamination of deep, penetrating wounds. Neonatal tetanus occurs in developing countries, and is caused by contamination of the umbilicus.

Incubation period
Usually 3–21 days.

Control
Clean wounds thoroughly. Routinely immunize children and following laceration injuries if the immune status of the child is in doubt or if the wound is particularly dirty. Booster doses of tetanus toxoid are also necessary if 10 years have elapsed since the last dose.

Toxocariasis

A common roundworm infection (*Toxocara canis* and *T. cati*) of dogs and cats. It is acquired by children worldwide. Symptomatic disease is rare, but occurs particularly in children subject to pica. Diagnosis is by serology and biopsy.

Source and spread
Natural hosts are dogs and cats. Eggs that are excreted in faeces require a maturation period in soil. The eggs hatch in the intestine and larvae penetrate the intestine wall to enter the blood vessels. In puppies less than 5 weeks old, larvae migrate to the intestines via the lungs and complete their maturation. Dormant larvae in adult bitches reactivate during the dogs' pregnancy, and migrate to cross the placenta or may infect puppies via milk. Larvae excreted in faeces by puppies may mature in the bitch once ingested.

Humans are infected by ingesting eggs from contaminated soil and grass. Children with pica are at greatest risk.

Incubation period
Weeks or months.

Control
Teach children good hygiene and prevent access to dog faeces. Keep dogs away from children's play areas. Cover sand-pits when they are not in use. Clean up faeces when exercising dogs in public parks. Worm all dogs regularly. (For the control of dogs generally see Chapter 10.)

Toxoplasmosis/congenital toxoplasmosis

A common and usually asymptomatic protozoal infection of humans caused by *Toxoplasma gondii*. It occurs worldwide. Infection in the womb in humans can lead to serious brain lesions. Diagnosis is by serology. Antibiotic therapy may be effective.

Source and spread
Definitive hosts are cats, which are infected by eating raw meat, birds or mice which contain parasite cysts. Humans may be infected by eating raw or inadequately cooked meat (mainly sheep, pigs, cattle or goats), and unwashed salad vegetables, or by ingestion of faecal oocysts from cat litter. Congenital infection of the foetus occurs when the human mother acquires a primary infection in pregnancy.

Incubation period
Uncertain, but possibly 1–3 weeks.

Control
Pregnant women should avoid handling cat litter, and should wash their hands after handling raw meat. Freezing may kill cysts in meat, but thorough cooking is strongly recommended. Pregnant women should also avoid contact with lambing ewes.

Tuberculosis

A potentially severe chronic bacterial disease caused by *Mycobacterium tuberculosis* and *M. bovis*, and which occurs worldwide. *M. bovis* has been almost eradicated from the cattle of several developed countries, including the UK. *M. tuberculosis* is of increasing concern in association with the AIDS epidemic. Diagnosis is by sputum staining and culture. Treatment is with long-term antibiotics.

Source and spread
Man is the reservoir for *M. tuberculosis* and transmission is by direct contact and air-borne spread. Cattle are the natural reservoir of infection with *M. bovis*, and transmission to humans is via the consumption of raw milk.

Incubation period
4 weeks to several years.

Control
Identify and treat cases promptly. Screen contacts for infection and treat early. Heat-treat all milk. BCG vaccination in children.

Typhoid and paratyphoid

A severe infection with *Salmonella typhi* or *S. paratyphi* A or B, with a high mortality if untreated. Most UK cases are imported. Diagnosis is by the isolation of the organism from blood, faeces or urine. Treatment is with antibiotics.

Source and spread
Man is the definitive host for these species of salmonella. After infection, a person may remain a symptomless faecal or urinary carrier for months or years. Transmission occurs usually by faecal or urine contamination of food or water. Outbreaks may result from infected food handlers and from sewage pollution of water supplies. Cases may also occur by person-to-person spread within households.

Incubation period
1–3 weeks.

Control
Separation of water supply and sewage disposal. Infected food handlers should be excluded from work until at least six consecutive monthly faeces and urine samples are negative. Household contacts of cases and carriers should be screened, and food handlers excluded from work until two negative faeces and urine samples, at least 48 hours apart, have been obtained. Travellers to endemic areas should be immunized.

Viral hepatitis – hepatitis A

This is a common, enterically acquired infection of the liver, commonest in children who may often not have jaundice. It occurs worldwide. Diagnosis is by serological methods to identify specific antibodies against the virus. There is no specific treatment, but passive immunization with immunoglobulin confers protection for a limited period.

Source and spread
The reservoir of infection is man. The virus is excreted in faeces before the onset of symptoms. Transmission occurs commonly in families by direct contact, via the faecal–oral route and sometimes by food- and water-borne spread. Outbreaks may occur in nurseries and schools.

Incubation period
2–6 weeks.

Control
Strict personal hygiene and sanitary disposal of faeces. Schools should provide adequate hand-washing facilities. A food handler who is not immune and who has contact with cases, may be advised not to handle food for 4 weeks after his or her last contact with an infectious person, and may be given immunoglobulin. Family contacts and travellers to endemic areas may be given normal human immunoglobulin. Immunoglobulin is effective after exposure if given within 2 weeks.

Viral hepatitis – hepatitis B and C

These are less common than hepatitis A in the UK, but worldwide they are very common infections of the liver, which carry an increased risk of chronic liver disease and hepatic carcinoma. Diagnosis is by serological identification of viral antigens and antibodies. There is no specific treatment.

Source and spread

Humans are the reservoir. Hepatitis B and C are carried in the blood and body secretions. Infected people may remain carriers for months or years after an acute infection. Transmission occurs by sexual intercourse; from mother to baby at birth; blood contamination of shared needles, as in intravenous drug users, unhygienic tattooing, and blood transfusions.

Incubation period

2–6 months.

Control

Screen blood donors and exclude contaminated blood. Sterilization of intravenous needles and avoid sharing needles. Avoid unprotected sexual intercourse with carriers. Maternal to infant transmission of hepatitis B can be prevented by giving specific immunoglobulin and vaccine to the infant immediately after birth. A safe and effective vaccine for hepatitis B is now available and is recommended for all health care workers who may be exposed to blood, and to household and sexual contacts of cases.

Viral haemorrhagic fevers

A variety of viruses may cause severe, often fatal infection. These viruses are not endemic in the UK and are only a problem for people visiting exotic areas. For example, Lassa fever is endemic in rural parts of West Africa. Diagnosis is based upon serology and isolation of the virus from body secretions. Antiviral agents may be used in the treatment of the infection.

Source and spread

A variety of animals and birds may harbour the viruses. Wild rodents are the reservoir for Lassa fever. In Lassa fever, transmission occurs by direct or indirect contact with rodent urine, which may contaminate food. Person-to-person spread does occur in some circumstances, such as in hospitals by direct contact with blood, secretions and droplets of infected patients. Other viral haemorrhagic fevers may be transmitted by mosquito and tick bites.

Incubation period

Usually a few days to 3 weeks.

Control

Avoid endemic areas. Isolate suspected cases and take precautions to avoid respiratory spread. Disinfect contaminated objects, clothing, etc. Specific immunoglobulin may be used to prevent infection in contacts. Ribavirin is used to prevent Lassa fever spread. Close contacts of proven cases should be quarantined for 3 weeks after the last contact.

Viral gastroenteritis

Probably the commonest form of infective gastroenteritis, although not the most commonly reported. It is caused by a variety of viruses including small round-structured viruses (Norwalk-like) and rotavirus. Worldwide it is a major cause of mortality due to dehydration in young children. Diagnosis is by electron microscopy of faeces obtained within 48 hours of onset, or by serological identification of virus antigen in faeces.

Source and spread

Man is the reservoir and the virus is excreted in huge quantities in faeces and vomitus during the first few days of illness. Transmission occurs by direct contact; faecal–oral spread; from infected food handlers up to 2 days after recovery from illness; and indirectly when virus particles contaminating surfaces are transferred to food or

Table 18.2 Common childhood infections transmitted by close contact with saliva, respiratory secretions or air-borne droplets

Disease	Agent	Clinical features	Incubation period	Period of communicability	Control
Chickenpox	Virus	Fever, rash	Usually 13–17 days	5 days before rash to 5 days after first crop of vesicles	Specific immuno-globulin to high risk contacts; antiviral agents
Measles	Virus	Fever, rash, cough	Usually 10–14 days	Onset to 7 days after rash	Routine vaccination of all children; specific immuno-globulin to contacts in some circumstances
Mumps	Virus	Fever, parotitis	Usually 18–21 days	1 week before to 10 days after parotitis	Routine vaccination of all children
Rubella	Virus	Fever, rash	Usually 17–18 days	One week before to 4 days after rash	Routine vaccination of all children, and some women of child-bearing age
Scarlet fever	*Streptococcus*	Fever, rash, pharyngitis, tonsillitis	1–3 days	Several weeks if not treated	Penicillin to cases and possibly to contacts
Whooping cough	*Bordetella pertussis*	Fever, paroxysmal cough	Usually 10–14 days	3 weeks from onset	Routine vaccination of all infants; antibiotic treatment of cases and possibly contacts

fingers and then to the mouth. Secondary household transmission following food-borne outbreaks is common.

Incubation period
18–72 hours.

Control
Strict personal hygiene. Food handlers should exclude themselves from work immediately if they suffer from gastro-enteritis, and for at least 48 hours after symptoms subside. Disinfection of contaminated areas and surfaces.

Yellow fever

A severe, febrile, mosquito-borne viral disease leading to liver and kidney failure and death in many cases. It occurs as a zoonosis mainly in forest dwellers in the rain forest areas of northern South Africa, and Central and South America.

Source and spread
The natural reservoirs of infection are forest monkeys, marmosets and humans. Transmission among monkeys is by the bite of various species of mosquito in forests, and to people who enter or live near infected forests. There may also be an independent human/mosquito cycle in urban areas. The urban cycle has been almost eliminated by eradication of the mosquito vector.

Incubation period
3–6 days.

Control
Control mosquitoes and avoid their bites. Immunize the exposed population and travellers to ende-

mic areas. Immunization confers lifelong protection and is obtained from yellow fever vaccination centres. (For mosquito control generally, see Chapter 9.)

REFERENCES

1. Committee of Enquiry into the future development of the Public Health Function (1988) *Public Health in England*, HMSO, London, Cmnd 289.
2. Langmuir, A.D. (1963) The surveillance of communicable diseases of national importance. *N. Engl. J. Med.*, **268**, 182–92.
3. Palmer, S.R. (1990) Review article: epidemiology in search of infectious diseases: methods in outbreak investigation. *J. Epidem. Comm. Health*, **43**, 311–4.

FURTHER READING

Barker, D.J.P. and Rose, G. (1990) *Epidemiology in Medical Practice*, 4th edn, Churchill Livingstone, London.

Bell, J.C., Palmer, S.R. and Payne, J.M. (1988) *The Zoonoses*, Edward Arnold, London.

Benenson, Abram S. (ed.) (1990) *Control of Communicable Diseases in Man*, 15th edn, American Public Health Association, Washington.

Grist, N.R., Ho-Yen, D.O. Walker, E. and Williams, G.R. (1987) *Diseases of Infection*, Oxford University Press, Oxford.

Holland, W.W., Detels, R. and Knox, G. (1991) (eds) *Oxford Textbook of Public Health*, 2nd edn, Oxford University Press, Oxford.

Russell, A.D., Hugo, W.B., and Ayliffe, G.A.J. (1992) *Principles and Practice of Disinfection, Preservation and Sterilization*, Blackwell Scientific Publications, Oxford.

19 Environmental epidemiology

Richard T. Mayon-White

DEFINITION OF ENVIRONMENTAL EPIDEMIOLOGY

Epidemiological methods have an important place in the protection of people from environmental hazards. Epidemiology can show which environmental factors are causing disease or injury, even when the mechanism or precise factor is unknown. When the nature of the harm is understood, epidemiology can determine if the effects can be prevented or reduced to an acceptable level. If hazards have been identified and controlled, epidemiology can be used to monitor the process. In short, **environmental epidemiology is the measurement and evaluation of the health effects of environmental hazards**. In this chapter, the main epidemiological methods are described and illustrated with examples drawn from non-communicable diseases.

One of the characteristics about epidemiology is that it enables us to detect unexpected or uncommon effects. This may lead some people to disbelieve the findings of epidemiological studies, because they know of many people who are exposed to the hazard without falling ill. They dismiss the evidence as circumstantial, because the damage cannot be shown to be 'cause and effect' in laboratory experiments. This is pertinent in legal proceedings when lawyers are unfamiliar with statistical arguments. Therefore, we must expect to have to argue carefully and persistently to get public action to control the environmental hazards detected by epidemiology.

The epidemiological methods described here should be seen as a progression both in the time required and levels of certainty. The early recognition of an environmental hazard is likely to come from a descriptive study. This should be followed by testing the suspected causation with an analytical method (case-control and cohort studies). If the analysis confirms the suspicion, an intervention should obviously follow with a proper evaluation of its efficacy.

DESCRIPTIVE EPIDEMIOLOGY

The straightforward enumeration of cases is a familiar method in public health. Public health reports over the past century recorded the number of deaths from certain causes, of notifiable infections, of cancers and of respiratory conditions. The fact that these reports were regular (annual) and related to well-defined areas (countries, regions or counties, towns or rural districts), have lead to obvious ways of looking for environmental factors. The familiarity disguises the very real difficulties in collecting reliable data, but large differences between the incidence in different places are quickly followed by suggestions as to the causes and possible cures.

An example to illustrate this approach is provided by **malignant melanoma**, a cancer of the pigment-forming cells of the skin. The cancer may start in a mole (a benign, pigmented skin tumour), or in apparently normal skin. Once the

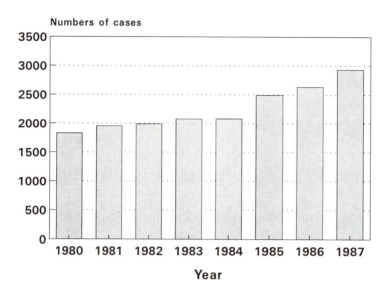

Fig. 19.1 Skin cancer incidence in England 1980–87. Malignant melanomas (ICD 172).

melanoma becomes cancerous, it tends to metastasize (spread to other parts of the body via the bloodstream) early, so that surgical treatment is not always effective. Consequently, the case-fatality rate of patients with malignant melanoma is high, and the death rate from this condition is a good indication of its incidence. The diagnosis of malignant melanoma is usually accurate in developed countries, because skin tumours removed by surgeons are checked by pathologists. This can lead to the diagnosis being recorded in a cancer register, so that all cases including survivors can be counted. As malignant melanomas occur in young and middle-aged adults, the diagnosis is likely to be made with particular care. For these various reasons, a high rate of melanomas in Queensland, Australia was an important observation. The best explanation is that sub-tropical levels of sunshine on fair-skinned people stimulate pigment cells to the point that some cells become malignant.

The incidence of melanomas is increasing in the UK (Fig. 19.1) and the USA, which reflects the popularity of holidays with lots of sunbathing. Melanomas are uncommon in black people, so there is clearly a genetic factor in the cause, in affording more tolerance of sunshine. But the environmental factor of this skin cancer is evident from the description of the geographical variation in incidence. The important part of the ultraviolet light spectrum is the B band (UV-B) from 280 to 320 nm. The carcinogenic potential of UV-B is not new information, but the link to a severe cancer like melanoma has raised public concern, leading to advice on prevention, both personal (care in sunbathing) and global (by the protection of the ozone layer in the lower stratosphere).

Changes in the incidence of a disease over a period of time is the essence of monitoring policies and programmes of prevention. The example of skin cancer has been chosen as one of the main targets in 'The Health of the Nation' programme of the British Government, with the aim of halting the rising incidence by the year 2005. Changes in incidence may also lead to the discovery of the cause. Usually, the change has to be an increase rather than a decrease in incidence in order to stimulate research. **Lung cancer** became more common in Britain in the first half of this century (Fig. 19.2). By 1950, there were a number of theories as to the cause of this increase, including the suggestion that environmental factors, like the exhaust fumes of cars and lorries, were the reason. The attraction of this theory was

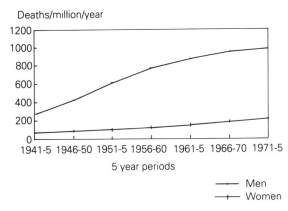

Deaths/million/year

Fig. 19.2 The increase in lung cancer deaths from 1941 onwards, mostly in men, provoked questions about environmental causes. The popularity of cigarette smoking had increased from 1914, so that men who started to smoke in their teens were at risk of long cancers in their forties. (Data from OPCS (1978) *Trends in Mortality*, DHI No. 3, HMSO, London.)

that the rise in the use and numbers of vehicles propelled by internal combustion engines ran in parallel to the rise in lung cancer mortality. However, as is now well known and widely accepted, the cause was part of the social environment: the increase in cigarette smoking. The association of lung cancer with tobacco was determined by a **case-control study**, of the type described later in this chapter. The annual average consumption of cigarettes has risen from 0.5 to 4.5 pounds weight per person between 1900 and 1947, followed by a tenfold rise in deaths from lung cancer in the same period.

Another illness and cause of death that has increased markedly in this century is **coronary heart disease**. There is a link to smoking, but other factors are also important. The study of coronary heart disease is complicated by the fact that it is part of a larger process of arterial disease, because the diagnosis is sometimes inaccurate, and because medical treatment affects the outcome. Despite these complications, there is consistent evidence of **geographical and temporal differences** in incidence. High rates of coronary heart disease correlate with high dietary consumption of saturated fats when the data from different countries are compared. The disease is

distinctly more common in men than in women, something that is not simply explained by theories about diet. So it is clear that coronary heart disease has multiple causes. Which causes are the most important cannot be resolved by descriptive epidemiology. Theoretically, the importance of the different possible factors can be calculated as relative risks in **cohort studies** described below. In practice, people are likely to be convinced only by studies in which the incidence of disease is reduced by removing one or more of the risk factors, that is, by conducting controlled trials of prevention, '**intervention studies**'.

The descriptive approach to environmental epidemiology can be summarized as:

1. Define who is to be counted as a case of the disease in question.
2. Find the cases from various sources of information (mortality statistics, hospital records, occupational health records and special surveys).
3. For each case, find the age, sex, place of residence, date when the disease started or was diagnosed or caused death, and any other factors that are deemed to be relevant.
4. Find the size of the population in which the cases have arisen.
5. Examine the data for patterns, calculate rates and compare with information about other populations.
6. See if there are correlations between disease and the attributes of different times and different places.
7. Think of the possible explanations of what has been found, but **be cautious about making any firm conclusions.**

The reason for the note of caution about firm conclusions is that descriptive studies are not very powerful tests of theories on causation, although they are essential in the formulation of ideas. In modern times, there are large computer banks of data on disease incidence and environmental factors. Remarkable coincidences are bound to be found when the computers are programmed to search through hundreds of combinations of disease and environmental factors. Not all the data are accurate and precise, particularly when they have been collected routinely for purposes other than epidemiological research.

CLUSTERS OF DISEASE

Coincidences are especially difficult to interpret when the number of cases is small, but significantly clustered in one place. The cluster of nine cases of childhood leukaemias in south-west Cumbria, near to, and possibly associated with, the nuclear processing plant at Sellafield, is one well-known example. But in other parts of the country, doctors can point to villages or small areas where there have been five or six cases of leukaemia when only one or two should be expected from the regional or national averages. In some cases, this added to the focus on nuclear installations, including the military establishments at Dounreay in Scotland and Aldermaston in Berkshire. There is another theory to explain these clusters of leukaemia, based on the influx of the workers and their families into areas that were previously much less populated. Viruses are a possible cause of leukaemia (at least in cattle and mice), and viruses spread more than usual when new populations are formed, in this case by industrial development. In such new populations, children would be likely to encounter more viral infections, and so might have an increased chance of getting leukaemia. This theory explains why leukaemia cases near Sellafield have not continued to be higher than the average, although improvements in radiological protection is an alternative explanation. Clusters of severe diseases like leukaemia and other cancers naturally excite local interest, resulting in all manner of hypotheses and rumours. With small numbers, it is practically impossible to prove or disprove the hypotheses. Their main scientific value is to promote and sustain large, well-designed studies, which may take several years to complete. In making such studies, it is wise to exclude the cases that have lead to the hypothesis and to look for cases arising later or in other places.

Suggestions of local environmental causes for clusters of diseases should not be made without careful thought to the fear that may arise, fear that is not easily dispelled by later research. An epidemiological study must contain a review of the various causes of bias that could have lead to the appearance of an unusual cluster. Has a single label, e.g. 'cancer', been attached to a mixed collection of diseases which are most unlikely to have a single common environmental cause? Have the cases been brought together by medical facilities, either for diagnosis (and hence registration) or for treatment, where the cluster has nothing to do with the cause? Has the cluster been formed by finding one or two cases, looking for more and stopping when, and only when, the incidence appears to be abnormal? Is the ascertainment of cases more complete in the area of the cluster than elsewhere? Has publicity affected the evidence submitted by people involved?

These critical questions may give to local people an impression that the epidemiologist does not understand their fears of a local cause. This impression is, of course, strengthened by statements about the unreliability of small numbers and the necessity of further studies. There is no easy answer to avoid this tension between understandable anxieties and the scientific approach, so caution is needed in reporting clusters of non-infectious disease. Standing back from the immediate concern may give a new perspective: when considering the cause of the nine cases of leukaemia near Sellafield that occurred on a 30-year period, one should remember that there were 16 500 cases elsewhere in Britain.

Once the cause of a disease is known, clusters of patients with the condition take on an entirely different significance. As with outbreaks of infectious disease, clusters of a non-infectious disease point to the need for more public health action. **Lead poisoning** causes anaemia and neuropathy. The clinical disease is well defined, and readily confirmed by blood tests, which can show not only highly abnormal levels of lead, but also the metabolic disturbances caused by lead. Lead is an accumulative poison, so prolonged exposure increases the risk of disease, in contrast to an infectious agent which would normally stimulate immunity or tolerance. In houses fitted with lead pipes in soft water areas, children are at more risk if their furniture and toys are painted with lead-based paints and if the streets are filled with cars emitting lead from petrol. There are two epidemiological methods to apply to this problem. The first is to set up surveillance to monitor the incidence of lead poisoning seen in clinical practice, so that every detected case is followed up with checks on the home, and the place of work of adult patients. The other method is by a prevalence survey, aimed at detecting over-exposure before clinical disease has reached the stage of frank poisoning.

PREVALENCE (CROSS-SECTIONAL) SURVEYS

The **prevalence** of a condition is the proportion of people in a given population who have the condition. It is not the same as the **incidence**, which is the proportion who develop the condition in a given period of time. The two terms are often confused. A **prevalence survey** is an obvious method for counting diseases or conditions that are chronic. In a chronic condition, some people may not seek medical advice until late, while others may stop attending doctors when they find that treatment does no more than palliate the condition. For both these reasons, medical records will underestimate the number of people with the condition. Yet other people may have sub-clinical effects, i.e. will have no symptoms despite detectable pathology.

Following on with the example of lead poisoning started above, a prevalence survey could be the collection of symptoms and blood samples of a sample of the population in a town with a soft water supply. The purpose of the survey would be to find parts of the town, types of houses, age groups and social factors which were associated with abnormal lead levels and related illness. It would then follow that the resources to find and treat cases, and to repair the defects in the environment, were concentrated on the areas of greatest need. It should be stressed that it would be unethical to make such a survey, with the intrusion into the lives of the people in the sample, unless it was expected that the survey could find a health problem and that the problem

could be corrected. As prevalence studies are not powerful methods of determining the cause of disease, their main use is in translating the knowledge about a cause into public health action.

In the example of a whole town being the population under consideration, it is likely to be more efficient to study a sample instead of every resident for a prevalence survey. A study of road traffic pollution and chest diseases in Munich, Germany looked at children aged about 10 years old. The sample was children who were in one grade in the local schools and who had lived in the area for 5 years. The study found higher rates of respiratory illness and reduced lung function at the schools in districts with more car traffic. In other cases, like the work force of a factory making lead batteries, there may strong arguments for studying everyone. The decision on whether to survey a sample or the whole population must be made with statistical advice on the appropriate numbers of people to study. If a sample will give sufficient numbers, further statistical advice should be taken on the selection of a sample that properly represents the population under consideration.

CASE-CONTROL STUDIES

In a case-control study, all the cases of the disease in question are taken and their histories of exposure to the possible environmental factor compared with the rate of exposure in controls. The controls are selected to be people who, before the start of the enquiry, might have the same chance of exposure as the cases. The history of exposure is often found by asking cases and their controls the same questions, either by interviews or by written questionnaires.

As mentioned above, tobacco smoking was suspected as a cause of lung cancer in Britain and the USA in 1947. Since the original case-control study that demonstrated the association between tobacco smoking and lung cancer 40 years ago, there have been questions about the cause of lung cancer in people who do not themselves smoke. One possibility has been that at least some of these non-smoker cases have been exposed to other people's tobacco smoke, and thus have been at risk, so-called '**passive smoking**'. Lung cancer in non-smokers is rare, but case-control studies are suitable in this situation. In the case-control studies on passive smoking, the groups of cases have been formed by taking patients with a proven diagnosis of lung cancer, but who have never smoked. In some studies, controls were chosen from among patients in hospital with other diseases, to be of about the same age and to have the same proportion of men and women. In other case-control studies on passive smoking, the controls were drawn from a sample of the population, and were not confined to hospital patients. Exposure to an environment of tobacco smoke was defined as living with a smoker (usually having a spouse who smoked). More of the patients with lung cancer than other people had lived with cigarette smokers. The difference is not very large, as living with a smoker increases this risk of lung cancer by about 30%. Nevertheless, this level of risk is sufficient to cause more than 200 deaths from lung cancer in non-smokers a year in Britain. If any domestic product or industrial air pollutant had this effect, there would be urgent action to control it. What has occurred is a slow but determined public health movement to reduce the exposure to other people's tobacco smoke.

A single case-control study finding this level of increased risk may not be very convincing on its own. Whenever possible, a second case-control study should be conducted on a different population by another team of investigators. This is exactly the same process as applies in the physical sciences, when experiments are repeated before their results are accepted. In the example of passive smoking, there have been at least 10 case-control studies, and their combined results were used to make the estimate of increased risk given above. The pooling of the results of several studies is called **meta-analysis**. Meta-analysis is being used more widely in epidemiology, because it helps to estimate the risk of an environment factor more accurately than can be achieved from a single study.

In conducting case-control studies, the control group must be chosen carefully to avoid **bias**. If the controls or the people who interview them know what the suspected factor is and that they are controls, their answers are likely to reflect this knowledge. This may happen when the control group is formed and studied after the cases. Another bias is to include the early cases whose histories suggested a link between the factor, and the disease in the first place in a case-control study to test the hypothesis. The controls should be of the same age, sex and social background as the cases. Controls of this sort may be obtained by asking patients to name friends and neighbours. If there are several ways of choosing controls, e.g. other hospital patients and neighbours, the option of using more than one group of controls should be carefully considered. To do so may increase the work, but it may also improve the reliability of the result.

One problem that has to be guarded against is confounding. **Confounding** happens when the link between a disease and a supposed factor is not a direct cause, but is due to something else to which both disease and factor are linked. In some British cities, mothers belonging to ethnic minorities are more likely than other mothers to have babies of low birth weight. Ethnicity, the factor that is measured, is a confounder, because low birth weight is caused by other factors, which are, in turn, associated with immigration more than ethnicity. The cause is environmental and lies in the quality of antenatal care, diet and home conditions. Once confounding is suspected, it can be taken into account in the analysis and prevented from confusing the results of a study.

The difficulty in convincing people of risks on the basis of case-control studies should not be underestimated. The method is not familiar to the general public or politicians. Case-control studies have shown the causes of disease before the pathological mechanism is known and before the causative agent is precisely identified. The task is even more difficult because epidemiological evidence is unlikely to be available before a chemical, a product or physical process is in widespread use. So there will be an established lobby of producers and users to resist the allegations of a health hazard. The case-control method has advantages in determining the environmental causes of disease. Because it depends on cases that have already occurred, it can produce results relatively quickly. By concentrating on cases and a similar number of controls, it is relatively inexpensive.

DOSES OF ENVIRONMENTAL FACTORS

Another aspect of environmental epidemiology has been demonstrated by the case-control studies on lung cancer and tobacco smoke. This is the effect of **increasing dosage**. Logically, one would expect that the greater the exposure, the greater the chance of disease if it is true that the factor under study is the cause of the disease. If one found the inverse (higher dosage, less risk of disease), one could doubt that the association between the preceding factor, e.g. smoking, and the disease was a cause-and-effect relationship. With both smokers and non-smokers who live with smokers, the risk of lung cancer increases with the number of cigarettes smoked and the number of years exposed to tobacco smoke. So a **dose effect** is present.

Working in the other direction, one might ask if there is a dose below which there is no ill-effect, This appears to be so with some toxins and some infectious agents. When it is possible to collect information that measures the amount of exposure, this should be done because of the difficulties of removing substances that have been in common use. With saturated fats in the diet and the risk of coronary heart disease, the advice is to modify the diet without a total abstention from saturated fats. With carcinogens, the present view is that there are no thresholds of safety. The decision on 'safe levels' becomes a balance of risks between the use of carcinogenic substances, such as tobacco or asbestos, and radiation on the one hand, and the use of alternatives or doing without. In this decision, the calculation of risks needs to be accurate. One disadvantage of the case-control method is that the calculation of risks has to be made indirectly, in contrast to the next method described.

COHORT STUDIES

The limitations of the case-control method may be overcome, at least in part, by applying the **cohort or prospective method**. With this method, a group or a sample of a population are observed over a period of time, to see who becomes exposed to various environmental factors and who develops disease. The immediate advantages of this method are that one can plan to generate the required information instead of relying on existing records and the memories of the subjects. The level of exposure can be measured instead of estimated. There need be no anxiety about the possibility of bias in the choice of controls. The price to be paid for these advantages include the greater cost and organization employed in following up a large group of people, and the delay until the group has been exposed and the disease has had time to develop.

One example of a cohort study is the follow-up of adults who lived in the American town of **Framingham, Massachusetts, in 1950**. The purpose of this was to learn more about the causes and development of **coronary heart disease and hypertension**. The study was run for more than 30 years. At 2-year intervals, the adult subjects in the study were medically examined, measuring blood pressure and blood cholesterol levels, among other things. Admissions to hospital for, and deaths from, heart disease were recorded as outcomes. With the passage of time, it became clear that a high blood cholesterol at the start predicted an increased risk of a heart attack, especially in men. The increase in risk was shown to depend on the level of cholesterol. From this, doctors could calculate how much heart disease could be prevented by reducing cholesterol levels to normal levels in those most at risk. This result was only the end of the first stage in preventing heart disease, because the methods of reducing cholesterol by modifying diets still needed to be proved.

A drawback of the Framingham study was that a proportion of the subjects recruited at the beginning of the study moved away, or stopped being followed up for other reasons. This could seriously weaken the conclusions of a cohort study, partly because the size and so the power of the study falls, and partly because the people lost to follow up may be significantly different from those who stay. Therefore, there are advantages in using cohorts which are more likely than a sample of the general population to stay in the study. An example of such a cohort is the employees in a large organization. Their qualifications, their pensions and the occupational health services all help to keep the subjects known to the researchers. A generation of British doctors have been studied to relate their lung cancer rates to their smoking habits. Civil servants in Whitehall have been followed up like the citizens of Framingham, and have demonstrated the benefits of exercise in preventing heart disease.

Workers in nuclear installations provide another example of a group of people followed in a cohort study. They are monitored for their exposure to **radiation** (including measurements of dosage and frequency), and for their incidence of cancer. At Sellafield, there have been slightly more deaths in workers from myeloma than expected (7 instead of 4) and slightly more prostatic cancer deaths (19 instead of 16), but other types of cancer including leukaemia were rather less common. Staff exposed to radiation were not more likely to die early or get cancer than those who were unexposed. This helps to show that careful environmental practices can control hazards to acceptable levels of risk.

INTERVENTION STUDIES

The epidemiological methods discussed so far could be considered to provide circumstantial evidence rather than direct proof. Direct proof would be given by intervening to remove a suspected environmental cause of disease. The logic is that if factor X is truely a cause of disease Y, then intervening to remove X will reduce the incidence of Y. If Y does not fall with such an intervention, then X is not a cause. Of course, real life is not as straightforward as this logic, and attempts to reduce a disease may fail because the removal of the cause is more difficult than anticipated.

In medical practice, there has been a revolution of thinking in the past 50 years in how doctors decide between different drugs and other treatments. In the past, empirical choices were made, by which the treatments that appeared to work were used again, and passed on in conventional teaching. Perhaps because the treatments were not very powerful, and perhaps because there was greater respect for the 'experience of the master', the traditional system was used for centuries. Nowadays, new drugs are tested in **randomized controlled trials**, aimed at removing any bias. These trials come close to the standard of biological experiments in their objectivity, and they have set the pace for preventive medicine.

In intervention trials, it is essential to make the groups of patients given different treatments as equal as possible in all respects before treatment starts. This is best done by allocating patients to the different groups by randomization, which gives an equal chance to every patient of receiving any of the treatments being tested. This system of randomized allocation can be used in trials of vaccines or other prophylaxis that are given to individuals, although randomized trials of prevention require formidable numbers of subjects.

It is much more difficult to use randomization in designing intervention studies of environmental change. In most circumstances, the nature of the intervention is such that there has to be a deliberate choice as to which population is treated. It is tempting to assume that the incidence of disease in the treated population before and after the change will show whether the intervention works. But it is wise to have a contemporary untreated population as a control. A project in Finland to prevent heart disease illustrates this point. **North Karelia** was a Finnish community with a high incidence of coronary heart disease. The preventive strategy was aimed at the multiple factors of heart disease, including smoking, blood pressure and diet. A neighbouring and similar community, **Kuopio**, was selected as a control population. This proved essential to the interpretation of the effects. Although smoking was reduced and blood pressure was treated, similar improvements were observed in the country. Mortality from coronary heart disease fell in both North Karelia and Kuopio.

Table 19.1 Comparison of epidemiological methods

Useful for	Descriptive	Prevalence	Case-control	Cohort	Intervention
Rare diseases	Yes	No	Yes	No	No
Rare causes	Yes	No	No	Yes	Yes
Time relations	Yes	No	No	Yes	Yes
Clustering	Yes	Yes	No	Yes	No
Risk assessment	No	No	Yes	Yes	No
Quick results	Yes	Yes	Yes	No	No
Low resources	Decreasing from descriptive to intervention				
Scientific rigor	Increasing from descriptive to intervention				
Avoiding bias	Increasing from descriptive to intervention				

Fluoridation of the water supply has been restricted by pressure groups to a minority of households in Britain. This created a 'natural' experiment, whereby the intervention could be tested. The population of Birmingham and other places supplied with additional fluoride have enjoyed far less dental caries than elsewhere.

ASSESSMENT OF EPIDEMIOLOGICAL STUDIES

Epidemiology is often the first line of investigation of environmental hazards. The results of epidemiological studies may be, therefore, the first evidence on the risks involved. It is not difficult for the significance of the early evidence to be exaggerated in the excitement of the discovery, or to be underrated by those whose business or lifestyle is threatened by the findings. To assess early evidence, a checklist of questions may help.

1. Do you know that the authors of the report and editor of the journal in which it is published are trained to be objective and scientific?
2. Is the method used in the study adequately described? The possible weaknesses in the methodology should be discussed by the authors in their report.
3. How many subjects recruited into the study left the study before it was completed? Dropout rates of more than 30% are worrying.
4. If there is a control group, has it been chosen in a way that offers a fair comparison with the cases (case-control study) or treated group (intervention trial)?
5. If there is no control group, is there a reasonable estimate of what might have been found without the factor of treatment under study?
6. Is there a dosage effect, and do the conclusions make biological sense? There should be a plausible explanation as how the environmental factor causes disease, even if the detail is not yet known.
7. Is the association between the environmental factor and the disease a strong one? The association should be tested by conventional statistical methods, but a lay person's guide is to ask how many of the cases are explained by the supposed causative factor.
8. Is there supporting evidence from independent studies? This is a very important question.
9. Does the study lead onto further research, either by showing how it can be repeated elsewhere to gain independent confirmation, or to explore ideas and problems thrown up by the study itself?
10. Does the study lead to some practical means of preventing disease?

A comparison of epidemiological methods is shown in Table 19.1.

FURTHER READING

The British Medical Association Guide to Living with Risk (1990) Penguin, London.

Buck, C., Llopis, A., Najera, E. and Terris, M. (1990) *The Challenge of Epidemiology: issues and selected readings*, Sci. Pub. 505 Pan American Health Organisation

Holland, W.W., Detels, R., Knox, G. and Breeze, E. (1985) *Oxford Textbook of Public Health, Vol. 3: investigative methods in public health*

Investigating Environmental Disease Outbreaks – A Training Manual (1991) World Health Organization, Geneva, 1991. WHO/PEP/91.35.

Part Four

Housing and
Development Control

20 Housing: standards and enforcement

Neville Hobday

INTRODUCTION*

Local authority role (see also Chapter 1)

State intervention in housing dates back to the second half of the nineteenth century, when powers were given to the medical officer of health to demolish individual unsatisfactory houses. Not surprisingly, this power had only limited effect, and it was extended by the Artisans and Labourers Dwellings Improvement Act 1875 to include areas of housing which were not capable of attaining 'a proper sanitary standard'. The Public Health Act 1875 was the first to introduce controls over new buildings when local authorities were allowed to make bye-laws applicable to such matters as lighting, ventilation, drainage and water supply.

Once the principle of minimum standards had been established, it proved impossible for the private sector – which even up until the end of the First World War produced 90% of the country's housing stock for letting – to provide accommodation of an adequate standard at rents that people on low incomes could afford. Consequently, Housing Acts of 1890 and 1909 gave permissive powers to local authorities to build houses to let. Eventually in 1919, the Housing and Town Planning, etc. Act made it a duty of local councils – with the aid of a government subsidy – to provide or ensure the availability of adequate and sufficient housing.

From that time on, the local authority role in the provision of housing expanded until the 1980s, when government policy encouraged authorities to move away from their traditional role as direct providers of subsidized housing. As more people became owner occupiers or rented from private or housing association landlords, the government urged local authorities to adopt more of an enabling role: assessing the needs of their area, seeking to ensure that these needs were met, giving financial support and assistance to providers under a range of powers, but only rarely resorting to direct provision of new housing in their own management. Capital programmes were to be directed towards the renovation of the existing housing stock in the public and private sectors.

National housing strategy

Local authorities' housing capital programmes cover the provision and renovation of their own housing and support for the private sector, mainly through renovation grants and financing housing association developments. The government seeks in its capital resource allocation to enable authorities to carry out their statutory function, in par-

---

* Many of the statutory processes dealing with housing, including specialized forms, and covered by this chapter are analysed in *Environmental Health Procedures*. [1] In that book, interpretive procedure charts are included.

ticular, their duties towards homeless people in priority need and specifically to:

1. Ensure that housing in their ownership is renovated where necessary and efficiently managed and maintained.
2. Assist private owners who could not otherwise afford necessary repair or improvement.
3. Support and supplement housing association and private sector investment in their area where necessary to meet demand from people in need.

Resources for local authority capital expenditure are made up of:

1. Capital grants from central government in support of certain expenditures.
2. New borrowing authorized by credit approvals granted under the capital finance system.
3. Authorities' own capital receipts (net of amount set aside to repay debt) and contribution from revenue.

In the context of present policies, the housing function of the environmental health officer in local government continues to be of major significance. Traditionally involved in the enforcement of satisfactory standards of provision and repair in private sector housing, the reduction in capital resource allocations and the changes in the local authority housing role mean that EHOs have an important duty to perform in developing a local housing strategy.

Current housing position

In England and Wales there are, according to recent surveys about three quarters of a million more dwellings than households [2], although there are still serious imbalances in areas of high demand mainly in London, the south east and the larger cities. The amount of space per person is among the highest in Europe, and almost all houses now have the basic amenities. There are, however, some major problems of disrepair in the rented sector, both public and private, and particularly acute ones in some urban areas.

About two-thirds of houses in England and Wales are owner occupied, one of the highest percentages in the world, and the private rented sector has declined from about 90% of the total stock in 1914 to only 8% in 1991. Council-owned housing has increased from 10% of all housing before the Second World War to about 20%. This percentage has declined in recent years due to right-to-buy sales and large scale voluntary transfers to housing associations. The housing associations themselves have expanded their role so the number of houses they own now exceeds 60 000 – about 3% of the total stock.

Fig. 20.1 illustrates dwelling tenure changes in England between 1914 and 1991 [2].

The situation in any area is also affected by the size, type, location and condition of the houses, and whether they are suitable to meet the needs of different sections of the community including young people, single people, families, the elderly and the disabled. Demographic changes taking place in the population and the projected growth in the number of elderly households is of particular significance at the present time.

In those areas where there is an imbalance between housing need and availability, the shortage is demonstrated by:

1. insufficient rented accommodation in the private and public sectors;
2. high occupation densities with congestion and overcrowding;
3. constant pressure for rented accommodation;
4. poor quality accommodation;
5. multi-occupied houses with periods of occupation well beyond what might be considered reasonable;
6. high land and house prices and, consequently, a depressed housing market and difficulties for first-time buyers.

Inevitably, this situation results in an increase in the number of homeless people, many of whom approach the local authority for assistance (see below).

Local housing strategy

Each housing authority is required to submit annually to the Department of the Environment (DoE) a strategy which, among other things,

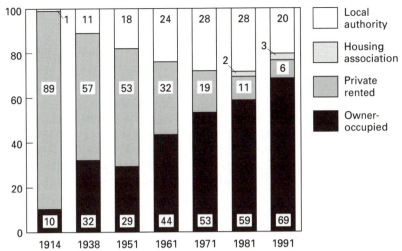

Fig. 20.1 Tenure change 1914 to 1991. Note: vacant dwellings are included within the tenure of their previous occupancy. (Source: DoE (1991) *English House Condition Survey 1991*, HMSO, London.)

should include a brief narrative description of its general housing policy setting out major aspects of the housing situation in its area, the overall aproach to those circumstances, and highlighting particular issues as appropriate. To achieve a consistent approach by local authorities the DoE produced a strategy guidance manual to be used in the 1995–96 Housing Investment Programme (HIP) process.

It is not possible for a local authority to make a once and for all housing policy. Changes in population, economic factors, social conditions and public expectation are all major considerations, as well as changing national political and financial stategies. An effective policy needs to be planned, programmed, regularly reviewed and monitored.

The environmental health officer not only plays an important part in helping to formulate the corporate housing strategy of the local authority, but also in framing the more detailed aspects of the policy dealing with the private – as opposed to the public – housing sector.

A local authority's policy for the private sector should refer to such matters as:

1. an integrated, planned and programmed approach to renewal areas, clearance, renovation grant aid and group repair schemes;

2. multi-occupied houses and tenanted properties;
3. enforcement policies;
4. vacant houses
5. housing aid and advice including harassment and eviction prevention;
6. design standards and open space provision;
7. the special needs of groups, such as elderly and handicapped people;
8. relationship with housing associations and voluntary organizations.

More specific guidance on local authorities' policies in the private sector is given by the Audit Commission [3]. The Commission emphasizes that authorities, rather than simply reacting to requests for service, should have a pro-active strategy which defines its priorities. Strategies should be based on information on the nature and scale of problems in the area and on the location of properties which need action. Councils should also pay close attention to the efficiency of their operation, setting target response times and adopting inspection procedures which ensure accuracy and consistency.

In addition, local authorities, as part of their corporate responsibilities, should establish a clear policy for dealing with complaints of disrepair from council tenants. It is wasteful of scarce resources to have both housing and environmental health departments pursuing routine complaints. The principle objective of such a policy should be for the housing department of the local authority to have a clear repair strategy with published response times for dealing with different items of disrepair depending on their urgency. The inclusion of an appeals procedure in cases of tenant dissatisfaction is also desirable. Such procedures should ensure the best use of staff and would involve the environmental health officer principally as an arbiter where there was disagreement over the cause or effect of any specific defects, or where a judgement on unfitness was required. (See also DoE Circular 21/84.)

THE CONTROL OF HOUSING STANDARDS

National house condition surveys

In order to provide the government with information on the condition of the housing stock right across the country, National House Condition Surveys are undertaken from time to time using sample survey methods. These surveys were first recommended by the Dennington Committee report, *Our Older Houses – A Call for Action*, in 1966 and the first was carried out in 1967. A second was undertaken in 1971, and others have followed at 5-year intervals since. The inspections are carried out by environmental health officers and other housing surveyors who are briefed and advised by the DoE. The reports based on these surveys form valuable information upon which to base national housing policy, and allow trends in unfitness, repair, improvement and overcrowding, etc., to be monitored.

The 1991 English House Condition Survey [2] found, among other things, that:

1. At the end of 1991 there were 19.7 million dwellings in England. A large part of the stock was old; a quarter of present dwellings was built before the First World War; 20% were built between the wars and the remaining 55% have been built since 1945.
2. 80% of dwellings were houses; 20% of dwellings were flats of which three-quarters were purpose built and one-quarter were conversions of older houses.
3. There were 75 000 (0.4%) houses in multiple occupation housing 275 000 households.
4. 517 000 (c. 3%) of households had less than the notional number of bedrooms they required.
5. By 1991 the number of dwellings with a missing basic amenity (e.g. a kitchen sink; a bath or shower in a bathroom; a wash hand basin; and cold water provided to each of these; and an indoor water closet) was 205 000 (1%). This compares with 463 000 (2.5% of the stock) which lacked basic amenities in 1986.
6. 711 000 rural dwellings were not on main drainage – 17% of the rural stock.
7. 90% of all houses with lofts had some form of insulation.
8. 70% of all dwellings required some work to the main external or internal elements of the building, rising to 90% for pre-1919 dwellings. The average cost of general repairs, i.e. those works needing to be done in the next 5 years, was £1,130.
9. 1.5 million dwellings were unfit, more than 50% of which were built before 1919.
10. 30% of the private rented sector was in the worst condition compared to less than 10% of the other tenures.
11. One-third of the 1.6 million houses, among the worst 10% of the stock, had neighbouring dwellings in the block also in poor repair. Most blocks in poor repair were privately owned pre-1919 dwellings.
12. Within the private sector there was a significant relationship between households' incomes and their housing conditions.

Housing assessments

Effective housing strategies cannot be developed without knowledge of the local housing conditions. Section 605 of the Housing Act 1985 – as substituted by paragraph 85 of Schedule 9 to the Local Government and Housing Act 1989 – requires local housing authorities at least once in each year to consider the housing conditions in their district with a view to determining what action to take in performance of their duties in relation to repair notices, slum clearance, houses in multiple occupation, renewal areas and renovation grants. Should he consider it necessary, the Secretary of State is empowered to issue direction as to the manner in which the duty to consider housing conditions should be undertaken.

Section 605 does not require a physical inspection of housing once a year but local authorities are expected to keep the information acquired on earlier comprehensive surveys up to date. Local housing market conditions, the demand for housing in relation to the existing supply, renewal and repair policies will all have had some effect over a 12-month period.

Types of local survey

House condition surveys can be grouped conveniently under three headings according to the purpose they are intended to serve:

1. strategy development;
2. action planning;
3. implementation.

Surveys falling into the first two categories aim to provide a statistical picture of housing characteristics sufficiently precise and reliable to be used for planning purposes. They do not however provide detailed specifications and costings of remedial work which could form the basis of a contract. This role is performed by the third category – the implementation survey.

Strategy development
These surveys are used to identify housing problems within a local authority to determine:

1. the nature and extent of the problems;
2. the appropriate levels of investment to tackle them;
3. priorities for action between tenures and between different locations within the district;
4. the effectiveness of decisions already taken and expenditure already committed, by measuring changes in the situation over time.

They may cover the whole of the stock or focus on a particular sector; for example, separate surveys may be conducted on public and private sector housing. They are sample surveys which take in a representative selection of dwellings from the stock rather than all dwellings. They are useful for:

1. the provision of information for the development of HIP (housing investment programme) strategy statements;
2. the provision of some of the data required in the HIP forms;
3. compliance with an authority's duty under section 605 of the 1985 Housing Act as amended by section 85 of Schedule 9 of the 1989 Local Government and Housing Act.

Action planning surveys
Such surveys are needed when an authority has already identified specific housing problems and decided the priority in tackling them. The next step is to design appropriate courses of action against the problems. These surveys could focus on:

1. The provision of information from which a range of costed options can be generated.
2. Determining the relationship between the housing problems and household circumstances, and establishing what solutions households would find appropriate.
3. The detailed description and understanding of particular problems in a specific sub-sector of the stock (e.g. HMOs, houses in multiple occupation).

They are normally confined to a relatively small geographical area or very specific sub-section of the stock. Information is needed about each of the dwellings in the defined population but not necessarily at the same level of detail for each. Examples of such surveys are those undertaken:

1. as part of a neighbourhood renewal assessment;
2. to develop an estate action programme;
3. to pursue an action programme involving HMOs.

Implementation surveys

Before beginning a programme of work on a stock of dwellings it is usual to draw up a schedule of work to identify precisely what is to be done to each individual property. The information required is collected in an implementation survey. Normally all dwellings to be included in the programme are surveyed.

House condition surveys tend to be labour intensive and therefore costly. It is important that an authority is clear about why it wants to conduct a survey and how it plans to use the information before embarking on the exercise.

A guidance manual produced by the Department of the Environment provides general advice on conducting surveys as well as detailed methodology to enable local authorities to carry out surveys using a tried and tested approach. The manual is based on experience gained during the English House Condition Survey and the production of the Neighbourhood Renewal Assessment Guidance Manual.

Inspection

An inspecting officer should have a means of identification. This should also clearly state the legislation, provisions and purposes for which the officer is authorized.

In all cases in which subsequent proceedings are contemplated, the names of the owner or owners are required. Powers of local authorities to require information as to ownership of premises, including houses, are now set out in section 16 of the Local Government (Miscellaneous Provisions) Act 1976.

Inspections under the Housing Act should be carried out in the knowledge that they may be the subject of examination at a public inquiry, in the County Court or by the Ombudsman, in the course of which every detail may be contested. The inspector's procedure must be correct, and his reports must be complete, accurate, and quite unassailable in the impressions they convey.

The undermentioned information should be recorded for each premises inspected:

    address
    date

brief description
owner agent
occupier(s)
commencement date of tenancy
rent

with necessary variations, and adaptation for multi-occupied premises.

It is important that inspections should be undertaken in a systematic way, taking the order of inspection in logically progressive fashion. As an illustration, the inspectation of a two-storey terraced house with single storey back addition should be examined in the following sequence:

Internal

1st floor:	front room
	rear room
staircase	
ground floor:	front room
	middle room
	rear room
facilities:	sanitary accommodation
	washing facilities
	water supply
	storage, preparation and
	cooking of, food
	internal drainage

Each room should be inspected in sequence, for example:

    floors
    walls
    ceilings
    windows
    doors
    lighting
    ventilation

In each case, a note must be made of the material used in construction and its condition, e.g. floor-concrete-extensive rising dampness.

Where houses are double handed, handing of each room should be done facing the front of the house, e.g. first-floor left or second-floor rear right.

External
    chimney

roof
walls
window/door woodwork
rainwater gutters and downpipes
yard paving
drainage

A systematic approach of this nature can be applied to the most complicated property and ensures that no important factors are missed.

The extent and, where possible, the effect of disrepair should be recorded and the use of the word 'defective' avoided if possible. More explicit terminology, such as rotting, leaking, sunken, uneven, bulged, cracked, fractured, etc., should be used.

Standard of fitness

For many years, conditions in individual houses have been considered in terms of fitness for human habitation. The first minimum standard of fitness was suggested in the *Manual on Unfit Houses* issued by the Minister of Health in 1919. A notable advance in the guidance offered to local authorities and their officers as to what should be regarded as a reasonable standard of fitness for habitation was made in the 'Report of the Standards of Fitness for Habitation Sub-Committee of the Central Housing Advisory Committee' dated October 1946.

In 1954 a standard of fitness in more negative form – specifying not what should render a house fit but what should be deemed to render it unfit for human habitation – was laid down. It became the first standard to receive statutory authority when it was incorporated in the Housing Act 1957. This standard – except for one or two minor amendments – remained in force for over 30 years until the Local Government and Housing Act 1989.

Paragraph 83, Schedule 9 of that Act substituted a new section 604 of the Housing Act 1985. The basis of the new standard remains the same in that it is a means of determining whether premises are fit for human habitation. The section stipulates that a house is fit unless it fails to meet one or more of the requirements in paragraphs (1) to (9) below, and by reason of that failure is not reasonably suitable for occupation.

1. it is structurally stable;
2. it is free from serious disrepair
3. it is free from dampness prejudicial to the health of the occupants (if any);
4. it has adequate provision for lighting, heating and ventilation;
5. it has an adequate piped supply of wholesome water;
6. there are satisfactory facilities in the dwelling for the preparation and cooking of food, including a sink with a satisfactory supply of hot and cold water;
7. it has a suitably located water closet for the exclusive use of the occupants (if any);
8. it has, for the exclusive use of the occupants (if any), a suitably located fixed bath or shower, and a wash basin, each of which is provided with a satisfactory supply of hot and cold water; and
9. it has an effective system for the draining of foul water and surface water.

Whether or not a dwelling house which is a flat satisfies the above requirements, it is unfit for human habitation if the building, or part of the building, outside the flat fails to meet one or more of the requirements in paragraphs (1) to (5) below, and by reason of that failure the flat is not reasonably suitable for occupation:

1. the building or part is structurally stable;
2. it is free from serious disrepair
3. it is free from dampness
4. it has adequate provision for ventilation; and
5. it has an effective system for the draining of foul, waste and surface water.

To encourage an objective interpretation of the standard, detailed guidance on its application is given in Annex A of DoE Circular 6/90. After quoting the statutory standard, the guidance starts with a general note on its overall application. For each of the requirements, the guidance provides general advice and lists the main items to which authorities are asked to have regard in forming their opinion of fitness. It then advises on the determination of fitness in respect of some of the more typical defects which are found. In deciding whether a dwelling house is or is not unfit, an authority should determine for each of the statutory requirements in turn whether or not the dwelling house is reasonably suitable for occupation because of a failure of that particular matter.

Subject to the location of defects, a dwelling house or building may fail to meet a particular requirement either due to the severity of a defect, or by reason of the extent of the defects. However, it is only unfit if, because of that failure, it is not reasonably suitable for occupation. In this respect, a dwelling would not normally be expected to be unfit for human habitation because of a minor defect. Such a defect might include an isolated area of damp, the odd missing or broken window pane, slipped or broken gutters in an otherwise adequate drainage system, and other comparable defects.

DEALING WITH UNFIT PROPERTIES

On identifying an unfit property, an authority is obliged to take action to deal with it. This might include:

1. a **repair notice**;
2. a **closing order**;
3. a **demolition order**;
4. including the property in a **clearance area**
5. **group repair**

A decision to include the property in a renewal area does not relieve an authority of this obligation, although the action taken is likely to form part of the authority's strategy for the area. In some cases, renovation will be the most satisfactory course of action, whether as part of action in a renewal area or otherwise. In other cases, demolition will be more satisfactory. Consideration should, however, intially be given to both on an equal basis and section 604A Housing Act 1985 requires authorities in reaching a decision to have regard to the 'Code of Guidance for Dealing with Unfit Premises' (Annex F of DoE circular 6/90) issued by the Secretary of State.

The Code recommends that authorities seek to reach a decision on individual premises in the context of overall strategies. Authorities will generally be expected to consider:

1. characteristics of adjoining properties to the unfit premises;
2. local accommodation needs; and
3. the impact of any decision on the local environment and community.

The Code also recommends that where authorities do not have sufficient information to make a decision in the context of an area strategy, they should conduct a survey and assessment using suitably modified Neighbourhood Renewal Assessment (NRA) techniques (see page 367). Annex G of DoE Circular 6/90 sets out how this might be done.

Under former housing legislation, considerable weight was attached to the cost of the various options. In the case of repair notices and demolition orders, this was the sole criterion. The Code stresses that economic factors should in future form only part of the matters to be considered. although authorities will be expected to make an economic assessment of the viable options. Paragraph 11 of the Code recommends the use of an economic formula to assist authorities in assessing the comparative merits of various courses of action. Examples are given in Annex H of DoE Circular 6/90.

The conduct of a survey and assessment will ensure that authorities are aware of the courses of action that may be open to them, and will provide a context for appraising those courses. The factors that an authority will consider it appropriate to take into account in arriving at a decision on the most satisfactory course of action will vary according to particular circumstances outlined in the Code.

Clearance areas

Where a local authority is of the opinion that the inclusion of the premises in a clearance area is the best course of action, it should proceed under section 289 of the Housing Act 1985. The wide-ranging factors in addition to those specified in the section which the authority is required to take into account are listed in the Code of Guidance.

A clearance area is an area which is to be cleared of all buildings in accordance with the section's provision. A local authority can declare an area after following the specified consultation and notification procedures if it is satisfied:

1. that the residential buildings in the area are unfit or by reason of their bad arrangement or the narrowness or bad arrangement of the streets, dangerous or injurious to the health of the inhabitants of the area;
2. that the other buildings in the area are for a like reason dangerous or injurious to health;

and that the most satisfactory course of action is the demolition of all buildings in the area.

The area should be defined on a map in such a manner as to exclude:

1. any residential building not unfit or dangerous to health;
2. any other building not unfit or dangerous to health;
3. any unfit residential building excluded from the area following the required consultations.

The authority should then forward to the Secretary of State a copy of the formal resolution, together with a statement of the number of persons occupying buildings in the area. Information on procedural requirements, etc., is contained in DoE Circular 77/75.

After the declaration of the area, the local authority must then purchase the land either by agreement or compulsory purchase order (CPO), and secure the demolition of the buildings (section 290 of the Housing Act 1985). It may also acquire added lands which surround or adjoin a clearance area and are needed to secure a clearance area of convenient shape and dimension. The guidance contained in Circular 5/93 should be followed when submitting clearance area CPOs for confirmation.

Formerly, compensation for unfit housing which was compulsorily acquired was restricted to site value. The Local Government and Housing Act 1989 repeals the relevant provisions of the 1985 Act, and ensures that in future compensa-

tion will be paid on the same basis as for fit houses, and assessed in accordance with the Land Compensation Acts. In practice, this means market value compensation.

Group repair procedures are dealt with in the section on Houses and Area Improvement.

Individual unfit premises

Where a local authority forms the opinion that a house is unfit for human habitation and should not be included in a clearance area, a decision needs to be made as to whether repair, closure or demolition is the correct option. In reaching this decision, regard must be made to the Code of Guidance for Dealing with Unfit Premises. An assessment of the costs of the various options is an important feature, but is only one of the elements which must be taken into account. Overall plans for the area in which the property is situated may influence decisions, and repair could be an option even if relatively expensive, if the rest of the immediate area is in good condition or is to be improved. Regard should also be had to such factors as the need for a particular type of accommodation in the area, the existence of a strong local community and the need and wishes of the owners and occupants of unfit dwellings.

Repair of unfit houses

Repair notices (section 189 of the Housing Act 1985) in respect of an unfit dwelling house (1) are served on the person having control of the premises, with a copy of the notice to any other person having an interest, and (2) must specify a date by which works should be started, as well as a time within which they must be completed. Works in default may be undertaken if either of these requirements is not observed or at any time after the start date if reasonable progress on the work appears not to be being made. There is a mandatory requirement (section 194) for a local authority to serve notice announcing intention to carry out works in default.

Paragraph 8, Schedule 15 of the Housing Act 1988 makes it an offence for anyone liable to comply with a notice to intentionally fail to do so. Prosecution may be instigated without prejudice to the power to carry out works in default and recover expenses. Notices are also registered as a local land charge. The effect of this is that the local authority does not need to serve a fresh repair notice if a transfer of the property takes place, and expenses can be recovered from the person having control of the property on whom the demand for expenses is made. Paragraph 6A, schedule 10 of the Housing Act 1985 empowers local authorities to sequester rents in recovering such expenses.

In assessing the fitness of a flat the section enables a local authority to have regard to the condition of the building containing it (section 604 of the Housing Act 1985 as amended).

The guidance on the fitness standard, Annex A of DoE Circular 6/90, makes specific reference to the difficulties which may be posed by **underground rooms**. Particular attention should be given to dampness, inadequate ventilation and light. Basements which are themselves dwelling houses will be subject to the separate application of the fitness standard. In the case of underground rooms which are part of a dwelling, consideration should be given to any defects which might cause the dwelling to fail the fitness standard and whether the dwelling is unsuitable for occupation because of those defects. In the case of underground rooms in a building containing one or more flats, the service of a closing order in respect of part of the building may be appropriate if that is the most satisfactory way of dealing with unfitness in a particular flat.

Having identified an unfit property, authorities are normally statutorily obliged to take some form of immediate action. Section 190A of the Housing Act 1985 provides an exception to this where the property is to be included in a group repair scheme within 12 months.

Appeals against a notice should be made within 21 days of its service. No grounds of appeal are specified except:

1. section 191(1A): that the works are the responsibility of someone else who is the owner (defined at section 207);

2. section 191(1B): that the service of a demolition or closing order would have been a more satisfactory course of action.

Section 189(2) clarifies the point that although notices under the section are referred to as 'repair notices', they need not be confined to works of repair and can include improvements.

In circumstances where a person served with a notice under section 189 has difficulty in finding a builder able to complete the work in the required timescale, section 191A allows the local authority to execute the works at the expense of the recipient and with his agreement.

Demolition and closing orders

For an individual unfit premises where the Code of Guidance has been taken into account, all the options evaluated and repair and improvement discounted, then a demolition or closing order will need to be made.

Sections 264 and 265 of the Housing Act 1985 empower local authorities to make such orders. Under section 264 an authority can close a house, a flat in a building or the whole or part of a building containing flats. Section 264 does not permit authorities to close part of a dwelling house or house in multiple occupation. The power to make partial closures is restricted to buildings which contain at least one flat, and the closing of any particular part of such buildings must be the most satisfactory course of action in relation to an unfit flat.

Under section 265, demolition orders cannot be served in respect of individual flats, but may be served in respect of the building containing them if some of the flats are unfit.

In view of the fact that the local authority will have had to reach a decision on the most satisfactory course of action before making an order and that this will almost certainly involve consultation with the owner, there is no requirement – as in earlier legislation – for a 'time and place' notice.

A demolition order requires premises to be vacated within not less than 28 days of the order becoming operative, and for demolition within 6 weeks of vacation. A closing order prohibits the use of the property for any purpose not approved by the authority (section 267). Section 268 requires that an order be served on any person who is owner of the premises and every mortgagee whom it is reasonably practicable to ascertain. A person aggrieved by a demolition or closing order may appeal within 21 days of its service to the County Court (section 269). The appeal can be made on the grounds that a repairs notice or a demolition or closing order – as the case may be – would have been more appropriate. When a demolition order has become operative, the owner of the premises should demolish them, and if he or she fails to do so the local authority can act in default, sell the materials and recover costs.

Section 584A of the Housing Act 1985 requires the owner of premises subject to a closing or demolition order to be compensated for any decrease, due to the order, in the compulsory purchase value of the property. The local authority has power to permit reconstruction of condemned premises. Under section 274 of the Housing Act 1985, the owner of premises in respect of which a demolition order has become operative or any other person who, in the opinion of the local authority, can put his or her proposals into effect may submit proposals for the reconstruction, enlargement or improvement of the premises. The authority may postpone the date fixed for demolition if it is satisfied that the work would produce premises fit for habitation. On completion of work, the Order may be revoked.

Repair of a house which is not unfit

Local authorities also have powers to require works to be carried out in premises which are in disrepair, but which are not unfit. In such cases where an authority is satisfied that:

1. a dwelling house is in such a state of disrepair that, although not unfit for human habitation, substantial repairs are necessary to bring it up to a reasonable standard having regard to its age, character and locality; or
2. a dwelling house is in such a state of disrepair that, although not unfit for human habitation, its condition is such as to interfere materially

with the personal comfort of the occupying tenant;

they may serve a repair notice on the person having control (section 190 of the Housing Act 1985). Section 190 notices may only be served in respect of an owner-occupied dwelling if the property concerned is in a renewal area.

The notice must specify a date by which work should be started, as well as a time within which it must be completed. The same rules apply regarding works in default, prosecution for non-compliance, land charges registration and recovery of costs as for section 189 of the Housing Act 1985 notices. In assessing the repair of a flat, local authorities are enabled to have regard to the condition of any part of the building containing it, and notices can be served where it is such as to affect the condition of the flat or to interfere with the personal comfort of the occupying tenant of the flat.

Appeals against a notice should be made within 21 days of the service. No grounds for appeal are specified, except section 191A that the works are the responsibility of someone else who is the owner (defined at section 207). Similar to the situation with section 189 notices, where a person served with a notice has difficulty in finding a builder able to complete the work in the required timescale, section 191A allows the local authority to execute the works at the expense of the recipient and with his or her agreement. Local authority enforcement options to improve a defective property are shown in Fig. 20.2.

Removal of obstructive buildings

An obstructive building is defined as, 'a building which by reason only of its contact with, or proximity to, other buildings is dangerous, or injurious to health'. (section 283 of the Housing Act 1985). If a building appears to the authority to be an obstructive building, it may proceed to order and secure its demolition.

The following are the steps that must be taken:

1. Serve upon the owner or owners notice of a time and place at which the question of ordering the building to be demolished will be

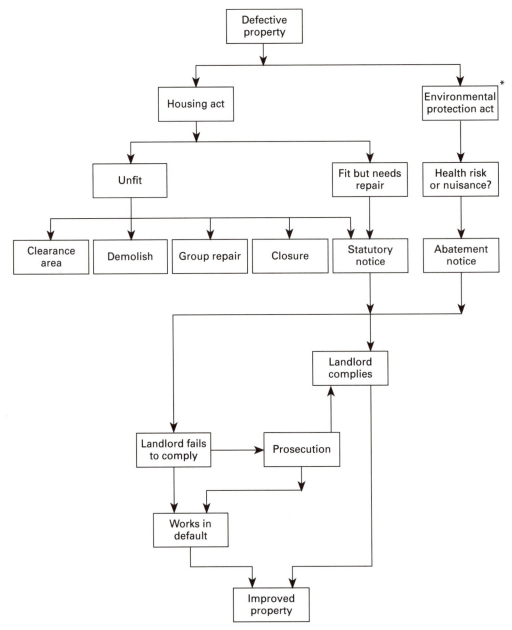

*Options under the Environmental Protection Act are dealt with in Chapter 33.
Fig. 20.2 Enforcement action to tackle poor condition housing: local authorities' options to improve a defective property. (Source: Audit Commission (1991) *Healthy Housing: the role of environmental health services*, HMSO, London.)

considered by the authority. (The owners are entitled to be heard when the matter is under consideration.)

2. If satisfied that the building is obstructive and it or any part of it ought to be demolished, make a demolition order accordingly.

3. Serve a copy of the order upon the owner or owners.

4. If requested to do so by the owners, purchase the building, the price to be assessed as prescribed by the Act, and as soon as possible after obtaining possession, carry out the demolition.

5. Alternatively, and in default of the owners themselves carrying out the demolition within a time prescribed in the order, the authority may enter and carry out the demolition and sell the materials rendered available thereby.

The expenses incurred by the authority and not covered by the sale of materials, may be recovered as a simple contract debt. The local authority must compensate the owner or owners in respect of loss arising from the demolition, the amount to be assessed as prescribed by the Act.

Cleansing of building before demolition

In order to prevent the migration of vermin from a building about to be demolished by reason of a demolition order, to other buildings adjoining it, and to prevent the sale of verminous building materials, local authorities are empowered by section 273 of the Housing Act 1985 to secure the disinfestation of any building before demolition.

The local authority may at any time between the date on which the order is made, and the date on which it becomes operative, serve notice on the owner of the building that they intend to cleanse it before it is demolished; it may then enter and carry out such work as it thinks requisite for the purpose of destroying vermin. The owner who has received such notice may require the work to be done within 14 days; at the expiration of that time he or she may proceed with the demolition.

HOUSE AND AREA IMPROVEMENT

Improvement policy

In its white paper *Housing: The Government's Proposals* [4], the government acknowledged that home ownership gave individuals the freedom to alter and improve their homes as they wished, and made a valuable contribution to improving the housing stock and allowing it to meet changing needs. However, emphasis was also placed on the fact that ownership carried with it the responsibility to keep the home in good repair.

The white paper stated that spending by individual owners through income, savings and loans, accounted for the vast majority of resources devoted to improving the private stock, but accepted that where owners were unable to afford the full costs of essential repairs and improvements, that help should be available through a reformed system of improvement grants.

The primary legislation used to introduce the revised grant system was the Local Government and Housing Act 1989. The underlying principle for all the grants is that of focusing assistance on bringing properties up to the standard of fitness. The main features of the 1989 Act can be summarized as follows (DoE Circular 12/90):

1. A **unitary renovation grant** which can be given for any works of improvement and/or repair to a dwelling, or for the provision of one or more dwellings by conversion.

2. **Mandatory and discretionary grants**. Renovation grants are mandatory when given towards eligible works required to make a house fit for human habitation, or to comply with a statutory notice, but discretionary for any other types of work.

3. **Test of financial resources**. The main determining factor for grant entitlement. The test takes different forms for owner occupiers, landlords and tenants.

4. **Classes of applicants**. Depending on the works required, owner occupiers are eligible to receive mandatory or discretionary grants. Grants to landlords are normally discretionary; grants are only mandatory towards the cost of bringing a dwelling up to the fitness standard where the works are required for compliance with a statutory notice. Only tenants with a repairing obligation under the terms of their tenancy are eligible to apply for renovation grants, although any tenant may apply for a disabled facilities grant. A land-

lord, other than a local authority, applying for a disabled facilities grant on behalf of a tenant, may be eligible for mandatory or discretionary grants.

5. **Common parts grants**. A unitary grant covering work of improvement and repair to the common parts of a building.
6. **Houses in multiple occupation (HMO grant)**. Landlords only are eligible to apply. A grant may be given for improvement or repair or both to make the HMO suitable for the number of occupants, or to make it fit or improve it above the fitness standard. A grant can also be given to convert a house to an HMO. Work required for compliance with a statutory notice attracts a mandatory grant.
7. **Disabled facilities grant** (DoE Circular 10/90 and 5/91). This complements the main renovation grant, and the requirements for the grant, such as the test of resources and the provision of certificates of future occupation, also apply. A mandatory grant is available for a broad range of essential adaptations, and a discretionary grant for other schemes.
8. **Group repair**. Individual grants may not be the most cost effective way of improving a block or terrace of houses. The 1989 Act therefore gives local authorities powers to carry out group repair schemes, enabling them to tackle blocks and terraces of run down private sector housing. Group repair is not a grant: individuals do not have to make an application.
9. **Minor works assistance** (DoE Circular 4/90). A new form of cash limited assistance targeted on low income groups and designed to cater particularly for elderly people who wish to remain in their homes and where, although repairs adaptations or improvements are required, full-scale renovation is considered inappropriate.
10. **Certificate of future occupation**. Applicants will normally have to provide an appropriate certificate and landlords will be bound by conditions as to the letting of grant improved properties. Clawback provision potentially applies to all applicants other than someone

with a tenant interest if a property is sold during the first few years after improvement.

Renovation grants

The undermentioned information applies – without qualification – to renovation grants and with various exceptions to other grants as well.

Applications

Section 102 of the 1989 Act requires that an application for a grant shall be in writing and shall specify:

1. The premises to which it relates.
2. Particulars of the work for which a grant is sought.
3. Unless the local authority directs otherwise, at least two estimates from different contractors.
4. Particulars of any preliminary or ancillary services and charges (Annex B, section 1 of DoE Circular 12/90, contains a specification of the fees and other charges which the Secretary of State has decided section 102(3) should be eligible for grant aid).
5. Other prescribed particulars. These particulars, including those necessary to apply the test of resources, are described by reference to the prescribed form. Applicants are therefore required to provide all the information requested in the forms.

Grant applications other than for disabled facilities grants may not be considered in respect of properties built or provided by conversion less than 10 years before the date of the application (section 103).

Section 104 of the Act specifies the interest a grant applicant needs to have in the property. Any person who has or proposes to acquire an owner's interest in all the 'land', on which it is proposed to carry out works, may apply. An 'owner's interest' is defined as either an estate in fee simple absolute in possession, or a term of years absolute of which not less than 5 years remain unexpired at the date of the application, and either interest can be held solely by the applicant or jointly with others. A tenant whose lease has at least 5 years still to run would be regarded as having an owner's interest for grant purposes. Different qualifying conditions apply for common parts grants.

A grant application from a tenant cannot be considered unless:

1. the terms of the tenancy require him to carry out the relevant work;
2. the application is for a disabled facilities grant.

Certificates and conditions as to future occupation

Section 106 of the Act deals with certificates and conditions as to future occupation. All applications for renovation and disabled facilities grants, except for certain types of ecclesiastical properties and charities, must be accompanied by a certificate of future occupation. There are three different types of certificates relating to renovation grants:

1. *Owner occupiers.* An owner occupation certificate certifies that the applicant has, or proposes to acquire, an owner's interest in the dwelling and that the or she or a member of his or her family intend to live in the dwelling as his or her only main residence for at least a year after the completion of work.
2. *Tenants.* A 'tenant's certificate' certifies that the applicant is a tenant of the dwelling, and that he or she or a member of his or her family intends to live in the dwelling as his or her only main residence.
3. *Landlords.* A 'certificate of intended letting' certifies that the applicant has or proposes to acquire an owner's interest in the dwelling, and intends to let the dwelling as a residence for a period of at least 5 years after the completion of work.

Owner occupiers and landlords who make a 'relevant disposal' of dwellings within 3 or 5 years respectively are required to repay grant to the local authority on demand. The amount to be paid is dependent on the period the dwelling is occupied after completion of grant work. The terms used to describe the different types of

disposal are 'relevant disposal' and 'exempt disposal' and are defined in section 124.

Mandatory grant

Where a local authority on receipt of a valid grant application considers:

1. that a dwelling is unfit for human habitation (section 604 of the Housing Act 1985 (as amended) and Annex A of DoE Circular 6/90); and
2. that completion of the relevant works will cause the dwelling to be fit; and
3. are satisfied that completion of the work is the most satisfactory course of action;

then a renovation grant is mandatory.

Notwithstanding this, a local authority is not under a duty to approve a grant if the application is a landlord's application unless the works are required by a section 189 Housing Act 1985 notice. Similarly, a grant need not be approved where the dwelling is scheduled to be included in a group repair scheme within 12 months (section 112). A grant to improve a dwelling above the fitness standard is normally discretionary, but where work is required to comply with a section 190 or section 352 Housing Act 1985 notice, then grant is mandatory (section 113).

Discretionary grant

Section 115 of the Act 1985 sets out a number of purposes for which works might be carried out and attract discretionary grant:

1. to put the dwelling in reasonable repair;
2. to provide the dwelling by conversion of a house or other building;
3. to provide adequate thermal insulation
4. to provide adequate facilities for space heating;
5. to provide satisfactory internal arrangements;
6. to enable the dwelling to comply with any requirements specified by the Secretary of State.

Grant approvals and payment

A local authority is required to notify grant applicants in writing not later than 6 months after the date of the valid application, whether or not the application is approved or refused. A grant can be paid after completion of the eligible work, or by instalments as the works progress. Payment is conditional upon work being completed to the satisfaction of the local authority, and on provision to the authority of an invoice demand or receipt for payment.

Test of resources for owner occupiers and tenants

The Housing Renovation, etc. Grants (Reduction of Grant) Regulations 1994 made under section 109 of the Act, provides for the determination of the financial resources and applicable amount (the assessment of needs and outgoings) in respect of applications for renovation grant or disabled facilities grant. Where an applicant's financial resources exceed the applicable amount, the regulations provide for a grant to be reduced by a sum equal to a notional 'affordable loan'. The regulations are also relevant to tenants' common parts applications, and to the determination of individual participant's contribution to the costs of group repair schemes.

The House Renovation Grant Limit Order – operative from January 1994 – restricts the upper limit for mandatory renovation grants to owners, tenants and landlords to £20 000.

Calculation of a grant for landlords

The amount of grant payable to landlords and charities is calculated in a different way from that payable to owner occupiers and tenants. Under section 110(2), local authorities are required to have regard to a number of matters:

1. the cost of the relevant works;
2. the amount of rent;
3. such other matters as the Secretary of State may direct.

In exercise of his powers under (3), the Secretary of State has directed that authorities shall take note of Annex B, section 2 of DoE circular 12/90, 5/91 and 7/93. These state that local authorities must have regard to the notional increase in rental income, which the relevant work would generate, to the amount of loan which would be raised from that increase over a 10-year repayment period at an interest rate of 3% above the bank base lending rate, and to the difference between the estimated expense and the amount of that loan. If the works are not expected to result in increased rental income, authorities are required to exercise discretion over the amount of grant paid to landlords. Each grant application must be examined on its merits and a blanket approach (such as the use of a standard percentage grant) avoided.

Rent officers are required to provide advice to local housing authorities by the Rent Officers (Additional Function) (No.2) Order 1990 (SI 1990 No.1068).

Common parts grant

The general framework for the operation of the grant is broadly as for renovation grants, but the detailed operation differs in a number of respects. A common parts grant application can normally only be made in respect of a building containing flats where at least three-quarters of those flats are occupied by 'occupying tenants'. An occupying tenant is a person who owns a flat (including a long leaseholder) or who is a tenant and whose flat is his or her only or main residence. There are two types of common parts grant application: the first is a landlord's application; the second is a tenant's application. For a landlord's application, the appropriate method of calculating a grant is the same as for any other landlord's application, and is governed by the provision of section 110. For tenants, the calculation of grant payable is based on the test of resources under section 109 – each applicant being individually tested in relation to his or her share of the cost of the works. The normal conditions as to the payment of a grant and completion of works apply to common parts grants, but there are no conditions as to the future occupation of a building. The repayment of a grant in the event of disposal of a building during the initial period applies to landlords' applications only.

Houses in multiple occupation (HMO) grant

The definition of an HMO for grant purposes is contained in section 100. It is the same as that contained in section 345 of the Housing Act 1985 – a house occupied by persons who do not form a single household – but excludes from the HMO any part of the house occupied as a separate dwelling by persons forming a single household. Further information on the definition and other aspects of HMOs is given in the DoE Circular 12/93 HMOs: Guidance on managing the stock.

An HMO grant is only payable to HMO landlords, and an applicant for a grant must provide an 'HMO certificate' stating that he or she has, or proposes to acquire, an owner's interest in the house in question (section 106(7)). A grant is calculated in the same way as other grants applied for by landlords, and is available towards eligible works required to make an HMO fit for human habitation, and for works to make it fit for the number of its occupants (section 352 (1A) of the 1985 Act as substituted by paragraph 49, schedule 9 of the 1989 Act). Fitness for the number of occupants relates to the provision of adequate cooking, food storage, washing and toilet facilities and to fire safety. DoE Circular 12/92 'HMOs: guidance on standards of fitness' gives comprehensive coverage of the subject matter. HMO grants are subject to the usual conditions as to the completion of works and payment of grant.

Disabled facilities grant

Section 101 of the 1989 Act provides for a 'disabled facilities grant' specifically for works to provide facilities and to carry out adaptations to dwellings, or to the common parts of buildings containing flats for the benefit of disabled people. Both mandatory and discretionary grants are available and DoE Circular 10/90, *House Adaptations for People with Disabilities* (HMSO, London), deals specifically with the subject. The works attracting mandatory disabled facilities grant are primarily aimed at facilitating access for the disabled person into and around his or her home, including access to or, in some cases, provisions of essential amenities such as toilets, bathroom and kitchen facilities, and adapting the controls of any heating, lighting or power supplies in order to make them suitable for use by the disabled occupant.

On receipt of an application, local housing authorities are required by section 114 to consult the appropriate welfare authority on whether the relevant works are 'necessary and appropriate' to meet the needs of the disabled person.

Group repair

Section 128 of the 1989 Act sets out the requirements which any group of buildings must fulfil in order to be included in a group repair scheme. Each scheme must have as its basis a 'primary building' which was constructed so as to include at least four separate houses. Additional 'qualifying buildings' may be added. No building may be included in a group repair scheme unless the whole or some part of its exterior envelope is not in reasonable repair, and the lack of reasonable repair has to affect at least 75% of the houses contained in the building. Paragraph 53 of the DoE Circular 12/90 states that for properties which are expected to have a long life, it would seem reasonable to allow for grant all repairs that would be likely to arise within a few years of the scheme, if not carried out as part of the scheme. Section 128(8) of the 1989 Act also adds that a building should not be regarded as being in reasonable repair unless the exterior is substantially free from rising or penetrating damp. Eligible works are limited to the exterior envelope of the building and associated works.

It is the responsibility of a local authority to initiate a group repair scheme, to make the necessary arrangements for the execution of, and payment for, the works required, and to collect contributions due from participants. No scheme can go ahead unless and until all participants have signified their agreement to take part (section 127). Authorities must undertake an economic appraisal of the options available to them, having regard to the advice set out in DoE Circulars 12/90, 5/91 and 7/93.

All the owners of properties included in a potential group repair scheme are eligible to participate as 'assisted' or 'unassisted' participants (section 127(3)). Unassisted participants who include local authorities, registered housing associations, etc., pay the full cost of the works; assisted participants in renewal areas are liable to contribute 25%, and those outside 50% of the costs of the work. Assisted participants, however, may be eligible for a reduction in the amount of their own contribution, possibly covering the full cost of the works by applying the appropriate test of resources (section 129(6)).

Annex B of DoE Circular 12/90 sets out the criteria specified in accordance with the provision of section 127(2), and any scheme which fulfils these criteria does not have to be submitted to the Secretary of State for approval. There may be circumstances where a scheme might be justified without satisfying the criteria. Such schemes should be submitted to the Secretary of State enclosing:

1. a plan showing the relevant properties;
2. a report on the proposed works;
3. detailed costings;
4. an appraisal of alternative courses of action considered;
5. justification for those aspects in which the scheme fails to meet the required criteria.

Section 130(2) of the Act requires a local authority to clawback a part of the costs if an assisted participant disposes of property within 3 years of completion of the scheme.

Minor works assistance

DoE Circular 4/90 give comprehensive guidance. Minor works assistance is intended to complement the mainstream grants available in the 1989 Act. It is primarily designed to streamline assistance with repairs and improvements to properties upon which only small scale work is required.

Section 131 of the Act (as amended) enables local authorities to provide minor works assistance by grant or provision of materials for:

1. the provision or improvement of thermal insulation;

2. works of repair to properties included in a clearance area or intended to be so included within 12 months;
3. repair, improvement or adaptation of a dwelling whose owner or tenant is 60 years old or more;
4. adaptation of a dwelling to enable a person who is 60 years old or more, and who is not an owner or tenant of the dwelling but is or proposes to be a resident, to be cared for
5. replacement of lead water service pipes.

Assistance cannot be given for works included in any other grant application under Part VIII of the Act. Help is available to an applicant who:

6. is wholly or mainly resident in the dwelling; and
7. has a sole or joint owner's interest in, or is a sole or joint tenant (i.e. private sector or housing association tenant) of the dwelling; and
8. is (or whose spouse is) in receipt of Income Support, or Council Tax Benefit, Family Credit or Disability Working Allowance; and
9. if the works are for the purpose set out in (3) and (4) above is 60 years old or more.

The total value of grant or other assistance given on any one application may not exceed £1080. More than one application can be submitted in respect of the same dwelling, but the total amount approved may not exceed £3240 in any 3-year period.

Full details are contained in the Assistance for Minor Works to Dwellings Regulation 1993 made under sections 131(3) and 137(2) of the Act and summarized in DoE Circular 4/90 and 7/93.

In 1991 the Energy Action Grants Agency introduced the Department of Energy's Home Energy Efficiency Scheme (HEES). This scheme is set up under the provision of section 15 of the Social Security Act 1990. Grants for loft, tank and pipe insulation, draughtproofing and energy advice are available to householders who are in receipt of specified benefits. As these grants are also available under Minor Works Assistance, HEES activity should be taken into account in local authority grant strategies.

Assistance for owners

The powers contained in section 169 of the Local Government and Housing Act 1989 enable local housing authorities to provide technical, professional and administrative services to assist owners to carry out relevant works. Works are relevant if they:

1. cause the dwelling to be fit for human habitation;
2. are eligible for a disabled facilities grant;
3. are eligible for a discretionary grant other than one for common parts (see section 115(3));
4. the works are for any of the purposes for which a common parts grant is available.

If the authority provides any assistance, it must decide whether to charge for it.

RENEWAL AREAS

The intention behind the provisions in the Local Government and Housing Act 1989 is to focus attention on the use of a new broader-based area strategy which includes environmental and socio-economic regeneration. The aim is to secure a reduction in the number of unfit houses whether by repair or demolition as part of such a strategy. Renovation grants and group repair schemes – linked as they are to the standard of fitness – should also form part of the strategy.

General Improvement Areas and Housing Action Areas, which were introduced by the 1969 and 1974 Housing Acts, provided a focus for local authorities' renewal strategies until the Local Government and Housing Act 1989 repealed them and introduced a new statutory concept of renewal areas (RAs). The Act encourages local authorities to assess the need for clearance and renovation on a systematic and area basis, and to declare RAs where concentrated action is required.

Section 89 of the Local Government and Housing Act 1989 states that a local authority, when being satisfied that:

1. the living conditions in an area are unsatisfactory, and

2. the conditions can best be dealt with by declaring the area to be a renewal area,

may pass a resolution declaring it to be so.

In order to satisfy themselves of (1) and (2) above, the authority needs to consider a report which it has commissioned, including particulars of the undermentioned matters:

1. living conditions in the area;
2. the ways in which the conditions may be improved;
3. the powers available to the authority if the area is to be declared an RA;
4. detailed proposals for the exercise of those powers;
5. the cost of the proposals;
6. the financial resources available;

and the report must contain a recommendation with reasons as to whether an RA should be declared.

Neighbourhood renewal assessments

In preparing the report, a local authority should base its decisions on the results of neighbourhood renewal assessment (NRA) on which detailed guidance is given in Annex B of DoE Circular 6/90.

The assessment process in Annex B includes:

1. an initial decision that areas of private sector housing could benefit from being declared an RA;
2. an approximate definition of the area;
3. setting up a core team of officers;
4. establishing aims and objectives;
5. generating options which should incorporate the view of members, residents, community groups, businesses, etc.;
6. information gathering from an environmental and housing survey and surveys of residents, landlords, commercial users, etc.;
7. an economic assessment of the various options;
8. options appraisal.

The success of the NRA process requires a corporate approach from the local authority. RAs are not just about housing, and an authority will need to consider the full range of disciplines that should be included in the assessment team. The NRA process is based on a series of logical steps which, when taken together, provide a thorough and systematic appraisal for considering alternative courses of action in an area. One of the main reasons for undertaking an NRA is to decide whether or not it is likely to be the right way of tackling a neighbourhood's problems.

The development and justification of a preferred strategy forms the crux of the NRA methodology, and it is essential that an authority should know exactly what it wants to achieve in an area, and why and how it can go about it before it embarks on the process and commitment of declaring a statutory RA.

Renewal area procedures

Before declaring an RA, a local authority must carry out the consulation and publicity set out in the direction at Annex E, paragraph 2 (section 89(5) of the Local Government and Housing Act 1989).

An area may not be declared to be an RA (Annex E, paragraph 3) without specific approval from the Secretary of State unless:

1. it contains a minimum of 300 dwellings;
2. 75% of the dwellings are in private ownership;
3. 75% of the dwellings are unfit, or could qualify for mandatory or discretionary grants;
4. 30% of the households in the area appear to be dependent to a significant extent on the receipt of specified social benefits.

The actions which a local authority is required to take after declaration of an RA are set out in sections 91, 92 and Annex E. Some of these need to be repeated at intervals not exceeding 2 years, in order to keep people in the area advised of progress.

The powers available to local authorities in RAs are contained in section 93 and Annex D to DoE Circular 6/90 and include:

1. acquisition of land and property
2. authority to carry out work or assist others to do so;

3. power to extinguish rights of way;
4. increased assistance to participants in group repair schemes

Under section 96(2), the Secretary of State can make contributions towards expenses incurred by local authorities under Part VII of the Act in carrying out environmental improvements. In Annex E, the Secretary of State has determined that the contribution shall not exceed 50% of the expenditure incurred based on a maximum eligible expense of £1000 per dwelling.

Matters eligible for contribution include:

1. street works;
2. landscaping
3. improvements to the exteriors and curtilage of dwellings;
4. community facilities;
5. miscellaneous environmental improvements.

The purpose in carrying out such work is for the authority to demonstrate its commitment to an area and its future, such that confidence will be increased and residents will be encouraged to invest in their own properties.

An RA will normally have a life of 10 years, and it is important that an authority should establish and implement monitoring and review procedures for the programme set at the start of the project.

HOUSES IN MULTIPLE OCCUPATION (HMOs)

Many households rely on HMOs to meet their accommodation needs. In 1985 the Department of the Environment commissioned a survey of HMOs which found, among other things, that housing in this sector was generally unsatisfactory: 'there are properties in poor physical condition, properties without adequate facilities and properties where the physical safety of tenants is at risk'. The survey highlighted particular shortcomings including:

1. poor standards of management;
2. lack of amenities;

3. defective or inadequate means of escape in case of fire;
4. poor repair.

The inhabitants of HMOs are often the more deprived members of society who either cannot, or choose not, to provide themselves with more adequate accommodation. The DoE survey also revealed that although the biggest concentrations of HMOs are in the inner cities and larger conurbations, over 40% are situated in the non-metropolitan districts.

Definition

The legislation covering HMOs is found principally in Part XI of the Housing Act 1985, as amended by Parts VII and VIII and Schedules 9 and 11 of the Local Government and Housing Act 1989. The Housing Act 1985 defined a house in multiple occupation as 'a house which is occupied by persons who do not form a single household', but this was extended by paragraph 44 of Schedule 9 of the 1989 Act to include a flat in multiple occupation. The term now encompasses any purpose-built or converted flat whose occupants do not form a single household. The CIEH has defined six categories of HMO:

1. houses divided into flats or bedsitters where some facilities are shared;
2. houses occupied on a shared basis where occupiers have rooms of their own;
3. lodging accommodation where resident landlords let rooms;
4. hostels, lodging houses and bed-and-breakfast hotels;
5. registered residential homes;
6. self-contained flats with common parts such as stairways.

Advice is also set out in DoE circular 12/93.

Registration*

Section 346 Housing Act 1985 allows local authorities to submit to the Minister for confirmation schemes or registration for houses in multiple occupation, which the minister may confirm with or without modification. Schemes may cover the whole or part only of the authority's administrative area and may include:

1. particulars to be kept in the register;
2. a restriction on the type of house in multiple occupation to be registered;
3. a requirement to register and notify any changes in registered particulars.

Local authorities can also exercise 'control provisions' whereby occupancy may be limited, and provision is also made for refusal or variation of registration where the authority considers the house in multiple occupation is unsuitable as the person managing the house is not thought to be a fit and proper person. Registration may also be conditional upon specified work being carried out.

Applications for registration or for variation not determined by the local authority within 5 weeks, are deemed to have been refused unless a longer period has been agreed in writing and appeal may be made to the County Court.

Regulations under section 150 of the Local Government and Housing Act 1989 empower local authorities for the first time to charge a fee for registering a property under a section 346 scheme. The fee is at the local authority's discretion, but is subject to a maximum charge. It is intended to cover the initial inspection and administrative costs of establishing the scheme, and should be set at a level no greater than that needed to fund the start up costs of the scheme. It is not annually renewable, nor is it intended to cover the general enforcement costs of action taken using Part XI powers.

Model schemes have been published by the DoE and advice on setting up an effective registration scheme can be found in DoE Circular 12/93. The procedure for submission and confirmation of schemes is described in DoE Circular 12/86.

* In November 1994 the Government issued a consultation paper on the Case for the Licensing of HMOs. This followed widespread concern over the generally poor condition of HMOs.

Standards of management

Problems can occur in multi-occupied houses, particularly in common areas and with shared facilities where no individual tenant has overall responsibility. Local authorities have powers to deal with unsatisfactory standards of management in order to tackle this problem. As from 1 July 1990, management regulations for HMOs made under section 369 of the Housing Act 1985 apply automatically to all HMOs. The Housing (Management of Houses in Multiple Occupation) Regulations 1990 make provision for ensuring that the person managing a house in multiple occupation observes proper standards of management.

Regulation 2 varies the definition of 'person managing' in section 398(6) of the Housing Act 1985, and that definition as so varied is used in these Regulations. The 'person managing' is referred to in the Regulations as 'the manager'.

The manager is required by the Regulations to ensure the repair, maintenance, cleansing or, as the case may be, good order of:

1. all means of water supply and drainage in the house (Regulation 4);
2. parts of the house and installations in common use (Regulations 6 and 7);
3. living accommodation (Regulation 8);
4. windows and other means of ventilation (Regulation 9);
5. means of escape from fire and apparatus, systems and other things provided by way of fire precautions (Regulation 10);
6. outbuildings, yards, etc. in common use (Regulation 11).

The manager is also required to:

1. make satisfactory arrangements for the disposal of refuse and litter from the house (Regulation 12);
2. ensure the taking of reasonable precautions for the general safety of residents (Regulation 13);
3. display in the house a notice of the name, address and telephone number, if any, of the manager (Regulation 14);

4. provide specified information to the local housing authority about the occupancy of the house where the authority gives him or her written notice to that effect (Regulation 15).

Regulation 16 imposes duties on persons who live in the house, for the purpose of ensuring that the manager can effectively carry out the duties imposed on him or her by the Regulations.

Under section 369(5) of the 1985 Act, knowingly to contravene, or to fail without reasonable excuse to comply with, any of these Regulations will be an offence punishable on summary conviction not exceeding level 3 on the standard scale.

Failure to comply with the Regulations is a criminal offence, and it is important that local authorities ensure that they are given extensive continuing publicity to allow those affected to make any necessary arrangements to check the management of their properties. Authorities should stress that the regulations are binding not only on managers, but also on the occupants, and that either could be liable for prosecution in the event of a breach. Enforcing authorities should also ensure that care is taken to establish where poor standards are due to management neglect or to misuse of the property by the occupants. Advice on the implementation of the regulations is given in the DoE Circulars 12/92 and 12/93.

Where a house does not comply with the management regulations, the local authority may serve on the manager a notice requiring him to execute any necessary work. The notice must specify dates for commencement and completion of the works (section 372 of the Housing Act 1985 as amended by Schedule 9 of the Housing and Local Government Act 1989). The commencement date must not be earlier than 21 days after the service of the notice. The time required for the work to be done must be reasonable, and the local authority may give written permission for this period to be extended. Any known owner or lessee must be informed of the notice.

As with repairs notices and section 352 notices, local authorities can serve notice of intention to carry out the remedial works themselves if reasonable progress is not being made, and recover their expenses under Schedule 10.

Any person served with a notice may appeal to the magistrates' court within 21 days on the grounds that:

1. the condition of the house did not justify the service of a notice;
2. there has been some material informality defect or error in connection with the notice;
3. the date specified for the beginning of the work is not reasonable;
4. the time allowed for doing the work is inadequate;
5. the works required are unreasonable in character or extent, or are unnecessary, or that the local authority has refused the execution of alternative works;
6. that some person, other than the appellant, is wholly or in part responsible for the state of affairs which necessitates the service of a notice, or will derive benefit from the work to be done as holder of an estate or interest in the premises.

HMOs – fitness standard for human habitation (section 604 Housing Act 1985 as amended)

The standard of fitness applies to HMOs by virtue of section 604(3) and (4) of the Housing Act 1985 as amended, and provides that an HMO is fit for human habitation unless, in the authority's opinion, it fails to meet one or more of the specified requirements in section 604(1) and by reason of that failure is not reasonably suitable for occupation.

Whether or not a house in multiple occupation which is a flat in multiple occupation satisfies those requirements, it is unfit for human habitation if, in the opinion of the local housing authority, the building or a part of the building outside the flat fails to comply with the requirements of section 604(2), and by reason of that failure the flat is not reasonably suitable for occupation.

Under section 604A of the 1985 Act, local housing authorities are required to consider the most satisfactory course of action for dealing with

such unfit HMOs in the context of Parts VI (repair notices) and IX (slum clearance), having regard to the statutory Code of Guidance for dealing with Unfit Premises (Annex H of DoE Circular 6/90). They are required to consider once a year the best means of discharging their functions under Part XI as under other Parts of the 1985 Act.

HMOs – standard of fitness for number of occupants (section 352 of the Housing Act 1985 as amended)*

Section 352 specifies the standard of fitness for the number of occupants of an HMO. An HMO does not meet the standard where in the authority's opinion it fails to meet one or more of the requirements mentioned below and, having regard to the number of occupants accommodated there, by reason of that failure it is not reasonably suitable for occupation by those occupants. The requirements are that the HMO has:

1. satisfactory facilities for the storage, preparation and cooking of food including an adequate number of sinks with a satisfactory supply of hot and cold water;
2. an adequate number of suitably located WCs for the exclusive use of occupants;
3. an adequate number of suitably located fixed baths or showers and wash hand basins, each provided with a satisfactory supply of hot and cold water for the exclusive use of the occupants;
4. adequate means of escape from fire; and
5. adequate other fire precautions.

Guidance on this new fitness standard for HMOs has been issued in DoE Circular 12/92.

Except in the instances referred to in the next paragraph, local authorities have the discretion to serve notice under section 352 as amended, to render the property fit for the number of occupants or take alternative action under section 354 – directions limiting the number of occupants.

---

* Also see 'Amenity Standards for HMOs', A Professional Practice Note. CIEH, September 1994.

Fire precautions

Section 352 enables an authority to require the installation of adequate other fire precautions, such as fire detection systems, fire warning systems and fire fighting equipment in appropriate circumstances, as well as means of escape. Where an HMO does not have adequate means of escape from fire, an authority may exercise its powers under section 368 – as amended by paragraph 55 of Schedule 9 – securing that part of an HMO is not used for human habitation as an alternative to the provision of a means of escape. However, for properties of at least three storeys high and 500 m^2 in floor space (Statutory Instrument 1981/1576) a local authority is obligated to exercise one of these powers.

The Secretary of State has the power in section 365(2A) to provide by order that an authority shall not exercise its powers under section 352 or section 368 in respect of a failure to provide adequate means of escape to specified categories of property. This power could be used where there was evidence that a local authority was concentrating on smaller properties where the risk was low at the expense of larger ones where the risk was greater.

Fire warning systems can make a valuable contribution to preserving life by giving people an early indication of a fire on the premises. Details of such systems for hostel type accommodation and houses converted into self-contained dwelling units are contained in DOE Circular 12/92. The circular provides an aid to the process of consultation between housing and fire authorities which is required by section 365(3) as amended.

If a local authority considers that there is a serious risk to life in the event of fire and is unable to take suitable action under housing legislation, it can ask the fire authority to use its limited prohibition powers under section 10 of the Fire Precautions Act 1971.

In the case of a multi-occupied flat, works – including means of escape – necessary under section 352 may only be required within the flat itself, and cannot be specified in respect of parts of the building outside the flat. If a flat is not large enough to accommodate the necessary work, then local authorities should consider the use of a Direction Order under section 354.

HMO notices

The single prescribed HMO notice can be used either where an authority decides that serving a repair notice under section 189 (unfitness for human habitation) is the most satisfactory course of action, or where work is required under section 352 (fitness for number of occupants), or both. The notice can be served on the person having control, or on the person managing the house.

Section 352(4) empowers the authority to specify dates for commencement and completion of works. The grounds of appeal are similar to those following service of a notice under section 372 of the Housing Act 1985 as amended.

The process for enforcing HMO notices is similar to the process for repairs notices under section 189 as amended by Schedule 15 of the Housing Act 1988 (DoE and Welsh Office Circular 1/89). Section 352 notices are local land charges thereby giving notice to subsequent owners that a notice requiring the carrying out of works has been served, and that new notices do not need to be served following a change of ownership.

The Housing Act 1985 generally requires an authority to inform owners and lessees of a property of action which it is taking on that property. The Local Government and Housing Act 1989 imposed three new requirements in respect of section 352 notices:

1. all occupants of the house must be informed when notices are served;
2. local authorities must keep a register of the notices served and make it available for public inspection;
3. local authorities must supply copies of notices, on request, to members of the public and may charge a reasonable fee for doing so.

Where no appeal is lodged against the reasonableness of the start date specified in section 352 or section 372 notices, work should be completed no later than the designated final date. If however, before this final date the local authority considers that reasonable progress is not being made towards compliance, it may decide to do the work itself. It must give the owner or recipient of the original notice not less than 7 days warning of its intention. The provisions of Schedule 10 of the Housing Act 1985 as amended apply where such notice is served, including where the work is then carried out by persons other than the authority, or someone appointed by the authority. Paragraph 13(3) of Schedule 15 to the 1988 Act introduced a ground of appeal where an authority undertakes work because reasonable progress is not being made. The appellant can argue that expenses should not be recovered because reasonable progress was being made. The right of appeal is only exercisable after the works have been completed.

Expenses are recoverable from the person having control of, or managing, an HMO at the time the demand for expenses is made. Paragraph 70(4) of Schedule 9 of the Local Government and Housing Act 1989 enables authorities to sequester rents in order to recoup the cost of works in default.

It is an offence for a person served with an HMO notice or a notice under section 372 to maintain proper standards of management willfully to fail to comply with the requirements of the notice. The maximum penalty on conviction is a fine not exceeding level 4 on the standards scale (section 37 of the Criminal Justice Act 1982).

HMO owners are entitled to a grant under section 113 of the Local Government and Housing Act 1989 where notice is served under sections 189, 190 or 352 of the 1985 Act to bring an HMO up to the fitness standards under both section 604 and 352 of the 1985 Act. Entitlement is subject to a test of resources. Grant remains discretionary when work is completed without service of a notice.

Direction to prevent or reduce overcrowding

As an alternative to or in conjunction with requiring work under section 352 of the Housing Act 1985, a local authority can issue a direction under section 354 limiting the number of occupants in an HMO. The direction may either:

1. specify a maximum number of individuals or households or both able to occupy the house in its existing condition; or
2. in conjunction with a notice requiring work to make the house fit for multi-occupation, specify the maximum number able to occupy the house after completion of the work.

The direction imposes an obligation on the occupier or any other person entitled to permit persons to take up residence:

1. to ensure that no person takes up residence to increase the number living there above the limit set; or
2. if the number already exceeds the limit, not to permit the number to increase further.

At least 7 days before giving a direction, a local authority must serve notice of its intention on the owner and all known lessees, and also post a notice in a part of the house accessible to all those living there. The person on whom the notice is served may make representation to the local authority, and the local authority must within 7 days of giving the direction, serve a copy on the owner and lessees and post a copy in the house.

A local authority may revoke or vary a direction upon application of any person having an interest or estate in the premises after having regard to any changed circumstances. If a local authority refuse an application for revocation, etc., or do not within 35 days of the making of the application notify the applicant of its decision, the applicant can appeal to the County Court.

At any time while a direction is in force, a local authority may serve on the occupier of an HMO notice requiring him or her to furnish within 7 days a statement showing the names and numbers of the people living in the premises and the rooms they occupy.

Overcrowding notices

Section 354 of the Housing Act 1985 deals with overcrowding in HMOs only as far as the number of occupants relates to the standard of fitness for multi-occupation, but further overcrowding provisions are included in sections 358 to 364.

In this case, if it appears to a local authority that an excessive number of persons is, or is likely to be, accommodated having regard to the rooms available, it must serve a notice on the occupier and/or person having control. The notice must state the maximum number of persons permitted to occupy each room for sleeping accommodation at any one time, or indicate that a particular room cannot be used for this purpose. The numbers to be fixed here are at the discretion of each authority, and will depend upon that authority's own housing circumstances.

Having specified the permitted occupancy, the notice can then require that either:

1. sleeping accommodation shall not be arranged other than in accordance with the overcrowding notice and in such a way that persons of opposite sexes over the age of 12 (other than husband and wife) do not share the same sleeping accommodation; or
2. that new residents will not occupy sleeping accommodation other than in accordance with the notice and in such a way that persons of opposite sexes over 12 share the same room.

Before serving the notice, the local authority must give 7 days notice to the occupier and person having control, and ensure as far as possible that each resident is informed of its intention giving an opportunity for representation to be made. Appeals against an overcrowding notice may be made to the County Court within 21 days by any person aggrieved, and the authority may at any time revoke or vary it so as to allow more people to be accommodated (but not less).

In order to determine the number of persons occupying the house at any time, the local authority may require the occupier to provide a written statement within 7 days specifying the mode of occupation. The local authority may on the application of a person having an interest or estate in the premises, revoke or vary the notice so as to allow more people to be accommodated. If such an application is refused or no decision is made within 35 days the applicant may appeal to the County Court.

It is an offence to fail to comply with an overcrowding notice (maximum fine not exceeding level 4 on the standard scale), or to fail to reply to a requisition or to knowingly give false information (maximum fine level 2 on the standard scale).

Control orders (sections 379–394 of the Housing Act 1985)

A local authority may make a control order in respect of a house in multiple occupation where they are satisfied that:

1. a notice has been or could be served under section 352 of the Housing Act 1985 as amended requiring works to make the house fit for the number of individuals or households in the house; or
2. a notice has been or could be served under section 372 requiring works to make good neglected standards of management; or
3. a direction has been or could be given under section 354 limiting the number of individuals or households to be accommodated

and living conditions in the house are such that an order is necessary to protect the safety, health or welfare of the residents.

A control order comes into force when it is made and, as soon as possible afterwards, the local authority must do what is necessary to protect the health, welfare and safety of the occupants, and must maintain proper standards of management.

As soon as possible after making the order, a copy of it, together with notices setting out the grounds for making the order, the effect of it and indicating the right of appeal, must be:

1. posted in the house; and
2. served on the person having control of the house and on any owner, lessee or mortgagee.

Compensation is payable quarterly to a dispossessed proprietor. After the order has been made, the local authority must prepare a management scheme and within 8 weeks after the order comes

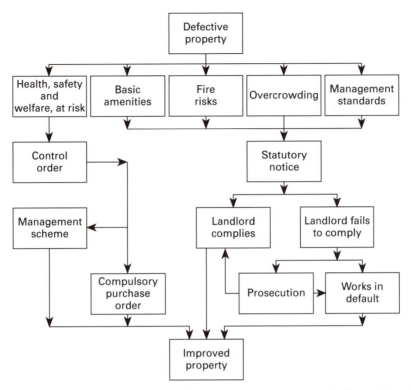

Fig. 20.3 Enforcement action on houses in multiple occupancy. (Source: Audit Commission (1991) *Healthy Housing: the role of environmental health services*, HMSO, London.)

into force serve a copy of it on the dispossessed proprietor, on the owner, lessee or mortgagee, and on any person who received a copy of the control order.

The scheme must give:

1. Particulars of works involving capital expenditure which the local authority would require under the Housing Act 1985, or other housing or public health legislation.
2. An estimate of the cost of carrying out the works.
3. The highest number of people or households which should live in the house from time to time, as works progress.
4. An estimate of the balances which, from time to time, will accrue to the local authority from the rent received after deducting compensation payable to the dispossessed proprietor and all expenditure (other than capital expenditure) and establishment charges.

A local authority may at any time vary the payment of surpluses on revenue account so as to increase them.

While the control order is in force, the local authority must keep full accounts in respect of the house and afford the dispossessed proprietor facilities for examining the account and inspecting the house.

If a control order is made in respect of furnished accommodation, the right to possession of the furniture will vest in the local authority for the time during which the order remains in force, and the authority may on written application by the owner of the furniture renounce its right to possession by giving him 2 weeks' notice. A local authority may fit out, furnish and supply a house subject to a control order with such furniture, fittings and conveniences as appear to be required.

At any time after the making of the order, but not less than 6 weeks from the date of the service of the copy of the scheme, a person having an estate or interest in the house or any other person who may be prejudiced by the making of the order may appeal to the County Court against the order.

Within 6 weeks from the date on which a copy of the scheme is served, any person having an estate or interest in the house may appeal to the County Court on the grounds set out in section 386(2) and Schedule 13 paragraph 3(1).

A control order ceases to have effect at the expiration of 5 years beginning with the date it came into force, but the local authority may on an application or on its own initiative revoke the order. The local authority must give at least 21 days' notice to occupiers, owners, lessees and mortgagees of its intention to revoke an order.

Within 28 days of the making of a control order, a local housing authority may make a compulsory purchase order for the acquisition of the premises under Part II of the 1985 Act. The duty to prepare and serve a management scheme is then suspended until the authority has been notified of the Secretary of State's decision.

The various forms of enforcement action on HMOs are illustrated in Fig. 20.3.

Other statutory powers

In respect of HMOs Housing Act legislation will nearly always be the most appropriate. However, there are certain instances when other statutory powers should be used to effect repairs and improvements. These powers include:

1. The statutory nuisance provisions contained in sections 79–81 of the Environmental Protection Act 1990.
2. The Health and Safety at Work Etc. Act 1974.
3. The dangerous building and drainage powers of the Building Act 1984 and Public Health Act 1961.
4. The Fire Precaution Act 1971.
5. Section 33 of the Local Government (Miscellaneous Provisions) Act 1976.

OVERCROWDING

The present overcrowding standards were first set down in the Housing Act 1935, and were re-enacted in 1985 despite the Minister of Health's statement when introduced over 50 years ago that:

> It is relevant to point out that the standard does not represent any ideal standard of housing, but the minimum which is in the view of Parliament desirable while at the same time capable of early enforcement.

Nevertheless, according to recent figures [3], under-occupation is considerably more widespread with overcrowding constituting only a small residual problem.

It should be noted that this section on overcrowding deals with the number of persons who may sleep in the space available in a dwelling house. Sections 354–357 of the Housing Act 1985 are referred to in the section on multi-occupation, where the number of occupants can be restricted having regard to the standard of fitness specified in section 352 as amended.

Where it appears to a local authority that there is need to prepare a report on overcrowding in its district or part of its district, or if the Secretary of State so directs, a survey must be made and details submitted to the Secretary of State on any proposal for providing new dwellings.

Overcrowding standards

The 1985 Act contains two principal overcrowding standards, both of which must be satisfied by all dwellings. These are:

1. proper separation of the sexes; and
2. the number and floor areas of the rooms.

The Act stipulates that a dwelling is overcrowded when the number of persons sleeping there:

1. is such that any two of those persons being 10 years old or more of opposite sexes and not living together as husband and wife must sleep in the same room (section 325); or
2. is in relation to the number and floor area of the rooms of which the house consists in excess of the permitted number of persons as defined in section 326.

In determining the number of persons sleeping in a house for the purpose of section 326, no account is taken of a child under 1 year old and a child between 1 and 10 is reckoned as one half of one unit.

The age limit set in (1) above is arbitrary and not based on a view of sexual maturity. The 1985 Act also deals with separation of the sexes at 8 years of age in the case of a local authority's own lodging houses (section 23(3)) and 12 years of age in multi-occupied premises (section 360(2)). In addition, in the case of common lodging houses the age of separation of the sexes is left to the discretion of the local authority (section 406), and for canal boats it is 12 years for females and 14 years for males (Canal Boat Regulations 1878 S.I. 1978 No.1878).

For the purpose of sections 325 and 326, the following definitions apply:

1. Section 343 'Dwelling' means any premises used or suitable for use as a separate dwelling. Under this definition any room – or part of a house – sublet to a tenant and occupied separately by him or her as a dwelling, constitutes a separate 'dwelling house'.
2. 'Room' does not include any room of a type not normally used in the locality, either as a living room or as a bedroom. Under this definition, in ordinary circumstances, rooms used as kitchens, sculleries, etc., must be excluded from calculations made under section 326.

Section 326 states that for the purposes of Part IV of the Act, the expression 'the permitted number of persons' means, in relation to any dwelling house, either:

1. the number specified in the second column of Table I in the Annex below in relation to a house consisting of the number of rooms of which that house consists; or
2. the aggregate for all the rooms in the house obtained by reckoning, for each room therein of the floor area specified in the first column of Table II in the Annex below, the number specified in the second column of that Table in relation to that area, whichever is the less:

provided that in computing for the purposes of the said Table I the number of rooms in a house, no regard shall be had to any room having a floor area of less than 50 sq ft.

The maximum or 'permitted' number of persons who may occupy any dwelling house is calculated from the two tables.

ANNEX

Table I		Table II	
Where a house consists of		Where the floor area of a room is	
1. one room	2	1. 110 sq ft or more	2
2. two rooms	3	2. 90 sq ft or more, but less than 110 sq ft	1½
4. four rooms	7½	3. 70 sq ft or more, but less than 90 sq ft	1
5. five rooms or more with an additional two in respect of each room in excess of five	10	4. 50 sq ft or more, but less than 70 sq ft	½
		6. under 50 sq ft	nil

Taking as an example a house of four rooms, the floor areas of which are, say, approximately 120, 100, 80 and 60 sq ft respectively, the permitted number of occupants under Table I would be 7½. Under Table II it would be 5; i.e. the rooms 120 sq ft – 2; 100 sq ft – 1½; 80 sq ft – 1; 60 sq ft – ½. As the number computed under Table II is the lower, viz. 5, this would be 'the permitted number of persons' who might occupy the house.

This standard is not satisfactory, and many authorities consider that a bedroom standard would be preferable to the prescribed general room standard, since under these present provisions all living rooms in addition to bedrooms are taken as being capable of providing sleeping accommodation.

Under section 330, licences to exceed the permitted number of a dwelling may be granted by a local authority to take account of exceptional circumstances. A licence remains in force for a maximum period of 12 months.

Rent book information

Section 4 of the Landlord and Tenant Act 1985 requires a landlord to provide a rent book for tenants whose rent is payable on a weekly basis. The rent book is required to state:

1. the name and address of the landlord (section 5 of the Landlord and Tenant Act 1985);
2. a summary of sections 324–331 of the Housing Act 1985 in the prescribed format; and
3. the permitted number of people that can live in the dwelling.

Occupiers must produce their rent books for inspection by any duly authorized officer. Local authorities must, upon application of the landlord or of the occupier, inform the applicant in writing of the permitted number of persons who may occupy the house.

Overcrowding notices

It is the duty of the local authority to enforce the provisions of the Act relating to overcrowding in dwelling houses in their districts (section 339). In such cases, the local authority may serve upon the occupier a notice requiring that the overcrowding be abated within 14 days and, if at any time within 3 months from the end of that time the dwelling is occupied by the same occupier or a member of his or her family and is overcrowded, the local authority may apply to the County Court for possession. On application, the Court must order possession be given to the landlord within a period of between 14 and 28 days.

The local authority may serve notice on the occupier of a dwelling requiring him or her within 14 days to provide a written statement of the number, ages and sexes of the persons sleeping in the dwelling. The situations under which the occupier and the landlord are guilty of committing an offence by causing or permitting a dwelling to be overcrowded are set out in sections 327 and 331 respectively of the Housing Act 1985.

Measurement of rooms

Rules for the measurement of rooms, etc., are laid down in the Housing Act (Overcrowding and Miscellaneous Forms) Regulations 1937 and state that:

1. measures are to be taken at floor level and to the back of any projecting skirting boards;
2. any part of the floor over which the ceiling height is less than 5 ft must be excluded;
3. the area covered by fixed cupboards or chimney breasts and within the area of any bay is to be included.

Other overcrowding provisions

1. A tent, van or shed or similar structure used for human habitation which is so overcrowded as to be 'prejudicial to the health of the inmates' is a statutory nuisance for the purposes of Part III of the Public Health Act 1936, section 268.
2. Common lodging houses – power to make bye-laws (section 406 of the Housing Act 1985). See also DoE Circular 12/86 (Welsh Office 23/86) paragraph 4.7.
3. Hop, fruit or vegetable picking – power to make bye-laws (section 270 of the Public Health Act 1936).
4. Canal boats – duty of the Secretary of State to make regulations (section 49 of the Public Health (Control of Disease) Act 1984).
5. Houses owned and managed by a local authority – power of an authority to make bye-laws for management, use and regulation.

THE LAW OF LANDLORD AND TENANT

Action by local authorities to improve conditions in the private housing sector can cause friction and disagreement between landlord and tenant. An officer carrying out a routine housing inspection of a tenanted dwelling needs to have some knowledge of the law of harassment and illegal eviction, and also of the various types of tenancies that exist. Local authorities should develop effective corporate policies to ensure that any action they take does not undermine a tenant's position, and that procedures are in place to deal promptly with harassment and threats of eviction.

Harassment

The law protects people living in residential accommodation from harassment and illegal eviction in two ways. Firstly, by making both a criminal offence and, secondly, by enabling someone who is harassed or illegally evicted to claim damages through the civil court. The law against harassment applies to all people living in residential property; it applies to them whether they have tenancies or licences, and it applies to the acts of anybody acting on behalf of a landlord, and, in some cases, to people who may or may not be connected with a landlord.

The Protection from Eviction Act 1977 as amended by the Housing Act 1988 makes it an offence to:

1. do acts likely to interfere with the peace or comfort of a tenant or anyone living with him or her; or
2. persistently withdraw or withhold services for which the tenant has a reasonable need to live in the premises as a home.

It is an offence to do either of the above having reasonable cause to believe that they would cause the tenant to leave his or her home or stop using part of it, or stop doing the things a tenant should normally expect to be able to do. It is also an offence to take someone's home away from him unlawfully. A conviction can lead to a fine and/or imprisonment.

In housing terms, harassment can cover a wide range of activities. It can take many forms short of physical violence, and it may not always be obvious to others that particular sorts of activity are intended to drive the tenant from the property.

The undermentioned are examples of harassment:

1. withdrawal of services like gas, electricity, water;
2. withholding keys;
3. anti-social behaviour by a landlord or his or her agent;
4. removing a tenant's belongings;
5. entering the tenant's accommodation without permission;
6. threatening language or behaviour;
7. failing to complete repairs.

Illegal eviction

A landlord normally cannot enforce his right to get his property back from a residential tenant or, in many cases, a licensee unless he does it through the courts. A landlord seeking possession from a periodic residential tenant (other than a tenant under the Housing Act 1988) or licensee must generally serve a written notice to quit giving at least 4 weeks' notice. A landlord seeking possession from an assured tenant under the Housing Act 1988 must tell the tenant of his intention to start court proceedings by serving a notice on him. Depending on the grounds on which the landlord is seeking possession, the period of notice will either be 2 weeks or 2 months, except in a few cases where the tenancy agreement allows for longer notice. The tenant is not required to leave the property until the notice expires and even then may not be evicted without an order of the court.

The Housing Act 1988 makes it a general requirement for a licensor to obtain a court order before he can evict a licensee. However, certain licences and tenancies are excluded from this requirement. They are broadly licences or tenancies granted on or after 15 January 1989:

1. by resident landlords to people with whom they or a member of the landlord's family share accommodation;
2. to trespassers;
3. to those occupying a property for a holiday or rent-free;
4. licences granted to the people living in certain publicly funded hostels.

However, although it is not necessary to get a court order to evict someone in the excluded categories, there is a common law requirement for a landlord to serve a periodic tenant with notice equivalent to the period of the tenancy. This means, for example, that if the tenancy was from month to month, the landlord must give a month's notice. (In the case of yearly tenancies, he must give 6 months' notice). At common law, a licensee must be given notice which is reasonable in all the circumstances.

Forms of tenure

The Housing Act 1988 created new forms of letting: the assured and assured shorthold tenancy, and the assured agricultural occupancy. These are now the standard forms of letting to new private tenants. However, tenants who were living in their present home before 15 January 1989, as well as tenants in unfurnished accommodation provided by a resident landlord under an agreement made before 14 August 1974, may very well have a regulated tenancy under the Rent Act 1977.

An **assured tenancy** is the standard form of tenancy for most new residential lettings made between private landlords and their tenants on or after 15 January 1989. A tenant cannot have an assured tenancy of a property which is not let as a separate dwelling, nor his or her only or main home.

Some new lettings will be assured shorthold tenancies. Although a shorthold tenancy is a form of assured tenancy, the rules, particularly about possession, are in some ways different.

An assured tenancy may be written, or there may be no written agreement, just a spoken agreement between the people concerned. They will agree the rent and other terms of the tenancy, such as whether the tenant may sublet, at the beginning. That rent will be whatever the landlord and tenant agree. The tenant will have long-term security of tenure, and he does not have to leave unless he wishes to go, or unless the landlord has grounds for regaining possession which he can prove in court.

The tenancy may in the first place be for a fixed number of months or years – a **fixed-term tenancy**. Or it may be granted for an indefinite period with payment of rent being made on a weekly or monthly (or other periodic) basis: this is a **contractual periodic tenancy**. If the tenancy is a fixed-term tenancy, when the term ends, the landlord and the tenant may agree to another fixed term, or to a periodic tenancy. If they do

not, then a periodic tenancy arises automatically. This type of tenancy is known as a **statutory periodic tenancy**.

If the tenant has a fixed-term tenancy, the agreement will normally provide:

1. either for the rent to be fixed for the length of the term; or
2. for it to increase one or more times, at regular intervals on a specified basis during the term.

If the tenancy is a contractual periodic tenancy, the landlord may propose a rent increase under the formal statutory procedure to take effect 1 year after the tenancy started, and at yearly intervals after the first increase.

If the tenancy is a statutory periodic tenancy, the landlord may propose a rent increase under the formal statutory procedure to take effect on the ending of the fixed term after which the statutory tenancy came into being, and at yearly intervals after the first increase.

He must propose the increase on a prescribed form, copies of which can be obtained from law stationers. He must give the tenant at least a month's notice if the period of the tenancy is monthly or less. If the period of the tenancy is more than a month, he must give the tenant notice equivalent to the period.

If the tenant agrees with the proposed increase, he need do nothing. It will take effect on the date specified in the notice. If the landlord and tenant mutually decide to come to some other arrangement as regards rent, they may do so. If the tenant does not agree with the proposed increase, he may refer the rent to the rent assessment committee. He must do this within 3 months.

The rent assessment committee is a body of independent people, some of whom have legal, surveying or other property or relevant expertise, and some of whom are lay people who have been appointed by the Lord Chancellor and the Secretary of State.

A **shorthold tenancy** is a kind of assured tenancy which offers the landlord a guaranteed right to repossess his property at the end of the tenancy. He does not have to prove one of the grounds described above. It has the following important features:

1. a first shorthold tenancy must be for a fixed period of at least 6 months;
2. the landlord must serve notice in a prescribed form before the tenancy is entered into that it will be a shorthold tenancy;
3. he must serve at least 2 months' notice to bring the tenancy to an end. It may have to be longer if the period of the tenancy is longer. Also, he could bring it to an end at 2 weeks' notice if he was relying on certain possession grounds.

The landlord and tenant can freely agree the rent and the other terms of the tenancy between them. However, the tenant does have the right in certain circumstances to refer the rent to the assessment committee, which is relevant if he is paying more than the market rent for the property concerned.

When the initial fixed term of the tenancy comes to an end, if the landlord has not served notice that he must leave, the tenant may stay in the property. Unless a new tenancy is agreed, a statutory periodic shorthold tenancy can arise. The landlord may at any time after the fixed term serve 2 months' notice (or longer in certain cases) to recover possession if he wishes: but the agreement can continue indefinitely if it suits both parties. The tenant will have certain rights to go to the rent assessment committee, like other assured tenants.

A tenant who is not able to afford the rent which he and a landlord agree between them for a property may be eligible for housing benefit towards that rent.

Most residential lettings by non-resident private landlords which began before 15 January 1989 will be **regulated tenancies** under the Rent Act 1977. It does not matter whether the letting is furnished or unfurnished. A few new lettings made after this date will also be regulated tenancies. A regulated tenant has certain important rights concerning the amount of rent he can be charged and security of tenure:

1. the landlord cannot evict the tenant unless he gets a possession order from the courts;
2. if the tenant dies, his spouse will normally take over the regulated tenancy – a family member who has been living in the home can take over an assured tenancy;
3. either the landlord or the tenant can apply to the rent officer for a fair rent to be registered;
4. once a rent is registered, it is the maximum the landlord can charge until it is reviewed or cancelled;
5. even if a rent is not registered, the landlord can only increase the rent in certain circumstances;
6. the landlord is usually responsible for major repairs;
7. the landlord, or in some cases the tenant, can ask the local authority for a grant towards certain repairs and improvements.

Some lettings will not be a tenancy but a 'licence to occupy'; e.g. where all the accommodation is shared with someone occupying it under a separate agreement or where the occupier has to live there because of his job. Licensees generally have fewer rights than tenants. The distinction between licences and tenancies is not straightforward. The exact position depends on the term of the agreement.

Bringing tenancies to an end

A landlord can get possession of his property from an assured tenant by serving notice that he wishes to have his property back and by going to Court. However landlords seeking possession of properties on shorthold or assured lettings from tenants unlikely to have a defence do not need to go to Court. The landlord must provide written evidence to support his claim and this must be served on the tenant at the outset of the proceedings. A judge decides whether to order possession on the basis of the papers.

In the case of a regulated tenancy the landlord must get a possession order from the Court before the tenant can be made to leave. This applies even if the tenancy agreement has come to an end. Possession can only be sought on one of the 19 grounds specified in the 1977 Rent Act.

Licensees have very limited security of tenure. If the landlord requires possession he need only serve a notice to quit. At least 4 weeks' notice normally has to be given. If the licensee does not move out the landlord still usually needs a Court Order.

Local authority powers to take legal proceedings

Where a local authority considers it expedient for the promotion of protection of the interest of the inhabitants of its area, it may prosecute or defend or appear in any legal proceedings, and in the case of civil proceedings may institute them in its own name (Local Government Act 1972 section 222). This power is used by district councils to take proceedings on behalf of tenants in relation to harassment and illegal eviction etc.

Implied and expressed condition of tenancy

Section 8 of the Landlord and Tenant Act 1985 provides that in contracts for the letting of certain small houses for human habitation, there are statutory implied terms to the effect that the house is at the commencement of its tenancy and during its continuance fit for human habitation. Subsection (1) of this section details the small houses to which the section applies which depends on the date the contract was made, the location of the house, the local authority, and the rent at which it is let.

The same implied condition of fitness and undertaking applies to the letting of houses to workmen engaged in agriculture as part of their remuneration or wages (section 9). The term 'house' in the above section includes part of a house.

Sections 11–17 impose burdens on landlords of dwellings subject to short tenancies, i.e. less than 7 years, where there are no specific repairing obligations on either side. The conditions implied as a landlord obligation are:

1. To keep in repair the structure and exterior of the dwelling house including drains, gutters and external pipes.
2. To keep in repair and proper working order the installations in the dwelling house:
   (a) for the supply of water, gas and electricity and for sanitation but not for the fixtures,

fittings and appliances for making use of the supply of water, gas or electricity; and
   (b) for space heating or heating water.

Section 14 limits the application of these provisions by excluding from them new leases granted to specified educational institutions, other specified bodies, housing associations, local authorities and the Crown, other than to the Crown Estate Commissioners.

Duty of care

Section 1 of the Defective Premises Act 1972 imposes a duty on persons building new dwellings, or converting or enlarging existing dwellings, to see that the work is done in a workmanlike or professional manner, with use of proper materials and so that the dwelling will be fit for human habitation upon completion. Section 2 excludes certain situations from the duty imposed in section 1 including where the building is undertaken with the benefit of a scheme approved by the Secretary of State, e.g. schemes approved by the National House Builders Registration Council.

Section 3 provides that the duty of care owed to persons who might reasonably be expected to be affected by defects in the condition of any premises arising from works or construction, repair, maintenance or demolition shall not be abated by the subsequent disposal of the premises by the person who owed the duty.

Section 4 imposes a duty of care on landlords for defects in the state of a premises which he or she has let under a tenancy where he or she has an obligation or right to remedy such defects.

Restoration of services to houses

Section 33 of the Local Government (Miscellaneous Provisions) Act 1976, (as amended), deals with the restoration or continuation of supply of water, gas and electricity, and allows a district or London borough council, at the written request of the occupier, to make such arrangements as it thinks fit with the undertakers for the supply to be either restored or continued where it has either been cut off as a result of the failure of the owner to pay for the supply, or when it is likely to be cut off as a result of such failure. Sums incurred by a local authority in restoring or securing the continuation of a supply of water, gas or electricity where these have been cut off are a charge on the relevant property.

HOMELESSNESS

Local housing authorities were made statutorily responsible for the homeless by the Housing (Homeless Persons) Act 1977, which is now consolidated as Part III of the Housing Act 1985. Previously, there was only a relatively limited duty placed on social service authorities by the National Assistance Act 1948 to provide temporary accommodation to persons in urgent need – being need which could not reasonably have been foreseen.

The 1977 Act resulted from a growing concern about the treatment which homeless people often received under the 1948 Act. The principal problems were the temporary nature of the provision; the shuttling of homeless people between authorities because of claims that they were ordinarily resident in some other authority's area, and the division of responsibilities between social services and housing authorities. The 1977 Act transferred to housing authorities more clearly defined duties to advise, assist and/or house homeless persons. The duty to accommodate or to secure permanent accommodation arises when an authority is satisfied that an applicant is:

1. homeless or threatened with homelessness; and
2. falls within one of the categories of priority need of accommodation; and
3. has not become homeless intentionally.

The legislation also contains a provision relating to 'local connection' which, in certain circumstances, enables authorities to shift the burden of housing to another authority. Comprehensive guidance on the legislation is given in DoE Circular 116/77 and the revised 3rd edition (1994) of the Code of Guidance.

The number of households accepted as homeless by local authorities doubled to over 126 000 – representing 300 000 or more people – between 1978 and 1989, but the full extent of homelessness is difficult to establish because authorities are statutorily required to find housing only for those homeless people defined as having a priority need. In addition, there are no reliable estimates of those who do not apply to local authorities.

Reasons for becoming homeless include:

1. dispute with family, landlord or friends;
2. landlord requiring property for own use;
3. loss or expiry of tenancy;
4. mortgage default or rent arrears;
5. fire, flood, etc.

With the growth of homelessness has gone a still more rapid growth in the use of temporary housing, including bed and breakfast accommodation. The significance of this for EHOs is that houses generally referred to as 'hostels', 'guest-houses', 'bed and breakfast accommodation' which provide shelter for people with no other permanent place of residence (as distinct from a hotel providing accommodation solely for visitors to an area who have another permanent home), are houses in multiple occupation. As such they should comply with both national statutory requirements and the amenity and space standards of the authority in whose area they are situated.

AGENCY SERVICES

An agency service can be defined as any service provided by an organization – whether public, private or voluntary – which gives assistance to clients to meet their needs or demands. In housing such services have been established and funded by a wide range of organizations including local authorities, housing associations, independent or charitable bodies, private companies, professional firms, etc. Agency services can be set up to help clients to obtain housing or to move to housing more appropriate to their needs, but the most common forms of service at the present time are those which aim to assist clients to repair, maintain, improve or adapt their homes – home improvement agencies.

The assistance provided by these agencies varies but can include:

1. general advice on housing options;
2. guidance on welfare rights;
3. financial advice;
4. assistance in obtaining a renovation grant, a loan from a bank or building society, or a grant or loan from the Department of Social Security;
5. technical advice on building problems;
6. aid in finding suitable builders;
7. supervision of work;
8. carrying out work.

Some home improvement agencies target a particular client group, such as elderly or disabled people, while others assist people living in a particular area. The early home improvement agencies were developed separately by some local authorities and voluntary sector organizations. Those organized by local authorities arose from the recognition of the fact that some households found difficulty in coping with renovation grant procedures. The objective of the agency service was the provision of technical help with the application, identifying a builder and carrying out work [5]. At the same time, organizations in the housing association and voluntary sectors were focusing on the housing needs of older people. Additional help was required in view of:

1. the ageing of the population and, in particular, the anticipated growth in the number of frail elderly from 6% at the present time to 11% (over 1 million) by the year 2000;
2. the rise in the level of owner occupation among older households;
3. the number of older people in houses in poor physical condition;
4. the general state of the housing stock.

The 1991 English House Condition Survey [2] found that:

1. It is lone, older householders in particular who are most likely to live in housing in the worst condition. They represent 12% of all lone older households, have usually lived in their homes for more than 20 years and are in the lowest income bands.
2. The oldest housing presents problems of upkeep for all older households in the owner occupied sector. Here, both lone and two-person older households are disproportionately represented in the worst condition of the pre-1919 stock, particularly where the homes are large.

In addition to the limited number of grant-based schemes run by local authorities, both Shelter and the Anchor Housing Trust established agency projects around the country. These aimed to provide help to older home owners to carry out repairs either of a minor nature, or to secure more significant repairs or renovations to enable them to remain in their own homes for as long as possible. The Shelter schemes were set up under an umbrella organization called Care and Repair, and Anchor's were known as Staying Put projects.

Some local authority schemes aimed to be self-financing on the basis of fees which were financed to a large extent by renovation grants. Few voluntary schemes charged fees, however, and most were reliant on funding from charitable sources, housing associations, the Housing Corporation or local authorities. Hence the financial position of most schemes, including those run by local authorities, was extremely precarious. In 1984, the Department of the Environment commissioned the first comprehensive review of the agency services that were operating at that time. This concluded that the services offered met a wide range of needs and were generally effective, but that they lacked the resources to reach their full potential [6].

To stimulate further development, to provide greater stability and continuity, and to provide more evidence on the type and volume of help that could be provided, the DoE in 1986 and 1987 made funding available to establish over 50 new projects. The basis of funding was that government finance should at least be matched pound for pound from other sources.

A report, *Monitoring Assisted Agency Services* [7], examined the performance of assisted schemes between January 1987 and December 1989. The report concluded, among other things, that:

1. The volume of work completed by different agencies varied but that this was not the only performance criterion, and on other measures relating to quality of work, impact on house condition, quality of advice and technical service, client satisfaction and the impact on property value most projects performed well.
2. Any future expansion of home improvement agencies should be based on a systematic analysis of levels of need in different districts, and resources should be directed at priority areas and client groups.
3. The most difficult issue for home improvement agencies is to secure their financial future.
4. Although voluntary and private sector contributions should continue to be encouraged, public sector funding is essential if agencies are to be established on a scale that would make the service available in the majority of areas. Section 169 of the Local Government and Housing Act 1989 gives local authorities the power to fund and provide agency services, but Exchequer support should be provided expressly for this purpose.

In response to this report the government agreed to continue to meet a proportion of the running cost of approved projects and set up a new national co-ordinating organization Care and Repair with a remit to develop new projects and to provide support to and monitor the progress of existing projects. By April 1993 about 150 home improvement agencies were operating in England, Scotland and Wales with government financial support and approximately 30 agencies were working independently.

Under section 4(3) of the Housing Association Act 1985, housing associations may also 'provide services of any description for owners or occupiers of houses in arranging or carrying out works of maintenance, repair or improvement or facilitating the carrying out of such works'. Local authorities can provide housing associations who have this as one of their objective with financial assistance. They may also provide such assistance

to any charity or other body specified by the Secretary of State. The authority must also encourage the association, charity or body to take such measures as are reasonably available to them to secure contributions from other persons. However, if any authority wishes to give financial assistance to a body other than a housing association or charity in connection with the provision of a home improvement agency for which no exchequer support is being paid, it will be first necessary to obtain the specific written consent of the Secretary of State (DoE Circular 5/91).

Local authorities considering whether to fund an agency either independently or in conjunction with the government or a housing association should take into account the:

1. housing needs of the residents;
2. aims and objectives of the scheme.
3. revenue and capital financial implications and the sources of available funds;
4. level and type of support required from the local authority.

Performance criteria will also need to be established with planned review periods and regular monitoring.

An example of a project's budgetary provisions includes:

1. salaries plus staff overheads;
2. office costs:
   (a) rent and rates,
   (b) heating, lighting, repairs, cleaning, etc,
   (c) furniture, equipment,
   (d) telephone,
   (e) stationery, postage, etc.;
3. travel;
4. publicity, advertising;
5. other expenses:
   (a) insurance,
   (b) training.

SPECIALIZED FORMS OF HOUSING

Temporary and moveable structures

The new fitness standard (see page 355) with its emphasis on the provision of fixed basic amenities cannot be applied to temporary and moveable structures, and the relevant sections of the 1985 Act have been repealed. The provisions of the Public Health Act 1936 continue to apply. In the case of caravans, site owners have powers under the Mobile Homes Act 1983 to require the removal from protected sites of residential mobile homes which have a detrimental effect on the amenity of the site.

Tents, vans, sheds, caravans, etc., used for human habitation

Tents, vans, sheds, and similar structures used for human habitation are by section 268 of the Public Health Act 1936, made subject to the provisions of that Act relating to nuisances, filthy or verminous premises, and the prevention of disease, as if they were houses or buildings used for human habitation. (For nuisances in tents, etc., see Chapter 7).

A local authority may make bye-laws for promoting cleanliness in, and the habitable condition of, tents, vans, sheds, and similar structures used for human habitation, and for preventing the spread of infectious disease and generally for the prevention of nuisances in connection therewith.

The principal provisions of the Model Bye-law Series XVII 1956 refer to:

1. weatherproofing, cleansing, etc.;
2. precautions in the case of infectious disease;
3. site maintenance by the owner including clearance of ditches, space between tents, etc.;
4. provision of sanitary accommodation and water supply;
5. waste water and refuse disposal.

Under section 269 (as amended by section 30 of the Caravan Sites Control and Development Act 1960) a moveable dwelling includes any tent, van or other conveyance whether on wheels or not, or any shed or similar structure used for habitation to which the building regulations do not apply. A local authority may grant:

1. licenses authorizing persons to allow land occupied by them within the district to be used as sites for movable dwellings: and

2. licenses authorizing persons to erect or station, and use, such dwellings within the district;

and may attach conditions concerning the number, type, space between, water supply, sanitary conditions, etc.

A person shall not allow any land occupied by him or her to be used for camping purposes on more than 42 consecutive days or more than 60 days in any 12 consecutive months, unless either he holds a licence from the local authority as in (1) above, or each person using the land as a site for a movable dwelling holds a licence as in (2) above.

A local authority shall be deemed to have granted a licence unconditionally unless within 4 weeks from the receipt of an application it gives notice to the applicant stating that it is refused, or stating the conditions subject to which a licence is granted, and, if an applicant is aggrieved by the refusal, or by any condition attached, he may appeal to a court of summary jurisdiction.

The section does not apply to a moveable dwelling which:

1. is kept by its owner on land occupied by him in connection with his dwelling house and is used for habitation only by him or by members or his household; or
2. is kept by its owner on agricultural land occupied by him and is used for habitation only at certain seasons and only by persons employed in farming operations on that land; or
3. is not in use for human habitation and is being kept on premises the occupier of which permits no movable dwelling to be kept thereon except such as are for the time being not in use for human habitation.

If an organization satisfies the minister that it takes reasonable steps for securing:

1. that camping sites belonging to or provided by it, or used by its members, are properly managed and kept in good sanitary condition; and
2. that movable dwellings used by its members are so used as not to give rise to any nuisance;

the minister may grant to that organization a certificate of exemption.

Caravan sites

Part I of the Caravan Sites and Control of Development Act 1960 (see also DoE Circulars 42/60, 75/77, 119/77 and 12/78) deals with the licensing conditions of caravan sites, their standards, registers of sites, consultation between planning and licensing authorities, power of entry, and the matters which principally concern the environmental health officer. The licensing system is administered by district councils. The minister has specified a 'Model Standard, 1989', with respect to the layout, provision of facilities, services and equipment to which local authorities must have regard in determining any conditions they wish to attach to a caravan site licence. Part II relates to the general control, development, planning and enforcement. Part III deals with repeals, financial provisions, interpretation, etc. Part I does not apply to London but, with certain modifications, it applies to Scotland.

In the interpretation of the Act:

1. **Caravan** means any structure designed or adapted for human habitation which is capable of being moved from one place to another and any motor vehicle, so designed or adapted, but does not include: any railway rolling stock and any tent (section 29 – as amended by section 13 of the Caravan Sites Act 1968).
2. **Caravan site** means land on which a caravan is stationed for the purposes of human habitation, and land which is used in conjunction with land on which a caravan is so stationed.
3. **Site licence** means a licence under Part I of the Act authorizing the use of land as a caravan site (section 1 (1)).
4. **Occupier** means, in relation to any land, the person who, by virtue of an estate or interest therein held by him, is entitled to possession thereof or would be so entitled but for the rights of any other person under any licence granted in respect of the land (section 1(3)).

Licensing of caravan sites*

No occupier of land may cause or permit any part of the land to be used as a caravan site unless he is the holder of a site licence. A penalty is provided (section 1). However, no site licence shall be required for the use of land as a caravan site in any of the circumstances specified in the First Schedule which include:

1. land for site incidental to its enjoyment as such of a dwelling house within the curtilage of which the land is situated;
2. land for a caravan for not more than 2 nights – provided no other caravan is situated there, and the land has not been used for stationing caravans for more than 28 days in the past 12 months;
3. holdings of 5 acres (2.02 hectares) or more if the 28 days use has not been exceeded and not more than three caravans were so stationed at any one time;
4. land which is occupied by an organization holding an exemption certificate;
5. land as respects which there is in force a certificate issued by an exempted organization if not more that five caravans are at the time used for human habitation on such land;
6. agricultural land for a caravan site for accommodation of persons employed in farming operations on land in the same occupation;
7. land used similarly for accommodation of forestry workers;
8. land for use as a caravan site which forms part of land on which building or engineering operations are being carried out, if that use is for the accommodation of persons employed in such operations;
9. land as a caravan site by a bona fide travelling showman;
10. land for use as a caravan site occupied by the local authority in whose area the land is situated.

Local authorities may apply to the minister for the withdrawal of any or all of the exemptions prescribed in the First Schedule. Generally, a site licence cannot be issued for a limited period. This is only possible where planning permission is for a

---

* Also see 'Licensing of Permanent Residential Mobile Home Sites', A professional practice note. CIEH, August 1994.

limited period and in these cases the site licence must expire at the same time (section 4).

A prerequisite to a site licence is the entitlement by the applicant for the planning permission for use of the land as a caravan site (section 3(3)). Conditions which may be attached to site licences are prescribed (section 5). Provision is made for appeal to a magistrates' court against conditions attached to a site licence or against alterations to such conditions. There is a time limit of 28 days after notification within which such appeals must be made.

Where an occupier of land fails within the time specified in a condition attached to a site licence held by him to complete to the satisfaction of the local authority any works required to be completed, the local authority may carry out those works, and may recover as a simple contract debt any expenses reasonably incurred by them (section 9).

Provision is made whereby transfer of licences can take place; the surrender of licences for alteration can be demanded, and the rights of occupiers of land subject to a licence or special tenancy are protected (sections 10, 11 and 12). Exemptions from the requirements of section 1 are provided for sites existing at the time of the Act coming into force. Restrictions are provided on any increase in the number of caravans on existing sites (section 16).

Local authorities are required to keep registers of the site licences issued for caravan sites in their areas. Local authorities, who have provided sites themselves, must make particulars of these sites available to people inspecting the statutory register (section 25).

Mobile home and caravan site standards

The Secretary of State for the environment has specified separate 'model standards' for mobile homes on permanent residential sites [8] and for static holiday caravan sites [9]. Where sites are mixed the standards for residential sites apply. Local authorities should have regard to the standards in deciding what conditions to apply to a site licence.

The model standards refer to such matters as:

1. density and space between caravans;
2. roads, gateways and footpaths;
3. hard standings;
4. fire-fighting appliances;
5. storage of liquefied petroleum gas;
6. electrical installations;
7. water supply;
8. drainage, sanitation and washing facilities;
9. refuse disposal;
10. parking;
11. recreation space;
12. notices.

The model standards represent the standards normally to be expected as a matter of good practice on sites for residential mobile homes or static holiday caravans or both. They are not intended to apply to other types of caravan sites. They should be applied with due regard to the particular circumstances of each case, including the physical character of the site, any services that may already be available within convenient reach and any other local conditions.

Consideration should be given to a carefully phased introduction of any new standards after consultation with site owners, the caravan occupiers and the fire authority as appropriate.

Section 7 of the Mobile Homes Act 1975 gives the Secretary of State power to prescribe minimum standards of layout, facilities, services and equipment for 'protected sites' under the Caravan Sites Act 1968, on which there are mobile homes occupied as an only or main residence. No such action has so far been taken. (See Caravan Sites Act 1968.)

Gypsy caravans

The application of the Public Health Act 1936 provisions dealing with tents, vans and sheds, etc., to gypsy caravans had long caused difficulties, not least because of the gypsies' nomadic lifestyle and special needs related to their business interests.

The Caravan Sites Act 1968, Part II (as amended by the Local Government Act 1972) made special provision for gypsy encampments and the provision of sites by local authorities. County and London borough councils had a duty to provide adequate accommodation in the form of caravan sites for the gypsies residing in, or resorting to, their area.

Outside London, the duty placed on county councils was to determine what sites were needed and to acquire or appropriate the necessary land; district councils then had the duty to provide services and facilities and to manage the sites subject to financial reimbursement by the county council. County councils were responsible for determining the rents to be charged by district councils.

However, despite the provisions of the 1968 Act, finding accommodation for gypsies and illegal camping continued to be a problem. As a consequence in November 1994 Parliament passed the Criminal Justices and Public Order Act which, among other things, repealed the duty of local authorities to provide and manage gypsy sites, although there is still a discretionary power to do so.

Local authorities have also been given increased powers to control unauthorized camping. Section 77 of the 1994 Act empowers a local authority to direct persons residing unlawfully in vehicles within the area of that authority on highway land, other unoccupied land or occupied land without the consent of the occupier to leave the land and remove their vehicles and any other property they have with them on the land.

Section 78 provides that a Magistrates Court may, on complaint by a local authority, make an Order requiring the removal from land of any vehicle and property and any person residing in it and authorizing an authority to enter the land and remove the vehicle and property.

The DoE Circular 18/94 recognizes that in some circumstances it may be in the public interest that where gypsies are camped unlawfully on Council land and are not causing a level of nuisance which cannot be effectively controlled, an immediate forced eviction might result in unauthorized camping elsewhere in the area which could give rise to a greater nuisance. Accordingly it is suggested that authorities should consider tolerating gypsies' presence on such land for short periods. The Circular also indicates that local authorities should also try to identify possible emergency stopping places as close as possible to the transit sites used by gypsies where gypsy families would be allowed to camp for short periods. Authorities should also consider providing basic amenities on these temporary sites.

Temporary buildings

The control exercised by local authorities over tents, vans, sheds and similar structures is strengthened by provisions for the control of buildings constructed of materials which are short-lived or otherwise unsuitable for use in permanent buildings. Section 19 of the Building Act 1984 allows local authorities to reject the plans for such buildings or fix a time within which the building must be removed.

Hop pickers, fruit pickers, etc. – accommodation

Under section 270 of the Public Health Act 1936, a local authority may make bye-laws for securing the decent lodging and accommodation of hop pickers and other persons engaged temporarily in picking, gathering, or lifting fruit, flowers, bulbs, roots or vegetables within its district.

The defects common to tents, vans, and sheds used for human habitation are those most common in connection with structures provided for the accommodation of hop pickers, etc. Complaints generally concern improper or insufficient sanitary accommodation, or inadequate arrangements for the storage and removal of refuse.

The principal provisions of the Model Bye-laws, Series XX, 1956 are as follows: any person who, for persons engaged in hop picking or in the picking of fruit and vegetables, provides any lodging not ordinarily occupied for human habitation must:

1. give to the council **28 days'** notice in writing of his or her intention to erect new lodging;
2. give **28 days'** notice in writing of his or her intention to reoccupy the lodging in any year after the first year of usage;
3. maintain the lodging in a clean, dry, and weatherproof condition at all times when in use;

4. new lodgings to be not less than **20** ft (6 m) apart at the front, and not less than **15** ft (4.5 m) apart elsewhere, and have an impervious path at least **30** ft (762 mm) wide along the whole front;

5. no obstruction to interfere with the access of air and light;

6. provide sufficient means of ventilation and natural light;

7. minimum floor space of **20 sq ft** (1.85 sq m) to each occupant (two children under **10** years to be counted as one person);

8. separation of the sexes;

9. provide suitable accommodation for cooking and drying of clothes (one cooking house for every **16** persons);

10. provide at all times a supply of good, wholesome water for domestic use in some suitable place (within **150 yds** (45.7 m);

11. provide clean, dry, suitable bedding;

12. cause walls and ceiling to be cleansed and/or limewashed **once in every year not more than 2 months before occupation**;

13. provide covered refuse bins, one for each **16** persons;

14. provide proper sanitary accommodation – separate for the sexes – not less than one for every **20** persons (including children) lodged.

(An illustrated booklet prepared for circulation by local authorities to hop growers, and explaining the byelaws, is obtainable on application to the DoE.)

Rooms unfit for occupation

The occupation of certain rooms is, by reason of their situation and irrespective of their condition, prohibited.

Under section 49(1) of the Public Health Act 1936, a room any part of which is immediately over a closet other than a water closet or earth closet, or immediately over a cesspool, midden or ashpit, shall not be occupied as a living room, sleeping room, or workroom. Any person who, after notice from the local authority, occupies or permits the occupation of such a room is liable to a penalty.

Common lodging houses

The necessity for special supervision of common lodging houses had been recognized from the earliest years in which legislation for the purpose of protecting the public health was enacted. Thus the Public Health Act 1848 required the Local Board of Health to 'cause a register to be kept in which shall be entered the name of every person applying to register a common lodging house kept by him or her, the situation of every such house, and also from time to time to make bye-laws for fixing the number of lodgers who may be received into each house, so registered, for promotion of cleanliness and ventilation therein and with respect to the inspection thereof, etc.' Any person keeping a common lodging house without having registered the same, and refusing to admit therein between the hours of 11am and 4pm any person authorized by the Local Board of Health was for every such offence liable to fine of 40 shillings (£2).

These provisions were re-enacted and extended by the Common Lodging Houses Acts 1851 and 1853, and it is of interest to note that the statutory provisions in force today with reference to common lodging houses are, in many respects, identical with the provisions of these old Acts.

Section 401 of the Housing Act 1985 defines a 'common lodging house' as a house (other than a public assistance institution) provided for the purpose of accommodation by night poor persons, not being members of the same family, who resort thereto and are allowed to occupy one common room for the purpose of sleeping or eating, and includes, where part of a house only is so used, the part so used.

A summary of the general provision relating to common lodging houses is contained in sections 402–416 of the Act. They include the power to make bye-laws. Copies of model bye-laws are kept by the Department of the Environment. However these have not been amended since 1938 and are outdated in many respects. The Department of the Environment recommends that instead of using bye-laws, local authorities use the houses in multiple occupation powers available to them as court decisions have indicated, among other things, that common lodging houses fall within the term 'house in multiple occupation'. Nevertheless, it should be noted that common lodging houses are excluded from the list of registrable premises in the DoE's model registration scheme for multi-occupied houses.

In 1993 the Department of the Environment began consultations on the repeal of the common lodging house provisions of the Housing Act and announced in January 1994 their intended repeal as part of the deregulation exercise.*

Canal boats

The Public Health (Control of Disease) Act 1984, sections 49–53, and the Canal Boats Regulations 1878, 1925 and 1931 require the owner of a canal boat who wishes to use the boat as a dwelling to apply for registration to a local authority whose district abuts the canal on which the boat is accustomed or intended to ply. These provisions do not apply, however, to boats carrying a cargo of petroleum.

A canal boat is defined as: 'Any vessel, however propelled, which is used for the conveyance of goods along a canal not being:

1. a sailing barge which belongs to the class generally known as 'Thames Sailing Barge' and is registered under the Merchant Shipping Act 1874–1928 either in the Port of London or elsewhere; or
2. a sea-going ship so registered; or
3. a vessel used for pleasure purposes only.'

Before registration can be effected, the boat must comply with the structural requirements laid down in the regulations. Provisions are also made to deal with the lettering, marking and numbering of registered boats, cleanliness and habitable condition and the spread of infectious diseases.

REFERENCES

1. Bassett, W.H. (1995) *Environmental Health Procedures*, 4th edn, Chapman & Hall, London.
2. Department of the Environment (1993) *English House Condition Survey 1991*, HMSO, London.
3. Audit Commission (1991) *Healthy Housing: the role of environmental health services*, HMSO, London.
4. Housing: the Government's proposals, Cmnd 214, HMSO, London.
5. Thomas, A.D. (1981) *Local Authority Agency Services: Their Role in Home Improvement 1981*, Research Memo No. 88, Birmingham CURS, University of Birmingham.
6. Leather *et al.* (1985) *Review of Home Improvement Agencies*, Bristol SAUS University of Bristol.
7. Leather, P. and MacIntosh, S., *Monitoring Assisted Agency Services*, Department of the Environment, HMSO, London.
8. Caravan Sites and Control of Development Act 1960, section 5, *Model Standards 1989: Permanent Residential Mobile Home Sites*, HMSO, London.
9. Caravan Sites and Control of Development Act 1960, section 5, *Model Standards 1989: Holiday Caravan Sites*, HMSO London.

FURTHER READING

Association of District Councils (1988) *The Challenge of Multiple Occupancy*, ADC, London.

Association of District Councils (1989) *A Time to Take Stock*, (recommendation to improve condition of the housing stock 1989), ADC, London.

Audit Commission (1989) *Housing the Homeless: the local authority role*, HMSO, London.

British Standards Institute (1990) *Guide on the Siting of Holiday Caravans and Park Homes* British Standard 6768, BSI, London.

Fire Spread Between Park Homes and Caravans (1989) HMSO, London.

Minor Works; a major step, Care and repair, Castle House, Kirtley Drive, Nottingham NG7 1LD.

---

* As of March 1993 these provisions were still in operation.

National Federation of Housing Associations (1984) *Inquiry into British Housing: The Evidence*, Information Paper 4, NFHA, London.

Ormandy, D. and Burridge, R. (1988) *Environmental Health Standards in Housing*, Sweet and Maxwell, London.

Rose Wheeler (1985) *Don't Move: we've got you covered*, Institute of Housing, London.

Thomas, A. and Hedges, A. (1986) *The 1985 Physical and Social Survey of Houses in Multiple Occupation in England and Wales*, DoE, HMSO, London.

21 The health effects of housing conditions

James Connelly

INTRODUCTION

It is a truism that establishing any particular thing as a **cause** of another thing is far from easy. Even constant conjunction – when in our experience B is always preceded by A – can simply be due to the fact that we have only limited time to observe. Such philosophical musing is always a possible rejoinder when a claim of causality is being made and is, so far, unanswerable. What, practically, can be done is to reason causality with reference to current conventions of evidence. A much used set of such criteria for causation is given by Bradford Hill [1].

Epidemiology is about observing whether certain things called 'factor(s)' (or 'exposure(s)') are connected ('associated') with certain problems (e.g. 'health states', 'diseases', 'disabilities'), and if association exists, **quantifying** the relationship. Further, it provides a framework for assessing whether such associations are causal in nature. This chapter is about the evidence that specific and general housing factors cause disease, or more generally ill health, where ill health unlike disease is defined entirely by the self-reported symptoms of the person themselves.

Three specific housing conditions will be discussed – dampness, cold housing and overcrowding – because these conditions have been studied by means of epidemiological methods using ecological (correlation) studies, cross-sectional studies (surveys) and, less frequently, case-control and longitudinal (follow-up) studies. In addition, the evidence that housing conditions affect mental health is discussed.

DAMP HOUSING

Studies using cross-sectional survey techniques have found significant associations between a variety of symptoms reported by adults regarding both their health and their children's health and damp housing conditions. A survey in a South Wales town found that those who reported a history of wheezing and breathlessness more frequently reported dampness in the home and were more likely to burn open coal fires throughout the year. These associations were not effected by smoking status or social class [2].

More recently, Hunt and colleagues from Edinburgh have considerably elaborated on such earlier findings with regard to children's health. Surveys were conducted in Edinburgh, Glasgow and London. The results showed that **children** in those homes classified as showing any degree of damp were reported by their parents as having significantly more vomiting, wheeze, irritability, fever and poor appetite [3]. The authors of this study also investigated whether the presence of mould growth in the home (observed during the assessment of damp by environmental health officers, who were unaware of the self-reported symptom findings) was associated with symptoms. In relation to the amount of visible mould, six symptoms – wheeze, sore throat, irritability, headaches, fever and runny nose – showed a 'dose–response' relationship, fulfilling therefore an important criterion for 'causality'. When the air spore count was considered there was a dose–response relationship with three symptoms: wheeze, fever and irritability. Multivariate analyses, taking account of possible confounding factors, showed that a significant effect of dampness/mould remained for wheeze, sore throat, headache and fever, other symptoms – vomiting and diarrhoea – were better explained by concomitant overcrowding; irritability was largely explained by parental unemployment and 'runny nose' was better explained by reports that the 'house was too cold' [3]. The authors concluded that their findings were consistent with the hypothesis that damp-associated fungi caused allergies or infections that produced four specific symptoms: wheeze, sore throat, headache and fever.

The interpretation of such survey results in relation to wheeze in children has been questioned by another Edinburgh group [4]. Parents of children aged 6–7 were surveyed for whether their child had experienced respiratory symptoms in the previous year and whether the home was affected by 'condensation or dampness on walls' and 'patches of mould or fungus'. Though the results of this survey showed that 'wheeze' and 'chesty colds' were around twice as frequent in children from homes reported to be affected by dampness or mould growth, compared to unaffected homes, the authors suspected that this result was due to biased reporting of wheeze, or home conditions, or both. They conducted further studies to obtain what they believed were more 'objective' measures: wheeze was taken as a central marker of asthma and was assessed by measured reduction in Forced Expiratory Flow in 1 second (FEV_1) after an exercise test; relative humidity in the child's bedroom was taken as a marker of 'dampness'. The results showed that there were no significant relationships between these objective measurements [4]. A later study reported that spore counts, measured monthly over 4 months, showed a large variation in concentration and did not relate to either reported 'mould' or to reported 'wheeze' [5].

Other relevant studies of home dampness with or without moulds and asthma include a case-control study which matched 72 adult asthmatics and 72 control subjects by age and sex. Nineteen asthmatics compared to nine controls reported visible mould on the walls of their homes (this difference was just outside conventional statistical significance); exposure was confirmed by a significantly higher proportion of asthmatics showing evidence of hypersensitivity to the fungi *Penicillium* [6]. A large recent study from North America largely confirms the findings and interpretation offered by Hunt and colleagues [7, 8] rather than the opposing view.

COLD HOUSING

The human physiological effects of cold temperatures or, more accurately, 'cold-stress' produced by an interaction between ambient temperature, prevailing airflow, air humidity and protection from clothing, are well documented [9, 10]. However, except for ecological level studies – studies which correlate outdoor temperature and all cause or cause-specific mortality rates for a given population – other types of more relevant epidemiological studies, relating house temperature and disease, are rare.

Nevertheless, there is a major argument in favour of an adverse effect of low housing temperature in the finding of **excess** winter seasonal mortality found in many temperate climate countries, this excess is especially prominent in the UK where around 40,000 excess deaths occur annually in England and Wales. The great majority of this excess occurs in older (65+) adults and the causes ascribed reflect the predominant general causes of death (cardiovascular, respiratory, accidents) with the notable exception of cancer. There is also around a two-fold seasonal variation in deaths attributed to Sudden Infant Death Syndrome (SIDS, 'cot-death'), with an inverse relationship between deaths and mean monthly temperature [10]. Though often highlighted, deaths from hypothermia are rare occurrences, comprising only around 1% of excess mortality, and only 0.05% if classifications only as the 'underlying cause' are counted. Though the excess mortality in the UK is showing a declining trend it is still, proportionately, much larger than that in North America and Scandinavian nations, where climate is more severe. The UK decrease appears to be confined to respiratory causes of death and seems to have accompanied the increase in central heating (which in Britain increased from 13% to 66%, 1964–84). The seeming paradox in the decline of respiratory deaths and the stability of cardiovascular deaths may be because cold housing is particularly important in the occurrence of respiratory causes but less important in cardiovascular causes of death. The winter excess in the latter is more dependent on episodic cold-stress exposures to outdoor climate. However, against this the marked decrease in cardiovascular deaths seen in Finland over the last 20 years have been ascribed to improvements in housing stock involving adequate affordable heating, increased insulation and appropriate ventilation.

Cold stress may increase the susceptibility of the human respiratory tract to infectious agents, the 'threshold' temperature, however, cannot be specified precisely – the lower the temperature the greater the risk. With regard to 'comfort', temperatures below 18°C have been found to invoke reports of 'discomfort' from most people, temperatures less than 16°C may begin to raise respiratory tract susceptibility, and at temperatures below 12°C there appear to be adverse effects on the cardiovascular system which become particularly marked at temperatures below 9°C, hypothermia becomes a major risk below 6°C. Domestic accidents are a major cause of morbidity and mortality especially at the extremes of age. There appears to be an increased susceptibility with decreasing indoor temperatures (Fig. 21.1), possibly due to depressed cerebral functioning.

OVERCROWDED HOUSING

The risk of transmission of infectious agents causing secondary cases spread via air (e.g. tuberculosis) or via the faecal–oral route (e.g. dysen-

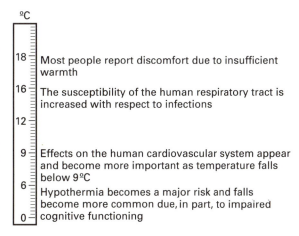

°C

18 — Most people report discomfort due to insufficient warmth

16 — The susceptibility of the human respiratory tract is increased with respect to infections

12

9 — Effects on the human cardiovascular system appear and become more important as temperature falls below 9°C

6 — Hypothermia becomes a major risk and falls become more common due, in part, to impaired cognitive functioning

0

Fig. 21.1 Physiological effects of low ambient temperature. Note: these effects relate to adults, infants have a different profile with respect to physiological response to ambient temperature, see [10].

tery) is, in part, dependent upon the number of people sharing living space. Crowding levels, measured as persons per room, have been shown in ecological level studies to correlate highly with both total mortality rates and particular non-infectious disease death rates. For instance, violent (including suicide) and accidental deaths are significantly associated with crowding (especially in males); peptic ulceration (particularly in females); myocardial infarction (heart attack) and stroke (particularly in males); bronchial carcinoma; cervical cancer; chronic bronchitis, asthma and emphysema all also show significantly high correlations with crowding, not explained by social deprivation factors or smoking [11].

Poor housing conditions for infants and young children, particularly crowding, have been implicated as a risk factor for the later adult occurrence of myocardial infarction and chronic obstructive lung disease (chronic bronchitis and emphysema), the observed adult social class mortality gradients for these diseases have been interpreted as reflecting the earlier social distribution of 'poor' housing [12]. Evidence from a UK prospective longitudinal cohort study, which followed up all babies born in a specified week in 1946, has demonstrated that adult chronic respiratory symptoms (chronic cough) and diminished lung function are positively associated with infant exposure to crowding. A possible explanation may be that crowding increased the risk of recurrent infant respiratory disease which caused structural pathological changes leading to morbid adult effects [13].

MENTAL HEALTH AND HOUSING

Characterizing 'mental health' or 'psychological well-being' is notoriously difficult, consequently its absence – mental disorder or psychological symptoms – is pragmatically investigated in studies of the psychological effects of housing. Moreover, isolating a **particular** housing factor and treating it as the 'exposure' in an epidemiological study presents even greater problems for outcomes of a psychological rather than a somatic (physical) type. Despite these difficulties research is beginning to reveal significant housing influences on psychological status [14].

After reviewing the empirical evidence (based on cross-sectional surveys), Freeman concludes that there is a likely adverse psychological effect of living in high-rise flats; however the relationship is not a simple cause–effect sequence. The relationship depends on a variety of other factors including: the perceived quality of the housing and the characteristics of its surrounding locality, the preferences of the occupants, the cultural meaning of 'high-rise' and the availability of socially supportive others [14]. Mothers of young children who live in flats have been shown to experience increased risk of depression due, in part, to loneliness and dissatisfaction with the accommodation. Moreover, depressed mothers were more likely to experience behaviourial problems in their children [15].

The specific factor of damp housing has been shown to be associated with increased levels of psychological symptoms. This influence is explained, in part, by the personal and social effects that such conditions engender: the continuous strain in trying to keep the house and clothing clean and fresh and the difficulties experienced in inviting others into the home. Overcrowded housing presents particular problems for

children and women. Children are denied adequate play space and this is possibly associated with later conduct disorders and decreased educational attainment [16]. Women, too, may be particularly vulnerable to overcrowded housing, not least because many are exposed for longer to the poor conditions and have less power in the domestic allocation of space [17].

CONCLUSIONS

Epidemiological studies of poor housing are beginning to reveal both **general** and **specific** health influences. It is also found that these adverse effects are concentrated, like poor housing itself, amongst lower-income and socially vulnerable groups – older people, children, women, ethnic minorities and the homeless. The task now is to begin to incorporate such research findings into building regulations and housing policy, with the goal of producing affordable health-promoting housing.

REFERENCES

1. Hill, A.B. (1977) *Short Textbook of Medical Statistics*, Hodder and Stoughton, London.
2. Burr, M.L., St Leger, A.S. and Yarnell, J.W.G. (1981) Wheezing, dampness and coal-fires. *Community Medicine*, **5**, 205–9.
3. Platt, S.P., Martin, C.J. and Hunt, S.M. (1989) Damp housing, mould growth and symptomatic health state. *British Medical Journal*, **298**, 1673–8.
4. Strachan, D.P. (1988) Damp housing and childhood asthma: validation of reporting of symptoms. *British Medical Journal*, 1223–6.
5. Strachan, D.P., Flannigan, B., McCabe, E.M. et al. (1990) Quantification of airborne moulds in the homes of children with and without wheeze. *Thorax*, **45**, 382–7.
6. Burr, M.L., Mullins, J., Merrett, T.G. et al. (1991) Indoor moulds and asthma. *Journal of the Royal Society of Health*, **108**, 99–101.
7. Dales, R.E., Zwanenburg, H., Burnett, R. et al. (1991) Respiratory health effects of home

dampness and mould among Canadian children. *American Journal of Epidemiology*, **134**, 196–203.

8. Dales, R.E., Burnett, R., and Zwanenburg, H. (1991) Adverse health effects among adults exposed to home dampness and moulds. *American Journal of Epidemiology*, **134**, 505–10.

9. Lloyd, E.L. (1991) The role of cold in ischaemic heart disease: a review. *Public Health*, **105**, 205–15.

10. Mant, D.C. and Muir Gray, J.A. (1986) *Building Regulations and Health*, Building Research Establishment DoE.

11. Kellet, J.M. (1989) Health and housing. *Journal of Psychosomatic Research*, **33**, 255–68.

12. Barker, D. and Osmond, C. (1987) Inequalities in health in Britain: specific explanations in three Lancashire towns. *British Medical Journal*, **294**, 749–52.

13. Britten, N., Davies, J.M.C. and Colley, J.R.T. (1987) Early respiratory experience and subsequent cough and peak expiratory flow rate in 36 year old men and women. *British Medical Journal*, **294**, 1317–19.

14. Freeman, H.L. (ed.) (1985) *Mental Health and The Environment*, Churchill Livingstone, London.

15. Richman, N. (1974) The effects of housing on pre-school children and their mothers *Developmental Medicine and Child Neurology*, **16**, 53–8.

16. Rutter, M. *et al.* (1974) Attainment and adjustment in two geographical areas III. Some factors accounting for area differences. *British Journal of Psychiatry*, 1974; **125**, 520–7.

17. Gabe, J. and Williams, P. (1986) Is space bad for your health? The relationship between crowding in the home and emotional distress in women. *Sociology of Health and Illness*, **8**, 351–71.

22   Housing hygiene

Ray Ranson

INTRODUCTION

Ever since the Stone Age, humans have been concerned with having adequate shelter to protect them from the elements and having a safe, healthy and comfortable housing environment in which to live. Unfortunately, most of the world's people do not live in housing which meets even basic health and safety requirements. Indeed, for increasing numbers, available shelter not only fails to protect against, but exposes them to, health risks that are for the most part preventable.

In the UK, housing and health was a major consideration of early public health legislation. Thus the early public health acts were aimed at improving sanitation and water supply, etc., in the crowded rookeries and tenements of the new industrial towns, which were the source of cholera and typhoid epidemics.

The Artisans and Labourers Dwellings Act 1848 marked the beginning of legislative intervention in the housing market. Early housing legislation made provision for clearance of slum and insanitary housing, introduced fitness standards and measures for dealing with overcrowding, partly to reduce tuberculosis. Building bye-laws (now regulations) were introduced to facilitate health and safety in the home through building construction standards. However, it was many years before local government was established on a firm enough footing for the effective implementation of public health or housing legislation.

CONTEMPORARY HOUSING AND HEALTH ISSUES

Since the Second World War, the initial response for dealing with the slums with all their attendant health problems was through slum clearance. However, since the late 1960s, there has been a move towards rehabilitation and area improvement. This was partly because of the failure of mass redevelopment schemes to provide housing in which people actually wanted to live, mainly because of poor design, environmental deprivation and social isolation, which is associated with much housing today.

With regard to health, numerous studies show some link between mental illness, stress and depression in families living in high-rise housing. Other studies have shown increased incidence of upper respiratory infections and accidents to children living in this type of accommodation. Studies have looked at the socially disabling effects which modern housing environments have had on the health of tenants. This is of particular importance to the elderly, women, single parents, the disabled, the long-term unemployed and chronically sick people who tend to spend a great deal of time at home, often isolated from the rest of the community. These same groups may have specialized housing and health needs. Other contemporary health issues related to housing include stress caused by lack of security on estates; illnesses related in some way to ineffective heating systems; home accidents caused by poor design;

noise-related stress; and the use of building materials that may affect health in some way, e.g. asbestos, formaldehyde products or materials that emit radon gas. This list is by no means exhaustive. Chapter 21 discusses the relationship between poor housing conditions and health in more detail.

These are problems for people with housing. Many others have no housing at all. According to the London Housing Unit between 2000 and 3000 mainly single people sleep rough in London every night [1]. For them shelter may be no more than a cardboard box under a railway arch. Many have health problems, such as alcoholism and psychiatric disorders. Some have chronic illnesses such as arthritis, diabetes, TB and bronchitis.

Health-related housing problems are partly caused by current policies for dealing with homeless people. This could be regarded as a minority public health problem, albeit an increasing one, particularly in the inner cities where it disproportionately affects black people, single parents, women, the unemployed and people surviving on social security payments. According to the National Audit Office, 126 000 families were accepted as homeless in 1989, and the number of households living in temporary accommodation quadrupled between 1982 and 1989 [2].

It is generally acknowledged by health professionals that temporary accommodation, including bed-and-breakfast hostels, is generally unsuitable for family housing on health grounds. A survey by the Health Visitors Association and SHELTER of homeless persons' accommodation showed widespread health problems associated with housing conditions. These ranged from infections associated with overcrowding, such as diarrhoea, vomiting, scabies, impetigo and chest infections, lack of facilities for preparing food and poor indoor air quality, to dietary problems associated with absence of cooking facilities [3]. Injuries to children are also high as a result of accidents associated with overcrowding or inadequate play facilities. The latter, if coupled with the mother's depression, can lead to slow child development. GPs and family practitioner committees have sometimes been reluctant to provide health care

for homeless families, which means that many homeless children are not immunized and receive no medication when sick.

As in the nineteenth century, it is thus against a background of multi-deprivation, poverty and discrimination that contemporary housing and health issues must be considered. Fortunately, increasing attention is currently being given to housing and health. Indeed, in the UK, local authorities are now required by law to consider the health and safety of occupants when deciding fitness. A background note to the Local Government and Housing Act 1989 [4] states that:

1. In deciding whether a dwelling-house is or is not unfit for human habitation, discomfort, inconvenience and inefficiency may be relevant factors but the primary concern should be in safeguarding the health and safety of any occupants.
2. The extent to which a building presents a risk to health and safety is governed by the nature of the defects present. However, the probability of accidents or damage to health may be increased either by the severity or extent of those defects. The location of defects may also be a material factor, as in some cases, may the persistence or duration of defects.
3. As a matter of general principle, the fitness standard should be related to the physical characteristics and condition of the dwelling-house and not to the particular current occupants or way that the house or flat is currently occupied. Thus, fitness under section 604 does not mean that the dwelling-house is necessarily 'fit' for the present type or number of occupants. For example, it may be fit, but wholly unsuitable for a particular disabled person or be statutorily overcrowded and have unfit and unventilated spaces currently used as bedrooms.
4. That said, to be fit for human habitation a dwelling-house must, by definition, be reasonably suitable for occupation – effectively for all household sizes and types of potential occupant who might reasonably be expected to occupy such property. Of the latter, the

elderly and young children are typically the most vulnerable to health and safety risks, not only because of their greater susceptibility, but because they tend to spend the greatest time in and around the home.

In addition, the introduction of neighbourhood renewal assessment in the same Act provides an opportunity to evaluate the wider aspects of housing and health within a particular area. This will inevitably mean that environmental health officers and housing officers will have to look much more closely at the physical and social environment when deciding whether to recommend clearance or improvement of housing. It will also mean taking a much more holistic view towards 'health', to include mental health and social well being and recognizing that housing hygiene is not just about buildings it is also fundamentally about people. (Statutory fitness standards and the assessment of required actions are covered in Chapter 20.)

PARAMETERS FOR HEALTHY HOUSING

As yet, scientifically determined parameters for healthy housing are generally unavailable, and there are difficulties in using empirical evaluation techniques for assessing the effects of housing conditions on health. Housing and health is not and never will be an exact science. The interrelationship between housing and physical and mental health is complex, and is invariably affected by extraneous variables, such as social class, poverty, state of nutrition and occupation or unemployment. Research studies have usually been unable to separate or explain the status of these various components.

However, the absence of definite measurements does not denote the absence of a relationship between housing and health, it just means that a relationship cannot always be proven. Fortunately, that does not stop us from suggesting parameters for healthy housing which reflect the considerable knowledge, experience and intuition of healthy housing needs. However, such para-

meters can only be generalized since it is recognized that particular groups within the community, (e.g. children, the elderly, disabled people and the chronically sick), may have different health and housing needs. The same is true of individuals within these groups.

It is partly for these reasons that healthy housing can only be tackled effectively if it forms part of a wider public health policy such as the WHO's 'Health for all by the year 2000' strategy, which has been formally adopted by most of the world's governments (see Chapter 12).

A number of targets relating to housing and health are included in the 'health for all' policy. For example, target number 24 states:

> By the year 2000, all people in each world region should have a better opportunity of living in houses and settlements which provide a healthy and safe environment.

This all-embracing goal has been criticized as being too idealistic. However, the intention of this target is to provide a focus for national and local authorities to consider what healthy housing initiatives can be achieved with the resources available.

To assist this process, the WHO (Euro) Region has produced housing guidelines which set out some of the basic principles and technical requirements for healthy housing [5]. The guidelines focus mainly on requirements in the home, i.e. shelter, and the immediate residential environment rather than in the wider macro-environment despite the obvious interrelationship between them. In this way, it is intended that the guidelines can be slotted into a wider environmental health programme when planning new housing settlements. They could also be used as a guide for assessing the hygienic quality of existing housing, e.g. fitness, and for professional and community education and training programmes. The following healthy housing parameters are a synopsis of the guidelines as based on WHO knowledge and experience of housing and health requirements across the world. The guidelines are applicable to a European context and not all are necessarily relevant to the UK situation.

WORLD HEALTH ORGANIZATION (EUROPE OFFICE) HEALTHY HOUSING GUIDELINES

Technical parameters

Housing layout requirements

1. **Provision of housing of suitable height to enable normal family life and social activities to be performed.**

   Many studies have shown that high-rise housing is unsuitable for family housing on health grounds, i.e. increased incidence of respiratory infections in young children and their mothers who may also exhibit mental disorders caused by social isolation and depression. Home accidents to children are higher than in traditional housing. Facilities for children's play is restricted which can affect child development and social interaction. Elderly and disabled people become more confined to the home and thus can become isolated. Indoor air quality and climate may be poor. Noise may cause stress. Insulating and fire-retardent materials, such as asbestos, may cause long-term health hazards. Such problems can be controlled by planning restrictions on storey height or allocation of families with young children to low-rise accommodation, provision of social and community facilities for residents and sensible internal design.

2. **Provision of housing and suitable dwelling size mix to enable community and social interaction.**

   The main advantage of mixed dwelling size development is encouraging diversification of residents in terms of age group interests and socio-economic and cultural backgrounds which, in the long-term, usually results in better community and social interaction. This point is particularly important to elderly or disabled people who are often housed in nursing homes or hospitals and effectively cut off from the wider community. It also permits better matching of housing to meet particular health needs.

3. **Provision of housing with sufficient space between building blocks so as not to intrude on view, privacy or impede isolation and air circulation.**

   The principal features of badly spaced housing includes intrusion of view and privacy (which can be important for mental health), overshadowing (which reduces sunlight and daylight) and, in some cases, reduction of air circulation around buildings (which could reduce ventilation to rooms). All these features may indirectly contribute to those diseases and conditions associated with poor natural lighting, sunlight deficiency and gloominess due to absence of view. Fire hazards may increase also.

4. **Provision for good orientation of buildings compatable with climate conditions.**

   In hot countries, correct orientation helps to ensure that buildings are not overheated by the sun and that at least one shady room is available in the house. Conversely, in cooler regions, radiation can be used to warm dwellings by facing them towards the sun. Orientation is important in relation to wind direction (which can adversely cool a building) and in preserving privacy from neighbouring buildings.

Space and density requirements

1. **Provision of housing built to suitable residential housing densities compatable with good environmental conditions and social and recreational needs.**

   High residential densities can be associated with congestion, overshadowing of buildings, lack of privacy, overloading of drainage systems and increased road accidents. Facilities for children's play and recreation may be restricted. Noise levels are often high. Residential density standards and planning controls should be adopted to regulate housing densities.

2. **Provision of housing of suitable size and sufficient usable floor area to satisfy human requirements for health, safety, family life, privacy, rest and domestic, recreational and social activities.**

Although indoor space requirements vary with culture, social and economic characteristics, over-crowding has been associated with spread of respiratory and enteric diseases; it affects educational attainment of school children, contributes to depression, annoyance and interpersonal conflicts and increased home accidents. The WHO Regional Office for Europe recommends that 12 m^2 of habitable space per person be provided in housing. However, this is not a health standard.

3. **Provision of sufficient open space for active and passive recreation and an aesthetically pleasing environment**.

Open space can provide some of the resources needed for active and passive recreation, and also can contribute to a sense of providing aesthetically pleasing settings. It can help to reduce residential densities; improves air quality; provides a noise barrier between residential areas and industry; and facilitates recreational activities.

Social requirements

1. **Provision of facilities for normal family life, hobbies, recreation and social activities**.

The shelter as a social setting has to accommodate individual and different interests and activities for family members including children's play, homework, sewing and reading, hobbies, entertaining friends and providing privacy when desired.

2. **Provision of facilities for normal community and wider social life**.

Housing residents are members of a wider community which people need to feel part of and able to relate to. Amenities, such as shops, schools and hospitals, need to be provided within easy reach of the residential neighbourhood. Where such amenities are not provided, people can feel cut off and isolated, which can put a strain on mental health and social well being.

3. **Provision of facilities to rest and recover from sickness or ill health.**

The home is not just a place to sleep in, but it is also a refuge from the rigours of work,

school or other activities and a place to recover from sickness or ill health.

Community facilities for people recovering from sickness or illness should be an integral part of any healthy housing policy. Good housing with family or community support provides a suitable environment for convalescence.

4. **Provision of reasonable conditions of privacy.**

People's reaction to privacy depends as much on their own attitudes as on physical facts.

Intrusion of privacy relates mainly to being seen, noise, social contact and communication. Some cultures prefer privacy for sleeping, washing and carrying out toilet activities, others do not.

5. **Provision of opportunity for achieving aesthetic satisfaction in the home and its surroundings.**

In terms of the housing surroundings, view is an important factor. Inside the house provision of furnishings and consumer appliances are important and relevant to aesthetic satisfaction in the home.

6. **Provision of opportunities to enable work activities to be carried out at home.**

The home is often used as a base for cottage industries. Housing may be unsuitable for some work activities depending upon the nature of work. Poisoning, asphyxiation or fire may present particular hazards. Indoor air quality and climate may be adversely affected by industrial processes carried out at home.

Shelter requirements

1. **Provision of suitable shelter to ensure that housing is wind and weathertight and otherwise protected from the external elements and other natural hazards.**

Geographical considerations and climate determine the degree of protection needed against the external elements and natural hazards. However, protection against rain and snow penetration is important in keeping the shelter free from dampness (which can adversely affect health), and the shelter must be able to moderate sunlight (which can adversely affect the indoor climate). The shelter should also be a safe refuge against earthquakes, volcanoes, cyclones, lightning, flooding, landslip and other natural hazards. In addition, frost, strong winds and subsidence can cause considerable damage to the hygienic integrity of the building structure.

2. **Provision for admission of direct sunlight and protection against excessive isolation.**
   Admission of sunlight provides significant physiological and psychological benefits to health and well being. In addition, it is a source of warmth but, in excess, can cause overheating of the building which can lead to fatigue and heat exhaustion. Design and construction measures should be used to optimize or moderate insulation in keeping with the climate.

3. **Protection against seismic activity.**
   Seismic activity causes loss of human life and property unless appropriate mesures are taken in the design of buildings. This is not a problem in the UK.

4. **Protection against external air pollutants.**
   The shelter must be able to help protect inhabitants from harmful pollutants in the outside atmosphere. These include suspended particulates, sulphur, carbon and nitrogen oxides, hydrocarbons, photochemical oxidants and lead. Such pollutants may contribute to bronchitis, pneumonia and other respiratory infections, or otherwise affect health. Planning and air pollution control measures can help to reduce the problem at source, although window and ventilator locations are also important.

5. **Protection against radio-active emissions.**
   There are a number of radio-active emissions in the atmosphere which, in low concentrations, do not affect health. However, radon gas, which is given off from the decay of uranium-238, can be found in much higher concentrations in indoor air. Radon exposure has been associated with increased incidence of lung cancer. Control measures relate to siting housing away from natural deposits in the ground, installing radon barriers to rooms, using radon-free building materials and in-

creasing ventilation to rooms. (See Chapter 42.)

6. **Protection against excessive noise and vibration from within and outside the dwelling.**
   The main consequences associated with noise include disturbance of sleep, annoyance and stress, all of which may affect mental health (see Chapter 40). Planning measures such as adequate separation of streets, traffic and industry from housing will all help to reduce noise levels. Design measures such as double glazing, noise insulation and internal layout of rooms will help to reduce noise nuisance from adjoining dwellings.

7. **Provision of suitable shelter against disease vectors, pests and vermin.**
   There are a number of insects and mammals which are of importance to housing hygiene and public health because of their ability to transmit disease, cause nuisance or otherwise affect health. These include houseflies, mosquitoes, cockroaches, bedbugs, fleas, mice and pigeons and other birds, which often infest lofts and dilapidated outbuildings. General control measures include sanitary design, housing maintenance and good housekeeping, as well as the elimination of breeding places, destruction of pests and preventing the vector from reaching human beings, i.e. through maintaining the integrity of the shelter against pest and vermin ingress. (See Chapter 9 for pest prevention and treatment.)

8. **Protection against intrusion by humans or dangerous animals.**
   Intrusion into housing by humans and dangerous animals can be a major health and safety hazard as a result of attacks or assault against the person. Poor security can lead to stress, particularly among elderly people living on their own. Such intrusion can be minimized by security measures and good design of the housing layout.

Design and construction

The detailed design and constructional requirements of housing hygiene encompasses all of the technical factors which relate to the shelter and the physical infrastructures which serve it.

1. **Provision of facilities which are designed to optimize performance of household tasks without causing undue physical or mental fatigue.**
   This is a generic requirement which is concerned with provision of environmental and housing facilities which meet general and individual physical and mental health requirements, as well as comfort and aesthetic considerations, sufficiency and layout of indoor space, use of building materials which are easy to keep clean, and provision of an indoor climate and indoor air quality which optimizes comfort in carrying out household tasks.

2. **Provision of a structure with sufficient strength, stability and durability of building components which are easy to maintain, repair and keep clean.**
   Good hygienic housing design and construction is necessary to enable effective cleaning and sanitary maintenance. Vital components in the structure include foundations, walls, floors and roofs. General hygiene considerations include strength, stability, durability, fire-resistance, protection against external elements and thermal and noise insulation.

3. **Provision of non-toxic or injurious building materials, furnishings and consumer goods.**
   There are a number of toxic chemicals and materials used in the construction of buildings, furnishings and consumer goods. Some may pollute indoor air, others are toxic through ingestion. Examples include lead or asbestos products, and polymers and toxins used in cleaning agents.

Sanitation requirements (the requirements for wholesome water and for the adequate collection and disposal of waste water are dealt with in Chapter 44)

1. **Provision of a sufficient clean, wholesome water supply reasonably accessible to the dwellings and protected against pollution from outside and within the dwelling.**
   The provision of potable and non-potable water supplies for drinking and washing purposes respectively, is a basic housing hygiene measure still denied to millions of people around the world, particularly in rural areas of developing countries. Clean water is not just necessary for drinking and food preparation, but is also vital for growing food crops. Qualitatively, water can become unfit for human consumption due to contamination from human or animal excreta, and toxic industrial effluent.
   Contaminants include water-borne pathogens, viruses, parasites, chemicals and heavy metals, all of which may cause intestinal illnesses. General control measures include water conservation and protection at source, during delivery and storage, treatment and purification, and monitoring and testing. In particular, water supplies must be protected from excreta contamination and chemical contaminants such as nitrates and land fertilizers.

2. **Provision of a sanitary means of disposing of waste and surface water.**
   The collection and sanitary disposal of domestic waste water is often neglected in many countries. Provision of piped water supplies to an area commonly causes a deterioration in existing health conditions until adequate waste disposal facilities have been installed. Inadequately disposed waste drainage can cause flooding of roads, wells and housing, creating further health hazards. To control this, waste-water collection/carriage systems should be installed as necessary for domestic and surface (i.e. rain) water.

3. **Provision of toilet facilities of such a nature as to minimize the danger of transmitting disease.**
   Insanitary toilet facilities encourage the spread of enteric diseases through the faecal–oral route or by flies. Where toilets are shared, the health risk increases. Appropriate toilet facilities in separate sanitary accommodation should be provided wherever practicable.

4. **Provision of sanitary arrangements for excreta disposal.**
   A number of epidemiological studies have been conducted into the significance of correct drainage and excreta disposal in preventing enteric and other diseases. Inadequate disposal can cause pollution of water courses, land and food crops. Flies and crawling insects

may transmit enteric disease. Parasitic diseases can be spread by food animals. Control measures include installation of piped water-carriage systems, on-site storage and treatment systems and pit latrines in appropriate cases. There are likely to be different solutions to this problem in urban vis-à-vis rural areas.

5. **Provision of sanitary arrangements for domestic washing and drying of clothes**.
   The washing and cleaning of vegetables, fruit, salads and other food with clean water helps minimize food poisoning. Similarly hot water and a sink is a basic provision for washing food utensils and washing of dirty clothes which may provide harbourage for fleas, bed bugs and lice.

6. **Provision of sanitary arrangements for personal washing and bathing**.
   Personal washing facilities are essential for effective personal hygiene as well as for personal self-esteem. It is particularly important to have personal hand-washing facilities available for after toilet use, and a bath or shower with hot and cold water supplies available for body washing. In all cases, there should be facilities for the sanitary removal of waste water.

7. **Provision of hygienic facilities for the storage, preparation and cooking of food**.
   Hygienic facilities for the storage, preparation and cooking of food play a major part in reducing food contamination and poisoning. This can be controlled by provision of hygienic food storage facilities with proper temperature control; elimination of practices leading to cross contamination between cooked and uncooked foods; provision of clean water supplies for washing, cooking and preparing food; provision of adequate personal and food washing facilities; eliminating contaminated food preparation areas and the eradication of animal and insect disease vectors.

8. **Provision of sanitary facilities for the storage, collection and disposal of solid and household waste**.
   The hygienic storage, collection and disposal of household refuse is an essential housing requirement, as well as being aesthetically and environmentally desirable. Health effects are generally related to nuisances from flies; harbourage of rats and mice; increased fire hazards; injuries from broken glass, tins, etc., particularly among children; inadequate collection, storage and disposal systems which cause additional problems from noise (refuse chutes) and nuisance from on-site refuse incinerators; and local air pollution. To overcome these, measures need to be taken to ensure the sanitary storage, collection and disposal of domestic refuse.

9. **Provision of separate sanitary arrangements for the housing of pets and domestic animals**.
   Domestic and pet animals can carry and transmit a number of diseases to man. In particular, salmonellosis is spread by a number of infected animals, including dogs. Domestic animals should be provided with housing separate from the dwelling. The control of communicable diseases from pet animals largely depends upon hygienic measures for the animals themselves, including veterinary care, suitable animal housing and health education of handlers.

Indoor air quality requirements

1. **Provision of an indoor atmosphere which is free from excessive toxic and/or noxious odours, chemicals, pathogens, water vapour and other air contaminants or pollutants.**
   In many cases, pollution concentrations can be higher inside housing than outside. More than 80 indoor air pollutants have varying adverse health effects, depending on toxicity, concentration and occurrence inside rooms. In terms of housing, the most common pollutants include carbon and nitrogen oxides, odours, formaldehyde, tobacco smoke, water vapour, air-borne allergens, asbestos and other mineral fibres, air-borne pathogens and toxic emissions from polymers and consumer goods.

   Although much is known about the toxicity of such gases as carbon monoxide, there is more doubt – even controversy – about the toxic effects of gases, such as nitrogen and sulphur gases, or tobacco smoke. There is similar uncertainty about the contribution of water vapour and air-borne mould spores to respiratory disease. In many cases, little or nothing is known about the toxicity of trace indoor pollutants.

Three main methods are used to control indoor pollutants: removing the source of the pollutants from the dwelling; controlling pollutant emissions at source; and expelling the pollutants from the dwelling through ventilation. In addition, in the case of condensation, a number of design and constructional measures relating to heating, thermal insulation and maintenance may need to be implemented.

2. **Provision of sufficient ventilation, so that air quality and hygro-thermal requirements maintain health and comfort conditions.**
   Good ventilation promotes physiological and psychological functioning of the human body, engendering a sense of well being and comfort. By contrast, deterioration in the physiochemical properties of the indoor atmosphere adversely affects the comfort and health of the occupants, depending upon the nature of the pollutant.

   The object of ventilation is, therefore, to provide a pure supply of air to occupied rooms, continually remove odours, vitiated or polluted air and to preserve an indoor climate that is dust free, at the correct temperature and humidity, and with adequate air movement conducive to health and comfort of occupants. Where possible, this is best achieved through natural ventilation, i.e. windows or airbricks, rather than mechanical means. Artificial ventilation is prone to breakdown unless periodically maintained. In some cases it may be a source of transmitting airborne pathogens, such as legionella. An optimum 18 m³/per hour ventilation rate is recommended in habitable rooms.

Indoor climate requirements

1. **Maintenance of a thermal environment which will not impose any significant strain on the thermo-regulatory mechanisms of the body, i.e. prevent undue heating or cooling of the body, and enable physiological functions to proceed at a level most favourable to rest and psychological comfort.**

Thermal comfort is important in assisting physiological functions to proceed at a level most favourable to rest, psychological comfort and the recovery of strength after previous exertions. From the point of view of health, it is the elderly and young children who have decreased thermo-regulatory functions. Conditions that lead to discomfort and disturb the body's heat regulating mechanism and equilibrium include pharyngitis and neuralgia through cooling or overheating of the body. Factors which affect thermal comfort include air temperature (optimum 20 to 22°C); mean radiant temperature, air movement (optimum 0.1 to 0.15 m/s) and humidity (optimum 30 to 60%); such conditions should be achieved through affordable heating, adequate thermal insulation and draught control.

2. **Provision of adequate daylight and artificial illumination and avoidance of glare.**
   The penetration of direct sunlight into living accommodation has favourable psychophysiological effects on both thermal comfort and biological activity of the body. It also has a bactericidal effect as well as psychological benefits. The visual function is adversely affected when light quality is poor, that is, when light reflections are suppressed or uneven. Such conditions can put additional strain on the eyes which may eventually affect eyesight. The aim of good lighting practice is, therefore, to ensure the most favourable conditions for the general and working capacity of the occupants by providing lighting that is both quantitatively and qualitatively adequate. Such provision should include some admission of natural lighting to all habitable rooms and, preferably, toilet/bathing compartments.

Home safety requirements

Interest in home safety has arisen partly because of changes in mortality patterns, which show that accidents to young persons and the elderly are now a major cause of deaths in many countries, and are often higher than infectious or parasitic diseases. It is a truism that safety is but one aspect of health, although it is often treated separately or disregarded altogether. To be effective, home safety policies should draw upon the results of epidemiology, safety design, education and legislative interventions.

1. **Protection of the neighbourhood against the hazards of motor vehicles.**
   Road accidents in residential areas cause a considerable number of deaths and injuries each year, particularly to young children. A balance, therefore, needs to be made between the layout of roads in relation to housing, in particular the degree of separation between pedestrians and motor vehicles, so that accidents are minimized.

2. **Avoidance of unsafe conditions in the housing environment, in outbuildings and surroundings of the home.**
   Although the home itself is the usual source of domestic accidents, a number of accidents occur in the immediate vicinity of the home. Older children, in particular, like to explore sheds, outbuildings and non-recreational environments. Accidents can arise from tampering with electrical installations, fires from inflammable substances stored in outbuildings and drownings in unprotected water sources. Any safety audit should include the examination and rectification of these areas.

3. **Protection against the risks and effects of falls.**
   The most important cause of accidental death in the home is falls. These cause up to two-thirds of all male accidental deaths in the home and up to four-fifths in women. Most fatalities are among the elderly. Stairs, ladders and furniture are the most common locations of falls. Control measures include the provision of non-slip floor surfaces, properly designed and balustraded staircases and balconies, avoidance of high-level cupboards, provision of safety catches to high windows, and provision of handrails to baths and WC compartments.

4. **Provision of adequate facilities enabling a means of escape in the event of a fire, and the control and removal of conditions likely to cause or promote fire.**

Fires are a common cause of death, particularly in housing which is inadequately protected and without a proper means of escape. In a burning building, smoke, fumes and heat constitute the most serious threat to occupants if they are unable to reach a place of safety quickly enough. The most common cause of fire deaths is asphyxiation from carbon monoxide poisoning. This and other toxic gases may be given off from building or furniture materials. Control measures include compartmentation of buildings and dwellings through fireproofing, ensuring an adequate means of escape, e.g. fire exits and protected staircases, the use of non-combustible building and furnishing materials, the provision of smoke detectors and fire extinguishers, and ensuring that heating appliances, open fires and fuel do not present a fire risk.

5. **Protection against burns and scalds.**
   Most burns and scalds occur in the vicinity of the home. These are mainly caused by touching and knocking over utensils filled with hot or boiling liquids.
   Hot water from heaters, geysers and boilers should be thermostatically controlled so that water is not delivered above 45°C. Work surfaces should be provided adjacent to cooking stoves. Kitchen areas should adjoin dining rooms where practicable.

6. **Provision against asphyxiation or gas poisoning from faulty heating and cooking appliances and services.**
   All fires and fuel-burning appliances need fresh air for correct combustion. In most cases, this is provided by natural means. Air deficiency can cause a dangerous building up of carbon monoxide, which can also be emitted if heating or cooking appliances are defective or if flue-ways are blocked. It is therefore important that these appliances are regularly serviced. Liquid petroleum gas (LPG) appliances, in particular, need special attention, and LPG cylinders must be correctly stored and handled. At all times, permanent and sufficient air supply must be provided to rooms containing heating and cooking appliances. Flues must be cleaned

regularly and kept free from obstructions. Gas pipes and tubing should be inspected regularly for leaks.

7. **Protection against electrical shocks from defective appliances and services**.

Defective electrical appliances, wiring and fittings commonly cause electrical shock and electrocution, particularly in children and the elderly. Many fatalities are caused each year by electrocutions. It is therefore important that new electrical circuits and appliances are installed in accordance with approved international safety standards. Old installations should be checked regularly for defects in wiring, earthing and electrical hazards. Residual circuit breakers should be installed in new housing.

8. **Protection against bodily injuries from lacerations and similar injuries.**

Lacerations by sharp tools and objects constitute the most common non-fatal type of injury in the home. Many involve accidents caused by broken glass in windows, glazed doors and panels. Glass should, therefore, not be used in doors or panels at the bottom of stairs or steps. Laminated or toughened glass should be used where there is a danger of impact damage, particularly at body level.

9. **Protection against poisoning from dangerous drugs, medicine and household chemicals**.

Many accidental poisoning cases occur each year from chemicals, drugs and medicines, particularly among children. Provision should, therefore, be made for adequate and secure storage facilities for these substances.

10. **Protection against poisoning from plants**.

Eradication and education measures should be instigated in areas where poisonous plants, berries, fruit and fungi are a problem.

Special housing requirements

The special housing needs of particular groups, such as children, the elderly, disabled and chronically sick, depend upon the health needs of these groups and the often varying needs of individuals within them. These needs should be considered as additional to the general requirements described elsewhere in these guidelines.

1. **Provision of housing suitably adapted to meet the needs of children, women with children and single parents**.

Children are especially vulnerable to enteric diseases, respiratory and chest infections, digestive disorders and also certain non-communicable diseases, such as lead poisoning and allergic conditions. Children living in poor housing are more susceptible to these diseases, and are more likely to be retarded in their development than children living in hygienic housing. Good child development requires access to open spaces, parks, and play and communal facilities, where children and their mothers can interact with others outside the home. High child densities, which are often a source of dissatisfaction to parents and children alike, should be avoided wherever possible in human settlements. Neither should families with young children be housed in high-rise housing. Inside dwellings, space is needed for play, and the design should ensure that home accidents are minimized. Avoidance of overcrowding will cut down the spread of respiratory disease, and proper sanitation will reduce the incidence of enteric diseases in children. In cold climates, children require a slightly higher indoor air temperature to compensate for impaired thermo-regulatory functions. Avoidance of lead paint and asbestos in construction will reduce the incidence of lead poisoning and the possibility of asbestos-related cancer.

The housing needs of mothers are often inextricably linked to the housing needs of their children. For example, the susceptibility of women to neurosis and depression may be aggravated by a poor housing environment, and this is likely to have a spin-off effect on their children.

Single parents have additional problems of finding the time to supervise children. This can result in increased child accidents and laxity in child hygiene practices. Special consideration needs to be given to help single parent families living in poverty. Community day nursery schemes can assist single working women with the task of supervising children.

2. **Provision of housing suitably adapted to meet the requirements of the elderly**.

The ageing process can make the elderly more susceptible to specific housing related conditions, e.g. reduction of mobility often means that the elderly spend more time in the home where they can soon become isolated. Psychological needs may also be different stemming from loss of job, friends and family. Hardening of the bones means that fractures are more likely following falls. Elderly people tend to need a room temperature 2 to 3°C warmer than young adults. Special housing for the elderly, such as warden-assisted sheltered homes which are integrated into the community, should be considered in any housing policy. Single storey accommodation can alleviate falls from stairs, and other measures should be taken to minimize home accidents. Special attention should be given to maintenance of heating appliances to reduce carbon monoxide poisoning. A noise-free environment will reduce stress.

3. **Provision of housing suitably adapted to meet the requirements of disabled persons**.

Disabled people should be integrated within the general population as much as possible. The built environment should not handicap those persons disabled by physical or mental impairment. However, the nature of preventative or remedial action depends upon the nature of the disablement. The most common disablement is impaired mobility. Ramps, adequately sized door openings and special adaptation of bedrooms, sanitary appliances and cupboards, etc., are examples of adaptations.

People with vision difficulties can be helped by the provision of colour, illumination and texture in building materials.

People with hearing and/or speech difficulties could benefit from noise-free and acoustically insulated housing. The mentally ill may benefit from communal housing with warden support (sheltered housing). Finally, people with allergies may be affected by housemites, moulds and certain building materials, which should be rectified in construction and dwelling maintenance.

4. **Provision of housing suitable for the chronically sick and others with special health needs**.

The house should provide an environment in which people can recuperate from illness. Indoor climate, air quality, privacy, noise insulation and community support are important factors to be considered when planning the housing of the chronically sick.

5. **Provision of housing suitable for the homeless, rootless and long-term unemployed persons**.

Many people are often forced to leave their villages and homes to seek work in the towns where they often end up unemployed and homeless. The long-term unemployed with housing spend more time in the house, which can place additional stress on the family and community infrastructures. Income support and provision of basic, affordable healthy housing with community, recreational and social facilities are examples of practical measures which can help this group.

Operational and organizational parameters

It is impossible to separate technical aspects of housing from policy considerations. This section suggests some of the factors which would need to be considered in formulating healthy housing policies if the WHO's strategy of 'health for all by the year 2000' is to be achieved. It is especially important that governments, local authorities and local agencies generate local programmes for achieving housing hygiene within their areas over a given time span. This policy should embody and inter-relate with other pursuant economic, social, cultural, health care and educational policies that impinge on housing hygiene, i.e. housing must be seen as part of a wider public health programme.

1. **The housing stock should be appraised regularly to ascertain hygienic quality.**

Periodic inspection of the housing stock is useful for ascertaining the state of repair or hygienic quality which is important for monitoring, preventive maintenance, rehabilitation and legal enforcement (see Chapter 20).

2. **Appropriate policies should be adopted for dealing with slum and insanitary housing.**

   Removal of slum or otherwise insanitary housing effectively eliminates associated conditions that are detrimental to the health, comfort and wellbeing of the occupants. The choices of action for dealing with insanitary housing include improvement of housing amenities and facilities by conservation measures, the upgrading of environmental amenities and services and clearance of slum housing with selective or comprehensive redevelopment action. There are advantages and disadvantages for each method. Much will depend upon available finance and cultural and historical considerations. However, it is important to take into account the wishes of the community. Also, much slum housing has been demolished only to be replaced by new slums which are often expensive to maintain, have been built on too large a scale, at a high density and are unpopular with residents.

3. **Adequate provision should be made for rehousing the homeless and persons from slum and insanitary housing.**

   The criteria for rehousing are usually determined by a points scheme for assessing housing need and the relative priority for rehousing. Rehousing could also be considered on medical grounds. Where there is a housing shortage, provision of prefabricated housing units, mobile homes and caravans could be considered as an interim step to long-term building programmes.

4. **Inter-sectoral co-operation should be adopted for corporate planning and management of housing hygiene policies.**

   Health and local authorities have a wide range of responsibilities in relation to housing. However, to be effective, the authorities must command the support of other agencies involved, and be able to co-ordinate inter-sectoral co-operation. This must include the participation of the community. A corporate approach that uses consultation and partici-

pation at the preplanning stage is one of the most important operational tools available for achieving healthy housing objectives.

5. **Basic housing standards, codes and legislation should satisfy fundamental human health needs.**

   Local housing codes and standards must reflect the prevailing economic, social and cultural background of the area if they are to be relevant. There must also be effective enforcement machinery for implementing them. Without legislation, one is left with education and persuasion, neither of which is very effective for ensuring that minimum healthy housing requirements are met.

6. **Physical planning policies should include consideration of environmental health and housing hygiene requirements.**

   Planning policies should be initiated which will promote the efficient management of environmental resources of an area in such a manner as to enhance health and avoid hazards. Planning policies should also allow the elimination or modification of present housing hazards resulting from past planning (or lack of planning) errors.

7. **Institutional, organizational and operational arrangements need to be adequate for implementing housing hygiene policies.**

   These arrangements vary considerably between housing agencies, particularly the balance between central and local control over administration of programmes. Theoretically, local authorities and housing associations are often best placed to implement programmes, but these are often poorly resourced. Housing functions may also be spread across a number of different local authority departments, necessitating a corporate approach to policy implementation.

8. **Adequate financial provision should be made available for sanitary housing provision.**

   Policy makers have to decide how best to share scarce public resources for a number of competing and, arguably, equally important needs. Housing must be seen as a long-term capital investment in a country's resources, but the progressive decay of old urban neighbourhoods cannot be halted without financial stimuli from the capital market. Public intervention is likely to be necessary at both central and local levels to assist with housing costs, e.g. through rent control, improvement grants and social housing provision.

9. **Suitably planned and routine repair and maintenance policies should be adopted for preventing insanitary housing.**

    Housing in disrepair, but which can be remedied at reasonable cost, should be repaired until it deteriorates to a state where it ceases to be cost effective to remedy. Planned maintenance programmes should be initiated before building components have reached the end of their useful life. This can be achieved through regular inspections of the housing stock and provision of effective machinery and resources, e.g. environmental health officers, to enforce repairs. In the end, prevention is always better and cheaper than cure.

10. **The involvement and participation of the community and women in housing hygiene policies should be maximized**.

    At its simplest level, community participation may simply be a communication exercise in getting feedback from the community on housing policy or planning options. At a more complex level, community participation can involve setting up housing co-operatives and self-build and other self-help schemes, sometimes with state help or supervision. The advantage of these schemes is that they allow people to design and build housing which they want and can afford.

    Women should be encouraged to participate in housing hygiene policies at every level since it is women who usually are responsible for bringing up children and attending to the family's health and education, and running the home. Their housing experience should therefore be exploited when embarking on new development or improvement schemes.

11. **Educational programmes should be implemented to support housing hygiene programmes**.

Education on housing hygiene can be conducted at a number of different levels. **Householders** are the largest group to be educated because families often build their own housing and, by definition, are the users of housing. **Architects and builders** require education in the hygienic design and construction of housing. **Health workers** need education in the health hazards of housing when conducting inspections or assessment; **policy leaders** and officials need clear information on the concepts and options for achieving healthy housing. A number of educational and publicity outlets (including television) should be used to promote the message.

Conclusions

Healthy housing is a basic human right, just as much as free access to health services and education. Yet despite this, housing hygiene is still denied to much of the population. The economic costs of this in terms of increased health care, time off from work, school and educational underachievement are considerable, but the human and social costs of poor housing should not be forgotten. It is recognized that insanitary housing is inexorably linked with poverty, culture and ignorance. However, these are not reasons for assuming that progress cannot be made towards the WHO's housing targets detailed in the 'Health for All by the year 2000' strategy. Many countries and communities have taken the opportunity to look at housing hygiene within the context of a wider public health policy, and have already achieved small but significant progress towards WHO targets. The challenge is not to complete the task but to at least begin it and this can only be accomplished if all the agencies and the community are working collectively together towards this goal.

APPRAISAL CRITERIA FOR HEALTHY HOUSING

The primary purpose of carrying out an individual housing inspection is to collect information relating to the condition of the property, e.g. state of repair, freedom from dampness, safety, layout and size in relation to occupancy; to ascertain the provision of amenities; and to assess compliance with housing and public health legislation, e.g. fitness for human occupation. Such inspections may follow a complaint, or they may be carried out as part of a more systematic survey.

The outcome of such inspections is usually to determine whether any legal action, i.e. service of a legal notice requiring works to be carried out, or other intervention, such as an award of a housing grant, is necessary. In the main, the choice is between rectification of any faults together with improvement, i.e. providing additional amenities, or closure and/or demolition in the case of the worst properties. In larger surveys, i.e. house-to-house or area surveys, such information is helpful in allowing policy makers to make wider decisions concerning possible intervention measures, such as declaration of improvement areas, provision of financial assistance, assessment for rehousing, rehabilitation, slum clearance and the establishment of special housing needs. It is also helpful in gaining some overview about the condition of the housing stock both locally and nationally. However, in the latter cases, it is usual to collect additional information relating to socio-economic characteristics, demographic profiles and occupancy, etc., e.g. residential density, number of persons per room, income, age and sex profiles, ethnicity and employment, etc. All of this is likely to be put into an economic planning and/or social perspective.

If local information on mortality and morbidity rates is available, it should also be possible to use an epidemiological approach towards housing options. However, morbidity is difficult to measure and data are often available only for specific population groups, such as school children or working people, and these data are subject to considerable error. In any case, there are methodological difficulties ascribing illnesses to housing conditions. However, the sort of relevant indicators which might be indicative of poor housing conditions include enteric infections, respiratory disease, physiological stress and accidental injury. If such health data are available, then they could be used as an aid to making informed choices for action. Collaboration with local GP practices, health clinics and the public health division of the local health authority, which might well have information about health patterns in the area, would be essential to this approach.

AUDITING HEALTH AND SAFETY OF HOUSING

Once a survey approach has been decided upon, it is usual to carry out a pilot survey of a defined housing sample. This may be randomized or stratified by housing type, area, or socio-economic characteristics. The choice of the area to be surveyed may be influenced by health and socio-economic data relating to the chosen area. For example, child density indices, numbers of elderly people, degree of unemployment, incidence of upper respiratory disease, enteric or home accidents may all be factors which would affect the selection of a housing sample. The size of the sampling frame will depend upon the degree of statistical accuracy required, available resources and size of area being surveyed. However, it is not unusual to inspect 10% of the housing stock during a pilot survey. This would then enable some priorities to be established for house-to-house inspections in a fuller survey.

However, before any survey work can get underway, it is necessary to decide what information is to be collected and, just as important **why** it is needed. If the health and safety audit is being conducted to determine the future action or requisite assistance, e.g. financial help or rehousing, then some attempt may be made to ascribe a score to various housing factors to establish the scale and priorities of particular housing conditions. Different scores can be given to individual items which reflect the health priorities for tackling them, e.g. the absence of water supplies to a house would have a higher points and priority rating than a house provided with inadequate water supplies; overcrowding coupled with absence of means of escape in case of fire in shared housing would be given a higher points rating and priority than a single occupied house with lower residential density (because the fire risk is lower). All these decisions are dependent upon having some rationale about the desired health outcome and the knowledge for achieving this through points ratings and priorities. Enforcement machinery, codes, legislation, finances and other resources need to be available if any meaningful outcome is to be gained. To achieve this, an audit of the policy, organizational, legal, financial, economic, educational and institutional framework for achieving housing hygiene objectives also need to be considered. This is especially relevant to the neighbourhood renewal and assessment approach advocated in the Local Government and Housing Act 1989.

At a technical level, a survey form or checklist is useful as a *aide-mémoire*, and avoids the frustration which every environmental health officer and surveyor feels when finding that he or she has missed a vital piece of information during the inspection, so necessitating a re-visit, admonishment in court or an ombudsman's enquiry.

REFERENCES

1. London Housing Unit (1988) *Another Disastrous Year for the Homeless*, LHU, London.
2. *Homelessness: Report by the Comptroller and Auditor General*, August 1990, HMSO, London.
3. Drennen, V. *et al.* Health visitors and homeless families, (1988) *Health Visitor 1986*, **59**, (11), 340–2.
4. Department of the Environment Circular (6)/90 (28 March 1990) *Local Government and Housing Act 1989 Area Renewal, Unfitness, Slum Clearance and Enforcement Action*, HMSO, London.
5. Ranson, R.P. (1988) *Guidelines for Healthy Housing*, Environmental Health Series EH13,

World Health Organization (EURO), Copenhagen.

FURTHER READING

Baltimore, M.D. (1962) *The Housing Environment and Family Life: a longitudinal study of the effects of housing on morbidity and mental health*, Johns Hopkins University Press.
Benson, J. *et al* (1980) *The Housing Rehabilitation Handbook*, The Architectural Press, London.
Ineichen (1991) *Housing and Health*, E. & F.N. Spon, London.
Littlewood, J. *et al Families in Flats*, HMSO, London. World Health Organization (1961) *Health Aspects of Housing*, WHO Technical Report Series No.225, WHO, Geneva.
Ormandy, D. and Burridge, R. (1988) *Environmental Health Standards in Housing*, Sweet & Maxwell, London.
Ranson, R. (1992), *Healthy Housing – A Practical Guide*, World Health Organization and Chapman and Hall, London.
World Health Organization (1965) *Environmental Health Aspects of Metropolitan Planning and Development*, Report of an Expert Committee, Technical Report Series No.297, WHO, Geneva.
World Health Organization (1974) *Use of Epidemiology in Housing Programmes and in Planning Human Settlements*, Report of an Expert Committee, Technical Report Series No.544, WHO, Geneva.
World Health Organization (1977) *Development of Environmental Criteria for Urban Planning*, Technical Report Series No.51, WHO, Geneva.
World Health Organization (1979) *Health Aspects Related to Indoor Air Quality*, EURO Reports and Studies No.21, WHO, Geneva.
World Health Organization (1983) *Indoor Air Pollutants: exposure and health effects*, EURO Reports and Studies No.78, WHO, Copenhagen.

23 Development control

Neville Hobday

PLANNING

Effective planning is essential to control the building of houses, shops, offices, factories and roads; to encourage sensitive development; to guide it carefully to chosen areas; and to make good use of land within towns. Care needs to be exercised between the competing claims of different land so that development fits well into the local scene. Planning shapes, manages and conserves the environment and helps to protect against damaging change while promoting new projects and developments.

The planning system works mainly through central government, county councils and district and London borough councils. Planning legislation and national guidance from central government are provided principally through the Department of the Environment. Major national issues like motorway schemes, airports, and nuclear power stations are usually decided after local public enquiries. County councils prepare structure plans that give broad, long-term guidance for development and conservation. District councils prepare local plans that show detailed land use and environmental proposals. They also undertake most development control to decide planning applications submitted for development (these responsibilities are subject to the Local Government Review which is currently taking place). Planning permission is usually required before any development can be carried out. Development is described legally in the Town and Country Planning Act 1990 as:

1. the carrying out of building operations, engineering operations, mining operations or other operations in, on, over or under land; or
2. the making of any material change in the use of building or land.

To avoid applying for planning permission in respect of minor proposals, certain activities are permitted by the Town and Country Planning General Development Order. This allows modest extensions to the side or rear of domestic property and certain works at factories, farms and by statutory undertakers.

Planning applications showing all the work proposed are known as 'full applications', and must be taken up within 5 years of permission being granted. Applications usually for more difficult or contentious proposals are submitted in principle. These are known as 'outline permissions'. They also last for 5 years, but within 3 years of the initial approval, full details known as 'reserved matters' must be submitted to, and approved by, the local authority.

A local authority has 8 weeks in which to decide on an application. A number of consultations on each application will take place before the proposal is decided. These consultations might involve:

1. neighbours;
2. parish councils;
3. statutory bodies;
4. Department of Transport – for applications affecting a major road;

5. internal consultations, such as the environmental health officer, on noise, safety and pollution problems.

Certain types of application require more intensive publicity, where either the applicant or the Council publicize either by a notice on the site or more usually by advertising in the local press. These proposals include:

1. 'Bad neighbour' proposals such as sewage works.
2. Conservation areas – proposals which materially affect the character of a conservation area.
3. Listed buildings – application for alteration, internal or external, or even demolition are given added publicity.

After all the consultations and negotiations have taken place, the application is ready to be determined. Decisions fall within three basic groups:

1. unconditional permission;
2. permissions subject to conditions; and
3. refusals.

An applicant has the right of appeal to the Secretary of State.

The Town and Country Planning Act 1990 makes provision for the enforcement of planning control. If a business or a building is commenced without first obtaining planning permission or conditions on an approval are not being complied with, then a local authority can serve an enforcement notice prohibiting the work or use continuing, and take steps to restore the land and buildings to their original state.

If land has been used for a particular purpose without planning permission, or conditions have not been complied with since before 31 December 1963 and the use has continued ever since then, an Established Use Certificate can be applied for. This gives security to the land without the need to obtain planning permission. The onus of proof rests with the applicant.

BUILDING CONTROL

Where building work is to be carried out it is likely that approval under the Building Regulations 1991 will be required. This is notwithstanding that planning consent may have been received or is not required for the purpose.

The Regulations, together with associated codes of practice and other standards, set down requirements for ensuring that building work is weathertight, insulated to the minimum standard, adequately fire protected, drained satisfactorily and is structurally sound so that each part performs the function for which it was designed. Some works, including small detached dwellings and minor building extensions, are exempt from the Building Regulations.

The Building (Approved Inspectors, etc.) Regulations 1985 give a developer the option of either applying to a local authority for Building Regulation consent, and using its building control officers for supervision, or of engaging an approved inspector for supervising the work. With the local authority option proceedings can commence either by the deposit of a full plans application or by the giving of a Building Notice. The building control officer inspects the work at various stages of construction. In the case of non-compliance with regulations, a local authority can take formal proceedings.

CONSERVATION

Planning law allows for the protection and preservation of whole areas of historic or environmental character, as well as individual buildings and trees.

The Planning (Listed Buildings and Conservation Areas) Act 1990 gives local planning authorities powers to declare Conservation Areas: 'areas of special architectural or historic interest, the character or appearance of which it is desirable to conserve or enhance'. Once a Conservation Area is declared, the local authority has special powers to protect the buildings within it and to control new development. Apart from a few minor exceptions, no building can be demolished without prior approval, and all trees are subject to similar protection.

Designation as a Conservation Area does not mean that there can be no change, but local authorities should ensure that new buildings are compatible with others in the area, and that careful attention is paid to the use of building materials.

The Department of the Environment compiles a list of buildings of architectural or historic interest – commonly referred to as listed buildings. Local authorities keep a complete record of these buildings available for inspection. Broadly speaking alterations, extensions or demolitions affecting them require special permission, known as 'Listed Building Consent'. It is a local authority's responsibility to ensure that, wherever possible, listed buildings are retained and properly maintained.

A local authority's main aim should be the continued viable use of a listed building, and should look favourably on any reasonable proposal or use that would ensure protection.

Trees are an important part of the landscape in many areas, and a number have been lost in recent years due to disease and changes in agricultural practice. A local authority can make Tree Preservation Orders on trees of high value either individually or in groups. The Order prohibits the removal, topping, lopping or wilful destruction of such trees without approval. Where a protected tree is felled, a local authority will usually require a suitable replacement. All trees in Conservation Areas are subject to similar protection. A list of Tree Preservation Orders is kept available for inspection.

PLANNING AND THE PUBLIC

In recent years, it has been widely recognized that public opinion is of the utmost importance in the making of planning decisions, whether in respect of application for planning permission, appeals or the preparation of structure and local plans. There is now much more public interest and involvement in planning, and local authorities should ensure that all persons affected have the chance to express their views on a particular matter.

A local authority is required by law to keep registers of planning applications received and the decision made. There is a legal requirement to advertise certain applications in the local press – those affecting listed buildings; development which would have a significant impact on a Conservation Area; major alterations to approved development plans; and applications which are considered to be 'bad neighbour' developments, e.g. a slaughterhouse or public convenience. It is also usual practice to consult the immediate neighbours about planning applications.

A local authority's local plans are also subject to publicity in an attempt to involve the public. Exhibitions and public meetings are normally held during the period of plan preparation, and all objections and comments are considered. If objections cannot be satisfactorily resolved, the persons involved may have a right to make their case at a public local inquiry.

PLANNING AND ENVIRONMENTAL HEALTH

Clearly, there are areas of mutual interest between the planning and environmental health functions where co-operation and liaison by the appropriate officers is essential if a corporate approach is to be achieved in development and enforcement policies. In normal circumstances, the planners consult all departments of the local authority in preparing the local plan, and environmental health comments are relevant on such matters as:

1. industrial development and problems with existing commercial and industrial concerns;
2. air pollution and noise;
3. condition of the private sector housing stock;
4. situation of possible housing development in relation to industry and roads;
5. contaminated land use.

Liaison and consultation is also necessary on planning applications for development and change of use. Issues such as possible nuisances from noise can often be resolved at the application stage, so preventing frustration and annoyance later. PPG24 planning and noise deals specifically with this issue (see Chapter 40). There may also be a need for co-operation between enforcement officers where conditions attached to a planning approval are breached or where a development has taken place without consent, and the activity is creating a nuisance.

The necessity for a corporate involvement in renewal areas is referred to in Chapter 20 on housing condition, and is stressed in DoE Circular 6/90. Environmental health and planning officers will need to liaise on such matters as:

1. housing, commercial and industrial redevelopment;
2. environmental improvements; and
3. traffic management schemes and car parking provision.

Useful guidance on the government's policy on planning and industrial development is given in DoE Circulars 22/80 and 16/84. It is acknowledged that structure and local plans have a central part to play in facilitating appropriate industrial development, but that there may be potential for conflict between approved and adopted plans, and the present needs of industry. The view is expressed that this conflict will be minimized if local plans are realistic, up to date, and make adequate provision for current and likely future industrial development. Paragraph 13 of Circular 16/84 states that while it may be right to prevent expansion of some industries within residential areas – and to plan for moving noxious or bad neighbour ones out – light industry and many forms of small business can often be accommodated within residential areas without creating unacceptable traffic, noise or other adverse effects and without detriment to the amenity of the area. However, in order that planning permission can be given, it may be necessary to impose conditions designed to make a proposed development acceptable in its local context. The conditions must be confined to what is strictly necessary.

On housing, DoE Planning Policy Guidance 3 states that new sites should be well related in scale and location to existing development. Schemes should also be well integrated with the pattern of settlement and surrounding land uses. In order to meet the requirements for new housing and at the same time maintain conservation policies, the document emphasizes the importance of full and effective use being made of land within existing urban areas. DoE Circular 22/80 states that when considering a planning application for a particular site, the character of the site and its surroundings, together with the design and layout of the proposed development and the marketing possibilities, need to be taken into account, as well as any density policies for the area as a whole. Conventional density requirements may not be a reliable guide for:

1. low cost starter homes;
2. small redevelopment sites;
3. infill sites.

Housing is clearly one of the key development activities in most local authorities and the role of the Local Plan is important. The Plan should ensure that sufficient housing land is provided and that the type of housing built meets the requirements of a local authority's residents. It is also important to ensure that the character and amenity of existing housing areas are maintained.

ENVIRONMENTAL ASSESSMENT*

The assessment of environmental quality as part of the formal planning process, or in considering improvement or enhancement schemes, is all embracing, and includes not only those matters with which the environmental health officer is familiar as part of day to day routine such as:

1. air pollution;
2. noise;
3. house conditions, design and space standards;
4. overcrowding

but also other matters such as:

1. street cleansing and litter;
2. pavements and roads;

---

*Also see PPG23 1994, planning and pollution control.

3. street furniture;
4. traffic management and parking;
5. open space provision;
6. commercial and industrial uses.

In evaluating the conditions, some of the matters listed above are of more significance than others, and it is necessary to weight the more important criteria.

The principle of environmental quality assessment is used in the National House Condition Survey where noise, air pollution and outlook are evaluated on a 1 to 4 scale. It is also an integral part – together with a social survey – of the Neighbourhood Renewal Assessment procedures introduced in the Local Government and Housing Act 1989 (see Annex B of Circular 6/90). Unsatisfactory environmental conditions could justify action by a local authority under housing or planning legislation.

As part of the planning process and of examining the impact of a major development, environmental assessment has taken on greater significance following the implementation of European Community Directive No. 85/337 by the Town and Country Planning (Assessment of Environmental Effects) Regulations 1988 (as amended 1994). These require the assessment of the effects of certain public and private projects on the environment.

Projects of the types listed in Schedule 1 to the Regulations are subject to environmental assessment in every case. Projects of the types listed in Schedule 2 are subject to assessment when their characteristics so require, i.e. where there are likely to be significant effects on the environment. In cases to which the requirement applies, the information to be provided by the developer in his or her environmental statement is brought together in Schedule 3 to the Regulations. This information is published, and authorities with relevant environmental responsibilities and the public are to be given an opportunity to express an opinion about the project. These views are taken into consideration in the decision-making process. Further background information and guidance is contained in DoE Circular 15/88 and 7/94.

PLANNING BLIGHT

Planning blight is the expression used to define the detrimental conditions which arise in an area – usually as a result of delay in implementation – when redevelopment is proposed. Houses and commercial premises become difficult to sell, roads, foootpaths, public buildings are not maintained, and residents' confidence in the area diminishes because uncertainty prevails.

If an owner occupied premises or an agricultural unit is already affected by a local planning authority's proposals, a Blight Notice can be served requiring the authority to purchase the premises at market value. The local authority can object to the notice and, if necessary, the claimant can refer the matter to the Lands Tribunal for determination.

The owner occupier must demonstrate that:

1. all or some of the land comes within the descriptions specified by section 149 of the Town and Country Planning Act 1990;
2. the interest to be sold must be one qualifying for protection; and
3. a genuine attempt has been made to sell, but without success, the property at a reasonable figure in the open market.

The effects of planning blight can be reduced by:

1. local authorities adopting a corporate planned approach to area renewal or redevelopment programmed over a reasonable period of time;
2. the implementation of defined plans in consultation with residents, commerce and industry;
3. Co-ordinated action by local authorities, statutory bodies and public utilities;
4. the proper management of redevelopment sites so as to minimize adverse environmental effects.

Part Five

Occupational Health and Safety

24 Legislative and administrative framework

Paul C. Belcher
and John D. Wildsmith

BACKGROUND

In 1970, the government appointed the Committee on Safety and Health at Work (**Robens Committee**) [1] and this was formed with the following terms of reference:

> To review the provision made for the health and safety of persons in the course of their employment (other than transport workers whilst directly engaged on transport operations and who are covered by other provisions) and to consider whether any changes are needed in:
>
> (a) the scope or nature of the relevant enactments;
> (b) the nature and extent of voluntary action concerned with these matters, and to consider whether any further steps are required to safeguard members of the public from hazards, other than general environmental pollution, arising in connection with activities in industrial and commercial premises and construction sites, and to make recommendations.

The Robens Committee report was published in July 1972 (Command 5034; HMSO), and made the following recommendations:

1. the creation of a more unified, integrated system to increase the effectiveness of the state's contribution to health and safety at work;
2. the creation of conditions for more effective self-regulation by employers and employees;
3. the establishment of a Health and Safety Commission with an executive arm called the Health and Safety Executive;
4. a continued enforcement role for local authorities which should be ultimately extended to cover the whole of the non-industrial sector.

THE HEALTH AND SAFETY AT WORK, ETC. ACT 1974 [2]*

This Act broadly implemented the recommendations of the Robens Committee and was brought into force over a period of 6 months commencing on 1 October 1974.

General purposes

The objectives of the Act are set out in section 1 and are:

1. securing the health, safety and welfare of persons at work;

---

*For a discussion of the current legislative system of Health and Safety Control in the UK, see 'Review of Health and Safety Regulations', HSC 5/94.

2. protecting persons other than persons at work against risks to health or safety arising from work activities;
3. controlling explosive, highly flammable or dangerous substances;
4. controlling the emission of noxious or offensive substances from prescribed classes of premises;
5. to enable the previously existing health and safety legislation to be progressively replaced by a system of regulations and approved codes of practice operating in combination.

Scope

All persons at work, with the single exception of people employed as domestic servants in private households, are covered by the Act (section 51). Section 52 makes it clear that the Act includes self-employed persons. The effect of this legislation was to bring some eight million people within the scope of this Act who were not covered by previous health and safety legislation. Emphasis is now placed upon people and their activities rather than specified premises and processes. In addition to people at work, the general public are protected against risks to their health or safety caused by work activities.

General duties

Sections 2 to 7 inclusive of the Act set out a series of provisions placing upon both employers and employees general duties in relation to their activities, and these provisions form the main thrust of the Act. All of the requirements are qualified by the provision that they are to be applied '**so far as is reasonably practicable**'. See 'A Guide to the Health and Safety at Work Act 1974' HSC 1990 HMSO. Also Edwards VNCB (1949) IKB 704 at 712 (1949) 1 A11 ER 743 at 747, CA per Asquith L.J.

Employers' duties to their employees (section 2)

1. To ensure their health, safety and welfare at work.
2. Provide and maintain plant and systems of work that are safe and without risks to health.

3. Ensure safety and absence of risks to health in the use, handling, storage of articles and substances.
4. Provide necessary information, instruction, training and supervision.
5. Maintain workplaces under their control in a safe condition without risks to health, and provide and maintain safe means of access and egress.
6. Provide a safe working environment without risks to health together with adequate welfare arrangements and facilities.

Provisions are also contained in the Health and Safety (Information for Employees) Regulations 1989. It should be noted that the terms 'health', 'safety' and 'welfare' are not defined in the Act.

Duties of employers and the self-employed to persons other than their employees (section 3)

1. Conduct the undertaking in such a way that persons not in his employment are not exposed to risks to their health and safety.
2. Self-employed persons must ensure that both himself, and other persons not employed by him, are not exposed to risks to their health and safety.
3. If prescribed by regulations, to give persons not employed by them, information about how their health and safety could be affected by his undertaking.

Duties of persons concerned with premises to persons other than their employees (section 4)
Take measures to ensure that in respect of non-domestic premises, all means of access and egress, and plant and substances in the premises, are safe and without risks to health.

Duties of persons in control of premises in relation to harmful emissions into the atmosphere (section 5)

1. For classes of premises prescribed by regulations, to prevent the emission into the atmosphere of noxious or offensive substances.
2. Properly use, supervise and maintain plant provided to control these emissions.

(See also the Health and Safety (Emissions to the Atmosphere) Regulations 1983 [4].)

Duties of manufacturers, etc., as regards articles and substances for use at work (section 6)
During inspections environmental health officers will become aware of matters which contravene the requirements of this section. In such cases, the case should be referred to the Enforcement Liaison Officer of the Health and Safety Executive for action.

1. Designers, manufacturers, importers and suppliers of any article for use at work must:
   (a) ensure that it is designed and constructed to be safe and without risks to health when properly used;
   (b) carry out such examination and testing as may be necessary;
   (c) ensure that adequate information is available about the use and testing of articles, and about any conditions necessary to ensure that it will be safe and without risks to health when it is put into use.
2. Designers and manufacturers must carry out research with a view to the discovery and elimination or minimization of any risks to health and safety.
3. Persons who erect or install articles for use at work must ensure that it is not done in a way which makes it unsafe or a risk to health when properly used.
4. Manufacturers, importers and suppliers of any substance for use at work must:
   (a) ensure that it is safe and without risks to health when properly used;
   (b) carry out such testing and examination as necessary;
   (c) make available adequate information about the results of relevant tests.
5. Manufacturers of substances for use at work must carry out necessary research with a view to the discovery and elimination or minimization of risks to health and safety which the substances may give rise to.

(See also the Health and Safety (Leasing Arrangements) Regulations 1992 [5].)

Section 6 was modified by the Noise at Work Regulations 1989 [6] (Regulation 12) so that the duty imposed under subsection (1) 'shall include a duty to ensure that where any such article is likely to cause any employee to be exposed to the "first action level" (i.e. a daily personal noise exposure of 85dB(A) or above) or to the "peak action level" (i.e. a level of peak sound pressure of 200 Pascal or above) then adequate information must be provided concerning the level of noise likely to be generated.'

With regard to this area of work, reference must also be made to the Supply of Machinery (Safety) Regulations 1992 [7] which implement Council Directive 89/392/EEC 'on the approximation of the laws of the Member States relating to machinery' (the Machinery Directive) [8] as amended by Council Directive 91/368/EEC. The Regulations mean that 'relevant machinery' (defined in Regulation 3) cannot be supplied unless it satisfies the relevant essential health and safety requirements laid down in the regulations, and also the appropriate conformity assessment procedure must have been carried out.

The Health and Safety Executive is made responsible for these Regulations (Part IV and Schedule 6) in relation to relevant machinery for use at work.

Duties of employees (section 7)
Employees while at work must:

1. take reasonable care for the health and safety of himself and other persons who may be affected by his acts and omissions;
2. co-operate with their employers and others who may have legal responsibilities under the Act.

Self-regulation

The Act lays great emphasis upon the principle of 'self-regulation' of the workplace by the employer and the employees, and the main thrust is set out in section 2(3) in the requirement that each employer must:

'prepare and as often as may be appropriate revise a written statement of his general policy with respect to the health and safety at work of his employees and the organization and arrangements for the time being in force for carrying out that policy, and to bring the statement and any revision of it to the notice of his employees'.

The Employer's Health and Safety Policy Statement (Exceptions) Regulations 1975 [9] release employers with less than five employees from this general obligation.

The objective of this provision is to ensure that each employer systematically evaluates the premises, operations, processes and practices, and produces systems of work and organizational and other arrangements to deal with them in such a way that hazards to health and safety are eliminated or minimized.

It is not desirable to issue a 'standard health and safety policy' document as this would negate the evaluation process. It is, however, possible to produce general guidance on the main elements, which should be:

1. **General statement:** a declaration of the employer's intention to seek to provide, so far as reasonably practicable, safe and healthy working conditions. The statement should be signed by the person in the most senior executive position in the company, and should give the name of the person who is responsible for fulfilling the objectives in the policy.

2. **Organization:** following an evaluation of the business, this part of the statement should indicate in detail the degree of health and safety responsibility appropriate to the various levels of management. It should name the key posts in the organization, and define their responsibilities, including line management, supervisors and health and safety specialists. The arrangements for joint consultation on health and safety matters should be set out, including the names of any appointed union safety representatives and the terms of reference and arrangements made for any joint health and safety committees.

3. **Arrangements:** this part should follow a comprehensive study of the full range of work activities to include:

(a) procedures for dealing with common and special hazards;
(b) safe systems of work;
(c) accident reporting and investigations;
(d) provision and use of protective clothing and equipment;
(e) procedures for introducing new machinery, processes and substances;
(f) emergency procedures including fire and explosion 'drills';
(g) arrangements for informing staff about health and safety issues;
(h) health and safety training provisions;
(i) safety inspections, audits, etc.

It should be noted that the involvement of employees in occupational health and safety in the workplace is encouraged. This is particularly stated in section 2 of the Act, which allows the appointment of 'safety representatives' by recognized trades unions in accordance with regulations drawn up by the Secretary of State (The Safety Representatives and Safety Committee Regulations 1977) [10]. Employers have a duty under this section to consult with such safety representatives. In prescribed cases or when safety representatives request it, employers are obliged to formalize the relationships by establishing 'safety committees'.

ADMINISTRATION

As suggested by the Robens Committee, the Act established both a **Health and Safety Commission** (HSC) and the **Health and Safety Executive** (HSE), the detailed provisions being set out in sections 10 to 14 inclusive and Schedule 2.

The main functions of the HSC include:

1. making general arrangements for the implementation of Part 1 of the Act and providing assistance to others concerned;
2. carrying out and encouraging research, publishing results and providing and encouraging training and information;
3. information and advisory services to all concerned with or affected by the Act;

4. preparing and submitting to the Secretary of State proposals for new regulations and approving codes of practice and guidance notes;
5. directing the executive to investigate major accidents or occurrences or other relevant issues.

The Commission is serviced by the Executive, which is also its main operational arm. The HSE has direct duties in relation to the enforcement of the Act, but it also provides research and laboratory facilities. It also provides the use of such services and other information to local authorities, to assist them with their enforcement of the Act.

Knowledge of the current guidance available on any topic is essential for any inspector enforcing this legislation.

The Employment Medical Advisory Service (EMAS) was continued by Part 2 of the Act, but now it operates as the 'medical arm' of the HSC. The services of EMAS can also be made available to local authorities.

ENFORCEMENT

Responsibilities for enforcing the Act are shared between the HSE and local authorities, and enforcement responsibilities are allocated on the basis of the 'main activity' carried on at each premises to which the Act applies. Currently, the arrangements are made according to the Health and Safety (Enforcing Authority) Regulations 1989 [11]. Schedule 1 (see below) lists those main activities which determine whether the local authority is the enforcing authority, while Schedule 2 lists activities for which, wherever they are carried on, the HSE is the enforcing authority, e.g. fairgrounds.

The Health and Safety (Enforcing Authority) Regulations 1989, Schedule 1

1. The sale or storage of goods for retail or wholesale distribution except:
   (a) where it is part of the business of a transport undertaking;
   (b) at container depots where the main activity is the storage of goods in the course of transit to or from dock premises, an airport or a railway;
   (c) where the main activity is the sale or storage for wholesale distribution of any dangerous substance;
   (d) where the main activity is the sale or storage of water or sewage or their by-products or natural or town gas;
   and for the purpose of this paragraph where the main activity carried on in premises is the sale and fitting of motor car tyres, exhausts, windscreens or sunroofs, the main activity shall be deemed to be the sale of goods.
2. The display or demonstration of goods at an exhibition for the purpose of offer or advertisement for sale.
3. Office activities.
4. Catering services.
5. The provision of permanent or temporary residential accommodation, including the provision of a site for caravans or campers.
6. Consumer services provided in a shop except dry cleaning or radio and television repairs and in this paragraph 'consumer services' means services of a type ordinarily supplied to persons who receive them otherwise in the course of a trade, business or other undertaking carried on by them (whether for profit or not).
7. Cleaning (wet or dry) in coin-operated units in launderettes and similar premises.
8. The use of a bath, sauna or solarium, massaging, hair transplanting, skin piercing, manicuring or other cosmetic services and therapeutic treatments, except where they are carried out under the supervision or control of a registered medical practitioner, a dentist registered under the Dentists Act 1984, a physiotherapist, an osteopath or a chiropractor.
9. The practice or presentation of the arts, sports, games, entertainment or other cultural or recreational activities, except where carried on in a museum, art gallery or theatre or where the main activity is the exhibition of a cave to the public.

10. The hiring out of pleasure craft for use on inland waters.
11. The care, treatment, accommodation or exhibition of animals, birds or other creatures, except where the main activity is horse breeding or horse training at a stable, or is an agricultural activity or veterinary surgery.
12. The activities of an undertaker, except where the main activity is embalming or the making of coffins.
13. Church worship or religious meetings.

In order to secure a degree of uniformity in the application of this legislation, both the Commission and the Executive issue a considerable amount of guidance to both enforcement authorities and to employers.

Liaison between local authority staff and HSE staff is achieved in several ways such as:

1. the establishment of a national Health and Safety Executive/Local Authority Liaison Committee (**HELA**);
2. local arrangements made through the appointment of an enforcement liaison officer (**ELO**) within each area office of the HSE.

For a discussion on the principles and approach to the enforcement of environmental health law generally including health and safety see Chapter 8.

Every enforcing authority may appoint such inspectors, having such qualifications as it thinks necessary (section 19). Each appointment must be made in writing, specifying which of the powers conferred upon inspectors (section 20) are conferred upon the person appointed.

It should be noted that it is **the inspector**, and not the enforcing authority, who has a number of powers conferred upon him, the principal ones of which are:

1. **Improvement Notice (section 21)**. Where an inspector is of the opinion that a person is contravening one or more of the 'relevant statutory provisions' listed in Schedule 1 of the Act, or has contravened one or more of those conditions in circumstances that make it likely that the contravention will continue or be repeated, he may serve upon him an Improvement Notice stating the particulars and his opinion, and requiring that the stated matters must be remedied within a specified period (not less than the period allowed for appeals).
2. **Prohibition Notice (section 22)**. This applies to any activities that are being or about to be carried on by or under the control of any person, which involve or will involve the risk of serious personal injury. A Prohibition Notice must specify the matters that cause the inspector to form his opinion, and directs a person not to carry out the specified activities. Such a notice may come into effect immediately where the risk is imminent, or it may be deferred, to come into operation after a specified period where circumstances allow this course of action.

A number of supplementary provisions relating to Improvement and Prohibition Notices are given in section 23, which state for example that notices may included directions as to the measures to be taken to remedy matters to which the notice relates, and also, that such directions may be framed by reference to any Approved Code of Practice.

Notices which do not take immediate effect may be withdrawn by an inspector at any time before any time period specified in the notice, and the period specified may be extended at any time when an appeal is not pending against the notice. This allows considerable flexibility in ensuring compliance with notices.

Arrangements for **appeals** against Improvement and Prohibition Notices are dealt with in section 24 of the Act. Appeals are normally made to **industrial tribunals**, which are independent judicial bodies, created to adjudicate in certain matters of dispute in the employment field in a speedy, informal and informed way. After its adjudication, the tribunal will issue written decisions which are binding upon the parties concerned. It should be noted that an appeal automatically suspends the operation of an Improvement Notice, but not a Prohibition Notice. However, this type of notice may be suspended by the tribunal after due consideration. The tribunal may cancel, modify or confirm any notice.

Where it is considered that there has been some administrative defect, a tribunal may be requested to review its decision. An appeal may be made to the High Court on a point of law.

Many additional powers are available under section 20, however, one important feature of this legislation is the power to deal with the cause of any imminent danger under section 25, where the inspector may seize any article or substances and '**cause it to be rendered harmless whether by destruction or otherwise**'.

The procedures for dealing with Improvement and Prohibition Notices and for the seizure of articles and substances are detailed in *Environmental Health Procedures* [12] by the use of flow charts.

Offences

Section 33 lists those matters which are considered to be offences under the Act, and these include:

1. failure to comply with the general duties under sections 2 to 7;
2. contraventions of health and safety regulations;
3. contraventions relating to statutory enquiries;
4. contraventions of Improvement and Prohibition Notices;
5. obstructing an inspector;
6. refusing to reveal information;
7. misusing or wrongfully revealing information obtained under statutory powers;
8. making false statements, entries in registers and forging documents;
9. failure to comply with court orders under section 42.

Where an offence is committed by one person but is due to the act or default of another person, that other person may be charged with the offence either in addition to, or in substitution for, the original person (section 36). Where offences are committed by corporate bodies, directors, managers, secretaries and others may be prosecuted if it can be proved that the offence was committed with their consent, connivance or that any neglect can be attributed to them

(section 37). The combined effect of these two sections is to render liable to prosecution any person with designated or implied health and safety responsibilities within an organization.

EUROPEAN INITIATIVES

One of the subsidiary aims of the European Economic Community was to improve the quality of the working environment. In the early years between 1957 and 1974 the newly formed Community concentrated upon the problems of occupational illness and disease. Following the adoption of the Social Action Programme in 1974 a number of Directives were introduced to approximate the laws of member states on issues such as safety signs [13] and exposure to vinyl chloride monomer [14].

As with other aspects of the Community, 'Action Programmes' were developed and implemented in 1978 and 1984, however since 1988 the approach adopted to regulate health and safety at work has been via the enactment of the 'Framework Directive' on the introduction of measures to encourage improvements in the safety and health of workers (89/391/EEC) [15].

Under this 'Framework Directive', a number of 'Daughter Directives' have now been adopted by Member States. At the present time, those of note include:

1. on the minimum safety and health requirements for the workplace;
2. on the minimum safety and health requirements for the use of work equipment by workers at work;
3. on the minimum health and safety requirements for the use by workers of personal protective equipment;
4. on the minimum health and safety requirements for the manual handling of loads where there is a risk particularly of back injury to workers;
5. on the minimum safety and health requirements for work with visual screen equipment.

The Daughter Directives are of real significance in the UK as they have lead to the development of a variety of new Regulations, commonly referred to as the 'Six Pack', which are listed below. Each of the new provisions is dealt with in subsequent chapters. A useful reference text on the social legislative background of European health and safety legislation has been produced by Neal and Wright [16].

The 'Six Pack'

The Management of Health and Safety at Work Regulations 1992. (Amended 1994.)

The Workplace (Health, Safety and Welfare) Regulations 1992.

The Provision and Use of Work Equipment Regulations 1992.

The Manual Handling Operations Regulations 1992.

The Health and Safety (Display Screen Equipment) Regulations 1992.

The Personal Protective Equipment Regulations 1992.

REFERENCES

1. The Committee on Safety and Health at Work (Robens Committee) (1972) Command 5034, HMSO, London.
2. The Health and Safety at Work etc. Act 1974. 1974 c.37. HMSO, London.
3. The Health and Safety (Information for Employees) Regulations 1989. S.I.1989. No.682, HMSO, London.
4. The Health and Safety (Emissions into the Atmosphere) Regulations 1983. S.I. 1983. No.943, HMSO, London.
5. The Health and Safety (Leasing Arrangements) Regulations 1992. S.I.1992 No.1524, HMSO, London.
6. The Noise at Work Regulations 1989. S.I.1989 No.1790, HMSO, London.
7. Supply of Machinery (Safety) Regulations 1992. S.I. 1992 No.3073.
8. Council Directive 89/392/EEC 'on the approximation of the laws of the Member States relating to machinery'. OJ No.L183, 29.6.89, p9.
9. The Employer's Health and Safety Policy Statement (Exceptions) Regulations 1975. S.I.1975 No.1584, HMSO, London.
10. The Safety Representatives and Safety Committee Regulations 1977. S.I.1977 No.500, HMSO, London.
11. The Health and Safety (Enforcing Authority) Regulations 1989.S.I.1989 No.1903, HMSO, London.
12. Bassett, W.H. (1995) *Environmental Health Procedures*, 4th edn, Chapman & Hall, London.
13. Council Directive on the approximation of the laws, regulations and administrative provisions of Member States relating to the provision of safety signs at places of work (77/576/EEC) as amended by Directive 79/640/EEC.
14. Council Directive on the approximation of the laws, regulations and administrative provisions of the Member States on the protection of the health of workers exposed to vinyl chloride monomer (78/610/EEC).
15. Council Directive on the introduction of measures to encourage improvements in the safety and health of workers (89/391/EEC).
16. Neal, A.C. and Wright, F.B. (eds) (1992) *The European Communities' Health and Safety Legislation*, Chapman & Hall, London.

25 The working environment

Paul C. Belcher and John D. Wildsmith

Whilst one can lay great emphasis on the responsibility of the individual worker to ensure that their health, safety and welfare is maintained, one must never forget the responsibility that rests upon the employer to provide a safe working environment. This chapter looks at some of the factors that help to ensure that the workforce has a workplace that does not present a risk to their health, safety and welfare, or does not impose undue stress on the worker.

WORKPLACE STRESS

Stress can occur in a variety of forms. Some would argue that it is a desirable part of our everyday existence. However, prolonged exposure to stress can be extremely harmful leading to coronory heart disease, hypertension and gastro-intestinal disorders. At a social level, excess stress can result in the disruption of relationships. Within the workplace, a person suffering from stress may be more likely to lose concentration, possibly at vital moments, thereby increasing the risk of death by injury to either themselves or to a fellow employee.

Given that stress can be extremely harmful to many people, it is important for both employers and enforcement officers to recognize those factors, including those physical factors discussed below, that may result in stress.

WORKPLACE HEALTH, SAFETY AND WELFARE

As far as local authority enforcing officers are concerned, control over workplace health and safety can now be thought of as being embodied in the Health and Safety at Work Etc. Act 1974 and in the new Workplace (Health, Safety and Welfare) Regulations 1992. These new Regulations implement most of the requirements of the Workplace Directive (89/654/EC) which is concerned with minimum standards for workplace health and safety. In most cases the Regulations bring together the legislative controls that existed prior to the 1974 Act.

The Regulations have different commencement dates. Workplaces that existed prior to 1 January 1993 will be brought within their control on 1 January 1996. For new workplaces taken into use after 1 January 1993, and for workplaces modified, converted or extended after that date, the Regulations came into operation on 1 January 1993. It is suggested that many employers and enforcing authorities should now be working towards full compliance with the new Regulations, even where compliance is not a legal requirement. Detailed guidance on the Regulations is contained in the Approved Code of Practice [1].*

The Regulations contain a general requirement for every employer and others to ensure that any

* HSE has also issued guidance, particularly for small firms – 'Workplace Health, Safety and Welfare', IND (G) 170L 1994, HSE Books.

workplace under their control, and where their employees work, complies with any applicable requirement. This duty is extended to those who have control of a workplace in connection with any trade, business or other undertaking (whether for profit or not).

Maintenance of workplace, equipment, devices and systems

Regulation 5 requires that the workplace and certain equipment, devices and systems be regularly maintained in an efficient state, in efficient working order and in good repair. The equipment etc. covered by this Regulation is that equipment etc., a fault in which is liable to result in a failure to comply with any of the Regulations.

The Approved Code of Practice [1] suggests that any system of maintenance should ensure that:

1. regular maintenance (including, as necessary, inspection, testing, adjustment, lubrication and cleaning) is carried out at suitable intervals;
2. any potential dangerous defects are remedied, and that access to the defective equipment is prevented in the meantime;
3. regular maintenance and remedial work is carried out properly; and
4. a suitable record is kept to ensure that the system is properly implemented and to assist in validating maintenance programmes.

The frequency of any maintenance should clearly depend on the nature of the equipment and its age. Regard should be had to advice from, for example, the manufactures and the Health and Safety Executive.

Examples of equipment covered by this Regulation include emergency lighting, fencing, fixed equipment used for window cleaning, anchorage points used for safety harnesses, escalators.

Ventilation

By virtue of Regulation 6 every enclosed workplace must be ventilated by a sufficient quantity of fresh or purified air. This requirement does not extend to work carried on in confined spaces where breathing apparatus may be necessary. In most cases, openable windows or other openings will provide satisfactory ventilation. However, if found to be necessary, mechanical ventilation should be provided. It is important that such systems be regularly maintained, especially due to possible risk of legionnaire's disease.

Temperature in indoor workplaces

Many working environments can be uncomfortable due to either excessive heat or cold. In cases of extreme heat or cold it is possible for workers to suffer from heat or cold stress. Regulation 7 requires that during working hours, the temperature in all workplaces inside buildings should be reasonable. The Approved Code of Practice [1] suggests a sedentary minimum temperature of 16°C, and 13°C where their is severe physical effort. The only exception to this rule is where processes such as cold storage require lower temperatures. In such circumstances the employer should take all reasonable steps to provide protective clothing, and sufficient rest periods for employees.

The Regulations also contain a general requirement for employers to provide a sufficient number of thermometers to enable employees to ascertain the temperature.

Gill [2] argues that to obtain a correct assessment of the thermal environment, four parameters need to be measured together:

1. The air dry bulb temperature.
2. The air wet bulb temperature.
3. The radiant temperature.
4. The air velocity.

A whirling hygrometer can be used to measure wet and dry bulb temperature whilst a simple globe thermometer can be use to measure the radiant temperature. To measure the air velocity either a kata thermometer or an airflow meter can be used. A detailed description of how to used these measurements to assess the thermal environment is found in Gill [3]. In addition, there are now on the market 'thermal comfort meters' which are not only able to carry out many of these measurements automatically, but are also capable of being linked to recorders and computers to enable rapid analysis of findings.

Lighting

Adequate lighting is an important prerequisite for ensuring the safety and comfort of people at work. Whilst natural light is the most desirous form of lighting, in many work situations this has to be either supplemented or completely replaced by some form of artificial lighting.

Suitable and sufficient lighting is required in Regulation 8. In addition, emergency lighting must be provided where failure of any artificial lighting could pose a risk to health and safety.

The amount and type of lighting provided in any work situation quite clearly depends upon the type of work being carried on there. The Health and Safety Executive have suggested levels of lighting for different work environments [4]. In addition, the Chartered Institute of Building Services Engineers have also produced a code for interior lighting [5].

Measurement of lighting levels can be simply carried out using a proprietary light meter. Where possible a light meter with a remote sensing device should be used, as this removes the risk of readings being affected by shadows from the operator.

Cleanliness

Every workplace, and the furniture, furnishings and fittings contained in it are to be kept sufficiently clean (Regulation 9). In addition, the surfaces of the floors, walls and ceilings of all workplaces shall be capable of being kept sufficiently clean, and all waste material must be kept in suitable receptacles.

It is important to bear in mind that only an adequately thought out planned cleaning programme will satisfy this general requirement.

Space

Regulation 10 requires that every room where persons work shall have sufficient floor area, height and unoccupied space for the purposes of health, safety and welfare.

The Approved Code of Practice [1] establishes that personal space should be at least 11 cubic metres. In calculating personal space it is assumed that there is a minimum notional ceiling height of 3 metres. For existing workplaces covered by the provisions of the Factories Act 1961, there is a requirement to comply with the specification contained in Schedule 1 Part 1 of the Regulations.

Workstations and seating

Workstations must be arranged so as to be suitable for any person who is likely to work there, and for any work likely to be done there (Regulation 11). For those workstations that are located outside, there must be protection from adverse weather conditions. These workstations must also be arranged so as to enable swift means of escape in cases of emergency.

Where necessary a suitable seat must be provided. Suitability is defined as being not only suitable for the operation being carried on, but also for the person for whom it is provided. Where necessary a footrest must also be provided.*

Workstations where visual display units, process control screens, micro-fiche readers and similar display units are used are covered by the Health and Safety (Display Screen Equipment) Regulations 1992 (see below).

Conditions of floors and traffic routes

Floors and traffic routes should be of sound construction and must be constructed so as to be suitable for the purpose for which they are used (Regulation 12). Traffic route is defined in the Regulations as:

a route for pedestrian traffic, vehicles or both and includes any stairs, staircase, fixed ladder, doorway, gateway, loading bay or ramp.

The Regulations specify that there should be no holes or slope or unevenness or slipperiness which

* See also 'A Pain in the Workplace – Ergonomic Problems and Solutions'.

could pose a risk to health or safety. In addition, such routes should be kept free from obstruction, and where necessary sufficiently drained.

Handrails should be provided where necessary. Open sides to staircases should be protected by an upper rail at 900 mm or higher, and a lower rail.

Falls or falling objects

In many workplace situations, e.g. construction sites, factories, offices, work has to take place at height. Such work will involve activities such as maintenance operations, installation of plant and equipment, window cleaning. The risk of falling, with often fatal results, is a common hazard of such operations. Dewis and Stranks [6] recognize that there are two outstanding causes of this type of accident. These they see as relating to firstly the means of access to the work situation, and secondly to the system of work adopted once the working position is reached.

In many cases employers will have considered the risks to employees of working at height. Exercises such as risk assessments, safety surveys and safety audits will reveal hazards, and meetings of safety committees and discussion with safety representatives will also lead to the establishment of safe systems of work (see chapter 27).

When considering the risks of working at height factors such as the provision of safety harnesses and belts, including the necessary anchorage points for their safe use, and the provision of protective clothing such as suitable headcovering, gloves and safety footwear for employees need to borne in mind.

The provisions of Regulation 13 extend this consideration to not only prevention of falls but also the protection of persons from being struck by a falling object likely to cause personal injury. In addition, every tank or pit shall be securely fenced, and every traffic route, where there is a risk of falling into a dangerous substance, shall also be securely fenced. The Regulations define dangerous substance as:

1. any substance likely to scald or burn;
2. any poisonous substance;
3. any corrosive substance;
4. any fume, gas or vapour likely to overcome a person; or
5. any granular or free-flowing solid substance, or any viscous substance which, in any case, is of a nature or quantity which is likely to cause danger to any person.

The Approved Code of Practice [1] suggests that fencing should be provided at any place where a person might fall 2 metres or more. Such fencing, where provided for the first time, should be at least 1100 mm above the surface. The fencing should also prevent objects being knocked off the surface.

Where fixed ladders are provided they should be of sound construction. If they are at an angle of less than 15 degrees to the vertical and more than 2.5 metres high, they shall be fitted with suitable safety hoops or other fall arrest systems. The Code of Practice [1] gives guidance on such ladders.

Of particular concern are racking systems, particularly those found in warehouses. The Code of Practice suggests that certain precautions be taken to ensure the minimization of risk to health and safety. In addition the Health and Safety Executive has published guidance on warehouse stacking [7].

Windows, transparent or translucent doors, gates and walls

All windows, doors, gates, walls and partitions glazed wholly or partially so that they are transparent or translucent must, where necessary for health and safety, be of safe material and be appropriately marked (Regulation 15). The Code of Practice [1] defines safety materials as:

1. materials which are inherently robust, such as polycarbonates or glass blocks; or
2. glass which, if it breaks, breaks safely; or
3. ordinary annealed glass which meets the thickness criteria laid down in the Approved Code of Practice.

As an alternative to using safety materials, transparent or translucent surfaces may be protected by the use of screens or barriers.

Regulation 15 further requires that windows, skylights or ventilators which can be opened, should not expose any person opening them to a risk to their health and safety, and when opened such windows, etc. should not expose any person to a risk to their health or safety.

Finally, Regulation 16 deals with the cleaning of windows and skylights in workplaces. With regard to the advice that should be given to those employed in cleaning windows, attention is drawn to the guidance given by the Health and Safety Executive [8] and the contents of the relevant British Standard [9].

Organization of traffic routes, etc.

Regulation 17 deals with the safe circulation of pedestrians and vehicles in the workplace. There must be sufficient separation between vehicles and pedestrians. All routes must be adequately signed.

All doors and gates are to be suitably constructed to include the fitting of any necessary safety devices (Regulation 18). In particular the Regulations require that:

1. any door or gate has a device to prevent it coming off its track during use;
2. any upward opening door or gate has a device to prevent it falling back;
3. any powered door or gate has suitable and effective features to prevent it causing injury by trapping any person;
4. where necessary for reasons of health or safety, any powered door or gate can be operated manually unless it opens automatically if the power fails; and
5. any door or gate which is capable of opening by being pushed from either side is of such a construction as to provide, when closed, a clear view of the space close to both sides.

Regulation 19 requires that all escalators and moving walkways function safely, be equipped with any necessary safety device, and be fitted with sufficient emergency stop controls. There is guidance issued by the Health and Safety Executive [10,11].

Welfare facilities

Regulations 20–25 deal with the provision of sanitary conveniences, washing facilities, adequate wholesome drinking water, suitable and sufficient facilities for changing clothing and suitable and sufficient facilities for rest and to eat meals. The Approved Code of Practice [1] gives details as to the minimum number of sanitary conveniences, etc. With regard to rest areas, both the Regulations and the Code of Practice stress the need to have regard to the risks of passive smoking, and employers are required to ensure that suitable arrangements are made so as to ensure no discomfort occurs [12].

Display screen equipment

Display screen equipment (DSE) is now covered by a specific set of Regulations, The Health and Safety (Display Screen Equipment) Regulations 1992. The Regulations implement a European Directive (90/270/EEC) on DSE.

There is some degree of overlap between this set of Regulations and the Management of Health and Safety at Work Regulations 1992, particularly with regard to issues such as risk assessment. The Guidance on the Regulations [13] points out that employers are required to comply with both the specific requirements of the DSE Regulations, and the general requirements of the Management Regulations. However, carrying out a risk assessment on a workstation under Regulation 2 of the DSE Regulations will also satisfy the requirements of the Management Regulations, but only for that workstation.

Health effects of display screen equipment

DSE has been blamed for a whole range of adverse health effects. One of the most spectacular is the effects of radiation emitted from the equipment on pregnant women. However, there is some epidemiological evidence to suggest that DSE can have some impact on health status. Generally, these effects are linked to the visual system and working posture. The effects include:

1. repetitive strain injury, or work-related upper limb disorders;

2. eye or eyesight defects;
3. epilepsy;
4. fatigue and stress.

For a detailed consideration of the health effects of DSE, attention is drawn to a number of publications from the Health and Safety Executive [14–16]. The International Labour Office in 1994 published *Visual Display Units: radiation protection guidance*, available from ILO publications, CH-1211, Geneva 22, Switzerland.*

The requirements of the Display Screen Equipment Regulations

DSE is defined as 'any alphanumeric or graphic display screen, regardless of the display process involved'. An operator or user is someone who 'habitually uses display screen equipment as a significant part of his or her work'. The Regulations suggest that generally an individual will be classified as a user or operator if most or all of the following apply:

1. the individual depends on the use of DSE to do the job, as alternative means are not readily available for achieving the same results;
2. the individual has no discretion as to use or non-use of the DSE;
3. the individual needs significant training and/or particular skills in the use of DSE to do the job;
4. the individual normally uses DSE for continuous spells of an hour or more at a time;
5. the individual uses DSE in this way more or less daily;
6. fast transfer of information between the user and screen is an important requirement of the job;
7. the performance requirements of the system demand high levels of attention and concentration by the user, e.g. where the consequences of error may be critical.

The Guidance document [13] gives the following examples of users:

1. word processing operators;

2. secretaries or typists;
3. data input operators;
4. journalists;
5. air traffic controllers.

Regulation 2 requires every employer to carry out a suitable and sufficient analysis of workstations used by users or operators, to assess the possible risks to health and safety. The assessment must be reviewed if there is a significant change or if the assessment is no longer valid. The employer, having identified the risks, is then required to reduce them to the lowest extent reasonably practicable.

Regulation 3 requires that all new workstations meet the detailed requirements of the Schedule to the Regulations. Existing (i.e. pre 1993) equipment is required to comply by the end of December 1996. The Schedule deals with issues such as the display screen, the keyboard, the work desk or work surface, the work chair, space requirements, lighting, reflections and glare, noise, heat, radiation, humidity and the interface between the computer and the operator/user. The Guidance document gives detailed advice on the interpretation of the Schedule.

Regulation 4 requires employers to plan the activities of users so as to ensure that sufficient rest periods are provided. The Guidance document suggests that short frequent breaks are more satisfactory than longer breaks. For example 5–10 minutes every 50–60 minutes working.

There is a general provision made in Regulation 5 for eye and eyesight tests to be made available on request, and at regular intervals. If any 'special corrective appliances' (generally speaking these are spectacles/lens) are required, then currently these have to be paid for by the employer.

Regulation 6 makes it a requirement for the provision of health and safety training for DSE users. In addition Regulation 7 requires employers to make available for users information about breaks, eye and eyesight tests and training both initially and when the workstation is modified.

---

* The NRPB has reviewed the health effects related to the use of VDUs – Vol. 5, No. 2, 1994.

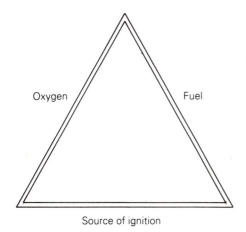

Fig. 25.1 Fire triangle.

FIRE

The 'fire triangle' is perhaps the most convenient way of studying the fire situation (Fig. 25.1). It is argued that fuel, oxygen and a source of ignition are needed in order for any fire to be sustained. As a result, in most cases, the removal of any one of these components of the triangle results in either the fire being extinguished, or fire prevention if no fire is occurring.

Classes of fire

Fires may be broken down into four main classifications:

1. Class A. These are fires involving solid materials of a cellulosic nature such as wood, paper, cardboard, coal and natural fibres. The risk of fire is at its greatest when the material is finely divided, e.g. wood shavings.
2. Class B. Fires involving liquids or liquefiable solids. With regard to liquids, one can further divide the classification into:
   B.1 those liquids that mix with water, e.g. methanol, acetone and acetic acid;
   B.2 those liquids that do not mix with water, e.g. waxes, fats, petrol and solvents.
3. Class C. Fires involving gases or liquefied gases in the form of liquid gas spillage or gas leaks. Examples are methane, propane and butane.

4. Class D. Fires involving certain flammable metals such as aluminium and magnesium.

Electrical fires

This classification is no longer used. They are often caused by the arcing or overheating of conductors. The problem with this type of fire is that often the electrical apparatus remains alive, causing a further risk to those involved in fighting the fire.

Dealing with fires

In order to extinguish a fire, one must have a knowledge of the combustion process. For the combustion reaction to proceed, the concentration of fuel to air must be in the flammable range, and the mixture must receive a certain amount of energy. Therefore, the reaction will cease if one or other of these criteria is not met.

One can employ this knowledge and deal with fires in one of three ways:

1. **Starvation**: by this is meant reducing the concentration of the fuel. This can be achieved by, for example, switching off the gas supply or building fire breaks.
2. **Smothering**: limiting the concentration of air. This can be achieved by allowing the fire to consume all the oxygen in the air while at the same time preventing any further air flow. Examples of this type of approach are the wrapping of a person whose clothes are on fire with a rug or covering fires with sand.
3. **Cooling**: this means reducing the energy input. This is by far the most common method of dealing with fires. By using water, the fire is put out because of the cooling effect of the water.

Fire-fighting agents

By applying the principles of extinction outlined above it is clear that, in the main, any fire-fighting agent will be used either to cool the fire or to starve the fire of oxygen. The most commonly used fire-fighting agents are:

Water

As outlined above, water is an extremely efficient cooling agent. It is generally applied to the fire either in the form of a fine spray, or as a jet. Application by use of a spray is more effective than a jet, and more heat can be absorbed by the drops in the spray than by the bulk flow in the jet. However, with large fires, heavy jets are needed to provide the necessary quantities of water.

Foam

Foam consists of a mass of small bubbles which form an air-excluding and cooling blanket over the fire. There are two basic types of foam: chemical and mechanical. Chemical foam is produced by the mixing of two chemicals, usually sodium bicarbonate and aluminium sulphate. This can be represented by the following equation:

$$6NaHCO_3 + Al_2(SO_4)_3 \rightarrow 2Al(OH)_3 + 3Na_2SO_4 + 6CO_2$$

Sodium bicarbonate + aluminium sulphate gives aluminium hydroxide + sodium sulphate + carbon dioxide

Mechanical foam is produced by the release of a foam solution via a self-aspirating nozzle.

Carbon dioxide

Carbon dioxide acts by diluting the oxygen content of the atmosphere surrounding the fire. It is contained in a liquid form under pressure, and boils off to gas when released.

Vapourizing liquids

These are halogenated hydrocarbons, which inhibit the spread of the fire by excluding air. All of the liquids used are extremely toxic, and care should be exercised in their use.

Dry powders

Finely reduced sodium bicarbonate or ammonium phosphate have been found to be extremely effective fire fighting agents when applied as a concentrated cloud.

Table 25.1 Classification of fire for portable extinguishers

Class of fire	Description	Extinguisher
A	Solid materials	Water, foam, dry powder, vapourizing liquid and CO_2
B	Liquids and liquefiable solids:	
	B.1 miscible with water	Water, foam, CO_2, dry powder, vapourizing liquid
	B.2 immiscible with water	Foam, dry powder, vapourizing liquid, CO_2
C	Gas or liquefied gas	—
D	Metals	—
—	Electrical equipment	Dry powder, vapourizing liquids, CO_2 (not computers)

Choice of portable extinguisher

Waterhouse [17] defines the type of fire extinguisher to be used by the class of fire (see above) that is being dealt with (Table 25.1).

Means of escape in case of fire

As mentioned above, it is imperative that all workplaces have a clearly defined procedure for ensuring that people know what to do and where to go in the case of a fire. To this end, all fire escapes should be clearly marked in accordance with the relevant British Standards, and all routes out of the workplace should also be protected in from fire. In addition staff, particularly new members of staff, should practise fire drills regularly.

REFERENCES

1. Health and Safety Executive (1992) *Workplace Health, Safety and Welfare – Approved Code of Practice to the Workplace (Health Safety and Welfare) Regulations 1992, L21*, HMSO, London.

2. Gill, F.S. (1986) Workplace pollution, heat and ventilation, in Ridley, J. (ed.) *Safety at Work*, 2nd edn, Butterworths, London.

3. Gill, F.S. (1980) Heat physics and measurement in Harrington, M.J. and Waldron, H.A. (eds) *Occupational Hygiene*, Blackwell, Oxford.

4. Health and Safety Executive (1987) *Lighting at Work HS(G)38*, HMSO, London.

5. Chartered Institute of Building Services Engineers (1989) *Lighting Guide*, The Industrial Environment LG1, London.

6. Dewis, M. and Stranks, J. (1988) *Tolley's Health & Safety at Work Handbook*, 2nd edn, Tolley Publishing Company, Croydon, Surrey.

7. Health and Safety Executive (1992) *Health and Safety in Retail and Wholesale Warehouses HS(G)76*, HMSO, London.

8. Health and Safety Executive (1992) *Prevention of Falls to Window Cleaners, Guidance Note GS 25*, HMSO, London.

9. British Standards Institute (1991) *BS 8213 Part 1 Windows, Doors and Rooflights: code of practice for safety in use and during cleaning of windows*, BSI, London.

10. Health and Safety Executive (1983) *Safety in the Use of Escalators PM34*, HMSO, London.

11. Health and Safety Executive (1984) *Escalators: periodic thorough examination PM45*, HMSO, London.

12. Health and Safety Executive (1992) *Passive Smoking at Work IND(G)63L*, HMSO, London.

13. Health and Safety Executive (1992) *Display Screen Equipment at Work, Guidance on Regulations L26*, HMSO, London.

14. Health and Safety Executive (1992) *Working with VDU's IND(G)36L*, HMSO, London.

15. Health and Safety Executive (1991) *Seating at Work HS(G)57*, HMSO, London.

16. Health and Safety Executive (1990) *Work Related Upper Limb Disorders: a guide to prevention HS(G)60*, HMSO, London.

17. Waterhouse, P. (1986) Fire, in Ridley, J. (ed.) *Safety at Work*, 2nd edn, Butterworths, London.

26 Protection of persons

Paul C. Belcher and
John D. Wildsmith

THE PERSONAL PROTECTIVE EQUIPMENT REGULATIONS 1992

These regulations came into force on 1 January 1993. They effectively replace all prescriptive legislation made prior to the Health and Safety at Work etc. Act 1974 and implement the requirements of a European Directive. With the Regulations came a set of Guidance Notes published by the Health and Safety Executive [1].

The Regulations place duties on employers and the self-employed, providing a framework for the provision of personal protective equipment (PPE) in circumstances where any assessment has shown a need for such protection. The Regulations do not apply to the provision of most respiratory protective equipment, ear protectors and some other types of PPE because there are already requirements laid down in Regulations such as the Control of Substances Hazardous to Health Regulations 1994, the Noise at Work Regulations 1989 and the Asbestos at Work Regulations 1987 which cover the use of PPE in particular circumstances. The main aim of the 1992 Regulations is to ensure the proper provision of PPE following a risk assessment.

In the Regulations, PPE is defined in Regulation 2 as:

> all equipment (including clothing affording protection against the weather) which is intended to be worn or held by a person at work and which protects him against one or more risks to his health or safety, and any addition or accessory designed to meet that objective.

As well as there being specific legal requirements, one must not forget the general duty of care owed to every employee by an employer. All employers must protect their workforce from the risk of reasonably foreseeable injury. Therefore as part and parcel of this general duty, it is reasonable to suggest that not only must such PPE be provided free of charge (see section 9 of the Health and Safety at Work Act 1974), it must also be readily available at all times.

In the Guidance to the Regulations [1] PPE is seen as a last resort. Rather, employers should seek to introduce changes to the process or safe systems of work in an effort to reduce the risk to the health and safety of their employees. (See Chapter 27 for a fuller discussion of risk assessment techniques.)

Any PPE provided by the employer must be 'suitable'. The Regulations state that PPE shall not be suitable unless:

1. it is appropriate for the risk or risks involved and the conditions at the place where exposure to the risk may occur;
2. it takes account of ergonomic requirements and the state of health of the person or persons who may wear it;
3. it is capable of fitting the wearer correctly, if necessary, after adjustments within the range for which it is designed;
4. so far as is practicable, it is effective to prevent or adequately control the risk or risks involved without increasing overall risk;
5. it complies with any enactment (whether in an Act or instrument) which implements in Great

Britain any provision on design or manufacture with respect to health or safety in any relevant Community directive listed in Schedule 1 which is applicable to that item of personal protective equipment.

Before choosing any PPE, Regulation 6 states that any employer or self-employed person must carry out an assessment to ensure that the proposed PPE is suitable. This assessment follows on from, but does not duplicate, the risk assessment requirement of the Management of Health and Safety at Work Regulations 1992,* which are concerned with the whole range of hazards present in the workplace and the evaluation of the extent of any risks involved. The assessment shall include:

1. an assessment of any risk or risks to health or safety which have not been avoided by other means;
2. the definition of the characteristics which personal protective equipment must have in order to be effective against the risks referred to in sub-paragraph (a), taking into account any risks which the equipment itself may create;
3. comparison of the characteristics of the personal protective equipment available with the characteristics referred to in sub-paragraph (b).

A specimen risk survey table is contained in Appendix 1 of the Guidance to the Regulations [1].

The Regulations go on to require that all PPE be maintained and that those who use it are adequately trained in its use, and the limits of the PPE involved. Furthermore, employers are under an obligation to ensure that employees use any PPE provided in an approved way. Finally, employees are under an obligation to notify their employer of any shortcomings with the PPE that they have been provided with.

RISKS TO HEALTH AT WORK

It may be convenient to divide the hazards to health into three categories. These are physical, chemical and biological hazards. Atherley [2] suggests a four-fold division along the lines of chemical substances, energies, climates and micropredators. However, the distinctions are somewhat arbitrary, and it may be easier to think of the three-fold division already suggested.

Physical hazards

These include the well documented hazards produced by, for example, light, heat, cold, noise and vibration. In addition, it may also be convenient to think of hazards such as ultra-violet and infra-red radiation and ionizing radiation under this heading.

Chemical hazards

This heading includes the whole range of substances and compounds found in organic and inorganic chemistry. Atherley [2] divides these substances into two headings: nutrients and non-nutrients. By the term nutrients, he refers to those substances that are required by the human body for 'the production of energy and the synthesis of tissue'. Under this heading may be found compounds such as proteins and common metals.

Having described the term 'nutrients' it will be quite clear that 'non-nutrients' are those substances not required by the body, either in excessive amounts, such as certain heavy metals, or not at all, such as some organic and inorganic substances and materials such as as asbestos.

Biological hazards

Those at risk may be involved in the handling of bacteria, viruses, plants, animals or animal products. More recently, there has been concern expressed about those who come into contact with those infected with HIV. In this case, attention is drawn to the Chartered Institute of Environmental Health handbook of advice. [3]

TOXICITY OF SUBSTANCES

Having made this distinction generally between various hazardous substances, and more particu-

---

* Amendment Regulations of 1994 extended the requirements to cover new and expectant mothers at work.

larly between nutrients and non-nutrients, it should be made clear that the toxicity of any substance depends upon a number of factors such as:

1. the nature of the substance;
2. the amount taken into the body compared to the weight of the body;
3. the physical condition and age of the body when exposure takes place;
4. the sex of the worker exposed to the substance.

Therefore, before one can attribute the term toxic to any substance, and hence determine the need for protection of any worker against exposure to that substance, one must establish some of the factors listed above.

Modes of entry of harmful substances

Having established some of the nature and range of harmful substances that can affect the human body, it is now necessary to look at the ways in which these substances can gain access to the body. It is convenient to think of these 'modes of entry' as falling under four main headings, although it should be borne in mind that some substances may have more than one mode of entry.

(1) Inhalation

A wide range of substances are carried into the human body on the breath. While the nose, airways and lungs behave as a fairly efficient filter against many substances, there is a critical size range where penetration can occur along the complete length of the respiratory tract.

Coates and Clark [4] estimate that particles larger than 10 μm in diameter are filtered off by the nasal hairs. Particles which are between 5 μm and 10 μm tend to settle in the bronchi and bronchioles, are then moved upwards to the throat by ciliary hairs, and are then coughed out. Particles which are smaller than 5 μm are able to reach the lung tissue. Coates and Clarke point out that fibres, which predispose to disease, have a length to diameter ratio of at least 3:1, and a diameter of 3 μm or less. Therefore the longer the fibre the more damaging it may be.

(2) Ingestion

Again many substances are passed in the body via the digestive system. If the substance is absorbed into the body, then it may be passed to the liver where it is rendered less toxic (detoxification) before being excreted. Some substances, such as bacteria and some chemicals, however, can cause harm without leaving the digestive tract.

(3) Entry through the skin

The skin is a very substantial defence against many substances. However, there are some substances that are able to pass directly through the skin and into the underlying tissue leaving the skin intact. In other cases, the substances pass into the epidermis but not through it, resulting in conditions such as dermatitis and some forms of cancer. Some substances, particularly solvents, are able to reduce the ability of the skin to protect the body against attack.

(4) Irradiation

This is the term used to describe the exposure of the body to both ionizing and non-ionizing radiation. Exposure may result in body surface penetration. This topic is dealt with in detail in Chapters 30 and 31.

Defence against harmful substances

As well as the protective equipment available to protect the worker, the body also possesses its own defence mechanisms. These are:

1. respiratory filtration;
2. cell defence mechanisms;
3. inflammatory response;
4. immune response;
5. thermoregulation;
6. metabolic transformation.

It is suggested that the reader should refer to more specific texts dealing with human physiology for a comprehensive discussion of these factors.

PRINCIPLES OF PROTECTION

As has already been made clear, the use of PPE to give protection against a particular hazard should not be seen as a substitute for other methods of dealing with the danger. For example, at a drilling machine with an exposed rotating spindle where there is a risk of entanglement, the aim should be to eliminate the risk by proper guarding of the machine, and not to rely on the operative wearing suitable head covering.

Having said this, is should be borne in mind that personal protection is not an easy option, and it is important that the correct protection is given for a particular hazard. In addition, one must be satisfied that the equipment being used is of sufficient quality in order to afford the worker with the required protection.

If one is to fulfil legal and moral obligations, it is essential that a programme of looking at all aspects of the provision and use of personal protective equipment is in place. Else [6] gives three key elements of information required for a personal protection scheme. These are:

1. the nature of the danger;
2. performance data of personal protective equipment;
3. the acceptable level for exposure to danger.

Nature of the danger

It is important that some details relating to the hazards to be faced are known. For example, with regard to a physical hazard such as noise, one would need to know the sound level and frequency characteristics of the noise. In addition, information could be gained from recorded accident/incident experiences, safety representatives, safety audits or surveys and medical records.

Performance data of personal protective equipment

The choice of equipment is extremely important. Its quality, durability, suitability, and lack of interference with the user's faculties and movements are important considerations affecting choice. In the UK the British Standards Institute (BSI) has traditionally conducted assessment of equipment and produced British Standards. It should be noted however that over the next few years many of the existing British Standards will be replaced so as to ensure harmonization with European Standards or 'Norms' (ENs).

As a consequence of the Personal Protective Equipment (EC Directive) Regulations 1992, which came into force on 1 January 1994, the Personal Protective Equipment Product Directive was implemented. This is effect requires that all PPE supplied for use at work must be independently assessed so as to ensure that it meets basic safety requirements. Satisfaction of this testing results in a certificate of compliance, and entitles the manufacturer to display the 'CE' mark on their product. The other effect of these Regulations is that it will now be illegal for any supplier to sell PPE unless it carries the 'CE' mark.

Acceptable level for exposure to danger

This factor is extremely important. Quite clearly for some dangers, such as exposure to potential carcinogenic substances, the only acceptable level can be zero. Both the employer and the enforcing officer must have a sound working knowledge of fixed legal standards, such as 'hygiene limits', and also of those standards of protection that are merely advisory in nature.

These suggested considerations must be viewed in conjunction with the general requirement to engage in a risk assessment contained in the Management of Health and Safety at Work Regulations 1992, and the more specific requirements with regard to PPE contained in the Personal Protective Equipment at Work Regulations 1992.

SELECTION OF PERSONAL PROTECTIVE EQUIPMENT

The general discussion of the Personal Protective Equipment at Work Regulations 1992 above has highlighted the need for any PPE chosen to be both 'suitable' and capable of protection against those risks to health and safety identified. Part 2 of the Guidance [1] lays down some general principles as to the way in which equipment should be chosen. In addition reference should be made to information available from suppliers. Again it should be remembered that all PPE purchased after 1 January 1994 must carry the 'CE' mark.*

Types of personal protection

PPE may be divided into the following broad categories:

1. Hearing protection.
2. Respiratory protection.
3. Eye and face protection.
4. Protective clothing.
5. Skin protection.

Hearing protection

Hearing protection can be divided into two main types: (a) earplugs and (b) earmuffs. Earplugs are designed to be inserted into the ear canal. Those which are designed to be disposed of after use are usually made from either mineral down, which is an extremely fine glass down, or from polyurethane foam. Re-usable earplugs are made of soft rubber or plastic. They must be thoroughly washed after use. Re-usable plugs in the first instance should be fitted by a trained person who should provide advice to the wearer on the correct method of inserting the plugs. Part 2 of BS6344: 1988 [6] gives an appropriate specification for earplugs.

Earmuffs are designed to cover the external ear. They consist of rigid cups which fit over the ear and are sealed to the head with soft cushion seals. They have several advantages over earplugs. One size will usually fit a wide range of people, they tend to offer greater protection, and they are easy to remove and replace. However, they are not without their disadvantages. They have a tendency to make the ears hot and are rather bulky. Part 1 of the BS6344: 1989 [7] deals with the required specification for earmuffs.

It is imperative that any type of hearing protection is of sufficient quality to reduce the noise level at the wearer's ear to below any recommended limit. The use of data from octave band analysis should be compared to design data provided by the manufacturer in order to ensure maximum protection. In 1983, the BSI produced a standard method for the measurement of sound attenuation of hearing protectors [8].

The Noise at Work Regulations 1989 lay down a requirement for employers to provide hearing protection in certain circumstances (Regulation 8). The advent of the Regulations has resulted in the Health and Safety Executive producing a series of Noise Guides. Paragraph 59 of Noise Guide No.1 [9] specifies five criteria for the selection of hearing protection. It states that attention should be paid to:

1. the level and nature of the noise exposure;
2. the job and working environment;
3. compatibility with any other protective equipment or special clothing worn;
4. the fit to the wearer;
5. any difficulty or discomfort experienced by the wearer.

Attention is also drawn to *Noise Guide No. 5* [10] which deals in detail with the selection of hearing protection.

Respiratory protection

As has already been emphasized, personal protection is a form of last resort protection. In the case of respirable dusts and fumes, every effort must be made to try and enclose the process and provide exhaust ventilation. Where this is not possible, then suitable protection must be provided.

Respiratory protective equipment may be divided into two broad categories: respirators which purify the air by drawing it through a filter thereby removing the contamination, and breathing apparatus which supplies clean air from an uncontaminated source.

Respirators
There are five basic types of respirator:

1. **Dust respirators** are the most commonly available form of respirator available. They afford protection against solid particles of matter or aerosol sprays, but not against gases. They

---

* HSE has also published 'A Short Guide to the Personal Protective Equipment at Work Regulations 1992'. ING (G) 174L, HSE Books. This is specifically aimed at advising small firms.

generally cover the nose and mouth of the wearer. BS 4555: 1970 provides a specification for dust respirators.

2. As well as dust respirators, there are light, simple **face masks** which protect the wearer from the effect of nuisance dusts or non-toxic sprays. It should be remembered that while these are a very popular form of respirator, they do not offer the wearer any real protection.

3. **Cartridge type respirators** give protection against low concentrations of relatively non-toxic gases and vapours. This is achieved by the use of replacement filter cartridges. Care should be taken to change the cartridge regularly to ensure maximum protection.

4. **Canister type respirators** incorporate a full face piece connected to a replaceable filter canister. This type of respirator offers far more protection than the cartridge type respirator. It is important that the correct canister is fitted to the equipment to ensure maximum protection to the wearer.

5. **Positive pressure powered respirators** can either cover the nose and mouth or the whole of the face. Air is drawn in through a battery powered suction unit, through filters and fed to the face piece at a controlled flow. The excess of air escaping around the edges of the face piece prevents leakage inwards. The BSI in BS4558: 1970 gives a specification for these respirators. This type of protection is mainly used when working with disease producing dusts, e.g. asbestos.

Breathing apparatus

The choice of breathing apparatus is extremely complex and should be made by those well versed in the use and limitations of such equipment. BS4275: 1974 [11] gives advice on the selection, use and maintenance of such equipment. There are three basic types of breathing apparatus.

1. **Closed circuit systems** which supply either oxygen or air from a cylinder carried by the wearer. Part 1 of BS 4667: 1974 [12] gives a specification for this type of apparatus. The air is supplied via a demand valve. The system gets its name from the fact that the wearer breathes the same air over and over again. When the wearer exhales, the exhaled air is purified and passes into a breathing bag where it is enriched with fresh oxygen from the cylinder. This results in the apparatus being suitable for use over a longer period of time.

2. **Open circuit systems** provide compressed air or oxygen from a cylinder worn by the worker. However, there is no breathing bag, hence the wearing time is greatly reduced. Part 2 of BS 4667: 1974 deals with this type of apparatus.

3. **Air line breathing apparatus** has a full face piece connected to a source of uncontaminated air by a hose. The equipment allows the operative to work in most types of toxic atmospheres, but the trailing tube can limit the movement of the wearer. Part 3 of BS 4667: 1974 provides a specification for this form of breathing apparatus.

It should be emphasized that although breathing apparatus provides the most effective protection against risks, because of their complexity their use requires specialized training and supervision. Detailed guidance has been published by the Health and Safety Executive [13] on the selection and use of respiratory protective equipment.

Eye and face protection

Eye injuries are extremely common. The main hazards are solid particles, dust, chemical splashes, molten metal, glare, radiation and laser beams. Injuries often result in severe pain and discomfort and, in many cases, long-term impairment of vision. It is extremely important that hazards are fully examined before any form of eye protection is chosen.

It is required that industrial eye protectors, such as goggles, visors, spectacles and face screens, satisfy the minimum requirements of BS 2092 (1987) [14]. This will be replaced eventually by BS EN 166, 167 and 168. BS 7028 (1988) gives advice on the selection, use and maintenance of eye protection [15]. In addition, part 2 of the Guidance to Personal Protective Equipment at Work Regulations 1992 [1] gives some advice on the choice of eye protection.

Protective clothing

There is currently a wide range of protective clothing available for use in most industrial situations. This ranges from well-known items such as safety footwear and overalls, to the more specialized gloves and aprons worn in certain work situations.

There is a whole range of British Standards and proposed European norms dealing with the full range of protective clothing. Once again the HSE Guidance [1] is useful in appreciating the criteria to be employed in selecting protective clothing.

It is important, as pointed out above, that those who wear protective clothing should be fully aware of the limitations of its use.

Skin protection

In some circumstances, it may not be possible or desirable to use gloves. In such situations, a proprietary barrier cream may be an alternative. Hartley [16] divides skin protection preparations into three broad groups:

1. **Water miscible** – protects against organic solvents, mineral oils and greases, but not metal-working oils mixed with water.
2. **Water repellant** – protects against aqueous solutions, acids, alkalis, salts, oils and cooling agents that contain water.
3. **Special group** – cannot be assigned to a group by their composition. They are formulated for specific applications.

It should be remembered that these creams are of only limited use as they are rapidly removed during the working day.

REFERENCES

1. Health and Safety Executive (1992) *Personal Protective Equipment at Work, Guidance on Regulations L25*, HMSO, London.
2. Atherley, G. (1978) *Occupational Health and Safety Concepts*, Applied Science Publishers, London.
3. Institution of Environmental Health Officers (1991) *Acquired Immune Deficiency Syndrome: guidance notes for environmental health officers*, CIEH, London.
4. Coates, T. and Clarke, A.R.L. (1986) Occupational diseases, in *Safety at Work* 2nd edn, (eds J. Ridley), Butterworths, London.
5. Else, D. (1981) *Occupational Health Practice*, 2nd edn. Butterworths, London.
6. BS 6344 (1988) *Industrial Hearing Protectors Part 2, Specification for Ear Plugs*, British Standards Institute, London.
7. BS 6344 (1989) *Industrial Hearing Protectors Part 1, Specification for Ear Muffs*, British Standards Institute, London.
8. BS 5108 (1983) *British Standard Method for the Measurement of Sound Attenuation of Hearing Protectors*, British Standards Institute, London.
9. Health and Safety Executive (1989) *Noise Guide No.1, Legal Duties of Employers to Prevent Damage to Hearing*, HMSO, London.
10. Health and Safety Executive (1989) *Noise Guide No.5, Types and Selection of Personal Ear Protectors*, HMSO, London.
11. BS 4275 (1974) *Recommendations for the Selection, Use and Maintenance of Respiratory Protective Equipment*, British Standards Institute, London.
12. BS 4667 (1974) *Specification for Breathing Apparatus*, British Standards Institute, London.
13. Health and Safety Executive (1990) *Respiratory Protective Equipment: a practical guide for users*, (HS(G)53), HMSO, London.
14. BS 2092 (1987) *Specification for Eye Protection for Industrial and Non-industrial Uses*, British Standards Institute, London.
15. BS 7028 (1988) *Guidance for the Selection, Use and Maintenance of Eye Protection for Industrial and Other Uses*, British Standards Institute, London.
16. Hartley, C. (1986) Occupational Hygiene, in *Safety at Work*, 2nd edn. (eds J. Ridley), Butterworths, London.

27 Plant and systems of work

Paul C. Belcher and
John D. Wildsmith

DANGEROUS MACHINES

Many serious accidents at work involve some type of machinery and, therefore, most machinery must be regarded as being intrinsically dangerous. A helpful guide which summarizes many of the key points which must be considered by employers, employees and enforcement officers, entitled, *Essentials of Health and Safety at Work*, was published by the Health and Safety Executive in 1990 [1].

TYPES OF INJURY

Injuries may result from any of the following:

1. (a) Trapping between moving parts and fixed parts, e.g. guillotine blades, garment pressers and sliding tables.
   (b) Trapping between moving parts, e.g. rollers, cogs, drive belts, food beaters and mixers. This category includes trapping by entanglement of hair or clothing, resulting in part of the body being brought into contact with the dangerous machine part.
   A common source of injuries of this type are '**nips**' and '**pinches**'. Of particular concern are '**in-running nips**'.
   Examples of this form of trapping and other hazards posed by a wide variety of dangerous machinery can be found in *British Standard Code of Practice for the Safety of Machinery, BS5304: 1988* [2].

2. Contact with moving parts, e.g. cutting blades, abrasive wheels, gear wheels – even slowly rotating parts must be considered to be potentially dangerous. This is particularly true in the case of gears or beaters as found in food processing machinery.
3. Burns, e.g. from hot exhausts and deep fat fryers.
4. Electrocution, e.g. from exposed electrical conductors.
5. Contact with moving workpieces, e.g. lathe.
6. Strike by machine parts or workpieces thrown from the machine, e.g. fractured abrasive wheels and insecure cutter blades.

Other non-mechanical hazards and environmental considerations are dealt with in the following chapters.

PRINCIPLES OF MACHINE GUARDING

The principles of guarding machinery were established as a result of the introduction of the Factories Act 1961 [3] and the Offices Shops and Railway Premises Act 1963 [4]. The established standards were supported by a considerable body of case law.

More recently the Provision and Use of Work Equipment Regulations 1992 (PUWER) [5] have amplified the requirements for the guarding of equipment and applied them across all industrial, commercial and service sectors. PUWER comes into force on 1 January 1993, although many of the provisions in so far as they apply to work equipment first provided for use in premises or undertakings before 1 January 1993 come into force on 1 January 1997. This will generally mean that older or poorly maintained equipment may need to be upgraded to meet the requirements of this new legislation.

The Offices, Shops and Railway Premises Act 1963 is most commonly enforced by environmental health officers, therefore the requirements of that legislation are given in the following section.

Offices, Shops and Railway Premises Act, 1963

(In Northern Ireland refer to the Offices and Shop Premises (Northern Ireland) Act 1966 as amended by the Office and Shop Premises Act (Repeals and Modifications) Regulations (Northern Ireland) 1979.)

This Act is enforced under the provision of the Health and Safety at Work, etc. Act 1974 [6], where it is described as a relevant statutory provision under Schedule 1 of that Act.

The Offices, Shops and Railway Premises Act 1963 applies to a variety of '**office premises**', '**shop premises**' and '**railway premises**', in which people are employed to work. These terms are defined in section 1 of the Act.

Fencing of machinery (section 17)

(Note: this section will be repealed when PUWER comes fully into force on 1 January 1997 for work equipment first provided for use in premises or undertakings before 1 January 1993.)

Every dangerous part of machinery used as, or forming part of, the equipment of premises to which this Act applies **shall** be securely fenced, unless it is in such a position or of such construction as to be as safe to every person working in the premises as it would be if securely fenced.

Guards must be of substantial construction, properly maintained and kept in position while the parts required to be fenced are in motion or in use.

Where the nature of the operation makes the provision of a fixed guard impracticable, a device may be provided that prevents the operator from coming into contact with dangerous machine parts.

Exposure of young persons to danger in cleaning machinery (section 18)

No '**young person**', i.e. a person who is under 18 years of age, must **clean** any machinery if, by doing so, they are exposed to risk of injury from a moving part of that or any adjacent machinery.

Training and supervision for working at dangerous machines (section 19)

No person shall work at any machine, which is prescribed by Order as being dangerous, unless they have been fully instructed as to the dangers arising in connection with it and the precautions to be observed, and either they have received sufficient training in work at the machine, or are under the supervision by a person who has a thorough knowledge and experience of the machine.

The Prescribed Dangerous Machines Order 1964 [7] lists the machines to which this section applies under the Offices, Shops and Railway Premises Act 1963, and under the Factories Act 1961; similar controls are exerted by the Dangerous Machines (Training of Young Persons) Order 1954. This legislation compares closely with provisions of the Factories Act 1961. It should, however, be noted that these provisions were designed to protect persons at work. Such guarding requirements may also be required under the provisions of the Health and Safety at Work, etc. Act 1974, where non-employees are exposed to a risk to their health and safety arising from an employer's undertaking.

The Health and Safety at Work, etc. Act 1974 does, however, incorporate a general duty of employers to provide plant and systems of work that are, as far as reasonably practicable, without risks to health.

THE PROVISION AND USE OF WORK EQUIPMENT REGULATIONS 1992

This legislation requires employers to ensure that work equipment (which may include second-hand, hired or leased equipment) must be so constructed or adapted as to be suitable for the purpose for which it is used or provided (Regulation 5). All such equipment must also be kept in an 'efficient state', in good repair, and where a maintenance log exists, that log must be kept up to date. The Health and Safety Executive have published guidance on the interpretation and application of the Regulations [8].

With specific regard to 'dangerous parts of machinery' (a term which is well established in health and safety law) new requirements are introduced (Regulation 11).

Measures must be taken to prevent access to any dangerous part of machinery or to any rotating 'stock-bar' ('any part of a stock-bar which projects beyond the head-stock of a lathe') or to stop the movement of any dangerous part or rotating stock-bar, before any person enters a 'danger zone'.

The term 'danger zone' means any zone in or around machinery in which a person is exposed to a risk to health or safety from contact with a dangerous part of machinery or a rotating stock-bar.

The required measures that must be taken are in the form of a hierarchy of four levels which are:

1. Fixed enclosing guards.
2. Other guards or protection devices.
3. Protection appliances such as jigs or push-sticks.
4. The provision of information, instruction, training and supervision.

All guards and protection devices must be suitable for the purpose for which they are provided, of sound construction and in good repair. Such devices must not unduly restrict the view of the operating cycle of the machinery and must not give rise to any increased risk to health or safety. The protection devices or guards must not be capable of being easily bypassed or disabled, which is an interesting development. Finally they must be situated at a sufficient distance from the danger zone although they can be designed so as to allow replacement of parts and maintenance work to be carried out without having to disable the device.

In addition to the guarding requirements, measures must be taken to prevent exposure to a number of specified hazards including:

1. articles or substances falling or being ejected from work equipment;
2. rupture or disintegration of parts of work equipment;
3. work equipment catching fire or overheating;
4. the unintended or premature discharge of any article or of any gas, dust, liquid, vapour or other substance which is produced, used or stored in the work equipment;
5. the unintended or premature explosion of the work equipment or substance produced, used or stored in it.

These Regulations also introduce specific requirements concerning the provision of a variety of controls and control equipment, including emergency stops and means of isolation from sources of energy. Finally work equipment must be clearly marked with any marking or warning which is appropriate for reasons of health and safety.

It should be noted that in addition to the Code of Practice for the safety of machinery, a number of European standards in support of the EC Machinery Directive have been produced [9–11].

MACHINERY PROTECTION

There are three basic principles of machinery protection which should be taken into consideration when applying occupational safety legislation.

Intrinsic safety

Intrinsically safe machinery is that which is safe without any further additions or alterations. This means, for example, that when dangerous parts are in motion or in use in some other way, they are not accessible to the operator or any other person.

This principle cannot always be applied. However, it is essential that potentially dangerous machinery should be made intrinsically safe wherever possible by virtue of design. This is an important aspect of *British Standard Code of Practice for Safety of Machinery, BS5304: 1988.*

Safety by position

Great care should be taken concerning this aspect of machine safety. A machine should not be assumed to be safe because of its position, for example, just because it is only approached infrequently. In such cases, a judgement must be made in the particular circumstances involved, bearing in mind the requirements of the Health and Safety at Work, etc. Act 1974, which can be more onerous than the requirements of the relevant statutory provisions.

Fencing or guarding of machinery

Ideally, guards should be designed with the machine and not added on as an afterthought. Essentially, fixed guards must be robust, to withstand severe treatment, adjustable and safe to use. They should also be capable of protecting operators or people in the vicinity against injury. This may mean that as well as forming a physical barrier, the guard may have additional functions, such as assisting the removal of toxic fumes or reducing noise to a safe level.

Many different types of guard are available but, in general, there is an order of preference, which is as follows:

Fixed guard

This type of guard is usually preferable, as it is securely attached to the machine and permanently guards the dangerous part or parts. The guard should be sufficiently large so as to stop anyone reaching over it, and it should be sufficiently distant from the dangerous parts so that it does not form a trapping zone between itself and any moving parts.

This type of guard is not suitable in many circumstances, e.g. where workpieces have to be inserted and removed regularly, or where regular maintenance is necessary.

It is often designed with a necessary opening in it, e.g. for a workpiece to contact a cutting blade. In such circumstances, the opening must be as limited as possible. In some circumstances, the operator is removed from the dangerous part by the incorporation of a sleeve or tunnel guard. This topic is dealt with in greater detail in *British Standard Code of Practice for Safety of Machinery, BS5304: 1988.*

When examining fixed guards, a number of points should be considered. The guard must be of sound and substantial construction, in good repair, and trapping or entanglement should not be possible. Any openings should be accepted only if the trapping area is not accessible through them.

Interlocked guard

There are two types of interlocked guard.

1. **Electrical interlock**. This consists of an electrical switch mechanism, which can be installed in a variety of ways. In one form, when the guard is moved, to give access to the dangerous parts, then the power to the machine is cut off, thus rendering the machine relatively safe. This is not acceptable if a dangerous part such as a cutting blade can still be contacted. By corollary, if such a guard is open, then the machine cannot be started up.

   It is important that if such systems fail, then they **'fail to safety'**, i.e. the electrical interlock will ensure that the machine remains incapable of being operated until the interlock is replaced or repaired.

2. **Mechanical interlock.** This is a moveable guard where, when it is open, the machine cannot be operated, and when the machine is in motion, it is not possible to open the guard. An interlock guard should satisfy the tests for a fixed guard referred to above. In addition, the extent to which the guard can be opened can be examined. Also, as the guard is closed, the operation of any limit switches should be noted, i.e. the extent to which the guard is in its correct position, before the machine will operate. Because it is a moveable guard, signs of wear should be looked for.

Automatic guard

This type of guard is one where the dangerous parts are enclosed while the machine is prepared for operation. The guard may open to an extent where the work can be removed when a work cycle is completed. When the work is removed, the guard closes again. Normally, the guard is closely fitted around the workpiece.

Examination of this type of guard should extend again to the tests for fixed guards. In addition, when the moving part of the guard is closed, it should not be possible to reach the dangerous parts. Finally, the extent of wear of any of the guard components should be assessed.

Trip guard

These may be moveable mechanical guards, which are operated when a person approaches a dangerous machine beyond a safe distance. A variation on this is where the guard incorporates either photoelectric cells, where a light beam can be disrupted, or a induction field detection coil, where the presence of a person will alter an electrical field. In both cases, when the sensor device is triggered, the machine can be shut off, to render it safe. Trip guards must satisfy the tests outlined above for the other guards.

It should be remembered that machine safety does not stop with the presence of a guard. Any guards must be made from suitable materials, and must be maintained regularly. If maintenance can only be carried out by removing guards, consideration must be given to ensuring some other form of protection to ensure a safe system of work.

All machine controls must be located in such a position that they cannot be operated unintentionally. Also, emergency cut-off switches should be clearly identified, readily accessible and in working order.

Persons operating machines should understand any risks involved, and be capable of rendering the machine safe in any emergency situation.

A common source of potentially dangerous machines are commercial kitchens. The hazards associated with a variety of machines, including food slicers, food processors, planetary mixers and waste compactors, pie and tart-making machines, incorporating some of the devices referred to above, can be found in two Health and Safety Executive publications: *Health and Safety in Kitchens and Food Preparation Areas*, HS(G)55 [12]; and *Pie and Tart Machines* HS(G)31 [13].

Lift trucks

Fork-lift trucks represent a special type of mobile machine which has become commonplace in factories, warehouses and large shops. They are especially useful for moving and storing goods, but they do feature predominantly in accident statistics. Every year about 6000 reportable accidents are recorded involving fork-lift trucks (HSE 1988). Some of these injuries are fatal. The key aspects involved in the safe use of these machines are dealt with in the Health and Safety Executive publication, *Safety in Working with Lift Trucks* [15].

Frequently, fork-lift truck accidents are associated with a lack of suitable operator training. Therefore, the need for employers to provide suitable training in this field should be recognized in order to comply with their legal duties under the Health and Safety at Work, Etc. Act 1974.

It is important to appreciate the characteristics of fork-lift trucks, so that the hazards that arise during their operation can be understood. It is also important to ensure that the racks used to store and unload many of the materials where lift trucks are employed are capable of carrying imposed loads, are in a good state of repair and are fixed securely in position.

Fork-lift trucks are designed to lift relatively heavy loads, most commonly, at the front of the vehicle, although there are some side-loading lift trucks. If the load is too heavy, then the truck can be tipped over. Also, if the vehicle is unevenly loaded or driven on sloping or uneven ground or cornered at excessive speed, then the stability of the vehicle can be affected, resulting in either shedding of the load, or turning over of the truck.

The truck is more likely to turn over if the load is raised to a high level, as the centre of gravity of the vehicle is raised.

The construction and use of fork-lift trucks is controlled by a variety of British Standard specifications, some of which are listed at the end of this chapter. Operators and inspectors should be familiar with the information that is required to be displayed on fork-lift trucks, which is as follows:

1. the manufacturer's name;
2. the type of truck;
3. the serial number;
4. the unladen weight;
5. the lifting capacity;
6. the load centre distance;
7. the maximum lift height.

These details must be recorded when investigating any accident or dangerous occurrence involving fork-lift trucks. Lift trucks are mobile machines, powered either by electric batteries or internal combustion engines. There are risks associated with each of these types.

Electric batteries have to be recharged, and this process involves the liberation of hydrogen gas. Battery charging should, therefore, only be carried out in a well-ventilated area where smoking is prohibited.

In buildings where fork-lift trucks are driven by internal combustion engines, effective ventilation is necessary in order to remove exhaust gases, which are toxic. In addition, areas used for refilling vehicles with petrol or diesel fuel should be located in the open air. Liquefied petroleum gas (LPG) cylinders should also be changed in a well-ventilated area. There must be no ignition sources in the vicinity of refuelling areas.

Because of the risk of causing an explosion, fork-lift trucks should not be used in premises where flammable vapours, gases or dusts are likely to be present, unless they have been specially protected for such use.

Operator training

Because of the extent and nature of accidents involving fork-lift trucks, the Health and Safety Commission, with the consent of the Secretary of State for Employment, under its powers contained in section 16(1) of the Health and Safety at Work, Etc. Act 1974, approved a Code of Practice entitled *The basic training of operators of*

rider operated lift trucks. This Code of Practice came into effect on 1 April 1989. Essentially, this document, incorporated into a more general training publication, *Rider Operated Lift Trucks – Operator Training. Approved Code of Practice and Supplementary Guidance* [15], provides practical guidance to employers with regard to their duties under section 2 of the Health and Safety at Work, etc. Act 1974;

'to provide such information, instruction, training and supervision as is necessary to ensure, so far as is reasonably practicable, the health and safety at work of his employees'.

One important point of this Code of Practice is that operator training must only be carried out by instructors who have themselves undergone appropriate training in instructional techniques and skills assessment.

The training provided should be largely practical in nature, and should be provided 'off-the-job', so that trainees and instructors are not diverted by other considerations.

Testing of trainees should be carried out by continuous assessment as well as a test or tests of the skills and knowledge required for safe lift-truck operation. The employer should keep records of each employee who has completed the basic training and testing procedure. The availability of this type of record in the case of an accident could be helpful to the outcome of the investigation.

LEGIONNAIRES' DISEASE
(see also Chapter 18)

Legionnaires' disease is a pneumonia-like condition caused by the bacterium *Legionella pneumophila*. In fact this organism produces a number of conditions, one of which is referred to as 'Pontiac fever'. This is a milder condition than legionnaires' disease, with an incubation period of between 5 hours and 3 days, and symptoms usually lasting for up to 5 days. The symptoms are similar to those of influenza: headache, nausea, vomiting, aching muscles and a cough. No fatalities have been reported from this condition [16].

Legionnaires' disease was first identified after an outbreak of pneumonia among delegates attending an American Legion Convention for service veterans, in Philadelphia in 1976, hence the name. Diagnostic tests were developed, and by testing stored specimens it was discovered that the disease could be traced back to the 1940s. The infection had escaped detection because the causative organism did not grow on conventional culture media.

Infection is caused by inhaling droplets which contain viable *L. pneumophila* organisms, and are fine enough to penetrate deeply into the lungs. There is no evidence that the disease can be transmitted from person to person, nor is the dose required to infect a person known. Males are more likely to be affected than females, and most cases have occurred in the 40 to 70 year old age group.

During the past few years, there has been a growing awareness of this condition, and some highly-publicized cases have heightened public awareness. In England and Wales, about 200 to 250 cases of legionnaires' disease have been reported each year, of which between 10% and 20% have been fatal. The Health and Safety Commission have estimated that the overall cost to society of legionellosis (excluding that attributable to foreign travel) is between 10 and 15 million pounds [17].

This infection has caused much concern because of its association with hot water systems and cooling towers of air conditioning and industrial cooling systems, where there is a generation of fine water droplets. The organism may, therefore, be present in a large number of workplaces and any risk of infection is clearly within an employers' duties to employees and non-employees under sections 2 and 3 of the Health and Safety at Work, etc. Act 1974.

It is, therefore, important to ensure that any high-risk areas in workplaces, such as cooling towers, are inspected on a regular basis, to ensure that they present no risk to health and safety as far as is reasonably practicable.

The procedures for the identification and assessment of risk of legionnellosis from work activities and water sources as well as the meas-ures to be taken to reduce the risk from exposure to the organism are explained in an Approved Code of Practice *The Prevention or Control of Legionnellosis (Including Legionnaires' Disease)*, which came into effect in January 1992 [18].

Procedures for the sampling of water services in all types of building, including domestic, commercial and industrial premises are provided in British Standard 7592: 1992 'Methods for sampling for *Legionella* organisms in water and related materials' [19]. This includes sampling for a variety of water services such as hot water services, cold water services, cooling systems and associated equipment. It should be noted that the British Standard is not applicable for sampling potable-water services or vending machines. Research work in this field continues, and it should be noted that at the present time, the British Standards Institution have produced a 'Draft for Development' culture method for the isolation of *Legionella* organisms and estimation of their numbers in water and related materials [20].

Where a potential risk exists, it is essential that cooling towers and associated water systems are subject to routine sampling as part of the general water treatment programme. Records of the analytical laboratory employed, the source of the sample, and the results obtained should be kept readily available for inspection.

Many systems are colonized by legionella bacteria without being associated with infections. The risk of infection can be minimized by good engineering practice in the design, construction, operation and maintenance of water installations.

In the case of those systems that are liable to produce a spray or aerosol in operation, or where a spray could be generated incidentally during the cleaning or maintenance, additional precautions should be taken by the person who has responsibility for the plant under the Health and Safety at Work, etc. Act 1974.

Cooling towers are of particular concern, and it is important that all parts of the system are thoroughly cleaned and disinfected normally twice per year (in spring and autumn). In order to achieve adequate disinfection, sodium hypochlorite solution may be used to give a concentration of at least 5 parts per million (5 ppm) of free available chlorine. Water should be sampled periodically near to the circulation return point. Chlorine levels can be determined using kits that are used to test swimming pools. (See Chapter 11.)

Regular chlorination of 1 to 2 ppm is normally advocated, but this is not appropriate in all cases as it may react adversely with other water treatments. Some biocides are known to be effective against legionella bacteria although resistance has been known to develop. In such cases, shock dosing using chlorination of 25 to 50 ppm of free chlorine is effective. A level of at least 10 ppm should be maintained in the system for 12 to 24 hours. The use of biocides can be alternated with the use of chlorination to achieve a satisfactory level of disinfection.

In view of the risk of legionnellosis, the Notification of Cooling Towers and Evaporative Condensers Regulations 1992 [21] requires any person who has, to any extent, control of non-domestic premises to notify the local authority that such plant is situated on those premises, giving information set out in the Schedule to the Regulations. This should assist environmental health officers in ensuring that appropriate, effective treatment and control systems are in place, as well as being vital in the case of any outbreak.

It is important that a safe system of work is devised in all premises where cleaning, maintenance and testing of the type of plant discussed above is carried out. This system of work, as well as any instruction and training necessary, must be made known to the personnel involved. For example, it is recommended by the Health and Safety Executive that suitable respiratory equipment, such as a high-efficiency, positive-pressure respirator with either a full face piece or a hood and blouse, is used. Also, such operations must be carried out in such a way as to avoid risks to other people working in the vicinity or members of the public.

In addition to its occurrence in cooling systems and water services, it should also be noted that spa baths have been linked with various infections, including legionnaires' disease. These are small pools where water is vigorously circulated by means of water and or air jets. The water is usually quite warm (typically above 30°C), and it is not changed between bathers as it is in the case of whirlpool baths. Careful water treatment is, therefore, needed in the case of spa baths.

In the case of a suspected outbreak of legionnaires' disease, past cases are a valuable source of reference. One useful publication is the *Broadcasting House Legionnaires' Disease* investigation, carried out by Westminster City Council in 1988 [22].

ELECTRICAL SAFETY

Every year about 50 people are killed by electric shocks in the workplace. In addition, poor electrical standards lead to the occurrence of many fires, for example, by overheating electrical conductors. Also, electrical installations and appliances can act as ignition sources and lead to explosions. It must be noted that in the case of flammable atmospheres, static electricity from movement of plant, materials or even clothing can be a potentially great hazard.

It should also be noted that where a person is suffering from an electric shock, employees with a basic first-aid training can, by prompt action, save his or her life. The Health and Safety Executive publish an *Electric Shock Placard*, which can be displayed in potentially dangerous areas and brought to the attention of employees.

In order to ensure that precautions are taken to prevent injury or fatality, The Electricity at Work Regulations 1989 [23] came into effect in April 1990. These Regulations are made under the Health and Safety at Work, etc. Act 1974. In order to assist those persons with duties under the Act and Regulations, the Health and Safety Executive has published a *Memorandum of Guidance on the Electricity at Work Regulations 1989*, HS(R)25 [24]. The guidance is designed to assist engineers, technicians and managers to understand the nature of the precautions to be taken. However, it is also of great use to those enforcing the provisions.

When dealing with electrical installations, reference is frequently made to the Institution of

Electrical Engineers Regulations for Electrical Installations (IEE Regulations). These are non-statutory regulations evolved by the IEE which relate to the design, selection, erection, inspection and testing of electrical installations. They form a code of practice which has been widely recognized and accepted in the UK and compliance with them is likely to achieve compliance with the statutory regulations.

In addition to the guidance memorandum, the Health and Safety Commission and the Health and Safety Executive have published a number of guidance notes on various aspects of electricity supplies and specific items of plant. Some of these are listed below:

1. PM32, *The Safe Use of Portable Electrical Apparatus*.
2. PM37, *Electrical Installations in Motor Vehicle Repair Premises*.
3. PM53, *Emergency Private Generation: Electrical Safety*.
4. GS27, *Protection Against Electric Shock*.
5. GS37, *Flexible Leads, Plugs, Sockets, etc*.
6. GS38, *Electrical Test Equipment for use by Electricians*.
7. HS(G)13, *Electrical Testing*.
8. HS(G)22, *Electrical Apparatus for use in Potentially Explosive Atmospheres*.

While carrying out an inspection of a premises, the electrical installation and the electrical supply to both fixed and portable machines should be examined. It may be that the inspector can recognize simple visual faults that may indicate that the electrical system requires examination by a competent electrician. It is stressed that such an examination must be carried out without risk to other employees or non-employees. Depending upon the circumstances, the employer may be required to provide an electrician's report, or the inspector may engage his own electrician.

Consideration must be given to ascertaining whether or not a particular business involves the use of portable electrical equipment. If such equipment is used, then its condition should be ascertained, and enquiries made as to how often the equipment is tested, the standards used, and any records kept should be examined. Where

portable equipment is used outside, then an isolating transformer or residual current circuit breaker should be used to protect operators and others in the case of an emergency. Some equipment can run on lower voltage supplies than mains voltage. In the case of some parts of electrical installations, e.g. display lighting, supplies can be as low as 12 volts.

Some basic points that should be considered are listed below.

Flexible leads and cables

The correctly rated 'flex' or cable should be used for the application. Flexes and leads should be positioned and fixed correctly, and in good repair.

Common faults are incorrect fixing to plugs (flex) or equipment, and damaged insulation, e.g. cuts, abrasions or heat damage. Joints should always be made using a suitable connector or coupler – joints made with insulating tape or 'block connectors' are normally dangerous. Care must be taken to ensure that cables are joined up with the correct polarities in each half of the connector.

Electrical socket outlets

Sockets should be sufficient in number and they must be positioned correctly to avoid tripping hazards from trailing flexes and overloading of the circuit due to the use of multi-point adapters.

Plugs

The flexible lead must be held firmly in the grip or clamp incorporated into the plug, and the individual wires must be connected firmly to the correct plug terminals. A suitably rated fuse must be installed.

Some tools and lamps are 'double insulated', and these have only two wires in the flex. Such appliances are recognized by the box-in-box symbol marked on them.

Switches

Every fixed machine must have a switch or isolator beside the machine which can switch off the

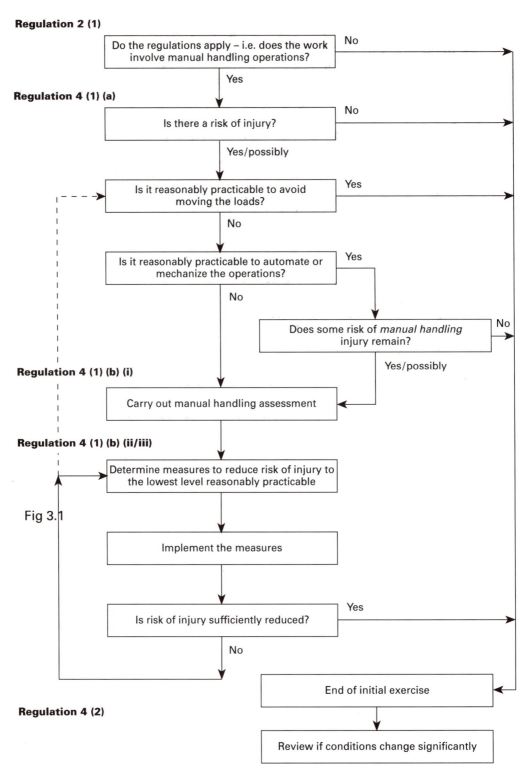

Regulation 2 (1)

Do the regulations apply – i.e. does the work involve manual handling operations? — No

Yes

Regulation 4 (1) (a)

Is there a risk of injury? — No

Yes/possibly

Is it reasonably practicable to avoid moving the loads? — Yes

No

Is it reasonably practicable to automate or mechanize the operations? — Yes

No

Does some risk of *manual handling* injury remain? — No

Yes/possibly

Regulation 4 (1) (b) (i)

Carry out manual handling assessment

Regulation 4 (1) (b) (ii/iii)

Determine measures to reduce risk of injury to the lowest level reasonably practicable

Fig 3.1

Implement the measures

Is risk of injury sufficiently reduced? — Yes

No

End of initial exercise

Regulation 4 (2)

Review if conditions change significantly

Fig. 27.1 How to follow the Manual Handling Operations Regulations 1992. (Source: Health and Safety Executive (1992) *Manual Handling – guidance on regulations*, L23, HMSO, London.)

power in an emergency. Power cables to machines must be armoured or heavily insulated, or installed in conduit.

Explosive atmospheres

Where the atmosphere of a work station is either dusty or potentially flammable, then specially protected equipment must be used. Inspectors must consider this risk, for example, where they are taking monitoring equipment into premises.

The Health and Safety Executive has produced a guide for those people who are seeking certification for the use of electrical apparatus for use in flammable atmospheres, *Electrical Equipment Certification Guide* 1982 [25].

MANUAL HANDLING

The Manual Handling Operations Regulations 1992 [26] came into force on 1 January 1993, as a result of the EEC legislation mentioned above. In the Guidance on the Regulations issued by the Health and Safety Executive [27] it is claimed that more than a quarter of the accidents reported to the enforcing authorities each year are associated with manual handling (i.e. the transporting or supporting of loads by hand or bodily force). Although manual handling accidents are rarely fatal, the majority are major injuries such as fractured arms, and they account for 6% of all major injures reported in 1990/91.

Sprains and strains arise from the incorrect application or prolongation of force, and poor posture and excessive repetition of movement can be important factors in their development. The main sites of injuries are the back (45%), finger and thumb (16%) and arm (13%). It should be noted that the injuries may occur over a considerable period of time.

The Regulations establish a clear hierarchy of measures which, in the first case, require that employers should, as far as reasonably practicable, avoid the need for employees to undertake any manual handling operations at work which involve a risk of their being injured. This may require the re-designing, automation or mechan-

ization of tasks. In order to comply with this requirement, a 'general assessment' carried out under the Management of Health and Safety at Work Regulations 1992 must be carried out, however, under these Regulations there is an additional, specific duty to carry out risk assessments of all manual handling operations where it is not reasonably practicable to avoid them.

Also, where manual handling operations cannot be avoided, the employer must take appropriate steps to reduce the risk of injury to the lowest level reasonably practicable.

The flow chart in Fig. 27.1 illustrates how to follow the Regulations.

REFERENCES

1. Health and Safety Executive (1990) *Essentials of Health and Safety at Work*, revised edition, HMSO, London.
2. British Standard Code of Practice for Safety of Machinery. BS5304: 1988, British Standards Institution, London.
3. The Factories Act (1961). 9 & 10 Elizabeth 2, c34, HMSO, London.
4. The Offices, Shops and Railway Premises Act (1963). 1963, c41, HMSO, London.
5. The Provision and Use of Work Equipment Regulations 1992. S.I. 1992 No. 2932, HMSO, London.
6. The Health and Safety at Work etc. Act (1974). 1974, c37, HMSO, London.
7. The Prescribed Dangerous Machines Order (1964). S.I. 1964 No. 971, HMSO, London.
8. Health and Safety Executive (1992) *Work Equipment – guidance on regulations*, Safety Executive L22. HMSO, London.
9. BS EN 292 (1991) *Safety of Machinery. Basic concepts, general principles for design. Parts 1 and 2: 1991*, British Standards Institution, Milton Keynes.
10. BS EN 294 (1992) *Safety of Machinery. Safety distances to prevent danger zones being reached by the upper limbs*, Milton Keynes, British Standards Institution.

11. BS EN 60204–1 (1992) *Safety of Machinery. Electrical equipment of machines. Part 1. General requirements*, British Standards Institution, Milton Keynes.
12. Health and Safety Executive (1990) *Health and Safety in Kitchens and Food Preparation Areas*, HS(G)55, HMSO, London.
13. Health and Safety Executive (1986) *Pie and Tart Machines*, HS(G)31, HMSO, London.
14. Health and Safety Executive (1979) *Safety in Working with Lift Trucks*, HS(G)6, HMSO, London.
15. Health and Safety Commission (1988) *Rider Operated Lift Trucks – Operator Training. Approved Code of Practice and Supplementary Guidance*, HMSO, London.
16. Health and Safety Executive (1987) *Legionnaires' Disease, Guidance Note EH48*, HMSO, London.
17. Health and Safety Commission (1989) *The Control of Legionellosis – Proposals for Statutory Action*, HMSO, London.
18. Health and Safety Commission (1991) *The Prevention or Control of Legionnellosis (Including Legionnaires' Disease). Approved Code of Practice*, HMSO, London.
19. British Standard 7592 (1992) *Methods for Sampling for* Legionella *Organisms in Water and Related Materials*, British Standards Institution, London.
20. Draft for Development DD211 (1992) *Method for Detection and Enumeration of* Legionella *Organisms in Water and Related Materials*, British Standards Institution, London.
21. Notification of Cooling Towers and Evaporative Condensers Regulations 1992. S.I. 1992 No.2225, HMSO, London.
22. Westminster City Council (1988) *Broadcasting House Legionnaires' Disease*.
23. Electricity at Work Regulations 1989. S.I. 1989 No.635 HMSO, London.
24. Health and Safety Executive (1989) *Memorandum of Guidance on the Electricity at Work Regulations 1989*, HS(R)25, HMSO, London.
25. Health and Safety Executive (1989) *Electrical Equipment Certification Guide*, HSE(M), Health and Safety Executive Electrical Equipment Certification Service, HMSO, London.
26. Manual Handling Operations Regulations 1992. S.I. 1992 No. 2793, HMSO, London.
27. Health and Safety Executive (1992) *Manual Handling – Guidance on Regulations*, L23, HMSO, London.

28 Toxic and dangerous substances

Paul C. Belcher and John D. Wildsmith

CLASSIFICATION OF HAZARDOUS SUBSTANCES

There are many substances used in the workplace, some of which may be obviously dangerous, but many more of which are not obviously hazardous. These hazards may be biological, physical or chemical.

Control of the hazards posed by dangerous substances has been developed to comply with the provisions of a number of EC directives:

1. Council Directive 67/548/EEC (OJ No. 196 16.8.67) as amended (for the 7th time) by Council Directive 79/831/EEC (OJ No. L154 5.6.92) in relation to the classification, packaging and labelling of dangerous substances.
2. Council Directive 78/631/EEC (OJ No. L204 2.7.78) on the classification, packaging and labelling of dangerous substance (pesticides).
3. Council Directive 88/379/EEC (OJ No. L187 16.7.88) as amended by Council Directive 90/492/EEC (OJ No. L275 5.10.90) on the classification, packaging and labelling of dangerous preparations.
4. Council Directive 91/155/EEC (OJ No. L76 22.3.91) on the system of specific information relating to dangerous preparations (Safety Data Sheets).

These Directives are now implemented by the Chemicals (Hazard Information and Packaging) Regulations 1994 [1] – the CHIP Regulations – which impose requirements upon the suppliers of 'substances or preparations which are deemed to be dangerous for supply and carriage' with the exception of substances defined in Regulation 3. The CHIP Regulations are operative from 1 September 1993.

The CHIP Regulations replace the Classification, Packaging and Labelling of Dangerous Substances Regulations 1984, and provide an improved system designed to protect people (and the environment) from the ill-effects of chemicals. Fundamentally, they still require the suppliers and consigners of chemicals to label and package them safely but in addition they require an initial 'classification' of the substances and the provision of safety data sheets for dangerous chemicals.

The fundamental requirement of CHIP is for a supplier to make an initial decision as to whether or not the chemicals involved are dangerous. If they are, then a decision has to be made concerning the type of hazard which must then be described using one of the appropriate '**risk phrases**' (which must be then used on labels and safety data sheets). This process is referred to as 'classification'.

Under Regulation 5, a substance is defined as '**dangerous for supply**' if they are so classified in the '**approved supply list**' which is the document entitled 'Information Approved for the Classification and Labelling of Substances and Preparations Dangerous for Supply' (2nd edn) [2], which

Table 28.1 Schedule 1: Classification of Substances and Preparations Dangerous for Supply. Part I: Categories of Danger

Column 1 Category of danger	Column 2 Property (see Note 1)	Column 3 Symbol-letter
Physico-chemical properties		
Explosive	Solid, liquid, pasty or gelatinous substances and preparations which may also react exothermically without atmospheric oxygen thereby quickly evolving gases, and which under defined test conditions detonate, quickly deflagrate or upon heating explode when partially confined	E
Oxidizing	Substances and preparations which give rise to a highly exothermic reaction in contact with other substances, particularly flammable substances	O
Extremely flammable	Liquid substances and preparations having an extremely low flash point and a low boiling point and gaseous substances and preparations which are flammable in contact with air at ambient temperature and pressure (see Note 2)	F+
Highly flammable	The following substances and preparations, namely – (a) substances and preparations which may become hot and finally catch fire in contact with air at ambient temperature without any application of energy, (b) solid substances and preparations which may readily catch fire after brief contact with a source of ignition and which continue to burn or to be consumed after removal of the source of ignition, (c) liquid substances and preparations having a very low flash point, or (d) substances and preparations which, in contact with water or damp air, evolve highly flammable gases in dangerous quantities (see Note 2)	F
Flammable	Liquid substances and preparations having a low flash point (see Note 2)	None
Health effects		
Very toxic	Substances and preparations which in very low quantities cause death or acute or chronic damage to health when inhaled, swallowed or absorbed via the skin	T+
Toxic	Substances and preparations which in low quantities cause death or acute or chronic damage to health when inhaled, swallowed or absorbed via the skin	T
Harmful	Substances and preparations which may cause death or acute or chronic damage to health when inhaled, swallowed or absorbed via the skin	Xn
Corrosive	Substances and preparations which, may on contact with living tissues, destroy them	C
Irritant	Non-corrosive substances and preparations which, through immediate, prolonged or repeated contact with the skin or mucous membrane, may cause inflammation	Xi

Table 28.1 continued

Column 1 Category of danger	Column 2 Property (see Note 1)	Column 3 Symbol-letter
Sensitizing	Substances and preparations which, if they are inhaled or if they penetrate the skin, are capable of eliciting a reaction by hypersensitization such that on further exposure to the substance or preparation, characteristic adverse effects are produced.	
Sensitizing by inhalation		Xn
Sensitizing by skin contact		Xi
Carcinogenic (see Note 3)	Substances and preparations which, if they are inhaled or ingested or if they penetrate the skin, may induce cancer or increase its incidence	
Category 1		T
Category 2		T
Category 3		Xn
Mutagenic (see Note 3)	Substances and preparations which, if they are inhaled or ingested or if they penetrate the skin, may induce heritable genetic defects or increase their incidence	
Category 1		T
Category 2		X
Category 3		Xn
Toxic for reproduction (See Note 3)	Substances and preparations which, if they are inhaled or ingested or if they penetrate the skin, may produce or increase the incidence of non-heritable adverse effects in the progeny and/or an impairment of male or female reproductive functions or capacity.	
Category 1		T
Category 2		T
Category 3		Xn
Environment Dangerous for the environment	Substances which, were they to enter into the environment, would present or may present an immediate or delayed danger for one or more components of the environment	N

Notes: 1. As further described in the approved classification and labelling guide.
    2. Preparations packed in aerosol dispensers shall be classified as flammable in accordance with the additional criteria set out in Part II of this Schedule.
    3. The categories are specified in the approved classification and labelling guide.
    4. (a) In certain cases specified in the approved supply list and in the approved classification and labelling guide substances classified as dangerous for the environment do not require to be labelled with the symbol for this category of danger.
       (b) This category of danger does not apply to preparations.

is approved by the Health and Safety Commission. They are also 'dangerous for supply' if they have the properties described in Schedule 1 (Table 28.1).

As in the previous legislation, substances which are dangerous for supply must be marked with appropriate 'indications of danger' which include 'hazard warning signs'. Indications of danger and the associated hazard warning sign are given in Schedule 2 of the Regulations (Table 28.2).

Regulation 7 provides that substances and preparations are 'dangerous for carriage' if they are so classified in the 'approved carriage list' which is the document entitled 'Information Approved for the Classification, Packaging and Labelling of Substances Dangerous for Carriage' [3], also approved by the Health and Safety Commission or if they have the properties described in Schedule 2 (Table 28.2).

Safety data sheets must be provided for dangerous chemicals (Regulation 6) by the supplier, for the information of the recipient of the substance or preparation. The information provided must be given using the following obligatory headings, as required by Schedule 5:

1. Identification of the substance or preparation and the company or undertaking.
2. Composition/information on ingredients.
3. Hazards identification.
4. First-aid measures.
5. Fire-fighting measures.
6. Accidental release measures.
7. Handling and storage.
8. Exposure control/personal protection.
9. Physical and chemical properties.
10. Stability and reactivity.
11. Toxicological information.
12. Ecological information.
13. Disposal considerations.
14. Transport information.
15. Regulatory information.
16. Other information.

The objective is to provide the recipient with sufficient, accurate date to enable them to take any necessary measures relating to the protection of health and safety at work and relating to the protection of the environment. It should be noted that safety data sheets are not required to be provided when these materials are sold to the public from shops.

Suppliers are required by CHIP to exercise all due diligence in complying with the requirements, therefore if a particular supplier wishes to use a classification assigned by a manufacturer or supplier high up the supply chain, they will be expected to have made appropriate enquiries to ensure that the classification is appropriate. Where reliable, reputable suppliers are used the checks required will normally be quite simple, however evidence may be sought by enforcement officers that appropriate enquiries have indeed been carried out.

In order to provide further guidance, the following Approved Code of Practice is available:

The Approved Code of Practice on Regulation 6. 'Safety data sheets for substances and preparations dangerous for supply' (2nd edn) [3].

THE CONTROL OF SUBSTANCES HAZARDOUS TO HEALTH REGULATIONS 1994 [4]

These Regulations, which came into effect on 16 January 1995, made under the Health and Safety at Work, etc. Act 1984, are generally regarded as representing a considerable improvement in the systematic control in the use of a wide variety of hazardous substances in the work environment. They are commonly referred to by the acronym of COSHH.

This legislation has been updated to comply with EC Directives relating to the importation, supply and use at work of benzene and substances containing benzene, and the protection of workers from risks related to exposure to carcinogens at work, respectively.

The COSHH Regulations apply to substances that have already been classified as being very toxic, toxic, harmful, corrosive or irritant under the provisions of the CHIP Regulations as outlined above. They also apply to:

1. substances that have specified 'maximum exposure limits' (specified in Schedule 1), or 'occupational exposure standards';
2. substances that have chronic or delayed effects, such as carcinogenic, mutagenic or teratogenic substances;
3. a substantial concentration of dust of any kind;
4. a micro-organism which can cause illness;
5. any other substance which is not listed in any of the above categories, but which has similar potential effects.

It must be noted that not all substances that can be a hazard to health are controlled by these Regulations. Some examples of these 'exempted' substances include:

1. lead – so far as the Control of Lead at Work Regulations 1980 (as amended) apply;
2. asbestos – as far as the Control of Asbestos at Work Regulations 1987 (as amended) apply;
3. substances that are only hazardous because of any one or any combination of the following:
   (a) explosive properties;
   (b) flammable properties;
   (c) high pressure;
   (d) high temperature;
   (e) low temperature;
   (f) radioactivity;
4. asphyxiants, if they are non-toxic.

There are a number of substances which are 'prohibited' under these Regulations. The substances and the extent to which they are prohibited are contained in Schedule 2 of COSHH, but the prohibition extends generally to the importation and supply for use at work (including articles).

The critical point of these Regulations is that an employer shall not carry on any work which is liable to expose any employees to any substance hazardous to health unless he has **made a suitable and sufficient assessment of the risks and of the steps that need to be taken to meet the requirements of the Regulations**. Such assessments must be reviewed where a significant change in work occurs or the original assessment becomes invalid for any other reason.

The assessment itself must include:

1. an assessment of the risks to health; and
2. the steps that need to be taken to achieve adequate control of exposure to hazardous substances; and
3. identification of any other action necessary to comply with the Regulations.

The assessment should consider what types of substances employees are liable to be exposed to, and this must include consideration of the consequences of the possible failure of measures provided to control exposure and the form in which the substances may be present and their effect upon the body. Of great importance is a consideration of the extent to which other workers or other persons (including non-employees) are likely to come into contact with the hazardous substances being assessed.

The employer must make an estimate of exposure levels and compare these to any available valid standards. If the assessment indicates that control is, or is likely to be, inadequate, then the employer must determine the steps that must be taken to obtain adequate control. It should be remembered that COSHH Regulations require that personal protective equipment should be used as a method of exposure control only after all other methods have been employed as far as reasonably practicable. This is a considerable diversion from previous thinking with regard to the protection of people at work.

An assessment can be considered to be suitable and sufficient if the detail and expertise with which it is carried out are commensurate with the nature and degree of the risk involved with the work.

In some circumstances, it will only be necessary to read manufacturers' or suppliers' safety information sheets to ensure that current working practices are satisfactory. In other cases, considerable atmospheric monitoring may be necessary before true exposure levels can be ascertained.

In addition to making an assessment of risks, employers are also required to ensure that the exposure of employees to substances hazardous to health is either prevented or, where this is not reasonably practicable, adequately controlled (by

Table 28.2 Schedule 2: Indications of Danger and Symbols for Substances and Preparations Dangerous for Supply

Regulation 2(1)

Column 1 *Indication of danger*	Column 2 *Symbol-letter*	Column 3 *Symbol*
Explosive	E	
Oxidizing	O	
Extremely flammable	F +	
Highly flammable	F	
Very toxic	T +	
Toxic	T	

Table 28.2 continued

Column 1 Indication of danger	Column 2 Symbol-letter	Column 3 Symbol
Harmful	Xn	
Corrosive	C	
Irritant	Xi	
Dangerous for the environment	N	

means other than personal protective equipment).

Where an employer provides any control measure to meet the requirements of these Regulations, they are also required to ensure that those measures are maintained in an efficient state, in efficient working order and in good repair. Thorough examination and testing of engineering controls is required.

Where monitoring is carried out or is specifically required to be carried out, then record of that monitoring must be kept, and the record itself or a summary must be kept available. Where the record is representative of the personal exposures of identifiable employees, this must be kept for at least 30 years. In any other case, the record must be kept for at least 5 years.

Where it is appropriate for the protection of the health of employees who are, or are liable to be, exposed to a substance hazardous to health (this includes work in processes specified in the Regulations), the employer must ensure that those employees are subject to suitable health surveillance, including biological monitoring.

An additional requirement of these Regulations is that where any employee is exposed, or may be exposed, to substances hazardous to health, then the employer must provide the employee with such information, instruction and training as is suitable and sufficient for that employee to know:

1. the risks to health created by such exposure; and
2. the precautions that should be taken.

This would include the disclosure of the results of any monitoring of exposure in the workplace and information on any collective health surveillance (so presented that it cannot be related to any individual).

It can, therefore, be seen that the Control of Substances Hazardous to Health Regulations 1994 provide a comprehensive set of measures that will act to improve the health and safety at work of employees and others affected by work activities. The Health and Safety Commission has approved two codes of practice which are published together, *Control of Substances Hazardous to Health; Control of Carcinogenic Substances* [5]. Also, the Health and Safety Executive has produced a very practical, basic guide, *Introducing Assessment – A Simplified Guide for Employers*, IND(G)64L [6].

Occupational exposure limits

For some years now, the adequacy of the control of inhalation of substances hazardous to health has been assessed by reference to the concentration of those substances in air inhaled as a result of work activities. These concentrations of hazardous substances are now referred to as occupational exposure limits (OEL) rather than the older and less accurate term of threshold limit values. These OEL figures are reviewed normally each year by the Health and Safety Executive in the form of a Guidance Note, Environmental Hygiene Series EH40 [7]. It should be noted that this guidance does not extend to detailed considerations of asbestos and lead exposure levels, where specific legislation exists, nor does it cover situations where work is below ground or exposure to micro-organisms. These OEL standards have been evolved along with the development of the concept of the COSHH Regulations.

Maximum exposure limit

The maximum exposure limit (MEL) is defined in the COSHH Regulations by reference to Schedule 1 which sets out the name of the substance, its chemical formula and the concentration of the substance (in air), which must not be exceeded

for one or both of two specified '**reference periods**' over which the exposure is averaged. The concentrations are expressed normally in both parts per million (ppm) and milligrams per cubic metre ($mg\ m^{-3}$). Concentrations of mineral fibres are expressed as fibres per millilitre of air (fibres ml^{-1}). Table 1 of Guidance Note EH40 reproduces the list of substances contained in Schedule 1 of the Regulations, with additional explanation relating to the application of these limit values and some advice on assessment and control of hazardous substances.

The significance of the MEL is that where an exposure limit has been specified in the Regulations, the control of exposure by inhalation can only be considered to be adequate where the level of exposure is reduced so far as reasonably practicable and, in any circumstances, below the prescribed MEL.

Occupational exposure standards

An 'occupational exposure standard' (OES) is also a concentration of an air-borne substance averaged over a reference period. Substances are assigned an OES on approval by the Health and Safety Commission after consideration of the available scientific data by the Working Group on the Assessment of Toxic Chemicals. In the case of these substances, concentrations are such that there is considered to be no evidence that the substance is likely to be injurious to employees if they are exposed to that concentration day after day. If exposure by inhalation exceeds the OES, then control is normally considered to be adequate as long as the employer has identified the reason that the OES has been exceeded, and that suitable steps are being taken to reduce exposure to achieve the OES as soon as is reasonably practicable.

Reference periods

Substances that are considered to be hazardous to health may cause adverse effects, ranging from irritation of the skin or mucous membranes, through to death. The effect may be produced either over a very short exposure period or over a

Table 28.3 Results of monitoring an employee to substances hazardous to health

Work period	Exposure (mg m^{-3})	Sample
07.30–09.30	0.24	2.00
09.30–09.45	0	0.25
09.45–12.30	0.18	2.75
12.30–13.00	0	0.50
13.00–15.00	0.34	2.00
15.00–15.15	0	0.25
15.45–17.00	0.65	1.25

much longer period. It is, therefore, important to develop exposure limits that reflect these differences, and this has been done with regard to both MELs and OESs. These are listed in the COSHH Regulations and EH40 as either 'long-term exposure limits' (8-hour time-weighted average reference period) or 'short-term exposure limits (15-minute reference period).

(a) Long-term reference period
The 8-hour reference period refers to a well-established procedure whereby the sum of individual occupational exposures over a 24-hour period are treated as being equivalent to a single, uniform exposure for an 8-hour period. This is known as the '8-hour time-weighted average (TWA)' for the exposure.
This may be represented mathematically by:

$$\frac{C_1 \times T_1 + C_2 \times T_2 + C_3 \times T_3 + \ldots \ldots \ldots C_n \times T_n}{8}$$

where C_1, C_2, C_n, etc, are the individual, measured occupational exposures, and T_1, T_2, T_n, etc, are the corresponding times for each exposure period.

EXAMPLE A person works in a premises performing a variety of different jobs, in some of which they are exposed to substances hazardous to health. Monitoring is carried out to give the results in Table 28.3.

Exposure is known to be zero during breaks or activities carried out in other parts of the premises; this exposure may also have to be measured in practice.
The 8-hour TWA is therefore:

$$\frac{0.24 \times 2 + 0.18 \times 2.75 + 0.34 \times 2.00 + 0.65 \times 1.25 + 0 \times [0.25 + 0.50 + 0.25]}{8}$$

$$= \frac{0.48 + 0.50 + 0.68 + 0.81 + 0}{8}$$

$$= 2.47 \text{ mg m}^{-3}.$$

(b) Short-term reference period
Here exposure should normally be measured over the prescribed period for the hazardous substance concerned: this is normally 15 minutes. Measurements for periods greater than 15 minutes should not be used to calculate the short-term exposure.

Long-term exposure limits are thus designed to protect against the effects of long-term exposure, while short-term exposure limits are designed to avoid acute effects of toxicants. Eight hours was selected to reflect the typical exposure during one working shift averaged over a 24-hour period, while the 15 minute period represents any 15 minute period during the working day. Where only short samples are taken, information such as short-term peak concentrations may be missed, whilst if a long-term sample is taken, significant high peak concentrations, which could be harmful, might not be detected as the result is averaged over that longer period. Monitoring systems and equipment must, therefore, be carefully selected and positioned in order to ensure that the data gathered can be usefully interpreted in the light of the available standards and guidance.

MONITORING STRATEGIES FOR TOXIC SUBSTANCES

Carrying out monitoring can be an expensive and time-consuming exercise, therefore some form of monitoring strategy must be applied in order to gain sufficient data for the purpose of the exercise, in as cost-efficient a way as possible. The data must, however, be accurate and reliable so that the requirements imposed by any health and safety legislation can be fulfilled. Suitable advice is contained in the Health and Safety Executive's Guidance Note EH42, *Monitoring Strategies for Toxic Substances* [8]. This document discusses the factors that influence air-borne concentrations of hazardous substances, and urges that a structured approach be taken. This procedure involves a number of distinct phrases for the monitoring work:

1. initial appraisal;
2. basic survey;
3. detailed survey;
4. routine monitoring.

With regard to these types of monitoring, a decision has to be made concerning the level of sophistication that the survey requires, both in terms of the quantity and quality of the data collected. The Guidance Note proposes a three-level approach to the carrying out of such an exercise. Finally, advice is given concerning the interpretation of results. It is essential that anyone carrying out or recommending an assessment under COSHH is familiar with this document.

Various other documents produced by the Health and Safety Executive are of significance when considering this topic, such as:

1. GS5: *Entry into Confined Spaces*, HSE 1980.
2. EH10 (rev): *Asbestos – Control Limits and Measurement of Air-borne Dust Concentrations*, 1988.
3. MDHS14: *General Method for the Gravimetric Determination of Respirable and Total Inhalable Dust*, 1993.
4. MDH70. *General Methods for Sampling Gases and Vapours* 1990.

Any person carrying on a work activity must understand the nature of any hazards associated with the materials being used. It is essential that when acquiring potentially hazardous materials, a hazard data sheet is obtained from the supplier. This data must be read and understood and kept in a readily accessible place. The contents of such data sheets will form the basis of instructions and training given to employees, as well as the selection and provision of any necessary protective equipment.

Safe arrangements must be made for the reception, storage and use of such materials and, as far as reasonably practicable, emergency procedures should be designed – in liaison with agencies such as the Health and Safety Executive, local authority and fire authority as necessary.

Finally, suitable arrangements should be made for any medical examinations (including health surveillance) required or deemed necessary, and first-aid facilities should be made available to the standard required by the Health and Safety at Work, Etc, Act 1974 enforcing authority.

Asbestos

The Control of Asbestos at Work Regulations 1987 [9] as amended [10] implement EC Directive 83/477/EEC 'on the protection of workers from the risks related to exposure to asbestos at work' and EC Directive 76/769/EEC as amended by EC Directive 83/478/EEC 'on restrictions on the marketing and use of certain dangerous substances and preparations' with regard to the labelling of products for use at work containing asbestos.

When considering the problems associated with exposure to asbestos, it is important to understand the concept of 'the fibre'. This term is defined in the 'European Reference Method for the determination of personal exposure, using the membrane filter method'. The principle of this method is that a measured volume of air is drawn through a membrane filter, which is subsequently rendered transparent and mounted upon a microscope slide. Fibres on a known fraction of the filter are counted under phase contrast microscopy, and the number of fibres in unit volume of the air can be calculated and compared to the standards indicated below. Details of the method are given in Health and Safety Executive publication MDHS 39 'Asbestos fibres in air' [11].

In this document the definition of a 'fibre' is given as 'particles with a length greater than five micrometres, a maximum width of less than 3 micrometres and a length to width ratio of greater than three to one'. These are the particles which are counted, but it should be noted that, as it is not possible to identify the chemical nature of the fibres collected, all 'fibres' are counted as being asbestiform and used in determining whether control limits and action levels have been exceeded.

The key features of the Regulations are:

(a) Assessments

Work with asbestos must be adequately assessed by an employer to determine the nature and degree of any exposure, and the steps which must be taken in order to prevent or reduce that risk. In the case of work consisting of the removal of asbestos a suitable, written 'plan of work' must be prepared which must include details of:

1. the nature and probable duration of the work;
2. the location of the place of work;
3. the methods to be applied;
4. the characteristics of the equipment to be used for the protection and decontamination of those carrying out the work and the protection of other persons on or near the worksite.

Employers are required to identify the type of asbestos involved in the work, or to assume that it is brown (amosite) or blue (crocidolite) the most hazardous types.

Employers must generally provide the enforcing authority with the particulars specified in Schedule 1 of the Regulations at least 28 days before commencing the work, unless the enforcing authority agree to a shorter period.

(b) Prevention of exposure

Employers have a duty to prevent or reduce the spread of asbestos from a workplace to the lowest level reasonably practicable. They must also prevent or reduce employees' exposure by means other than the use of respiratory protective equipment.

Other related duties include the need to monitor the air for asbestos fibres and to provide information and training relating to the risks involved and the precautions which must be taken.

(c) Control limits

These represent a level of asbestos in the air above which respiratory protective equipment must be worn.

The limits refer to one of the following concentrations of asbestos in the atmosphere when measured or calculated by a method approved by the Health and Safety Commission:

1. For chrysotile (white asbestos):
   (a) 0.5 fibres per millilitre of air averaged over any continuous period of 4 hours;
   (b) 1.5 fibres per millilitre of air averaged over any continuous period of 10 minutes.
2. For any other form of asbestos, either alone or in mixtures with any other form of asbestos:
   (a) 0.2 fibres per millilitres of air averaged over any continuous period of 4 hours;
   (b) 0.6 fibres per millilitre of air averaged over any continuous period of 10 minutes.

(d) Action level

This represents a cumulative exposure level over a period of 12 weeks. If an action level is likely to be exceeded then the work must be reported to the Health and Safety Executive, 'asbestos areas' must be designated, medical surveillance of workers must take place and health records kept.

The limits are:

1. Where the exposure is solely to chrysotile, 96 fibre-hours per millilitre of air; or
2. where the exposure is to any other form of asbestos either alone or in mixtures including mixtures of chrysotile with any other form of asbestos, 48 fibre-hours per millilitre of air; or
3. where both types of exposure can occur separately during the 12-week period, a proportionate number of fibres per millilitre of air.

A number of Approved Codes of Practice have been issued in relation to working with asbestos, such as 'The Control of Asbestos at Work' [12] and 'Work with Asbestos Insulation, Asbestos Coating and Asbestos Insulating Board [13]. A further useful publication from the Health and Safety Executive is Guidance Note EH10 'Asbestos: exposure limits and measurement of airborne dust concentrations' [14]. This document gives good practical advice on the measurement of airborne asbestos and the associated calculations of fibre levels. Of particualr importance is the methodology for '**clearance monitoring**' which must be carried out before a site is handed back to the control of its occupiers after asbestos removal operations. Using the specified method, the lowest fibre level which can reliably be detected above background levels, in a 480 litre sample, is about 0.01 fibres per millilitre, and therefore this level is taken as the '**clearance indicator level**'. Sites should not be considered to be satisfactory until such a test has been successfully completed. EH10 also gives further reference to other guidance notes, videos and other material that will be useful in dealing with asbestos in a variety of work situations.

Reference should be made to the Control of Asbestos in the Air Regulations 1990 [15] which prescribe a limit value for the discharge of asbestos from outlets into the air during the use of asbestos. These Regulations also provide for the regular measurement of asbestos emissions from specified types of premises. Provision is also made for the control of environmental pollution by asbestos emitted into the air resulting from the working of products of from the demolition of buildings, structures or installations containing asbestos. Finally the Asbestos (Prohibitions) Regulations 1992 [16] implement EC Directive 91/659/EEC 'on restrictions relating to the marketing and use of dangerous substances and preparations (asbestos)'. These regulations repeal similar provisions made in 1985 and basically extend the prohibition on the import of crocidolite and amosite, to all forms of 'amphibole asbestos', namely crocidolite, amosite, fibrous anthophyllite and fibrous tremolite and mixtures containing any of those minerals.

REFERENCES

1. Chemicals (Hazard Information and Packaging) Regulations 1994. SI 1994 No. 3247.
2. Health and Safety Executive (1993) *The Approved Supply List: information approved for the classification and labelling of substances and preparations dangerous for supply*, 2nd edn, HMSO, London.
3. Health and Safety Commission (1993) *The Approved Code of Practice on Regulation 6. Safety data sheets for substances and preparations dangerous for supply*, HMSO, London.
4. Control of Substances Hazardous to Health Regulations 1988. S.I. 1988 No. 1657, HMSO, London.
5. Health and Safety Commission (1988) *Approved Code of Practice: control of substances hazardous to health – control of carcinogenic substances*, HMSO, London.
6. Health and Safety Executive (1988) *Introducing Assessment – a simplified guide for employers*, IND(G) 64(L), HMSO, London.
7. Health and Safety Executive (1994) *Occupational exposure limits 1994*: Guidance Note EH40/94, HMSO, London.
8. Health and Safety Executive (1989) *Monitoring Strategies for Toxic Substances*, Guidance Note EH42, HMSO, London.
9. Control of Asbestos at Work Regulations 1987. S.I. 1987 No. 2115, HMSO, London.
10. Control of Asbestos at Work (Amendment) Regulations 1992. S.I. 1992 No. 3068, HMSO, London.
11. Health and Safety Executive (1990) *Asbestos Fibres in Air: Determination of personal exposure by the European Reference version of the membrane filter method. Methods for the Determination of Hazardous Substances*: MDHS 39, HSE, London.
12. Health and Safety Commission (1993) *Approved Code of Practice. The Control of Asbestos at Work*, HSC, London.
13. Health and Safety Commission (1993) *Approved Code of Practice. Work with Asbestos Insulation, Asbestos Coating and Asbestos Insulation*, HSC, London.
14. Health and Safety Executive (1990) *Asbestos: exposure limits and measurement of airborne dust concentrations*, Guidance Note EH10.
15. Control of Asbestos in the Air Regulations 1990. S.I. 1990 No. 556, HMSO, London.
16. Asbestos (Prohibitions) Regulations 1992. S.I. 1992 No. 3067, HMSO, London.

29 Accident prevention and investigation

Paul C. Belcher and
John D. Wildsmith

In 1956 the then Ministry of Labour postulated six principles of accident prevention [1]. These are:

1. accident prevention is an essential part of good management and of good workmanship;
2. management and workers must co-operate whole-heartedly in securing freedom from accidents;
3. top management must take the lead in organizing safety in the works;
4. there must be a definite and known safety policy in the workplace;
5. the organization and resources necessary to carry out the policy must exist,
6. the best available knowledge and methods must be applied.

It is interesting that it was 18 years later, with the advent of the Health and Safety at Work, etc. Act 1974 and the attendent regulations, that these important principles received legislative support.

Before beginning to look at the whole process of accident investigation and prevention, it is necessary to examine what is meant by the term accident.

The Oxford English Dictionary definition of accident is: 'an event without apparent cause, unexpected event, unintentional act, mishap'.

An early definition was put forward by Lord MacNaughton in *Fenton v Thorley & Co Ltd* [1903] AC 443 where 'accident' was defined as:

'some concrete happening which intervenes or obtrudes itself upon the normal course of employment. It has the ordinary everyday meaning of an unlooked for mishap or an untoward event, which is not expected or designed by the victim.'

The thinking behind such a statement has greatly influenced the actions of those involved in accident prevention. However, this definition can be seen as being somewhat narrow in that it lays emphasis on the actions of the worker, and that it seems to infer that all accidents result in injury which is evident at the time of the incident.

Bamber [2] offers a wider definition of accident when he says that an accident is:

'an unexpected, unplanned event in a sequence of events, that occurs through a combination of causes; it results in physical harm (injury or disease), to an individual, damage to property, a near-miss, a loss, or any combination of these effects'.

This is a far more satisfactory definition of accidents in that it recognizes a wider view of the causes and effects of accidents.

CAUSES OF ACCIDENTS

Accidents don't just happen, they have a cause. Once this principle is accepted, then the whole notion of accident prevention and investigation takes on a new dimension. In addition, one must accept that the cause of the accident may not be immediately obvious, and that the employee or employees involved may not be primarily responsible for the accident occurring. The Health and Safety Executive [8] emphasize this point when they state that:

> the majority of accidents and incidents are not caused by 'careless workers', but by failures in control (either within the organisation or within the particular job), which are the responsibility of the management.

Therefore, whilst on the surface the accident investigation may identify certain factors that led to the accident or incident occurring, the primary causes, they must be seen as symptoms of more fundamental underlying causes which allow these factors to exist or persist, the secondary causes.

Examples of such primary causes include:

1. working without authority;
2. using defective equipment;
3. horseplay;
4. failing to wear personal protective equipment;
5. inadequate or missing guards to machines.

Secondary causes may include:

1. financial pressures;
2. lack of policy;
3. lack of commitment;
4. lack of knowledge.

As the Health and Safety Executive [8] make clear, failure at this level can lead to:

> unrealistic timescales for the implementation of plans which put pressure on people to cut corners and reduce supervision; . . . job and control systems which failed to recognise or allow for the fact that people were likely to make mistakes and might have difficulties communicating with each other.

A fuller discussion of the theory of accident causation can be found in studies carried out by Gordon [4], Heinrich [5], Bird and Loftus [6], Hale and Hale [7] and Petersen [8].

ACCIDENT NOTIFICATION

There should be an efficient and effective system of accident notification in any industrialized society. The reasons for putting forward this view include:

1. to ensure compliance with current legislation;
2. to assist in the monitoring and development of health and safety policies;
3. to provide a feed-back mechanism which will assist in the development of safe systems of work;
4. to provide information to enforcing authorities so as to enable the refining of hazard analysis and inspection strategies.

The current legislation dealing with the notification of accidents can be found in the Reporting of Injuries, Diseases and Dangerous Occurrences Regulations (RIDDOR), which came into force on 1 April 1986. These Regulations replaced the Notification of Accidents and Dangerous Occurrences Regulations 1980. A significant change in the notification system that the introduction of RIDDOR required was the notification of accidents involving certain trainees, particularly those on government sponsored work experience schemes. Detailed guidance relating to the regulations is contained in a booklet published by the Health and Safety Executive [9].

The effect of this legislation is that it places a duty on all employers and other 'responsible persons' who have control over employees and work premises to report to the relevant enforcing authority accidents, both fatal and non-fatal, which occur in the workplace. This notification must take place immediately by the quickest practicable means, and must be reported in writing within 7 days to the relevant 'enforcing' authority. Regulation 10 details the exceptions to this requirement.

Regulation 3(1) lists those accidents which are reportable. As well as including accidents that result in physical injury, the Regulations require the notification of other incidents that result in, for example, decompression sickness, loss of consciousness resulting from lack of oxygen, and acute illnesses that are the result of exposure to harmful substances, pathogens or infected material.

The Regulations also require the notification of occupational diseases, such as poisoning, skin diseases, lung diseases, infections and some cancers (see Schedule 2, columns 1 and 2).

In addition to requiring the notification of accidents and occupational diseases, the Regulations also require the notification of 'dangerous occurrences'. These include explosion of pressure vessels, the release of more than one tonne of flammable liquid and the partial or total collapse of a building. The full list of defined dangerous occurrences can be found in Schedule 1 of the Regulations.

These provisions are currently being reviewed by the Government. As part of the drive to deregulate industry it is proposed that RIDDOR will be modified from 1 April 1996. The draft new RIDDOR provisions:

1. Clarify that injuries caused by deliberate acts of violence arising from or in connection with work are reportable.
2. Modify lists of dangerous occurrences which should be reported and include, in particular, certain dangerous situations on railways, which would satisfy requirements set out in the King's Cross and Clapham Junction Inquiry Reports.
3. Change the definition of a major injury to exclude incidents which had the potential to cause major injury – these would be reclassified as dangerous occurrences.
4. Revise the lists of reportable occupational diseases in line with the DSS list of diseases which qualify for Industrial Invalidity Benefit and the European Schedule of Occupational Disease.
5. Introduce a requirement to report communicable diseases offshore.

When the revised Regulations first come into force – scheduled for 1 April 1996 – fatalities, major injuries and dangerous occurrences will be reportable forthwith by the quickest practicable means (normally by telephone), supplemented by a written report within 10 days (14 days for gas incidents). All other reportable injuries and disease cases must be reported in writing within 10 days of them coming to the employer's attention.

A fuller description of the required notification procedures together with a flow-chart can be found in *Environmental Health Procedures* [10].

INVESTIGATION OF ACCIDENTS

Having been informed of an accident or dangerous occurrence, it is incumbent upon the enforcing authority to investigate the incident as quickly as possible. In the case of serious or fatal injuries, an investigating officer should preferably be at the scene within the hour.

Under the provisions of the Health and Safety at Work, etc. Act 1974, an inspector has the power to ask questions, the answers to which may be written down in the form of a statement. The investigating officer must ensure that all such questioning and statement collection is carried out in accordance with the provisions of the Police and Criminal Evidence Act 1984 (see Chapter 8).

In addition to taking statements, the inspecting officer may also take away documents, for example, safety policies, and may take photographs at the scene of the accident. The object of the investigation is to establish as clearly as possible the sequence of events that lead up to the accident, and to subsequently consider any recommendations that could be made to ensure that the incident does not reoccur.

As soon as possible after the investigation has taken place, the investigating officer should prepare a written report. Such report should be concise and, where necessary, should be supported by sketches, photographs and statements. It should be borne in mind that any report may not only be required in a criminal action, but may also be requested in any claim for damages taken through the civil courts.

As to any subsequent action that may be taken, this matter is often taken out of the hands of the investigating officer. However, in deciding what course of action should be taken regard should be had to:

1. the seriousness of any contravention;
2. the degree of risk present at the time;
3. the means available to remedy the situation.

ACCIDENT PREVENTION

Quite clearly, any accident warrants full investigation, not only to establish the exact cause of the accident, but also to establish ways in which a similar incident can be prevented from happening again. An important underlying principle of the Health and Safety at Work, etc. Act 1974 is that any employer should provide a safe place of work and safe systems of work.

In their publication *Successful Health and Safety Management* [3] the Health and Safety Executive argue that:

> all accidents, ill-health and incidents are preventable.

If any employer is to realize this ideal within their workplace then due consideration must be given to the systematic development of accident prevention strategies.

Typically, accident prevention strategies include: hazard analysis safety inspections, accident investigations, checking of safety devices, publicity, training and education and safe systems of work. Some of these principles will now be examined.

Hazard analysis

Central to the whole notion of accident prevention is the identification of all potential hazards in the workplace. A hazard may be thought of as [3, p. 66]:

> the potential to cause harm, including ill health or injury; damage to property, plant, products or the environment; production losses or increased liabilities.

To some extent this exercise will have already been carried out in many workplaces in order to ensure compliance with the Control of Substances Hazardous to Health Regulations 1994 (COSHH).

This principle has been extended by the Management of Health and Safety at Work Regulations 1992 (amended 1994). These Regulations require every employer and self-employed person to carry out a suitable and sufficient assessment of the health and safety risks to employees and others not in their employment arising out of or in connection with their operation (Regulation 3). There is also a requirement for those who employ five or more persons to record any 'significant findings' from such an assessment. The Approved Code of Practice [10] suggests that any such record should contain a statement of significant hazards identified, the control measures in place and the extent to which they control the risk, and the population exposed to the risk.

There are several ways in which the existence of hazards may be established. These include:

1. workplace inspections;
2. analysis of production/work programmes;
3. analysis of individual job specifications.

Risk assessment

Once an analysis of potential hazards has been carried out, it may then be possible to evaluate the potential risk of the individual operations within the workplace, and also to identify those parts of the process which are particularly hazardous.

Risk may be thought of as [3, p. 66]:

> the likelihood that a specified undesired event will occur due to the realisation of a hazard by, or during, work activities or by the products and services created by work activities.

Within the Approved Code of Practice [11] a more concise definition of risk is presented as:

> the likelihood that the harm from a particular hazard is realised.

Any evaluation carried out will ultimately lead to the establishment of a hazard rating for that particular premises and/or the particular operation(s) carried on at the premises. Such a hazard rating could be used to prioritize the inspection regime to be used by the enforcing authority.

There are a number of ways in which such a hazard rating can be developed. Most are based on the simple formula:

RISK = SEVERITY ESTIMATE × LIKELIHOOD OF OCCURRENCE

Examples of such estimating techniques can be found in *Successful Health and Safety Management* [3].

Risk control

Having established the potential hazards within a workplace, the next step is to establish systems to either eliminate or reduce the potential risk to the worker. Bamber [12] suggests a gradation of measures from long term (permanent) to short term (temporary). He presents the grading as such:

Long term 1. Eliminate hazard at source
2. Reduce hazard at source.
3. Remove employee from hazard.
4. Contain hazard by enclosure.
5. Reduce employee exposure to hazard.
Short term 6. Utilize protective equipment.

Such a system of grading is extremely useful, not only with regard to the reduction of physical hazards, but also of chemical hazards. It may also be regarded as being an order of priority, in the sense that the long-term aim must always be to eliminate the hazard at source, but while achieving this more short-term actions may be employed.

A similar hierarchy of control is proposed by the Health and Safety Executive [3].

There are various ways in which hazards may be controlled. For example, guarding of machines, efficient ventilation of the workplace, monitoring of the use of hazardous substances and the use of protective equipment. However, as indicated, the use of protective equipment must always be seen as the short-term solution to the controlling of hazards within the workplace.

Having engaged in such activity it is vital that monitoring and review of both hazards and risks and of any control measures introduced is carried out. To this end the Management of Health and Safety at Work Regulations 1992 require that not only must employers plan and implement such a review process (Regulation 4), but also imposes on employees a duty to inform their employer of any shortcomings in health and safety arrangements (Regulation 12). This point is reinforced by the Approved Code of Practice [11] where the Health and Safety Executive state that:

> the avoidance, prevention and reduction of risks at work needs to be an accepted part of the approach and attitudes at all levels of the organisation and apply to all its activities, i.e. *the existence of an active health and safety culture affecting the organisation as a whole needs to be assured.*

Safe systems of work

Safe systems of work are fundamental to the whole notion of accident prevention. They have been defined by the Electrical, Electronic, Telecommunications and Plumbing Union (EETPU) [13] as a:

> laid out and considered method of working that takes proper account of the potential hazards to employees and others in vulnerable situations, and provides a formal framework to ensure that all of the steps necessary for safe working have been anticipated and implemented.

Consideration of this definition reveals that any safe system of work that has been properly thought through will of necessity form part of the 'arrangements' section of any safety policy (see below).

Any safe system of work will include a consideration of some of the following issues:

1. assessment of the task;
2. hazard identification and risk assessment;
3. the safe design, installation, and use of all plant tools and equipment;
4. effective planned maintenance of plant and equipment;
5. a safe working environment;
6. suitable and sufficient training for all employees;

7. compliance with safety policy;
8. adequate consideration of vulnerable employees, e.g. young persons, pregnant women and disabled persons;
9. regular reviews of all procedures employed within the workplace to ensure maintenance of high standards.

In certain circumstances, it may be necessary to employ a **permit to work** system. This is, in essence, an extension of the principle of a safe system of work, and requires written permission before a particular job may commence. The permit is a written document identifying the plant to be worked on and details the precautions to be taken before work can commence.

Permit to work systems are required by legislation in certain circumstances, e.g. entry into confined spaces. They may also be advisable in circumstances such as maintenance work on machinery, work in high-risk fire areas, working with asbestos and work with corrosive or toxic substances.

Safety training

Section 2 of the Health and Safety at Work, etc. Act 1974 places a duty on an employer to provide such information, instruction, training and supervision as is necessary to ensure, so far as is reasonably practicable, the health and safety at work of employees.

It is essential that training be seen as being necessary for all employees, that is, from manager to manual worker. In addition, training courses should reflect the individual needs of the workforce, e.g. driver training for fork-lift truck drivers, safe use of personal protective equipment, fire safety training.

The need for training presents the enforcing authority with an ideal opportunity to enter the workplace in a 'non-threatening' capacity, enabling them to win the confidence of not only the management, but also of the general workforce.

There are a number of different options available for meeting training needs. The introduction of National Vocational Qualification (NVQs) will allow for workplace assessment of competence in health and safety matters. In addition there are the Basic and Advanced Certificates in Health and Safety at Work offered by the Chartered Institute of Environmental Health. For managers it is possible to link health and safety training in the Management Charter Initiative (MCI). The Health and Safety Executive [3] lay down some guide-lines for the assessment of training needs.

SAFETY POLICIES AS AN AID TO ACCIDENT PREVENTION

The Health and Safety at Work, Etc. Act 1974 places employers under a general duty to prepare a written statement of health and safety policy. The only exception from this general rule is where there are less than five persons employed on the premises. The Health and Safety Commission have published advice on the preparation of safety policies [14].

In essence there are three parts to any safety policy. These are:

1. a general statement of intent;
2. organization;
3. arrangements.

These provisions have been expanded by the Management of Health and Safety at Work Regulations 1992. The risk assessments and significant findings discussed above will form an essential part of the safety policy, as they form the basis of the control measures to be implemented and the responsibilities within the organization.

The general statement of intent outlines in broad terms the organization's overall philosophy in relation to the overall management of health and safety.

Such statements should set the direction for the organization and should ideally identify ways in which health and safety can contribute to overall business performances. As the Health and Safety Executive [3] make clear:

> health and safety and quality are two sides of the same coin.

Part two of the policy statement outlines the chain of command in terms of health and safety management. It indicates those persons who have positions of responsibility or accountability, and their sphere of operation. It will also contain details of how the implementation of the policy is to be monitored. This section will contain information of the role and function of safety committees and safety representatives. A full discussion of this aspect of health and safety policies is contained in *Successful Health and Safety Management* [3].

The final section of the policy deals with the practical arrangement by which the policy will be effectively implemented. This will include details relating to safety training, safe systems of work, machine/area guarding, housekeeping, noise control, radiation safety, dust control, health checks, fire precautions, accident reporting and investigation systems, emergency procedures, and workplace monitoring. Many of these will be identified by the risk assessments undertaken as a requirement of the Management of Health and Safety at Work Regulations 1992 (see Chapter 27). It should be emphasized that this is only an indicative list. Each safety policy is a unique document, which should be tailored to the circumstances of each workplace.

Quite clearly, the health and safety policy is an extremely important document. A well-written policy will enable the inspecting officer to be able to identify all potential risks and hazards within the workplace. It will also enable officers to assess the organization's perception of the risks that exist, and enable him to tailor the inspection and subsequent recommendations accordingly.

An essential feature of the Robens Report was that health and safety was everyone's business. This has received renewed emphasis by the Health and Executive [3] and the introduction of the Management of Health and Safety at Work Regulations 1992. In order to hammer this point home, Robens suggested that there must be the participation of all employees in the making and monitoring of arrangements for safety and health in the workplace. It is, therefore, not surprising that one of the important features of the health and safety policy is the use of safety committees and safety representatives.

The Safety Representatives and Safety Committees Regulations 1977 gave statutory effect to this requirement for joint consultation. To complement the regulations, a Code of Practice has been prepared and this is supplemented by Guidance Notes. The three documents are contained in one publication published by the Health and Safety Commmission [15].

REFERENCES

1. Ministry of Labour and National Service (1956) *Industrial Accident Prevention*, Report of the Industrial Safety Sub-Committee of the National Joint Advisory Council, HMSO, London.
2. Bamber, L. (1986) Principles of accident prevention, in *Safety at Work*, 2nd edn (ed J. Ridley), Butterworths, London.
3. Health and Safety Executive (1991) *Successful Health and Safety Management*, HS(G) 65, HMSO, London.
4. Gordon, J.E. (1949) The epidemiology of accidents. *American Journal of Public Health*, **39**, 504–15.
5. Heinrich. H.W. (1959) *Industrial Accident Prevention*, 4th edn, McGraw-Hill, New York.
6. Bird, F.E. and Loftus, R.G. (1976) *Loss Control Management*, Institute Press, Loganville, Georgia.
7. Hale, A.R. and Hale, M. (1972) *A Review of the Industrial Accident Research Literature*, Committee on Safety and Health at Work Research Paper, HMSO, London.
8. Petersen, D.C. (1978) *Techniques of Safety Management*, 2nd edn, McGraw-Hill, USA.
9. Health and Safety Executive (1986) *A Guide to the Reporting of Injuries, Diseases and Dangerous Occurrences Regulations* 1985, HMSO, London.
10. Bassett, W.H. (1995) *Environmental Health Procedures*, 4th edn, Chapman and Hall London.
11. Health and Safety Executive, *Management of Health and Safety at Work. Approval Code of Practice*, HMSO, London.
12. Bamber, L. (1986) Techniques of accident

prevention, in *Safety at Work*, 2nd edn, (ed J. Ridley) Butterworths, London.

13. Electrical, Electronic, Telecommunications and Plumbing Union (1979) *Safety, Health and Welfare: Code of Practice – Television and Audio Servicing Industry*, EETPU, London.

14. Health and Safety Executive (1986) *Writing your Health and Safety Policy Statement*, HMSO, London.

15. Health and Safety Commission (1977) *Safety Representatives and Safety Committees*, HMSO, London.

30 Ionizing radiation

Paul C. Belcher
and John D. Wildsmith

TYPES OF RADIATION

Environmental health officers may encounter problems with ionizing radiation when dealing with waste disposal matters or with the issue of radon gas and its radioactive 'daughter elements' in dwellings and, increasingly, in the workplace.

The atoms of some naturally-occurring substances are found to be 'unstable', and these will undergo a spontaneous transformation or decay process so that they achieve a more stable state. These substances are known as **radioisotopes**, and they reach their stable condition by emitting radiation, principally in the form of alpha particles, beta particles, gamma radiation and X-radiation. The transformation process is called **radioactivity**, and the emissions may be referred to collectively as **ionizing radiation**.

The time period for a radioisotope to undergo decay to form a new element (which itself may be radioactive) varies between materials. The indicator used to describe the rate of decay is the **half-life** ($T_{1/2}$). This is the time taken for half of the radioactive atoms present to decay from the original element.

The various forms of ionizing radiation are emitted with different energies and, as they are different in form, they have different properties. Some of the principal properties must be discussed so that the nature and effects of ionizing radiation can be understood.

Alpha radiation is mainly emitted by isotopes of heavier elements, and it consists of helium nuclei which are made up of two protons and two neutrons, which are tightly bound together to create a particle. This is a relatively large particle with a mass of 4 units, with 2 units of positive charge. Most of the transformations which result in the emission of alpha particles are accompanied by gamma radiation or X-radiation, which adjusts the energy balance of the emitter.

Beta radiation is mainly emitted by intermediate and lighter elements. It consists of high-speed electrons which originate in the atomic nucleus and have a mass of approximately 1/1840 mass units and carry 1 unit of negative charge. Most of the transformations which give rise to beta radiation also emit energy adjusting gamma radiation or X-radiation.

Gamma radiation is only emitted as a consequence of alpha or beta emissions. It is a form of electromagnetic radiation which consists of quanta of energy in the form of a wave motion. It is therefore non-particulate and uncharged.

X-radiation is electromagnetic radiation that differs from the other forms mentioned above in that it is non-nuclear in origin. It is normally electrically generated, although it can be generated when atomic electrons undergo a change in orbit, such as when beta particles react with other matter.

ENERGY TRANSFER

The energy contained in ionizing radiation is expressed in electronvolts. One electonvolt is the amount of energy gained by an electron when passing through an electrical potential of 1 volt. The energy of a particle depends basically upon its mass and its velocity and, therefore, this system can also be applied to the other forms of ionizing radiation. Because this is such a small unit it is usually expressed in kilo electronvolts (keV) or mega electronvolts (MeV).

Alpha particles typically have a charge of 2 to 8 MeV while beta particles have 1 keV to 5 MeV. Gamma radiation is typically in the range 1 keV to 6 MeV, while X-radiation can be much higher [1].

Another fundamental characteristic of the principal types of radiation is the ability to penetrate materials. Heavy, slow alpha particles will not penetrate a sheet of paper and have a range of a few centimetres in air. Because the radiation is particulate and charged, this means that alpha radiation interacts both physically and electrically with the media through which it passes and, as it is effectively 'stopped', it must be considered as giving up all of its inherent energy by transferring it to the interacting material. Normally, this energy excites electrons of the absorbing medium, and this can cause the electrons to be released from their atomic orbits, which produces ions. Therefore, the effect of alpha particles can be to ionize material which they contact, possibly with serious biological consequences.

Beta particles produce a similar ionization. However, they are much lighter and thus more penetrative than alpha particles. Beta particles will penetrate a sheet of paper and have a range in air of a few metres.

Gamma radiation and X-radiation have a very large range in air and are extremely penetrative. As they are non-particulate in nature, they interact with the electrons of matter by a series of different mechanisms. One mechanism is referred to as the 'photoelectric effect', where a gamma photon or X-photon is completely absorbed by an atomic electron, which is subsequently ejected from its atom. These electrons can then shed their energy to other atoms in the same way as beta particles.

Ionizing radiation is, therefore, of sufficiently high power to ionize various atoms of which living tissues are composed, including water content.

The rate at which radioactive particles lose their energy during their passage through matter can be described by the term '**linear energy transfer**' (**LET**), which is the average energy deposited per unit length travelled. Heavy, slow particles have a high LET, whereas light, fast particles have low LET.

EFFECTS OF IONIZING RADIATION

The potential for ionizing radiation to produce damage in living tissues is considerable. Essentially, in the case of humans, this can be considered in relation to two routes, i.e. whether the radiation source is either inside or outside of the body [2].

Alpha radiation is stopped quite easily, therefore any source outside of the body can be shielded and rendered safe. Because of its short range even in air, external sources should normally present very little risk from alpha particles. However, if an alpha emitter is in contact with the skin or taken into the body, then there will be a considerable energy transfer to the living tissues, and this will present a significant risk to health. When ionization occurs, the tissue close to the track of the energy deposition will contain large numbers of chemically active chemical species such as ions, free radicals and excited atoms. In these conditions, unconventional chemical reactions of an unpredictable nature take place. These unusual reaction products can produce adverse side-effects on the surrounding tissue. Also, DNA molecules are susceptible to alteration with potentially serious consequences.

Some protection to the effects of beta radiation is afforded by ordinary clothing, therefore the risks from external sources are slightly higher than for alpha particles. Also, because of their penetrative properties, beta emissions from inside the body may penetrate to the outside, and thus also pose less of a risk than alpha particles, although this may still be a significant risk.

Gamma radiation and X-radiation may pass through the human body depositing little energy on the way.

UNITS

There are a number of units which are used to describe the characteristics and effects of ionizing radiation. and the more common units used are explained below [3].

Radioactivity

This represents the 'activity' of a radioisotope in terms of the number of disintegrations occurring each second. The unit is referred to as the 'becquerel' (Bq), and is defined as:

$$1 \text{ Bq} = 1 \text{ atomic distintegration per second}$$

This is a rather small unit and is of dubious practical significance as it does not differentiate between the type of ionizing radiation and, therefore, it does not indicate anything about the biological effect of the radiation concerned.

Radiation absorbed dose

This is the amount of energy absorbed by a receiving medium per unit mass, from all sources. The unit of absorbed dose is referred to as the 'Gray' (Gy). The Gray is defined as:

$$1 \text{ Gy} = 1 \text{ joule kg}^{-1}$$

Absorbed dose is quite a useful physical concept, but as it does not differentiate between the different types of ionizing radiation, it is not a good indicator of damage caused to biological systems.

Radiation dose equivalent

The difference in the 'radiobiological effectiveness' of different types of radiation is taken into consideration by the development of a unit of radiation dose equivalent. This unit is referred to as the 'Sievert' (Sv). The Sievert is derived in the form of a weighted absorbed dose. Therefore, the absorbed dose (in Gray) is multiplied by a so-called 'quality factor' (Q), which is itself derived to account for the distribution of the absorbed dose. This product is further multiplied by a factor designated 'N', which can be used to take into account further modifying factors. In fact, the value of 'N' has been assigned a value of unity, and so the overall equation for radiation dose equivalent can be expressed as:

$$\text{dose equivalent (Sv)} = \text{absorbed dose (Gy)} \times Q \times N$$

The values assigned to the radiation types mentioned above are 20 for alpha particles and 1 for gamma radiation, X-radiation and beta radiation, reflecting the potential of these radiations to produce biological damage.

Dose rate

Both the Gray and Sievert are units which relate to an amount of energy which is received without reference to any time period. Radiation hazards may be assessed or controls applied either in terms of a simple dose, or in terms of a dose rate. The dose rate is expressed as either Gray per hour or Sievert per hour. The standards that must be applied may be derived, for example, from standards such as those contained in the Ionizing Radiation Regulations 1985.

CONTROL OF RADIATION EXPOSURE

Limits of radiation exposure are rather unusual in that they are agreed on an international level. The International Commission on Radiological Protection (ICRP) was formed in 1928 to perform this function. Since then, it has reviewed available scientific evidence relating to the effects of exposure to ionizing radiation and modified exposure limits where necessary. In the UK, a great deal of advice and a large variety of published material, as well as monitoring and advisory services, are available from the National Radiological Protection Board (NRPB).

One aspect of protection against ionizing radiation is that the biological damage may be confined to an irradiated individual or, depending on the site of the damage, adverse effects may be manifested in subsequent offspring, indicating a hereditary consequence. These types of effect are referred to as '**somatic**' and '**hereditary**' effects respectively. Occupational limits (discussed below) reflect this with particular regard to exposure of the abdomen of women [4].

There are two other expressions that are used by the ICRP in connection with the effects of radiation. An effect for which the probability of the event occurring, rather than its severity, is regarded as a function of received dose without a threshold or trigger level, is referred to as a '**stochastic**' effect. On the other hand, an effect for which the severity varies directly with the received dose, and therefore for which a threshold or trigger value may exist, is referred to as '**non-stochastic**' effect.

IONIZING RADIATION REGULATIONS 1985

These Regulations [5] are made under the provisions of the Health and Safety at Work, etc. Act 1974 to implement the basic requirements of European Directive 80/836/Euratom as amended by Directive 84/467/Euratom. They lay down basic standards for the protection of workers and the general public against the dangers arising from the use of ionizing radiation in work activities.

One of the basic requirements of the Regulations is that, with certain exceptions, employers and self-employed persons are required to notify the Health and Safety Executive that they are working with ionizing radiation.

As with COSHH, employers are required to take all necessary steps to restrict the exposure of employees and non-employees to ionizing radiation, so far as is reasonably practicable. Specific exposure limits are contained in Schedule 1 of the Regulations. These dose limits are listed for five different situations in terms of effective dose equivalents:

1. Dose limits for the whole body.
2. Dose limits for individual organs and tissues.
3. Dose limits for the lens of the eye.
4. Dose limit for the abdomen of a woman of reproductive capacity.

5. Dose limit for the abdomen of a pregnant woman.

In order to illustrate the way in which the standard is specified, the dose limits referred to in Part 1 are listed below:

1. for employees aged 18 years and over, 50 mSv in any calender year;
2. for trainees aged under 18 years, 15 mSv in any calendar year;
3. for any other person, 5 mSv in any calender year.

Areas where persons are more likely to receive more than specified doses must be designate as 'controlled' or 'supervised' areas, and access must be restricted. Employees who receive more than specified doses of radiation are required to be specially designated as 'classified persons'. The doses of radiation received by such persons must also be monitored and recorded by dosimetry services approved by the Health and Safety Executive. Also, certain employees must be subjected to medical surveillance. Radiation levels have to be monitored in controlled and supervized areas.

Finally, every employer who works with ionizing radiation is required to make an assessment of the hazards that are likely to arise from the work, and where more than specified amounts of radioactive material are involved, the assessment must be sent to the Health and Safety Executive.

In 1985, the Health and Safety Commission approved a code of practice entitled. *Protection of Persons against Ionizing Radiation Arising from any Work Activity* [6] as a practical guide to the Ionizing Radiation Regulations 1985.

DETECTION AND MEASUREMENT OF IONIZING RADIATION

As with many hazardous environmental agents, the presence of ionizing radiation must be discovered by employing some form of detecting device. This, as well as detection, may produce some form of measurement of radiation levels.

The commonly available instrumentation is based upon one or more of the following devices:

1. With the **ionization chamber**, a small voltage is applied between two electrodes situated in an air-filled chamber, and ions generated by the ionizing radiation flow towards either the anode or the cathode, depending upon their electrical charge. The ionization process, therefore, generates an electrical current which is in proportion to the radiation intensity, and measuring the current allows the radiation intensity to be measured.

2. The **Geiger-Müller Tube** also works on the principle of gas ionization. However, here a very high voltage is applied between the electrodes. This accelerates the electrons formed upon ionization, which themselves cause further ionizations and hence a multiplication of the current generated. Because of this form of amplification, a single ionization can generate a detectable pulse of current.

3. The action of the **scintillation counter** relies upon a solid material, the atoms of which can be excited by the ionizing radiation, thus storing energy. When the electrons return to their original energy state, the energy which was stored is lost, usually in the form of photons of visible light, hence the term 'scintillation'. The scintillations produced are detected and amplified by a photomultiplying device, and an electrical signal is produced which is proportional to the energy of the original ionizing radiation.

4. The **film badge** is the most common form of dosimeter, consisting of a small section of photographic film encased in a specially-designed holder. There are many different types, but essentially the film contains coatings of different sensitivities. The film is blackened by impinging radiation, and the degree of blackening (when referred to a standard) can be related to an approximate radiation dose. The holder is designed to contain a variety of sections with different screening or filtering properties, and therefore by comparing the blackening that occurs between different density screens, the nature of the radiation type can be assessed. These devices are used extensively for logging personal, whole-body exposure.

5. The **thermoluminescent dosimeter** is a device that uses the properties of certain materials to emit light photons in response to impinging ionizing radiation. These devices can give an electrical signal related to radiation dose, which can then be processed and stored on logging equipment.

Radon

Issues relating to the occupational exposure to radon are discussed in Chapter 42.

REFERENCES

1. Goldfinch, E.P (ed.) (1989) *Radiation Protection – Theory and Practice*, Institute of Physics, London.
2. Martin, A. and Harbison, S.A. (1986) *An Introduction to Radiation Protection*, 3rd edn, Chapman & Hall, London.
3. National Radiological Protection Board (1988) *Living with Radiation*, HMSO, London.
4. United Nations Environment Programme (1985) Radiation Doses, Effects, Risks, UNEP.
5. Ionizing Radiation Regulations, S.I. 1985 No. 1333, HMSO, London.
6. Health and Safety Commission (1985) *Protection of Persons against Ionizing Radiation Arising from any Work Activity*, HMSO, London.

31 Non-ionizing radiation

Paul C. Belcher and John D. Wildsmith

Non-ionizing radiation is generally regarded as being that part of the electromagnetic spectrum with wavelengths greater than 0.1 nm. Should radiation of this energy level impinge upon tissue, the energy imparted is not sufficient to produce excitation or ionization in the form described in Chapter 30. Non-ionizing radiation may still, however, be hazardous as it can cause tissue disruption by thermal damage, and there is a growing body of opinion as to a number of less tangible effects upon the human body which include a number of specific hazards in the workplace. There are many parts of the electromagnetic spectrum that should be considered under the heading of 'non-ionizing radiation'. These are identified under separate headings below. It must be appreciated that the radiations consist of part or parts of a continuous spectrum and, therefore, the divisions employed are somewhat artificial. They are, however, necessary to assist our understanding of this form of potential hazard.

The various types of radiation are described in an order ranging from the shorter wavelengths to the longer wavelengths. Devices such as lasers, which may emit more than one type of non-ionizing radiation, are then considered. The approximate wavelengths of the principal types of non-ionizing radiation are indicated in Fig. 31.1. It should be noted that most forms of non-ionizing radiation fall outside of the visible part of the electromagnetic spectrum and, therefore, the hazard created may not be detected until actual damage is done. This means that the potential

Wavelength

| 1nm | 100nm | 10fm | 1mm | 10m | 100km |

(ULTRA-VIOLET) (VISIBLE) (INFRA-RED) (MICROWAVES) (RADIOFREQUENCY)

Fig. 31.1 The electromagnetic spectrum.

risk posed by all sources of non-ionizing radiation must be understood and appropriate action, including surveys using appropriate monitoring equipment, must be carried out wherever a risk exists.

ULTRA-VIOLET RADIATION

This form of radiation is emitted naturally by the sun as well as a number of artificial sources such as insect killing devices, mercury discharge lamps, photocopiers and sunbeds. There are three principal classes of ultra-violet radiation which are broadly based upon the physical properties and biological effect of the radiation. These three classes are described as UV(A), UV(B) and UV(C).

UV(A): wavelength 315–400 nm.
UV(B): wavelength 280–315 nm.
UV(C): wavelength 100–280 nm.

The sun emits ultra-violet radiation in all of these classes, However, the atmosphere, particularly if pollution levels are high, will absorb most of the UV(A) and UV(B). Exposure to solar radiation is increasingly being associated with a growing incidence of skin cancer.

Biological effects of exposure

These depend on a number of factors, such as the energy of the radiation concerned, the dose received and the part of the body affected. This can produce both short- and long-term effects which are generally well understood.

Skin effects

Short-term effects are erythema (reddening of the skin), which is similar to sunburn, as the blood vessels are dilated and the blood supply to the affected tissues increases. UV(A) induces rapid tanning of the skin, whereby the existing pigmentation (melanin) is stimulated. This does not give a long-term tan. UV(B) and UV(C), which are of higher energy than UV(A), tend to produce a long-term tanning effect by actually increasing the activity of the melanin-generating cells in the skin. It should also be noted that UV(A) has greater penetrative properties and can, therefore, produce adverse effects in deeper tissues.

A further long-term effect is that of premature ageing of the skin. The skin becomes dry, cracked and thickened. A more serious effect is the induction of a variety of skin cancers, although the class of ultraviolet radiation which is most likely to induce such cancers is unknown.

The main conclusion of an HSE-funded report is that current recomendations on exposure limits to ultra-violet radiation (UVR) generally afford adequate protection against acute effects to the skin, but may not be adequate when considering eye data, particularly in the spectral region 310–340 nm. (See 'A Critique of Recommended Limits of Exposure to Ultraviolet Radiation with particular Reference to Skin Cancer' (1994.) NRPB for HSE, HSE Books, ISBN 0 7176 0749 6.)

Eye effects

The eye is affected in a number of ways by ultra-violet radiation. Inflammation of the cornea and conjunctiva can be induced, which are painful conditions although there are usually no permanent effects. This irritation may, though, have other safety consequences, e.g. when using dangerous machinery or handling hazardous chemicals in the workplace, or even driving motor vehicles or fork-lift trucks.

Ultra-violet radiation can also damage the retina if large doses are received, although this is not common as the lens and cornea tend to absorb the energy. Children are at particular risk as their eyes transmit much more UV(A) to the retina than older people.

The principal long-term effect that has been identified in connection with the eye is the production of opacity in the lens. This is known as cataract formation.

It should, therefore, be appreciated that any equipment considered to pose a risk to the health of workers or the public must be dealt with within the provisions of the Health and Safety at Work, etc. Act 1974. Welders, for example, should wear suitable goggles or a mask, and they must also ensure that any passers-by are not exposed to the ultra-violet radiation generated (in addition to other hazards).

Ultra-violet lamps must be of an appropriate type, e.g. in insect killing devices. Equipment such as photocopiers must be properly enclosed, and staff who use the equipment must be properly instructed in use of the machines and appraised of any risks involved.

One difficult area is the wide use of commercial ultra-violet tanning equipment. This is still very widely used and here people deliberately expose themselves to a source of ultra-violet radiation. The Health and Safety Executive has recognized this risk and have produced Guidance Note GS18, *Commercial Ultra-violet Tanning Equipment* [1], which gives the scale and nature of the risks and offers advice on how these risks can be minimized. One extremely important area, covered in this document, is the fact that customers must be given information before using this type of equipment so that they can evaluate the risks involved, and have freedom of choice to decide whether or not to use the equipment. It is, however, important that information that is provided is understood, and that the equipment is tested as far as is reasonably practicable, to ensure that it falls within the Health and Safety Executive guidance. Further examination or the risk of skin cancer (cutaneous melanoma) arising from exposure to fluorescent lights and ultra-violet lamps, can be found in the work of Swerd-low *et al*. [2]

VISIBLE LIGHT

The main problem associated with this form of non-ionizing radiation is usually the lack of visible light, which can render any workplace hazardous. The requirement to provide adequate levels of illumination is dealt with in Chapter 25.

It should, however, be noted that there are some additional hazards associated with visible light. One of the principal hazards is dealt with below in the section on lasers. Unsuitable forms of lighting can introduce an element of hazard, for example, when fluorescent lights are used to illuminate moving equipment. It is possible that since the fluorescent light will 'flicker' at a high rate that cannot be detected normally by the human eye, it may produce a stroboscopic effect on moving parts of machinery, giving the illusion that a rapidly spinning fan, for example, is static. Clearly, this could prove to be hazardous and, therefore, it is important to ensure that the type of lighting is suitable for the purpose.

Very bright lights as sometimes found in welding operations and in places of entertainment, can induce temporary blindness. People working in such situations must wear suitable forms of eye protection.

INFRA-RED RADIATION

All objects which have a measureable temperature emit infra-red radiation. Normally, the sensory mechanisms of the body will detect a build-up of heat before tissue disruption occurs. Infra-red radiation can produce effects similar to sunburn, i.e. a general irritation of exposed skin. It must be noted, however, that as with some other forms of non-ionizing radiation, the eye is particularly vulnerable to damage: parts such as the lens have no protective, cooling mechanism and, therefore as the heat builds up, damage such as coagulation of the proteins in the lens can occur, giving rise to cataract formation.

Quite a wide variety of infra-red sources are encountered in the workplace, such as lights (including some lasers) and heaters. The normal solution to the problem of exposure to infra-red radiation is to wear eye protection. This means that employers must be able to select and provide suitable protective equipment and supply adequate information to staff who may be exposed to this risk. British Standard BS1542: (1982) *Equipment for Eye, Face and Neck Protection Against Non-Ionizing Radiation Arising During Welding and Similar Operations* [3] provides further guidance on this subject.

MICROWAVES AND RADIOFREQUENCY RADIATION

These two types of non-ionizing radiation are very similar, and are often dealt with together. One way of defining each term is to call those radiations with wavelengths of between 10 m and 10^4 m 'radiofrequency radiation,' and those of wavelengths between 1 mm and 10 m 'microwave radiation'. For the purposes of control of this type of radiation in the working environment, the above figure should be regarded as a guide rather than a precise definition. A useful summary of the extent of exposure to both of these types of non-ionizing radiation can be found in the publication NRPB-R144, *Sources of Exposure to Radio-frequency and Microwave Radiations in the UK* produced by the National Radiological Protection Board in 1983 [4].

Microwave radiation

Microwave radiation is used principally in communications systems, heat-treatment processes in industry, ranging devices and devices for the heating and cooking of foodstuffs. The proliferation of such devices over a relatively short period of time has led to the need for an understanding of the biological effects of exposure to this type of radiation. Microwaves (as with other forms of non-ionizing radiation) can be generated as a continuous output, or in very short bursts of energy. This factor can be important, for example, when using detection devices, since the average power delivered from a pulsed system will be less than the peak power. A high peak power, delivered at a rapid pulse repetition rate, could cause significant tissue damage, while a continuous output of the same mean power may be far less damaging. This aspect of non-ionizing radiation is also mentioned in connection with lasers.

The development of exposure standards for microwave radiation in the UK is based upon the degree of thermal damage caused. This is not the same as in certain other countries where rather more subtle effects upon the human body are attributed to this form of energy. The current UK occupational exposure limit is 10 mW cm^{-2} for continuous generators with a lower limit of 5 mW cm^{-2}.

The most common source of microwave energy is probably from microwave ovens. It should be noted that the British Standard BS 3456: 1988 [5] allow such appliances to leak microwave energy to a maximum level of 50 mW cm^{-2} at a distance of 5 cm from any surface. Such equipment should be in a good state of repair and particular attention should be paid to the condition of the door seals. Accumulations of food debris can allow radiation leakage.

Research into other effects caused by microwaves, such as hormonal changes and effects upon the nervous system, continue. One useful source of reference on this issue is NRPB-R222, *Health Issues in the Siting of a Low Frequency Transmission Mast* [6], produced by the National Radiological Protection Board.

Radiofrequency radiation

Radiofrequency radiation is used principally for communications. However, it is also employed quite extensively in induction heating units for processing a wide variety of materials such as wood, plastics, paper, ceramics and textiles. Such units must be designed and sited correctly to ensure that stray energy is not allowed to affect workers or passers-by. This involves screening the radiofrequency generating unit efficiently, as at suitably high exposure levels, this form of non-ionizing radiation can produce deep-seated tissue damage.

In particular industries, there are more extensive problems, and the Health and Safety Executive have produced several Guidance Notes of some significance to environmental health officers including PM51: Safety in the Use of Radiofrequency Dielectric Heating Equipment [7].

They contain useful guidance on the monitoring equipment and techniques that should be used in the detection and control of radiofrequency radiation in the workplace.

The International Labour Office have published a practical guide: 'The Protection of Workers from Power Frequency Electric and Magnetic Fields' (1994) ILO Publication, CH-1211, Geneva, Switzerland.

LASERS

The word laser is an acronym for the term 'light amplification by the stimulated emission of radiation'. These devices produce a unique kind of non-ionizing radiation, usually with a very small range of wavelengths in the form of a collimated beam, i.e. a beam of energy that can be considered not to disperse as it moves through the environment, hence the energy is contained within the beam to a large extent, and can, therefore, be transmitted over great distances.

Laser radiation may be in the ultra-violet, infra-red or the visible part of the electromagnetic spectrum. The most common forms are visible lasers, and thus the radiation is normally referred to as laser 'light' (typically with wavelengths of 0.4 to 0.7 μm).

There are several principal types of laser device, based upon the lasing material. These are solid state (crystal), gas, semi-conductor and liquid dyestuffs.

Lasers are commonplace in work situations, such as product launches, discotheques, theatres, outdoor and indoor displays, supermarket check-out systems, beauty therapy studios and the repair of devices such as compact disc players.

General guidance concerning the assessment of safety is available in two significant documents.

European Standard EN 60825: 1991 *Radiation Safety of Laser Products, Equipment, Classification, Requirements and User's Guide* [8] (will have the status of a British Standard.)

This standard describes the biological effects of lasers and it includes details of how to assess the risk posed to the skin and eyes, in the form of a series of algorithms. It also classifies laser products into one of four basic types, based upon the power output to which a person has access (this is not the same as the maximum power of the laser unit).

Class 1

These are inherently safe laser products which are either very low-power devices, or high-power devices, which are designed in such a way that the power to which access can be obtained does not exceed the maximum permissible exposure level, e.g. by the use of interlocked enclosures.

Class 2

These are low-powered products emitting visible radiation. They are not inherently safe, however, a suitable degree of protection is normally provided by the body's normal aversion responses, including blinking of the eye.

Class 3

This class is divided into two sub-types, 3A and 3B. Type 3A have a power output of visible radiation of up to 5 mW for continuous lasers, and 5 mW peak power for pulsed and scanning lasers. The power classification is also limited to 2.5 mW cm^{-2}, and so protection is afforded to the eye by aversion responses. However, the use of common optical devices, such as binoculars, may prove to be hazardous unless they contain suitable filters.

Type 3B is more powerful and these lasers may be visible or invisible. Continuous lasers must have a maximum power of 0.5 W while the limit for pulsed lasers is specified and 10^5 Jm^{-2}. Direct viewing of laser beams of this intensity is hazardous, and reflection from mirrored surfaces (as may readily be found in places of entertainment) is also deemed to be hazardous.

Class 4

This class is the highest laser class which contains all lasers with an output which exceeds that specified for class 3B. In addition to biological hazards, this class may pose a risk of fire as the beam is so powerful. Where such systems are used to provide entertainment such as a public display, it is advisable that the Health and Safety at Work, etc. Act 1974 enforcing authority, the Public Entertainment Licensing Authority and the fire authority will usually need to liaise to ensure the safety of all associated with this activity.

Health and Safety Executive Guidance Note PM19, Use of Lasers for display purposes [9]

This document reiterates some of the basic information contained in the European Standard. It is, however, designed to cover the situation of indoor and outdoor laser displays, which are usually the situations where the most powerful laser products and the most dangerous systems in terms of additional hazards are encountered.

A helpful practical guide to the issues which must be considered by environmental health officers is included, and includes the following matters.

Prior to the public use of any display laser product, the operator of the system must supply the enforcing authority with sufficient information to assess the risks to employees and members of the public who may view the display. This information will include appropriate radiometric data shown on diagrams of the beam paths. Relevant calculations should also be provided before the display takes place.

Once the information is provided it can be used in conjunction with a series of tables which give Maxium Permissible Exposure Levels (MPE) for the eyes and skin and Accessible Emission Limits

(AEL) for the various classes of laser. The rather complex data in the various tables are converted into simple graphical representations which are easy to interpret. An example of the tabulated information along with the corresponding graphical data for the MPE for direct ocular exposure of the cornea to laser radiation is shown.

With regard to the operation of the laser system, the display area should be demarcated using the calculations made by the operator to ensure that the audience or the general public (as well as the operators and any performers) are protected from the laser radiation within the guide limits. The level of exposure should not exceed the MPE at any point where the public is permitted during the display and in addition, unless effective means are employed to prevent access to the laser beam(s), the MPE should not be exceeded at any point:

1. less than 3 metres above any surface upon which the audience or general public is permitted to stand, or
2. less than 2.5 metres in lateral separation from any position where a person in the audience or the general public is permitted during the display.

Where displays are outdoors, consideration must be given to those persons who are liable to view the beam directly within the normal optical hazard distance and also those who might view the beam or its reflections using optical aids. All publicity material including tickets and posters must contain appropriate warnings where relevant to ensure that viewing aids such as binoculars and telescopes are not used.

In the case of people who carry out maintenance work on all types of laser products, there may be a considerable risk. They must receive proper training and must be equipped with appropriate eye protection while carrying out maintenance operations. They must also ensure that safety interlocks are not overridden, and that passers-by are not affected when testing systems.

Finally, the risks posed to health and safety enforcing officers must not be ignored. It is important that where such persons are likely to be put at risk, they too are equipped with suitable forms of protection. They must also be supplied or should be able to obtain the use of a suitable form of measuring equipment.

A recent, further publication is 'The Use of Lasers in the Workplace: A Practical Guide' published in 1994, the International Labour Office Publications, CH-1211 Geneva 22, Switzerland.

REFERENCES

1. Health and Safety Executive (1982) *Commercial Ultra-violet Tanning Equipment*, Guidance Note GS18, HMSO, London.
2. Swerdlow *et al.* (1988) Fluorescent lights, ultra-violet lamps and the risk of cutaneous melanoma. *British Medical Journal*, **297**, 647–50.
3. British Standards Institution (1982) *Equipment for Eye, Face and Neck Protection Against Non-ionising Radiation Arising During Wedding and Similar Operations*, BS1542, BS1, London.
4. National Radiological Protection Board (1983) *Sources of Exposure to Radiofrequency and Microwave Radiations in the UK*, NRPB-R144, HMSO, London.
5. British Standard B.S. 3456. Part 102. Section 102.25. British Standard Specification for the safety of household and similar electrical appliances 1988, British Standards Institution, London.
6. National Radiological Protection, *Health Issues in the Siting of a Low Frequency Transmission Mast*, NRPB-R222, HMSO, London.
7. Health and Safety Executive (1986) Guidance Note PM51 *Safety in the Use of Radiofrequency Dielectric Heating Equipment*, HMSO, London.
8. European Standard E.N. 60825 (1991) *Radiation Safety of Laser Products, Equipment Classification, Requirements and User's Guide* British Standards Institution, London.
9. Health and Safety Executive (1980) Use of Lasers for Display Purposes, Guidance Note PM19 HMSO, London.

Part Six
Food Safety and Hygiene

32 Introduction to food safety

Mike Jacob

ORGANIZATIONS INVOLVED WITH FOOD HYGIENE AND SAFETY

The Ministry of Agriculture, Fisheries and Food (MAFF) and the Department of Health both have direct interests in all legislation relating to food. The MAFF Minister and the Secretary of State for Health act as joint signatories for food legislation, but lead responsibility for individual sections of this legislation is taken by the department most concerned.

MAFF has wide general interests in controls on food production and ultimate food quality. This includes a responsibility for ensuring that the public receives value for money in terms of correct labelling, the absence of adulteration and the presence only of essential and approved ingredients in food. MAFF also ensures the nation's food supply, and has major responsibilities for research and links with other countries exporting food to the UK. Early in 1990, MAFF formed its **Food Safety Directorate** as a separate and independent section of the Ministry from its commodity divisions. The Directorate comprises the Food Safety Group, Food Science Group, Animal Health and Veterinary Group, and the Pesticide Veterinary Medicines and Emergencies Group.

The purpose of the Food Safety Directorate was to answer criticisms of MAFF being too closely interested in the needs of farmers and food producers rather than consumers. The Directorate has the means to act independently and primarily in the safety interests of consumers.

The Department of Health is responsible for the health implications of the food consumed, but both departments work closely together on all aspects of food contamination. The Department of Health through its Health Aspects of Food Medical and Administrative Divisions and the Health Promotion Divisions, deal with all food health issues.

RELATIONSHIPS TO FIELD ORGANIZATIONS

The State Veterinary Service, which has the responsibility for animal health is an integral part of the MAFF. The Department of Health does not deal with food safety through a comparable, centrally employed food inspection service. Instead the Food Safety Act 1990 and the various Regulations which fall under it, are enforced by local and port health authorities, the authorized officers carrying out inspection and other duties under this legislation being environmental health officers with some technical assistance.

Environmental health statistics suggest that about 20 to 25% of technical and professional staff time in environmental health departments is devoted to food safety-related matters [1]. It is unlikely, therefore, that of the 6000 environmental health officers working in England and Wales, more than 1500 are at any one point in time involved in duties associated with food safety and hygiene legislation.* As regards this work, the local authorities have total autonomy and control in the way in which the enforcement duties are exercised. But as explained later, codes of practice under the Food Safety Act 1990 guide local authorities in this enforcement area. It is particularly important for each environmental health department to have at least one specialized food environmental health officer to oversee food inspection responsibilities.

NATIONAL HEALTH SERVICE – MEDICAL OFFICERS FOR ENVIRONMENTAL HEALTH OR CONSULTANTS IN COMMUNICABLE DISEASE CONTROL

Medical advice for local authorities is available from Directors of Public Health or consultants in communicable disease control (CCDC) responsible for the investigation and control of communicable disease, particularly food and water-borne disease. CCDCs act as local authority appointed 'proper officers' under the Public Health (Control of Disease) Act 1984, in regard to those functions carried out by the local authority where medical expertise is necessary. NHS Circular HSG(93) 56 deals with the role of the CCDC who is directly accountable to the director of public health for the control of communicable disease throughout the district of a health authority. (Chapter 16 deals with administration of communicable diseases generally.)

The Public Health Laboratory Service (see also Chapter 18)

The 52 regional and area laboratories of the Public Health Laboratory Service (PHLS) receive regularly samples of food and water supplies submitted by environmental health authorities for microbiological analysis. Prior to the Food Safety Act 1990 the PHLS had no statutory function in this respect (apart from the examination of milk samples), but the Act introduced the official role of '**Food Examiner**' representing an official laboratory recognized as the authorized centre for the examination of food for microbiological contamination. The PHLS now therefore performs a statutory role as Food Examiner. The PHLS is funded by the Department of Health.

In some areas, examination of food and water supplies may be carried out by laboratories attached to hospitals within the National Health Service, by local authorities' own 'in-house' laboratories, or private laboratories acting for them.

Since 1977, as well as the laboratories involved, the **Communicable Disease Surveillance Centre (CDSC)**, which is a part of the PHLS, has assisted in many outbreak investigations, providing support for medical officers and for environmental health officers. The CDSC has developed considerable expertise in epidemiological investigation, and the compilation of outbreak reports and can now provide a major source of information on outbreak investigation techniques, control measures and features of particular pathogens involved in outbreaks.

The CDSC publishes a weekly publication, the *Communicable Disease Report (CDR)*, which is now widely available. It provides information relating to communicable food and water-borne diseases, with details of epidemiology and special food investigations.

In addition to the routine examination of food and water samples submitted to the regional and area laboratories by environmental health officers, there has in recent years been an increasing amount of survey work undertaken by these laboratories in collaboration with the **Central Food Hygiene Laboratory** of the PHLS, which specializes in food contamination investigation and provides great expertise in the microbiology of food poisoning. Similarly, the **Laboratory of Enteric Pathogens** of the PHLS provides much information on specific enteric pathogens, such as salmonella, which is essential to outbreak investigation. The regional and area PHL directors routinely have direct links with local authority chief

---

* A LACOTS survey in 1993 in England, Wales and Northern Ireland showed 2171 fte working on food safety enforcement, 1403 EHOs and 768 technical officers.

environmental health officers, and CCDCs, rather than directly with the Department of Health. The Department, however, maintains close links with the Central Public Health Laboratory, the CDSC and the Food Hygiene Laboratory at Colindale. (For the investigation of communicable diseases including food poisoning, see Chapter 17.)

In the event of a national food hazard, there will be direct contacts between the laboratory, local chief environmental health officers, CCDCs and the Department of Health. In many cases, one of the central specialist laboratories of the PHLS will also be involved.

THE RICHMOND COMMITTEE

Future food microbiological surveillance

The Richmond Committee (chaired by Sir Mark Richmond, Vice Chancellor of Manchester University) was formed in 1989 to advise the Secretaries of State for Health, the Minister of Agriculture, Fisheries and Food and the Secretaries of State for Wales, Scotland, and Northern Ireland, on matters remitted to it by Ministers relating to the microbiological safety of food and on such matters as it considered needed investigation. The Committee produced its first report in February 1990 [2] in which it proposed a structure comprising a Steering Group on the microbiological safety of food to co-ordinate microbiological food safety and an advisory Committee on the health aspects of the microbiological safety of food.

The objective of the latter is to provide an independent expert view on the public health implications of food safety matters and in particular, upon the results of future surveillance. It also advises on the areas where surveillance on other government activities are needed. These two commitees were set up in June 1990.

Chemical surveillance

Surveillance of both microbiological hazards and chemical hazards are now therefore subject to central control and monitoring. The structure of chemical hazards comprises;

1. **A steering group on the chemical aspects of food surveillance** which oversees chemical safety and nutritional adequacy in the UK food supply. Ten working parties surveying foods for specific chemical substances work to it, covering nutrients, food additives and inorganic and organic contaminants ranging from heavy metals to veterinary drug residues.
2. **A food advisory committee** which assesses and advises on the risk to humans of chemicals which are used or occur in food and on the exercise of powers concerning labelling, composition and chemical safety. It examines and comments on reports of other relevant advisory committees before they are published.
3. Three **medical and toxicological advisory committees** set up by the Department of Health who advise on medical and toxicological aspects of chemicals in food. These committees consider the results of surveys produced by the steering group and advise the steering group on the public health implications.
4. **The Advisory Committee on Novel Food and Processes**, the **Veterinary Products Committee**, and the **Advisory Committee on Pesticides** also provide advice and guidance as necessary.

In the event of either a microbiological or chemical food hazard arising, the Department of Health and/or the MAFF take direct action to deal with it. The advisory committees above would not be involved.

Proposals for food law

The Richmond Committee was asked to look at specific questions relating to the increasing incidence of microbiological illnesses of food-borne origin, particularly from strains of *Salmonella, Listeria* and *Campylobacter* to establish whether this was linked to changes in agriculture and food production, food technology and distribution, retailing, catering and food handling in the home and to recommend action where appropriate. The Committee was later asked to consider the implications of the outbreak of botulism caused by the consumption of hazelnut yoghurt in June 1989, which occurred mainly in the north west of England. The Committee subsequently completed its work by 31 July 1990 and published the second part of its Report on 14 January 1991 [3]. This contained wide ranging recommendations, most of which were supported by the government [4].

Representations were sent to ministers regarding changes in the food safety law which were necessary. The work of this Committee has been a major influence in food safety policy. The greatest risk areas of the nation's food supply and all aspects of food handling in commercial distribution, retail, catering and in the domestic kitchen were analysed, with numerous recommendations being made.

The government responded through sections of the Food Safety Act 1990, and by setting up an **Implementation Advisory Committee** (now disbanded) to produce codes of practice for enforcement authorities. Additionally, the government put in hand new research, surveillance and advisory machinery to ensure that it is continually updated on the need for policy changes related to microbiological risks in food [5].

An important area arising from the Report will be the future action taken to ensure closer co-ordination between the collection of data on human food-borne disease, and the collection of information by the State Veterinary Service in relation to zoonoses and information in animal databases. One of the recommendations of the Committee was that existing links between veterinary and human systems should be strengthened by giving the PHLS a formal responsibility to collate information from human and veterinary sources, to give as complete a view as possible on the current state of microbiological contamination of humans and food animals, and of any developing trends. The government accepted this need in its response to the Committee's first report.

Public health in England (Acheson Report)

Recommendations of the Acheson Committee investigation, *Public Health in England* (the report of a committee of inquiry into the future development of the public health function set up by the Secretary of State for Social Services [6] – in 1986 (see also Chapter 16) are referred to in the recommendations of Richmond. One involves the need for training of both CCDCs and environmental health officers to enable them to take effective and coherent action to control food poisoning outbreaks. Training initiatives for environmental health officers, both through the CDSC and other training centres, follow from this recommendation. The Institute of Environmental Health was seen by Richmond as playing an essential role in ensuring that training courses for environmental health officers were uniform and sufficiently comprehensive in dealing with food safety issues.

Public Health in England reported on a need for a review of the law of infectious disease control, and Richmond recommended that both local authorities and health authorities should, in future, have a specific statutory duty to provide an infectious disease control service. (The Department of Health produced a consultation document on this subject in October 1989 [7] but no legislative changes have so far been made.)

At present, food- and water-borne disease outbreaks are mainly investigated by environmental health officers, but the investigations should be supervised by CCDCs under arrangements made at the time of local government and National Health Service reorganization in 1974. Richmond recommended that statutory responsibility for leading and co-ordinating the services should lie with the health authority, but that strong links are required with the local authority environmental health officers. For the future, it is not likely that environmental health officers would wish to relinquish this work as the investigation of outbreaks is linked directly to the need for enforcement action where outbreaks may have been caused by breakdown in food hygiene in the preparation or service of food. It is not likely either that staffing levels in health authorities will be substantially increased in future to do the work currently undertaken by environmental health officers in relation to food-borne outbreaks.

Other proposals

On food microbiology, the Richmond Report recommended that local authorities, the Department of Health and the Welsh Office, should encourage environmental health departments to target their future surveillance work more precisely and to carry out, whenever possible, well-founded surveys to provide good quality information as a sound basis for decision making. The government accepted this recommendation, and has taken forward proposals for environmental health officers' work in this area through the consideration of the Steering Group and codes of practice on enforcement duties including food sampling.

Other important recommendations of the Richmond Committee included the need for environmental health officers, through inspection activities, to promote the **hazard analysis critical control point principle (HACCP)** as a means of promoting food safety, and that professional staff in environmental health departments should be trained in HACCP as well as appropriate training in food microbiology, food technology and food control systems; where necessary environmental health officers should call in more expert sources of advice to advise on more complex food manufacturing processes; to achieve more adequate levels of monitoring than they do at present, specialist food technicians should be recruited by local authorities to assist environmental health officers.

The main purpose of the Acheson Committee investigation was to undertake a broad and fundamental examination of the role of public health doctors, including how such a role could best be fulfilled. The inquiry followed two major outbreaks of communicable disease, one of which was a major salmonella food poisoning outbreak at the Stanley Royd Hospital in Wakefield in August 1984.

One of the most important recommendations of this inquiry was that for the future, directors of public health in health authorities, and chief environmental health officers, should meet on a regular basis and establish channels of communication which encouraged collaboration between health authorities and local authorities (see Chapter 16).

Both in relation to the investigation of food-borne disease and dealing with any food hygiene problems in National Health Service (NHS) premises, liaison and close co-operation between health and local authorities is obviously highly important. Following the abolition of Crown Immunity in hospitals and other NHS premises, environmental health officers, directors of public health, CCDCs and senior management of NHS districts have increasingly been involved in close co-operation on the investigation of outbreaks, measures to promote better standards of food hygiene in NHS kitchens, and the training of employees in essential aspects of food hygiene.

The government is committed to changing the law in relation to infectious disease control. This, hopefully, will have the effect of cementing existing relationships and create a better overall structure for the investigation and control of communicable disease.

PERIOD OF CHANGE

The nature of the food industry, distribution, retailing and consumer preference is currently subject to major changes. There have been many and varied changes in the last 10 years in institutional, recreational, tourist and fast-food catering. More recently in the retail area, there has been a massive growth in a taste for chilled food with emphasis on 'fresh' and 'natural' products, free of additives, preservatives and any artificial ingredients. There has been a substantial growth in the number of multiple retailers selling such products. The storage, distribution and sale of such food puts heavy pressure on the integrity of refrigeration storage, speed of delivery and shelf-life of products.

Undoubtedly, many of the problems of salmonellosis, listeriosis and other infections have been related to these trends in marketing, but other factors, such as the increasing tendency of single households to eat out and the choice of convenience foods, have had a part to play.

The European Single Market, which came into existence on 1 January 1993, means that the inspection of food is now concentrated at the point of production within the Union. The free movement of food means the absence of discrimination between products produced in the UK or in any of the other European Union (EU) States.

There have been some fears that the lowest common denominator will, in future, apply insofar as inferior goods legitimately produced in any of the EU member states, according to the laws of those states, can move freely in the EU as a whole. This may mean that products of a quality unacceptable according to the domestic food legislation of the UK will, nevertheless, have to gain entry because of the EU rules. This is not likely to be a valid argument. Modern consumers are discriminating and have a wide range and choice of foods already available. EU legislation will increasingly focus attention on common, horizontal standards of labelling, consumer information, food hygiene, general inspection, sampling and analytical requirements for food on an EU-wide basis. Sub-standard foods will be identified and eliminated by this process, and imports of food from countries outside of the EU will be subject to ever-increasing scrutiny and controls.

The Channel Tunnel will also likely increase the volume of 'roll-on roll-off' imports to the UK with minimal inspection of food entering the UK due to the quantity of products involved.

These developments should not be seen in negative terms from the public health risks involved. They are the means of providing better services and availability of food supplies for consumers in a widening community, where the influence of EU-wide standards of inspection and emphasis on safe food of good quality will, in the future, play an increasing part in the advantages of living in Europe. The inspection system will however take time to develop on a 'European' basis. It is not likely that truly common standards of inspection and enforcement will apply across the EU by the end of 1996.

REFERENCES

1. Jacob, M. *et al.* (1989) The role of the Department of Health in the microbiological safety of food. *British Food Journal*, **91**, 8.
2. Committee on the Microbiological Safety of Food (1990) *The Microbiological Safety of Food, Part 1*, HMSO, London.
3. Committee on the Microbiological Safety of Food (1991) *The Microbiological Safety of Food, Part 2*, HMSO, London.
4. Ministry of Agriculture, Fisheries and Food (1991) *Report of the Committee on the Microbiological Safety of Food, Part 2. Recommendations and Government's Response*, HMSO, London.
5. Department of Health (1990) *Report of the Committee on the Microbiological Safety of Food, Part 1. Recommendations and Government's Response*, HMSO, London.
6. Committee of Inquiry into the Future Development of the Public Health Function (1988) *Public Health in England*, HMSO, London.
7. Department of Health (1989) *Review of the Law on Infectious Disease Control*, Consultation Document, HMSO, London.

33 Food safety law

Mike Jacob

LEGISLATION PRINCIPLES

Traditionally in the UK, the enforcement of food law has involved two basic principles:

1. the need to ensure food safety and to protect food from any microbiological, toxic or other contamination that can render it unfit for human consumption; and
2. to ensure that consumers of food are not fraudulently treated, and that food when purchased is of a nature, substance and quality as demanded by the purchaser.

In July 1989, the government issued a white paper, *Protecting the Consumer* [1] in which it set out its commitment to a food safety strategy for the future. The white paper stated that new legislation would be intended to:

1. ensure that modern food technology and distribution methods are safe;
2. ensure that food is not misleadingly labelled or presented;
3. reinforce present powers and penalties against law breakers;
4. ensure that new EC directives on food can be implemented;
5. streamline future legislation by combining the Acts which apply in England. Wales and Scotland;

and indicated that the maintenance of food safety depended on:

1. research to provide a sound up-to-date understanding of food safety;

2. expert advice to help the government decide on action in the light of scientific, technical and medical evidence;
3. legislation to set standards which lay down what the consumer has a right to expect, requiring how the standards should be met, and imposing penalties if they are not;
4. providing monitoring and surveillance of both food composition and its safety through taking samples for examination and testing;
5. enforcement – mainly through local authority action – to ensure that statutory provisions are met.

In 1992/93 it was anticipated that MAFF would commission some £18 million of research out of a total Government spend on Food Research of some £30.7 million [2]. Over 350 Government-funded projects are being carried out in laboratories in MAFF and by institutes such as the Institute of Food Research.

Research is essential to implement the aims of food safety and to create conditions for efficient agricultural, fisheries and food industry activity.

The typing of food poisoning bacteria is carried out by the Public Health Laboratory Service (PHLS) and this is part of its responsibilities which contributes to the diagnosis, treatment prevention and control of food borne illness.

Government research priorities for 1992/94 included work on the following topics:

1. The effect of processing conditions such as heat, cold, water activity, pH, atmosphere and packaging on the growth of pathogenic food micro-organisms.

2. The effectiveness of various processes in controlling microbial growth including microwave and ohmic heating, irradiation, aseptic processing, sous-vide and cook-chill operations.
3. The safety factors needed to ensure the safety of minimally processed foods.
4. Rapid methods for the detection of pathogenic micro-organisms or their toxins in food.
5. Improved methods for the isolation and concentration of micro-organisms from food.
6. Methods suitable for the screening of pathogenic micro-organisms (specific identification is not necessarily required).
7. Methods suitable for the specific detection of pathogenic strains of selected food organisms (the priority is not necessarily very rapid methods, specificity is more important).
8. Methods suitable for on-line detection.

Micro-organisms and subjects of particular interest are:

(a) pathogenic strains of *Salmonella;*
(b) pathogenic strains of *Campylobacter;*
(c) pathogenic strains of *Listeria;*
(d) *Yersinia;*
(e) *Aeromonas;*
(f) verotoxigenic strains of *E. coli,* including *E. coli* 0157;
(g) cross contamination during food-handling operations, including hygienic design and operation of equipment;
(h) efficacy and effects of cleaning or sanitizing of environments or equipment in which food is handled;
(i) growth in processing, packaging and distribution operation (e.g. vacuum packing);
(j) growth in food preparation operation (e.g. use of microwave ovens);
(k) growth in domestic and catering environments.

THE FOOD SAFETY ACT 1990

This Act, which implements the Government's strategy, received the Royal Assent in July 1990, and is the means of enforcement control through wide-ranging regulations and codes of practice.

The main provisions on food safety are contained in Part II of the Act and these are summarized briefly in this chapter. The various statutory procedures are dealt with in detail with the aid of flow diagrams in *Environmental Health Procedures* [3].

Section 7: rendering food injurious to health

Any person who renders any food injurious to health by means of any of the following operations:

1. adding any article or substance to the food;
2. using any article or substance as an ingredient in the preparation of food;
3. abstracting any constituent from the food;
4. subjecting the food to any other process or treatment with intent that it shall be sold for human consumption;

shall be guilty of an offence.

In determining for the purpose of this section whether any food is injurious to health, regard shall be had:

1. not only to the probable effect of that food on the health of the person consuming it; but
2. also to the probable cumulative effect of food of substantially the same composition on the health of a person consuming it in ordinary quantities.

'Injury' in relation to health, includes any impairment whether permanent or temporary and 'injurious to health' is to be construed accordingly.

This section therefore provides power to deal with manufacturing processes or procedures where, either by negligence or design, the safety of the food is undermined, either where the food could cause injury when eaten as a single item, or where consumed in small quantities as part of normal dietary intake over a period.

Section 8: selling food not complying with food safety requirements

This was a new, wide-ranging provision which defines that food fails to comply with food safety requirements if:

1. it has been rendered **injurious to health** by means of any of the operations mentioned in section 7;
2. it is **unfit for human consumption**; or
3. it is so **contaminated**, whether by extraneous matter or otherwise, that it would not be reasonable to expect it to be used for human consumption in that state.

Where any food which fails to comply with food safety requirements is part of a batch, lot or consignment of food of the same class or description, it shall be presumed for the purposes of this section until the contrary is proved, that all of the food in that batch, lot or consignment fails to comply with those requirements.

The question of fitness is a matter to be determined by the court on the basis of the circumstances of the particular case. Contamination could be such as to make the food unfit or unsound and unmarketable.

The presumption in this section that part of a batch, lot or consignment which is unfit or contaminated is representative of a larger quantity from which it derives, provides the power to deal with a larger consignment even where only a small proportion of it has been found to be unfit or contaminated on examination.

Section 9: inspection and seizure of suspected food

This provides power for an authorized officer of a food authority to inspect and seize suspected food. Where the authorized officer considers that food is likely to cause food poisoning or any disease communicable to humans, or otherwise not to comply with food safety requirements, he can order its detention in some specified place, or seize the food and remove it in order to have it dealt with by a justice of the peace. Where the food is detained, the officer must within 21 days determine whether or not he is satisfied that the food complies with food safety requirements, and either withdraw the detention or seize it within that period for it to be dealt with by a justice of the peace.

If a detention notice is withdrawn or a justice of the peace refuses to condemn it, the food authority will be liable for compensation to the owner of the food for any depreciation in its value arising from the activity of the officer.

Section 10: improvement notices

This provides the power for an authorized officer to serve an 'improvement notice' where he has reasonable grounds for believing that the proprietor of a food business is failing to comply with any regulations to which this section applies, e.g. Food Hygiene Regulations. Notices are subject to appeal procedure. (See also Code of Practice No.5 (revised April 1994), *Improvement Notices* and the Food Safety (Improvement and Prohibition – Prescribed Forms) Regulations 1991.)

The improvement notice:

1. states the officer's grounds for believing that the proprietor is failing to comply with the regulations;
2. specifies the matters which constitute the proprietor's failure so to comply;
3. specifies the measures which in the officer's opinion the proprietor must take in order to secure compliance;
4. requires the proprietor to take those measures, or measures which are at least equivalent to them, within such period (not being less than 14 days) as may be specified in the notice;
5. indicates that any person who fails to comply with an improvement notice shall be guilty of an offence.

The service of an improvement notice was an important new power, as no such notice was recognized or specified in previous Food Acts.

In accordance with new guidance contained in the revised Code of Practice issued in April 1994:

(a) the use of improvement notices should not generally be considered as the first option when breaches are found on inspection – officers should use informal procedures where it is considered this will secure compliance within a reasonable timescale; and
(b) notices may only be signed by environmental health officers, official veterinary surgeons (OVSs) and others where they possess a

degree in an appropriate science or technology.

Failure to comply with the improvement notice is itself an offence.

Section 11: prohibition notices

This section deals with 'health risk conditions' with respect to the operation of a food business. (See also Code of Practice No.6, *Prohibition Procedures*, and the Food Safety (Improvement and Prohibition – Prescribed Forms) Regulations 1991.) A health risk condition is one which involves the risk of injury to health.

The magistrate's court is able to apply a prohibition on the use of a process or treatment for the purpose of the business or the use of premises or equipment for the purpose of the business, where the risk of injury to health applies. A prohibition order can be applied by the court on the proprietor participating in the management of any food business, or any food business of a class or description specified in the order. An order can be applied to a manager of a food business as it applies in relation to the proprietor of such a business, providing the manager is a person who is entrusted by the proprietor with the day-to-day running of the business or any part of the business.

Where the health risk condition is no longer fulfilled regarding the business, the local authority is under an obligation to take action lifting the prohibition order.

Section 12: emergency prohibition notices and orders

This section provides important new powers for environmental health officers to take necessary and immediate action themselves, where health risk conditions are not fulfilled by food businesses. (See also Code of Practice No.6, *Prohibition Procedures*, and the Food Safety (Improvement and Prohibition – Prescribed Forms) Regulations 1991.)

A prohibition with immediate effect can be applied by the service of an emergency prohibition notice by the environmental health officer on the proprietor of the business. The service of such a notice may impose the appropriate prohibition on the use of a process or on the premises themselves.

The emergency prohibition notice must be followed up immediately by an application to the court for an emergency prohibition order. At least 1 day before the date of such an application, the food authority must serve notice on the proprietor of the business of the intention to apply for this order.

An emergency prohibition notice shall cease to have effect:

1. if no application for an emergency prohibition order is made within the period of 3 days beginning with the service of the notice, at the end of that period:
2. if such an application is so made, on the determination or abandonment of the application.

An emergency prohibition notice or emergency prohibition order shall cease to have effect on the issue by the enforcement authority of a certificate to the effect that it is satisfied that the proprietor has taken sufficient measures to secure that the health risk condition no longer applies to the business.

A food authority must apply for an emergency prohibition order within a period of 3 days beginning with the service of the emergency prohibition notice. If it does not, or if the court in considering the order is not satisfied on hearing the application that the health risk condition was fulfilled, it will be liable for compensation to the proprietor of the business for any loss suffered.

Section 13: emergency control orders

This section provides the power for a minister (at the Department of Health, MAFF, Scottish or Welsh Offices) to make an order prohibiting the carrying out of a commercial operation with respect to food, food sources or contact materials, which may involve imminent risk of injury to health. The minister may also give such directions as appear to him to be necessary or expedient related to the prohibition. If the minister has to do anything under this section in consequence of any person failing to comply with an emergency control order, or a direction under this section, the minister may recover from that person any expenses reasonably incurred by him.

This section provides substantial power to back up food hazards or emergencies to prevent food in national distribution which is known to be a hazard to health being consumed. Normally, these hazards are dealt with by voluntary co-operation by the parties involved, but where in future such co-operation is not forthcoming. the reserve power of an emergency control order will be available.

Section 14: consumer protection

This section provides that any person who sells to the purchaser's prejudice any food which is not of the nature or substance or quality demanded by the purchaser, shall be guilty of an offence.

Section 15: falsely describing or presenting food

This section provides offences for labelling or falsely describing food so as to mislead as to the nature or substance or quality of the food.

Sections 16–18: the power to make regulations dealing with food safety and consumer protection

Wide-ranging powers are provided in section 16 for ministers to make regulations regarding substances and composition of food; microbiological standards; processes or treatments in the preparation of food; the observance of hygienic conditions and practices in commercial operations; the labelling, marking, presenting and advertising of food; and other general regulations for the purpose of securing that food complies with food safety requirements, or in the interest of public health, or for the purpose of protecting or promoting the interests of consumers.

Regulations may also make provision for the hygiene of contact materials which come into contact with food intended for human consumption, and their labelling.

Section 17 allows ministers to make regulations to comply with EC obligations, and under section 18 ministers may make regulations regarding novel foods; genetically modified food sources or foods derived from such sources; and special designations for milk and the licensing of milk.

Section 19: registration of premises

Regulations made by ministers under this section deal with the registration by enforcement authorities of premises used or proposed to be used for the purpose of a food business, and for prohibiting the use for those purposes of any premises which are not registered in accordance with regulations. The Food Premises (Registration) Regulations 1991 were made under this power but are currently under review.

Section 21: defence of due diligence

The defence of due diligence replaces the strict liability offences under previous legislation. In proceedings under the Food Safety Act 1990, a defendant can plead a defence that he took all reasonable precautions and exercised all due diligence to avoid the commission of the offence by himself or by a person under his control.

What will constitute due diligence is, to a certain extent, defined in section 21. It is likely, however, that future case law will revolve around the extent to which an importer or food manufacturer exercises sufficient foresight in respect of the food imported or produced as regards the quality and safety control applied before the food is put on the market for consumers.

Most of the current authorities for due diligence decisions lie in actions relating to trade descriptions. The decisions made indicate that defendants need to have done some positive act to satisfy the defence, and where a system of inspection by some subordinate is applied, it may be necessary to show that the system is adequately supervised by senior management. Where senior managers may not be in a position to check the information, there may be a duty on such managers to find out from the persons who supplied the actual goods what system or systems they may have operated to ensure that no offences under the legislation were likely to take place. In some cases, however, there may be instances where the size and organization of a business is such that the requirement of supervision by a superior in a company is unnecessary and impracticable. (The subject of due diligence for food manufacturers is dealt with further on page 531.)

Section 23: provision of training by food authorities

This section provides the means for a food authority to provide either within or outside its area, training courses in food hygiene for persons who are, or intend to become, involved in food businesses, whether as proprietors or employees or otherwise.

The Government's proposals on food hygiene training are dealt with on page 506.

FOOD AND ENVIRONMENT PROTECTION ACT 1985

Part I of this Act deals with emergency orders in relation to major contamination risks to food production in agriculture or elsewhere from the release of toxic chemicals or other substances. Emergency orders may be made designating areas of land in the UK or of the sea within British fishery limits, or both of such land and of such sea, where the food deriving from such areas may be, or may become, unsuitable for human consumption. Ministers in such circumstances may make emergency orders which have to be laid before and approved by resolution of each House of Parliament.

In the event of particular emergencies, ministers may authorize investigating or enforcement officers who are not officers of ministerial departments, such as environmental health officers.

DEREGULATION AND FOOD LAW

As part of the Government's general initiative on deregulation, a detailed paper on deregulation and food law was produced by the MAFF Food Safety Group in February 1993. The consideration covered the whole area of policy related to food safety and quality legislation both within the European Union (EU) and national measures in the UK. The desire to implement subsidiarity within the EU links with deregulation to ensure that only laws which in future are strictly necessary for public health and consumer protection purposes are both introduced and enforced. Alternative measures which can be employed and which reduce burdens on industry are to be pursued in the future. In September 1993 a MAFF news release [4] set out a detailed plan for deregulation in the food law sector. The Deregulation and Contracting Out Act 1994 provides the means to abolish regulations seen as now being unnecessary or over-burdensome on industry.

The programme of action on food hygiene includes:

1. Simplification and consolidation of the Food Hygiene (General) Regulations 1970 (as amended) and associated regulations as part of the implementation of the new EC Hygiene of Foodstuffs Directive 93/43/EC (see page 504).
2. Amendment of the Fresh Meat (Hygiene & Inspection) Regulations to exclude from its scope depots handling packaged meat.
3. Establishment of a National Meat Hygiene Service in April 1995.
4. Consolidation and revision of regulations covering milk hygiene including implementation of the EC Directives on milk hygiene.
5. A review of provisions for temperature controls in various hygiene regulations.
6. A review of 'vertical' directives related to hygiene (i.e. those specific to a type of foodstuff) with a view to consolidation with the general hygiene of foodstuffs directive (conclusion of this is unlikely before 1996.)
7. Review and simplification of the Imported Food Regulations 1984.

Some deregulation policies have already been adopted by the Government – particularly in the development of the Directive 93/43 which has as one of its main themes a 'business friendly' approach. Emphasis is on the development and use of business guides to good hygiene practice backed up by enforcement procedures which concentrate on real food safety risks rather than the minutiae of structural and equipment standards in premises. The revised Food Hygiene Regulations to implement the directive will follow this policy.

Other deregulation policies in the food hygiene field which have already seen changes include the abandonment of the slaughter policy for egg laying flocks (introduced because of salmonella infections), the abandonment of proposed regulations on vacuum-packed foods, and changes in the registration requirements for food premises. It is anticipated that the Registration Regulations requiring the registration of food premises as a means of identification, will be withdrawn. The Government have also announced their intention to implement the meat hygiene Directives as lightly as possible for small businesses only trading on the local market and have modified their earlier proposals on food hygiene training so that the present simple requirement contained in Directive 93/43/EC that 'Food business operators shall ensure that food handlers are supervised and instructed and/or trained in food hygiene measures commensurate with their work activity' will be all that will be required (i.e. there will be no prescribed standards of training or targeted levels of achievement through training).

Environmental health officers and other enforcement officers will no doubt feel distinctly uneasy at the scope and scale of the Government's deregulation proposals. Much of the legislation now targeted for abolition was introduced because of known food safety risks. Although MAFF and the Department of Health have been at pains to stress that there is no intention of 'going soft' on food hygiene and safety, because of the complaints they have received, particularly from small businesses, of the draconian nature of food legislation and the unwelcome and frequent scrutiny they receive from officials, there is nevertheless a feeling that the Government is over-reacting. Support for food safety legislation and the work of environmental health officers has been welcomed from the major food producers who also have fears that the Government should not put at risk food safety standards by going too far with deregulation policy.

FOOD HYGIENE REGULATIONS

Directive 93/43 on the hygiene of foodstuffs

Some important provisions of the Directive are:

1. Hygiene conditions are outlined in relation to:
   (a) general requirements for food premises;
   (b) specific requirements for rooms where foodstuffs are prepared, treated or processed;
   (c) requirements for moveable and/or temporary premises (such as marquees, market stalls, mobile sales vehicles);
   (d) requirements for premises used primarily as private dwelling-houses, premises used only occasionally for catering purposes and vending machines;
   (e) transport;
   (f) equipment for food premises;
   (g) food waste;
   (h) water supply;
   (i) personal hygiene of employees;
   (j) specific provisions regarding food, e.g. foods known to be contaminated should not be accepted by food companies;
   (k) food hygiene training – there is a general requirement that employees should be supervised and instructed and/or trained in food hygiene matters commensurate with their work activity.

2. The Directive refers to the Commission, assisted by Member States and other interested parties, encouraging the development of guides to good hygiene practice to which food businesses may refer. These guides should be to the standards of the EN 29000 series where appropriate and should be based on the Recommended Code of International Practice, General Principles of Food Hygiene of the Codex Alimentarius (FAO/WHO – a United Nations Body). It will be for the food industry itself, not governments to produce these guides. Government help will be available however for caterers and retailers operating small businesses.

3. Article 1 of the Directive requires the Commission within 3 years of the Directive's adop-

tion, to examine the relationship between other Directives specifically dealing with commodities (e.g. milk and eggs) and 93/43 so that eventually the horizontal measures in the latter can replace those which are related, in the former.

4. In Article 3 food business operators are required to identify any step in their activities which is critical to ensuring food safety and ensure that adequate safety procedures are identified, implemented, maintained and reviewed on the basis (where practicable) of the system of HACCP (hazard analysis and critical control points).

5. Article 4 sets out provisions for microbiological and temperature control criteria for certain classes of foodstuffs which may be adopted after consultation with the Scientific Committee for Food set up by decision 74/234/EEC.

6. Article 7 states that Member States may maintain amend or introduce national hygiene provisions which are more specific than those laid down in 93/43 providing that they are not less stringent and do not constitute a restriction, hindrance or barrier to trade in foodstuffs.

7. Article 8 requires competent authorities to carry out a general assessment of the potential food safety hazards associated with businesses, paying particular attention to critical control points identified by those businesses to assess whether the necessary monitoring and verification controls are being operated.

Aspects of these provisions of Directive 93/43 are dealt with in more depth in later chapters. It is obvious from the text of the Directive, however, that the UK negotiating team exerted a major influence in the drafting. Many of the provisions follow a designed policy of emphasis on industry self-regulation and guides to good hygiene practice with enforcement being related to hazards and risks in food handling. If the Commission are successful in bringing commodity directives into line with 93/43 this should simplify the current mass of legislation which has emanated from the

EU in the last 5 years and should help to pursue the twin paths of deregulation and subsidiarity for the future.

The Food Safety (General Food Hygiene) Regulations 1995

These Regulations will come into force in 1995 and replace all the existing regulations relating to food hygiene (general, markets, stalls and delivery vehicles, docks, wharves and on ships) in England, Scotland and Wales.

The Regulations will not apply to any part of a food business which is subject to the requirements of other regulations referred to in Chapter 36, which implement EU product-specific Directives, e.g. meat and poultry meat, meat products, egg products, etc. However, where those regulations make no provision for the training of persons employed in the food business, the training requirements in these Regulations will apply.

The main obligations on proprietors of food businesses are:

1. **Hygienic operations** – the following operations must be carried out in a hygienic way: **preparation, processing, manufacture, packaging, storage, transportation, distribution, handling and offering for sale or supply, of food**.

2. **Staff illness** – The proprietor must notify the CCDC at the local environmental health department if any staff reports a food-borne illness or infection. This includes typhoid, paratyphoid, or any other salmonella infection or dysentery or any staphylococcal infection likely to cause food poisoning*.

3. **Staff training** – The proprietor must ensure that food handlers engaged in the food business are supervised and instructed and/or trained in food hygiene matters commensurate with their work activity.

4. **Identify critical steps to ensure food safety**:
   (a) consider the potential food hazards in the business operation;
   (b) identify the points in the operation where food hazard may occur;

---

* This original proposal is now being reviewed and may not be included in the regulations.

(c) decide which of the points identified are critical to ensuring food safety – the 'critical points';

(d) identify and put in place effective control and monitoring procedures at those critical points;

(e) periodically, and particularly when there are changes in food operations, key personnel or structural changes, new purchase of equipment, etc., review the potential food hazards, the critical control points, the control and monitoring procedures.

5. **Comply generally with the rules of hygiene** – Whether the premises are permanent, temporary or moveable, or include the use of vending machines; if transport is used to move food from one place to another, the basic requirements are the same. Care must be taken to prevent food handled being contaminated; supervision of staff is necessary to ensure they are handling food hygienically; premises vehicles and equipment must be structurally sound and in good working order, able to be cleaned effectively, and are cleaned effectively; washing facilities for the business operation and for staff hygiene, sanitary accommodation and waste collection and disposal must be adequate and hygienic.

The requirements are no more onerous than the similar requirements in previous Food Hygiene Regulations.

Food Hygiene Training

Of particular importance is the requirement in Schedule 1 Chapter X that food handlers are supervised, and instructed and/or trained in food hygiene matters commensurate with their work activity. There will be many instances, particularly in the case of small businesses, where proprietors are not sure what their obligations are regarding such supervision, instruction/training. Environmental health officers will be available to offer advice, but an assessment of staff training needs may be required and an examination of the options available for training, necessary.

Although detailed staff training plans are not required under the Regulations, proprietors may wish to consider such planning, together with appropriate qualifications desirable for employees at varying levels of seniority and responsibility within companies.

The main obligations on Food Authorities are:

1. **Assessing risks to food safety** – Enforcement officers will be under a duty to concentrate on matters of public health and to ensure that potential risks and food hazards are identified and brought to the attention of proprietors. They also have the responsibility to bring breaches of the Regulations to the notice of proprietors, particularly where such breaches could lead to formal notices and prosecution.

   After an inspection of food premises, the proprietor has the right to be informed of any adverse findings by the environmental health officer. Food Authorities have been advised by the Government that such informal advice, either in oral or written form, should precede the service of any formal improvement notice under Section 10 of the Food Safety Act 1990.

   When assessing risks to food safety, or wholesomeness of food, environmental health officers should have regard to the nature of the food, the manner in which it is handled and packed, any process to which the food is subjected, and the conditions under which it is displayed or stored. (See Revised Code of Practice No.9, *Food Hygiene Inspections*, page 520.)

2. **Regard to guidance on good hygiene practice** – A food authority must give due consideration to any **relevant** guide to good hygiene practice recognized by the Government, or any European guide, details of which have been published by the European Commission in the C series of the *Official Journal of the European Communities*. 'Relevant' means relevant to the food business in question.

   It is anticipated that the various sectors of the food industry will develop (with Government assistance), guides to good hygiene practice which will be mainly designed to inform and guide food companies as to the hygiene standards required for particular food operations. Environmental health officers will also be receiving advice on standards of reasonable hygiene requirements in food operations from LACOTS. When this guidance is in place, it should lead to improved common standards of hygiene for particular food sectors and common enforcement standards amongst environmental health officers. There should therefore be less reason in future, for argument as to whether environmental health officers requirements are reasonable or appropriate as guidance on interpretation of the Regulations will be widely available for both industry and enforcement personnel.

Temperature control

The Food Hygiene (Amendment) Regulations 1990 and 1991 introduced new controls over chilled foods accompanied by Department of Health Guidance [5,6] on the types of food to be held at the required temperatures and the guidelines to be followed on enforcement. These regulations have been the subject of much critical comment and new regulations on chill controls and hot holding are proposed for implementation on 15 September 1995. The main features of this proposal are:

1. A general requirement to keep foodstuffs likely to support the growth of pathogenic micro-organisms or the formation of toxins at temperatures which would not result in a risk to health, as in the EU Food Hygiene Directive.
2. A requirement to keep such foods at or below 8°C; there would be exemptions for foods where chill control is not necessary to prevent a risk to health;
3. A facility for upward variation from the maximum chill temperature.
4. Businesses manufacturing, preparing or processing food would be able to vary the 8°C maximum temperature upwards where this was justified by a scientific assessment of safety of the food at the new temperature, in conjunction with an assigned shelf-life. The higher

temperature would be communicated to other businesses in the food chain. Variations would be expected to apply mainly to short shelf-life products, where tighter chill controls are not a safety requirement.*

FOOD HYGIENE TRAINING – GENERAL ASPECTS

In 1989 during the passage of the Food Safety Bill through Parliament the Department of Health issued a Consultation Document on Hygiene Training. This discussed the options available in relation to the proposal to make regulations on Food Hygiene Training and referred to the National Council for Vocational Qualifications (NCVQ) initiatives to improve vocational qualifications. A further statement was issued in the Summer of 1992 and on 17 December 1992 the Department of Health released its amended proposals for food hygiene training, instruction and supervision.

Now that the Hygiene of Foodstuffs Directive 93/43/EC has been adopted the Government have made a requirement in the Food Safety (General Food Hygiene) Regulations 1995 for business operators to supervise, instruct and/or train their employees in food hygiene according to the work they do (see page 505). The operator will have to assess the different activities involved and choose which method of training (if this option is exercised) is suitable. There will be no requirement for company training plans, records or statutory training periods but the Government are initiating voluntary guides to good practice. Additionally a Code of Practice under Section 40 of the Food Safety Act 1990 will guide environmental health officers on enforcement aspects. Environmental health officers will not be responsible for deciding upon the level or the content of training. Any method of training is acceptable providing the right information relative to the tasks performed is conveyed. No examinations following the training are necessary.

---

* Before these proposals can be implemented in the UK they are subject to agreement by the Commission and the EU.

Environmental health officers, when giving companies advice on various training needs, must not identify with one particular type of training available, but should advise on the various training options on the market. Priority should be given to the high risk type of food operation in regard to training need and any prosecution should only take place where in addition to lack of training there is a significant breach of hygiene standards indicated by insanitary premises or a food poisoning outbreak arising from poor handling practices.

Where the food authority serves an improvement notice they must not invite the business to participate in their own training course. A criticism of the Department of Health's proposals is that there is little indication of what the training is intended to achieve. The 1989 Consultation Paper seemed to point the way for food hygiene training to be incorporated as an essential ingredient in food workers' vocational training and for appropriate standards of training to be enforced. It now seems that exhortation rather than strong enforcement is to be the means whereby effective training of employees is to be promoted. Voluntary guides to good practice are already in existence but the main problem is likely to be the number of small businesses which are still unwilling to undertake training unless compelled to do so.

It has been significant that since the Government indicated that it did not intend to press for compulsory training as indicated in 1989, there has been a substantial drop in the numbers of candidates presenting themselves for training courses operated by the various examining and training bodies. It is to be hoped that there will in future be continuing take-up of the basic food hygiene training administered by the Chartered Institute of Environmental Health, The Royal Society of Health, The Royal Institute of Public Health & Hygiene, The Royal Environmental Health Institute of Scotland and the Society of Food Hygiene Technology. It is likely that the courses run for the basic or primary level examinations of these various bodies will be of the standard recommended by industry guides. It is to be hoped also that even though it is not necessary under the Government's recent proposals for food handlers to pass the relevant examinations, they will continue to do so to at least indicate that a basic level of food hygiene awareness is being achieved.

EUROPEAN UNION LEGISLATION AND PROPOSALS

EC Directive 89/397/EC(C) on the Official Control of Foodstuffs is of major significance to future food law enforcement and was the first step in the development of EU policy on food safety and quality. The aim of the Directive is to lay down the EU rules to be followed when national authorities carry out controls on the conformity of foodstuffs and materials and articles intended to come into contact with foodstuffs, to ensure the protection of the consumer. The areas covered by the Directive include general monitoring of foodstuffs, sampling programmes throughout the distribution chain and in-factory enforcement and inspection. The Directive creates obligations for Member States and for the Commission to carry out investigations and make reports on:

1. Standards of training for food inspectors in the member States.
2. Quality standards for laboratories involved in inspection and sampling under the directive.
3. An EU inspection service.

Member States must draw up forward programmes laying down the nature and frequency of inspections to be carried out regularly in regard to food production, manufacture and import into the EU process, storage, transport, distribution and trade. Each Member State is obliged to report to the Commission on its programme of inspection in these areas carried out during the year. The Commission in turn transmits to the Member States a recommendation concerning a co-ordinated programme of inspections for the following year.

Under Article 15 each Member State must communicate to the Commission the names of the competent authority or authorities within their territory, their functions and the official laboratories or other laboratories authorized to carry out analyses and examinations in accordance with the requirements of the Directive.

Additional measures in Directive 93/99/EEC relating to this Directive were adopted by the Council in 1993. Member States will be required to ensure that their competent authorities have, or have access to, a sufficient number of suitably qualified and experienced staff, in particular in areas such as chemistry, veterinary medicine, food microbiology, food hygiene, food technology and law, so that controls under the Official Control of Foodstuffs Directive 89/397/EEC can be properly exercised. Member States must also take all measures necessary to ensure that the laboratories involved in control activities comply with the general criteria for the operation of testing laboratories laid down in European standard EN 45001 supplemented by Standard Operating Procedures and the random audit of their compliance by quality assurance personnel. Member States must also designate bodies responsible for the assessment of laboratories under Article 7 of 89/397/EEC.

The Commission will be appointing officials to co-operate with the competent authorities of the Member States to monitor and evaluate the equivalence and effectiveness of official food control systems which they operate. The Commission will report to the Member States on the work of officials employed by their competent authorities.

There is a proposal that each Member State designates a single liaision body to assist and co-ordinate communication and in particular, the transmission and reception of requests for assistance. A single liaison body will be important in future in dealing with queries regarding food imports and exports and disputes arising from products found to breach the Single Market standards.

The existence of single liaison bodies in the Member States will aid other EU and WHO initiatives regarding food research, the dissemination of information and the training of officials. In particular with the anticipated growth in the number of Member States in future, the new entrants to the Single Market will find the liaison arrangements of instant benefit.

One WHO initiative involves the up-dating of their European Food Safety Services Manual, containing information on all government departments involved with aspects of food safety in the WHO European Region (over 50 countries). In addition to a hard-copy publication, the information will form a computer database and will be 'business friendly' so that any government or local government official or food exporter/importer will be able to access information on the relevant government departments in the European Region. The liasion arrangements now proposed by the EU will fit well with this operation.

The Sutherland Report

In March 1992 the Commission appointed a high level group of six individuals to review progress in developing the single market and to make recommendations on its future. The group was asked to look specifically at five main areas, including the extent to which administrative mechanisms were adapting to the removal of frontiers, the area where acts or measures taken in one Member State could be recognized as equivalent to another and whether as a result there would be enough mutual confidence to satisfy producers, suppliers and consumers.

Amongst the findings and recommendations of this group the following are important in relation to food safety controls;

1. Although the single market rules have been discussed thoroughly at Member State level and within the European Parliament, efforts to provide information to consumers have had limited success and much more needs to be done to explain the need for and operation of the new Law. A communications strategy to make EU Law clear, more consistent and more effectively transposed at national level is required.

2. The challenge is to reassure the consumer and to capture the imagination of business, particularly of smaller firms, that the rules of a really frontier free market will be applied across the community.

3. In order to apply the principle of subsidiarity correctly the group suggest five criteria for

Community action – need, effectiveness, proportionality, consistency and communication.

4. On the issue of access to the Courts and legal redress and to ensure better application of EU remedies, Member States should appoint independent mediators to hear complaints.

5. A major problem in the enforcement of common rules is the difference in penalties awarded to similar offences in different Member States. This in itself could lead to competitive disadvantage for businesses. The European Court of Justice has ruled that penalties imposed must not go beyond what are strictly necessary and that control procedures must not restrict the freedom required by the Treaty. Nor must they be so disproportionate to the gravity of the offence that they obstruct that freedom. Further work therefore should be done on the harmonization of penalties.

6. The group considered five operational guidelines for cooperation as follows;

   (i) Each enforcing authority should accept a duty to cooperate with others through direct contact and via contact points. They should accept that they have community-wide responsibilities in that their functions directly affect EU citizens.

   (ii) Each Member State should appoint a central contact point for each broad field of the internal market.

   (iii) These contact points and information about relevant enforcement bodies should be notified to all other contact points and to the Commission. These will then form a contact group.

   (iv) Authorities should feed into the contact points regularly and not wait for specific enquiries to be made.

   (v) When an authority requests information from another for market control purposes this must be supplied rapidly and automatically with the receiving authority respecting the confidentiality of any commercial information.

The Group also recommended in the approach to EU legislation that where progress over several years has enabled a satisfactory degree of approximation to be achieved, Directives should be converted into directly applicable Regulations thereby giving consumers, businesses and enforcement authorities a single point of reference for EU legislation.

The Maastricht Agreement involves the ever closer political and economic union of the EU whereas the Sutherland Group has recognized the need to consolidate existing achievements and making sure the single market operates fairly and effectively in future [7].

QUALITY ASSURANCE

In September 1989, LACOTS (see Chapter 3) produced the publication *Guidance Notes on Inspection of Food Production Factories for Local Authorities* [8]. This was produced by a multi-disciplinary working party set up because of the future needs for **'in-factory' enforcement** arising from Directive 89/397/EEC (above) and the Food Safety Act 1990. The objective of the Guidance Notes is to assist local authority officers in their role of enforcing the provisions of the Food Act, particularly related to the manufacture of foods.

All producers of food will usually claim to have some system of control of the quality of their products. This may range from a system of simple quality control checks to a **quality assurance (QA) scheme** designed around the principles of British Standard BS5750: 1987 [9] and, in some instances, accredited to that standard.

Any food manufacturing QA scheme should be based on principles contained in the Institute of Food Science and Technology (IFST) guidance on good manufacturing practice [10].

The LACOTS guidance is designed to be capable of operation in any category of food factory, whether large or small and with or without a definable QA system. It covers aspects of the compositional requirements of food and hygiene of production, storage, distribution and product labelling. It is a very useful document to be used for multi-disciplinary inspection of food factories as envisaged in the EU Directive.

REFERENCES

1. Government White Paper (1989) *Food Safety Protecting the Consumer*, HMSO, London.
2. MAFF Food Safety Directorate, MAFF Food Food Research Strategy and Requirements Document, 1992–94, August 1991, Ministry of Agriculture, Fisheries and Food, Nobel House, 17 Smith Street, London SW1P 3JR.
3. Bassett, W.H. (1992) *Environmental Health Procedures*, 3rd edn, Chapman & Hall, London.
4. MAFF News Release, 299/93, 14 September 1993, 'Gillian Shepherd Announces Food Deregulation Plan'.
5. Department of Health, Environmental Health and Food Safety Division (1990) *Guide to the Food Hygiene (Amendment) Regulations 1990 – Temperature Controls*, HMSO, London.
6. Ministry of Agriculture, Fisheries and Food and Department of Health (1990) *Guidelines for Enforcement of Temperature Controls in the Food Hygiene (Amendment) Regulations 1990*, HMSO, London.
7. The Internal Market After 1992, Meeting the Challenge, London Office, European Commission, 8 Storeys Gate, London SW1P 3AT.
8. Local Authorities Co-ordinating Body for Trading Standards (1989) *Guidance Notes on Inspection of Food Production Factories for Local Authorities*, LACOTS, Croydon.
9. British Standards Institute (1987) *Quality Systems* BS 5750: 1987, Part 0, section 0.1 *(International Equivalent) ISO 9000 1987*, BSI, London.
10. Institute of Food Science and Technology, *Food and Drink Manufacture – Good Manufacturing Practice. A Guide to its Responsible Management*, 2nd edn, IFST, London.

34 Machinery of inspection and control

Mike Jacob

ENVIRONMENTAL HEALTH OFFICERS AND LOCAL AUTHORITIES

The environmental health officer acts as the authorized officer of his employing authority to carry out inspection and enforcement duties required in particular legislation. The Food Safety Act 1990 and the regulations made under it provide the main *vires* for the environmental health officer's powers of entry, and the inspection and enforcement duties which he carries out.

Local authorities are autonomous bodies insofar as they are not controlled directly by central government departments in their work on food safety. Although as explained in Chapter 33, EU legislation now requires central government co-ordination and direction of the work of environmental health officers in this field, the position is not similar to that of the State Veterinary Service, which is a direct enforcement organ of MAFF.

Inevitably within the European context where other member states look to central government to ensure the maintenance of standards over food production and exports, there must be government (through MAFF and the Department of Health) involvement by way of central authorization of manufacturing establishments and other control procedures in the food inspection work traditionally carried out by local government and environmental health officers. This, however, only affects the administrative structure of the work, not the nature of it or the ultimate degree of responsibility resting on the officer carrying out food and food premises inspection.

Local authorities act as 'competent' authorities for EU inspection duties. However the nature of these inspection duties is increasingly being prescribed in Government Codes of Practice.

CODES OF PRACTICE

Section 40 of the Food Safety Act 1990 provides for ministers to issue codes of recommended practice as regards the execution and enforcement of this Act and of regulations and orders made under it. Codes shall be laid before Parliament after being issued.

Every food authority must have regard to any relevant provision of any such code, and shall comply with any direction which is given by the ministers. Ministers are obliged to consult with organizations which appear to them to be representative of interests likely to be substantially affected before issuing the code.

An Implementation Advisory Committee (IAC) was set up in 1990 to advise Ministers on the development of Codes. In February 1993, the Food Minister decided, because of the expanded remit of LACOTS (the Local Authorities Co-ordination Body on Food and Trading Standards), that the IAC should be wound up. LACOTS (see Chapter 3) and the Scottish Food Co-Ordinating Committee now advise Ministers on new Codes of Practice.

At the end of 1994, the situation on codes of practice issued was as follows:

Codes issued:

No. 2, *Legal Matters*;

No. 3, *Inspection Procedures*;

No. 4, *Inspection, Detention and Seizure*;

No. 5, *Improvement Notices* (revised April 1994);

No. 6, *Prohibition Procedures*;

No. 7, *Sampling*;

No. 8, *Food Standards Inspections*;

No. 9, *Food Hygiene Inspections* (revised 1994);

No. 10, *Enforcement of the Temperature Control Requirements of the Food Hygiene Regulations*;

No. 11, *Enforcement of the Food Premises (Registration) Regulations*;

No. 12, *Division of Enforcement Responsibilities for the Quick Frozen Foodstuffs Regulations 1990* (revised February 1994);

No. 13, *Enforcement of the Food Safety Act in Relation to Crown Premises*;

No. 14, *Enforcement of the Food Safety (Live Bivalves, Molluscs and Other Shellfish) Regulations 1992*;

No. 15, *Enforcement of the Food Safety (Fisheries Products) Regulations 1992*;

No. 16, *Enforcement of the Food Safety Act in Relation to the Food Hazard Warning System*;

No. 17, *Enforcement of the Meat Products (Hygiene) Regulations 1994.*

As part of the Regulation Programme, the Codes are being reviewed.

FOOD SAFETY INSPECTION – INFRASTRUCTURE

Some district local authorities act as agencies for county councils in respect of work related to the compositional quality of food and labelling, and other local authorities, such as the London boroughs and metropolitan districts, are responsible for this work through environmental health departments. Other than in these specific cases, trading standards officers carry out the main functions relating to sampling and examination of food for composition and labelling, working with public analysts locally. Centrally, they link to the Food Standards Division of MAFF. The whole structure of local authorities will however be subject to change as a result of the proposed creation of unitary authorities in Scotland and Wales and some in the non-metropolitan areas of England.

LACOTS (the Local Authorities Co-ordinating Body on Food and Trading Standards

This organization is sponsored by the Association of County Councils, the Association of Metropolitan Authorities, the Covention of Scottish Local Authorities, the Association of District Councils and the Association of Local Authorites in Northern Ireland. The main function of LACOTS is to co-ordinate the practical aspects of enforcement work. It also advises Central Government and provides an effective channel for collection and exchange of technical information on food consumption, labelling and now also food hygiene matters. For this purpose it employs environmental health officers as well as trading standards officers and other staff.

LACOTS carried out a pilot exercise on extending its **'home authority' principle** (HAP) to food hygiene and microbiological safety [1]. Sixteen local authorities and a corresponding number of food trading enterprises were involved in this pilot which has been shown to successfully expand the home authority principle to food hygiene work. This principle has been a proven aid to effective enforcement based upon good practice and commonsense. Its main features are to prevent infringements by offering advice at source and by encouraging enforcement authorities and businesses to work in liaison with a particular authority called the Home Authority in order to minimize duplication and public expenditure. It is designed to assist businesses to comply with the law in a spirit of consultation rather than confrontation although nothing in the guidelines produced by LACOTS can remove from a business the onus of compliance; or the primary duty for the enforcement of laws from the authority in whose area a specific food contamination incident or breach of food hygiene law has taken place.

Under HAP the following definitions are important:

The Home Authority

This is the authority where the relevant decision-making base of an enterprise is located. It may be the place of the head office or factory, service centre or place of importation. In de-centralized businesses the role and location of the authority is a matter which may require discussion with other authorities, taking into consideration the views of the enterprise.

The Originating Authority

This term is used to refer to an authority in whose area a de-centralized enterprise produces or packages goods or services. The Originating Authority is one which will have a special responsibility for ensuring that goods and services produced within its area conform with legal requirements. Most enterprises in the UK operate from a single base and in these circumstances the functions of Home Authority and Originating Authority are combined.

The Enforcing Authority

This term refers to all other authorities undertaking inspections, receiving complaints, making enquiries or detecting infringements. It most commonly relates to enforcement in the 'market place' but can be extended to include enforcement throughout the distribution chain.

Under HAP a Home Authority should be willing to offer counsel and guidance on policy issues, compliance with the law, adherence to recognized standards and codes of good practice and advise on remedial actions.

The Home Authority is the primary link between enforcement authorities and originating authorities and enterprises which are based in the Home Authority area. The responsible officer within the Home Authority should be willing to advise colleagues and assist in the resolution of complaints and enquiries. Responsibility can be given to a named officer who should maintain a record of relevant incidents, company policies and diligence systems together with a record of significant advice offered to each business within the area.

Because of resource or other constraints, an authority may be unable to accept Home Authority responsibilities. It might however be able to suggest ways in which another authority or group of authorities might assume the responsibility.

Home Authorities should be notified by originating authorities of significant findings regarding manufacturing, packaging, servicing and hygiene problems together with details of companies' diligence procedures and commitment to quality assurance. There will likely be circumstances where an originating authority is able to undertake many of the functions of the Home Authority on issues which are straightforward.

Each local authority retains its statutory responsibility for the enforcement of the law. However it may be appropriate when infringements are detected for the enforcing authority to liaise with the Home Authority or the originating authority before embarking upon detailed investigations or legal actions. This may help to avoid unnecessary duplication, providing the investigating officer with essential background information on company policies or longstanding problems of which the Home Authority are well aware.

The Enforcing Authority should ensure that decisions to prosecute and the results of legal proceedings are notified to the Home Authority as routine. Professional judgement will determine whether brief details of administrative actions such as written warnings, suspension notices or improvement notices need to be referred to the Home Authority incident record. Minor corporate matters should be referred to the Home Authority to take whatever action it judges to be appropriate.

The local authority associations have resolved that LACOTS should receive reports of legal actions taken contrary to the advice of the Home Authority or the advice of a LACOTS National Panel.

LACOTS has advocated the development of HAP throughout the EU and the European Free Trade Area. The European Forum of Food Law Practitioners have adopted HAP and in the initial stages LACOTS is available to act as the link authority in dealings between the individual local authorities and food enforcement practitioners in other Member States.

LACOTS is generally providing a very valuable 'third force' between Government departments and the food authorities, liaising with both and co-ordinating advice, guidance and action in a number of important food hygiene areas. Through the issue of circulars, it is providing good advice on the interpretation of aspects of food hygiene requirements contained in Food Hygiene Regulations and the Hygiene of Foodstuffs Directive 93/43/EC.

In February 1994 LACOTS issued guidelines to environmental health officers on Food Safety

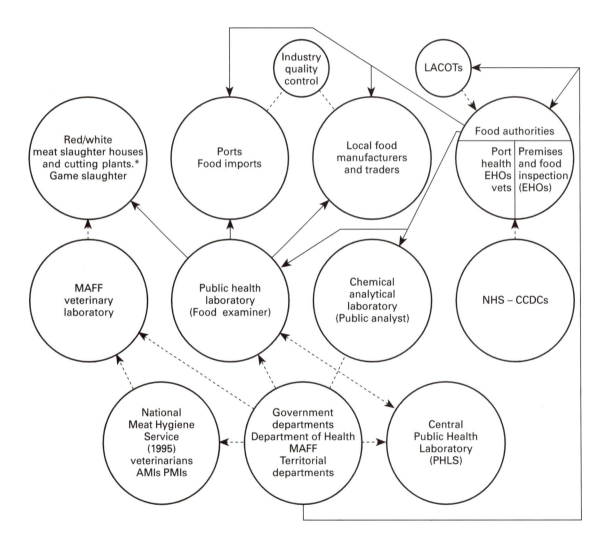

Fig. 34.1 Local food control infrastructures. EHOs = environmental health officers; CCDCs = consultants in communicable disease control; AMIs = authorized meat inspectors; PMIs = poultry meat inspectors; MAFF = Ministry of Agriculture, Fisheries and Food.

* From 1 April 1995 these premises will become the responsibility of the National Meat Hygiene Service, and thereby removed from local food control arrangements.

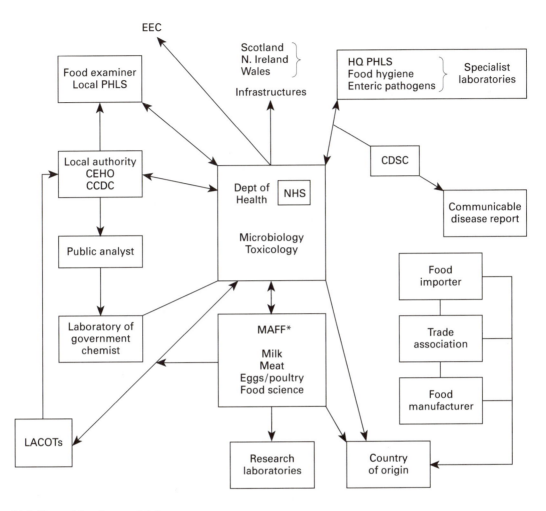

Fig. 34.2 Central food control infrastructure.

Enforcement Policies. This guidance focuses on the need for authorities to have a systematic approach to enforcement matters including:

1. a documented enforcement policy;
2. enforcement based on risk to public health;
3. commitment to statutory codes and LACOTS guidance;
4. commitment to local liaison groups and LACOTS collaborative procedures;
5. enforcement training;
6. identified decision makers with clear limits of authorization;
7. clarify informal and formal actions;
8. identify circumstances where formal actions are to be taken including formal cautions;
9. identify the criteria for prosecutions.

Figs 34.1 and 34.2 indicate the interrelationships between environmental health departments, the health authorities which employ consultants in communicable disease control, the PHLS and

* From 1 April 1995 responsibility for meat and poultry hygiene and inspection will be taken over by the National Meat Hygiene Service and will therefore become a part of the central food control infrastructure.

the Communicable Disease Surveillance Centre. MAFF, through the State Veterinary Service, provides controls over animal health and will also link with the National Meat Hygiene Service to be formed in 1995.

In the central food infrastructure, the Laboratory of the Government Chemist can be used for special examinations or as a reference laboratory in relation to public analysts' work. The government departments involved, the Department of Health and MAFF, link closely with trade associations representing sections of the food industry, either importers or UK food manufacturers, regarding legislation aspects and, particularly, when food hazards arise and action has to be taken either to stop food imports or to withdraw suspect foods from the UK market.

The Department of Health Food Hazard Scheme [2]

Fig. 34.3 illustrates the Department of Health Food Hazard Warning System, which shows the action taken, mainly on a voluntary co-operative basis, when a nationally distributed foodstuff is found to be hazardous and has to be withdrawn from the market. The emergency control order power now contained within section 13 of the Food Safety Act 1990, provides a statutory backup to the Department of Health action in regard to such hazards. However, it is likely that this power will only be used in an extreme situation where the voluntary co-operation of either a food importer or UK producer is not forthcoming when the evidence suggests that food nationally distributed presents a public health hazard. Emergency orders must be made by ministers.

The voluntary action comprises a six-stage procedure, with environmental health officers usually being requested to follow up on the withdrawal action instituted by the food industry, by ensuring that the suspect food has actually been removed from sale. This might require environmental health officers visiting wholesale, distribution, retail and catering outlets, or telephoning such outlets, and/or the use of local radio, TV and news media to publicize the scale of the problem.

The Department of Health Hazard Warning System has been in operation since 1979, and works well. From the moment that a central decision is taken to withdraw food from sale, the action of the importer or manufacturer and action by the Department of Health and local authorities who are contacted by the Department by fax or BT Gold, ensures the removal of suspect foods within 48 hours. It is not likely that any other country in the world possesses such an effective system. (See also Code of Practice No.16, on the Food Hazard Warning System.)

AUDIT COMMISSION REPORTS

In April 1990, a National Food Premises Condition Survey was organized by the Audit Commission in co-operation with the Institution of Environmental Health Officers. The survey covered over 5000 premises which were inspected by environmental health officers in nearly 300 local authorities in England and Wales. The Commission subsequently produced a report, *Environmental Health Survey of Food Premises* [3], and an additional report, *Safer Food. Local Authorities and the Food Safety Act 1990* [4].

The Audit Commission's study of this area of environmental health work arose from the increased interest nationally in food safety in 1989 and 1990, and the specific Audit Commission interests in the efficiency, effectiveness and economy of local authority work. Environmental health officers' responsibilities related to food inspection were critically examined as part of this exercise.

The results of the *Environmental Health Survey of Food Premises* indicated that almost one in eight food premises in England and Wales presented a significant or imminent health risk, one-third of these either warranting prosecution or being closed down. Large metropolitan areas had significantly more high-risk premises than the rest of the country.

Almost 46% of the food premises visited had not been inspected within the last year, a quarter of these had not been visited within the last 3 years, and a further 5% had never been visited at

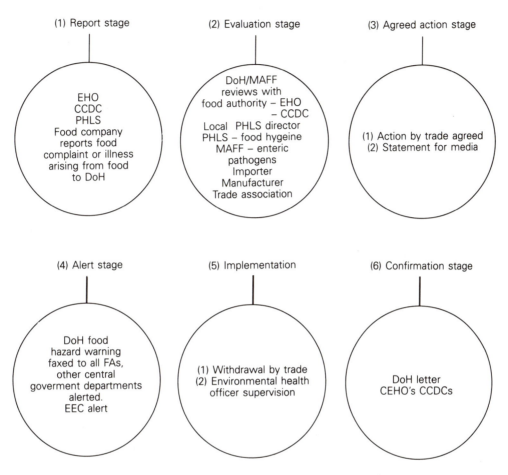

Fig. 34.3 Food hazard warning system. FA = Food Authority; other abbreviations as in Fig. 34.1.

all. Factors most commonly assessed as high health risks were ineffective monitoring of temperatures, poor staff hygiene awareness, cross-contamination resulting from poor practices, inadequate hand-washing facilities, and lack of management hygiene awareness. The survey raised a number of questions relating to the resources of environmental health departments to carry out effective food inspection work. The report, *Safer Food. Local Authorities and the Food Safety Act 1990*, which was published in December 1990, made suggestions and proposals for the future.

The Commission concluded that the extent of the current food industry had outpaced the regulatory regime in place to control it, and that changes were needed in four main areas:

1. A national co-ordinating body on enforcement was needed. A local authority sponsored body such as LACOTS could further develop the codes of practice. Such a body could be extended by a small body of skilled staff, including food technologists and legal experts, to provide support for local authorities in their work under the Food Safety Act 1990 and Directive 89/397/EC on the control of foodstuffs. The work of LACOTS was subsequently expanded into Food Hygiene as a result of this recommendation.
2. The increasing complexity of food production and the steps taken by food companies to protect their reputation is not matched by the resources or expertise of many small local authorities. The Food and Drink Federation

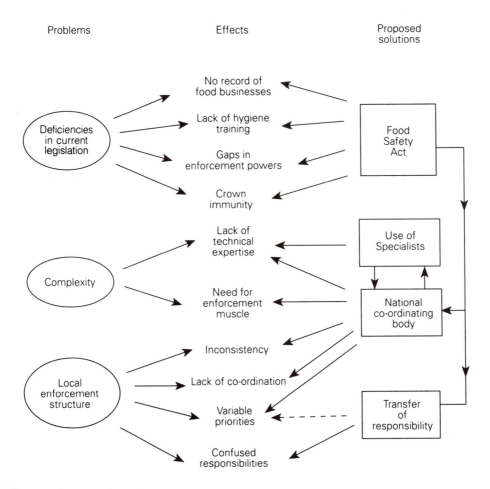

Fig. 34.4 Impact of proposed solutions.

and the British Retailers Association complained of inconsistent local, interpretation of legislation. The Codes of Practice under Section 40 of the Food Safety Act 1990 and guidance issued by LACOTS are now designed to meet this criticism.

3. Enforcement authorities must be able to match the expertise of the food industry. The training needs of inspectors, the development of specialisms for environmental health officers and others in areas of food law enforcement should all be reviewed.

4. The career structure of officers in local government food authorities should be reviewed,

affording opportunity for advancement to the chief officer posts to specialist technical officers other than for example, generalist CEHOs.

Problems perceived and solutions suggested by the Audit Commission are contained in Fig. 34.4.

The case for a central or independent enforcement body had been promoted during the parliamentary debate on the Food Bill, and had been rejected by the government. However, with the anticipated changes in local government organization, government deregulation policies and EU developments, a central body cannot be ruled out as a possible new agency to deal with complex aspects of food manufacture and technology in the future. There is, therefore, a need to upgrade and improve the level of training that specialist environmental health officer food inspectors receive in the areas of food science and technology. New MSc and other specialist food courses for environmental health officers have been available from 1991. Hopefully these will be fully taken up by environmental health officers.

REFERENCES

1. LACOTS (Local authorities Co-ordinating Body on Food and Trading Standards) Home Authority Principles, Pilot Project 1993, LACOTS PO Box 6, Robert Street, Croydon CR9 1LG.

2. Jacob, M., Billingham, V.S. and Rubery, E. (1989) The role of the Department of Health in the microbiological safety of food. *British Food Journal*, **9**, (1), 8.

3. Audit Commission (1990) *Environmental Health Survey of Food Premises*, Information Papers, No.2 June HMSO, London.

4. Audit Commission (1990) *Safer Food. Local Authorities and the Food Safety Act 1990*, HMSO, London.

35 General controls on food safety

Mike Jacob

ROLE OF INSPECTION

The environmental health officer as an enforcement officer under the Food Safety Act 1990 and regulations made under it is responsible for inspecting premises to check that compliance with the law is being achieved. The frequency of such inspections is usually determined on a priority basis and guidance on inspection frequency and the nature of inspection with regard to particular premises, is contained in the *Codes of Practice No. 3 Inspection Procedures* [1] and *No. 9 Food Hygiene Inspection* [2]. There has been much discussion on the point whether inspection in all cases, should be seen as an enforcement mechanism or whether it should contain a health education element. There is no doubt that an effective inspection should include a degree of education for proprietors and managers of food businesses who may be unaware of the standards required in regard to food hygiene for the operation of the business or particular aspects of it. In the autumn of 1993, the Government issued a document for proprietors of food businesses – 'Food Law Inspections and Your Business' [3]. This leaflet describes what proprietors should expect when a business is inspected under the Food Safety Act and advises what to do if the proprietor thinks the outcome of the inspection is wrong or not fair.

The introduction of new powers in the Food Safety Acts – improvement notices, prohibition orders and emergency prohibition notices – now provide substantial back-up powers to the environmental health officer's inspection. Although a purely informal visit with a health educative aspect remains a valued option for environmental health officers, the function of inspection is mainly for enforcement with breaches of legislation being identified, recorded and acted upon as necessary. An informal notice or letter may be sent by the environmental health officer following the inspection, identifying the problems which require remedial action and stating the date by which this should be achieved. The improvement notice formalizes the whole procedure and provides a prescribed period in which the defects noted by the environmental health officer must be remedied. The Government initiated changes to the relevant Codes of Practice to stress that informal procedures can still be employed and that environmental health officer's actions should be prioritized according to the scale of risks presented by particular hygiene situations Inspections of food premises are the essential element of enforcement. If informal procedure is to be employed by the environmental health officer there must be some confidence that it will produce the desired result. If an improvement notice is served, discretion can be allowed by the environmental health officer by the amount of time prescribed for necessary work to be carried out.

OVERZEALOUS ENFORCEMENT

During 1993 there was much media criticism of overzealous activity on the part of environmental health officers, in addition to general criticism about the extent of new regulatory controls over the food industry, which was one of the reasons for the Government's initiative on deregulation.

The Department of Health investigated each report of over-zealousness on the part of environmental health officers and found that virtually all of them were without foundation (see Chapter 8). In a few cases, however, it did appear that officers had been unreasonable. In the future it is essential that a clear distinction is made between what work or action is essential or mandatory to comply with food safety requirements and what is merely desirable (in the view of the environmental health officer or other officer) to comply with the law.

Advice on wall surfaces, cleaning routines and the adequacies of such things as washing facilities, although provided with the best of intentions to secure optimum conditions in premises, may be misconstrued by managers or proprietors of food businesses as being mandatory requirements.

Subsequently, LACOTS produced general guidance notes to assist food authorities undertaking programmed food hygiene inspections [4] and additionally began to develop circulars providing guidance on interpretation of requirements for food premises to meet the obligations imposed in Food Hygiene Regulations [5]. The aim of this guidance is to ensure the consistency of enforcement by environmental health officers and common interpretation of the legal requirements by environmental health officers across the country. Earlier the Department of Health had written to all chief environmental health officers drawing their notice to the essential need for environmental health officers to concentrate their activities on situations which indicated significant risks were present. [6]

In 1994 LACOTS issued further guidance to food authorities on food enforcement safety policies.

As a result of the Government's activity in the field of deregulation and its interest in over-zealous inspection complaints, environmental health officers and other enforcement officers have been subject to conflicting pressures. The Food Safety Act was seen as the answer to a deteriorating food safety situation – illustrated by increased incidence of salmonellosis, the botulism outbreak in north-west England in 1989 and action by environmental health departments under earlier legislation to close hundreds of food premises because of insanitary conditions, rodent and pest infestations. The present government policy is for exhortation, rather than strong enforcement, to be the means to secure higher food hygiene standards. The leaflet on Food Law Inspections referred to at the beginning of this chapter has as its final statement 'Closer partnership between food businesses and local authorities means better public protection and fair trading'.

Just what this closer partnership entails is not entirely clear, but taking the wording of the EU Hygiene of Foodstuffs Directive into account, it will likely mean that Guides of Good Hygiene Practice developed by the various food industry sectors, guidance from government departments and LACOTS will increase in future but regulations will be simplified and less in number. This policy does not necessarily mean that environmental health officers should reduce their inspection activity, but should result in the exercise of good judgment as to where and when to use the strong powers provided in the Food Safety Act 1990. Where it is possible to achieve the necessary compliance with the law by a harmonious relationship with a food business proprietor or manager and the use of informal action, this line should be pursued. There is no suggestion however that premises which pose risks to health should not be subject to strong enforcement procedures and prosecution where justified.

The highly important Code of Practice No. 9 on Food Hygiene Inspections [2] has been substantially revised to make it consistent with the philosophy of the Directive, in regard to industry self-regulation [Hazard Analysis Critical Control Points (HACCP) system], and concentration by enforcement officers on risk assessment. It now needs also to recognize the requirements of the recently agreed Official Control (Additional Measures) Directive which comes into force in 1995. This Directive requires the consistency in qualifications of officers employed for enforcement functions.

The Government now proposes that from 1995, only qualified staff will be able to carry out inspections of food premises. For lower risk categories of food premises, lower levels of qualifications of inspectors will be allowed and a timescale has been set for these to come into effect by mid-1999. The qualifications for carrying out inspections of lower risk categories of food premises are now being developed by the Environmental Health Officers Registration Board and the Institute of Food Hygiene and Technology.

The Government are also having more thoughts on the subject of HACCP and the fact that for small businesses there are dangers that the misguided may launch into full-blown HACCP systems, record keeping and monitoring arrangements which will be disproportionate to their needs. To avoid this, specific guidance on hazard analysis in small businesses is being developed (see page 597). This guidance together with the industry guides to good hygiene practice being formulated should mean that small businesses only apply the self-regulatory controls which are necessary. Food authorities are being advised that these developments will take time and they should make sure that the appropriate guidance is available for small businesses before pressing them on the need to apply HACCP principles.

On the subject of food hygiene training of food handling staff, the revision to Code of Practice No. 9 on Food Hygiene Inspections suggests that training requirements should be assessed by food businesses as part of a hazard analysis. This should be the means of relating training needs to risks in a business but not necessarily as part of a formal hazard analysis system. For the future, where potential food hazards are being properly assessed and controlled, there should be a changed approach to inspection on the part of the enforcement officer. It should not be necessary for the officer to assess training levels or levels of food hygiene awareness among staff, other than as confirmation of a discussion about the hazard analysis system with the proprietor. Guides to industry good hygiene practice may also provide some help in the assessment of training levels.

This recent Government advice, with the exception of prescribed qualifications of inspection staff following the Additional Measures Directive, follows the deregulation policy initiated last year. The likely effect on enforcement staff may not be what either the Government, or the food industry as a whole, would wish. There are already signs that following the 'overzealous' inspection publicity and its aftermath, the number of inspections of food premises has dropped. This does not present a problem if the industry self-regulatory measures now being promoted with such vigour by the Government ensure that good standards are being maintained. Experience with certain sectors and small businesses within them, however, suggests that there will always be a need for a regular external inspection presence, firm in character and certainly not 'underzealous' in application of food hygiene essentials.

MANAGEMENT CONTROLS

Food industry management have a responsibility to apply good manufacturing practice, which means that products are consistently manufactured to a quality appropriate to their intended use. Legal requirements of composition safety, hygiene and labelling have to be fulfilled. This is achieved by appropriate product specification and adequate supervision over all aspects of the food's manufacture, from the integrity of the in-coming raw materials, to the packaging and appropriate shelf-life of the product leaving the factory.

In catering operations, the responsibility of management includes adequate supervision over untrained staff carrying out basic food handling activities. This must in future include an element of training of such staff to inculcate in them the degree of necessary responsibility to ensure that food poisoning outbreaks do not occur from foods prepared and handled in the establishment. This often can be an extremely onerous task, but the management responsibility cannot be avoided.

Modern management includes responsibility over three main areas of operation:

1. to ensure that the premises in which the food is handled is structurally sound, clean and effec-

tive, and that the equipment provided is effective, sound and capable of doing the necessary task;

2. the employment of properly trained and responsible staff handling food at all stages of the operation, such handlers working to high standards of personal food hygiene;

3. to apply appropriate measures to protect food from contamination at all stages of the manufacturing chain, ensuring minimal cross-contamination risks, effective temperature control (adequate cooking and cooling practices) and ensuring that the appropriate shelf-life is applied to products.

Outside of the establishment, quality control checks should be applied to raw materials purchased and vehicles used for the distribution and sale of products.

The hazard analysis approach (HACCP)

HACCP [7,8] is being regarded as the modern concept for maximizing food safety and minimizing food hazards. It has been adopted and is being promoted by the UK Government, the EU, WHO and the International Commission for Microbiological Specifications for Foods. It can be applied equally to the food processing and food service industries, or to food preparation in the home in both developed and developing countries.

HACCP is a preventative system of control, particularly with regard to microbiological hazards. It consists of:

1. a hazard analysis which identifies the hazards associated with the growing, harvesting, processing, manufacturing, distributing, marketing, preparing or using a raw material or food product and assessing the associated risks;

2. determining the critical control points required to prevent or control any identified hazard;

3. establishing the appropriate preventative or control measures with criteria for measuring these controls.

4. monitoring the effectiveness of preventative or control measures at critical control points;

5. taking action to rectify any situation that is out of control.

The process should identify potentially hazardous raw materials and foods that may contain poisonous substances, pathogens or large numbers of food spoilage micro-organisms and/or that support microbial growth. It should also find sources, methods and specific points of contamination by observing each step of the food processing or preparation, and determine the potential for micro-organisms to survive or multiply during the production, processing, distribution, storage and preparation of food for consumption.

HACCP originated in the USA in 1969 in a National Academy of Sciences publication on salmonella. The US Food and Drug Administration later began to use the HACCP approach in its inspection programme for the manufacture of low acid canned foods.

Examples of HACCP application

*Canning**

Critical control points and examples of some of the aspects that must be monitored in canning include:

1. **Ingredients** (thermophilic spore-load): the relative proportion of various ingredients and effective changes in this on heat penetration characteristics, e.g. the bulking of a product or gelling which reduces heat penetration.

2. **Mixing and filling**: are these even and consistent? This is important where the contents are a mixture of solids and liquid, or contain chunks of various sizes.

3. **Sealing**: this is critical to prevent leakage. Appropriate procedures for seam checking are necessary. Double seams and overlaps require particular examination.

4. **Retorting**: operating parameters of the retort process need to be specified and monitored, e.g. the venting process time and temperature and associated F_0 value and cooling procedures.

5. **Cooling**: of main concern here is the microbiological quality of the cooling water and

*See also 'Guidelines for the Safe Production of Heat Preserved Foods', Department of Health 1994, HMSO, London.

associated chlorination. (The Aberdeen typhoid outbreak in 1963 was caused by contaminated cooling water gaining access to the interior of cans of corned beef in the cooling process.)

6. **Subsequent handling and storage of cans**: monitoring and recording of the results and the action taken on deviations are necessary. It is essential to ensure that cans are not handled when wet and still cooling as staphylococcal infection from hands may be drawn through can seams.

Food service

Critical control points for evaluation in food service activities are:

1. selecting and receiving raw materials;
2. storing, handling and preparing raw materials, including thawing and handling of frozen foods;
3. cooking – effective cooking temperatures;
4. handling after cooking, including further preparation, hot holding, cooling, reheating, serving and packing;
5. cleaning and sanitation of premises;
6. hygiene of workers;
7. training of employees in all steps of the procedure.

In some areas, the menu itself may be a critical control point. By excluding from menus high-risk foods that cannot be handled safely, hazards are identified and excluded from the food service.

In recent years, the microbiological monitoring of food has become an important part of the inspection role. The environmental health officer is primarily concerned with pathogens in food as these have a direct effect on safety and can render the food unfit for human consumption if they are not subsequently destroyed by any process of cooking or other treatment that will render them innocuous.

Microbiological monitoring in HACCP

In using HACCP, critical control points have to be identified and monitored. During monitoring, sampling of foods during preparation for microbiological examination may be useful in indicating contamination [9]. However, this is likely to be practicable only in large manufacturing or food service operations.

Microbiological monitoring with the setting of microbiological specifications or guidelines plays a major part in food manufacturing quality control. A systematic approach to controlling all aspects of an end product's safety and quality, from the moment the raw material arrives at the factory to the point in time when the packaged end product goes into the distribution network, can be achieved through microbiological checks.

EC Directive 93/43/EEC and HACCP

Article 3.2 of the above Directive requires operators to identify any step in their activities which is critical to ensuring food safety and to ensure that adequate safety precautions are identified, implemented, maintained and reviewed on the basis of principles used to develop the system of HACCP. These are:

1. analysing the potential food hazards in a food business operation;
2. identifying the points in those operations where food hazards may occur;
3. deciding which of the points identified are critical to food safety;
4. identifying and implementing effective control and monitoring procedures at those critical points;
5. reviewing the above periodically and whenever operations in the business change.

Article 3.2 does not mean that HACCP techniques as developed for large manufacturing companies must be applied to all food businesses, or that specialist HACCP teams and documented plans must be employed. The level of analysis, monitoring, and documentation must vary according to the risks, size and nature of the business.

FOOD EXAMINERS

The Food Safety Act 1990 places importance on the role of microbiological monitoring purposes.

The 'food examiner' performs the statutory function of microbiological examination of food. While providing the means for samples to be taken for microbiological examination, the Food Act 1984 made no reference to a statutory role for such an examiner. The PHLS, funded by central government, has traditionally performed the role of carrying out microbiological examination of food sampled by environmental health officers, and it is likely that the major role of food examiner will be performed by the PHLS. However, they may not carry out this function exclusively if local authorities set up their own private laboratory services, or employ independent microbiologists to perform the role. The qualifications of personnel and the accreditation of the laboratories must, however, comply with the Food Safety (Sampling and Qualification) Regulations 1990.

MICROBIOLOGICAL SURVEILLANCE OF FOOD

Following the recommendations contained in the report of the Richmond Committee, the Government have set up a national system for the microbiological surveillance of food. The Advisory Committee on the Microbiological Safety of Food advises Ministers and is supported by a Steering Group which is composed of representatives of Agriculture and Health Departments throughout the UK and from outside Government [10]. The Steering Group (SGMSF) has now been operating for over 2 years and work is well under way building up databases on the extent to which food is contaminated and the disease which is occurring and is perhaps attributable to that contamination. Working groups on a number of surveillance projects have been set up and are dealing with:

1. Infectious intestinal disease (IID).
2. Pathogens and indicator organisms in cream cakes and salad bars.
3. Ready to eat meats and meat products and the microbiological status of carcasses leaving abattoirs.

4. Types of *Clostridium botulinum* that can grow at refrigeration temperatures.
5. The survival in food of sublethally injured *Vibrio cholerae*.
6. The detection of salmonella in home-produced and imported eggs and in imported whole chickens.
7. Various *Campylobacter* studies and projects undertaken by professional groups in the PHLS, universities, research associations and food research associations on emerging pathogens and verocytotoxin producing *E. coli* (VTEC) and food-borne viruses.

Various environmental health departments are involved with the collection of samples and other investigation work concerned with these studies which are influenced also by EU measures under Directive 89/397/EEC.

In their general food inspection work environmental health officers have an important part to play in determining local risk factors relating to food production and sale. The incidence of food-borne disease and zoonoses locally makes working relationships important with CCDCs, the PHLS and the MAFF district veterinary officers to ensure full consultation on food contamination issues. The high costs of sampling and testing food now make microbiological monitoring an expensive exercise; in the food industry the use of complex sampling plans does not always result in a guarantee that sampling alone can guarantee the safety of a product. In some cases, unjustified feelings of security in those responsible for the interpretation of the results can follow. This situation has led to the use of HACCP as a preferred method of ensuring food safety, and environmental health officers should promote its use.

METHOD OF INSPECTION

Prior to Codes of Practice Nos 3 and 9, little had been written about the environmental health officer's method of inspection of food premises as part of his enforcement functions. It is accepted practice that such inspection is carried out without prior notice, and that it is comprehensive in nature, looking at all aspects of the premises' operations in regard to the legislation which might apply to those operations.

The method of inspection should particularly follow the guidance contained in Code of Practice No. 9 (revised April 1994). Potential risks arising from the activities carried on such as processing, cooking, handling and food storage, should be assessed*.

Additional assessment of the legislation applicable to the food preparation and manufacturing operation being carried out; the general hygiene of the premises as regards the structure, equipment and personnel employed are necessary. An audit of the company's quality assurance system may be appropriate, but the environmental health officer should concentrate on risk assessment.

Although a normal rule could be that inspection is carried out without notice, this might beneficially be varied on occasions. A formalized inspection of the premises when the environmental health officer is expected by the proprietor will usually result in the premises being prepared beforehand and presented for inspection in an optimum state of cleanliness as perceived by the proprietor or manager of the business. The environmental health officer can usefully use such a situation to illustrate to the proprietor either the adequacy or inadequacy of the proprietor's understanding of the legal requirements. The inspection, as well as being an enforcement measure, therefore, acts as an educational one in regard to the future standard of hygiene which needs to be maintained.

Inspection forms

In the USA and some other countries, an inspection form is often used as a checklist procedure. Simple ticks made on a checklist can serve as a record and enable the inspector to see fairly quickly any outstanding items from a previous inspection. The ticked inspection forms presented to the establishment proprietor or manager indicate defects that must be remedied. A type of

inspection form and notice used in the USA is shown in Fig. 35.1.

Where inspection forms are not used, the manner in which the environmental health officer carries out his actual inspection might be one of individual preference, but it is likely that the most comprehensive detail can be recorded by hand-written notes in a notebook or verbal dictation into a pocket recorder. The details obtained on an inspection may be highly significant in the event of the service of an improvement notice, an emergency prohibition notice, subsequent court proceedings for a prohibition order or in regard to a prosecution for offences under Food Hygiene Regulations. He might need to rely on his notes taken at the time of inspection in giving evidence and, therefore, the development of a comprehensive note-taking technique for the preparation of a detailed report, notice or letter to be written regarding the premises, is usually advisable. Of great importance is the fact that any report must be compiled immediately after inspection. Any delay in its preparation can make it invalid as evidence.

The inspection report needs to encompass a record of each and every part of the premises, including rear yard areas where refuse is stored and rooms for ancillary equipment, such as refrigeration machinery and the storage of cleaning materials. The inspection report should include a record of what the premises contains, the condition in which it is found, and the defects requiring attention; the number of personnel employed, particular aspects of their personal hygiene and protective clothing, and the degree to which they have received food-hygiene training; the storage facilities for in-coming food, chill storage facilities, food processing preparation and cooking equipment, the state of pots, pans, cutlery and crockery; and the particular practices related to the handling of food which might be observed during the inspection. Offences under the regulations should be verbally pointed out to the proprietor or manager, and confirmed later in an improvement notice or informal letter.

---

*In 1994, LACOTS issued a draft guidance note to local authorities on the application of risk assessment principles to food hygiene inspections.

FOOD COMPOSITION

EC Directive 89/397/EEC on the official control of foodstuffs

The composition of food produced and sold in the EU is governed by controls exercised by this Directive.

Article 2 of the Directive requires that member states shall ensure that products intended for consignment to another member state are inspected with the same care as those intended for marketing on their own territory. Article 4 goes on to require that inspections shall be carried out regularly where non-compliance is suspected, with inspection covering all stages of production, manufacture, import into the EU, processing, storage, transport, distribution and trade. As a general rule, inspections are to be carried out without prior warning.

As well as requiring hygiene inspection. Article 5 requires one or more controls of inspection, sampling and analysis, examination of written and documentary material, and examination of any verification systems set up by the undertaking and the results obtained.

Article 6 requires the following to be subject to inspection: raw materials, ingredients, technological aids and other products used for the preparation and production of foodstuffs; semi-finished products; finished products; processes used for the manufacture or processing of foodstuffs; labelling and preservation of foodstuffs; and preserving methods.

Article 7 states that samples of the products enumerated in Article 6 may be taken for the purpose of analysis, and these analyses shall be carried out by official laboratories.

Other requirements in the Directive refer to examination of the standards of training provision for food inspectors, the establishment of EU quality standards for all laboratories involved in inspection and sampling under the Directive.

Competent authorities of the member states are under an obligation to draw up forward programmes of inspection and sampling requirements with annual reports to the EU Commission on the activity being undertaken.

The requirements of the Directive have been met by various government initiatives including provisions in regulations.

The Food Safety (Enforcement Authority) (England and Wales) Order 1990

This Order assigns responsibilities for functions under the Act in regard to work related to food composition.

Ministers have also made a code (Code of Practice No. 1, *Enforcement*) [11] under their powers in section 40 of the Food Safety Act 1990, on the division of responsibility for enforcement of matters arising under sections 7, 8, 9 and 14 of the Act. Both the Order and the Code of Practice will be subject to necessary change as a result of the review of local authority organization currently being undertaken.

Basically, the Act provides that cases involving contamination by micro-organisms or their toxins, such as strains of *Salmonella, Listeria* or the bacterium *Clostridium botulinum* will be dealt with by district councils. Chemical contamination which poses no immediate risk to health will be dealt with by county councils, and they will undertake routine checks and analyses for chemical contamination. However, where there is evidence of gross contamination which potentially poses an immediate hazard to human health, the facts of the case should be passed on to the district council (environmental health department) for further action. Equally, if the district council discovers chemical contamination but the level is such that there is no immediate hazard to health, the information should be passed to the county council for further action. In both instances, the authorities concerned should liaise with one another so that knowledge about any particular case or set of circumstances can be pooled. Where imported foods are concerned, the port health authority should take the appropriate action in all cases.

As far as consumer protection is concerned, the code provides for county councils to use the powers in section 14 (selling food not of the nature or substance or quality demanded), which deals with compositional offences, adulteration

INSPECTION REPORT
FOOD SERVICE ESTABLISHMENTS

Permit No. _____

Type _____ NSD_____

| CITY, COUNTY OR DISTRICT | NAME OF ESTABLISHMENT | ADDRESS | OWNER OR OPERATOR |

Sir: Based on inspection this day, the items marked below identify the violation in operation or facilities which must be corrected by the next routine inspection or such shorter period of time as may be specified in writing by the health authority. Failure to comply with this notice may result in immediate suspension of your permit (or downgrading of the establishment). * An opportunity for an appeal will be provided if a written request for a hearing is filed with the health authority within the period of time established in this notice for the correction of violations.

SECTION B. FOOD
1. FOOD SUPPLIES

		Specify:	Bakery products	Poultry and poultry products	Meat and meat products	Frozen desserts	Shellfish	Milk and milk products	Demerit points
1	Approved source								6
2	Wholesome – not adulterated								6
3	Not misbranded								2
4	Original container; properly identified								2
5	Approved dispenser								
6	Fluid milk and fluid milk products pasteurized								6
7	Low-acid and non-acid foods commercially canned								6

2. FOOD PROTECTION

		Preparation	Storage	Display	Service	Transportation	Demerit
8	Protected from contamination						4
9	Adequate facilities for maintaining food at hot or cold temperatures						2
10	Suitable thermometers						
11	Perishable food at proper temperature						2
12	Potentially hazardous food at 45°F. or below, or 140°F. or above as required						6
13	Frozen food kept frozen; properly thawed						2
14	Handling of food minimized by use of suitable utensils						4
15	Hollandaise sauce of fresh ingredients; discarded after three hours						
16	Food cooked to proper temperature						6
17	Fruits and vegetables washed thoroughly						2
18	Containers of food stored off floor on clean surfaces						2
19	No wet storage of packaged food						2
20	Display cases, counter protector devices or cabinets of approved type						2
21	Frozen dessert dippers properly stored						2
22	Sugar in closed dispensers or individual packages						2
23	Unwrapped and potentially hazardous food not re-served						4
24	Poisonous and toxic materials properly identified, colored, stored and used; poisonous polishes not present						6
25	Bactericides, cleaning and other compounds properly stored and non-toxic in use dilutions						

SECTION C. PERSONNEL
1. HEALTH AND DISEASE CONTROL

26	Persons with boils, infected wounds, respiratory infections or other communicable disease properly restricted	6
27	Known or suspected communicable disease cases reported to health authority	6

2. CLEANLINESS

28	Hands washed and clean	6
29	Clean outer garments; proper hair restraints used	2
30	Good hygienic practices	4

SECTION D. FOOD EQUIPMENT AND UTENSILS
1 SANITARY DESIGN, CONSTRUCTION AND INSTALLATION OF EQUIPMENT AND UTENSILS

		Good repair; no cracks	No chips, pits or open seams	Cleanable, smooth	Approved material	No corrosion	Proper construction	Accessible for cleaning and inspection	Demerit Points
31	Food-contact surfaces of equipment								2
32	Utensils								2
33	Non-food-contact surfaces of equipment								2
34	Single-service articles of non-toxic materials								2
35	Equipment properly installed								2
36	Existing equipment capable of being cleaned, non toxic, properly installed; and in good repair								2

2. CLEANLINESS OF EQUIPMENT AND UTENSILS

37	Tableware clean to sight and touch	
38	Kitchenware and food-contact surfaces of equipment clean to sight and touch	4
39	Grills and similar cooking devices cleaned daily	
40	Non-food contact surfaces of equipment kept clean	2
41	Detergents and abrasives rinsed off food-contact surfaces	2
42	Clean-wiping cloths used; use properly restricted	2
43	Utensils and equipment pre-flushed, scraped or soaked	2
44	Tableware sanitized	
45	Kitchenware and food-contact surfaces of equipment used for potentially hazardous food sanitized	4
46	Facilities for washing and sanitizing equipment and utensils approved, adequate, properly constructed, maintained and operated	4
47	Wash and sanitizing water clean	4
48	Wash water at proper temperature	
49	Dish tables and drain boards provided, properly located and constructed	2
50	Adequate and suitable detergents used	2
51	Approved thermometers provided and used	
52	Suitable dish baskets provided	2
53	Proper gauge cocks provided	
54	Cleaned and cleaned and sanitized utensils and equipment properly stored and handled; uensils air-dried	2
55	Suitable facilities and areas provided for storing utensils and equipment	2
56	Single-service articles properly stored, dispensed and handled	2
57	Single-service articles used only once	
58	Single-service articles used when approved washing and sanitizing are not provided	6

SECTION E. SANITARY FACILITIES AND CONTROLS
1. WATER SUPPLY

59	From approved source, adequate, safe quality	6
60	Hot and cold running water provided	4
61	Transported water handled, stored, dispensed in a sanitary manner	6
62	Ice from approved source; made from potable water	6
63	Ice machines and facilities properly located, installed and maintained	2
64	Ice and ice handling utensils properly handled and stored; block ice rinsed	2
65	Ice-contact surfaces approved; proper material and construction	

*Applicable only where grading form of ordinance is in effect.

Fig. 35.1 Inspection form of the type used in the USA. (Source: US Department of Health, Education and Welfare (1962) Food Service Sanitation Manual, US DHEW, Washington DC.)

Page 2

	2. SEWAGE DISPOSAL	Demerit points	Item	SECTION F. OTHER FACILITIES 1. FLOORS, WALLS AND CEILINGS	Demerit points
66	Into public sewer, or approved private facilities	6	91	Floors kept clean, no sawdust used	2
	3. PLUMBING		92	Floors easily cleanable construction, in good repair, smooth, non-absorbent; carpeting in good repair	1
67	Properly sized, installed and maintained	2	93	Floor graded and floor drains, as required	2
68	Non-potable water piping identified	1	94	Experior walking and driving surfaces clean; drained	2
69	No cross connections	6	95	Exterior walking and driving surfaces properly surfaced	1
70	No back siphonage possible		96	Mats and duck boards cleanable, removable and clean	2
71	Equipment properly drained	2	97	Floors and wall junctures properly constructed	2
	4. TOILET FACILITIES		98	Walls, ceilings and attached equipment clean	2
72	Adequate, conveniently located, and accessible, properly designed and installed	6	99	Walls and ceilings properly constructed and in good repair; coverings properly attached	1
73	Toilet rooms completely enclosed, and equipped with self-closing, tight-fitting doors; doors kept closed	2	100	Walls of light color; washable to level of splash	2
74	Toilet rooms, fixtures and vestibules kept clean, in good repair, and free from odors	2		**2. LIGHTING**	
75	Toilet tissue and proper waste receptacles provided; waste receptacles emptied as necessary	2	101	20 foot-candles of light on working surfaces	
			102	10 foot-candles of light on food equipment, utensil-washing, hand washing areas and toilet rooms	2
	5. HAND-WASHING FACILITIES		103	5 foot-candles of light 30'' from floor in all other areas	
76	Lavatories provided, adequate, properly located and installed	6	104	Artificial light sources as required	2
77	Provided with hot and cold or tempered running water through proper fixtures	4		**3. VENTILATION**	
78	Suitable hand cleanser and sanitary towels or approved hand-drying devices provided	2	105	Rooms reasonably free from steam, condensation, smoke, etc.	2
79	Waste receptacles provided for disposable towels	2	106	Rooms and equipment vented to outside as required	2
80	Lavatory facilities clean and in good repair	2	107	Hoods properly designed; filters removable	2
			108	Intake air ducts properly designed and maintained	1
	6. GARBAGE AND RUBBISH DISPOSAL		109	Systems comply with fire prevention requirements; no nuisance created	2
81	Stored in approved containers; adequate in number	2			
82	Containers cleaned when empty; brushes provided	2		**4. DRESSING ROOMS AND LOCKERS**	
83	When not in continuous use, covered with tight fitting lids, or in protective storage inaccessible to vermin	2	110	Dressing rooms or areas as required; properly located	
84	Storage areas adequate; clean; no nuisances; proper facilities provided	2	111	Adequate lockers or other suitable facilities	1
85	Disposed of in an approved manner, at an approved frequency	2	112	Dressing roms, areas and lockers kept clean	2
86	Garbage rooms or enclosures properly constructed; outside storage of proper height above ground or on concrete slab	2		**5. HOUSEKEEPING**	
87	Food waste grinders and incinerators properly installed, constructed and operated; incinerators areas clean	2	113	Establishment and property clean, and free of litter	2
			114	No operations in living or sleeping quarters	2
	7. VERMIN CONTROL		115	Floors and walls cleaned after closing or between meals by dustless methods	2
88	Presence of rodents, flies, roaches and vermin minimized	4	116	Laundered clothes and napkins stored in clean place	2
89	Outer openings protected against flying insects as required; rodent-proofed	2	117	Soiled linen and clothing stored in proper containers	1
90	Harborage and feeding of vermin prevented	2	118	No live birds or animals other than guide dogs	2

MERIT SCORE OF THE ESTABLISHMENT_____

MARKS _____

_____

_____

_____

Date_____ Health Authority_____

Fig 35.1 continued

and misleading claims where these matters are not specifically provided for in regulations.

The code provides for district councils also to use section 14, but only in respect of foreign bodies and mould. Most of these cases should in future be brought under section 8(2)(c), but district councils may want to make use of existing case law on 'nature, substance or quality'. The code proposes that all foreign body work be undertaken by district councils (or leaving foreign body work to be organized by local agreement in the light of what makes best sense in the circumstances of the area).

SAMPLING AND EXAMINATION OF FOOD

Sampling programmes

Under the official Control of Foodstuffs Directive (89/397/EC) food sampling forms part of normal food enforcement activities. Member states have a duty to take the samples identified by the Commission and report back the results during the early part of the following year. However the EU does not stipulate how many samples should be taken, this is for Member States to determine. This is described as the EU Co-ordinated Food Control Programme.

In order to obtain a co-ordinated approach to all sampling, environmental health departments should plan their programmes through the local food liaison groups so that the EU programme requirements form part of each group's annual sampling programme.* Each year the EU's required programme is set out in an EU Recommendation, e.g. for 1994, EU Recommendation 94/175/EEC required a programme for the detection and enumeration of *Listeria monocytogenes* in meat-based patés sold in the retail sector. Sampling levels over and above those recommendations are at the discretion of the food authorities.

The Food Safety (Sampling and Qualifications) Regulations 1990

For the purposes of the Food Safety Act 1990, 'analysis' is defined in section 53 as any technique to determine the composition of food, and includes microbiological assay. 'Examination' is defined in section 28 as microbiological examination of food.

These Regulations set out the detailed procedure to be followed when an enforcement officer takes a sample of food for analysis, or where it is taken for examination. The Regulations do not include aspects of 'average' or 'acceptance' sampling procedure (sampling techniques based on statistical plans).

An important element of the Regulations is the certificates by analysts or examiners in regard to samples submitted to them. The certificates are for use by enforcement officers in any proceedings which might follow the taking of samples, analysis or examination.

Code of Practice No. 7, *Sampling* [12], deals with procedures for taking samples and for analysis and examination.

Qualifications of analysts and examiners

Consistent with the requirements of Directive 89/397/EEC on the official control of foodstuffs, the 1990 Regulations also require specified qualifications for analysts and examiners. Because of previous lack of statutory recognition of the role of microbiological examination of food, the arrangements for food examiners are transitional – there has been no one qualification which denotes the requisite academic attainment and practical experience in food microbiology which the Department of Health considered appropriate to satisfy a court of law as to the competence of an expert witness.

USE-BY DATES – THE FOOD LABELLING (AMENDMENT) REGULATIONS 1990

The above Regulations which implement EU Directives require perishable pre-packed foods to

---

*These programmes are now also influenced by LACOTS.

be labelled with 'use-by' dates. The decision whether to use a 'best before' or 'use-by' date remains with those responsible for the labelling of the product. In addition to the use-by date, the Regulations requires a description of the storage conditions which must be observed. The instructions must be simple and clear and, where appropriate, include the temperature at or below which the food should be kept.

The Regulations create offences for persons selling out-of-date use-by foods, and for anyone other than the person originally responsible for date marking of food to change the date mark. Responsibility for enforcement on selling expired use-by food is given to all food authorities, i.e. both trading standards officers and environmental health officers, since although food labelling legislation is enforced by trading standards officers, this offence is essentially a food safety measure, and it is more cost effective for environmental health officers to take action in this one specific labelling area when they are monitoring stock rotation and enforcing the food hygiene legislation.

MAFF Guidelines on use-by dates [13]

These guidelines advise when this type of date mark should be used and provide supplementary information on storage of the foodstuff concerned.

Emphasis is placed on 'best before' being the usual date mark unless the product is microbiologically unstable and likely to pose a threat to public health after a short period. In such circumstances a 'use-by' date is required.

Clarification is provided on the use of 'use-by' dates on vacuum-packed foods – this method of packaging is not in itself sufficient cause to attract a 'use-by date'. The product itself must be highly perishable and a potential public health risk.

The guidelines include advice on storage instructions where an exact temperature specification is not critical.

FOREIGN BODIES IN FOODS

Code of Practice No. 1, *Responsibility for Enforcement*, under section 40 of the Food Safety Act 1990 deals with powers under section 14 (selling food not of the nature or substance or quality demanded), and indicates that district councils should be able to use section 14, but only in respect of foreign bodies and mould in food. The code indicates that all foreign body work should be undertaken by district councils. In future, the government wishes enforcement authorities to make use of sections 7 and 8 of the Act, rather than section 14 wherever it is possible to do so, so as to build up a substantial body of case law on 'food safety requirements', which will include all aspects of contamination risk.

Foreign bodies can occur in foodstuffs accidentally, by negligence or intention. The use of blackmail or extortion through threats and the use of dangerous substances or objects can result in police action under Section 38 of the Public Order Act 1986. This makes it an offence to contaminate or interfere with food with the intention of causing any public alarm or anxiety. Action can also be taken under the Theft Act 1968 where there is intent to obtain gain from such action.

The prevention of foreign bodies in food

Section 21 of the Food Safety Act 1990 provides a defence of taking all reasonable precautions and exercising all due diligence. This defence may be particularly applicable to cases of foreign bodies in food. Manufacturers would need to show throughout the manufacturing process that:

1. potential foreign body hazards can be identified;
2. reasonable precautions exist to ensure that hazardous substances do not gain access to food and place consumers at risk;
3. procedures are well understood by staff and are well documented;
4. regular checks are carried out with appropriate records to demonstrate that the precautions are working;
5. corrective actions are taken and recorded where precautions fail; and
6. they keep a record of training of staff to prevent foreign body hazards.

The food manufacturer's responsibility is to produce a manufacturing system which makes deliberate contamination as difficult as possible, and employs a hazard analysis and a set of monitoring procedures which, together with staff training, reduces the involuntary addition of foreign bodies to food within the factory to nil.

Guidance has been issued by LACOTS to assist environmental health departments in handling food complaints. It encompasses best existing practices, promotes the home authority principle and builds upon the Codes of Practice [14].

REFERENCES

1. Food Safety Act 1990 (1990) *Code of Practice No 3 Inspection Procedures – General*, HMSO, London.
2. Food Safety Act 1990 (Revised 1994) *Code of Practice No. 9 Food Hygiene Inspections*, HMSO, London.
3. Department of Health (1993), Food Law Inspections and your Business, MAFF leaflet FL1.
4. LACOTS, Guidance on Food Hygiene Inspections, General Guidance Notes to Assist Local Authorities Undertaking Programmed Food Hygiene Inspections, June 1993, LACOTS, PO Box 6, Robert St, Croydon CR9 1LG.
5. LACOTS, Chief Officer Circular 25 June 1993, Contents FS 6 93, General, Food Hygiene (General) Regulations 1970 (As Amended).
6. Letter from the Department of Health to Chief Environmental Health Officers in England 6 May 1993, Overzealous Enforcement of Food Hygiene Legislation.
7. International Commission for Microbiological Specifications of Food, *HACCP in Microbiological Safety and Quality*, No. 4., Application of the Hazard Analysis Critical Control Point (HACCP) System to Ensure Microbiological Safety and Quality, Blackwell Scientific Publications, Oxford.
8. Munce, Dr Barbara A. (1988) *Hazard Analysis and Food Safety*, Paper given at Inaugural World Congress and Environmental Health, Sydney, Australia, 26–30 September.
9. (1988) *Micro-organisms in Food, Sampling for Microbiological Analysis; Principles of Specific Applications*, 2nd edn, Blackwell Scientific Publications, Oxford.
10. Steering Group on the Microbiological Safety of Food and the Progress of Surveillance Studies (1992) Department of Health Bulletin for Environmental Health Departments Vol. 1, No.5.
11. Food Safety Act 1990 (1990) *Code of Practice No. 1, Responsibility for Enforcement of the Food Safety Act 1990*, HMSO, London.
12. Food Safety Act 1990 (1990) *Code of Practice No. 7, Sampling for Analysis or Examination*, HMSO, London.
13. MAFF Guidelines on Use-by Dates, November 1993, Copies available free from MAFF Consumer Protection Division, Room 30A, Ergon House, c/o Nobel House, 17 Smith Square, London SW1P 3JR.
14. Guidance on Food Complaints, January 1994, LACOTS, PO Box 6, Robert St, Croydon CR9 1LG.

FURTHER READING

Sprenger, R.A., *Hygiene for Management, A Text for Food Hygiene Courses*, Highfield Publication, Rotherham.
Aston, G., Tiffney, J. and Knight, Charles, *The Essential Guide to Food Hygiene*, Tolley, Croydon.
Food Hygiene, NHS Health Service Catering, HMSO, London.

36 Food safety – controls over risk foods

Mike Jacob

FRESH MEAT

The Single Market Directive on fresh meat 91/497/EEC has been implemented in Great Britain by the Fresh Meat (Hygiene and Inspection) Regulations 1992.* Fresh meat intended for human consumption must be obtained from or stored in slaughterhouses, cutting premises, cold stores, farmed game handling and processing facilities. The proposals seek to be as non-prescriptive as possible but with premises licensed by MAFF. Initially, local authorities through the appointed official veterinary surgeons (OVSs) will have responsibilities for supervising premises and making decisions on the fitness of carcases (but see National Meat Hygiene Service below). The Fresh Meat Regulations do not apply to premises where meat is cut or stored for sale to the final customer.

Wild game is to be subject to separate regulations to implement Directive 92/45/EEC which regulates hygienic production and distribution of wild game.

The main provisions of the Fresh Meat Regulations are:

1. the licensing of slaughterhouses, cutting premises and cold stores;
2. the supervision and control of premises;
3. conditions for the marketing of fresh meat;
4. the admission of and detention in slaughterhouses of animals and carcases;
5. the construction, layout and equipment in premises;
6. hygienic requirements;
7. ante-mortem inspection;
8. slaughter and dressing practices;
9. post-mortem inspection and health marking/certification;
10. cutting practices, wrapping and packaging of fresh meat;
11. storage, freezing and transport of fresh meat.

POULTRY MEAT

The Poultry Meat, Farmed Game Bird Meat and Rabbit Meat (Hygiene and Inspection) Regulations 1994* came into operation on 1 May 1994 and implement Directives 71/118/EEC, 91/495/EEC, 91/494/EEC [1].

The regulations apply to slaughterhouses, cutting premises, cold stores and re-wrapping centres. Poultry means domestic fowls, turkeys, guinea fowl, ducks and geese whilst farmed game birds means birds other than poultry, not generally considered to be domestic but which are bred, reared and slaughtered in captivity. Rabbit means domestic rabbit.

---

* Both sets of Regulations are to be replaced in 1995 and will provide for the transfer of regulatory powers from local authorities to the Minister, who will delegate responsibility to the NMHS.

The main provisions of these regulations:

1. prohibit the use of any premises as a slaughterhouse, cutting premises, cold store or re-wrapping centre unless they are licensed and make provision for the issue, on application, of licences by the Minister (Regulation 4);
2. provide for the revocation of licences (Regulation 5);
3. provide for an Appeals Tribunal to hear appeals against refusals to licence, conditions imposed on the grant of licences, and revocations of licences (Regulation 6);
4. subject to a specified exemption, prohibit the use of a slaughterhouse for slaughtering a bird or rabbit not intended for sale for human consumption (Regulation 7);
5. require the appointment of inspectors to supervise licensed premises (Regulation 8);
6. provide for the designation by the Minister of OVSs, the revocation and suspension of such designations, and specify the powers of official veterinary surgeons (Regulations 9 and 10);
7. provide for the authorization by the Minister of persons as plant inspection assistants and for the revocation and suspension of such authorizations (Regulation 11);
8. require the carrying out of pre-slaughter health inspections and post-mortem health inspections of birds and rabbits and also make provision in relation to the application of the health mark, and prohibit the use of a mark resembling a health mark likely to deceive (Regulation 12);
9. prohibit the slaughter of a bird or rabbit for human consumption without giving the food authority at least 72 hours, or other shorter period as agreed, advance notice except where such slaughter is at a fixed time and day in accordance with a regular practice (Regulation 13);
10. specify the conditions to be complied with in relation to the sale of fresh meat for human consumption and, subject to specified exceptions, prohibit the sale of such meat unless those conditions are complied with (Regulation 14);
11. specify the documents necessary when transporting fresh meat (Regulation 15);
12. enable an OVS or inspector to prohibit slaughter in specified circumstances and provide for authorization of slaughter subject to conditions (Regulation 16);
13. require official veterinary surgeons to keep specified records and also require them to notify the presence of specified diseases, and require food authorities to keep specified records and supply copies to the Minister on request (Regulation 17);
14. specify the duties of occupiers and producers (Regulations 18 and 19);
15. create offences and prescribe penalties (Regulation 20);
16. enable food authorities to recover specified costs from producers (Regulation 21);
17. require food authorities to supply specified information to the Minister (Regulation 22);
18. provide defences in relation to exports (Regulation 23);
19. specify the enforcement authorities and make provision for the application of various provisions of the Food Safety Act 1990 (Regulations 24 and 25);
20. amend specified Regulations (Regulation 26).

Circular FSH 1/94 from MAFF gives guidance on these regulations. A significant change from earlier provisions is that hygiene controls will be operated by the industry through a system of poultry industry assistants (PIAs) under the supervision of OVSs. Such arrangements are to be agreed with MAFF and are to be subject to audit rather than intensive supervision. Therefore, where companies provide appropriate guarantees and trained staff, they will be able to carry out post-mortem inspection of poultry themselves under supervision by the OVS. Where the company cannot provide this role, inspection will be carried out by the OVS assisted by PMIs (poultry meat inspectors).

The control of poultry supply farms, the enforcement of animal welfare laws and the licensing of poultry slaughtermen will pass to the National Meat Hygiene Service (NMHS) on the 1

April 1995 (see below). Licensing of premises covered by the Regulations falls to Agriculture department staff.

Appointment of inspectors

The qualification of inspectors to be appointed as authorized officers to act on behalf of local authorities are specified in Schedule 22 of the Fresh Meat (Hygiene and Inspection) Regulations 1992 and Schedule 16 of the Poultry Meat, Farmed Game Bird Meat and Rabbit Meat (Hygiene and Inspection) Regulations 1994.

NATIONAL MEAT HYGIENE SERVICE (NMHS) [2]

The Deregulation and Contracting Out Act 1994 makes provision for the creation of this new service which will replace the existing local authority-based inspection services for meat and poultry. The NMHS is to be established as an agency of MAFF in April 1995. It will take over from about 300 local authorities hygiene, inspection and welfare of animals responsibilities in licensed fresh meat plants in Great Britain.*

The decision to set up the service follows earlier reviews of the existing inspection regime, pressures brought about the European Single Market and a detailed investigation by a team from MAFF, the Department of Health and Price Waterhouse Management Consultants. Ministers were convinced that a single agency was the best of the options available to manage resources and staff and provide a consistent and cost-effective service.

The NMHS will have four core functions which will be undertaken by plant-based staff and monitored/administered by regional and headquarters staff. These are:

1. To ensure compliance with hygiene rules in licensed fresh meat (red, poultry and game meat) premises including:

(a) maintenance and improvement of hygiene standards;
(b) monitoring water quality;
(c) enforcement of unfit meat rules.

2. To provide a meat inspection service in licensed fresh meat (red, poultry and game) premises (including poultry supply farms) through:
(a) ante- and post-mortem inspections;
(b) health marking;
(c) reporting to the State Veterinary Service diseases subject to national control programmes, e.g. tuberculosis;
(d) keeping records of ante and post-mortem inspections, water testing and condemnation data.

3. The enforcement of hygiene controls in meat product plants which are integrated or co-located (on the same site) as licensed fresh meat plants.

4. The enforcement of welfare at slaughter rules in licensed red and poultry meat slaughterhouses through:
(a) monitoring of handling, stunning, slaughter and bleeding;
(b) licensing of red meat and poultry meat slaughterman (including certificates of competence for poultry slaughtermen).

MAFF's State Veterinary Service (SVS) will monitor and audit the work of the NMHS in plants; the SVS will continue to be responsible for the licensing of plants.

Additional functions being considered for the NMHS are:

1. the collection and despatch of samples for statutory veterinary medicines residue testing;
2. the submission of samples on behalf of the SVS for examination and testing for certain diseases, e.g. brucellosis;
3. the enforcement in slaughterhouses of legislation governing controls on veterinary drugs residues, including powers to detain and sample suspect animals and carcasses.

---

* These include slaughterhouses, cutting plants and cold stores and also certain meat products plants where these are in the same complex as a licensed fresh meat or poultry meat plant.

The advantages of the NMHS compared with the present system are stated as:

1. consistency of supervision and enforcement of a single agency when compared with inspectors and veterinarians employed by 300 local authorities;
2. a single organization is better able to manage future changes following from rationalization of the meat industry;
3. the new service will be in a better position to seek and encourage higher standards in the industry, thereby benefiting consumers.

Transfer arrangements will allow existing local authority staff to work for the NMHS but the long-term role of the environmental health officer in meat inspection now appears dubious. Qualification requirements in EU legislation means that environmental health officers can only act as non-veterinary auxiliaries and it is not likely that many environmental health offices will therefore see a future for themselves specializing in meat inspection duties. Current training courses require meat inspection work under the supervision of an OVS so that environmental health officers can be employed in slaughterhouses.

It is still important for this training in meat inspection to continue. Knowledge of animal anatomy and physiology is important in all areas of food inspection related to meat products and processed foods. The microbiological aspects of foods of animal origin are essential elements of training courses for environmental health officers to enable comprehensive understanding of foodborne diseases which originate in foods derived from animals. Currently there are no plans to expand the role of the NMHS beyond the areas listed above. For the future, however, the existence of a centrally based veterinary controlled inspection service responsible for a large sector of the nation's food supply could raise future questions regarding its expansion into a central 'food inspection agency'. The proposed changes in local government structure in Great Britain and the establishment of the NMHS presents dangers to the role of the environmental health officer in food inspection work, particularly if this work is lacking in specialism and expertise. It is essential that the initial and in-service training of officers in this area matches European requirements so that in future Ministers continue to endorse the local authority functions for food inspection carried out by environmental health officers.

Knackers' yards

Currently, knackers' yards remain the responsibility of local authorities regarding inspection and licensing. However, EU proposals, if agreed, will see this responsibility transferring to the State Veterinary Service. Existing knackers' yards have until 31 December 1995 to comply with EC hygiene standards under the newly adopted Directive 90/667/EEC on the disposal and prevention of animal waste and the prevention of pathogens in feeding stuffs. This new directive does not cover compound feeding stuffs containing animal and vegetable products for which there will be separate provision at a later date. The disposal of high-risk material under the Directive's requirements entail treatment to a core temperature of at least 133°C for 20 minutes at a pressure of 3 bar. Annex 2 to the Directive contains microbiological standards for salmonellae (absence in 25 g) and enterobacteriae, which must be met by end products.

Animal By-Products (Identification and Movement Control) Regulations (expected to be implemented in 1995).

These Regulations will replace legislation dating from the 1980s which sought to exclude unfit meat or animal products not intended for human consumption from the market place.

Occupiers of slaughterhouses or animal by-products premises such as knackers' yards must sterilize and stain the material concerned either immediately, or after a short period of storage on the premises. Poultry meat is included within the scope of the Regulations and is subject to controls other than sterilizing and staining.

Catering refuse containing meat and animal waste is not covered.

Local authorities will be responsible for enforcement outside of licensed plants but the main enforcement agency will be the NMHS.

Animal health aspects of meat hygiene

The Zoonoses Order 1989 designates *Salmonella* and *Brucella* strains as a risk to human health. This designation is a procedure provided for in the Animal Health Act 1981, enabling control powers in the Act to be used to deal with risk to human health as well as those to animal health. The State Veterinary Service must be notified when these organisms are isolated from samples taken from farm animals and carcases, products or the farm environment.

Powers under the 1989 Order have been used to apply strict control to the production of processed animal protein and animal feed. The Zoonoses Order 1989 and the Processed Animal Protein Order 1989 require (since March 1989) positive isolations of strains of *Salmonella* in processed animal protein and in animal feed, to be notified to the State Veterinary Service who have extended power to prohibit their movement.

Processed animal protein processors are obliged to have a sample tested on each day that they consign finished products from their premises, and for a period of 28 days to withhold processed animal protein from incorporation into animal feedingstuffs if a sample proves positive for *Salmonella* species. Processors are obliged to register with MAFF, and only laboratories authorized by MAFF are allowed to carry out the statutory tests. The frequency of MAFF inspections of plants processing animal proteins has been increased from 10 to 20 times per year.

New more rigorous licensing controls were introduced in 1989 under the Importation of Processed Animal Protein Order 1981 for imported fish or animal protein. The EU has adopted the Zoonoses Directive 92/117/EEC which will be influential in any future UK controls.

Trade terms for animals

Cattle
Bull, entire male; **ox, steer**, castrated male; **stirk**, cattle about a year old, male or female, entire or not; **bull calf**, entire calf; **heifer calf**, female calf; **heifer**, young cow before calving; **cow**, female after calving.

Sheep
Ram, entire male; **tup**, entire young male; **wether or widder**, castrated male; **ewe**, female after lambing; **gimmer**, female before lambing; **ewe lamb**, young female; **teg**, young sheep either sex, entire or not.

Pig
Boar, entire male; **hog**, castrated male; **porker**, young pig, either sex, entire or not; **sow**, female after having had a litter; **gelt or gilt**, female, no litter.

Goat
Billy, entire male; **wether or hog**, castrated male; **nanny**, female; **kid**, young of either sex.

Horse
Mare, female; **filly**, young mare; **stallion**, entire male; **gelding**, castrated male; **mule**, hybrid horse/ass.

General
Store cattle, **sheep or pigs**; animals kept for breeding or, if for market, not yet fatted.

INSPECTION OF ANIMALS

The inspection of animals before slaughter is essential. From the point of view of early segregation and, when necessary, notification of diseased or suspected animals, the importance of detecting any sign of disease in the living animal is important.

The meat inspector should be quick to notice signs of disease or unsatisfactory condition in the living animal in order that he may be guided in any special respect in the post-mortem examination.

The coat of the sick animal is rough or 'staring'; the nostrils may be dry or covered with foam; the eyes are heavy; the tongue protruding; respiration laboured; movements slow and difficult. There may be diarrhoea, or blood-stained urine. Usually, a sick animal will isolate itself.

A healthy animal in good condition is easy of movement; the eyes are bright and quick; the muzzle is cool, moist, and of healthy appearance; the tongue does not protrude; the respiration is easy and regular, and expired air is free from colour.

Temperature and pulse

Temperature: horse, 38°C; ox, 38.6°C; pig, 39.4°C; sheep, 39.4°C; birds, 42°C (average).

Pulse-beats vary according to conditions – temperature, excitement, etc: horse, about 37; ox, 40; dogs, 70 to 80; and sheep, 70 to 80. The pulse is taken at the back of the fetlock, or outside edge of the jaw in an ox; the inside edge of the jaw in a horse; and on the femoral artery in smaller animals.

The carcase and organs

A carcase of meat consists of the skeleton with its muscles and membranes and also the kidneys and fat surrounding them. The offal includes the head, tongue, feet, skin and all internal organs except the kidneys.

The carcase is separated internally into two parts by the diaphragm, a strong tendinous and muscular organ, which extends across the body from above the sternum (breast bone) to immediately below the kidneys. The diaphragm – known to butchers as the 'skirt' – is pierced by the oesophagus or gullet, and large blood vessels. The fore part of the carcase (the thorax, thoracic cavity or chest) is lined by a thin, transparent serous membrane – the parietal pleura. A similar membrane lines the hind part (abdomen, abdominal cavity, or belly) and is known as the parietal peritoneum. In healthy animals, these membranes are smooth and glistening, free from inflammation or adhesions of any kind.

The comparative anatomy of animals presented for slaughter is given in Table 36.1.

Thorax

The thorax or chest contains the lungs, gullet (oesophagus), wind-pipe (trachea), heart, pericardium and visceral pleurae.

1. Healthy **lungs** of properly bled animals are light red in colour, and the surface is smooth and glistening. On palpatation, their substance should be found spongy and homogeneous – free from any solid parts, lesions, inflammation, tubercles or cysts. During life, the lungs of a healthy animal expand to occupy practically the whole of the chest cavity. After death, healthy lungs collapse.

2. The **oesophagus or gullet** passes from the pharynx between the large lobes of the lungs and continues through the diaphragm into the stomach.

3. The **trachea or windpipe** begins at the lower border or the larynx and on reaching the lungs branches into the left and right bronchi.

4. The **heart** lies somewhere to the front and rather to the left side of the middle line behind the sternum and having on each side of it a lobe of the lungs. It is somewhat pear-shaped, its apex being the pointed end. In health it is brownish-red in colour and its covering membrane – the epicardium – is smooth and glistening. In properly bled animals the ventricles contain only a small quantity of coagulated blood.

5. The **pericardium** is the sac or bag (serous membrane) in which the heart lies.

6. In healthy animals, the **visceral pleura** is a thin, transparent, glistening membrane which covers the whole of the organs in the chest cavity.

Abdomen

The abdomen contains the stomach, liver, pancreas, spleen, omentum, mesentery, intestines, kidneys and, in female animals, the ovaries and uterus.

Table 36.1 Comparative anatomy

Teeth			***Liver*** cont.	
Bovine	No incisors on upper jaw		Pig	Five long, thin lobes; fine interlobular or mottled appearance on its surface; weight up to 1.8 kg
Horse	Six incisors on each jaw			
Sheep	Four pairs of incisors on lower jaw			
Pig	Three pairs of incisors and one pair of canines or tusks on lower jaw		**Kidneys**	
			Bovine	Distinctly lobulated; right is bean shaped; left is three sided (appears twisted)
Tongue				
Bovine	Thick at base; pointed; firm in texture; upper surface rough and bristly; several circumvallate papillae on each side; epiglottis thick and broad, sometimes partly black		Horse	Non-lobulated; right is heart shaped; left is long and narrow
			Sheep	Bean shaped, non-lobulated; shorter, rounder, and thicker than those of the pig
Horse	Flattened and broad at its free extremity – like a palette-knife; has only two well-marked circumvallate papillae; the epiglottis is pointed; texture is soft, not firm like that of bovines		Pig	Flat and haricot bean shaped
			Spleen	
			Bovine	Extended oval in shape; firm and convex when healthy
Sheep	Thick at its base, broad at its tip; has a deep middle furrow and a thick, strong sheath		Horse	Long and scythe shaped
			Sheep	Oyster shaped, reddish-brown, elastic
Pig	Smooth with no dorsal ridge; one well-defined circumvallate papilla on each side; tip is rounded		Pig	Long, narrow, bright red strip with one edge sharp and the other thick and round
Ribs			**Pluck**	
Bovine	Thirteen pairs, flat, broad		Bovine	Lungs, trachea, heart (heart usually sold separately)
Horse	Eighteen pairs, round rather than flat in section		Horse	Lungs, trachea, heart
Sheep	Thirteen pairs		Sheep	Lungs, trachea, heart, liver, spleen
Pig	Fourteen pairs		Pig	Lungs, trachea, oesophagus and larynx (no spleen), liver and heart
Lungs			**Stomach**	
Bovine	Left: three lobes Right: four and sometimes five lobes		Bovine and ruminants	Four compartments
Horse	Left: two lobes Right: three lobes		Horse	Simple stomach
			Pig	Simple stomach
Sheep	Similar to bovines; texture very firm		**Heart**	
Pig	Left: two or three lobes Right: three or four lobes; tissue is very soft and breaks down under pressure		Bovine	More pointed than in the horse; has two bones in the partition between the auricles; hard, white fat at its base; three grooves on its exterior
Liver			Horse	Less conical than in bovines; no bone, two grooves on exterior
Bovine	One large and one small lobe (or thumb piece); gall bladder is attached; weight up to 4.5 kg		Sheep	Similar to bovine but no bone; fat is white and very firm
Horse	Usually four lobes two middle lobes shortened; dark, no gall bladder		Pig	Round at its apex; fat is softer than in sheep
Sheep	Two large lobes and a small triangular thumb piece; weight up to 1 kg			

1. In ruminants, the **stomach** consists of four compartments; the rumen or paunch, the reticulum or honeycomb, the omasum or manifold, and the abomasum, reed or rennet – the true stomach.

2. The **liver** is situated towards the right side and touches the diaphragm. The gall bladder is attached to it and close to portal space. (The horse has no gall bladder.) After removal from the animal, it becomes reddish-brown in colour. The substance of the organ should be moderately firm; the blood vessels should not be congested with blood; the bile ducts should not be hard or prominent; and it should be free from abscesses, nodules, cysts, or discoloured areas.

3. The **pancreas** (gut bread) is an irregularly shaped glandular organ attached to the liver.

4. The **spleen** (milt) is a flat, reddish-brown organ, that lies along, and is attached to, the stomach. It has a high blood content. Its external membrane should be free from inflammation. It should maintain its shape after removal from the animal. Failure to do this, or any abnormal softening of the substance, is indicative of disease.

5. The **omentum** (caul) consists of two layers of the visceral peritoneum, having between them a varying quantity of fat. It envelops the abdominal organs. The surfaces should be smooth and glistening.

6. The **mesentery** is a fold of the peritoneum containing fat, which forms the medium of attachment between the intestines. The surface should be as described above.

7. The **intestines** lie posteriorly to the stomach. They are convoluted, and contained by the mesentery from which they are separated after removal from the animal. Their surfaces should be as described above.

8. The **visceral peritoneum** is similar to the visceral pleura, except that the organs covered are those in the abdomen.

Lymph glands or nodes

Lymph glands are nodular in form – and for that reason are often referred to in meat inspection as 'nodes' – varying in size from a pin's head to a hen's egg. They may be round, flattened, oval, or kidney shaped. They are supplied with afferent and efferent vessels. Afferent vessels convey lymph directly from the various tissues to their respective lymph nodes. After traversing a node, the composition of the lymph is altered and it leaves the gland or node by the efferent vessels, which convey it back to certain circulatory ducts or veins. They are adjuncts to the vascular system. While the lymphatic system may protect the body from disease, it may also furnish a route of entry for disease. Each gland functions for a certain region and is named after that region. Lymphatic glands are of great importance in meat inspection. On section, they should be quite smooth, although they vary in colour. Glands may be darkened in colour by normal pigment or particles of carbon; such glands are not diseased.

It should be noted that there are other glands, such as the salivary and thyroid glands and the pancreas, which are secreting glands only. These are irregular in shape, and may be distinguished from lymph glands by the fact that they are lobulated.

Names and positions of the most important lymph glands
The approximate positions of the glands to be found in the carcase of bovines and swine when dressed, and which are important in meat inspection, are indicated in Figs 36.1 and 36.2.

1. The **submaxillary** gland is placed superficially in the lower part of the jaw, one on each side between the maxillary (jaw) bone and the submaxillary salivary gland, i.e. just in front of the jaw bone, where it curves abruptly upwards. These glands are generally removed with the tongue.

2. The **retro-pharyngeal** gland – there is one on each side of the posterior wall of the pharynx – at the base of the tongue bones.

3. The **parotid** glands. A pair of glands situated one on each side of the cheek near the junction of the upper and lower jaws, partly embedded in the parotid salivary glands.

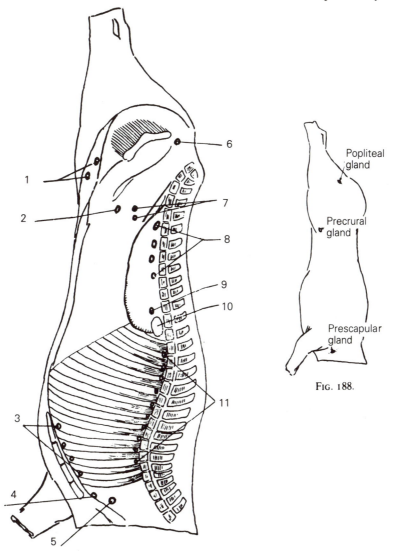

Popliteal
gland

Precrural
gland

Prescapular
gland

FIG. 188.

Fig. 36.1 Position of the lymphatic glands (bovine). (1) Supra-mammary in the female, or superficial-inguinal in the male. (2) Deep inguinal. (3) Supra-sternal. (4) Pre-sternal. (5) Pre-pectoral. (6) Ischiatic. (7) Internal and external iliacs. (8) Lumbar. (9) Renal gland (ductless: not a lymph gland). (10) Renal capsule. (11) Thoracic or sub-dorsal.

4. The **gastro-splenic** glands. In cattle these are located in the folds between the second compartment (reticulum) and the fourth or true stomach (abomasum). In swine, they are three or four in number and are situated under the pancreas. The splenic glands lie in a fissure of the spleen close to the stomach, and when the spleen is removed the glands are very often left on the stomach.

5. The **mesenteric** glands lie between the folds of the mesentery adjacent to the intestines. They consist of a continuous chain situated along and near the serrated edge of the mesentery.

6. The **hepatic** or **portal** glands are located on the posterior surface of the liver around the portal fissure. In swine, they are usually removed with the intestines.

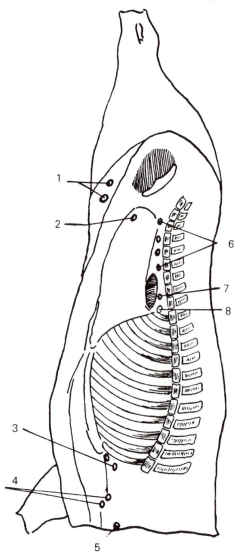

Fig. 36.2 Position of lymphatic glands (swine). (1) Supra-mammary in the female, or superficial-inguinal in the male. (2) Iliac. (3) Pre-pectoral. (4) Cervical. (5) Retro-pharyngeal. (6) Lumbar. (7) Renal gland. (8) Renal capsule.

7. The **renal** glands are situated in the fatty tissue on the course of the renal artery close to the second lumbar vertebra.

8. The **adrenal** or **supra-renal capsules.** These are two in number, situated one above each kidney and embedded in the fatty tissue (kidney fat) close to the first lumber vertebra. They are reddishbrown in colour. On section,

each gland is found to be composed of two distinct portions, the outer cortex is darker in colour than the inner portion – the medulla. *Note*: The adrenals are ductless glands not connected with the lymphatic system – they are not, therefore, lymph glands. They may, however, be affected by disease and their examination should form part of all routine inspections of carcases.

9. The **bronchial** glands are located in the fat on each side of the trachea at the top of the lungs.

10. The **mediastinal** glands (usually three or four in number) are located in the fat between the two large lobes of the lungs.

11. The **superficial-inguinal** glands (in the male) or **supra-mammary** gland (in the female). In the male animal, this is found in the fat at the neck of the scrotum; in the female animal, behind and above the udder.

12. The **lower cervical** and **pre-pectoral** glands are located in the fatty tissue on the lower side of the entrance to the thorax.

13. The **pre-sternal** gland is located against the first bone of the sternum and first rib. (This gland is superficial, and is known to butchers as the inspector's gland.)

14. The **supra-sternal** glands are located along the course of the internal thoracic vein and artery and covered by muscular tissue. They lie in the spaces between the ribs close to the point of junction with the sternal cartilages.

15. The **thoracic** or **sub-dorsal** glands are located in the spaces between the ribs embedded in the intercostal muscles along each side of the dorsal vertebrae.

16. The **pre-scapular** gland is located above and inward from the shoulder joint embedded in fat and covered by muscular tissue (it is incised from the outside).

17. The **iliac** (internal) gland is a large gland found in the loin fat (suet) on each side of the pelvic region.

18. The **lumbar** glands are embedded in the fat bordering the large blood vessels beneath the lumbar vertebrae.

19. The **pre-crural** glands are large glands, one on each side, in the flanks at a point where

the butcher separates the thin and thick flanks (they are incised from the outside).

20. The **popliteal** gland is a deep-seated gland situated in the fat in the silver-side (it is incised from the outside).

21. The **ischiatic** gland is a deep-seated gland adjacent to the external surface of the ischiatic bone, and is frequently seen when the butcher separates the rump from the aitch bone.

DISEASES IN RED MEAT ANIMALS

The following notes relate to some of the more important diseases and conditions which may render a carcase or its organs, or part of them unfit for human consumption.

Actinomycosis and actinobacillosis

These are two closely related diseases which affect cattle and pigs. The lesions of actinomycosis are usually found in the bones, and those of actinobacillosis in the softer tissues such as the tongue, lips, palate and lymphatic glands.

In cattle, the lesions of actinomycosis are usually found in the head, generally the lower jaw, which gives rise to the condition known as lumpy jaw. The bone becomes thickened and honeycombed and there is a quantity of yellow, glandular pus. In pigs, actinomycosis is usually found in the udder, in either the form of ulcers or thickening and hardening of the udder tissue together with thick-walled abscesses.

The thickening of the masseter muscles in bovines is usually due to actinobacillosis, as is the hardening and enlargement of the tongue known as wooden tongue. The lesions may take the form of ulcers together with the development of fibrous tissue.

Anthrax

A disease communicable to man (malignant pustule) and notifiable under the Animal Health Act 1981.

Anthrax may occur in all food animals, sheep and bovines being particularly susceptible. The disease is caused by entry into the body by ingestion, inhalation or inoculation, of the anthrax bacillus or its spores. The spores form only in the presence of oxygen, and may remain alive in air, e.g. on a pasture, for long periods of time – even for years. The course of the disease is rapid: the first indication may be the finding of the animal dead. In such cases, the oozing of blood or blood-stained fluid from the natural openings should be regarded with suspicion.

In a carcase that has been opened, indications of anthrax are dark discoloration or tarry condition of the blood and, in particular, distinct enlargement of the spleen, the pulp being soft and dark – sometimes described as resembling blackcurrant jelly. The muscular tissues, glands, organs, and membranes are dark and haemorrhagic. The carcase putrefies rapidly.

Under the **Anthrax Order 1938**, whenever anthrax is suspected, notification must be made at once to the police and to the veterinary inspector, and all further procedures should be carried out under official direction.

If the disease is confirmed, the whole carcase, including the hide, is condemned and must be destroyed, preferably by incineration on the spot, or if no more ready means is available, in the nearest incinerator – the carcase being properly disinfected and the openings plugged before transport. Alternatively, the carcase must be buried at least 6 ft (1.8 m) deep surrounded by quick lime 12 in (31 cm) thick at a spot not accessible to cattle, etc, away from any dwelling, and at such distance from any well, etc, to preclude risk of contamination of any water supply. All infected articles must be thoroughly disinfected – steeping in hot 5% solution of caustic soda is suitable – or burnt.

The premises on which anthrax has occurred become an 'infected place', and thorough disinfection must be carried out in a manner set out in detail in the Order.

Braxy

An acute infective disease of sheep occurring mainly in cold winter conditions. The course of the disease is rapid: frequently, affected animals are found dead. The flesh gives off an offensive odour and putrefies rapidly. All such carcases should be considered unfit for human consumption.

Caseous lymphadenitis

This disease resembles tuberculosis, and is of bacterial origin. The most common mode of infection is through a skin abrasion. It has been found in every kind of tissue in affected animals, muscles, bones, serous membranes, lymph glands, and organs. The lesions vary in size from a mere speck to that of a hen's egg, and are encapsulated. They are caseous, greenish in colour, and may be of the consistency of clotted cream, or more solid with an appearance like a cut section of an onion.

Cysticercus bovis (measly beef)

This has become common in Great Britain during postwar years. The cysticerci vary in size from a pin's head to that of a pea, and may be somewhat elongated. They are macroscopic and should be sought for in the muscles of the cheeks, tongue, cervical region and thorax, heart, diaphragm, and other musculature. The actual situation of the cysticerci is in the connective tissue between the muscle fibres. The parasite is encapsulated. It is the immature form of *Taenia saginata* in man – one of the largest of the tape-worms. In cases in which the infection is only localized, carcases may be made safe by cold storage.

Cysticercus cellulosae (measly pork)

This is not common in Britain. The cysticerci are about the size of a grain of wheat, but vary in size and are white in colour. They are macroscopic and are found particularly in the cheek muscles, tongue, heart, diaphragm, and the cervical and sternal muscles. Other muscles may be affected. The cysticerci lie in the connective tissue between the muscle fibres, and are encapsulated. Progenitor of *T. solium* in man.

Decomposition

This is a question of fact. The meat may be dry and almost black on the exterior surfaces, yet not bad. A greenish colour denotes advanced decomposition. Meat is tested for decomposition by thrusting long skewers deep into different parts, particularly in the vicinity of the deep-seated bone joints. If decomposition is present in any degree, the characteristic odour is conveyed when the skewers are withdrawn.

Dropsy

A dropsical condition is not a disease in itself, it is caused by disease in the liver, heart or kidneys. There is an increase in the watery content of the blood. The musculature is flabby, soft, and contains an excess of moisture.

Osteitis

The bones are enlarged and the sheaths surrounding them inflamed. The muscular tissue around may atrophy and show lesions of inflammation. Affected parts should be condemned and the rest of the carcase passed if otherwise sound.

Osteo-myelitis

In this disease, there is a purulent condition of the bone marrow. The condition may be considered a special form of pyaemia, and affected carcases, together with their organs, should be condemned.

Swine erysipelas

A disease, chiefly of adult swine, characterized by dark red discoloration – in the early stages as spots, and when advanced as a generalized condition – over the skin. The heart and liver show signs of degeneration, the spleen and kidneys are enlarged and dark – the latter when incised may exude a dark red fluid – the pleura and peritoneum are haemorrhagic. In chronic cases, there may be wart-like vegetations on the valves of the heart. The carcase sets badly and putrefies rapidly.

Swine fever

A disease notifiable under the Animal Health Act 1981 (also known as hog cholera and pig typhoid). Most frequently attacks young pigs and spreads rapidly. A red rash appears on the skin, especially at the base of the tail, under the belly, on the inside of the thighs and on the ears. Rounded, ulcer-like projections develop on the intestine, particularly in the vicinity of the ileocaecal valve, a typical 'ulcer' being about the size of a one pence piece. The mucous membrane of the intestines is more or less inflamed. The lymphatic glands present a 'strawberry' appearance and there may be haemorrhages in the kidneys.

Swine vesicular disease

A notifiable disease which affects pigs only. Caused by an entero-virus which may be carried by faeces and swill and on vehicles, boots and clothing. The signs are similar to those of foot-and-mouth disease, i.e. anorexia, fever, lameness, and with vesicles in the interdigital clefts and on the coronary bands. Smaller vesicles sometimes occur on the snout, hocks and knees. When an outbreak occurs, control measures similar to those for foot-and-mouth disease are put into operation.

Trichinosis

Occurs in man and other animals as a result of the ingestion of pork, etc, containing trichinae – the larvae of the parasite *Trichinella spiralis* – a nematode. The parasite is developed in the intestines from larvae swallowed in infested meat. The muscles gradually affected are the diaphragm, tongue, and larynx. Sections of these muscles should be examined under a microscope.

Trichinella spiralis is conveyed by rats, and it is thought that pigs become affected by eating infested carcases of these animals. Dogs may also be affected.

Tuberculosis

At one time this was commonly found in bovines and swine, but following the Tuberculosis Eradica-

Table 36.2 Common cestode infections

Parasite	Host	Immature form of parasite	Intermediary hosts
T.marginata	Dog	C.tenuicollis	Pig, sheep, and all ruminants
T.echinococcus	Dog	Echinococcus veterinorum	Pig, sheep, and all ruminants
T.caenurus	Dog	C.cerebralis	Sheep, bovines, and ruminants
T.senella	Dog	C.ovis	Sheep
T.serrata	Dog	C.pisiformis	Hare, rabbit

tion Scheme is now rarely seen. It is characterized by the formation of tubercles in or upon various parts of the carcase (principally the serous membranes and lymph glands) and in the organs. The tubercles vary in size from mere specks to that of a hen's egg. In section, they are purulent, caseous (cheesy) or calcareous. On the serous membranes (pleura and peritoneum), tubercles may be found clustered together and resembling bunches of grapes.

Urticaria

A mild form of swine erysipelas, in which there is an eruption on the skin of haemorrhagic areas which are diamond shaped, hence the butcher's term 'diamonds' for this condition. If the carcase sets well, it should be passed after affected portions of the skin have been removed.

PARASITIC DISEASES

Cestodes (tape-worms)

In addition to those already mentioned, the cestodes in Table 36.2 are commonly met with.

Trematodes

The only trematodes which are of importance in meat inspection in this country are 'flukes' (*Distoma hepaticum* and *D. lanceolatum*). They are flat in shape similar to a flounder fish, up to three-quarters of an inch (19mm) long and half as wide. Their habitat is the bile ducts of the livers of sheep, cattle, and pigs (much less common in the last). The bile ducts of affected livers are visibly distended and thickened ('pipey livers'), and from these, flukes may easily be extruded. Frequently, the carcases of affected animals are in good condition, but if the liver functions have been seriously interfered with, as sometimes happens in sheep, the carcases may be anaemic, emaciated, hydraemic, and in consequence unfit for human consumption. In minor cases, only affected livers – or parts of them – are condemned.

Nematodes

Strongylus micurus infests bovines; *S. filaria* and *S. rufescens* infests lambs and sheep; and *S. paradoxus* infests pigs. These are small worms whose habitats are the lungs of animals. Small nodules and pneumonic areas are set up in the lungs. Affected organs should be condemned.

Ascarides

Ascarides are long cylindrical worms which infest the small intestines of sheep, pigs, and calves. Heavy infestation causes an unpleasant odour in the flesh which may render the carcase unfit for human consumption. The intestines should be destroyed in all cases in which ascarides are present.

EMERGENCY SLAUGHTER

Extreme care must be taken in the inspection of animals brought into a slaughterhouse for emergency slaughter. Such animals which are known or suspected to be diseased must be slaughtered either at a different time or in a different place from other animals. Where, after inspection, the condition causing the emergency slaughter is not evident, or in the case of any doubt, samples should be submitted for laboratory examination. In the absence of such facilities at the slaughterhouse, examination will be carried out by either the PHLS or the local Veterinary Investigation Centre of the MAFF. A certificate from a veterinary surgeon should always accompany any animal submitted for emergency slaughter stating what, in his opinion, the animal is suffering from and details of any medicines prescribed.

POULTRY INSPECTION

Definitions

1. **Petit poussins.** Young chickens weighing 227–454g (8–16 oz).
2. **Spring chicken.** About 3 months old; weight about 0.9–1 kg (2–21/2 lb).
3. **Roasting chicken.** Includes year-old cockerels, pullets, young hens, usually about 3–6 months old; weight 1.36–1.8 kg (3–4 lb).
4. **Capon.** Male birds which have been 'de-sexed', usually by implanting in the neck a pellet of stilboestrol (usually done at 9–11 weeks) and the bird is killed at 11–13 weeks, giving a good quality fattened chicken of 1.8–2.27 kg (4–5 lb).
5. **Boiling fowls.** Hens which have laid eggs and are generally over 2 years old.
6. **Broilers.** These are young chickens or fowls reared intensively for the table and killed at 9–12 weeks with a live weight of 1.36–1.8 kg (3–4 lb). This method of poultry production has become very popular and is probably the main source of supply of table poultry in this country.

The birds are housed in a 'broiler house', which consists of a low-roofed insulated building with a floor area of approximately 450 sq m and able to accommodate about 7000 chicks. The house is usually covered with 10–15 cm of wood shavings, which are left in position for the whole of the time the one batch of chicks is being reared. Day-old chicks become ready for killing in about 70 days, but during this period something over 4% will have died.

At the packing station, everything is arranged on a 'line' system dealing with something like 25 000 carcases a day. Briefly, the procedure is as follows: birds are received and then suspended by the legs ready for killing. After electrical stunning, killing is usually done by the cutting of the jugular vein. The bird then passes through the bleeding tunnel and on to the plucking machine. In the wet plucking machine, the birds are immersed for 1–3 minutes in water at a temperature of about 51.6°C. Rubber flippers on a rapidly revolving drum then strike the birds, and the feathers, other than stub and wing feathers, are removed. Stub and wing feathers are removed in another machine.

After removal of the feet and head, the birds are eviscerated in a separate evisceration room. They are afterwards drained and dried, packed, weighed, packaged and placed in a cold store. If the birds are to be held in store for a few months, the temperature is about −9.4°C, but if they are being held for only a short period higher temperatures are usual.

During the processing operation, inspection points should be established at the reception area; after plucking – for whole bird inspection; and the evisceration point – for full inspection.

7. **New York dressed.** (NYD) Uneviscerated, fresh, chilled or frozen birds.
8. **Oven ready.** (OR) Eviscerated, frozen birds.
9. **LL 'long legs'** and **TD 'tied down'** indicates presentation of NYD carcases.

Inspection

Age
Young birds are usually identified by the pliability of the posterior end of the breast bone, the smooth legs and smooth, glistening feet. In the older birds, the legs are rough and the feet hornier.

Freshness
When fresh, the eyes are bright and prominent, and the feet moist and pliable. The flesh gives easily when pressed. Later, the eyes become dark and sunken, the feet hard and stiff, and at a later stage the carcase becomes greenish at the tail vent, followed successively by greening of the abdomen, back, ribs and neck. The carcase gives off an offensive odour.

Diseases

The abnormal conditions most commonly found in the inspection of poultry are infection of the liver, emaciation, decomposition, and oedema.

The liver is examined in an undrawn bird by pulling back the left leg and making a 5 cm incision in the flank, parallel with the last rib. The aperture is enlarged as necessary with the fingers and the liver examined. If it is found to be abnormal, the bird should be drawn and the viscera examined. If the liver and viscera are diseased, the bird should be condemned.

Salmonellosis
From the point of view of public health, this is probably one of the most important diseases. It is a disease of baby chicks, and the organisms of the *Salmonella* group which cause the greatest concern to public health officers are *S. enteriditis* and *S. typhimurium*, which in young chicks give a mortality rate of 80–90%. It is thought that many chickens which survive become carriers and harbour the organism in the intestinal tract and gall bladder, so that infection can be readily transferred to a packaging station with the possibility of widespread dissemination.

The carcase will probably show no lesions and bacteriological tests will be necessary. Several carcases should be sent to the bacteriologist.

Escherichia coli septicaemia
A disease of young chickens almost exclusively confined to the broiler house. It occurs either as a septicaemic disease in young birds, or as granulomatous lesions in the intestines of old birds. A postmortem examination reveals fibrinous pericarditis when usually a mass of pus is seen around the heart; the carcase may be emaciated. The strains of organism which cause the disease in poultry are unlikely to affect man, but if the carcase is emaciated or if there is pus around the heart, the carcase should be condemned.

Infectious synovitis and arthritis
Infectious synovitis is now fairly common among broiler-house birds and is characterized by swelling of the hock joints, foot pads, sternal bursa, and sometimes the wing joints. The swellings contain grey viscous fluid, often with spots of pus, and the liver and spleen are usually swollen and congested. Septic arthritis also causes an accumulation of pus around the hock joints.

Parasitic conditions
None of these are transmissible to man and judgement of the carcase will depend on the degree of emaciation.

Tuberculosis
Avian tuberculosis is a chronic infectious disease, but owing to the long incubation period is unlikely to be seen in broilers. The casual organism is the avian type of tubercle bacillus (*Mycobacterium tuberculosis avium*). Cattle, pigs, and man are susceptible to the avian bacillus. Emaciation is a characteristic feature of the disease, and the liver is usually enlarged and studded with white or yellow nodules from a pinpoint to 13 mm in diameter. Similar lesions may be found in the spleen, intestines, bone marrow (usually femur and tibia), and lungs.

Avian leucosis complex
The leucosis which can affect adult poultry can produce anaemia, emaciation, and weakness. On post-mortem inspection, the liver is usually found to be much enlarged and friable. Fowl so affected are unfit for human consumption.

Blackhead
An infectious disease of turkeys, particularly young ones, and occasionally chickens, pheasants, partridges, etc.

A post-mortem examination shows degenerate circular, yellowish areas up to 2.5 cm diameter on the liver, and enlargement of the caecal tubes which often contain a solid white core. Peritonitis may also be present.

Tumours
These are of various kinds and are usually seen as swellings in the flesh, skin, bones, or organs. The most frequent sites are the breast, liver, skin, leg and wing bones, and ovaries.

Egg peritonitis
Inflammation of the abdominal cavity and its contents owing to the presence of egg yolk or even shelled eggs free in the abdominal cavity.

Internal laying
Yolks deposited in the abdominal cavity owing to some abnormality.

Impaction of the oviduct
The oviduct is the tube that carries the developing egg from the ovary to the cloaca. In some cases, the oviduct is distended and completely impacted with large masses of cheesy egg material laid down in concentric rings.

Degeneration of the ovary
This, with rupture of one or more ova, causes the release of yolks into the abdominal cavity. Sometimes, rupture of a blood vessel in a degenerated ovary causes death from internal haemorrhage.

MEAT PRODUCTS

The Single Market Directive on meat products (92/5/EEC) was implemented by the Meat Products (Hygiene) Regulations 1994 and Code of Practice No. 17, which deals with their enforcement.

Operating procedures and hygiene standards during the manufacture, distribution and storage of meat products are covered and other products of animal origin such as meat extracts, rendered animal fats, greaves and intestines are subject to legal controls.

Meat products are any products from or with meat which have undergone treatment such that the cut surface shows that the product no longer has the characteristics of fresh meat. Such treatments include heating, smoking, salting, marinating, curing or drying. Products such as raw sausages and mince meat are covered by a further

Directive 88/65/EEC. Controls do not apply to premises supplying the final consumer (i.e. retailers or caterers).*

The above Directives require enforcement by 'Competent authorities' which means that local authorities and environmental health officers are responsible for enforcement. Detailed advice for the food industry on the new controls has been produced by MAFF and guidance for environmental health officers by the Department of Health [3,4].

General meat products

There are a large variety of meats produced in various pack sizes and enclosures within the UK. There are an estimated 20 000 premises, both large and small, producing for local, regional or national distribution. Additionally, there is a large volume of imported canned meat and products in hermetically sealed containers – vacuum packs and packs providing anaerobic environments.

Risk assessment of both home products and imported products depends on knowledge of methods of manufacture, storage conditions, particularly the storage temperature, and shelf-life. The nature of products, the pH, the degree of water activity (aw), and the presence of preservatives are all influential factors related to safety.

As a general safety rule, a minimum temperature–time treatment should be achieved during cooking, followed by sufficiently rapid cooling to minimize the growth of surviving organisms. The relationship between cooking temperature and tenderness is complex. Many methods are available for cooking, e.g. plate, infra-red and microwave cookers, and for cooling, e.g. plate, spray and cryogenic processes. Cooling can result in the growth of bacteria, perhaps derived from spores that survived the cooking process. Difficulty may be caused in cooling a large joint (exceeding 5 cm thick) and therefore portioning of hot or partially cool joints may be necessary. It is generally recommended that joints of meat should not exceed 2.5 kg.

In catering, meat should be cooled from 50 to 10°C in less than 5 hours, and subsequently cooled to and maintained below 5°C.

Department of Health ten-point plan for cooked meat products

In August 1990 the Department of Health issued a ten-point plan [5] following information on a number of food poisoning outbreaks in 1989 related to meats cooked in small establishments and mostly due to *Salmonella typhimurium*. The recommendations on cooking and cooling are as follows:

1. **Cooking.** The centre of the meat must reach a core temperature of at least 70°C for 2 minutes or the equivalent. Assurance that cooking equipment can achieve this performance consistently should be sought. The cooking process must be monitored, records of core temperatures (using a probe thermometer) of at least one item from every cook should be obtained. The probe thermometer must be washed and disinfected after each use, and the accuracy of the thermometer checked regularly.
2. **Cooling.** The product should be cooled as soon as possible. Products should be cooled through the temperature zone of 10–55°C. Cooked products should be stored at 5°C or less in a designated refrigerator.

Other precautions listed in the ten-point plan include hygiene principles to reduce cross-contamination risks, cleaning and personal hygiene.

Mechanically recovered meat (MRM)

MRM is used in the manufacture of meat products and, potentially, can be hazardous through the presence of bacteria. Generally, MRM preparation should be carried out in ambient temperatures not greater than 10°C. Bones should be passed through the meat recovery system immediately after removal from the carcase or held below +5°C if they are to be used within 24 hours.

---

* UK regulations dealing with minced meat and meat preparations are to be drafted in 1995 for implementation in January 1996.

If bones are not to be used within this time, they should be frozen and held at −10°C.

Comminuted meat must be chilled to not more than 2°C and used within 48 hours. If it is not used within this period, it must be cold stored at −18°C. It is essential to ensure that equipment used in this process is kept in a clean condition with effective cleaning being carried out between operations.

Blood products

Fresh blood must be used very quickly as it deteriorates within 24 hours. If blood is stored, the addition of salt is recommended. Dried blood can be used as an alternative. Blood used in edible products should only be used from healthy animals, must be collected hygienically in sterile containers and cooled immediately.

Jellying

Jelly prepared from gelatine and water is an ideal medium for bacterial growth. Jellying operations should be carried out in an area specially provided for the purpose. All equipment used must be kept as clean as possible throughout the work shift, and cleaned between shifts.

Regular microbiological monitoring of the jelly solution is desirable to ensure that the operation is being effectively controlled. Prepared jelly solutions must be held at a minimum temperature of 70°C, and any jelly left over at the end of the work day or which has been allowed to cool must be discarded.

Vacuum packing

Large quantities of whole and sliced cooked and uncooked cured meats and cooked uncured meats are packed and distributed in various vacuum packs. These packs can pose a danger through the growth of anaerobic food poisoning organisms. A strict hygiene regime involving equipment, the environment and personal hygiene is necessary. Special areas or rooms for vacuum packing operations and for controlling temperatures during slicing and packing to prevent the temperature of products rising above 7°C are necessary. For distribution purposes, products should be cooled as near to 0°C as is possible. (See Chapter 38 for more detail on vacuum-packed products.)

Department of Health Advisory Memorandum on the processing of pasteurized large canned hams

The Department issued this advice in 1972 [6], based on guidance provided by the Committee on Medical Aspects of Food Policy (the COMA Committee). The guidance which is still valid was provided because ham was a meat product which had specified limits for the preservatives nitrate and nitrite. The Committee recognized that in order to avoid excessive loss of weight and to preserve quality, it was necessary to cook large canned hams and shoulders, i.e. those above 2 lb (1 kg) in weight in temperatures which did not sterilize the meat. These hams are described as 'pasteurized'. While the minimum heat process is sufficient to destroy vegetative bacteria normally present, it is not severe enough to destroy with certainty all bacterial spores which the meat is liable to contain. Good commercial practice is relied on to produce a palatable, safe and stable product depending on factors related to spore load, salt, nitrate and nitrite content and the pH value.

For pasteurized hams, it is customary to heat them at a temperature of between 65 and 70°C, the choice depending on the relative importance attached to the cooking out loss and probability of spoilage. As regards their effect on bacterial spores, in particular those of *Clostridium botulinum*, there is no reason to believe that treatments differ significantly. They are, however, important in relation to the conditions of storing after processing. Spores of *C. botulinum* cannot readily develop in these products at temperatures of 15°C or below. Pasteurized canned ham should always, therefore, be stored under cool conditions. A product which receives a lighter heat treatment near to 65°C, and which will be stored for a long period, is likely to require a much lower keeping temperature than one which receives the more severe heat treatment near to 70°C.

For both home-produced and imported products, it is important that pasteurized canned hams are kept under refrigeration up to the time of opening. Blown cans are sometimes a common experience during the summer due to the distribution and storage of products at high ambient temperatures rather than under refrigeration. Aerobic spore-forming species of bacillus can form gas from nitrate and carbohydrate, and hence 'blow' cans. Most gas-forming bacillus are non-pathogenic. However, anaerobic spore-forming species of *Clostridium* can usually form gas in meat and blow the can. In addition, they often produce foul odours and flavours that are off. *C. sporogenes* and, sometimes, *C. perfringens* may be present and can suggest that *C. botulinum*, which is fortunately far more rare, may be present. This organism has not, however, been found in canned ham. Heat resistant faecal streptococci do not blow cans, but their presence is revealed by off odours or discoloration after the can is opened. These organisms are commonly found on the surface of cured meats.

The blowing of cans through the formation of gas can serve as a useful indicator of potentially dangerous products, and they should be withdrawn from sale immediately.

Canned meats

Detailed and comprehensive controls on all aspects of canning are necessary to ensure a safe system of food production (see page 523).

Handling of empty cans
The control of the can seaming process requires frequent checks on seaming and seaming equipment. Pressure testing of cans is highly important. For can filling, no autoclaving, cooking, heating or retorting processes should be carried out in any room where cans are filled with a cold meat product, or where cans are closed and seamed. In establishments where cans are filled with a hot meat product, there must be sufficient separation between precooking areas, areas in which cans are filled and sealed, and areas in which cans are sterilized. Ventilation systems must effectively prevent condensation, and hygiene standards must also be high. There must be a logical product flow with no backtracking or line crossing.

Processing
Detailed process checks are necessary. Automatic time and temperature recording devices must be fitted to each retort or tank, and records must be kept and retained for a minimum period of 3 years from the date of production. Additionally, retorts and processing tanks must be fitted with direct reading control thermometers. Retorts must also be fitted with pressure gauges.

For can cooling and drying, considerable control over can cooling water must be exercised. Cooling water must be protected against contamination with proper chlorination procedures. Cans must not be handled when wet after retorting, and other general post-process procedures must be effectively applied.

During processing, the requirements for process lethality is a highly critical factor in ensuring safety. Where environmental health officers are responsible for canning operations within their districts, they must be fully familiar with the guidance procedure for the canning industry contained in the Guidelines on the Safe Production of Heat Preserved Foods, produced by the Department of Health [7].

Salmonella enteritidis poultry and eggs

During 1987, *Salmonella enteritidis* became the most frequently reported *Salmonella* serotype in poultry and, by 1989, the problem also became severe in eggs. As a result of much media attention, an investigation by the House of Common Select Committee on Agriculture followed. Government department and industry investigations resulted in the development of a comprehensive package of control measures to deal with the problem.

The Zoonoses Order 1989
Under this Order laboratories are required to report the results of tests which demonstrate the presence of salmonellas in food animals and live

birds. Other samples may be taken for diagnosis, movement restrictions may be imposed and compulsory slaughter with compensation for infected poultry flocks may be applied. Premises can be cleaned and disinfected, as can vehicles.

Earlier control measures were modified in February 1993 after publication of the report of the Advisory Committee on the Microbiological Safety of Food on 'Salmonella in Eggs' [8] and the adoption by the Council of Ministers of the EC Zoonoses Directive 92/117/EEC laying down harmonized rules for the control of salmonella in poultry.

Breeding flocks of domestic fowl comprising 250 or more birds have to be tested every 4 weeks by the owner, with official samples being taken every 8 weeks. Flocks infected with *S. enteritidis* or *S. typhimurium* have to be slaughtered. The Directive does not include harmonized measures for the control of salmonella in commercial egg laying flocks. After considering the findings of the ACSMF report the Government considered that there was no longer a need to monitor laying flocks or to require the compulsory slaughter of those fowl found to be infected with *S. enteritidis.**

The Processed Animal Protein Order 1989

This Order is concerned with protein of animal origin which is processed for use in animal or poultry feed. Products must be tested for salmonella and no contaminated material may be used for poultry feed.

Importation of Processed Protein Order 1981

Licences are required under this Order to import processed animal protein intended for use in animal (including poultry) feed. Consignments are sampled for salmonella at ports of entry. Controls have been imposed on those countries whose products are frequently found to be contaminated.

In addition to the above controls, MAFF has introduced codes of practice to give positive guidance on the control of salmonella at all stages of the poultry production chain – in rendering plants during storage, handling and transportation of raw materials for incorporation in feed, in feed mills, in breeding flocks and hatcheries and in broiler houses. As a programme of concerted control of salmonella in poultry, the UK approach is the most comprehensive in the world.

Eggs and salmonellosis

In August 1988 the chief medical officer at the Department of Health issued a general warning to the public [9] to avoid eating raw eggs following numerous outbreaks of *S. enteritidis* and some outbreaks of *S. typhimurium* where the epidemiological evidence showed a strong association with eggs. Particularly, *S. enteritidis* phage type 4 was consistently shown to be associated with egg, and subsequent research and investigation indicated the particular invasive nature of *S. enteritidis* phage type 4 and its transfer of infection from the chicken to the egg through the trans-ovarian route.

The measures outlined earlier in relation to poultry aimed at reducing salmonella infection also address the problem of salmonella contamination levels in eggs, but until the evidence indicates that the levels of salmonella found in eggs and egg products are diminishing, the Department of Health's warning stands.

In terms of the UK consumption of around 30 million eggs a day, the incidence of known infection is quite small. However, environmental health officers should continue to warn consumers to avoid eating raw shell eggs. This warning applies also to their use in uncooked foods, such as home-made mayonnaise, mousses and ice-cream, as well as to egg drinks. Vulnerable groups were advised that whole shell eggs should be cooked until they were hard rather than runny.

Normally, commercially produced products are manufactured with bulk pasteurized egg and so are safe. No additional precautions are needed in the cooking of eggs, providing the cooking is adequate.

---

* Following a survey, ACMSF reported in 1995 a downward trend in the prevalence of *Salmonella* in UK-produced raw chicken (see MAFF/DoH Food Safety Bulletin No. 57, January 1995).

The following simple hygiene measures are advised for the storage and use for the storage and use of eggs:

1. Eggs should be stored in a cool, dry place, preferably under refrigeration (at 8°C as below).
2. They should be stored away from possible contaminants like raw meat.
3. Stocks of eggs should be rotated.
4. Hands should be washed before and after eating eggs.
5. Cracked eggs should not be used.
6. Preparation surfaces, utensils and containers should be regularly cleaned and always cleaned between the preparation of different dishes.
7. Egg dishes should be consumed as soon as possible after preparation or refrigerated if not for immediate ate use.
8. Egg dishes to be eaten cold should be refrigerated.

In their report on 'Salmonella in Eggs' the ACMSF Committee considered that while eggs must be regarded as an important source of human salmonella infection, the contribution they made to current levels of human salmonellosis could not be quantified precisely. Only a small percentage of eggs were considered to be contaminated with *S. enteritidis* and studies indicated that the number of organisms they contain when laid is very low. It is recommended that eggs should be consumed within 3 weeks of lay and that 'use-by' dates should be provided on egg packs and the eggs themselves; that industry and retailers should draw up Codes of Practice for the storage and handling of eggs; and that once purchased, eggs should be stored in the refrigerator. The Government is considering the recommendation on 'use-by' dates and has taken up the other recommendations [10].

Eggs and mayonnaise

Outbreaks of salmonella food poisoning have been associated with contaminated mayonnaise. The low pH and presence of organic acids, in particular acetic acid, normally make it an unfa-vourable environment for the survival or growth of most bacteria. Salmonellae, however, may survive but not multiply in mayonnaise for at least 24 hours.

The ability of mayonnaise to kill salmonellae more rapidly at room temperature than in the refrigerator has been recognized. The US Food and Drug Administration recommends that the pH in mayonnaise should be 4.1 or less, and that the product should be held at 18 to 22°C for at least 72 hours before use unless pasteurized egg is used. In Denmark, an outbreak of 10 000 cases of salmonellosis due to contaminated mayonnaise in 1955, led to the Danish administration recommending a holding period of 4 days at room temperature or 2 hours at 40°C. These recommendations are contrary to general guidance on food handling practices in the UK, although pasteurized egg is used in the commercial production of mayonnaise.

It is likely that recent outbreaks of salmonellosis associated with mayonnaise were most likely due to contaminated raw egg being used, but mishandling of products in the early stages of preparation may also be a contributing factor.

Pasteurization of eggs

The EC Directive on Hygiene and Health Problems Affecting the Production and the Placing on the Market of Egg Products (89/437/EEC) sets out detailed requirements for the processing of egg products. This Directive is implemented by the Egg Products Regulations 1993. 'Egg Products' are defined as products obtained from eggs, once the shell and outer membrane have been removed. These may be made from fresh whole egg, yolk, whole egg and yolk, or albumen. The definition includes liquid, concentrated, crystalized, frozen, quick frozen, coagulated or dried egg products to which some other foodstuff or additive has been added. Boiled eggs are excluded.

'Egg' includes eggs laid by hen, duck, goose, turkey, guinea fowl or quail. Incubated, pulled (from carcase) or broken eggs may not be used.

The process of pasteurization is specified as 2.5 minutes at 64.4°C for whole egg and yolk, but there is provision for food authority approval of alternative, equivalent heat processes. No time/temperature parameters are specified for the treatment of albumen – food authorities must be satisfied by the operators of businesses of the effectiveness of proposed processes and the degree of expertise involved.

Detailed guidance for enforcement officers was published on the Regulations and sent to all chief environmental health officers in England by the Department of Health in August 1993 [11].

The Ungraded Eggs (Hygiene) Regulations 1990

These Regulations prohibit the retail sale by producers of cracked eggs at the farm gate, in local markets and by door-to-door selling because of the hygiene risks they represent.

The eggs must be visibly cracked and are such that the producer could reasonably have been expected to have identified and removed them from sale. It includes leaking eggs and eggs in which the shell, when viewed in the ordinary light by the naked eye, are visibly cracked. Enforcement responsibility for these Regulations lies with environmental health officers.

OTHER ANIMAL INSPECTION

Farmed, wild game and rabbit are now covered by EC Directives 91/495/EEC, 91/497/EEC and 92/45/EEC and the Poultry Meat, Farmed Game, Bird Meat and Rabbit Meat (Hygiene and Inspection) Regulations 1994 (see page 533).

Rabbits

The principal conditions which lead to condemnation of rabbits are injury, decomposition, moulds, and fungi. These conditions are most common in imported frozen rabbits.

The diseases common in rabbits are parasitic, namely *C. serialis, C. pisiformis*, and *Coccidiosis*.

C. serialis are large cysts containing a watery fluid, and may easily be found by palpatation. *C. pisiformis* are small cysts, about the size of a pea, containing a watery fluid and a white spot – the head of the parasite – in the abdomen. Coccidosis

is caused by the protozoa known as Coccidia. They are microscopic. The parasites multiply rapidly in the intestines and the disease may spread to the liver and lungs, where it may be recognized by the whitish or yellowish, irregularly shaped areas or nodules it creates. Affected rabbits are usually emaciated and should be condemned.

Myxomatosis is a disease of rabbits which is prevalent in Australia, and serious outbreaks of which have occurred in England. The condition affects mainly the eyes (causing blindness) and the respiratory organs. There is usually a mucopurulent conjunctivitis associated with periorbital oedema, and there may be cutaneous tumours about the ears, nose, and feet. The disease is not thought to be communicable to man, but carcases affected should be condemned.

Hares

These are not condemned when in a 'high' condition, but when putrid should be seized. Hares are classed as game.

Game

Animals and birds pursued or taken in field sports or in the chase are classed as game. Legally, hares, partridges, pheasants, grouse, moor-game, black-game, and bustards are game. Game and wild birds can be taken legally only in their proper seasons. The close seasons are: hares, 1 March to 31 July; grouse, 11 December to 11 August: partridges. 2 February to 31 August; pheasants. 2 February to 30 September; wild birds, 2 March to 31 July. This relates to home game only – foreign game may be dealt with at any time.

Only licensed dealers may legally sell game. Game is not usually sold or eaten in fresh condition. Hanging increases its gastronomic and digestive qualities. Great care should be exercised before seizing it for its condition, but if putrid it is unfit for food.

MILK AND MILK PRODUCTS

Directive 92/46/EEC covers all community production of raw milk, heat-treated milk and milk-based products, from cows, ewes, goats and buffaloes intended for human consumption. Member States are required to implement this Directive from 1 January 1994 (Draft Regulations and Codes of Practice have been published and it is proposed that these will be finalized for implementation during 1995). This will mean that UK producers of sheep and goats' milk and milk products will be subject to detailed controls for the first time. Existing Milk Hygiene Regulations relating to cows' milk will be repealed and replaced by the Regulations. The Directive however, will not affect national rules on the direct sale to the consumer of raw milk and raw milk products. The Directive sets microbiological product standards and hygiene standards for production and processing plants and rules for packaging, transport, storage and labelling.

Milk pasteurization

The high temperature short time (HTST) is a well proven system. The flow of milk through a HTST plant is as follows. The raw milk is tipped into a weighing tank, weighed, released into a receiving tank, and then pumped into a storage tank. From the storage tank it flows to the balance tank (where the level is maintained by a float valve), and from this tank it is pumped, at a regulated rate, to the regenerative section of the heat exchanger. Here it is preheated by the pasteurized milk leaving the holder and then passes through the filter to the heating section, where its temperature is raised to just above the legal minimum by the circulation of hot water. The heated milk flows from the heat exchanger to the holder, during its passage through which it is held for the prescribed period at the required temperature, and from the holder it is fed via the flow diversion valve, back to the heat exchanger for cooling and, later, chilling.

After processing, the milk gravitates, or is pumped to a bottle filler which fills and caps bottles fed to it by conveyor from a bottle-washing machine. Sometimes the milk is filled into cartons. Modern sophisticated milk pasteurization techniques are becoming more common. The ALPAST Milk Pasteurization Line (Fig.

36.3) and the ALCOPE Pasteurizer Control Panel (Fig. 36.4) are illustrations of improved technologies.

Sterilized milk

Sterilized milk is preheated to a temperature of between 43 and 49°C, and is either filtered or clarified by passing it through a centrifugal clarifier. The milk is again heated to a temperature of 66–71 °C, and then homogenized at about 122 060 kg per sq m (2500 lb per sq in). This process ruptures the fat globules which allows them to remain in suspension in the milk.

The hot homogenized milk is then filled into hot sterile bottles, which are then sealed with a 'crown' cap.

The bottles are then processed, either in a batch retort or a continuous retort, where they are heated at approximately 104°C for 30 minutes. The bottles are then cooled, and are ready for sale. An alternative method is used whereby the milk may be sterilized by a continuous-flow method and then put into aseptic containers in which it is to be supplied to the consumer.

Ultra-high temperature (UHT) treatment

The first UHT process was developed in Switzerland by a firm by the name of Alpura Ltd who gave the name of uperization to the process.

In this process, the milk is pumped into a preheater which consists of a double pipe coil, where the milk is preheated to 78°C; it is then transferred to the uperization unit, where it is heated to 150°C and held at this temperature in a timing tube for 2.4 seconds, which is considered necessary to ensure absolute sterilization. By this method, water is incorporated in the milk, and the water is removed by pumping the milk through an expansion nozzle at a reduced pressure, and through a centrifugal separator.

The water-free milk passes to a sterile homogenizer and then to a cooler, where the milk is cooled to a temperature of approximately 15.6°C, when it is aseptically filled into cartons.

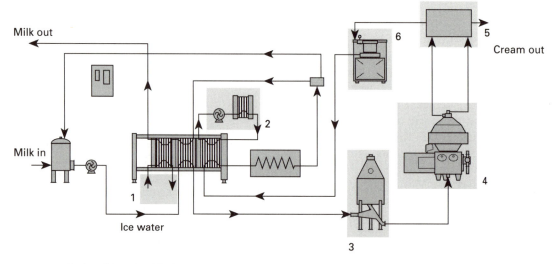

Optional function blocks

1. Ice water control
2. Hot water generation
3. Deaeration/deodorization
4. Separation
5. Standardization
6. Homogenization

Process Description for ALPAST with Local Automatic Control

Pasteurization Module

Milk enters the buffer tank via a float valve, which regulates the milk level. A low level switch is used to control tank emptying during sequence changes. The tank is automatically cleaned via a sprayball.

Milk is pumped from the buffer tank to the regeneration section of the plate heat exchanger and then heated to pasteurization temperature using hot water as the heating medium. A mechanical device maintains a constant flowrate. After pasteurization at the required temperature the milk passes to a holding cell, before being cooled by regeneration and ice water to the required outlet temperature. Pasteurized milk is maintained at a higher pressure than unpasteurized milk by means of a booster pump and constant pressure valve.

If the temperature falls below the preset pasteurization temperature forward flow is automatically broken and milk circulated to the buffer tank.

During start-up the regeneration section is by-passed to minimise the warming up period.

Ice Water control (optional)

An automatic valve initiates ice water supply, the temperature being regulated by a manually set regulation valve in the ice water return line.

Hot Water Generation (optional)

Hot water heating medium is generated in a steam/water heat exchanger, the temperature being accurately controlled by means of an automatic steam regulating valve.

Deaeration and Deodorization (optional)

Air and/or volatile flavours are removed under vacuum before the milk is heated to pasteurization temperature.

Separation and Standardization (optional)

Milk is separated and can be standardized in-line before being heated to the final pasteurization temperature. If a deaerator is included in the line, it is positioned before the separator for optimum separation efficiency and reduced "burn-on" of milk product.

The separator is automatically by-passed during start-up.

Homogenization (optional)

Milk is homogenized prior to heating to final pasteurization temperature. Full or partial homogenization is used dependent on the product requirements. An open by-pass of product from the outlet to the inlet of the homogenizer ensures that the homogenizer does not cavitate.

The homogenizer is positioned after deaeration, separation and standardization, if these have been selected.

Basic Version

The same functionality is achieved with Basic control, but all operations, except low temperature diversion, are manually initiated. No facility exists in the Basic version to maintain a higher pressure on the pasteurized milk side.

Fig. 36.3 ALPAST Milk Pasteurization Line. (Courtesy of Alfa Laval Food and Dairy Engineering and Tetra Pak UK.)

Working Principle

The control panel features the following functions/controls:

- Operating power on/off switch.
- Six start/stop buttons with signal lamps for process line units, such as feed pump, hot water pump, and other pumps.
- Temperature controller, with a range of 0–100°C, regulation commencing automatically as the hot water pump is started.
- Recorder for the temperature (0–100°C) and return valve (V1) position, starting automatically as the feed pump is started; the recorder draws a temperature graph and also marks the chart whenever the return valve (V1) changes over from Forward Flow to Return (recirculation) or vice versa; the recorder incorporates a temperature monitor, actual temperature dropping below setpoint causing the return valve (V1) to change over to recirculation and an alarm to be triggered.
- Alarm beacon, flashing red when an alarm is triggered.
- Alarm Reset switch; in Forward Flow mode, an alarm is triggered by temperature dropping below setpoint or level in the inlet balance tank dropping below the actuation point of the level switch; in Return mode, reaching correct temperature or level is indicated by an alarm.
- Manual/automatic/remote control selector switch for the return valve function mode; with signal lamp.
- Automatic control of the external recirculation valve (V2) by means of a low-level switch in the inlet balance tank; too low a level causes the valve to change over in order to prevent the plant to be starved of product, thus retaining it in production mode; an alarm is also triggered.
- Manual/automatic/remote control selector switch for the external recirculation valve function mode; with signal lamp.
- Selector switch, with signal lamp, for an additional unit, e.g. regenerative section by-pass valve (V3).
- Facilities for valve position (V1 and V2) indication by means of microswitch feedback.

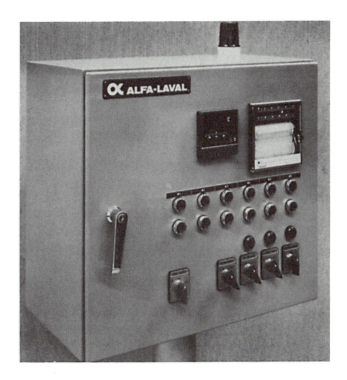

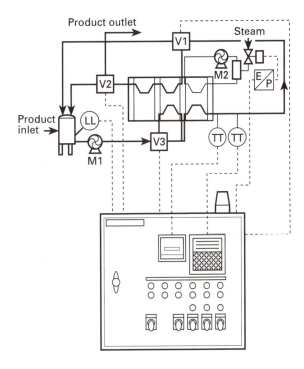

Fig. 36.4 Alcope Pasteurizer Control Panel. (Courtesy of Alfa Laval Food and Dairy Engineering and Tetra Pak UK.)

There are two further methods of UHT treatment, one known as the Alfa-Laval Process, and the other as the APV Process.

In the Alfa-Laval Process, the milk is heated by direct steam injection, and in the APV Process by hot water and steam circulation.

The system developed by Alfa-Laval Ltd, known as VTIS (vacu-therm-instant-sterilizer), is as follows:

From the storage tank milk enters the float hopper, is pumped to the plate heat exchangers, where its temperature is raised to 75°C, partly by regeneration with flash vapour from vacuum vessels and partly by live steam. A high-pressure pump pumps the preheated milk through a steam injector and in a fraction of a second the steam heats the milk to 140°C. In the pipe, the milk is held under pressure at 140°C for 4 seconds. The milk, now sterile, continues through the flow diversion valve to a vessel in which a constant vacuum is maintained. Here the temperature of the milk falls instantly to 76–77°C, and exactly the same amount of water vapour flushes off as was injected by steam heating. The vapour is condensed in the plate heat exchangers, partly by input milk and partly by cooling water. The milk is drawn from the vacuum vessel by pump and passed to an homogenizer and then to a cooler in which its temperature is lowered to about 20°C, or lower if wanted. The milk is now ready for packaging.

If milk is insufficiently heated in the steam injector, due to steam or electric power failure, a thermosensitive element instantly actuates the flow diversion valve. The milk is then diverted to another vacuum vessel from which the pump returns it to the float hopper via the plate heat exchanger, where its temperature is lowered to 20°C. This diversion arrangement prevents insufficiently heated milk from contaminating the aseptic parts of the plant.

The complete VTIS plant includes a built-in cleaning and sterilization operation under the control of an automatic timer, which in turn is built into the instrument panel.

It is, therefore, only necessary for the operator to set the plant to 'cleaning', and press a starting button to ensure the whole plant is cleaned by the circulation of acid and detergent, and is subsequently raised to a temperature of 130°C for complete sterilization. For a process such as this, chemical sterilization is considered to be inadequate.

Sterilization of heat-treatment plant

This is an important aspect of the efficient processing of milk [12], consists of two operations, namely cleaning followed by sterilization. Sterilization may be carried out by hot water, steam, or one of the approved chemical agents.

Cleaning

Subject to minor alterations, depending on the type of plant, the usual procedure followed is:

1. preliminary rinse;
2. washing or scrubbing with detergent;
3. final rinse.

The preliminary rinse removes all loose residues and the detergent is intended to remove all hardened residues, which have not been removed by the preliminary rinse. The final rinse clears the plant of detergent and freed residues, and leaves the surfaces clean for sterilization. The preliminary rinse should be carried out as soon as possible after the day's work, in order to prevent milk residues drying and hardening, and the detergent solution then used at the recommended concentration. In the case of HTST plant it is usually circulated at a temperature of 72°C for 40 minutes and the plant is then dismantled, scrubbed, and rinsed.

Sterilization

Generally, when using hot water, the plant surfaces should be held at a temperature of 85°C for 10 minutes and in the case of steam 99°C for 5 minutes. The sterilants permitted are approved brands of sodium hypochlorite and chlorine, or quarternary ammonium compounds. It is generally accepted that where residues remain on the plant surfaces. heat is more effective, but if the plant has been effectively cleaned beforehand, chemical sterilization can be just as good.

'In place' cleaning

Because the cleaning and sterilization of dairy plant is time consuming and arduous, and there is always the risk of recontamination during reassembly, the technique of 'in place' cleaning has been developed. The system involves cleaning and sterilization (it is sometimes possible to carry out both operations simultaneously), which is done without the complete dismantling of the plant.

As the nature of the residue varies in different parts of the plant, e.g. in the parts dealing with raw and heated milk, different detergents are necessary and, in order to avoid the wasteful application of chemicals and risk corrosion in parts of the plant, it is usual to divide the plant into circuits for the purpose of cleaning. Also in the case of larger plants, division into circuits enables cleaning to be carried out in the sections which have been cleared of milk while milk is still being processed or bottled. A typical circuit arrangement for a HTST plant would be:

1. raw milk reception and ancillary pipes;
2. tanks;
3. pasteurizing equipment.

A suitable cleaning procedure for that part of the plant containing raw milk would be:

1. cold water rinse: 5 minutes;
2. hot detergent: 10–20 minutes;
3. cold water rinse: 5 minutes;
4. sterilization by hot water or chemicals: 15 minutes;
5. cold rinse: 5 minutes (only after chemical sterilization).

For the pasteurizing equipment, the method usually used is, first, a cold-water rinse followed by the circulation of a detergent to soften the water and attack inorganic constituents of the deposits. A second detergent wash to remove the organic matter is then applied and this is followed by sterilizing and rinsing.

Enclosed tanks are usually cleaned and sterilized by the application of the various solutions to the inside of the tank by the means of pressure sprays.

The failure of heat-treated milk to satisfy the prescribed tests should be followed by repeat sampling and examination of the thermograph charts with, if necessary, the swabbing and test rinsing of the plant.

Swabbing

The apparatus consists of a piece of stainless steel wire about 350 mm long formed into a loop at one end and notched at the other to hold either a wad of cotton wool, or some unmedicated ribbon gauze.

Where possible, an area of 930 sq cm should be examined. The sterile swab is received from the laboratory in a test tube containing quarter strength Ringer's solution and plugged with cotton wool. Before use, the excess liquid is squeezed out of the swab by pressing it with a rolling motion against the inner surface of the tube, and it is then rubbed with a fairly heavy to and fro motion over the area being examined. The area should be covered twice, the swab being rotated to ensure all parts make contact with the surface being tested. After use, the swab is replaced in the tube, the tube plugged with cotton wool, and taken to the laboratory.

Rinsing

For utensils such as bottles, etc, rinsing is more satisfactory, but care must be taken to see that the rinse solution comes into contact with all parts of the utensil. One-quarter strength Ringer's solution is used, the quantity depending upon the capacity of the vessel. For all sizes of bottles, 20 ml is used, the bottle being rotated about 12 times.

Liquid milk

Under the proposed Dairy Products (Hygiene) Regulations 1995 the detailed requirements, including microbiological specifications, are contained within 12 schedules. Previously, to aid enforcement in the sampling and testing of pasteurized milk for the purpose of the Milk (Special Designation) Regulations 1989, the Institution of Environmental Health Officers, the PHLS, the Milk Marketing Board, the National Farmers' Union and the Dairy Trade Federation jointly produced guidelines on sampling and testing [13]. These guidelines have no statutory authority, but are aimed at the sensible application of the 1989 Regulations. Directive 92/46/EEC has detailed requirements for conditions of raw milk prior to admission to treatment establishments; the hygiene of the production holding; hygiene of standardization centres; microbiological standards to be met on admission to heat-treatment establishments; special requirements for the approval of treatment establishments; registration of collection centres and standardization centres; hygiene requirements relating to the premises' equipment and staff of establishments; standards relating to heat treatment, packaging and labelling of final heat-treated products; the storage of pasteurized milk; and transportation after heat treatment.

The UK should have no difficulty in meeting the microbiological standards as domestic milk production already conforms to the higher step two requirements of the earlier EC heat-treated milk directive 85/397 repealed on 1 January 1994. Standards in the 500 or so farm pasteurization plants within the UK may be variable, however, and require constant monitoring.

British Standard Code of Practice for the Pasturization of Milk on Farms and in Small Dairies

The British Standards Institution (BSI) produced this Code of Practice in 1994 [14] which provides a new standard for farm pasteurization plants. The BSI Committee which considered the code of practice had a substantial environmental health officer input, and the code is of benefit to both farmers, milk producers and environmental health officers carrying out enforcement inspection.

Milk products

As a result of Directive 92/46/EEC there will be new general hygiene requirements for these products, including animal health requirements on raw milk, hygiene of the dairy holding, microbiological standards for raw milk, microbiological standards for milk-based products and conditions governing labelling. Of particular importance is

the fact that the words 'made with raw milk' must appear clearly in the labelling of milk-based products manufactured from raw milk, whose manufacturing process does not include heat treatment. A large proportion of all imported Continental cheese of the soft and mould ripened variety is made from untreated milk. Similarly, UK cheese production of products made from cow's, sheep and goat's milk may not involve pasteurization of the milk as part of the manufacturing process.

Cheese

The Consumers Panel set up by MAFF in 1990 considered the question of labelling for cheese made from unpasteurized milk. The evidence, however, does not suggest a problem from this cheese similar to that of risks of salmonellosis and campylobacter arising from liquid untreated milk. The development of acidification, the ripening process, and the pH of end products has considerable influence on the likely survival of pathogens if carried over from the use of untreated milk in cheese manufacture.

Two important outbreaks of food-borne disease arising from the consumption of cheese made from unpasteurized milk occurred in 1989. In one, 155 persons were made ill (vomiting within 6–24 hours) thought to be caused by an undetectable staphylococcal enterotoxin (no organism was found). In the other out break. 39 persons were ill from *Salmonella dublin* in an imported cheese from the Republic of Ireland.

In both these incidents, the cheese producers subsequently decided to introduce pasteurization of the milk during the manufacture of their cheese. Apart from these outbreaks, the safety record of cheese has been good and, in general, has not led to a conclusion that a higher risk is attributable to cheese made from unpasteurized milk compared with that made from pasteurized milk. This is particularly the case with strains of *Listeria*, where the evidence suggests that the main risk is to end products contaminated by post-process handling in dairies.

The dairy industry has addressed these contamination risk problems. The Dairy Trade Federation has produced comprehensive guidelines to cover the manufacture of dairy-based products. The Creamery Producers Association has produced guidelines for large cheese plants [15] and the Milk Marketing Board has produced similar guidance for the manufacture of cheese in small dairies and 'on farm' plants particularly related to *Listeria* risks [16]. The Specialist Cheese Makers Association has also introduced a hygiene standards scheme which has as its main objective, to achieve good hygienic practice in the manufacture of speciality cheese in the UK [17].

UK cheese manufacture represents 21% of the total UK milk utilization, and the modern trend to reduce the content of preservatives relying only on temperature control and shelf life to inhibit bacterial risks means that cheese, if improperly manufactured and controlled, could represent a substantial risk to consumers.

ICE CREAM

Unlike much Continental ice cream, most ice cream produced in the UK has a vegetable rather than a dairy fat base. Dairy-fat based ice cream is also popular in the UK however. Its manufacture will in future be covered by Directive 92/46/EEC and the Dairy Products (Hygiene) Regulations 1995. Ingredients used in the manufacture of ice cream are required to be pasteurized by one or other of three specified methods, or sterilized and thereafter kept at a temperature below 7.2°C until the freezing process has begun. It is an offence to sell or offer to sell ice cream which has not been so treated (except in the case of certain water ices and ice lollies), or which has been allowed to reach a temperature exceeding −2.2°C without again being heat treated.

In the pasteurization process, after the ingredients have been mixed, the mixture shall not be kept for more than 1 hour above 7.2°C before being raised to, and kept at, a temperature of pasteurization (normally 71.1°C for 10 minutes, or 79.4°C for at least 15 seconds). It must then, within 1 hour 30 minutes, be reduced to not more than 7.2°C and kept there until freezing has begun.

Alternatively, processing of ingredients can also be safeguarded by sterilization; the mixture must be raised and kept to a temperature of not less than 148.9°C for at least 2 seconds. A mixture so sterilized need not be cooled as for pasteurized products, provided it is immediately canned under sterile conditions.

Any ice cream which has an elevated temperature above −2.2°C must be subject to a reheating process prior to sale.

Soft ice cream

Soft ice cream is made from either powder or liquid mixes, which have previously been heat processed. The mix is tipped into a hopper in the dispensing machine where it is fed by means of a drip feed or pump into the freezing compartment. Air is introduced during freezing to improve texture and to reduce the shock to the tongue when the ice cream is eaten. It also increases the bulk (over-run). The mixture is then frozen in the freezer barrel and delivered to the service nozzle at a temperature of −5°C. 'Thick shakes' served in fast-food restaurants use similar equipment. The food contact parts of the machinery may be complex and somewhat difficult to clean; complete dismantling is necessary in order to clean and disinfect individual components. Where the machine is located in a mobile vehicle, cleaning and disinfection facilities may not always be readily at hand. Manufacturers' instructions on the use of machines must be followed, and personal hygiene of operators is very important, both during the dispensing of soft ice cream and cleaning operations.

Self-pasteurization machines

A fairly recent innovation has been the introduction of self-pasteurizers for dispensing soft ice cream. These employ a pasteurization cycle after business is completed for the day in which any liquid mix stored in the machine and all food contact parts are heated to pasteurization temperatures to eliminate any build up of contamination. However, this pasteurization is for the purpose of cleaning, not to safeguard the ice cream itself.

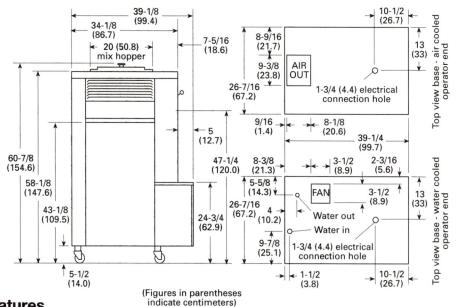

(Figures in parentheses indicate centimeters)

Features

Freezing Cylinder
Shake side, 7 quart (6.6 litre). Soft serve side, 3.4 quart (3.2 litre).

Mix Hopper
Two, 20 quart (18.9 litre) mix hopper capacity. The insulated reservoirs are refrigerated during normal and standby operation to maintain the mix below 40°F (4°C).

Indicator Lights
A warning light flashes alerting operator of insufficient mix level. When the mix out light flashes, the unit automatically is placed in the 'Standby' mode, protecting the freezer from damage.

Electronic Controls
The software in the Universal control is programmed to monitor all modes of operation. Product viscosity is continually measured to assure consistent quality at all times.

Auto Dispensing
Shake side: One dispensing spout provides four separate flavours. Flavours are selected from conveniently located touch pads at the front of the unit. Solid state portion control automatically closes draw valve at proper fill level and prevents syrup carry over. Syrup calibration is microprocessor controlled and aids the operator to accurately set the proper syrup flow.

Power Interrupt and Lock-Out
This computer based safety feature is programmed to alert the operator if product reaches unsafe temperatures as a result of power loss. If Heat Treatment features are improperly used, the unit automatically locks all freezer functions until proper measures are taken to ensure health codes are met.

LCD Readout
To assure proper performance, the LCD (Liquid Crystal Display) readout will identify temperatures in the hopper or freezing cylinder at any point of operation. Can also provide history of temperatures and times during last 13 heat cycles.

Thorough Agitation
Product is continually blended in the hopper during the Heat Treatment cycle, and maintains the mix at or below 40°F (4°C) in 'Auto' or 'Standby'.

Air/Mix Pump
Coaxial air/mix pumps are located in the refrigerated hoppers providing consistent overrun and fast ejection.

Self-Contained Syrup Compartment
Lower, front compartment contains four, individually regulated, 1 gallon (3.8 litre) syrup tanks. (A self contained air compressor is located in the freezer.) Use only single strength syrup that is free of pulp and seeds.

Syrup Rail
Four compartment syrup rail is recessed in front of freezer: two heated and two room temperature. The 2 quart (1.9 litre) reservoirs serve a wide variety of syrups and toppings.

Fig. 36.5 Shake and Soft Ice Cream Freezer. (Courtesy of Taylor Freezer UK.)

In February 1984, representatives of the DHSS, the Department of Agriculture for Scotland, DOE Northern Ireland and the Welsh Office had discussions with manufacturers and importers of three types of soft ice-cream machine, each employing a self-pasteurizing technique. [18] The meeting considered the machines' operations. Self-pasteurization temperatures (65.5–76°C for up to 35 minutes) are followed by the machine being kept at 4°C until freezing recommences. This self-pasteurizing process at the end of working periods is an alternative to dismantling and cleaning the machine frequently. Periods of 2 weeks to 1 month were considered as acceptable intervals between the time of dismantling and thorough cleaning of the individual components and internal surfaces of the machine. These claims were subsequently tested by the PHLS. Using sterile mixes, grade 1 results on methylene blue tests were produced for up to 1 month's operation without cleaning. Later in the summer of 1990, a self-pasteurizer ice-cream machine was tested for *Listeria* species by an independent laboratory, and was found satisfactory in eliminating the organism by the self-pasteurization process.

From the information to date, therefore, it appears that the manufacturers' claims for these machines are justified, and that they can, under normal commercial conditions, be operated safely for a period of 2 weeks with self-pasteurization being applied at the end of each working period. At the end of the 2-week period, however, the machines should be dismantled for thorough and effective cleaning, similar to other soft ice-cream machines.

The Ice Cream Federation and the Ice Cream Alliance have produced a code of practice on the hygienic retailing of ice cream [19].

Fig. 36.5 provides an illustration of one of the latest shake and soft ice-cream freezers using a self-pasteurization technique. Model PH 90 has an on-board computer and a refined monitoring system. It can disable or 'lock-out' a machine if a correct heat cycle has not been completed within the last 24 hours. It will also 'lock-out' if a complete disassembly and brush clean is not carried out after the 13th heat cycle. A Liquid Crystal Display readout will identify temperatures in the hopper or freezing cylinder at any point of the operation. It can also display information on the previous 14 heat cycles. It has a fault diagnostic system with an audible alarm to alert the operator if a fault occurs.

FISH AND SHELLFISH

EC Directives now control the hygiene of production and distribution of fish and shellfish in the EU. The Directives are:

1. 91/493/EEC on Health Conditions for the Production and Placing on the Market of Fishery Products.
2. 92/48/EEC on Hygiene Aboard Fishing Vessels.
3. 91/492/EEC on Shellfish Hygiene.

These Directives have been implemented by respectively:

1. The Food Safety (Fishery Products) Regulations 1992.*
2. The Food Safety (Fishery Products on Fishing Vessels) Regulations 1992.*
3. The Food Safety (Live Bivalve Molluscs and other Shellfish) Regulations 1992* (see also Codes of Practice Nos 14 and 15).

Hygiene requirements are set for the handling of all seawater and freshwater fish and their roe, farmed fish and crustacea at all stages from catching to processing; processed shellfish, i.e. smoked, frozen or cooked. These requirements are contained in the Fishery Products Regulations.

The Live Bivalve Molluscs and other Shellfish Regulations cover oysters, mussels, cockles and farmed scallops and gastropods such as whelks and winkles. Microbiological end-product standards together with a system of classification of shellfish harvesting areas according to the levels of microbiological contamination of the shellfish are pre-

---

* These regulations were amended in 1994 mainly to implement Community hygiene conditions for the importation of fishery products and live shellfish from third countries.

scribed. Gatherers of shellfish must complete a Movement Document to accompany shellfish from harvesting areas to retail sales. Each consignment of live bivalve molluscs or other shellfish leaving a dispatch centre must have attached to it a health mark.

A coastal fisherman who sells a small quantity of either fish or shellfish direct to the final consumer is exempted from the above Regulations. (Small quantities are defined in the appropriate Regulations.) These transactions are however still caught by general Food Hygiene Regulations.

These Regulations, and in particular the Food Safety (Live Bivalve and other Shellfish) Regulations 1992 have considerable implications for local authorities and environmental health officers in coastal areas. The identification, policing and microbiological monitoring of shellfish harvesting and relaying areas and purification plants requires considerable inspection resources – disproportionate to the size of the industry, but nevertheless important because of the health risks from these products. In British coastal waters it is almost impossible to find molluscs which can be taken direct from harvesting areas and pass the end-product standard of less than 300 faecal coliforms or less than 230 *E. coli* per 100 grammes of mollusc flesh and intra-valvular liquid. This means that products must be either relaid, or sent to depuration plants for purification – or possibly both, depending on their contamination levels. These are labour-intensive and time-consuming activities for the fishermen involved, all of which require some degree of supervision by environmental health officers. The position is complicated also by MAFF controls in regard to parasites which may be found in shellfish such as oysters, requiring restrictions on the movement of products in and out of controlled areas where parasitic infection is known to be present.

The Department of Health has issued advisory leaflets for the fish and shellfish industries on the requirements contained in the new legislation [20, 21] and have also published a guidance package for environmental health officers on the Shellfish

and Fish Hygiene Directives and relevant legislation [22].

Scombroid poisoning (see Chapter 17)

Fresh fish does not normally present a major public health problem, and fish, because of its rapid decomposition rate, tends to become spoiled and inedible before becoming a risk to health. There is an exception with species of scombroid fish, e.g. tuna and mackerel, where early decomposition in the fish is associated with scombroid poisoning in humans. However, providing the fish are placed as soon as possible after catching under ice with the temperature being kept as far as possible below 8°C, no problems occur. Incidents in the UK have been associated with smoked mackerel and canned scombroid species of fish, such as tuna, and also in non-scombroid species such as sardines where the problem is related to delays in canning the fish and retaining its quality after catching. However, scombroid poisoning is not usually serious, normally resulting in a rash, diarrhoea, flushing and headache among people affected with recovery within 24 hours. The presence of histamine (caused by prolonged storage of fish at elevated temperatures) in samples of suspected fish is usually indicative of a problem. Of fish samples with more than 20 mg histamine/100 g, 94% were from incidents in which scombrotoxic symptoms were characteristic, but where fish had 5–20 mg/100 g, only 30% of incidents were clinically distinctive. Histamine is produced in the fish by the action of bacterial decarboxylase enzymes on the amino acid histidine, which is present in dark-fleshed fish [23].

Shellfish toxins (see also Chapter 17)*

In May 1990, Paralytic Shellfish Poisoning (PSP) risks arose on the north-east coast of England and Scotland when high levels of toxins were discovered in molluscs. In the light of known risks to public health. the government issued an immediate warning to the public to refrain from eating all shellfish harvested between the Humber and

---

* In June 1994 PHLS reported the first cases of diarrhoeic shellfish poisoning (DSP) in the UK, which was contracted from imported mussels. It is a separate and less serious condition than PSP.

Montrose in Scotland. PSP results from a build up of toxin in shellfish. The sources of the toxin are the dinoflagellate species, the most common being *Protogonyaulux tamarensis* and *Gyrodinium auveolum*. Particular problems arise due to exceptionally high growth – a 'bloom' of one of these algal microorganisms. These blooms are difficult to predict. Bivalve molluscs are a hazard to health because they accumulate and concentrate toxin by continuously filter feeding minute particles from the sea.

A previous major occurrence of PSP in Britain was in 1968, when 78 people in the north east of England were affected. Routine monitoring for toxin in mussels on the east coast was instigated after this outbreak. The action level for PSP toxin in mussels is 400 mouse units per 100 g of mussel tissue (a mouse unit being the amount of toxin required by injection to kill a mouse in 15 minutes). Levels detected in mussels in May 1990 were up to 20,000 mouse units. By July 1990, however, levels had fallen substantially.

Fish and shellfish inspection

The supervision of fish and shellfish constitutes an an important part of the duty of any environmental health officer. For the efficient performance of this duty, the inspector must possess knowledge of the distinguishing features of the various species of edible fish, the law relating to the marketing of fish, and a familiarity with trade practices. He must possess an intimate knowledge of the signs of freshness and staleness in fish, and of the methods by which various kinds of fish may be examined.

Fish is one of the most quickly perishable of foods. In order to be of good quality, it must be fresh and 'in season'. Fish are in best condition prior to spawning. The spawn is produced at the expense of flesh and tissue. After spawning, fish appear ill fed, the flesh is soft and flabby and will not keep.

Distinguishing features of fish (Fig. 36.6)

Round fish

1. **Cod.** Body: cylindrical, thick and rounded near the head. Colour: greenish or brownish-olive in colour with yellowish or brown spots; under parts white; white curved lateral line. Upper jaw longer; long barbel on chin. Fins: 3 dorsal, 2 pectoral, 2 ventral, 2 anal. Length: up to 90 cm.

2. **Haddock** (Fig. 36.7). Similar to, but smaller than a cod; black, curved lateral line with a blackish spot above the pectoral fin (called finger and thumb marks). Short barbel on chin. Colour: greenish bronze above, under parts white. Fins: 3 dorsal, 2 ventral, 2 pectoral, 2 anal. Length: up to 60 cm.

3. **Whiting** (Fig. 36.8). Smaller than a haddock; head pointed; well marked, curved lateral line, no barbel. Colour: greyish yellow with silvery under parts; black spot on the upper side of the root of the pectoral fin. Fins: 3 dorsal, 2 pectoral, 2 ventral, 2 anal. Length: up to 40 cm.

4. **Coalfish.** Larger fish than whiting, dark slate-blue in colour, almost black on back and sides. Lower jaw slightly longer than upper, small barbel. White, straight lateral line. Fins: 3 dorsal, 2 ventral, 2 pectoral, 2 anal. Length: up to 90 cm.

5. **Pollack.** Similar to the coalfish, but has no barbel. Dull green in colour; under parts whitish. Lower jaw protrudes. Dark lateral line well curved over pectoral fin. Fins: 3 dorsal, 2 ventral, 2 pectoral, 2 anal. Length: about 90 cm.

6. **Ling** (Fig. 36.9). Elongated fish with very small scales. Colour: usually grey with white under parts. Lateral line: not prominent; long barbel. Fins: 2 dorsal (the first high and short, the second extending almost to the tail), 2 pectoral, 2 ventral, 1 anal, 1 caudal. Length: up to 90 cm.

7. **Hake.** Body: long and slender, large scales, large mouth but no barbel. Colour: dark grey on back and slightly lighter on under parts. Lateral line: dark, slightly curved. Fins: 2 dorsal, 2 pectoral, 2 ventral, 1 anal. Length: up to 90 cm.

8. **Catfish.** Elongated and cylindrical body. Colour: bluish grey with dark broad bands down the sides. Smooth skin. Head resembles an ugly cat, with long canine teeth. Lateral line:

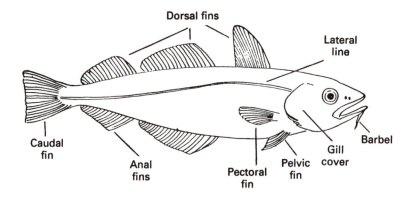

Fig. 36.6 Distinguishing features of a fish.

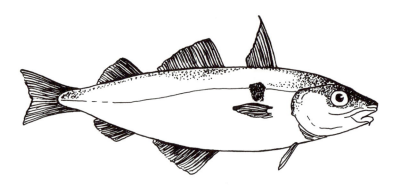

Fig. 36.7 Haddock.

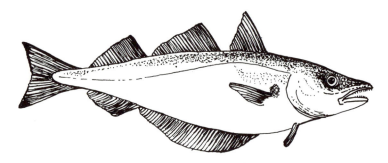

Fig. 36.8 Whiting.

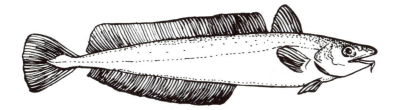

Fig. 36.9 Ling.

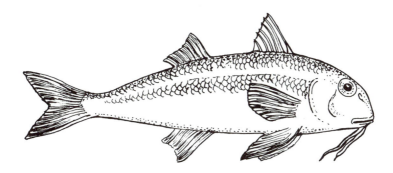

Fig. 36.10 Red mullet.

straight, not prominent. Fins: 1 long dorsal, 2 pectoral, 1 anal. Length: usually 60 cm. Another specimen of catfish is light grey in colour with large black spots covering the body. Black bands absent.

9. **Grey mullet**. Rounded body; large, round smooth scales. Colour: silvery grey. No lateral line. Fins: 2 short dorsal, front one composed of four spins, 2 pectoral, 2 ventral, 1 anal, 1 caudal. Length: up to 45 cm.

10. **Red mullet** (Fig. 36.10). Rather round body. Colour: bright red. Head has a front surface sloping down to the flat under-surface and the jaws and mouth are at the lower part. Two long, stiff barbels. Lateral line: straight. Fins: 2 dorsal, 2 pectoral, 2 ventral, 1 anal, 1 caudal. Length: up to 45 cm.

11. **Grey gurnard** (Fig. 36.11). Colour: grey with white spots. Head: strongly armoured with bony plates, and has an angular wall-sided shape; spines along lateral lines and base of dorsal fins. Fins: 2 dorsal, 2 pectoral, 2 ventral, 1 anal, 1 caudal; three lowest rays of the pectoral fins separate and independently movable. Length: up to 45 cm.

12. **Mackerel**. Body: cylindrical. Colour: green shot with blue, with dark, vertical wavy bars on sides; under parts silvery. Lateral line: straight. Fins: 2 dorsal, followed by 5 finlets, 2 pectoral, 2 vental, 1 anal. Length: up to 45 cm.

13. **Herring**. Colour is more greenish blue than in the sprat, silvery, and iridescent on sides and underparts. Lateral line: not continuous. Fins: 1 dorsal, 2 pectoral, 2 ventral, 1 anal, 1 caudal (ventral fins behind the commencement of the dorsal). Spines on the belly weak: edge of the belly rather blunt. Length: up to 30 cm.

14. **Sprat**. Colour: green-blue back, silvery sides and under parts. Smaller than the herring and dorsal fin a little farther back than in the herring. Lateral line: straight, not continuous. Ventral fins slightly in front of commencement of dorsal. Edge of the belly very sharp; spines on it strong. Length: up to 15 cm.

15. **Pilchard or sardine**. Colour: olive green above, silvery below. Belly: rounded with weak spines: body rounder and less deep than the herring or sprat. Lateral line: not continuous: straight. Fins: 1 dorsal, 2 pectoral, 2 ventral, 1 anal, 1 caudal; dorsal fin nearer the

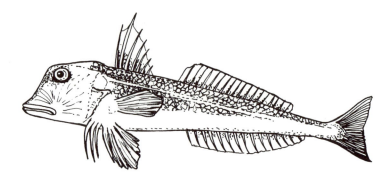

Fig. 36.11 Grey gurnard.

snout than tail. Ventral fin behind the commencement of the dorsal. Length: up to 22 cm.

16. **Salmon**. Long, round, fish. Colour: bluish black on the back with black spots above lateral line and on head; white under parts. Lateral line: straight. Fins: 1 dorsal, 1 adipose dorsal, 2 pectoral, 2 ventral, 1 caudal. Length: up to about 1.2 m.

17. **Common trout**. Colour: yellowish or reddish brown: cheeks and sides grey or a rich yellow; dark spots over upper part; red spots along lateral line; white below. Dorsal fin and gill covers; spotted. Fins: 1 dorsal, 1 adipose dorsal, 2 pectoral, 2 ventral, 1 anal, 1 caudal. Length: up to 70 cm.

18. **Eel**. Long, flexible body. Colour: dark olive green above and whitish or yellowish below. Fins: dorsal, caudal, and anal fins join, forming one long fin, extending from about a quarter of the length of the body from the snout to the middle of the body underneath. Lower jaw projects. Length: up to about 90 cm.

19. **Conger**. Body like that of eel, long, slender, flattening towards the tail. Colour: dark above, whitish beneath; dorsal fin edged with black. Fins: 2 pectoral. Dorsal fin commences close behind the pectoral fin and continues into the anal region, round the end of the tail. Mouth: wide, upper jaw slightly longer than lower. Length: up to 2.75 m.

Flat fish

1. **Turbot** (Fig. 36.12). Diamond shape with blunt, bony tubercles on the top side. Colour: mottled and speckled brown above, whitish below. Distinguished from brill by greater breadth in proportion to length and the presence of the tubercles. Lateral line: strong and arched. Length: up to 90 cm.

2. **Brill**. Like a turbot, but without tubercles. Longer than turbot in proportion to its width. Colour: mottled brown above, lower side white. Lateral line: strong and arched. Length: up to 60 cm.

3. **Halibut** (Fig. 36.13). Body thick and narrow, approaching the shape of an upright fish. Colour: olive or dark brown on the right side, white and sometimes mottled on left. Smooth skin, lateral line arched. Eyes: on right side. Length: 1.8–3.6 m.

4. **Sole** (Fig. 36.14). Narrow, oval shape. Mouth: not at end of snout but below it. Jaws: curved. Colour: brown or greenish brown, with rows of darker blotches along the centre of upper side and along base of fins. Lateral lines: straight. Length: up to 45 cm.

5. **Plaice** (Fig. 36.15). Shape: oval. Lower jaw longer than upper. Colour: brown with orange or red spots on the right hand side. Skin: smooth. Lateral line: nearly straight. Rough bony knobs on head. Eyes: on right side. Length: up to 45 cm.

6. **Witch** (Fig. 36.16). Body: long oval, very thin and flat. Colour: pale brown on one side, smokey white on the other. Head and mouth: smaller than plaice. Lateral line: straight. Eyes: on right side. Length: up to 45 cm.

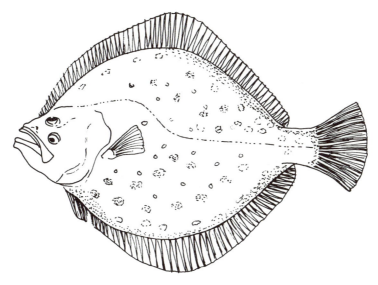

Fig. 36.12 Turbot.

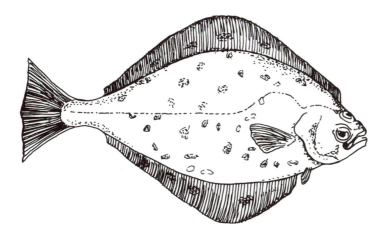

Fig. 36.13 Halibut.

7. **Dab** (Fig. 36.17). Shape: similar to plaice but usually smaller. Colour: light brown; no spots on the back. Lateral line: curved above pectoral fin. Skin: rough. Eyes: on right side. Length: up to 30 cm.

8. **Lemon sole or lemon dab** (Fig. 36.18). Shape: oval, small head and mouth. Skin: smooth and slimy. Colour: rich brownish yellow on right side, with round and oval spots of a darker colour; underside white.

Lateral line: straight. Eyes: on right side. Length: up to 45 cm.

9. **Megrim** (Fig. 36.19). Narrow, thin body. Eyes on left side. Colour: pale brownish yellow spotted with brown; dirty white underside. Lateral line: well marked and curved. Length: up to 60 cm.

10. **Flounder** (Fig. 36.20). Shape: like plaice. Colour: upper side brown, sometimes nearly black: underside brilliant white. Row of spiny

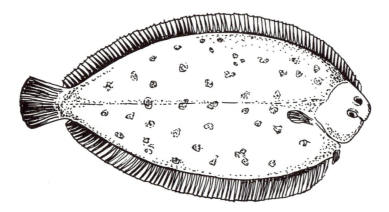

Fig. 36.14 Sole.

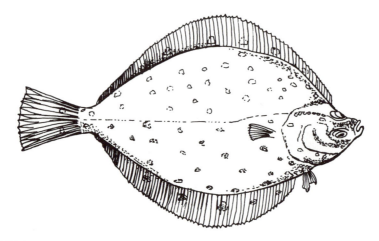

Fig. 36.15 Plaice.

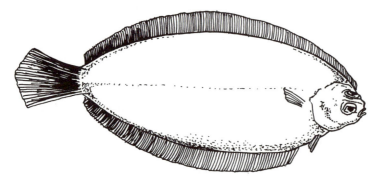

Fig. 36.16 Witch.

scales from head to tail along the middle of the dark side. Lateral line: straight. Eyes: on left side. Length: up to 33 cm.

Symmetrical flat fish

John Dorey (Fig. 36.21). Body: thin, deep, short with smooth skin. Colour: brownish with round

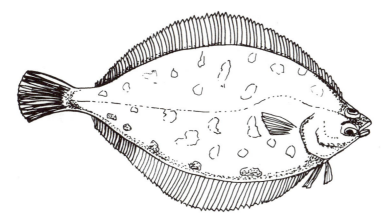

Fig. 36.17 Dab.

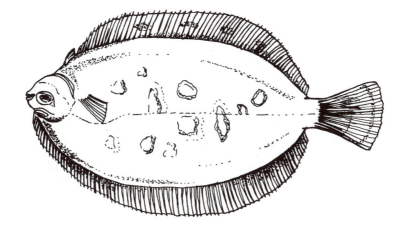

Fig. 36.18 Lemon sole.

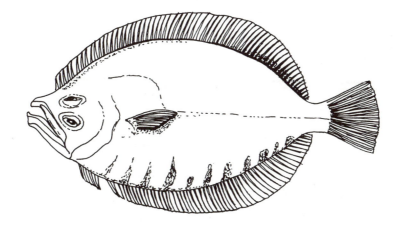

Fig. 36.19 Megrim.

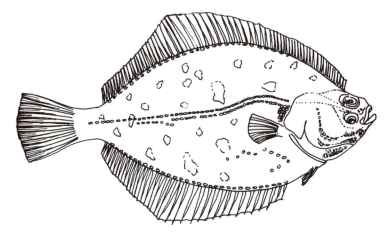

Fig. 36.20 Flounder.

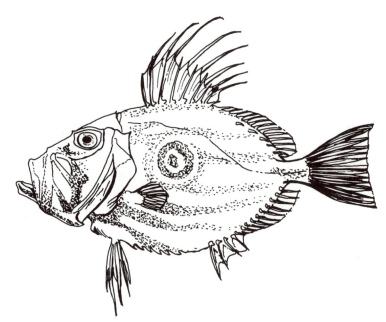

Fig. 36.21 John Dorey.

black spot in the centre. Fins: 2 dorsal, 2 pectoral, 2 ventral, 1 anal, 1 caudal, first dorsal fin with spines. Length: up to 60 cm.

Skate family (body vertically flattened)
Skate (Fig. 36.22). Rhomboid shape with tail not as long as body. Colour: grey or brown with blackish grey underside. Smooth skin with spines running down centre of body and tail. Length: up to 1.8 m.

Processed fish

Finnan haddock
The fish are beheaded, split, the air bladder removed, and then steeped in 70 to 80% brine for 3 to 15 minutes the time depending on the size and fattiness of the fish. They are then hung to drip (the longer the better), and smoked over soft wood and peat or oak sawdust from 4/6 hours. The temperature of the kiln should not exceed

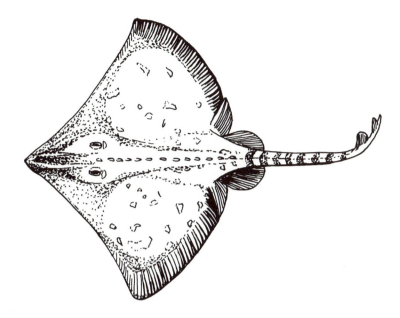

Fig. 36.22 Skate.

26.5°C. A golden yellow colour is regarded as desirable, and this is obtained by adding a dye to the brine.

Red herrings

For export, the whole fish is dry salted in concrete tanks (about 1 tonne of salt to 10 000 herrings) and left there for 14 days or longer. They are then smoked for a period of 2/3 weeks. For home consumption, the fish are kept in brine from 2/5 days when smoked over small fires of oak chips and sawdust for a fortnight or longer.

Golden cutlets

Small whiting and haddock are usually block filleted, although whiting may be skinned. After thorough washing, they are weakly brined in a solution containing a dye, and the lightly smoked for 2/3 hours.

Bloaters

Prepared from whole herring slightly salted (usually mixed with salt and left overnight), washed, then threaded on speats and smoked for 4 hours at 29 to 32°C.

Fillets

Fresh haddock, cod, ling, pollack or coalfish are filleted and most of the lug removed; cod fillets are normally skinned. They are put in 70 to 80% brine for 4 to 10 minutes; dye is added to the brine bath and fish allowed to drip for at least 2 hours and then smoked for 2 to 5 hours according to their size.

Buckling (hot smoked herrings)

Herrings are usually beheaded and gutted, and then immersed in 70 to 80% brine for 1 hour. They are then hung up to drip, and then smoked for 1 hour at a temperature of 32°C, followed by a second hour at 44 to 49°C, and a third hour at 71 to 77°C.

Smokies

Haddock or whiting which have been beheaded and hot smoked.

Kippers

These are prepared from herrings which are washed, split down the back and gutted, and brined for anything up to 30 minutes depending on their size and fattiness. Dye is added to the brine; they are hung up to drip for at least 1 hour and then smoked at a temperature not exceeding 30°C (usually about 4 hours for dyed and 6 hours for undyed fish).

For the smoking of fish see below.

Smoked mackerel

The fish are headed and gutted. The gut cavity is cleaned and the black belly wall lining is removed. They are then soaked in 75% brine for 1 to 1½ hours before being hung up to drain for a similar period. The fish are then threaded on to speats and smoked at 30°C for 1 hour, the temperature being raised to 50°C for the second hour. The fish are then turned and smoked for a further 1 to 1½ hours at 75°C before being removed and cooled.

Kippered mackerel

Gutted mackerel may be split down the back in the same way as herring are prepared for kippering, or block fillets may be cut from the fish. The fish are then soaked in 75% brine for 12 minutes (7 minutes for fillets), drained for about 2 hours and cold smoked in a mechanical kiln at 30°C. Fillets require about 2½ hours, split fish about 4 hours.

Curing of fish

Smoking of fish

The reason for smoking fish is to impart a more tasty flavour and to ensure some degree of preservation. The smoking processes involve the use of a cold or a hot smoke, the cold smoke cure being the one most usually used in this country, the smoke being generated from hardwood sawdust.

Usually, the fish is first soaked in brine to reduce the moisture content, allowed to drain, and then smoked in a kiln which is either a brick chamber connected to a chimney, or a mechanical kiln such as the Torry. In the Torry kiln, the smoke is led into the chamber by ducts, heating being provided by electric steam or hot water heaters, which permits the kiln to be operated at a controlled temperature. The warm smoke is blown over trolleys on which the fish is hung, and the trolleys may be interchanged to ensure that the fish nearest the incoming duct is not excessively dried. A proportion of the smoke is continuously vented to the atmosphere and replaced by fresh smoke. A kiln of this type gives a more uniform product, more quickly and with less labour than the traditional kiln.

In hot smoking, the fish is cooked as well as smoked. The method is used for eels, sprats, buckling and Arbroath smokies.

Salt curing

Common salt is used for this, the purpose being to delay, or even prevent the growth of spoilage organisms, partly by the withdrawal of moisture. The two types of cure are known as 'dry' and 'pickling'.

The absorption of salt depends on many factors, one being the fattiness of the fish so that the dry cure is usually used for white fish such as cod, and the pickle for such fish as herring and mackerel.

There are two types of dry cure, the heavy or hard cure and the Gàspe or light cure, in which the fish is not exposed to the action of the salt for such a long period.

In the heavy cure, the fish, after being beheaded, gutted and split, are stacked with alternate layers of salt. It is kept like this for about a fortnight, but may be more, during which time the liquor is allowed to escape. It is now said to be lying in wet stack, and periodically the fish is restacked to produce an even cure.

PINK. If the fish lie in wet stack for too long, spoilage occurs, and one group of causative organism imparts a pink colour to the fish. In the early stages, this can be removed by scrubbing and washing. If left too long, the flesh becomes brown, soft, offensive and unfit for consumption.

In the pickling process, the fish are packed, alternating with layers of salt, in closed barrels, the pickle being formed by the salt dissolving in the body fluids.

The purity of the salt is an important factor in the dry cure, and it appears that the bacteria which cause pink are actually in the salt, and while causing putrefaction of the fish, are harmless to humans.

DUN. The lighter cure is not usually attacked by pink because the salt content is inadequate for the growth of the organism, but spoilage known as 'dun' does occur. This is a grey, black or fawn mould which first appears as small spots. It gets unsightly but does not render the fish unsafe or inedible and can be removed by wiping.

Examination of fish

The general condition as to the freshness of fish may usually be obtained by superficial examination. Fresh fish is bright in appearance, as if it were alive. The eyes are bright and full, and the pupil black; the gills are bright red in colour; the flesh is firm to the touch and the body is stiff; the abdominal cavity is clean and free from offensive colour.

A stale fish has eyes that are dull and sunken, and the pupils grey; the flesh is soft and limp, the body is flabby, not stiff; the gills are dark red, grey, brown or green in colour, the walls of the abdomen are discoloured and the smell is offensive.

If a more complete examination is necessary, the fish must be split. If stale, the flesh leaves the bone easily. A pink colouring along the backbone is a sure sign of decomposition. The membrane below the backbone in the abdominal cavity (sometimes known as the 'sound') should be examined. In fresh fish, the blood is a natural red colour and of normal consistency. If stale, it is dark, thick, and may be offensive.

Points in connection with the special examination of various fish are as follows:

1. **Cod.** As above. In salted cod, pink patches or spots are a first sign of decomposition.
2. **Haddock.** Cured haddock should 'handle' dry and be bright yellowish in colour.
3. **Herring.** Suspend the fish – head upward – between the finger and thumb. In this position, pressure upon the gill covers will, if the fish is fresh, cause a stream of bright red blood to

exude, of normal consistency and free from offensive odour. If stale, the blood is scarce, thin, dark in colour and may be offensive.
4. **Spray.** Test as with herring.
5. **Mackerel.** Test as with herring. The fish should be stiff, and the eyes bright. The first sign of decomposition is the soft, jellified condition of the abdominal walls. The fish decomposes readily.
6. **Smelt.** When fresh, it exudes an odour like that of a cucumber.
7. **Skate and dogfish.** A strong smell of ammonia in the early stages of decomposition.

Diseases and conditions of fish

Wet fish is a valuable and safe source of protein food, which is generally free from abnormality or disease. There are, however, a few conditions which may become evident during processing.

Parasites
1. **Roundworms** are the most common parasites found in fish, tapeworms and flukes being much less common, many worms only affect the viscera and are therefore removed by gutting.
2. *Anisakis simplex* is similar to the codworm (see below) which is white in colour and therefore difficult to detect. Judgment is as with the codworm.
3. *Chloromysciumthyrsites* is a protozal infection which affects the hake in particular. Enzyme actions are produced by the organism, which severely soften the flesh a few days after they are caught. Fish affected are often termed 'milky' hake.
4. *Dibothriocephalus latus* is a tapeworm which can infect humans who have eaten infected fish which has been undercooked. Pike, cod, grayling and, perch and salmon have been found to harbour cysts of the adult worm, which are readily recognised as a white body in the flesh of fish. Affected fish are unfit for human consumption and may be seized.
5. *Grillitia ermaceus* is found in its adult stage in roker fish, but the halibut is the host for the

completion of the larval stage. It is harmless to man.

6. *Phocanema* (**codworm**) (previously *Porrocaecum decipiens*) is a round worm commonly found in cod. It is up to 2.5 cm long and varies in colour from creamy white to dark brown. The worm is found mostly in the liver and around the gut, but when infestations are heavy, worms penetrate the flesh where they often become coiled and encased. The worms eventually die but can survive in an active state for years. There is no evidence to suggest that the worm causes illness in man. They are killed by freezing and cooking, although they may survive the curing process.

   Since these worms are often embedded deeply in the flesh, superficial inspection of fillets is not enough, but a large proportion can be detected if the fillets are candled. Although harmless, fish severely affected should be rejected on aesthetic grounds.

7. *Sarcotases* is a parasite which penetrates the musculature or visceral cavity of fish and grows to a length of several centimetres. It is repulsive in appearance as its gut consists of a bag filled with black fluid (digested blood); it is often buried deep in the muscle of the fish.

Diseases

1. **Furunculosis** is an infectious condition caused by the bacillus *Salmonicida* which affects many species of freshwater fish, including salmon and trout. Affected fish develop nodules beneath the skin which burst or discharge fluid. Affected fish should be regarded as unfit for human consumption as this is a highly contagious disease.

2. **Salmon disease** (salmon plague) affects fish of the salmon family, which results in white patches which grow to cover the fish and kill it. This is another highly contagious disease, and it is recommended that affected fish are burnt to destroy the causative organisms.

3. **Tuberculosis**, in the form of nodules within the flesh or gut, is occasionally found in fish. The lesions result from infection by *Mycobacterium*

tuberculosis, but the condition is not communicable to man.

4. **Tumours** occur in fish and may be malignant or benign, particularly sarcomata. They appear as fibrous growths in almost any location, with osteomatas running down the radial bone of the fish. Halibut are often affected and catfish and cod are affected to a lesser degree. Localized lesions may be trimmed, but badly affected fish should be rejected as unfit for consumption.

5. **Ulcerative dermal necrosis (UDN)** causes an ulcerative condition of the gills and head of salmon. It is a viral disease which is often associated with a secondary fungal infection, which gains access through damaged tissue.

Other conditions

1. **Colour abnormalities** may be seen occasionally, e.g. red cod or green flounder. These fish are usually rejected as unmarketable, though they may be fit for consumption.

2. **Damage** is caused by careless handling on vessels and in docks and in nets. Soft fleshed fish are particularly vulnerable, and many fish have to be rejected because of damage which makes them unsuitable for processing.

3. **Emaciation** in fish (or 'slinkers') is normally found around spawning time. The flesh is flaccid and watery, and the condition results in fish of poor quality. It is an offence to sell freshwater fish in this condition.

4. **Weedy fish** often have an iodine-like smell and are sometimes referred to as 'stinkers'. The peculiar smell is caused by the fish eating a pteropod, *Himacina helicine*, which is found in northern waters (Barents Sea). The smell does not render the fish unfit for food, but a retailer might find it unsaleable.

Bacterial conditions

Fish are by no means a common source of food-borne infections. However, the common types of food poisoning organisms grow on seafoods if allowed suitable conditions.

1. *Clostridum botulinum* occurs naturally in the marine environment, the type E strain being

usually associated with fishery products. Several deaths per year are caused throughout the world, and are usually attributable to under-processed fish or faulty canning techniques. Large numbers of this organism have been found in commercial trout farms and, therefore, strict attention to all stages of production to ensure the organism is not given a chance to produce its potent neurotoxin. (See DHSS guidance note, *Recommended Practices for the Processing, Handling and Cooking of Fresh, Hot-smoked and Frozen Trout* [24], and MAFF Guidance on the Microbiological Safety of Smoked Fish [25].)

2. **Salmonellae** and *Staphylococcus aureus* are not regular inhabitants of either the fresh or salt-water environments. Fishery products can, however, become contaminated during processing.

3. *Vibrio parahaemoliticus* occurs naturally in fish and is a major cause of gastroenteritis in Japan, where fish forms an important part of the diet. The organism is generally killed by cooking and most outbreaks result from under-processed or cross-contaminated products.

4. **Scombroid poisoning**, see Chapter 17.

Distinguishing features of shellfish

The term shellfish includes creatures of the orders mollusca, which can be subdivided into bivalves (mussels, oysters, clams, cockles, scallops), univalves (periwinkles and whelks) and crustacea (crabs, lobsters, crayfish, prawns, shrimps, etc.) (see Fig. 36.23).

Molluscs

1. **Cockle *(Cerastoderma edule)*.** Roughly circular concave shells having ribs radiating from the hinge. The colour of the shell is usually cream or fawn with some darker markings. Size: up to 4 cm diameter. The flesh is partly grey, partly yellow with occasional orange patches.

2. **Clam *(Venus merceneria)*.** Harplike symmetrical shells with clear concentric growth lines. The colour of the shells is a pale fawn to a yellowish brown. The flesh varies from cream to a yellowish beige in colour. The syphon is black and there is a small purple patch on the otherwise white interior of the shell.

3. **Escallop *(Pecten maximus)*.** Two concave, tightfitting, fan-shaped shells which possess distinctive ribs. The upper shell is flat and the lower concave. The shell is pink or orange brown. Size: approximately 10 cm. The flesh is white (adductor muscle) and the roe orange. When prepared for sale, the other organs are removed.

4. **Mussel *(Mytilis edulis)*.** Two smooth, concave, symmetrical shells. The colour of the shells being blue-black. Size: approximately 7.5 cm long and 2.5 cm wide. The flesh is beige and orange in colour.

5. **Oysters.**
   (a) Native oyster *(Ostrea edulis)*. A roughly circular, thin upper shell with a slight protrusion at the hinge or heel. The lower shell is deeper and heavier. Colour: varies from pale beige to greenish brown, but annual growth rings are always visible on the shell. The adductor muscle is a pinkish or yellowish beige white, the surrounding cillae and alimentary system is somewhat darker. Oysters from certain areas possess a greenish tinge.

   (b) Portuguese oyster *(Crassostrea angulata)*. The shell is in two parts, the upper flatter than the lower, which is concave. Both shells are more irregular and longer than the shells of the native oyster. The shell is flint like and greenish grey in colour. The flesh is a pale greenish white.

   (c) Pacific oyster *(Crossostrea gigas)*. Two roughly triangular shells, the upper flatter than the lower, having a frilled appearance derived from the irregular annual shell growth, which protrudes from below that of the previous year. Colour varies from bluish grey to dark green if covered with marine organisms. The flesh is cream-beige.

6. **Periwinkle *(Littorina littorea)*.** A small, compressed, thick spiral shell which is almost spherical. The entrance is bluish white and is guarded by a blackfoot, but the shell is black

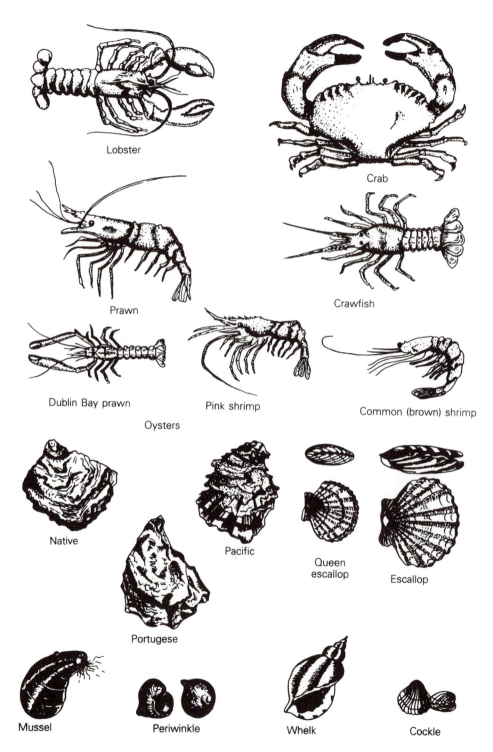

Lobster

Crab

Prawn

Crawfish

Dublin Bay prawn

Pink shrimp

Common (brown) shrimp

Oysters

Native

Pacific

Queen
escallop

Escallop

Portugese

Mussel

Periwinkle

Whelk

Cockle

Fig. 36.23 Shellfish.

or grey black. Size: approximately 2.5 cm. The flesh is dark grey to black in colour.

7. **Queen escallop *(Chlamys opercularis)*.** Very similar to the escallop but both shells are concave and smaller than the escallop. The colour is usually pink, red-brown or yellow marked with white. Size approximately 9 cm. The flesh is white with a smaller orange roe than the escallop. (Where the fish are mechanically processed the roe is removed with the other viscera.)

8. **Whelk *(Buccinum undatum)* ('buckie').** A strong, thick spiral shell which is pale sandy-brown in colour with lighter and darker markings. The entrance may be closed by the extension of the 'foot', a round bony plate. Size: approximately 7.5 to 10 cm. The flesh is dull yellow with darker coloured viscera and is long and thin.

Crustacea

1. **Crab *(Cancer pagurus)*.** A roughly oblong carapace with rounded corners. When alive the upper surface is brownish red and the underside yellowish white. The first pair of legs are modified into heavy, black claws, each with a moveable pincer. The shell surface is minutely granulated and the front margin is divided into lobes. After boiling, the colouring lightens and becomes more red than brown. Size: across the back up to 30 cm. The white meat, muscle, is removed from the claws and brown meat, liver and gonads, is found in the carapace. Sexual difference: the tail or apron of the female is heart shaped and broad, while in the male it is narrow.

2. **Crawfish *(Palinurus elephas)* 'spiny lobster', 'langouste').** The carapace is reddish brown and spiny with two strong spines protecting the eyes, which are large and globular. The tail is cylindrical with sharp-edged bony plates on the flanks and ends in a bony fan. There are single acting claws on the first pair of legs, and the antennae are long with spiny bases. Size: up to 45 cm. The flesh of the tail is used for food and is similar to that of the lobster.

3. **Dublin Bay prawn *(Nephrops norvegicus)* ('scampi', 'Norway lobster', 'langoustine').**

The body and tail are narrow and cylindrical. The first pair of legs is slender and long with unequal claws, each having one moveable pincer. The eyes are large and the rostrum is long and has three teeth on each side. It has four short and two long antennae. The colour is pale flesh, darker in parts, which becomes a more opaque orange after boiling. Length: up to 20 cm. The tail meat is white with some pale pink bands.

4. **Lobster *(Homarus gammarus)*.** The carapace is cylindrical with a well-developed rostrum. The tail segments taper only slightly and terminate in a broad fan of overlapping shell segments. The claws are very large, unequal in size and each has a moveable pincer. The remaining legs are round and weak. It has four short and two long antennae. The colouring is blue-black on the back and flanks with a little creamy or orange spotted colouring on the underside. When boiled it becomes bright scarlet. Length: up to 45 cm. The male has five body segments and relatively heavier claws. The female has seven body segments. The tail meat is pinkish white. That of the claws is covered with a pinkish orange skin.

5. **Prawn *(Pandalus borealis)*.** The carapace has a long, slightly upward curved rostrum, and the antennae are long and pink and the eyes are large. It has a series of sharp points along the head. When fresh, the prawn is translucent grey, spotted, and lined with purplish grey. When boiled, prawns turn pinkish red. Length: up to 10 cm. The meat of the tail is pinkish white and segmented.

6. **Shrimps.**

(a) Brown shrimp *(Crangon crangen)*, (common shrimp). The brown shrimp has no rostrum, the forward edge of the carapace having a series of serrations. The eyes are conspicuous and close together. It has two long and four short antennae with scales on the base of the first pair. The first pair of legs is robust, smooth and strong and form small claws. Length: up to 6 cm. It is almost colourless but develops its colouring when boiled.

(b) Pink shrimp (*Pandalus montagui*). The rostrum is long and almost straight with a slight curve upwards at the extremity. There are 7 to 8 teeth on the upper side, and three on the underside. It has large eyes and long antennae, and the first pair of legs are short. It is almost colourless but develops its colour when boiled. Length: up to 5 cm.

Examination of shellfish

Bivalves should be alive before processing, and this can be readily checked by ensuring that the shells are closed, or close quickly if tapped. The shells should sound like hard pebbles when tapped together, the body being firm and rigid. After death, the flesh of the animals decays rapidly, becoming soft and damp with a characteristic foul odour. They may become unfit within an hour or so. A bag or sack of mussels, when shaken, should have a solid sound, whereas there would be a hollow or rattling sound should they be unfit. Two exceptions to this rule are the escallop and the queen escallop, which may well keep for several days after death.

The operculum of univalves should be moist, tight closed and fresh looking in a sound specimen. The flesh should be firm and fresh, with a minimum of slime and should have a pleasant smell. As the animal begins to decay, the operculum becomes open or loose. The shell gives a dull sound on tapping and the body becomes soft, sticky and slimy and has an offensive odour.

Lobsters and crabs are cooked before consumption and turn pink on boiling. The animal should still be alive or should have been boiled while still fresh. The tightness of joints and compactness of limbs indicate it was killed by immersion in boiling water or, in the case of crabs, was killed immediately before boiling. The shell is crisp, bright and dry in the case of boiled lobster, and has a pleasant, slightly sweet smell.

Decay causes a stale, sticky exudate to be emitted from between the joints of the limbs and tail, giving off an offensive odour (particularly under the apron of crabs and the carapace of lobsters), and a discoloration from pink to grey-green or brown if severe.

Prawns and shrimps should be crisp, dry and clean, with a fresh, sweetish, slight iodine-like smell. During the decay process, the shells become soft and wet and soapy to the touch. Heat is produced when these animals decompose and ammonia is produced. It is possible to plunge a hand in a bag of prawns or shrimps in order to determine fitness by reference to temperature.

Conditions and diseases of shellfish

The majority of shellfish are eaten raw or only partially cooked. They are rarely completely sterilized by cooking, and if derived from layings polluted by sewage. there is a real danger of their being the means of conveying water-borne diseases. Many outbreaks of typhoid or enteric fever and other gastro-intestinal infections have been traced to the consumption of polluted shellfish.

Shellfish layings are generally situated in estuaries where the danger of sewage pollution is high. Certain shellfish, e.g. cockles, mussels and winkles, occur principally on mud banks and are collected at low tide when the danger of pollution is at its height.

1. **Salmonellae** may be found in molluscs and crustacean shellfish taken from polluted coastal waters, or contaminated during handling. Although only small numbers are found on fresh shellfish, poor storage and handling can allow the organism to multiply.
2. *Vibrio parahaemolyticus* is a naturally occurring organism, and is widely distributed in the marine environment. It is more commonly found in crustaceans, but has been recorded in molluscs. Food poisoning from this organism is likely to occur only when shellfish are incorrectly processed under conditions whereby the vibrio can proliferate.
3. **Erythematous** is an allergic condition sometimes known as musseling or mussel poisoning. A severe allergic effect is produced on persons who have a natural susceptibility to it.
4. **Paralytic shellfish poisoning** can result from eating mussels which feed on planktonic proto-

zoa, principally on the genus *Gonyaulax*. These produce a potent neurotoxin (see page 564).

5. **Viral hepatitis type A** is a serious disease for which shellfish have been shown to be a source of infection. Because of the lack of suitable methods for isolating viruses, and because the incubation period is long, the role of shellfish is not fully understood. There is evidence that virus particles can remain viable in sea water for longer periods than faecal bacteria, and under certain conditions viruses may be retained in molluscs after they have been subjected to purification processes. Mussels, oysters and clams from various parts of the world have been shown capable of accumulating entero-viruses from the water in which they have been feeding.

6. **Parasitic organisms** may be present where shellfish are exposed to sewage. However, the present role of shellfish in the spread of parasitic disease appears to be limited. (There is evidence that lung fluke infection caused by *Paragonimus westermani* may be due to the consumption of raw, freshwater crab.)

7. The regular consumption of large quantities of shellfish containing accumulated **chemical substances** such as heavy metals, may lead to chronic intoxication of the consumer.

REFERENCES

1. Letter from MAFF Jun–13.42.14 July 1993, Implementation Of New Poultry Meat Hygiene Directive, MAFF Public Consultation Document Jun–5.16, Implementation of EC Directive 92/116/EEC and Parts Of 91/495/EEC and 91/494/EEC in Great Britain.

2. 'The National Meat Hygiene Service.' *Environmental Health*, **101/102**, 76–90.

3. Meat Products 1992, Advice For The Meat Products Trade, Food Sense, MAFF/HMSO, 51 Nine Elms Lane, London SW8 5DR.

4. Department of Health Information. A Guide to Single Market Hygiene Controls for Food Businesses, Department of Health, Skipton House, 80 London Road, London SE1 6LW.

5. Department of Health and Ministry of Agriculture Fisheries and Food (1990) *Ten Point Plan For Safer Cooked Meat Production*, HMSO, London.

6. Department of Health and Social Security (1972) *Processing of Pasteurized Large Canned Hams*, Advisory Memorandum, HMSO, London.

7. Department of Health. Guidelines for the Safe Production of Heat Preserved Foods, 1994. HMSO, London.

8. Advisory Committee On The Microbiological Safety Of Food (1993) *Report on Salmonella In Eggs*, HMSO, London.

9. Department Of Health (1988) Avoid Eating Raw Eggs, Press Statement August, Department of Health, Skipton House, 80 London Road SE1.

10. Advisory Committee On The Microbiological Safety Of Food (1993). *Report on Salmonella In Eggs, Recommendations And Government's Response*, Microbiological Safety Of Food Division, MAFF, Room 515a, Ergon House, 17 Smith Square, London SW1P 3JR.

11. Department of Health, Guidance For Enforcement Officers On The Egg Products Regulations 1993, Department of Health, Skipton House, 80 London Road, SE1 6LW.

12. Ministry of Agriculture Fisheries and Food (1975) *A Guide To Clean Milk Production*, BS 5226: 1975, HMSO, London.

13. Institution Of Environmental Health Officers (1989) *Guidelines for the Sampling and Testing of Pasteurized Milks for Enforcement Purposes*, IEHO, London.

14. British Standards Institute (1990) *British Standard Code of Practice for the Pasteurization of Milk on Farms and in Small Dairies*, DAC 17, BSI, London.

15. The Creamery Proprietors Association (1988) *Guidelines For Good Hygienic Practice In The Manufacture Of Soft Fresh Cheeses*, Creamery Proprietors Association, London.

16. Milk Marketing Board (1989) *Guidelines for Good Hygienic Practice for the Manufacture of Soft and Fresh Cheeses in Small Farm Based Production Units*, MMB, Thames Ditton.

17. Specialist Cheese Makers Association, *Hygiene Standards Scheme*, Specialist Cheese Makers Association, Thames Ditton.

18. Correspondence (1984) Self pasteurizing soft ice cream machines – 'Carpigiami' 'Coldelite' and 'Luna-Ice'. *Environmental Health* **92** (2).

19. Ice Cream Alliance, The Ice-Cream Federation in Association, Institution of Environmental Health Officers, Department of Health and Milk Marketing Board, *Code of Practice for the Safe Handling and Service of Scoop and Soft Serve Ice Cream*, Ice Cream Alliance, 90/94 Grays Inn Rd, London WC1X 8AH.

20. Department of Health, EC Directives on Fish (EC/Fish) 10/92.

21. Department of Health, EC Directive on Shellfish (EC/Shellfish) 10/92.

22. Department of Health, Shellfish Hygiene Directive and Fish Hygiene Directive, EHO Guidance, Package 1994.

23. Bartholomew, B.A. (1987) Scombrotoxic fish poisoning in Britain: features of over 250 suspected incidents from 1976 to 1986. *Epidemiology and Infection*, 775–82.

24. Department of Health and Social Security, *Recommended Practices for the Processing, Handling and Cooking of Fresh, Hot-smoked and Frozen Trout*, HMSO, London.

25. Microbiological Safety of Smoked Fish, MAFF Food Sense, London SE99 7TT.

FURTHER READING

Bacon and Meat Manufacturers Association, *Code of Practice for the Hygienic Manufacture of Meat Products*, BMMA, London.

APPENDIX

Table of EC Food Hygiene Directives and UK Implemented Regulations (as at September 1994): Vertical/ Horizontal Food Hygiene Directives

EC Directives	Adopted	UK Regulations	Implemented
Fresh (red) meat			
1. Council Directive 64/433/EEC on health conditions for the production and marketing of fresh meat	26 June 1964		
2. Council Directive 91/497/EEC amending and consolidating Directive 64/433/EEC on health problems affecting intra-Community trade in fresh meat to extend it to the production and marketing of fresh meat	19 July 1992 for implementation no later than 1 January 1993	The Fresh Meat (Hygiene and Inspection) Regulations 1992*	1 October 1992 – Regulations 4, 5, 6, and 9
3. Council Directive 91/498/EEC on conditions for granting temporary and limited derogations from specific community health rules on production and marketing of fresh meat	29 July 1991 for implementation not later than 1 January 1992		
Poultrymeat			
4. Council Directive 71/118/EEC on health problems affecting trade in fresh poultry meat	15 February 1971		
5. Council Directive 92/116/EEC amending and updating Directive 71/118/EEC on health problems affecting trade in fresh poultry meat	17 December 1992 for implementation not later than 1 January 1994	The Poultry Meat, Farmed Game Bird Meat and Rabbit Meat (Hygiene and Inspection) Regulations 1994*	1 May 1994
Wild game			
6. Council Directive 92/45/EEC on public and animal health problems relating to the killing of wild game and the placing on the market of wild game meat	16 June 1992 for implementation not later than 1 January 1994	The Wild Game (Hygiene and Inspection) Regulations	in draft
Rabbit meat and farmed game			
7. Council Directive 91/495/EEC concerning public health and animal health problems affecting the production and placing on the market of rabbit meat and farmed game meat	27 November 1990 for implementation not later than 1 January 1993	See Poultrymeat	

* To be replaced by new regulations in 1995.

EC Directives	Adopted	UK Regulations	Implemented
		Meat products	
8. Council Directive 77/99/EEC on health problems affecting intra-Community trade in meat products	21 December 1976		
9. Council Directive 92/5/EEC amending and updating Directive 77/99/EEC on health problems affecting intra-Community trade in meat products and amending Directive 64/433/EEC	10 February 1992 for implementation no later than 1 January 1993	The Meat Products (Hygiene) Regulations*	in draft
10. Proposal for a Council Directive amending 77/99/EEC on health problems affecting the production and marketing of meat products and certain other products of animal origin	in draft	The Products of Animal Origin (Import and Export) Regulations 1992	1 January 1993
Commission Decision laying down special conditions for approval of rewrapping centres referred to in Directive 77/99/ EEC, and for the marking of products therefrom	in draft		
Proposal for Commission Decision on the conditions and criteria to be applied to establishments manufacturing meat products without an industrial structure or production capacity	21 April 1994		
		Minced meat and meat preparations	
11. Proposal for an EEC Council Directive laying down the health rules for the production and placing on the market of minced meat and meat preparations	in draft		

* Now the Meat Products (Hygiene) Regulations 1994.

EC Directives	Adopted	UK Regulations	Implemented
Balai			
12. Council Directive 92/118/EEC laying down animal health and public health requirements governing trade in and imports into the Community of products not subject to the said requirements laid down in specific Community rules referred to in Annex A(I) to Directive 89/662/ EEC and, as regards pathogens, to Directive 90/425/EEC	17 December 1992 (for implementation by 1 July 1994)		
Commission Decision on the marketing and imports of eggs	in draft		
Note *Further decision on gelatins for human consumption, frogs legs and snails to be decided*			
Fishery products			
13. Council Directive 91/493/EEC laying down the health conditions for the production and the placing on the market of fishery products	22 July 1991 for implementation not later than 1 January 1993	The Food Safety (Fishery Products) Regulations 1992	1 January 1993 – Regulations 9(1) parts, 9(2), 8, 10
Note *Provisions of Directive (91/493/ EEC) to be re-examined before 1 January 1998 by the Council acting on proposals from the Commission on the basis of experience gained*			15 January 1993 – remaining Regulations
		The Food Safety (Fishery Products) (Import Conditions and Miscellaneous Amendments) Regulations 1994	in draft (planned 1 July 1994)
		The Food Safety (Fisheries Products) (Derogations) Regulation 1992	1 July 1992
Commission Decision 93/140/ EEC laying down the detailed rules relating to the visual inspection for the purpose of detecting parasites in fishery products	19 January 1993	The Food Safety (Fishery Products) (Import Conditions and Miscellaneous Amendments) Regulations 1994	in draft (planned 1 July 1994)

EC Directives	Adopted	UK Regulations	Implemented
Commission Decision 93/185/ EEC laying down transitional measures concerning the certification of fishery products from third countries in order to facilitate the switch over to the arrangements laid down in Council Directive 91/493/EEC	15 March 1993	The Food Safety (Fishery Products) (Import Conditions and Miscellaneous Amendments) Regulations 1994	in draft (planned 1 July 1994)
Council Decision 93/383/EEC on reference laboratories for the monitoring of marine biotoxins	14 June 1993		
Council Decision 93/351/EEC determining analysis methods, sampling plans and maximum limits for mercury in fishery products	19 May 1993		
Commission Decision (94/—) laying down the rules for the application of the second subparagraph of Article 6(i) of Directive 91/493/EEC	(at SVC 20/21 April 1994)		not yet published
Commission Decision 93/140/ EEC laying down the detailed rules relating to the visual inspection for the purpose of detecting parasites in fishery products	19 January 1993	The Food Safety (Fishery Products) (Import Conditions and Miscellaneous Amendments) Regulations 1994	in draft (planned 1 July 1994)
Commission Decision 93/185/ EEC laying down transitional measures concerning the certification of fishery products from third countries in order to facilitate the switch over to the arrangements laid down in Council Directive 91/493/EEC	15 March 1993	The Food Safety (Fishery Products) (Import Conditions and Miscellaneous Amendments) Regulations 1994	in draft (planned 1 July 1994)
Council Decision 93/383/EEC on reference laboratories for the monitoring of marine biotoxins	14 June 1993		
Council Decision 93/351/EEC determining analysis methods, sampling plans and maximum limits for mercury in fishery products	19 May 1993		
Commission Decision (94/–) laying down the rules for the application of the second subparagraph of Article 6(i) of Directive 91/493/EEC	(at SVC 20/21 April 1994)		not yet published

EC Directives	Adopted	UK Regulations	Implemented
Live bivalve molluscs			
14. Council Directive 91/492/EEC laying down the health conditions for the production and the placing on the market of live bivalve molluscs	15 July 1991 for implementation not later than 1 January 1993	The Food Safety (Live Bivalve Molluscs and Other Shellfish) Regulations 1992	1 January 1993 – Regulations 1–5, 7–9 and 14.
Note *Provisions of Directive (91/492/ EEC) to be re-examined before 1 January 1998 by the Council acting on proposals from the Commission on the basis of experience gained*			15 January 1993 – remaining Regulations
		The Food Safety (Live Bivalve Molluscs) (Derogations) Regulations 1992	1 July 1992
		The Food Safety (Live Bivalve Molluscs and Other Shellfish) (Import Conditions and Miscellaneous Amendments) Regulations 1994	in draft (planned 1 July 1994)
Milk and milk-based products			
15. Council Directive 92/46/EEC laying down the health rules for the production and placing on the market of raw milk, heat-treated milk and milk-based products	16 June 1992 for implementation not later than 1 January 1994	The Dairy Products (Hygiene) Regulations	in draft
16. Council Directive 92/47/EEC on conditions of granting temporary and limited derogations from specific community health rules on production and placing on the market of milk and milk-based products	16 June 1992 for implementation not later than 1 January 1993 – Article 2(2); 1 January 1994 – remaining provisions.		
Commission Decision on general hygiene conditions in sheep and goat's milk productions holdings	in draft		
Commission Decision laying down rules for TB checks for goats kept with cows	in draft		
Commission Decision amending article 5.9 of Directive 92/46 with regard to freezing point of milk	20 April 1994		

EC Directives	Adopted	UK Regulations	Implemented
Commission Decision establishing maximum residue content of pharmacologically active substances in milk	in draft		
17. Council Directive amending 92/46/EEC laying down health rules for the production and placing on the market of raw milk, heat-treated milk and milk-based products (COM (93)715)	in draft		

Eggs and egg products

EC Directives	Adopted	UK Regulations	Implemented
18. Council Directive 89/437/EEC on the hygiene and health problems affecting the production and placing on the market of egg products	20 June 1989 for implementation not later than 31 December 1989		

Note

The Commission to report to the Council with proposals for amending the annex of Directive (89/437/EEC) to take account of experience gained and scientific and technological developments by 31 December 1994

EC Directives	Adopted	UK Regulations	Implemented
19. Council Directive 91/684/EEC amending Directive 89/437/EEC on the hygiene and health problems affecting the production and placing on the market of egg products	19 December 1991 for implementation not later than 31 December 1991	The Egg Product Regulations	14 July 1993

Hygiene of foodstuffs

EC Directives	Adopted	UK Regulations	Implemented
20. Council Directive 93/43/EEC on the hygiene of foodstuffs	14 June 1993 for implementation not later than 30 months after date of (14 January 1996)	The Food Safety (General Food Hygiene) Regulations	Regulations out for consultation

Note

The Commission to examine the relationship between this, and the product specific Directives and, by 14 June 1996, make any appropriate proposals in the interests of compatability

37 Food hygiene

Mike Jacob

CONTROLS OVER FOOD HANDLING PERSONNEL

Major risks of food contamination can lie with food handlers, depending on their degree of conscientiousness in handling the food which other people will eat, the amount of training which they have received and the degree of supervision applied in the particular establishment. Organisms of the genera *Salmonella* and *Campylobacter*, and the bacterium *Staphylococcus aureus*, may be transmitted by food handlers through cross-contamination of food and food surfaces. Given the right conditions within the food premises, these organisms may multiply to an infective dose causing an outbreak of food poisoning when food from the establishment is consumed.

Food handlers may acquire contamination from the food they handle in any particular establishment. This can apply particularly to processing factories where large quantities of poultry cuts, mincemeat, etc., may be handled by numerous employees. Management should be aware of such risks and take adequate screening precautions and protective measures to avoid employee contamination in this way. Additionally, where employees suffer personal symptoms of gastro-intestinal disease, perhaps after holidays abroad, they should have sufficient awareness of the significance of these symptoms in relation to their tasks as food handlers.

This is a matter primarily of effective training in food hygiene, which is the only way to achieve long-term high standards of food handling habits among personnel in food premises.

Protective clothing

Management should set an example by always wearing protective clothing in food handling areas, as should all visitors to premises. This particularly applies to environmental health officers when entering food handling areas.

Clothing should be light in colour, changed frequently, and made of a material that can be easily washed and kept clean. Protective clothing should adequately protect the food and the wearer. Cooks and those engaged in preparing and serving food should have white or light-coloured overalls that ensure that food will not come into contact with clothes worn underneath. Head coverings to protect the food from hair, as well as to protect the hair and scalp from the effects of steamy heat, fat vapours and flour, should be worn. For heavy duty work, e.g. preparing vegetables and cutting meat, rubber aprons are recommended.

First-aid equipment

Adequate and easily accessible bandages, dressings and first-aid equipment are required under the food hygiene regulations. Cuts or scalds should be covered with protective waterproof dressings so that any infection does not spread. Blue waterproof dressings are preferable as they can be easily seen if they get into food. One member of staff trained in first aid should be available whenever employees are on duty in the kitchen or food processing area. Names of such staff should be clearly displayed within the work area.

Anti-microbial effectiveness of handwashing in food establishments

The epidermal layer of the skin contains many cracks, crevices and hollows favourable to bacterial growth. Bacterial flora can also become established in the hair follicles and the sweat and sebaceous glands. High humidity can create a moist and nutritious environment causing a rapid growth of micro-organisms.

Persons who work in environments that have high temperatures and humidity, such as a kitchen in a restaurant, can develop a very dense microflora on their skin. Total bacteria counts, the number of Enterobacteriaceae, *Salmonella*, *Escherichia coli* and *Staphylococcus aureus* on the hands and forearms, are dramatically affected by where a person works. For those workers in meat, poultry and egg processing operations there will likely be regular and heavy contamination of hands from such organisms as *Escherichia coli* and *Staph. aureus*, and species of *Salmonella*.

Personal hygiene is highly important in any food establishment. Bathing and handwashing should follow any act that offers even a remote possibility that the hands have picked up contamination; the covering of cuts and abrasions and designated areas only for smoking, are principles to be applied.

Hand soaps containing antimicrobial agents and alcohol applications may be used, but what should be stressed in food service establishments is proper and frequent handwashing. Any handwashing and hand treatment must kill a broad spectrum of micro-organisms, especially pathogenic bacteria, while also maintaining a residual effect on the skin without causing irritation [1].

Health surveillance

A WHO consultation document [2] concluded that routine medical laboratory screening of food handlers is of no particular value. Such examination can only reveal the health status of the worker at the time of the examination, and cannot take into account later bouts of diarrhoea or other infectious conditions. Medical examinations are also unreliable in the detection of

carriers of pathogens who, in most cases (with the possible exception of those excreting *S. typhi*), are unlikely to transmit gastro-intestinal organisms. Food handlers should, however, be encouraged to report any illness immediately.

There is no evidence that food handlers infected with human immunodeficiency virus (HIV) transmit the virus through food. Therefore, routine serological testing for HIV is not relevant. A commonsense approach to monitoring the health of staff is recommended with special arrangements for contract staff who visit food handling areas, e.g. to clean or service food vending machines.

Questionnaires should be completed by all job applicants and then looked at by a doctor acting on behalf of the food service establishment. The doctor can assess from the questionnaires whether further examination or treatment is necessary. In some cases, it may be decided that because of the medical history, individuals should not be employed at all in food handling.

Food handlers should be encouraged to adopt a code of personal hygiene embodied in a leaflet or booklet given to them when they take up employment. This should make reference to the need for food handlers to report infections to their employers and information regarding visits to doctors when ill, to alert such doctors that the patient is a food handler. Workers employed in NHS catering establishments are provided with such a book, *Clean Food* [3].

EU requirements on medical examination of food handlers

EC directives on poultry, meat, fresh meat and meat products require medical examination before staff commence work on food handling and the medical certificate must be renewed annually. The Directive on the Hygiene of Foodstuffs (93/43/EEC) however merely has the following requirements:

No person known or suspected to be suffering from, or to be a carrier of, a disease likely to be transmitted through food or while afflicted for example with infected wounds, skin infections, sores or with diarrhoea, shall be permitted to work in any food handling area in any capacity in which there is any likelihood of directly or indirectly contaminating food with pathogenic micro-organisms.

This provision clearly places the responsibility on proprietors or managers of food businesses and the employees themselves to ensure food handling personnel are medically fit to handle food. Proprietors and managers may therefore require medical examinations of employees to ensure compliance with this requirement.

The future will likely see the provisions on personal health of food handlers in all the commodity Directives and those in Directive 93/43, brought into line making a consistent requirement on fitness to handle food applicable to all food sectors.

MICROBIOLOGICAL RISK ASSESSMENT

Many food premises in which food is manufactured stored or sold are not purpose built. Buildings that are planned and designed to optimize natural lighting, ventilation and other environmental conditions, and with new facilities, will promote higher hygiene standards. Where buildings are non-purpose built, management and employees have to be aware of the hazards which might arise because of poor design, and difficulties in cleaning, storage of raw materials and waste disposal.

Microbiological aspects of food poisoning are minimized by good quality control procedures over all aspects of handling. There must be an understanding of the risks that can arise from handling raw food materials, including cross-contamination. Effective cleaning of surfaces, equipment and the structure of premises, the general cleanliness and conscientiousness of the employees in food handling, adequate cooking and cooling and other temperature control arrangements, effective and secure packing and final storage before despatch or service to customers are other important elements of quality control.

Fresh thinking has had to be applied and cleaning arrangements in the light of problems associated with *Listeria monocytogenes*. Unlike species of *Salmonella*, which up to now has represented the main pathogenic risk in food-handling situations, organisms can grow at temperatures as low as 3°C (temperatures lower than most domestic and commercial refrigeration equipment is able to achieve under normal circumstances).

In catering and retailing, even under cool, ambient conditions, it is not likely that refrigeration and storage cabinets are generally able to achieve temperatures lower than 5°C. For the food manufacturer, in large or small operations, this means that it is highly important that food susceptible to listeria growth, such as patés, soft cheeses and cooked chicken dishes, leave the manufacturing or process areas free of listeria. Where a product is contaminated prior to distribution, the organisms proliferate at the temperatures normally found at the retail outlet.

Pathogens like wet environments and listeria is no exception, being commonly found in drains and wet areas of processing factories. Wood surfaces and hard cold surfaces susceptible to condensation are likely to harbour *Listeria* organisms, and if these cannot be avoided, cleaning systems have to be devised effectively to reduce contamination risks. Experience in the US dairy industry suggests an effective policy appropriate in dairy environments is to assume the presence of listeria within food process areas, but to establish the exact location of the bacteria by a series of precise sampling investigations [4]. When positive areas of listeria presence have been established, the cleaning schedules that are devised and the protective measures that are employed provide an effective guarantee of success in eliminating the organisms.

The use of high-pressure sprays within process areas should now be avoided wherever possible, because water droplets increase the likelihood of spreading *Listeria* organisms from one area to another. The use of colour-coded brushes and other cleaning equipment, and effective isolation of wet process areas from dry in, for example, milk powder manufacturing plant, are other important measures for reducing listeria risks.

Handling foods likely to be contaminated by viruses

Viruses are living organisms that are smaller than bacteria. They have been recorded as causing outbreaks of intestinal illness even though they cannot multiply in foods, only in certain living tissues. The spread of viruses from the hands of human carriers and from water to food is important. Molluscan shellfish grown in sewage-polluted water may be significant in causing viral illness. Fruit and vegetables contaminated by faeces and various types of salad prepared under unhygienic conditions have also been involved in outbreaks of viral contamination.

Viral contamination risks in foodstuffs, therefore, are usually due to contamination of the foods while they are growing or during harvesting or preparation.

Outbreaks of illness associated with small, round viruses have been common in molluscan shellfish, and an outbreak of viral hepatitis was traced to frozen raspberries picked in Scotland where the pickers contaminated them in the field through lack of proper sanitary accommodation being provided [5,6].

Consumers should be aware of the sources of foods and the hygiene of production methods. For example, it should be known that shellfish products, such as oysters, clams and mussels, have originated from clean seawater sources, or have been subject to purification; and that other molluscs, such as cockles, have been heat processed to ensure that a centre temperature of 90°C has been achieved for at least one-and-a-half minutes.

Critical Use of Water in the Food Industry

Environmental health officers should be aware of the risks posed by the use of water by the food industry. Where chlorinated mains water is used the efficacy of chlorination in removing contamination should not be taken for granted and frequent in-plant checks should be carried out. Where secondary water storage takes place within food factories further chlorination or other treatment of water may be necessary and tanks should be checked regularly for dead rodents or birds. The use of river water or private boreholes for cooling or washing purposes should be investigated thoroughly, particularly where large volumes of water are being used by high throughput factories.

Purposes for which water may be used in food production

FOR COOLING PURPOSES (not in contact with the product)

- Milk heat exchangers – cold or chilled.
- Condensers (refrigerating plant and evaporators) compressors, etc.
- Cooling sterilized can products – potentially in contact with products.

FOR HEATING PURPOSES

- Heating section of HTST plant, etc.
- Boiler feed.
- Heat recovery from hot condensates, etc.

FOR CLEANING PURPOSES

- Rinsing churns and other plant.
- Chemical cleaning solutions.
- Washing of yards and floor areas.
- Flushing toilets.

USED AS INGREDIENT OR OTHERWISE IN CONTACT WITH PRODUCTS*

- Liquid drinks, cottage cheese, butter wash water, watering concentrates, baby foods.
- Follow-through water in pasteurizing plant; pre-rinse of other plant when rinsings are saved.
- Bottle washer final rinse.
- Rinsing plant after cleaning and chemical sterilization.
- Canteen, drinking water, wash basins, sinks.
- Crop irrigation.
- Transportation medium (fruit, vegetables, fish).

For standards applicable: for the use of water in food production, see Chapter 44.

* High risk use.

CATERING PREMISES

Problems associated with catering hygiene standards in the UK mainly concern the use of non-purpose-built kitchens, the employment of untrained staff, poor supervision and inadequate knowledge in dealing with pathogenic risks that can arise during the preparation and serving of foods. A detailed examination of these aspects is contained in Chapter 9 of Part II of the Richmond Report [7].

Effective temperature controls for foods and the provision of appropriate cooking and cooling equipment are essential prerequisites for good catering operations. The reduction of cross-contamination risks can be achieved by designing effective handling procedures with line arrangements that ensure that raw materials pose no threat to foods under preparation or service by cross-contamination. In an ideal situation, persons handling raw materials should be separate from those handling cooked foods, but the scale of many small catering operations means that in the course of a working day, supervisors, managers and employees may be involved in numerous tasks involving the handling of both raw and prepared foods. This does not necessarily pose problems provided the personnel involved exercise proper precautions and have been appropriately trained as to the risks involved.

Thorough cooking should kill the bacteria present in raw foods. Although some bacteria can give rise to spores that can survive cooking, problems will only arise if the cooling of cooked food takes place too slowly, or if, after cooking, the food is stored at kitchen temperatures for excessive periods. Meat and poultry obviously need the most care, especially if joints of meat or birds are large. Meat and poultry should be cooked so that an internal temperature of 70°C is reached in the deepest part of the bird or joint for 2 minutes. Internal temperature checks of meat and poultry using probe thermometers are recommended.

A wide variety of kitchen equipment is currently used in catering operations. There is no central approval system for the hygiene and appropriate nature or design of appliances used for preparing and cooking foods in the UK. Some of this equipment may not be easily cleanable, and frequent inspection of the appliances may, therefore, be necessary. Environmental health officers often experience difficulties in requiring the dismantling of complex machinery for the purposes of cleaning, and it may be necessary to use the powers in the Food Safety Act 1990 for serving improvement and emergency prohibition notices for specific items of dirty and uncleansed equipment of this type. A particular problem is the continued and ongoing use to which such equipment is put over long working periods with little respite for cleaning, and to remove grease and food debris. This can lead to a build-up of food residues and pest infestation in catering establishments. Initiatives on European food equipment standards are currently being considered in response to EC Directive 89/392/EEC. which will apply to food machinery including catering equipment. Work in this area is being undertaken by the British Standards Institute.

The Directive covers both safety and hygiene requirements, dealing with such aspects as surfaces; assembly; ease of cleaning; and, if necessary, disinfection; prevention of the entry of pests or accumulation of waste food in areas which cannot be cleaned, and the provision of suitable instructions [8].

The Directive has led to European Working Groups being formed under CEN Technical Committee 153 to draw up standards. National Panels set up under BSI include membership drawn from industry, HSE, food research associations and environmental health officers from the Department of Health, the CIEH and the Royal Environmental Health Institute of Scotland. Working groups and national panels cover the following machinery:

Food Processing (MCE/3/5)
Bakery Machinery (MCE/3/5/1)
Meat Processing (MCE/3/5/2)
Food Slicing (MCE/3/5/3)
Catering (MCE/3/5/4)
Edible Oils and Fats (MCE/3/5/5)
Pasta Processing (MCE/3/5/7)
Bulk Milk Coolers (MCE/3/5/8).

Methods of cooking

Quick, high-temperature cooking is the best for food safety. Steam under pressure, thorough roasting of small quantities of meat, and grilling and frying are the best means to achieve thorough cooking. In convection ovens, air is circulated by a fan to improve the transfer of heat and to make cooking faster, more even and effective than in conventional ovens. Vegetative bacterial cells are killed in such ovens, but not necessarily spores. In pressure steamers, food can be cooked to order within minutes. They create good conditions for the destruction of bacteria and spores by the combination of pressure and heat. In hard water areas, it is usually necessary to install a water-softening plant to treat the water to be used for steam generation.

Microwave ovens

Microwave ovens have in recent years undergone much scrutiny, and the performance standards of a number of ovens have been found unsatisfactory when subjected to critical testing and laboratory examination. A number have been removed from the market as a result of this exercise. A new system for classifying domestic microwave ovens to improve and simplify cooking instructions has been agreed [9]. The UK Association for the Manufacture of Domestic Electrical Appliances (AMDEA) announced that from 1 September 1990, all the ovens marketed by their members in the UK would be rated for power output according to the procedure described in the international standard IEC 705.

Microwaves heat food by agitating the molecules, especially water molecules. The main disadvantages of microwave cooking are poor heat distribution and the inability to brown joints of meat. To overcome these problems, some ovens have forced air convection currents and infra-red sources so that they can roast, bake, fry and grill in the same way as conventional ovens. 'Standing times', i.e. the time that the food should be allowed to stand after being removed from the microwave oven, must be observed. A survey carried out by environmental health officers in 1990 found that about half the microwave ovens used by caterers were domestic models. Sustained use of a domestic microwave oven can lead to a build-up of heat in the magnetron, which results in a significant reduction in power output. The Ministry of Agriculture, Fisheries and Food (MAFF) requested the Institution of Environmental Health Officers to encourage the use of catering microwave ovens rather than domestic models in commercial premises, and has written to organizations in the catering industry on similar lines. In addition, MAFF has commissioned research into the variability of performance of microwave ovens for catering purposes.

Hazards in catering

Slowly cooked rare beef has been the cause of many outbreaks of salmonellosis and *Clostridium perfringens*, and is due to the ineffectiveness of the time/temperature combination to destroy these organisms present in the meat. An internal temperature of 70°C must be achieved to provide an effective thermal kill.*

Restrictions on the use of unpasteurized milk, shell eggs and egg products due to salmonella risks are other areas for environmental health officer investigation in catering practices. Additional responsibilities concerned with storage temperatures involve frequent checks on perishable foods requiring storage at 8°C and under.

Reheating

It is common practice to cook large joints of meat or poultry and then to slice them ready for reheating after a period of refrigeration or storage at ambient (room) temperature. This practice should be discouraged as it prolongs the time the meat is kept within a temperature range suitable for the multiplication of bacteria, particularly salmonella and *C. perfringens*. Where meat is stored overnight under refrigeration prior to

---

* Recent evidence suggests that 'cold spots' on kitchen griddles can result in coliforms in meat not being destroyed. Illness caused by *E. coli* 0157:47 has been reported (*E. coli* 0157:47. Human illness in North America. *International Food Safety News*, Feb. 1993, Vol. **2**, 15–16.

reheating next day, it should be sliced and stored in shallow trays in refrigerators operating at or below 5°C to ensure that all the meat being stored is effectively chilled.

Wherever possible, environmental health officers should advise proprietors, particularly of small catering establishments, to keep meat raw and preferably cold overnight, and to cook it thoroughly on the day it is required. If reheating before serving is unavoidable, an internal temperature of 70°C must be achieved.

Temperature checks with probe thermometers should be used as a routine. Stews, curries, soups, mincemeat, gravies and sauces are common causes of food poisoning. On reheating, the middle of the mass of food may not reach a high enough temperature to kill bacteria. Such dishes should be cooked and eaten on the same day, but if reheating is unavoidable they should be heated throughout to a temperature of at least 70°C, and maintained at that temperature for at least 2 minutes before consumption. Any liquid or solid prepared dishes should never be reheated more than once, i.e. they should not be heated more than twice in total.

Cook-freeze and cook-chill systems

Detailed guidance on these systems are contained in the Department of Health guidelines on cook-chill and cook-freeze catering systems [10]. Both cook-freeze and cook-chill systems have advant-

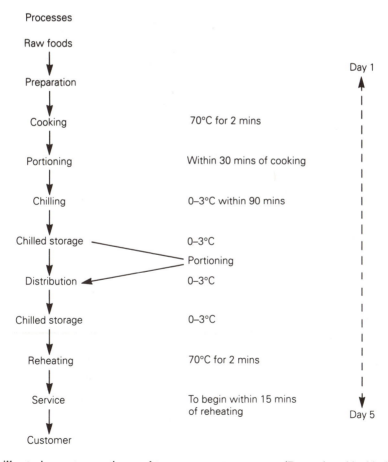

Fig. 37.1 Cook-chill catering systems – time and temperature parameters. (Reproduced by kind permission of Mrs A. West, Huddersfield Polytechnic, and the Campden Food and Drink Research Association, Chipping Campden. Source: see Fig. 37.2.)

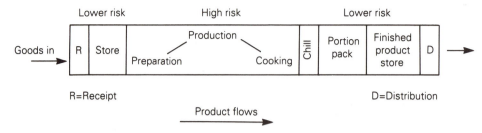

Fig. 37.2 Cook-chill catering system – design for linear flow. (Reproduced by kind permission of both Mrs A. West, Hotel & Catering Research Centre, Huddersfield Polytechnic from her paper 'Design Requirements of Cook-Chill', and the Campden Food & Drink Research Association, Chipping Campden, Gloucestershire. Source: Campden Food & Drink Research Association (1989) Hygiene – The Issues for the '90s, *Campden Food and Drink Research Association Symposium Proceedings 7–8 November*, 1989, pp. 142–8.)

ages for catering. Stores can be centralized, staff time saved and portions controlled. However, in both systems, a mistake in the preparation of batches of food could possibly lead to large-scale outbreaks of food-borne disease. Recent concerns have centred on listeria risks associated with cook-chill foods, but surveys of products, particularly supplied to the National Health Service, have confirmed that even though *L. monocytogenes* can grow at 3°C, the organism is rarely found in cook-chill foods.

A comprehensive approach to hygiene control is required in these type of operations, a highly important element being that after initial cooking, the temperature range at which surviving organisms can grow (7°C to 60°C) must be spanned as rapidly as possible to minimize growth during cooling after cooking and during thawing or reheating (see Figs 37.1 and 37.2.) [11].

Cook-freeze
This system of catering is a method of preparing and cooking food in economic quantities, retaining it in a state of suspended freshness by rapid freezing and freezer storage, and serving it when and where required from finishing kitchens which require relatively low capital investment and minimal staffing.

Fig. 37.3 shows a simplified arrangement by which the benefits of a factory scale operation become possible. On a smaller scale, using a conventional cooking area, meat, fish, vegetables, sweets and pastry would be produced on a batch basis, one at a time.

Generally speaking, three kinds of initial storage are required: frozen storage for vegetables and dairy products, and dry storage for dry goods. The size of the stores is dictated by the frequency of deliveries and production demand.

The normal food preparation equipment is used during production, but it is vital that it is of sufficient rating to ensure it meets the output demanded of it. As much of the equipment is in use throughout the day, it is important that it is easy to clean and maintain. Indeed, it is essential that the working conditions of a cook-freeze kitchen are maintained at a high standard. Control of bacterial contamination and multiplication, is achieved by initial quality control and batch checks. In large factory style production, full-time quality control staff will be needed, although for smaller operations environmental health departments will be able to offer assistance.

Food control temperature chart

Fig. 37.4 shows the main examples of the critical temperatures in relation to general handling of foods and the various process controls.

Assured Safe Catering

The Department of Health has recently produced guidance for caterers – referred to as 'Assured Safe Catering' – which is based on the application of hazard analysis principles [13]. In addition to

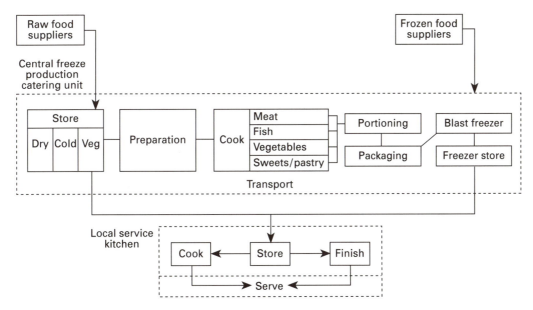

Fig. 37.3 Diagram to illustrate the main features of the cook-freeze process.

the comprehensive advice contained in this publication, a summary of the main points are published separately in a leaflet [14].

Assured Safe Catering looks at the catering operation step by step, from the selection of the ingredients right through to the serving of food to the customer. By analysing each step of the operation, anything which might affect the safety of the food is identified. The caterer is then able to decide when and how to control these identified hazards.

Essential elements in the process are:

Stage 1: planning. Planning and preparation are necessary before developing the system. Staff must be fully briefed and kept up to date on proposed changes in the management of the catering operation. Too much must not be attempted at once. A staged control programme is advised.

Stage 2: getting organized. A decision on how many people are necessary to operate a control system is necessary. This obviously will vary according to the size of the business. In large businesses it may be justifiable to set up a team. Persons able to recognize biological, physical or chemical hazards must be included and abilities to

identify control measures and critical points are also essential.

Stage 3: drawing up a flow diagram (Fig. 37.5). This needs to show each step of the operation from purchase of ingredients to food service to the customer. Once the diagram has been prepared it needs to be checked to ensure that all foods produced in the establishment are covered.

Stage 4: listing the hazards and introducing the controls. This stage is the essential one to ensure that the catering operation is a safe process. It has six sub stages:

(a) Listing the hazards – if staff members are unable to recognize hazards, external help should be sought. A hazard is defined as anything that can harm a consumer.

(b) Identify the control measures – actions necessary to remove the identified hazards or reduce them to safe levels. Control measures must be able to be carried out in the kitchen where they are to be operated.

(c) Critical Control Points – these are the steps in the food preparation routine which have to be carried out correctly to make sure that hazards are removed or reduced to safe levels, e.g. cooking or cooling to appropriate temperatures.

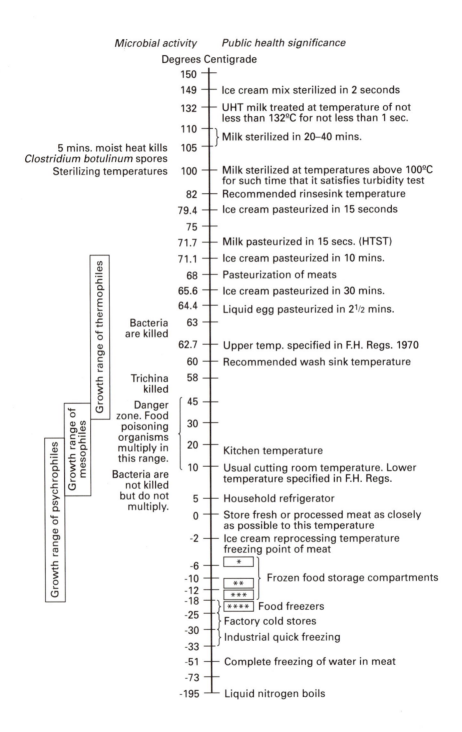

Microbial activity　　*Public health significance*

Degrees Centigrade

	150	
	149	Ice cream mix sterilized in 2 seconds
	132	UHT milk treated at temperature of not less than 132ºC for not less than 1 sec.
	110	} Milk sterilized in 20–40 mins.
5 mins. moist heat kills	105	
Clostridium botulinum spores		
Sterilizing temperatures	100	Milk sterilized at temperatures above 100ºC for such time that it satisfies turbidity test
	82	Recommended rinsesink temperature
	79.4	Ice cream pasteurized in 15 seconds
	75	
	71.7	Milk pasteurized in 15 secs. (HTST)
	71.1	Ice cream pasteurized in 10 mins.
	68	Pasteurization of meats
	65.6	Ice cream pasteurized in 30 mins.
	64.4	Liquid egg pasteurized in 2½ mins.
Bacteria are killed	63	
	62.7	Upper temp. specified in F.H. Regs. 1970
	60	Recommended wash sink temperature
Trichina killed	58	
Danger zone. Food poisoning organisms multiply in this range.	45	
	30	
	20	Kitchen temperature
	10	Usual cutting room temperature. Lower temperature specified in F.H. Regs.
Bacteria are not killed but do not multiply.	5	Household refrigerator
	0	Store fresh or processed meat as closely as possible to this temperature
	-2	Ice cream reprocessing temperature freezing point of meat
	-6	[*]
	-10	[**] } Frozen food storage compartments
	-12	[***]
	-18	[****] Food freezers
	-25	Factory cold stores
	-30	Industrial quick freezing
	-33	
	-51	Complete freezing of water in meat
	-73	
	-195	Liquid nitrogen boils

Growth range of thermophiles

Growth range of mesophiles

Growth range of psychrophiles

Fig. 37.4 Food control temperature chart.

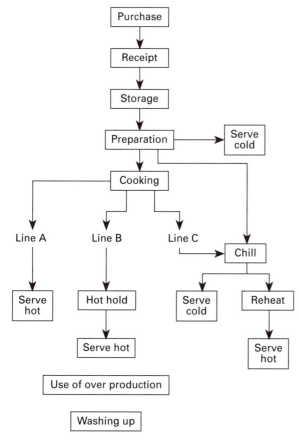

Fig. 37.5 Assured safe catering: flow diagram of any catering operation.

(d) Decisions on how to check, and if necessary record, that controls have been applied – checks should be kept as simple as possible, e.g. that knives, chopping boards, etc., are properly cleaned before use; – records should indicate that the food safety controls are adequate and work effectively.

(e) Putting the system into action – preparation of record sheets; instructions for staff on controls and checking procedures. These should say:

What is to be done
How it is to be done
When it is to be done
Where it is to be done
Who is to do it.

(f) Checking the system – once the system is in place for the first step of the operation, it should be checked through to ensure that it is running as planned; e.g. checking of the critical points is satisfactory.

Stage 5. A repeat of stage 4 for each step of the catering operation.

Stage 6: a full system check. Once the system has been set up for all the steps on the flow chart a check is necessary that the whole system is working as intended. This means making sure that the critical points identified are:

being applied correctly;
being checked as often as necessary;
accompanied by adequate instructions.

Stage 7: full system review. After the system is up and running, changes may be made in the nature of the business, the premises or the staff. A review of the system may then be necessary to make sure that it is still working as originally designed.

Assured Safe Catering could perhaps be alternatively named 'Applied common sense in catering', as the principles of risk assessment and management supervision over critical aspects of food production should have no mystique about it. The HACCP discipline does however require perhaps more than usual management consideration of the step by step approach and ability of staff to assess risks and understand the controls. Hopefully these recent Department of Health publications will be effective in making catering operations safer and better managed in the future.

Hygiene of premises

Layout

Food premises must be designed so as to produce a logical flow of work in such a way as to separate different work processes, particularly those where cross-contamination is possible, e.g. preparation and cooling areas (see Fig. 37.6). Regard must also be paid to providing adequate space for activities to be undertaken and to the ease with which cleaning can be carried out. Particular care needs to be taken when existing premises are to be adapted for use, since problems of layout are often difficult in these circumstances. Fig. 37.7 shows a diagrammatic layout of a school meals kitchen.

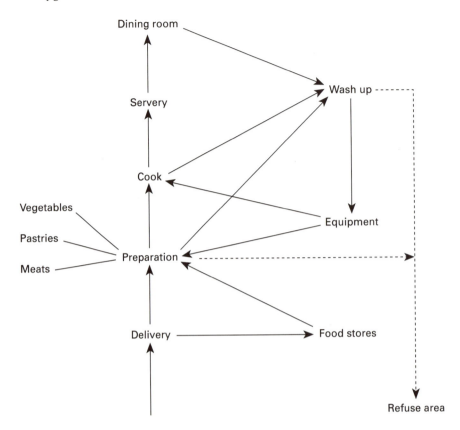

Fig. 37.6 Work flow in catering premises.

Floors

These must be constructed of a hard, impervious material which is relatively smooth but which is not slippery even after wetting. Care must be taken in the use of jointed materials to avoid crevices in which grease might accumulate. Hard tiles of quarry, terrazzo or granolithic types are excellent. In areas subject to heavy wear by trolleys, etc., carborundum strengthened tiles should be used. Wherever possible, floor construction should be solid and not suspended. Joints between floor and wall surfaces should be coved to facilitate cleaning.

Walls

Again hard, smooth finishes are essential with any joints being flush and narrow. Ceramic tiles are excellent, although difficulties can occur where heavy use is envisaged, e.g. around machinery.

Laminated or stainless-steel sheeting may also be used, but particular attention needs to be given to jointing and to avoiding gaps between the back of the sheeting and the wall surface where insect infestations can occur. Hard plaster surfaces finished with gloss paint are also acceptable.

Light-coloured finishes are essential, not only to highlight dirt but also to assist in the overall lighting of the room. Obstructions to access to wall surfaces such as that which might be provided by plumbing and ductwork should be avoided. These should either be let in floors, walls or ceilings or should be contained in casing which can be constructed at the floor/wall or wall/ceiling junction.

Ceilings

Surfaces need to be carefully chosen in order to avoid condensation problems. Plasterboard with

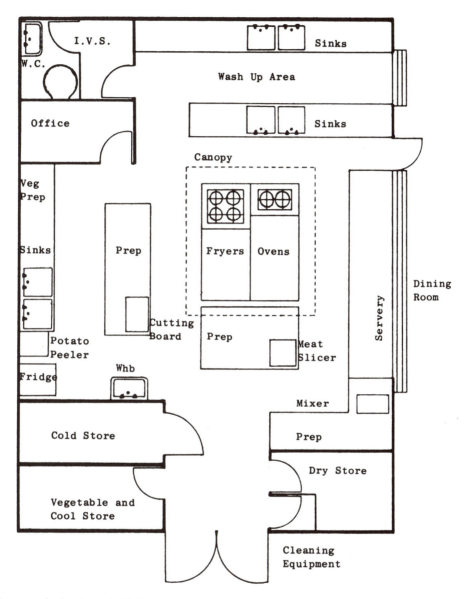

Fig. 37.7 Layout of school meals kitchen.

emulsion paint is satisfactory in most situations. Suspended ceilings provide harbourage for rodents and insects. Light colours are required to finishes.

Lighting
Adequate lighting is essential in order to provide safe working conditions and to aid cleansing. Fluorescent fittings are preferable to tungsten.

Ventilation
Particular attention needs to be paid to areas where cooking and equipment washing is taking place, since inadequate ventilation in these areas can lead to excessively high working temperatures and the creation of stress conditions. It is doubtful whether natural ventilation can ever be satisfactory in these situations and mechanical ventilation should, therefore, always be incorporated.

Design is assisted if all cookers and washing operations are grouped together so that steam and vapours can be collected at one point in each case and transferred to the atmosphere via exhaust ventilation. In many circumstances, particularly in congested urban areas, some form of odour treatment is necessary, and this can be effectively provided by the use of carbon filter units.

Refuse

The amount of refuse stored within the premises must be restricted to the minimum, and should be restricted to the use of paper/plastic sacks or plastic bins with lids for the reception of waste in preparation areas. and these should be replaced as frequently as possible. Refuse storage should be provided externally in an area properly paved and drained to a trapped gully. Hosing facilities are desirable. The type of container provided will depend upon the needs of the particular premises, but can include plastic or galvanised bins with tight-fitting lids, or galvanised bulk containers (1 cu m). Collection should be frequent and in all catering premises this should be daily.

The storage of bulky, dry waste creates considerable difficulty, particularly in premises with restricted outside space. The use of a small, commercial compactor can be beneficial in these circumstances.

Equipment

A wide range of equipment will be found in food premises but there are general rules which can be applied. It must be:

1. constructed so as to facilitate ease of cleaning and be free from inaccessible points;
2. non-absorbent;
3. placed in such a way that cleaning is possible on all sides.
4. well maintained.

Cleansing

The fundamental objective in food premises is the killing of pathogenic organisms and the elimination of situations in which they might thrive.

PLANNED PROGRAMME The cleaning of the structure, equipment and working surfaces should be on a planned programme basis devised for the particular premises and based on a principle that cleaning should, as far as possible, be undertaken on a 'clean as you go' basis. Cleaning programmes should be in written form and agreed with the staff and the environmental health officer. An example is shown in Table 37.1.

CLEANSING TECHNIQUES . These must incorporate the proper use of the various chemical formulations available:

1. Detergents reduce surface tension and remove grease, thus enabling sterilants to act effectively. They do not destroy bacteria.
2. Sterilants or disinfectants kill bacteria and the main types are:
   (a) **Hypochlorites** are probably the cheapest and most common anionic disinfectants used in food premises. They possess a wide antimicrobial activity, being effective against both Gram-positive and Gram-negative bacteria including some spores. Having little taste or smell, they be used with confidence where food is handled but their chief disadvantage is that they fairly easily inactivated by organic material. Metallic materials or equipment may be corroded by prolonged immersion in hypochlorite solution. Examples are Chloros and Domestos.
   (b) **Iodophors** are more expensive than hypochlorites but are very similar in action, though they do tend to be less sporicidal. Generally, iodophors all incorporate a detergent. They show little inactivation by materials, other than those of an organic nature. Examples are Vanodine and Wescodyne.
   (c) **Quarternary ammonium conpounds (QAC)** have a more limited range of antimicrobial activity than those above, but remain a popular cationic disinfectant for food premises. They are good in alkaline solutions against Gram-positive bacteria and also against most moulds. They do, how-

Table 37.1 Cleaning schedule – school kitchen

Description	Product	Concentration % solution per gallon	Method	Frequency
Floor – kitchen	Bactericidal detergent	0.5 (¾ fl oz) (as specified by manufacturer)	Fill bucket or container from tap proportioner; wash or scrub manually with scrubbing brush, mop or squeegee; final rinse with clean cold water;	At least daily – at end of day
			Supplement with sweeping	As often as necessary
Floor – pantry, larder, vegetable store			Sweep with brush; wash (as above)	Daily/weekly
Walls – tiled to 4′	General detergent for general cleaning or as above	1.2 (2 fl oz)	Apply manually with low-pressure spray; final rinse with clean water (heavy soiling areas); dust accessible fixtures	Once a week — Each working day
Ceiling, light fittings, ventilation hoods (exterior) etc.			Brush or sweep manually; vacuum clean if possible	Once a week
Ventilation hood, hood (interior)	General detergent	As specified	Wipe with cloth	Once a week
Drainage – open channel	Sodium hypochlorite solution for sterilizing and stain removing	1.4 (2 fl oz)	Pour solution down head of drains at end of cleansing procedure to disinfect and deodorize	Each working day
Utensil sinks	Bactericidal detergent	0.5 (¾ fl oz)	Fill bucket or container from tap proportioner; wash or scrub manually; final rinse with clean cold water	Daily
Wash hand basins (if glazed stoneware)	Fine abrasive powder containing chlorine based bleach e.g. Vim, Glitto	Neat	Sprinkle on surface; wipe with damp cloth; rinse off with clean water; wipe dry	Each working day
Refrigerators	Bactericidal detergent	0.5 (¾ fl oz)	Wash or scrub manually; final rinse with clean water	As required
Stainless steel tables	Bactericidal detergent	0.5 (¾ fl oz)	Wipe with a clean cloth; re-rinse with water; apply with cloth, mop or brush; ideally, use a warm solution, leave for approx. 10 minutes; final rinse with clean water	After each use
Framework, including underside of table			Wash or scrub manually	At least once a month

Table 37.1 continued

Description	Product	Concentration % solution per gallon	Method	Frequency
Machinery – parts which come into contact with food	Bactericidal detergent		Wipe clean of all food particles and, where possible, detach and wash with cloth or brush in a hot solution; leave for approx. 10 minutes; final rinse with clean water.	After each use
Mechanical parts which do not come into contact with food	Bactericidal detergent		Wipe clean of all food particles and apply detergent solution with a cloth; rinse cloth and wipe off	Daily
Structural or covering members	Bactericidal detergent		Dust with a brush; wash clean with a cloth; ideally use a hot solution, leave for 10 minutes and rinse with clean water; dry and polish with a clean dry cloth	Daily/once a week
Ovens and cookery equipment – tops, sides, shelves	Powdered detergent for cleaning all metal surfaces	0.4 (2/3 oz)	Spray or brush on solution; ideally, use hot solution (60–70°C); leave for 10 minutes; scrub or wash thoroughly; final rinse with clean water	Daily
Insides	As above	As above	As above	Weekly

Safety Instructions
It is important for safe handling of chemicals to follow any instructions specified in product literature.

Removal of gross soiling
As a prerequisite to cleaning, gross soiling matter should first be removed. This will ensure maximum effectiveness of the detergent/disinfectant.

General housekeeping
The necessity of 'cleaning as you go' is emphasized as this will minimize the extent and degree of soiling necessary for a cleaning programme. Supplement daily cleaning with a thorough cleaning once a week and take the opportunity to remove any articles which have no business in the kitchen.

Temperature of detergent solution
Wherever possible, hot detergent solution should be used to achieve the quickest and best results.

Contact time
The efficient use of a detergent depends on the time allowed for it to be in contact with the soiling matter. It is essential that contact times are adequate.

Cleaning utensils
These should be kept clean. Cloths, dishcloths, etc. should be boiled in soap and water after each day's use. Scrubbing brushes must be washed clean in hot water and detergent and rinsed in clean water after each use. Scrubbing pails should be rinsed in hot water and stood upside down after use.

ever, tend to be inactivated by organic material, soap, hard water, wood, cotton, nylon, cellulose sponge mops and a few plastics. Some bacteria will even grow in QAC solutions and, therefore, special care is needed when preparing and using solutions. Examples are Hytox and Nonidet.

(d) There are several types of **phenolic disinfectants**, but their main disadvantage is that many brands possess a very strong smell and they are inactivated by some plastics and by rubber. The white fluid phenolics and the clear soluble type have a range of antimicrobial activity similar to that possessed by the hypochlorites and iodophors, and they are less easily inactivated by materials of an organic nature. The chloroxylenol phenolic disinfectants show a reduced range of antimicrobial activity and organic material will more readily inactivate them. Examples are white fluid phenolics: Izal and White Cyllin; clear, soluble fluid phenolics: Clearsol and Stericol; choroxylenol phenolics: Dettol.

(e) **Ampholyte disinfectants** are also good detergents, but they are fairly expensive. Their range of antimicrobial activity is narrow and many materials, such as hard water, organic material, wood, rubber, cotton, nylon, cellulose sponge and some plastics, will readily inactivate them. Example: Tego.

When a chemical disinfectant rinse is incorporated in a cleansing schedule and it follows a detergent wash, it is very important to ensure that compatible products are in use. Anionic disinfectants, such as hypochlorites and phenolics, are compatible with anionic detergents, but deactivated by cationic detergent. Similarly, cationic disinfectants such as QAC are compatible with cationic or non-ionic detergents, but inactivated by anionic detergents.

CROCKERY AND UTENSILS. Hand washing should be carried out in sinks constructed of stainless steel, a suitable method is illustrated in Fig. 37.8. Food waste should first be taken off and the crockery washed in the sink containing detergent in water which should be at a temperature of approximately 60°C. The crockery is then transferred to the second sink where the temperature of the water should be not less than 80°C, and in which the crockery or equipment is rinsed and sterilized. If water temperature of this order cannot be achieved, a chemical sterilant should be used. The crockery etc. can be placed into the second sink having been stacked in crockery trays, thus enabling a higher water temperature to be used than would be the case if the hands had to be immersed. Drying should be done in these trays and not by the use of cloths.

In many of the larger catering establishments, machines are used for dishwashing. These machines include detergents and rinse sprays, the temperatures of which can be controlled at about 50–60°C and 66–82°C respectively. In some machines, an added refinement is the provision of a hand-held or foot-operated spray, which is used to remove gross soiling by food particles.

The plates or articles to be washed are loaded onto carrier racks and, as they pass through the machine, are subjected to wash and rinse sprays; the whole washing processing is completed in about 1 minute.

The wash water which contains the detergent may be continually used in the larger machines so it is necessary to top up the detergent regularly. The rinse water is taken direct from the mains and is usually recirculated to the wash tank. The washed crockery should be delivered hot and steaming so that it can be air dried, thereby eliminating the need for the use of dishcloths and reducing the risk of cross-contamination.

The efficiency of dishwashing machines depends on the use of a good detergent at the right concentration and the maintenance of the wash and rinse sprays at the correct temperature. If machines are used carelessly, poor results will follow. The smaller types of machine incorporate the wash and rinse sprays in one unit. On these machines, articles to be washed are placed on racks and hand fed into the machine. Generally, the sprays are selected manually and the timing of the wash is not automated.

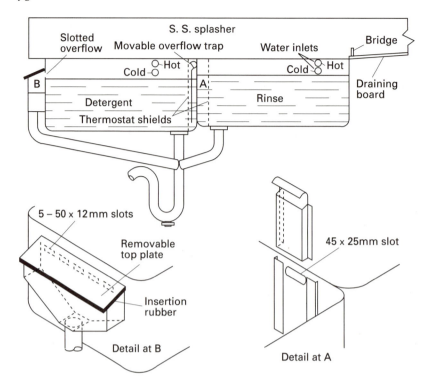

Fig. 37.8 Twin washing and rinsing sink, especially suitable for use in catering establishments.

On inspection of food premises, environmental health officers should check cleaning schedules being used. Nominated personnel should be responsible for ensuring effective cleaning in all food handling and non-handling areas.

Cleaning schedules should be seen as part of a total system of cleaning and maintenance, including decoration and repair. This should be part of a long-term policy of maintaining a clean environment for food safety and for aesthetic reasons.

OUTDOOR CATERING

Much outdoor catering is carried out in the UK, either at regular events, such as race meetings, regattas, and other sporting events, or for one-off occasions, such as pop festivals.

Guidance notes [12] to cover these situations have been produced by the Chartered Institute of Environmental Health following consultation with organizations having experience of large outdoor events. Trade organizations, particularly the National Outdoor Catering Association, have participated in developing these standards. The guidelines deal with planning for events, general food safety and service provision, and should be used by environmental health officers in all situations where outdoor event catering occurs.

MARKETS AND STALLS

Street markets are a traditional feature of British life, and although the nature of market sites and stalls is not conducive to the best standards of hygiene, good hygiene controls over perishable foods are possible by appropriate separation of cooked foods from uncooked foods, and the wrapping of particular food items. Central toilet and washing facilities, both for washing equipment and food items, such as fruit and vegetables, and personal hand washing facilities should adjoin market sites. Many of these facilities require updating and improvement consistent with present-day trading conditions. Revision of the Food Hygiene (Markets, Stalls and Delivery Vehicles) Regulations 1966 will be necessary in the light of the Hygiene of Foodstuff Directive, and these are included in the draft Consolidated Food Safety (General Food Hygiene) Regulations 1995.

Traditional market trading is not likely to disappear from the British scene – traders in permanent premises welcome the addition of markets to central commercial areas as they tend to result in increased trade for all. Legislation requirements in regard to food labelling and hygiene standards, necessitate regular surveillance over street markets by environmental health officers. The new standards being applied to fixed premises as a result of the Food Safety Act 1990, regulations, and codes of practice must be applied equally to all sites where food is being produced, handled and sold, irrespective of whether they are temporary in nature or only operating on specific days, such as street markets.

Mobile traders

Powers under the Food Safety Act 1990 allow environmental health officers to cross the borders of their own districts where necessary, to follow up suspected breaches of the Act or Regulations by mobile traders.

There are many new designs of purpose-made mobile food vehicles on the market but unfortunately, there are also many old buses, vans and other vehicles which have been adapted for selling food, with inadequate facilities and poor hygiene standards. Chapter 111 of the Annex to Directive 93/43/EEC covers the hygiene requirements for vehicles generally.

REFERENCES

1. Restaino, L. and Wind, C.E. (1990) Antimicrobial effectiveness of handwashing for food establishments. *Dairy Food and Environmental Sanitation* **10**, (3), 136–41.
2. World Health Organization (1989) *Health Surveillance and Management Procedures for Food Handling Personnel*. WHO Technical Report Series No. 785, WHO Geneva.
3. Department of Health, *Clean Food NHS Catering*, HMSO, London.
4. Fuqua, R.G. (1988) A practical environmental sampling plan for dairy processing plants. *Dairy and Food Sanitation*, **8** (10), 521–3.
5. Noah, N.D. (1981) Foodborne outbreaks of hepatitis A. *Medical Laboratory Sciences*, **38**, 428.
6. Reid, T.M.S. and Robinson, H.G. (1987) Frozen raspberries and hepatitis A. *Epidemiology and Infection*, **98**, 109–12.
7. Report of the Committee on the Microbiological Safety of Food, *The Microbiological Safety of Food, Part II*, Chairman Sir Mark Richmond, HMSO, London.
8. Council Directive Relating to Machinery (89/392/EEC), Department of Health Bulletin for Environmental Health Departments, Vol. 1, No 4, August 1992.
9. MAFF Food Safety Directorate News Release, FSD 57/90, 7 August 1990, 'New Power Rating System for Microwave Ovens'.
10. Department of Health, *Chilled and Frozen. Guidelines on Cook Chill and Cook Freeze Catering Systems*, HMSO, London.
11. West, A., Hotel and Catering Research Centre, Huddersfield Polytechnic (1989) Design requirements for cook chill. Paper at Campden Food and Drink Association Symposium, 7–8 November.
12. Institution of Environmental Health Officers, *National Guidelines for Outdoor Catering*, IEHO, London.
13. Department of Health (1994) *Assured Safe Catering – A Management System for Hazard Analysis*, HMSO, London.
14. Leaflet on Department of Health Assured Safe Catering, A Summary of the Main Points from the Department of Health Publication, BAPS Health Publication Unit, DSS Distribution Centre, Heywood Stores, Manchester Road, Heywood, Lancashire 0110 2PZ.

FURTHER READING

Jacob, M., *Safe Food Handling – A Training Guide for Managers of Food Service Establishments*, WHO, Geneva/HMSO, London.

38 The preservation of food

Mike Jacob

INTRODUCTION

Most foods intended for human consumption are of biological origin, except for the obvious exceptions of salt, water, etc., and it is important that this basic fact should not be forgotten. Biological systems are seldom inert; during the course of life, the metabolism of the living organism proceeds continuously to produce the end product of the adult animal, or the leaves, tubers, buds and seeds of the plant. Pick an apple, net a herring or pod a pea, and you will halt the metabolic processes. The animal or plant will die and so cease to grow. During its life, it possessed a complicated and highly efficient mechanism of protection from bacteria, yeasts and moulds. With death, this mechanism no longer operates. The condition of the living plant or animal will change over time but, after death, changes occur which are likely to be cumulative, irreversible and largely deteriorative unless steps are taken to halt them. It has always been one of the primary objectives of research in the food industry to develop and perfect techniques for arresting these changes during the necessary periods of distribution and storage. The preservation of food can be effected in a number of ways, e.g. smoking, salting, pickling, drying, canning or freezing. All of these methods achieve a temporary cessation of deteriorative changes, some at the expense of many of the characteristics of the fresh food.

MICROBIAL FOOD SPOILAGE

Foods are not stable commodities and when they have to be imported or transported over long distances, as much of our food is, it may deteriorate very quickly. This deterioration is brought about by a combination of physical damage, chemical breakdown or contamination, insect or rodent activity, enzyme breakdown or spoilage caused by micro-organisms, whose access is aided by many of these causes. Changes in taste, smell, colour, texture and appearance are the main features of microbial spoilage. Some of these changes being very distinct, such as the 'sulphur stinker' spoilage of canned foods, or the production of 'ropiness' in bread.

The pattern of spoilage will depend upon the microbial load of the particular foodstuff and is governed to a large degree by the type of food and its origin. Even so, the load will still be subject to change as a result of the storage, handling and processing to which the food is subjected, thus allowing selected categories of organisms to become dominant. For example, during the process of pasteurization, heat-sensitive bacteria, yeasts and moulds may be destroyed, but heat-resistant spoilage organisms remain, and food stored under chilled conditions, while inhibiting the growth of mesophiles, still allows psychrophiles to grow unhindered.

The main groups of organisms involved in food spoilage are moulds, yeasts and bacteria. Generally, moulds affect the surface of foodstuffs when their spores are able to germinate. They produce a mycelium which gradually penetrates the food, producing the familiar fluffy whiskers which have a distinctive colour. The food may also eventually become musty, softer and sticky or slimy. As well as spoiling the more common perishable foods, they are capable of affecting foods containing high sugar and salt contents and 'dry' foods, which may become damp as a result of bad storage.

Yeasts will grow in aerobic and anaerobic conditions which have acid or high sugar concentrations. They may be the fermentative type which break down sugars to produce alcohols, carbon dioxide and acids, or of the oxidative type which oxidize sugars, organic acids and alcohol, raising the pH in the process. Some osmophilic yeasts can spoil dried fruits and concentrated fruit juices, being able to tolerate conditions of low Aw (0.60) (Aw is a measure of the availability of water for microbiological growth) while others can tolerate high salt contents and may contribute to the spoilage of foods preserved in this manner.

Although bacteria are simple, single cell organisms which occur widely and cause spoilage under many conditions, they are limited by a low Aw (0.91) and do not feature in the spoilage of dried foods. However, in other foods which provide a suitable nutrient environment, they are able to bring about several types of spoilage. Bacteria growing on moist surfaces of meat, fish and vegetables will not only produce taints and odours, but can also bring about a degeneration of the food to produce slimes which, in turn, may produce pigments capable of bringing about colour changes, e.g. *Pseudomonas fluorescens* (fluorescent green) and *Serratia marcescens* (red). A wide variety of organisms are capable of producing a viscose, sticky material (rope), which can affect soft drinks, wine, vinegar, milk and bread, e.g. *Bacillus subtilis*. Some bacteria possess the ability to ferment carbohydrates. Homofermentative lactic acid bacteria produce lactic acid, whilst heterofermentative produce butyric and propionic acid in addition to the gases carbon dioxide and hydrogen. Foods which have been improperly processed and packaged so as to give

anaerobic conditions may be tainted with hydrogen sulphide, ammonia amines or other foul-smelling products, produced as a result of putrefaction by the anaerobic decomposition of protein. While aerobic hydrolysis of proteins may produce bitter flavours, these may in some cases enhance the palatability of certain foods and are, therefore, not always detrimental. Rots of many soft fruit and vegetables may be caused by bacteria such as the genus *Erwinia*. These activities can be slowed or arrested by killing the bacteria (by sterilization as in canning), depriving the bacteria of essential water for their metabolic activities (as in smoking and drying), altering the pH (as in acid pickling), effectively depriving the bacteria of available water by increasing the osmotic pressure of the surrounding medium (by the addition of sugar, etc.), or by sharply reducing the temperature below that at which bacteria can grow and multiply (as in freezing).

Although these treatments are designed to achieve a complete cessation of the biological activity, limited enzymic activity is inevitable and, over long periods, will cause deteriorative changes. With efficient preservation, however, it may take years before these deteriorative changes can be recognized by taste or appearance. When dried foods become moist, canned foods are punctured, or quick-frozen foods raised in temperature, the familiar pattern of spoilage reasserts itself.

DEHYDRATION

Drying deprives bacteria of the moisture necessary for their growth and reproduction, and also has the advantage of reducing the activity of enzymes which cause ripening and, ultimately, the rotting of foodstuffs.

The preservation of food by drying goes back thousands of years and fruit, fish, meat, etc., are still dried in the sun and provide the diet for millions of people. Sun-dried foods are subject to contamination by insects, birds and air-borne infection. Because of the limitation of this traditional method, most foods are now dried by artificial methods.

Solid foods

Today, 'solid' foods usually undergo some treatment prior to dehydration, e.g. vegetables are usually blanched by steam or hot water to inactivate enzymes; hot alkaline dips are used to remove wax from the surface of fruits and meat; fish and poultry are usually pre-cooked, but this cannot be relied upon to remove pathogens.

An essential of the dehydration process is efficient contact between the product and the hot air, together with the quick removal of moisture. Various techniques are used.

The fluidized bed dryer is a common type of dryer which has proved particularly useful for drying vegetables. It consists of a series of several perforated beds with fans underneath. The food, e.g. peas, is held in suspension by the upward blast of the hot air, which also provides the lateral movement. As the product drops from one bed to another, the temperature is increased (from 40°C to a maximum of 55°C at the end) and the moisture content is reduced from 80 to 50%.

The peas are then subjected to a further form of treatment in another type of dryer – a hot-air bed where moisture falls to approximately 20%. The hot-air bed dryer is a chamber in which the product is placed on perforated trays, through which hot air is passed from below, but there is no fluidization. Peas then receive a further treatment in dryers until the moisture content falls to approximately 5%.

These hot-air systems can give rise to undesirable effects due to the reactivation of enzymes and an alternative is vacuum drying.

Liquid foods

These are usually dried by:

1. Spraying a thin film of the liquid food on to heated rollers, e.g. potato flakes, tomato paste, instant breakfast cereals and animal foods. The food is scraped from the rollers in flakes and is then powdered. Drum dried foods are generally not as satisfactory as spray dried foods as they possess a more cooked character and do not reconstitute as well.

2. Spraying the liquid food through an atomizer into a heated chamber, e.g. milk, egg products, tea and coffee powders. A development of this involves the injection of a gas into the feed line which produces a foam which dries more rapidly.

Since these products are hydroscopic, it is essential that they are kept dry and correctly packaged so as to prevent contamination.

Freeze drying

This is the most advanced technique for eliminating the water contained in foodstuffs. The product to be dried is first frozen and then exposed to a vacuum of not less than one Torr (mmHg). The water contained in the product in the form of ice is directly sublimated into vapour, avoiding the liquid phase. The vapour is then eliminated by condensers. Freeze drying is also described as drying by sublimation, or lyophilization. The shape, colour and taste of the original product is preserved and freeze-dried foodstufs are easily rehydrated, instantly regaining their original properties, even when adding cold water. The process is carried out either in steel cabinets or in long, insulated tunnels fitted with vacuum locks and gates for continuous operation.

Due to the development of more efficient methods of heat transfer, accelerated freeze drying (AFD) was developed, which has given rise to the 'instant meal' which consists of pre-cooked freeze-dried foods to which is added hot water about 15 minutes before serving. Foods dried by this method do not distort but take the form of a spongy mass which can be quickly reconstituted. It is used to dry a variety of foods including meat, poultry, fish, shellfish, vegetables and fruit.

Freeze dried foods are stable at room temperatures but for long storage they should be refrigerated. They are usually vacuum packed or packed with an inert gas to prevent oxidation.

Infra-red drying

This is a system, using high-powered sources of radiation, which has been used in the dehydration of fruit, vegetables, meat, fish and cereals.

Use of solvents

Yet another method of dehydration is the use of a solvent such as ethyl acetate which forms a low boiling point mixture with water which can be removed by distillation, the residual solvent being removed by vacuum drying.

With all drying methods, it is important to remember that the microbiological load in the product will depend upon the initial load before dehydration, and that when water is added to effect reconstitution, the organisms commence growth. Even with AFD methods, few bacteria are killed and food must, therefore, be processed under strict hygiene conditions.

REFRIGERATION

Refrigeration has long been used for the preservation of food (see also temperature control chart, Fig. 37.4). There are three basic categories of refrigerated food: chilled food, frozen food and quick-frozen food. Chilled food is held at a temperature slightly above 0°C where no ice crystals form in the food and where either ice or mechanical refrigeration is used to achieve the desired temperature. Examples of this include wet fish; bacon, pies and sausages, which are sold from a refrigerated display cabinet; vegetables which are hydro-cooled by immersion in an ice-water slush and spray tank between picking and transport to market.

Chilling

This is an imprecise term, the temperature of which tends to vary with the product. It can mean any reduction in normal temperature. It varies because different foods deteriorate at different temperatures, e.g. fruit (apples will brown if the temperature is low).

Refrigeration temperature is usually taken to be below 5°C, and is the temperature which inhibits the growth of pathogens, though, of course they still remain viable. *C. botulinum* will, however, grow and produce toxin between 3 and 4°C, so temperatures are best kept at below 3°C.

Frozen food has its temperature maintained at around −10°C, and this includes most of the frozen meat sold in this country. Quick-frozen foods pass through the zone of maximum crystal formation (0 to −5°C) within a very short time, which is never more than 3 hours, and are held at a temperature of −18°C, although some sensitive food such as fish (if stored for a long time) should be maintained at −29°C or even lower if the texture is not to be damaged. (For Sous-Vide System for chilled meals see page 619).

Quick freezing

The conventional method of quick-freezing is by plate frosters. Here the product is pre-packed in packages which are as slim as is practical and is held in contact under pressure between upper and lower freezing plates, through both of which a refrigerant is circulated. The plates are on an hydraulic ram which allows contact to be maintained during the inevitable expansion during freezing. At the end of the freezing time, the product is removed from contact with the plates and placed in cold store. This method is suitable for products which take a long time to freeze, i.e. meat and fish. A method of quick-freezing which has gained acceptance, particularly for a free-flowing product such as peas, is that of air blast freezing. This method can be continuous as opposed to the batch process of plate freezing and consists of cascading the product onto a belt which moves through a freezing tunnel. Air is circulated in the tunnel either around and across the belt, or the belt is dispensed with and an upward flowing cushion of refrigerated air carries the product up and forward in a 'fluid-bed' technique. This method is suitable for freezing vegetables incuding peas and beans.

A further method (cryogenic freezing) involves contact of the food with a non-toxic refrigerant such as liquid nitrogen or oxygen. Freezing in this case can be accomplished in seconds rather than hours, and this can give quality advantages to delicately textured products. Most freezers used commercially for this method are spray freezers, which consist of an open-ended insulated freezing tunnel through which the food passes on a belt

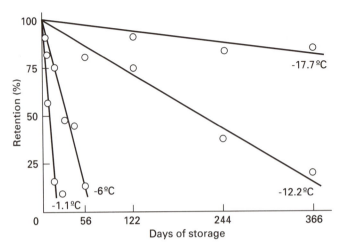

Fig. 38.1 Effect of temperature on ascorbic acid retention in peas.

conveyor. At the exit of the tunnel there are the liquid nitrogen sprays. Passing through the tunnel (about 6 minutes) brings the product close to its freezing point and the sprays effect freezing in 1–1½ minutes. Liquid nitrogen boils at −196°C and boiling occurs when the food is immersed due to rapid heat transfer. The method is used for foods such as strawberries and raspberries.

Foods may also be quick frozen by immersing in very cold fluids, such as invert sugar solutions or brine.

In the pulse method, the wrapped food is placed in an insulated chest into which liquid nitrogen is sprayed intermittently, the temperature of the food being allowed to equilibrate between each pulse. More recently, 'freon' has been approved in the USA for direct contact freezing of food.

In addition to the maintenance of the correct temperature (−18°C) of quick-frozen foods, it is important also that the original packaging of the food is kept intact as a barrier to moisture vapour, and oxygen. Intense illumination should also be avoided for long periods where green vegetables in translucent wrappings are concerned, as this may lead to loss of colour.

In judging the fitness of quick frozen foods for human consumption, it is important to distinguish between loss in quality and hazard to health. Quick-frozen foods which have been allowed to

thaw are not necessarily unfit for human consumption and they should therefore be judged on the same basis as any other perishable foods.

Although microbiological growth virtually ceases at temperatures below −10°C, and a percentage of vegetative cells may be destroyed by freezing, it cannot be relied upon to prevent food poisoning, as once the food is thawed the micro-organisms will grow. Freezing has little effect on spores and viruses and toxins are stable in this position. There is even a species of yeast which will grow at temperatures as low as −34°C. Nutritional loss, by protein denaturation and rancidity, as well as dehydration by sublimation, can occur at lower temperatures. Fig. 38.1, shows the rate of loss of vitamin C (ascorbic acid), the vitamin most sensitive to high storage temperatures. Fig. 38.2 illustrates the temperature range of growth of food poisoning organisms and psychrotrophic organisms. Both of these diagrams demonstrate the importance of maintaining quick-frozen foods at −18°C at all times. It follows that in assessing the fitness of quick-frozen foods which have suffered temperature fluctuations, both the period and the degree of fluctuation are vital factors.

While the loss of quality may not necessarily be evident to the eye or by taste, the physical appearance of a quick-frozen product can sometimes indicate whether or not it has been subjected to temperature fluctation. Loss of colour in

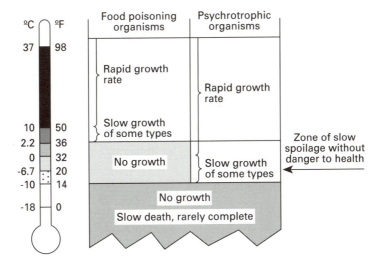

Fig. 38.2 The temperature range of growth of food-poisoning organisms and psychotropic organisms.

green vegetables, a darkening of the surface area on poultry, a lightening of the surface area of other meat products, can all indicate that temperature fluctuations may have occurred. While these are generalizations, they can be useful indicators. It is important to realize that changes caused by temperature fluctuations are irreversible and cumulative. Successive large fluctuations lead to sublimation of moisture from the food and may well, over a long period, give rise to loss of weight as well as loss of quality, all of which will occur more rapidly where permeable or defective packaging materials are used.

The Quick Frozen Foodstuffs Regulations 1990

Quick-frozen foods are perceived to be of a higher quality than ordinary frozen foods, hence the reason for the EC Directive and the Regulations. Environmental health officers and trading standards officers are responsible for enforcement.

These Regulations apply to food which has undergone 'quick-freezing' whereby the zone of maximum crystallization is crossed as rapidly as possible.

Products must be suitably pre-packaged so as to protect them from microbial and other contamination and dehydration and must remain so packaged until sale.

Products available for sale must be labelled with:

1. indication of the date of minimum durability;
2. an indication of the maximum advisable storage time;
3. an indication of the temperature at which and the equipment in which it is advisable to store it;
4. a batch reference; and
5. a clear message not to refreeze after defrosting.

Quick frozen foods must be stored at or below −18°C.

Provisions controlling the monitoring of temperature during transport and for sampling and analysing the temperature of quick frozen foodstuffs will be applied as a result of new EC Directives on this subject.

Code of Practice No. 12 (revised February 1994) under the Food Safety Act 1990 provides advice on the division of enforcement responsibilities between environmental health officers and trading standards officers for these Regulations.

The Code also makes it clear that quick frozen foods (QFF) temperature monitoring should not be a high priority for food authorities, since the principal objective of producers is to make available high quality products – the temperature parameters are concerned with food quality not food safety. Most monitoring is likely to be carried out by the Home Authority on out-going products at the factory or distribution warehouses of haulage companies, and retail store QFF temperature checks will mainly occur during the course of programmed visits or as a result of complaints.

These checks are not only concerned with actual recorded temperatures, but with positioning and operation of the manufacturers' and distributors' own temperature monitoring equipment and records.

Cabinet hygiene

The proper and efficient use of the retail cabinet can only be achieved by following the principles laid down in the code of practice issued by the UK Association of Frozen Food Producers [1]. This code should be studied by everyone concerned with the handling of quick-frozen foods.

FERMENTATION

The process of anaerobic respiration, or fermentation, is utilized to preserve several types of food and to produce many others. For example many short-life vegetables can be preserved by the addition of acids, and in some products these conditions are allowed to develop naturally as a result of the growth of organisms which produce lactic acid. Pickled cabbage (sauerkraut) and olives are examples of food preserved in this way. Many others (onions, cauliflowers and walnuts) may depend on lactic acid production before other preservatives, such as vinegar, are added.

BIOTECHNOLOGY IN FOOD PRODUCTION

Biotechnology has been used in food production and processing for thousands of years. Almost every ingredient used in the production of food has as its source a living animal, plant or micro-organism. Food sources available to early humans, both plant and animal, evolved through the process of natural selection. Genetic diversity arising from spontaneous genetic changes was first exploited when farmers saved the seeds from their best crops for later sowings and used their best animals for breeding.

New techniques have brought about significant advances in animal breeding. Hormones to increase ovum production, followed by artificial insemination, can provide up to a dozen or so embryos which can then be implanted into surrogate mothers.

Genetic modification techniques can also be applied to the micro-organisms that produce fermented foods, including those involved in bread and beer production. For example in bread making, a more efficient system for metabolizing maltose can reduce bread making time. In the dairy industry, lactic acid producing bacteria can be genetically modified to produce strains with improved phage resistance or bacteriocin or flavour production. Single cell (bacterial or fungal) protein has been developed as a source of human and animal food. The organism *Fusarium graminearum* is grown on hydrolysed starch. The most abundant renewable biomass on earth is cellulose, an estimated 5–15 tons being produced per capita per year. Much of the cellulose is bound physico-chemically to lignin. Some higher fungi, including some edible species, can be used to convert ligno cellulose directly into fungal protein suitable for human consumption.

The use of rennet, the common milk clotting preparation, to produce cheese and other dairy products is by far the largest single use of enzymes by the dairy industry. Extra-cellular fungal proteinases can serve as rennet substitutes.

Bacteria, viruses, fungi, nematodes and insects can be used as biological control agents in pest control. Various toxins produced by organisms are also used. Many viruses pathogenic to insects are now being developed commercially and fungal insecticides have been used successfully since the beginning of this century.

In food analysis the application of biotechnology has resulted in the development of rapid and sensitive analytical methods which may have many applications in food analysis. For example the use of DNA probes and immuno-assay methods are expected to prove useful in improving the detection of food contaminants.

The Food and Agriculture Organization (FAO) and WHO have examined the safety of foods produced by biotechnology. The prime consideration is to ensure that pathogens should not be introduced into foods by the process. In the evaluation of foods produced by biotechnology, databases are required on:

1. nutrient and toxicant contents of food;
2. the molecular analysis of organisms used in food production;
3. the molecular nutritional and toxicant content of genetically modified organisms intended for use in food production.

FAO and WHO also recommend the need for consumers to be provided with sound scientifically based information on biotechnology in food production [2].

FOOD IRRADIATION

The process of food irradiation involves the exposure of food to ionizing radiations such as gamma rays, x-rays or electrons [3]. Gamma rays and x-rays are forms of radiant energy just as sunlight or radio waves. But only the high energy forms of radiation are ionizing. Ionizing radiation interacts with the material being irradiated by transferring some of its energy to particles in the molecules of the material, producing electrically charged particles called ions. The energy transfer causes transfer between the different molecules. These reactions destroy or prevent organisms, such as species of *Salmonella*, multiplying. The technique of irradiation of food has been approved for use in some countries for over 20 years, and is currently used in 21 countries including Belgium, France, the Netherlands and the USA. In the UK, irradiation has been used for over 30 years to sterilize medical equipment, certain pharmaceuticals, cosmetics and packaging.

The need for food irradiation arises from the fact that fresh foods deteriorate during storage and can be contaminated resulting in the growth of micro-organisms that can cause food-borne disease. Indeed, some food can contain food poisoning organisms among their microbial flora, and these organisms may also be present in the environment.

Food spoilage can be caused by the action of micro-organisms, or the over-ripening of fruits, or sprouting of vegetables or grains. Traditional methods of preservation, such as drying, salting, fermentation, pickling and smoking, have been supplemented with freezing, chilling, canning, pasteurization and treatment with chemical preservatives. Food irradiation is an additional method of preservation, and for some products offers a successful way of reducing spoilage and enhancing safety by controlling bacterial levels, while having minimal effects on the nature and quality of the food.

For the future, the main use of irradiation is likely to be in reducing the number of harmful bacteria, such as species of *Salmonella, Listeria*, and *Campylobacter*, that can be present in certain foods, such as poultry, prawns or shrimps. For produce such as dried herbs and spices, irradiation could be used to destroy insects, pests and bacteria in place of the existing chemical fumigation method. However, irradiation is not suitable for use on all foods – some fruits, for example, are softened by irradiation, and some fatty foods develop a rancid flavour.

Irradiation cannot make bad food good, and it cannot improve the appearance or taste of the food, or mask unpleasant odours.

All food carries a low level of natural radioactivity, and there is no measurable increase in the level of radioactivity after food is irradiated under approved conditions. Over the last 40 years, food irradiation has been studied more than any other process. The UK Advisory Committee on Irradiated and Novel Foods, WHO, the FAO Joint Expert Committee on Food Irradiation, and the EU Scientific Committee for Food have all concluded that there is no hazard associated with food that has been exposed to doses of ionizing radiation up to an overall average dose of 10 kilograys (10 kGy is the amount of energy required to raise the temperature of 1 kg of water by 2.4°C), and irradiation introduces no significant nutritional or microbiological problems.

Following the government's decision to proceed with making irradiation an accepted process of food treatment in the UK, the proposals for legislation follow those recommended by the CODEX Alimentarius Commission, a joint WHO/FAO body set up to prepare international food standards. In 1983, the Commission adopted both a general standard for irradiated food and a code of practice for the operation of food irradiation facilities. This is the basis of the controls adopted for the UK. The important elements include:

1. a maximum limit on the irradiation dose that may be applied;
2. licensing on a product-by-product and irradiation plant-by-plant basis;
3. regular inspections of irradiation plants by expert central government staff;
4. microbiological testing to ensure that only food of normal sound quality is irradiated;
5. controls over imported irradiated food through official verification that the controls and standards achieved by exporting countries are equivalent to those in the UK;
6. full labelling of irradiated foods so that consumers can make a choice whether or not to buy irradiated food, compared with non-irradiated food available.

These principles are embodied in the Food (Control of Irradiation) Regulations 1990 and the Food Labelling (Amendment) (Irradiated Food) Regulations 1990 which came into effect on 1 January 1991.

The government has commissioned research into the development of suitable detection tests for irradiated food. However, the government believes that with an effective control and labelling system, it is not essential to have detection tests to identify irradiated foods. These tests are difficult to develop as the effects of irradiation on food are small and, in many instances, simply mirror the effects produced by other processing, including cooking, but several lines of research into detection tests are showing promise.

The Government's continuing programme of dietary monitoring will be used to assess the contribution of irradiated foods to our diets and,

linked with this, measurements will continue to be made of the impact of irradiation on the nutrient content of individual foods.

WHO has recognized the benefits of irradiating food to reduce the numbers of bacteria in foods and, in fact, has recommended in its ten *Golden Rules for Safe Food Preparation* [4] to the consumer that people should select irradiated fresh or frozen poultry wherever possible.

The general conclusion is that food irradiation is a safe process proven over four decades of research and by the independent review of a number of expert committees including the UK independent expert group, the Advisory Committee on Irradiated and Novel Foods.

PROCESSED AND PRESERVED FOODS

Foods processed in anaerobic environments present an ideal medium for the growth of bacteria if the heat process is inadequate to destroy all pathogens and spoilage organisms within the pack, or the closure of the can or pack is not effective in stopping the entry of micro-organisms. Further hazards may arise from improper handling of products during processing, which cause damage and subsequent contamination of the internal contents of the can or pack.

C. botulinum represents the major risk to such foods because of its heat resistance. The bacterium will not grow below a pH of 4.5. All foods with a pH of less than 4.5 are known as acid foods, and those with a pH of more than 4.5 are termed low-acid foods. The acid foods, such as fruit conserve, only receive a relatively low heat process. Meats and vegetables with a much higher pH are given a process known as a botulinum cook to render them commercially sterile. Process time and temperature is determined for each pack of low-acid food, and will depend on such things as composition, weight, headspace, the viscosity of contents, the presence of preservatives and intended storage conditions. Scheduled processes for all low-acid products have been established and must be adhered to by canned food manufacturers [5].

They must be sufficient to ensure the destruction or inactivation of all pathogens. Certain heat-resistant, spore-forming spoilage organisms which may be present, e.g. *Bacillus stearothermophilus*, are more resistant than *C. botulinum*, the most heat-resistant, toxin-producing pathogen; so by ensuring the destruction of spores of the former the latter is also destroyed and the food made safe.

CANNED FOODS

It is the canners' aim to produce a 'sterile' product, one in which all micro-organisms are destroyed. In some instances, however, it is not practical to achieve this and, in these situations, the storage temperature or the acidity of the contents are relied upon as being sufficiently adverse to the small numbers of heat-resistant spores which remain to prevent their growth. The food is then considered commercially sterile. As micro-organisms capable of causing spoilage at pH below 4.5 are generally of low-heat resistance, acid and high-acid canned foods are subjected to a less severe heat-treatment process than the medium–low-acid canned foods. With the medium and low-acid canned foods, it is essential that they are heated sufficiently to destroy the heat-resistant spores of *C. botulinum*. Where low-acid canned foods, e.g. canned meats, incorporate curing salts which are also microbial inhibitors, they can be given milder heat treatments. Such commodities as large canned hams and luncheon meats are, in effect, only pasteurized, and must not be considered as sterile. The heat treatment given is sufficient to destroy vegetative cells and limit the number of heat-resistant spores to no more than 10 000 per g. In view of their limited treatment, such products should be stored under refrigeration. After the heat-treatment process, great care is exercised to ensure that products are not recontaminated with pathogens or spoilage organisms. The entry of food poisoning organisms is prevented by ensuring that there is no human handling while seals are wet, and that the disinfection of cooling water is adequate. Spoilage is prevented by attention to proper sealing, avoidance of damage while seals are set, rapid drying of containers and adequate cleaning and disinfection of all wet, post-processing handling equipment and cooling waters.

There have been outbreaks of food poisoning associated with canned meats and fish, where contamination of the product has arisen during the cooling process by way of contaminants in cooling water and the canning environment finding a way through the seams during expansion/contraction. Bacteria involved have included *Staph. aureus. S. typhi* and *C. botulinum*.

Spoilage of canned foods

In canned foods, spoilage is generally indicated by a 'blown' condition of the cans. The contents of cans in this condition are more or less decomposed and are unfit for human consumption. The principles of sterilization are now so well understood that faulty cans, rather than understerilization, are the most frequent cause of spoilage.

Certain canned fruits, notably plums, cherries, raspberries, loganberries, and blackcurrants can have a blown appearance, which makes them unmarketable, even though the fruit itself is both sound and sterile. The gas producing the pressure by which the cans are blown is found on analysis to consist largely of hydrogen, and in consequence this type of failure has come to be known as 'hydrogen swell'. The cause of the trouble is principally the action of the fruit acids upon the tin-plate. In the course of time, the action results in perforation of the can. The action occurs principally along the seams and other parts of the can which are subjected to severe strain during manufacture, and where the protective lacquer coating is defective. Cans lacquered after manufacture are rarely affected. Hydrogen swell occurs only in cans containing fruit, and is unlikely to occur in cans that have been sealed for periods of less than 12 months.

Taints and catty odours, so called because they resemble the odour of cats' urine, onion or garlic, have occasionally plagued the food industry in several countries. Such objectionable odours and flavours usually affect canned meat and vegetables and obviously make the food unacceptable to the consumer. Investigations carried out by British Food Manufacturing Industries Research Association demonstrated that contamination of the food by mesityl oxide, an unsaturated ketone, can give rise to these odours, particularly where it is able to react with hydrogen sulphide.

Examination of canned foods

The routine methods of examination of cans containing food are: inspection, pressure, percussion or tapping, and shaking.

Inspection reveals evidence of blowing, damage, e.g. indentation or leakage, and excessive rusting. Dented cans resulting from rough handling are always suspect, particularly if they are damaged on a seam, which may result in its opening and air being admitted to the can. Occasionally, end seam defects such as false seams and irregularities such as wrinkles and pleats (where the metal folds back over itself during the first operation of seaming) will become apparent during inspection, Uniform, light-coloured rust spots on the labels seldom indicate leakage. However, if any of the spots have a darker inner area, then the can may be perforated.

The terminology used in conjunction with defects in cans is as follows;

1. **Flipper.** A slight positive pressure inside the can, due to the production of gas, such as hydrogen or CO_2, which is usually due to chemical or microbiological activity such as that produced by sacharrolytic strains of clostridia which not only produce acid but also quantities of gas. It can be demonstrated by striking the can against something solid when one end bulges out. When the end returns to its original shape it is known as a Flipper.
2. **Springer.** Greater gas pressure causes a springer. In this condition, one end is permanently bulged and if this is pushed in the other end bulges. Both flippers and springers suggest incipient spoilage.
3. **Soft swell.** This is the term given to the condition where both ends are bulged but will move slightly under the pressure of the thumb,

and in the case of hard swell the pressure is sufficient to prevent the pushing in of the ends. The condition indicates spoilage. (But see note on tinned coffee, below.)

4. **Flat sour.** No gas in the tins but the contents have an unpleasant odour and flavour and are inedible. In medium- and low-acid canned foods, *Bacillus stearothermophilus* and *B. coagulans* ferment carbohydrates and cause flat sours giving the contents an unpleasant odour.
5. **Hydrogen swell.** This is due to the action of acid in the contents acting on the tin. The gas burns on ignition and the condition is usually associated with fruit.
6. **Sulphur stinker.** Spoilage is produced by organisms of the clostridia group which produce the gas hydrogen sulphide. This defect is nowadays relatively rare. Slime and ropiness can be caused in acid and high-acid canned foods by strains of the organism *Leuconostoic*. Canned soft fruits may occasionally be found to be soft and pulpy as a result of spoilage from heat-resistant moulds (*Eyssochlomys fulda*).
7. **Sulphiding**. This is a purple stain on the inner surface of cans of food containing sulphur, e.g. fish and meat. It is due to hydrogen sulphide being formed due to the breakdown of sulphur-containing proteins. A thin layer of sulphide is formed inside the tin, and this attacks the mild steel from which the can is made. Iron sulphide is formed causing discoloration of the meat or fish where it is in contact with the metal. The staining can be removed by trimming.

In the case of blown tins of coffee, it should be remembered that all freshly roasted and ground coffee gives off CO_2 (carbon dioxide) and when it is packed in an airtight, tin-plated container the pressure of the CO_2 inside may cause the tin to bulge. Only a container made of material so thick as to resist the internal pressure could prevent this from happening, and since the CO_2 expands more readily in warm weather, the bulging of tins is more likely to occur in summer months.

When the ground coffee ceases to exhale CO_2 and begins to absorb moisture from the atmosphere, it becomes stale. Therefore a 'blown' tin of coffee is proof that the coffee was freshly roasted, ground and packed, in the first instance that the tin is airtight, and that it is holding the fresh coffee with its natural exhalation of CO_2 in the finest possible condition.

Cans of salmon and other sea foods are sometimes found to contain crystals which resemble glass. They are in fact crystals of magnesium ammonium phosphate, a normal product of the digestive system of the fish and are quite harmless.

Crystals of calcium tartrate have been reported in canned cherries and crystals of potassium hydrogen tartrate in canned grapes. All these crystals, with the exception of potassium hydrogen tartrate, will dissolve in vinegar.

CHEMICAL PRESERVATIVES

Certain chemicals have been found to interfere with the principal agents that cause deterioration in food. They possess the ability to slow or arrest microbial growth by interfering with cell permeability, enzyme activity or with their genetic mechanism.

The traditional substances, such as salt or sugar, which have been in use for thousands of years, exert a preservative effect by dissolving in the water of the food, and forming a concentrated solution in which spoilage organisms are unable to live. The concentrated aqueous solution is able to exert a strong osmotic pressure and the cells are consequently deprived of available water. Brines utilize salt to preserve meats, whereas sugar acts as a preservative in such products as jam, syrup and honey.

Many permitted preservatives, such as sulphur dioxide and proprionic, benzoic and sorbic acids, exert their effect by virtue of their acidity and are also important mould inhibitors. Some preservatives occur naturally, such as benzoic acid (found in cranberries), and these tend to be more effective against moulds and yeasts. In addition to exerting a preservative effect, some chemicals may also be of benefit in helping to maintain colour in ingredients which are going to be processed.

THE SOUS-VIDE SYSTEM FOR PREPARING CHILLED MEALS

This system involves a vacuum-packed product designed to retain the quality of food while at the same time enabling an improved shelf-life for a chilled product. It is particularly suited to the hotel and restaurant sector of the catering industry, and was developed in the mid 1970s in France. It is being used in hundreds of restaurants in France and the rest of Europe. In its simplest form the system involves:

1. the preparation of high quality raw ingredients;
2. precooking, e.g. browning if necessary;
3. placing the food into special heat-stable air and moisture high barrier plastic bags or pouches;
4. creating a vacuum and sealing the pouch;
5. either steam cooking at specific times and temperatures to ensure pasteurization of the food, or cooking the food for immediate consumption;
6. rapid chilling to reduce the temperature to 0–3°C within 90 minutes from the end of cooking;
7. labelling and controlled refrigerated storage within this temperature range until required for consumption within 5 days of date of production.

It is claimed that the aroma, flavour and texture of the food is preserved and maximized due to the construction of the pouch. No natural flavours are lost, but the product does rely on high quality original raw ingredients.

Only small regeneration kitchens are necessary to reheat the food – minimal equipment and less skilled manpower are required compared with a conventional restaurant.

The problem with the system is that the creation of the anaerobic environment inside the pouch increases the risk of food poisoning from *C. botulinum, C. perfringens* and other pathogens. The whole system depends heavily on the integrity of the process and the knowledge of all the operatives involved in ensuring safety. Internal temperature checks by thermocouples or thermistors can check centre temperatures of food before vacuumization. Temperature monitoring devices should be independent of the oven to enable the product sample to be monitored throughout its cooking and chilling cycle. Ideally, temperature printouts of cooking, chilling, and storage cycles should be made [6].

The SVAC (Sous Vide Advisory Committee) has produced a Code of Practice on the use of Sous Vide [7].

ANAEROBIC FOOD PACKS

Following the outbreak of *C. botulinum* from yoghurt in the north west of England in the summer of 1989, the Department of Health sent a letter to all chief environmental health officers [8] asking for appropriate checks to be made on producers of foods produced in anaerobic environments. The increasing use of vacuum packs in small manufacturing and retail premises to preserve the quality and shelf-life of foods does represent a substantial risk factor, and the points made by the Department of Health in its letter requested CEHOs to identify other food processors who may be using processes that have not been subjected to a hazard analysis. In the Department's view, it was likely that such producers would be the smaller manufacturers, particularly those who had commenced food manufacture recently, or who had made changes to their products/processes without expert advice.

Developments in food processing that could introduce hazards are the increasing use of vacuum packing, reduction in preservatives (particularly salt and nitrites), reduction in sugar content to produce a lower calorie product, and the tendency to use lower cooking temperature to reduce loss of yield and improve the colour and texture of products. Environmental health officers were asked as a matter of urgency to carry out an assessment of the safety of all types of food processes undertaken within their districts where the foods produced were packaged anaerobically. These included heat-treated, cured, smoked or fermented products in metal enclosures or vacuum packs, or other forms of packaging. The

food processors concerned were asked to supply evidence of the scientific and technical evaluation of the safety of their process. If they were unable to do so, this was taken as an important indicator of possible hazards in the process. If there was any doubt, the companies were asked to obtain an expert evaluation of their process and to submit it without any delay to the local environmental health department. A list of organizations expert in food safety assessment to which companies could be referred was given in the annex to the Department of Health letter.

Chief port health officers were also asked to draw the attention of importers to the letter. Imports of all foods in anaerobic packs were reviewed. Where necessary, particularly with new products in non-traditional containers, importers were asked to produce evidence that the safety of these foods had been evaluated by experts.

In carrying out an assessment of food processes within districts, the following questions are highly important. Environmental health officers should be able to judge whether potential hazards exist as a result of the answers:

1. What are the range of products produced, the pack size and the number of different variations in each product?
2. Are technical personnel employed or retained by the company, and what are the training and background of those personnel?
3. What are the pH, salt and sugar levels of the products and their water activity? (If the processor is unable to provide satisfactory answers to these questions and seems unaware of their significance in relation to product safety, this should alert environmental health officers to potential defects in the process.)
4. What is the total product life of all products? What are the storage temperatures required to achieve the prescribed product life and how has the life been technically determined?
5. How is the product packaged and what steps are being taken to ensure container/packaging integrity?
6. To whom are the products supplied and for what purpose (i.e. retail sales or as ingredients of other manufactured products)? What advice

is given to customers for the storage and use of the products?

7. What evaluation has been made of raw materials and their suppliers? How is the safety of the raw materials determined?

8. What records are kept and what is the system for tracing of product and recall procedures? What codes are applied?

9. What is the system for action in the event of process deviations from production schedules?

ADVISORY COMMITTEE ON THE MICROBIOLOGICAL SAFETY OF FOOD

The Advisory Committee on the Microbiological Safety of Food (ACMSF) held an initial review of the microbiological aspects of the safety of vacuum-packed and other hermetically sealed foods in June 1991. The Committee concluded that a careful assessment was needed of the action that might be required to protect the public from any risk of botulism or other dangers. A Working Group was set up to carry out a detailed investigation. The Group presented its report to the Committee in September 1992 [9]. The Government undertook to take these recommendations forward [10]. It now appears unlikely, however, that new controlling Regulations will be introduced to cover these processes. Among the important recommendations contained in the Report were the following;

1. Because of the changes taking place in food production technology, food manufacturers should critically assess all new food process procedures to ensure elimination of risk of botulism.

2. Home preservation methods such as home canning or bottling of low acid products such as vegetables and meats and home vacuum packaging (except for frozen products) should not be encouraged.

3. In addition to chilled temperatures of 10°C, prepared chilled foods with an assigned shelf-life of more than 10 days should contain one or more controlling factors at levels to prevent the growth and toxin formation by strains of psychrotrophic *C. botulinum*.

4. Cooking or reheating of food alone should not be relied upon to destroy any botulinum toxin present in foods but other controlling factors should be used in foods susceptible to the growth of psychrotrophic *C. botulinum* in order to prevent growth and toxin production by psychrotrophic strains of *C. botulinum*.

5. In addition to chilled temperatures maintained throughout the chilled chain, the following controlling factors should be used singly or in combination to prevent growth and toxin production by psychrotrophic *C. botulinum* in prepared chilled foods with a shelf-life of more than 10 days:

   (a) a heat treatment of 90°C for 10 minutes or equivalent lethality;
   (b) pH of 5 or less throughout the food and throughout all components of complex foods;
   (c) a minimum salt level of 3.5% in the aqueous phase throughout the food and throughout all components of complex foods;
   (d) an aw of 0.97 or less throughout the food and throughout all components of complex foods;
   (e) a combination of heat preservative factors which can be shown consistently to prevent the growth and toxin production by psychrotrophic *C. botulinum*.

6. The risk of *C. botulinum* hazard in chilled food must be addressed by manufacturers, caterers and retailers. Examples include smoked salmon and trout cuisine, sous vide products and modified atmosphere packaged sandwiches.

7. Food manufacturers and caterers should ensure that they have a thorough understanding of the operational capabilities of vacuum packaging machines, that the appropriate pouch or tray materials are used and that the machinery used for establishing the vacuum function is to required specification.

8. Vacuum packaging machine manufacturers should alert users to food safety hazards and the risk from organisms such as *C. botulinum*.

9. Cooking of sous vide products should not be undertaken unless operators have available

the technical expertise to ensure that pasteurization equipment and operating procedures are adequately designed and tested to give a uniform and known heat load to all containers during each cycle.

10. Information should be made available to consumers on correct handling practices with regard to vacuum modified atmosphere packaged foods.

11. Foods sent by mail order should be subject to controlling factors in addition to temperature to prevent the growth of pathogenic microorganisms including pyschotrophic *C. botulinum*.

12. There should be a comprehensive and authoritative Code of Practice for the manufacture of vacuum and modified atmosphere packed chilled foods with particular regard to the risks of botulism. It should include guidance on:

(a) raw material specifications;
(b) awareness and use of HACCP;
(c) process establishment and validation (including thermal process);
(d) packaging requirements;
(e) temperature control through production, distribution and retail;
(f) factory auditing and quality management systems (including awareness and use of HACCP);
(g) thorough understanding of requirements to establish a safe shelf-life;
(h) thorough understanding of the control factors necessary to prevent the growth of and toxin production by psychrotrophic *C. botulinum* in chilled foods;
(i) application of challenge testing;
(j) equipment specifications particularly with regard to heating and refrigeration;
(k) training.

TRENDS

A major trend in food processing has been the development of convenience foods. This has led to cook-chill ready meals, a huge growth in sandwich sales, together with continuing development of dairy products, particularly desserts and gâteaux, and many other products that busy consumers would prefer to buy rather than make at home. The development of high-quality nutritious snacks has resulted in people eating fewer regular meals and a decrease in the formal family meals.

The desire to have foods 'additive free' has resulted in increased pressure on food manufacturers to reduce or eliminate preservatives, synthetic colours and anything else associated with 'E' numbers. Increased public knowledge of nutrition issues has raised the profile of such food ingredients as salt, sugar, cholesterol, fats and fibre, and has resulted in the increased development of products with specific claims in these areas. As part of the increased nutrition awareness, low-fat products in the dairy sector have flourished. An increase in the popularity of ethnic foods, different packing forms and cooking methods, such as microwave ovens has widened the technological base of convenience foods available for consumers.

The removal of preservatives from a wide range of products has increased the risk of premature yeast and mould problems for manufacturers, as well as increasing the potential for pathogen growth. Increasing emphasis on process control, pack integrity and chill chain control must be part of the food manufacturers' present policy. The Chilled Food Association has issued guidelines for good hygienic practice in the manufacture of chilled foods other than those produced by catering operations. [11] Four categories of prepared, chilled food are covered:

1. those prepared from raw components;
2. those prepared from cooked and raw components processed to extend the safe shelf-life;
3. those prepared from only cooked components;
4. those cooked in their own packaging prior to distribution.

The guidelines are intended to ensure that the cooking processes are sufficient to destroy vegetative pathogens, in particular *Listeria monocytogenes*.

COLD CHAIN VEHICLE DISTRIBUTION

Temperature-controlled vehicles

There are several types of vehicles designed and built to **maintain** temperature, not to change the temperature of either chill or frozen foods. Within the UK, as in some other EC countries, there is no legislation to control the thermal efficiency of insulation other than on international journeys, where the carriage of international foodstuffs comes under the ATP Regulations. These lay down minimum values of insulation efficiency and are only valid for a certain period during which the container requires certification.

The various refrigeration systems employed in vehicles include:

1. **Water ice systems** with temperature parameters 3–10°C (very few systems are in operation at the present).
2. **Total loss systems** using either carbon dioxide (dry ice) or liquid nitrogen. The former skips the liquid phase altogether, and by a process of sublimation vaporizes directly from the solid state.
3. **Liquid nitrogen**, carried in vacuum-insulated tanks on the vehicle, boils at −196°C. It is the gas which via solenoid valves is piped into the container through a number of spray headers. This system is silent, has a high degree of reliability, and has the ability to pull down the box temperature very rapidly. However, local areas of under cooling can still occur.
4. **Eutectic** systems use either roof-mounted tubes or plates, which are fitted to the front bulkhead or side walls of the vehicle and are filled with brine solution which is cooled by freon passing through pipes within the plates or tubes. Similar to the nitrogen system this system does not have forced air circulation. Cooling can be provided for a finite period, that is until all the eutectic has melted. The system is very inflexible, providing either frozen only or chill only.
5. **Vapour compression systems**. This is commonly known as mechanical refrigeration and is driven by either hydraulic motors, electric motors or diesel engines. It is very flexible,

capable of temperatures between +20°C to −30°C. Its flexible temperature capability coupled to the type drive unit makes it the most common transport refrigeration unit. They may switch between heating and cooling automatically in response to the thermostat in order to maintain present load space temperature, irrespective of whether the outside is at a higher or lower temperature.

Vehicles are now being designed for the carriage of multi-temperature perishable foodstuffs. These have the ability to divide frozen products from chilled, and also to control the chill product air temperatures and split certain chill products into two different temperature bands. Position switches are accessible to the driver so that each temperature position can be preset and then locked. Temperatures can be preset to whatever parameters the retail customers require foods to be delivered at.

Containers must be precooled before carrying either frozen or chilled food. If containers have not been precooled, problems can arise in shrink-wrapped products and maintaining the quality of perishable foods inside the container. Temperature monitoring equipment is now an essential modern component of such vehicles. The position of sensors is in the warmest part of the container. Electronic data collection coupled with on-board printers and the means to put the data into a personal computer are developments coming into the industry [12].

PACKAGING OF FOOD

The Materials and Articles in Contact with Food Regulations 1987 implement requirements regarding materials and articles which come into contact with food, including packaging.

The essential requirements of a packaging material are:

1. it should be inert toward the food product;
2. it should protect the product from adverse environmental conditions;
3. it should present the product to the consumer in an appealing manner;
4. it should be easy for the consumer to use.

The Materials and Articles in Contact with Food (Amendment) Regulations 1994 deal with:

(a) purity standards for regenerated cellulose film,
(b) residues migrating into foodstuffs, and
(c) administrative amendments to bring the 1987 Regulations into line with the single market.

The type of packaging chosen for a particular foodstuff depends on a number of factors, not the least important of which is the nature of the goods to be packaged, especially if it is moist or greasy. Dry goods, such as flour or sugar, can be packed in simple materials such as paper, but foods such as coffee or biscuits, which are susceptible to humidity changes, must be packed in moisture-proof packages to keep them in a saleable condition. In turn, greasy foods require greaseproof packaging and moist goods, moisture-proof packages. Having considered the nature of the goods, a number of packaging materials may present themselves as suitable. The final choice will then be based on the physical requirements of the pack to enable it be stored and distributed in good condition.

When comparing the availability of materials, one of the main considerations (apart from cost) is that of compatibility. There are subtle considerations such as the elimination of odour, dye or solvent contamination, and the matter of aesthetic appeal.

Clingfilms

Small amounts of chemicals may possibly transfer foods from tightly wrapped clingfilm under certain circumstances. MAFF's Food Safety Directorate issued advice in November 1990 following media interest and concern over the use of clingfilms with food [13]. The advice covered **all plastic** food wrapping films, which have a 'cling' property, whatever their composition and whether used in the home or in shops. The advice does not cover the thicker, non-cling plastic wrapping often used by retailers and manufactures.

Plastic packaging materials such as clingfilms confer many benefits. In particular, they assist in preventing contamination of food by micro-organisms. Clingfilms also provide considerable benefits of convenience to consumers, but it is known that small amounts of chemicals can transfer into foods from such wrapping under certain circumstances. There is **no** evidence to suggest that the use of these chemicals has caused harm to health and clingfilms remain suitable for most foods uses.

Following earlier work, the government issued general advice in 1986 concerning the use of clingfilms in cooking. Further work discussed in a report (MAFF Food Surveillance Paper No. 30) has shown that chemicals in clingfilms tend to transfer most into high-fat foods such as cheese, and government experts have advised that clingfilms should not be used to wrap foods of this type. Advice to consumers is as follows:

1. Do not use clingfilms in conventional ovens.
2. In a microwave oven, use clingfilms for defrosting or reheating foods; when cooking, use them for covering containers, but they should **not** come into contact with food or be used for lining dishes.
3. Do not use them in a way that makes them come into contact with high-fat foods. If in doubt, use an alternative wrapping material – there are many to choose from.

Manufacturers are recommended to label packs along the above lines, and retailers are recommended to follow the advice given in point (3) above.

Paper

This is probably one of the oldest and most common packing materials; it is not only cheap and easily disposed of, but is also easily printed and may be allowed to come into contact with food. However, it is clear that in its usual form it is only suitable for dry goods or, for example, as outer wrappers for confectionery.

Waxed paper

This has been found suitable for wrapping bread and protecting sliced loaves from disintegration and loss of moisture. It is not possible to wrap bread in a completely waterproof material as it is liable to become soggy and mouldy. Bread is, therefore, cooled (to reduce condensation), wrapped in wax paper and the ends heat sealed. The seal is 'loose' enough to allow some moisture to escape and gives the sliced loaf a more acceptable shelf-life and keeps it clean. Waxed paper, or light gauge card, is familiar as a material for forming disposable liquid cartons, such as milk cartons. It is also extensively used for frozen products, where it gives mechanical protection to the contents.

The tetra-pak

This is an irregular-shaped pack used to contain UHT milk and is formed from a paper base and polythene liner. The polythene allows the ends to be sealed.

Polythene

Being moisture proof, but not entirely vapour proof, polythene is put to innumerable uses. Being a thermoplastic it is useful for heat sealing and may be over-printed to a degree. Its main use is as a bulk, cheap package and shrinkwrap material for fruit and vegetables. Polythene packed meats, such as hams and large cuts of bacon, may be scalded after packing to shrink the packing material into intimate contact with the surface. This will kill heat-sensitive, surface organisms but, even with highly salted foods, bacterial growth may continue at a slow rate unless the products are refrigerated.

Polystyrene

Although brittle, polystyrene can be extruded and this makes it suitable for forming containers for cream, yoghurt, milk, etc. In its foamed form, it is extensively used for meat trays, insulated cups and egg containers.

Pliofilm

This is a chlorine rubber product, similar in appearance to polythene. It is widely used for meat packaging as it is heat shrinkable and mois-

ture proof. It is also permeable to oxygen and this quality allows the surface of packed meats to stay fresh and red.

Nylon and PVC

These are usually used in combination with cellophane, to produce vacuum-pack envelopes, the layers of substances being bonded together with adhesives, with a thermoplastic layer being placed internally, to allow the pack to be heat sealed. These containers are suitable for conditions where it is essential that no air or moisture gets into the pack and no grease gets out. Crisps may be packed in this way with an inert atmosphere of dry nitrogen to keep them crisp and prevent rancidity. Nitrogen packs are also used for products such as dried milk and coffee and dehydrated goods.

Cellulose

Cellulose materials used in combination with other materials is another form of transparent packaging, but may not be moisture or gas proof, although it can be reasonably greaseproof. It is ideal for packaging bread, confectionery, sausages, meats and cheese and, although not thermoplastic and therefore heat sealable, it allows moisture to evaporate without condensing and encouraging mould growth.

Aluminium

This has the disadvantage of being expensive, opaque and will not heat seal, but as a metal it is both moisture and gas proof and has good heat reflective qualities. It is ideal for packing dairy goods, such as cheese, and being malleable makes ideal tops for milk bottles, jam jars, yoghurt containers, etc. Used as a laminate, it is useful for sacheting liquids and dehydrated foods. Used to nitrogen pack goods, it gives great strength and long-term gas permanence to the package.

Glass

Glass, in the form of jars or bottles with hermetically sealed covers, makes a most suitable food preservation container. The material possesses advantages over tinplate as there is no risk of metallic poisoning, it is always possible to see the condition of the contents, and the costly vacuum sealing machinery necessary for cans is not needed. On the other hand, it can be easily broken or splintered and is more costly. Because of the danger of breakage, lower temperatures and longer exposures are necessary when treating the contents.

The Materials and Articles in Contact with Food Regulations 1987 control the use of the materials intended to come into contact with food. The basic aim of the Regulations is to establish a general standard for the manufacture of articles and materials which come into contact with food by requiring these goods to be made in such a manner that they do not transfer any of their constituents to the food, thus making it harmful or unacceptable to the consumer. The protection extended to the consumer prohibits the importation, use or sale for food (Food Safety (Exports) Regulations 1991) or the use of any material which does not satisfy the standard. (See also Directives 89/109/EEC and 80/590/EEC.)

Gas packing

Many foodstuffs are so sensitive to oxygen that the only way to ensure an adequate shelf-life is the complete removal or exclusion of the oxygen. Ways of doing this are to:

1. pack the container so tight that there is little room for air; or
2. evacuate the air; or
3. remove the air and replace it with a non-oxidizing gas.

It is now possible to pack foods in atmospheres known to inhibit deteriorative changes. The technique has been used successfully for meats, vegetables and dairy products, and has also proved effective for fish. For each type of food it is necessary to determine the optimum mixture of gases. Thus for meat it is necessary to increase the level of oxygen to maintain the desirable red colour but, for nuts, oxygen should be excluded to prevent oxidative rancidity. With fish the rate

of bacterial spoilage can be slowed down by increasing the level of carbon dioxide.

The required atmosphere is carefully controlled at the time of packing and hence the description, controlled atmosphere packaging (CAP). An alternative description for the same process is modified atmosphere packing (MAP), as the atmosphere within the pack will change during storage. It is necessary to distinguish between this technique and the more complicated system of controlled atmosphere storage, in which the individual gases of the atmosphere are monitored continuously and maintained at predetermined levels throughout storage.

A number of machines providing different degrees of sophistication are now available for CAP. With the simplest machines the product is placed in a plastic sleeve, flushed with a gas mixture and then sealed. More sophisticated machines provide an integrated packaging system. These machines will thermoform base trays from a roll of plastic film into which the product is placed. The loaded trays pass along the machine to be evacuated and then are filled with the required mixture of gases. A second roll of film is heat sealed to the top edges of the trays and the finished packs pass out of the machine.

The advantages of these packs include extension of shelf-life if stored under carefully chilled conditions: the containment of odour and drip for products such as fish; the packs can be attractively labelled; and a wide variety of products can be displayed by retailers without the need for specialist skills.

For fish particularly, loss of freshness is caused by autolytic deterioration brought about by enzymes naturally present in the flesh, followed by the invasion of spoilage bacteria. The autolytic changes commence on the death of the fish and result in a breakdown of the compounds responsible for the sweet and desirable flavours. During this period, bacteria found on the surface of the fish start to invade the flesh and their growth causes a breakdown of the tissues. The effect on the cooked product is the gradual development of increasingly undesirable flavours. At the surface, the effects of bacterial growh are seen as the development of a slime. With fatty species, a further undesirable change occurs due to the development of rancid flavours.

In using CAP for fish, the gases carbon dioxide (CO_2), nitrogen (N_2) and oxygen (O_2) are commonly used. Extensive trials show that CO_2 inhibits bacterial activity, but autolytic changes proceed. Nitrogen is an inert gas included in the gas mixture to offset the adverse effects of high levels of CO_2 by maintaining the shape of the pack. Oxygen appears to reduce the amount of drip from white fish, but this gas may be beneficially omitted from packs of fatty fish to delay the onset of oxidative rancidity. Inclusion of O_2 does not overcome the potential hazard of toxin production by *C. botulinum*. Thorough bacteriological testing has shown that toxin production is primarily dependent on temperature and that maintaining the fish at 4°C or below is the best preventative measure. Thus packing fish in a controlled atmosphere presents no more danger than other forms of packaging fish with a potential botulinogenic hazard, providing chill temperature storage is maintained. To obtain the maximum benefit from packing in a controlled atmosphere, it is recommended that the temperature of packs is accurately maintained at 0–2°C throughout production, distribution and retailing [14].

REFERENCES

1. The UK Association of Frozen Food Producers, *Recommendations for the Handling of Quick Frozen Foods, Production, Distribution, Retailing, Freezing and Storage in the Home*, Code of Practice UK AFFP, London.
2. Strategies for Assessing The Safety of Foods Produced by Biotechnology, Report of a Joint FAO/WHO Consultation, World Health Organization, Geneva.
3. Ministry of Agriculture, Fisheries and Food (1990) *Food Irradiation, Some Questions Answered*, MAFF Food Safety Directorate Information Issue No. 2, HMSO, London.
4. World Health Organization, *Golden Rules for Safe Food Preparation*, WHO, Geneva.
5. Department of Health, *Guidelines for the Safe Production of Heat Preserved Foods*, 1994, HMSO, London.
6. Schafheitle, J.M., The sous-vide system for preparing chilled meat. *British Food Journal*, **92**(5), 23–7.
7. SVAC (Sous Vide Advisory Committee) (1991) Code of Practice For Sous Vide Catering Systems, Sous Vide Advisory Committee, Tetbury, Glos.
8. Department of Health letter to CEHOs and chief port health inspectors, 29 August 1989. *Guidance for Environmental Health Departments on the Prevention of Botulism*, reference EL(89)P145.
9. Advisory Committee On The Microbiological Safety Of Food, Report On Vacuum Packaging And Associated Processes, January 1993, HMSO, London.
10. Advisory Committee On The Microbiological Safety Of Food, Report on Vacuum Packaging And Associated Processes, Recommendations and Government's Response, MAFF, Room 515a, Ergon House, Smith Square, London SW1P 3JR.
11. Chilled Food Association (1989) *Guidelines For Good Hygienic Practice in the Manufacture of Chilled Foods*, Chilled Foods Association, London.
12. Slocum, P. (1990) Cold chain distribution and other transport matters. Paper given at the Leatherhead Food RA Symposium on Food Safety Legislative Aspects, 7 November.
13. Ministry of Agriculture, Fisheries and Food (1990) *Cling Film*, MAFF Food Safety Directorate Information Issue Number 7.1, Special Edition, HMSO, London.
14. Seafish Industry Authority (1985) *Guidelines for the Handling of Fish Packed in a Controlled Atmosphere* SFIA, Edinburgh.

Part Seven
Environmental Protection

39 Introduction to environmental protection

Martin J. Key

This chapter considers the reasons for the recent elevation of environmental concern among both the general public and politicians; the effect that this increased awareness is having on current and developing pollution philosophies; the economic aspects of pollution control; the future challenges and problems likely to be faced in the environmental arena; and briefly examines the subject of radiation in the environment.

INTRODUCTION

'Perpetual twilight reigns during the day, and during the night fires on all sides light up the dark landscape with a fiery glow. The pleasant green of pastures is almost unknown; the streams, in which no fishes swim, are black and unwholesome; the natural dead flat is often broken by huge hills of cinders and spoil from the mines; the few trees are stunted and blasted; no birds are to be seen, except a few smoky sparrows, and for miles and miles black waste spread round where furnaces continually smoke, steam engines thud and hiss, and long chains clank, while blind gin horses walk their doleful round.'

This was the description of the industrial Black Country in the Midlands in 1851. The Industrial Revolution was responsible for prolific industrial growth, but at what cost to the environment?

It has been said that the latter part of the 1980s has seen the start of the 'Green Revolution'. However, the first concerted effort to deal with this environmental destruction was taken in 1863 when the first Alkali, etc. Works Regulation Act was passed, which required extensive reductions in offensive emissions, and established the Alkali Inspectorate to enforce this requirement. Since that date, environmental protection legislation has developed steadily, but it is true to say that it was only in the late 1970s that public and, perhaps more importantly, political attention was focused on environmental problems. There is now common agreement between international bodies that concerted multilateral actions are required to achieve the necessary protection of the environment.

The environment is a complex interaction of many ecosystems, and it therefore follows that measures to control man's impact on the environment will similarly be a complicated mixture of actions and policies. While severe environmental damage can be caused by relatively short-term activities, the effect of these activities and measures to rectify the environmental damage are very much long-term problems. Policies and controls in place now will not start to have a noticeable effect until after the turn of the century, thus failure to act now may be irrevocable. It is also of paramount importance to remember that environmental effects are global, therefore unilateral action to rectify this damage will fail – it requires international co-operation and clear, targeted global action.

REASONS FOR CURRENT ENVIRONMENTAL CONCERN

It has long been recognized that public concern plays a major role in the development of environmental legislation. For example, public complaint in the 1860s concerning emissions from alkali works resulted in a parliamentary enquiry which led to the Alkali, etc. Works Regulation Act 1863 being enacted. The great London smog of 1952, which was responsible for 4000 extra deaths as the direct result of 5 days of smog aroused intense public outrage. The result was a detailed study of air pollution by the Beaver Committee, which led to the enactment of the first Clean Air Act of 1956. More recently, we have seen the publication of a major government white paper on the environment [1], which details an environmental strategy into the next century. The first direct legislation arising from this broad view of government policy in the environmental field is the Environmental Protection Act 1990, which sees a long awaited overhaul of environmental protection in Britain, particularly in the area of pollution control.* This has arisen as a result of increasing environmental awareness among the public, and greater demands and expectation concerning environmental quality.

This public realization has indeed been a very rapid process and the following are some of the main reasons for this awakening:

1. Disasters such as the gas cloud escape at Bhopal and the nuclear reactor failure at Chernobyl highlight the dramatic effects of environmental incidents, and illustrate both the local and global implications of such environmental disasters.
2. Better economic growth has led to higher standards of living and consequently greater demands and expectations concerning the 'quality of life', such as healthy living, clean air and water, and enjoyment of natural environmental amenities.
3. The realization that the world cannot accommodate pressures of increasing population and rapid technical growth without an effect.
4. The speed and complexity of change in technology appears to be outstripping the development of prediction and control measures.
5. The realization that global problems are in effect a summation of national and international pollution, and that while global actions are needed to control pollution, these cannot be fully implemented without national commitment to pollution control.
6. The wish to leave our children a world worth inheriting, indeed many people fear that we have already caused irrevocable damage, e.g. global warming and stratospheric ozone depletion.
7. More co-ordinated efforts by the green movement and pressure groups, e.g. Greenpeace and Friends of the Earth, and their more dramatic use of the media in their campaigns.
8. Less local dependency on industry; whereas in the early part of this century people living around factories were commonly employees at the factories and, therefore, were more prepared to accept poor environmental standards knowing that their livelihood depended on continued operation of the factory, this is no longer such a major constraint.

The sudden appearance of the Green Party in the late 1980s in mainstream politics again reinforces how important public perception of environmental concerns are. This resulted in the so called 'greening' of the main political parties, and has now firmly established environmental protection policies high on the agenda. It is also important to realize the effect of international co-operation on environmental matters, in particular, the extensive activities of the EU in this area.

WHAT IS POLLUTION?

Releases into the environment can result in a wide range of environmental effects. In order to consider these effects further, it is perhaps neces-

---

* Now to be followed by the Environment Bill, due to be enacted in 1995.

sary to consider what the term **pollution** means. There are a number of proposed definitions, however, the most recent definition used in the Environmental Protection Act 1990 defines pollution in terms of the capability of a substance to cause harm to man or other living organisms supported by the environment. The term **harm** can be further defined as:

> harm to the health of living organisms, interference with ecological systems of which they form part or offence caused to any sense of man or harm to his property.

Thus it can be seen that the term pollution takes into account physical risk, ecosystem damage, damage to property and somewhat aesthetic considerations of offence to senses.

POLLUTION CONTROL STRUCTURES

Pollution control responsibilities are currently split between central and local government, although the bulk of industrial processes are subject to local government control. The Environmental Protection Act 1990 implemented a number of major changes in pollution control strategy and structure in Britain, particularly in the fields of air pollution, waste disposal and noise control. The following is an overview of the current structure of pollution control, which is examined in greater detail in following chapters.

Air pollution control

Responsibility for air pollution control has traditionally been split between Her Majesty's Inspectorate of Pollution (HMIP) and local authorities. IIMIP was formed in 1987 within central government by the amalgamation of the Alkali Inspectorate, the Radiochemical Inspectorate and the Hazardous Waste Inspectorate.

The larger industries with potentially major environmental impact had been under the control of HMIP subject to a prior approval system for a considerable period of time. This system was based upon a preventative approach which sought to apply pollution controls at the design stage of process planning to maximize the environmental

controls in an economically viable manner. Part I of the Environmental Protection Act 1990 updated this approach and replaced the historical industrial pollution control system for other processes based upon statutory nuisance control under the Public Health Act 1936 (now replaced by Part III of the Environmental Protection Act 1990). The previous local authority controls were based on reactive controls, that is the powers were available to deal with pollution episodes once they had been caused.

There are two fundamental principles of Part I of Act, which are:

1. Processes prescribed by regulation must not be operated without an authorization from the relevant enforcement agency (HMIP or the local authority in whose area they are located).
2. The authorization issued must contain specific conditions which are designed to achieve the objectives of the Act, the principal relevant objective is that the process must operate using the best available techniques not entailing excessive cost (BATNEEC) to prevent or, where not practicable by such means, to minimize emissions of prescribed substances and to render harmless any substance which may be emitted.

There is still a large number of industrial and commercial processes not prescribed which are subject to the reactive statutory nuisance provisions of Part III of the Act.

Water pollution control

Prior to 1989, the control of discharges to water was the remit of the water authorities. However, with the implementation of the Water Act 1989 (now consolidated in the Water Resources Act 1991 and the Water Industry Act 1991) and the privatization of the water supply industry along with the formation of the National Rivers Authority (NRA), the current control system is relatively complex. Control of discharges to water is currently undertaken by three organizations:

1. HMIP controls the discharge of substances prescribed by the Trade Effluents (Prescribed Substances and Processes) Regulations 1989,

the prescribed substances being the so-called 'red list'.

2. NRA controls the discharge of pollutants to controlled waters, including rivers, watercourses, lakes and groundwater.

3. The Water Service Companies control the discharge of trade effluent to sewers by both trade effluent discharge consents and trade effluent discharge agreements.

Waste disposal

The regulation of waste disposal is currently undertaken by local government, the responsibilities being divided between metropolitan districts and boroughs, and non-metropolitan county councils. The control was exercised by the issue of waste disposal licences under the Control of Pollution Act 1974. In addition, regulations made under this Act, defined 'special wastes', the movement of which to disposal sites needs to be covered by prior notification of intended movements to the waste disposal authority. HMIP also has a role in waste disposal, which currently is an overview of the arrangements including an audit of the performance of waste disposal authorities. There have been a number of problems in the waste disposal field which generally revolve around inadequate legislation. Primarily, there is currently no detailed control over former landfill sites producing landfill gas and, secondly, the licensing legislation did not permit adequate enforcement of licence conditions. The Environmental Protection Act 1990 included a number of new provisions which go some way to addressing these problems, including separating operational waste disposal functions from regulatory authorities by the formation of 'arms length' companies, creation of a duty of care for all links in the waste disposal chain, and the requirement that holders of waste management licences are 'fit and proper persons'.*

The implementation of Part II of the Environmental Protection Act 1990 in 1994 replaced the old waste management licensing system through the Waste Management Licensing Regulations 1994.

Noise control

The control of noise is regulated by local authorities under the provisions primarily of the Environmental Protection Act 1990. There is a growing problem of community noise, particularly in towns and cities, again where public tolerance will no longer permit noisy behaviour of neighbours. The Noise and Statutory Nuisance Act 1994 introduced new controls over noise in public places.

Emissions of radioactive substances†

Control of the release of radioactive substances is the responsibility of HMIP who enforce the provisions of the Radioactive Substances Act 1993. This legislation covers registration of sites keeping radioactive substances, and licensing of the discharge of radioactive waste to air, water and solid waste disposal routes. The principal problem is the lack of availability of disposal methods and facilities for medium- and high-risk radioactive waste.

Planning

One common theme among all pollution control activities is the importance of planning. Enforcement of planning controls under the Town and Country Planning Act 1990 is a local authority responsibility, and environmental matters are central to the decision-making process of planning new development. One of the more recent initiatives in the planning field was the development of the environmental impact assessment for larger proposals, particularly industrial processes with significant pollution potential, and the subject of environmental impact assessment is considered further in the next section.

Recent guidance from the government in Planning Policy Guidance Note No. 23 1994, Planning and Pollution Control, offers advice on the interface between planning controls and environmental protection controls. It suggests that with the new powers being implemented for environmental

---

* Proposals to deal with former landfill sites are included in the Environment Bill due to be enacted in 1995.
† See 'The Review of Radioactive Waste Management Policy – Preliminary Conclusions'. August 1994, DoE.

regulation, the use of planning powers to control environmental pollution should not be necessary. Where there are relevant controls which are enforced by a pollution control regulatory body, the control of pollution issues should be left to the relevant controls of that body and not incorporated into the planning discussions. The planning issue legitimately considers land-use planning issues.

Environment Agency

The government have announced their intention to form a new Environment Agency to provide for an integrated enforcement and advisory agency on environmental issues operating at arms-length from government departments. The aim is to ensure that the Agency is independent and can critically assess effectiveness of legislation. The legislation to form the agency is due in 1995, but the framework is likely to be based upon an amalgamation of the National Rivers Authority and HMIP. In addition, the local authority waste regulatory functions under Part II of the Environmental Protection Act 1990 are expected to be brought into the agency. The Agency will operate from April 1996.

NEW PHILOSOPHIES IN POLLUTION CONTROL AND THE EUROPEAN DIMENSION

Initiatives taken in the EU have had an important role in shaping new pollution control approaches now being carried through into national legislation within Britain. However, it is also fair to say that the UK is itself developing new international initiatives in pollution control, particularly in relation to cross-media pollution problems by developing the **'integrated pollution control'** approach which seeks to apply the **'best practicable environmental option (BPEO)'**. This section will examine the basis of EU environmental programmes, the impact of these programmes on UK legislation and practice, and the way that these concepts have been developed into more wide-reaching environmental control strategies.

European Union actions

The UK joined the EU in 1973. The Treaty of Rome created the EU (then known as the European Economic Community, EEC) in 1957, and one of the fundamental objectives was the creation of a 'Common Market'. The Single European Act, which came into effect on 1 July 1987, expanded this concept to create an 'internal market' without internal frontiers to allow the free movement of goods, persons, services and capital, and set a target date of 31 December 1992 for these initial measures to be in place. In order to achieve these aims, it is necessary to harmonize legislation through the EU, and this includes extensive harmonization of environmental legislation.

However, the EU has not only attempted harmonization, but also has produced a number of programmes to improve environmental standards throughout the EU. The first step in this action was again due to public opinion on environmental matters and developments in other international organizations, which led to the European Commission preparing a programme for action. The first Programme of Action on the Environment was produced in 1973, and detailed the objectives and principles of a Community environmental policy, and described the measures to be taken to reduce pollution and nuisances and to improve the environment. There followed three further action programmes in 1977, 1983 and 1987, and the recent fifth programme.

The most recent of these, the fifth action programme, is concerned with a number of issues, namely climate change, acidification, air and water pollution and waste management, aimed at achieving sustainable development. This issue is considered further later in this chapter.

It also proposes the adoption of an **'integrated substance orientated approach'**, which is similar in effect to the new integrated pollution control concept included in the Environmental Protection Act 1990.

It is, however, directives which have a more active effect on policies and legislation in member states. These directives are not themselves legislation, but are required to be implemented by national legislation. While it is not possible here to examine in detail all directives with relevance to the environment, the following examples illustrate how wide reaching these EU measures have been in respect of their impact on UK environmental strategies.

1. Directives which set statutory air quality standards, including 80/779/EEC on sulphur dioxide and suspended particulates, 822/882/ EEC on lead in air and 85/203/EEC on nitrogen dioxide in air. Directive 84/360/EEC, the so-called 'framework directive', which required the use of BATNEEC to control air pollution from certain prescribed processes.
3. Specific directives setting control standards for certain types of industrial process, e.g. 88/609/ EEC on large combustion plant and 89/369/ EEC on municipal waste incinerators.
4. Directives relating to the treatment and trans-frontier shipment of hazardous wastes, particularly 78/319/EEC on toxic and dangerous waste, and 84/631/EEC on the trans-frontier shipment of hazardous wastes within the EU.
5. A directive on pollution caused by certain dangerous substances discharged into the aquatic environment (76/464/EEC), which resulted in the so-called 'red list' substances falling under special controls.
6. A directive concerning the assessment of the environmental effects of certain public and private projects (85/337/EEC), which has led to the implementation under town and country planning legislation of the requirement to undertake environmental impact assessments of certain types of development capable of causing environmental harm (Town and Country Planning (Assessment of Environmental Effects) Regulations 1988 (SI 1199)).

The role of the EC has recently been expanded by the agreement to form the **European Environmental Agency**, which will have a remit to collect data concerning environmental standards within the EU and examine compliance with directives issued by the EU. Whether in the long-term this organization will have a wider brief other than collection of data is still unclear, although many believe that this could be the start of a European pollution control enforcement agency. However, the difficulties already encountered in finding common ground for agreement on location, structure and brief of the Agency does not suggest that extending the remit is a feasible proposition currently.

Best available techniques not entailing excessive cost (BATNEEC)

The EU's directive on the combating of air pollution from industrial plants (84/360/EEC), the so-called 'framework directive', required that member states took all necessary measures to require operators of certain categories of industrial processes to seek prior authorization, and required the use of all appropriate preventive measures against air pollution, including the application of BATNEEC. A lengthy consultation process undertaken by the Department of the Environment resulted in the implementation of these requirements in the Environmental Protection Act 1990. However, it was felt that the word technology did not impart the necessary control philosophy, and therefore in the Act the requirement is that processes use the best available techniques not entailing excessive cost (BATNEEC) for preventing the release of substances to any environmental medium, or where it is not practicable by such means, for reducing the release of such substances to a minimum and for rendering harmless any substances which are released. The subtle difference between the word 'technique' and 'technology' is that technique implies not only the hardware used to control emissions, but the way that hardware is operated, including the number, qualifications, training and supervision of staff and the design, construction and maintenance of equipment.

The true interpretation of the term BATNEEC will be revealed in the long term, when cases are taken through the legal system and individual circumstances are subjected to detailed legal consideration. However, the intention is that BATNEEC should be interpreted as meaning the following:

1. 'Best' should mean the most effective in preventing, minimizing and rendering harmless

polluting emissions, and there may be more than one set of techniques which can be termed 'best'.

2. 'Available' should mean procurable by any operator of the class of process in question. It should not imply that the technique is in general use, but it does require general accessibility.

3. 'Techniques' includes the process and how the process is operated, including the concept and design of the process and staff numbers, supervision, training and working methods.

4. 'Not entailing excessive cost' needs to be taken in two contexts, depending upon whether it is applied to a new or an existing process. The presumption will be that the best available techniques will be used, although that can be modified by economic considerations where the cost of applying the best available techniques would be excessive in relation to the environmental protection achieved. In applying the not entailing excessive cost test for existing processes, the intention is that these processes will be upgraded to the standards applicable to new processes in the same category and, therefore, the cost consideration is essentially concerned with the timescale for this upgrading programme. EC Directive 84/360/EEC allows for the following matters to be taken into account when determining the timescale for upgrading existing processes:
   (a) the plant's technical characteristics;
   (b) its rate of utilization and length of its remaining life;
   (c) the nature and volume of polluting emissions from it;
   (d) the desirability of not entailing excessive costs for the plant concerned, having regard in particular to the economic situation of undertakings belonging to the category in question.

The principle in the application of BATNEEC is, therefore, the use of the most efficient pollution control technique, having regard to a balance between the economic costs and environmental costs. A later section of this chapter considers how the environment can be costed, and how a financial approach can therefore be taken to balancing the true cost of environmental degradation.

In determining what particular control strategy will fulfil the BATNEEC objective, a systematic and analytical approach must be taken. Once the pollutant produced by a process has been identified, it is relatively simple to produce a list of available control techniques. The next step is then to systematically assess each of these control techniques and examine how efficient and effective they are in relation to control of the particular pollutant in the particular circumstances of its production in the process concerned. The next stage is then to consider the relative cost of each of these control techniques, including both capital and running costs, and then to compare how the efficiency of pollution control and costs correlate. In most cases, the more efficient the arrestment technique, the most expensive it will be to provide. The difficult stage is then to determine where the balance lies between the cost and the environmental protection achieved, and this should relate to a number of parameters including:

1. any air quality guidelines that exist for the pollutant concerned;
2. the ecotoxicity of the pollutant concerned;
3. whether the pollutant concerned has any nuisance potential, for example, odour;
4. any additional environmental problems and supplementary costs incurred by particular arrestment equipment, e.g. the production of liquid waste or solid waste which will then require further treatment and disposal.

The final stage in the decision-making process is the evaluation of all of the data to determine which technique provides the best environmental protection in relation to the nature and hazard of the pollution concerned, and incurs realistic and commensurate costs having regard to the economic position of the industry sector. It is also likely that an additional consideration will be a comparison of the range of techniques used elsewhere in the world, particularly in Europe, as in line with the harmonization ideals of the EU

BATNEEC should receive similar interpretations across the EU.

It is likely that with the enforcement of the BATNEEC requirements, particularly the substitution of the word 'technique' for 'technology', the UK will once more become one of the leaders in environmental protection practice. The BATNEEC approach has been somewhat extended by the Environmental Protection Act 1990, which introduces for the larger polluting industries the concept of 'integrated pollution control', which is examined in detail below.

Best practicable environmental option (BPEO)

The Royal Commission on Environmental Pollution has been the driving force behind the promulgation of the BPEO concept. This Royal Commission is in effect, a 'think tank' appointed by the government to advise on matters, both national and international, and is charged with considering the pollution of the environment, adequacy of research in this field, and the future possibilities of danger to the environment, and the reports which it produces are independent of government control. The Royal Commission's twelfth report issued in 1988 entitled *Best Practicable Environmental Option* [2], proposed the following explanation of the term:

> 'A BPEO is the outcome of a systematic consultative and decision making procedure which emphasizes the protection and conservation of the environment across land, air and water. The BPEO procedure establishes, for a given set of objectives, the option that provides the most benefit or least damage to the environment as a whole, at acceptable cost, in the long term as well as in the short term.'

The concept of BPEO is instrumental in the current changes and administration of pollution control in Britain.

Historical development of BPEO
While the practice of considering BPEO for pollution from processes is currently being implemented in the Environmental Protection Act 1990, the concept is not new. BPEO was first used in the Royal Commission on Environmental Protection Fifth Report, Air Pollution Control: An Integrated Approach, published in 1976 [3].

In the fifth report, the Commission highlighted that pollution could not be considered as an individual, media-related problem, but that there was a complex interaction between air, water and land and that all pollutants could potentially be transferred between the different media. The Commission examined the concept of **best practicable means (BPM)**, which has been central to the control of industrial air pollution since the late nineteenth century. The BPM approach takes account of controlling pollution by means which are reasonably practicable with regard to local conditions, financial implications and the current state of technical knowledge.

It was therefore proposed that the logical extension of the BPM approach would take account of the need to control all forms of pollution from a process to minimize the damage to the total environment, and as an initial means of achieving this aim a unified inspectorate was proposed to regulate industrial pollutants released to air, water and land.

The government's response to the fifth report, while accepting the importance of the need to control pollution taking account of the whole environment, did accept the need to establish the unified pollution inspectorate to promote this concept. The Royal Commission, concerned that its recommendations had not been implemented, reiterated the need for a multi-media approach in both its tenth report *Tackling Pollution – Experience and Prospects* [4] published in 1984, and eleventh report *Managing Waste: The Duty of Care*, published in 1985 [5].

This resulted in the establishment of the unified pollution inspectorate, Her Majesty's Inspectorate of Pollution, in 1987. Subsequently, the BPEO concept has been included in the Environmental Protection Act 1990 by means of the term 'integrated pollution control', which is discussed later in this chapter.

Evaluation of BPEO
The definition above states that a BPEO is a systematic consultative and decision-making procedure, it is therefore necessary to initially

identify the objective of the study. In addition, a careful and imaginative examination of alternative ways of achieving this objective (the options) should be produced. It is more cost effective to take account of environmental considerations early in the planning process for any project, and this may lead to a more acceptable environmental solution involving careful selection of the project operation rather than simply applying an 'end of pipe' solution. The term 'practicable' relates, among other matters, to the financial implication of the consideration of environmental effects, both capital and running costs. There is an element in BPEO assessment of balancing the financial costs with the environmental effects of applying different options in achieving the objective.

It is unlikely that any solution to a BPEO study will be the absolute best, as the other considerations in the study will interpret and evaluate the balance between cost and environmental effect. In addition, it is likely that any BPEO solution will be time related and, as further research and technological developments are made, the BPEO may change. It is therefore important that in any BPEO assessment a mechanism is put in place to review regularly the decision making process. It is therefore necessary during the initial BPEO study to provide a clear audit trail of the decisions taken and the justification for arriving at these decisions.

The Royal Commission's twelfth report [2] included a summary of the steps to be taken when evaluating a BPEO study and this is produced at Table 39.1. In addition, the report included a list of ten principles which are critical to reaching the correct decision. These are:

1. Environmental considerations should be introduced into project planning at the earliest possible stage.
2. Alternative options should be sought diligently and imaginatively in order to identify as complete a set as is possible.
3. The identification of potential damage to the environment should be done in such a way as to uncover the unusual and improbable as well as the familiar and likely.

Table 39.1 Summary of steps in selecting a BPEO.

Step 1: Define the objective
State the objective of the project or proposal at the outset, in terms which do not prejudge the means by which that objective is to be achieved.

Step 2: Generate options
Identify all feasible options for achieving the objective: the aim is to find those which are both practicable and environmentally acceptable.

Step 3: Evaluate the options
Analyse these options, particularly to expose advantages and disadvantages for the environment. Use quantitative methods when these are appropriate. Qualitative evaluations will also be needed.

Step 4: Summarize and present the evaluation
Present the results of the evaluation concisely and objectively, and in a format which can highlight the advantages and disadvantages of each option. Do not combine the results of different measurements and forecasts if this would obscure information which is important to the decision.

Step 5: Select the preferred option
Select the BPEO from the feasible options. The choice will depend on the weight given to the environmental impacts and associated risks, and to the costs involved. Decision-makers should be able to demonstrate that the preferred option does not involve unacceptable consequences for the environment.

Step 6: Review the preferred option
Scrutinize closely the proposed detailed design and the operating procedures to ensure that no pollution risks or hazards have been overlooked. It is good practice to have the scrutiny done by individuals who are independent of the original team.

Step 7: Implement and monitor
Monitor the achieved performance against the desired targets especially those for environmental quality. Do this to establish whether the assumptions in the design are correct and to provide feedback for future development of proposals and designs.

Throughout Steps 1 to 7: Maintain an audit trail
Record the basis for any choices or decisions through all of these stages, i.e. the assumptions used, details of evaluation procedures, the reliability and origins of the data, the affiliations of those involved in the analytical work and record of those taking the decisions.

Note: The boundaries between each of the steps will not always be clear-cut: some may proceed in parallel or may need to be repeated.

Source: Royal Commission on Environmental Pollution (1988) *Best Practicable Environmental Option*, 12th report, HMSO, London.

4. The context within which items (1) to (3) are considered should be sufficiently extensive to cover all the significant aspects of the project, whether local or remote, short or long term, and having regard to the people affected.
5. The documentation associated with each project should be structured to make it possible to trace decisions back to the supporting evidence and arguments, so providing an audit trail.
6. The documentation should include the origins of data used with any relevant information concerning the procedures used for the evaluation of risks and the reasons for the decisions based on those evaluations.
7. In order to assist in taking decisions having social and political implications, the scientific evidence must be presented objectively.
8. The determination of acceptable cost should take full account of any damage to the environment in addition to monetary cost. Financial considerations should not be over-riding.
9. There must be appropriate and timely consultation with people and organizations directly affected. The circle of those involved in taking decisions should be appropriately wide.
10. The procedure should be adaptable to incorporate innovations in methods of analysis and decision making by a feedback system.

In conclusion, BPEO is an assessment based on precautionary principles, wherever possible adopting low pollution or clean technology. The difficulty in fully evaluating a BPEO is likely to lie in attempting to determine the effect of pollutants being released into the environmental media to determine which options have the most beneficial environmental effects. It is likely that decisions made in the short term based on current knowledge may well have to be rectified at a later date when more research and information is available on the environmental impact of releasing the same substance into the different environmental media. This is one of the reasons for taking a precautionary approach in asssessing BPEO.

Integrated pollution control (IPC)

The Environmental Protection Act 1990 provides a regulatory strategy for requiring the adopting of the best practicable environmental option. This is achieved by the requirement that where a process is designated for central control by HMIP, and is likely to involve the release of substances into more than one environmental medium, BAT-NEEC will be used for minimizing the pollution which may be caused to the environment taken as a whole by the releases, having regard to the BPEO available. This procedure is termed 'integrated pollution control'.

The Royal Commission on Environmental Pollution's fifth report [3] proposed the integration of pollution control on a multi-media basis, and the seven main objectives of integrated pollution control are:

1. To develop an approach to pollution control that considers discharges from industrial processes to all media in the context of the effect on the environment as a whole.
2. To improve the efficiency and effectiveness of HMIP.
3. To streamline the regulatory system clarifying the roles and responsibilities of HMIP, other regulatory authorities, and the industries which they regulate.
4. To contain the burden on industry.
5. To maintain public confidence in the regulatory system by producing a clear, transparent system that is accessible and easy to understand and clear and simple in operation.
6. To ensure that the system will respond flexibly, both to change in pollution abatement technology and the new knowledge of the effects of pollutants.
7. To provide the means to fulfil international obligations relating to environmental protection.

An example of the IPC and BPEO approach is the consideration of sulphur dioxide emissions from large combustion plant. There are principally four options relating to the environmental release of sulphur dioxide from such processes:

1. the emission of sulphur dioxide to air;

2. the arrestment of sulphur dioxide by a wet method resulting in an acidified liquid discharge;
3. the arrestment of sulphur dioxide by a dry method resulting in a solid waste for disposal;
4. a change in feedstock to the combustion process reducing the sulphur content of the fuel burned, thus minimizing sulphur dioxide emissions.

The relative efficiency of each of these methods has to be considered along with the financial, social and political costs of adopting any of the four options. The balance of environmental effect is similarly very complex, as although reduction in emissions of sulphur dioxide to the air is of importance, the production of an acid-bearing liquid effluent or solid waste for subsequent disposal will also have an environmental effect. The balance of the overall costs and environmental implications requires detailed and careful consideration.

Environmental assessment

Environmental assessment, also known as **environmental impact assessment**, is a systematic procedure for collecting, analysing and presenting environmental data to ensure that the likely effects of a new development on the environment are fully understood and taken into account before the develoment is commenced. The concept was enacted by the EC Directive, *The Assessment of the Effects of Certain Public and Private Projects on the Environment* (85/337/EEC), which came into effect in July 1988. The requirements of this Directive have been implemented by the issue of a number of sets of regulations, including the prime instrument the Town and Country Planning (Assessment of Environmental Effects) Regulations 1988 (as amended 1994). The environmental assessment procedure is now integrated into the town and country planning process.

The aim of an environmental assessment is for the developer to provide the necessary information and undertake assessment of this information to enable scrutiny of the project and also to enable the predicted effects, and the methods for modifying or mitigating them, to be properly evaluated by the planning authority before a development decision is given. The decision-making network in an environmental analysis for an industrial process will, in many ways, be complementary to a BPEO study. The environmental assessment is the full information collection and decision-making process and is supported by an environmental statement, which is the developer's own assessment of the likely environmental effects of the project.

The legislation applies the environmental assessment technique to two separate lists of projects, the first in which an environmental assessment is required in all cases, and the second list where the project is likely to give rise to significant environmental effects. Those processes for which an environmental assessment is required in all cases are as follows:

1. crude oil refineries;
2. installations for the gasification and liquefaction of 500 tonnes or more of coal or bituminous shale per day;
3. combustion processes with a heat output of 300 megawatts or more;
4. installations for the storage or disposal of radioactive waste;
5. integrated iron and steel works;
6. installations for extracting and processing asbestos;
7. integrated chemical installations;
8. construction of motorways, express roads, railway lines and airports;
9. trading ports and inland waterways;
10. installations for the incineration, chemical treatment or landfill of special waste.

The exact content of an environmental statement is largely dependent upon the type of project [6,7] and scale of the project. However, all environmental statements should include the following information:

1. A description of the proposed project, including the site location, design, size and scale of the development.

2. Information about likely environmental effects, including expected residues and emissions.
3. A description of the likely effects on the environment, on:
   (a) human beings
   (b) fauna
   (c) water
   (d) climate
   (e) material assets
   (f) flora
   (g) soil
   (h) air
   (i) landscape
   (j) cultural heritage.
4. Where significant environmental effects are identified, the statement should include a description of the measures proposed to avoid, reduce or remedy these adverse effects. This should include an outline of the alternatives considered and the reasons for the choice with justification in relation to the environmental effects.

An environmental assessment and statement is very much a public document and, therefore, should include a non-technical summary. An important part of an environmental assessment is a continuation beyond the construction period to actually investigate the real environmental effects in terms of, for example, air quality and water quality, and a comparison with the predicted effects to enable both an assessment of the accuracy of the original statement and to aid future environmental assessments in identifying shortcomings in the assessment process and technique.

ECONOMIC ASPECTS OF POLLUTION CONTROL POLICIES

The economical and technological aspects of pollution control are inextricably linked. The economic aspects of pollution control range from the central philosophy of the polluter pays principle, upon which all pollution control legislation is based, and which is a central consideration in enactment of BATNEEC and BPEO, through to direct economic policies involving taxation and charges for pollution. This section examines the polluter pays principle, methods of charging for the environment, the concept of sustainable development and compensating for pollution related environmental damage.

The polluter pays principle

The polluter pays principle is central to the whole subject of economic measures as a mechanism for achieving environmental protection. It originates from a UN conference in 1972, was incorporated in the EC First Action Programme on the Environment in 1973 and was laid down in detail by the OECD Council in 1974. The central theme to the principle is that environmental resources are limited and while their use is not given a direct value, the misuse of such resources is not reflected in the market. It therefore seems reasonable to expect that the cost of pollution prevention control measures should be reflected in the cost of goods and services which cause the pollution either in production or consumption in order that the rational and careful use of environmental resources is encouraged.

There are three main options for enforcing the polluter pays principle, which are:

1. By setting standards, either of emission or environmental quality, and the cost of achieving these standards is wholly borne by the producer.
2. By instigating a system of pollution charges or taxes on the product resulting in environmental damage, or on the use of certain harmful materials in a process.
3. By initially setting national mass ceiling standards, and issuing tradeable pollution permits in amounts consistent with those ceiling standards.

One very important factor in assessing the success of the polluter pays principle, is who eventually meets the cost. It is usual when production costs are increased for these costs to be passed directly on to the consumer and, therefore, it is the consumer rather than the initial polluter who bears the cost. While at first sight this may seem inequitable, it reflects the true philosophy of market force environmental protection measures. The consumer who demands the product is encouraging the pollution and should, therefore, bear the overall costs, and be aware of the environmental element in order to allow a choice of paying the increased cost or changing demand for more environmentally benign products.

The Earth Summit

The International actions on global environmental issues are beginning to take shape. The most recent of these major International initiatives was the United Nations Conference on Environment and Development (known as the Earth Summit) which took place in Rio de Janeiro in 1992. The conference was a result of the Brundtland Report (Our Common Future) of 1987 which identifed the need to achieve sustainability in development.

The Earth Summit was attended by World leaders and officials from over 160 countries. The result of the summit were the following initiatives:

1. The production of a Framework Convention on Climate Change – this is aimed at stabilization of greenhouse gases, primarily carbon dioxide, at 1990 levels by 2000.
2. The production of a Convention of Biological Diversity – the aim of this is to protect and preserve endangered plants and species on land and in the oceans.
3. The establishment of Agenda 21, which is a detailed document setting out guidance for governments on establishing environmental policies to meet the needs of sustainable development.
4. A statement of principles for the management, conservation and sustainable development of all the world's forests.

The UK Government has ratified these conventions, along with over 150 other signatories. As a result of the UK involvement, the Government issued in 1994 four major documents outlining their plans to meet the objectives of the Conventions. These documents were:

1. Sustainable development: the UK strategy.
2. Climate change: the UK Programme.
3. Biodiversity: the UK Action Plan.
4. Sustainable forestry: the UK Programme.

Sustainable development

There is no simple or clear definition of the term 'sustainable development', and it could be said that it means all things to all men. The concept of sustainable development, however, is relatively straightforward. It assumes that the environment is a limited resource and, therefore, any activity which consumes the resource is depleting future availability. The idea of sustainability is that any activities undertaken should not reduce the availability of the resource in the future, i.e. no depletion of the resource should occur in the short or long term. It is tied also to the term 'development', which is a complex mixture of social and economic considerations including economic growth and quality of life. Therefore, it could be said that sustainable development is the increase of capital wealth and quality of life without the depletion of environmental wealth or resources.

There are three critical considerations to sustainable development, which are:

1. There needs to be a value given to the environment, including natural, built and cultural environments. Environmental quality is seen as an important characteristic of quality of life, and unless real value is given to environmental resources, the current practice of treating them as a free sink for wastes and by-products of production will result in long-term deterioration of available environmental resource.
2. Sustainable development concerns both short- and medium-term time horizons, and should also take account of predicted longer-term trends, perhaps 100 years or more.
3. Behind the theory of sustainable development is emphasis on equity, both within our existing society to ensure the availability of resource to the least advantaged, and also equity to future generations to ensure that they are left with equivalent natural wealth.

There are two alternate views on what can be considered sustainable development. The first is that by providing a method of valuing the environmental resource, as long as succeeding generations are left with the equivalent capital wealth, that is, taking account of the environmental resources by allocating a monetary value, the concept of sustainable development has been met. The second is that compensation for the future should focus not only on capital wealth, but more on environmental wealth and that future generations must inherit no less environmental capital than the current generation inherited. It is obvious from these two considerations that environmentalists would side with the second interpretation of sustainable development, while industrialists and economists would largely favour the first interpretation. It is interesting to note that the policy on future environmental controls proposed by the current government favour the second approach, i.e. that the environmental capital should not be reduced from one generation to another.

The UK approach to implement a policy structure to accomodate sustainability is dealt with in four strategy documents produced by the government in 1994 as a result of the Earth Summit.*

The role of economic measures in environmental protection

There are a number of different economic measures which can be used to reflect and encourage environmental protection measures. These include charges and levies, tradeable quotas and liability and compensation schemes. The principle behind the economic measures is that if a market-based approach to the environment is taken, consumers and producers are given clear indications of the cost of using environmental resources, and this is clearly in line with the polluter pays principle. It is important to realize at the outset that even if economic instruments were to be more widely used, there is still a central role for regulation and enforcement and monitoring of performance to determine compliance with standards. The simplest of the charges is the one that is included in the Environmental Protection Act 1990, i.e.

charges to recover the cost of enforcement and regulation. The remainder of this section considers in more detail alternate economic measures.

Levies and deposit refund schemes
One possibility where a material or product proves costly or dangerous to handle at the end of its operational life, e.g. tyres, is that the consumer should meet the cost of this disposal in accordance with the polluter pays principle. One method would be to charge a levy on the original product which would be returned through a central scheme to organizations undertaking the final disposal of the waste at the end of its operational life. Another method is to use a deposit and refund which encourages consumers to return materials or products which can be recycled. This scheme has had previous widespread use, e.g. in soft drink bottles where a deposit and refund scheme was operated to encourage the return and recycling of glass bottles.

Charges based on damage to the environment
The use of a charge which reflects the environmental costs of using resources or releasing wastes to air, water or land appears very sensible. It would encourage industry to review its operations and either choose to pay the charge and use the environmental resource, or more likely invest in cleaner technology to reduce its overhead cost for environmental matters. The main problem with this approach still relates to how to assign value to the environment.

Charges or taxes on products and materials
This option involves adding an environmental charge or tax directly to the price of materials or services offered to reflect the environmental damage caused. The most widely considered of these is the use of a carbon tax to encourage the reduction of carbon emissions. These proposals appear to have merit for further consideration; however, it is impossible to unilaterally adopt these taxes as they would have a devastating industrial, economic and social impact. Another variation of this taxation method is to use differ-

* Also see the 5th EC Environment Action Programme: Towards Sustainability – Government Action in the UK (1994), DoE.

ential rates to encourage the use of cleaner techniques or cleaner materials. This is used with unleaded petrol, where a tax differential results in unleaded petrol being considerably cheaper than the more polluting leaded variety.

Tradeable quotas

This approach is based upon determining a permitted ceiling for total emissions and then producing tradeable quotas in discrete blocks of permitted discharge 'units', which could be bought and sold within the industry sectors. The difficulty in this case is initially setting the total permitted amount, and also the fact that there would still need to be regulatory control to ensure that emissions were within the quota values. There is currently detailed consideration being given to implementation of a quota system for SO_2 emissions from power generating plants.

Liability and compensation

This approach is based upon the theory that if a polluter is liable for the environmental damage caused, it will encourage more careful behaviour and a reduction in the release of substances which may have such environmental effects. One of the problems with this approach is that it may be difficult to obtain insurance for such strict liabilities for certain environmental risks. This again has more wide reaching industrial and economic effects, and unilateral implementation of such measures would have a marked effect on the industrial competitiveness of UK industry.

In most cases, the charge-based approach using economic measures would still require fairly extensive regulatory control. This would effectively increase the overall burden on industry and may limit performance of UK industry in the European and on the worldwide market. The selection of the most equitable economic measure is very much process and market specific, and it is likely that in future an integration of economic and regulatory controls will be implemented once further research has identified the most effective methods of ensuring transparent and fair economic systems. The question of liability for environmental damage is considered further in the later section on 'Future policies in environmental protection' below.

Assigning value to environmental resources

The concept of allocating a value to air quality or water quality poses a number of very difficult problems. If you assume that the current wave of environmental awareness is a preference for cleaner air and water and generally a more attractive and enjoyable environment, this can be compared to the demand for, and selective purchase of, materials, goods and services, and therefore is very much an economic consideration. Therefore, an improvement in environmental quality is also an economic improvement. One of the difficulties however, is that many environmental resources cannot be costed – you cannot price the existence of a certain fish species in a water course, for example. In addition, there is no clear market because nobody purchases environmental improvement. The absence of either a direct or indirect market further complicates the economic evaluation of environmental resources.

It is, however, important that the approach to allocating values to environmental resources is further developed. At least with monetary values being assigned it gives a clear indication that the utilization of environmental resources is not free, that is to say, because nobody purchases or can claim exclusive rights to clean air that does not mean that industry has the right to pollute it. In addition, the decision-making process which would result in the evaluation of environmental values will at least identify the gains and losses of environmental quality, and will lead to the realization of the true value of environmental resource.

The valuation of the environment would certainly assist with decision-making processes related to the interpretation of BATNEEC and BPEO, as this would enable a true cost benefit analysis to be undertaken of environmental cost against capital cost for environmental control strategies and measures.

RADIATION IN THE ENVIRONMENT

Radiation is one of the pollutants about which the general public express great concern. It is invisible and cannot be detected by any of the other human senses, and is associated by many people with bombs, nuclear reactor failures and the causation of cancer. However, radiation is not only linked to the generation of nuclear power, but is a natural phenomenon which always has and always will be present in the environment due to naturally radioactive materials. There is no difference between the effects caused by 'artificial' radiation or 'natural' radiation. The public awareness of radiation in the environment was heightened by the nuclear reactor accident at Chernobyl in Western Ukraine in 1986, and which lead to contamination of water, soil, plants and food animals in the UK. The physics of ionizing radiation is described in Chapter 30.

Effects of radiation (see also Chapter 28)

The biological effects of exposure to radiation are due to the deposition of energy from radiation to any tissue through which it passes. One of the main effects in the tissue is localized ionization of cells due to electrical interaction. This may result in changes to the chemical nature of cell and can alter the rate of growth of the cell and result in a tumour. The types of effect produced can be divided into two categories: **somatic** which only affects the irradiated person due to cell depletion by cell death or prevention of division; and hereditary effects which damage the reproductive cells causing genetic mutations. In addition, the effects may be classed into two other categories: **stochastic** (effects which either happen or do not happen, such as hereditary defects and cancer), or **non-stochastic** (the severity is dose related, e.g. cataract formation).

Sources of ionizing radiation

The sources of ionizing radiation which cause general exposure of the public can be classified into natural sources and artificial sources. The following is a brief list of sources.

Natural radiation

COSMIC RADIATION. Cosmic rays come to earth from outer space and the sun. The cosmic rays from the sun are generally given off in bursts during solar flares. Cosmic rays are affected by the earth's magnetic field, and are absorbed by the atmosphere so that the dose of radiation decreases as the altitude decreases.

GAMMA RAYS. These are gamma rays emitted from the earth's crust which contains radioactive materials such as uranium, thorium and potassium 40. An additional source of this exposure is from mined building materials which contain quantities of these radioactive materials.

RADON DECAY PRODUCTS. Radon is a gas produced by decay of uranium, and a similar gas (thoron) is produced from naturally occurring thorium, which is present in rocks and building materials. The role of radon as an indoor air pollutant is discussed in Chapter 42.

INTERNAL EXPOSURE. This is mainly exposure from diet, and principally involves potassium 40.

Artificial sources of radiation

EXPOSURE FROM MEDICAL TREATMENT. There are two uses of radiation in medicine, firstly for diagnostic purposes and, secondly, for treatment, particularly of cancer. Diagnostic X-rays account for 93% of the collective dose from medical sources. Medical doses will vary between individuals dependent upon their state of health. The use of radiation in the treatment of disease is usually either by radiotherapy (treatment with X-rays or gamma rays to target tissue), or nuclear medicine involving the introduction of radioisotopes into the body.

NUCLEAR WEAPON TEST FALLOUT. The dose from nuclear fallout arising from atmospheric testing of nuclear weapons, particularly in the early 1960s, is very low. There has generally been a large reduction in atmospheric testing of nuclear weapons since the limited ban imposed in 1963.

RADIOACTIVE DISCHARGES. Releases of radioactivity into the environment occur to all three environmental media. These releases originate from nuclear power generation, defence establishments, research organizations, hospitals, radioactive waste disposal and the non-nuclear industry (the most important non-nuclear source being the combustion of coal). These releases are regulated by HMIP.

OCCUPATIONAL EXPOSURE. This can originate from both natural and artificial radiation exposure during occupational activities. The artificial sources include the nuclear fuel cycle, medical, dental and veterinary practice, usage in research and in general industry, e.g. for process and quality control. Exposure to natural radiation occurs in, for example, miners and aircraft staff due to exposure to radon and cosmic rays respectively (see also Chapter 30).

CHERNOBYL ACCIDENT. The Chernobyl accident led to substantial quantities of radionuclides dispersed over Europe. Within the UK, the contamination was largely corresponding to areas of high rainfall, thereby promoting wet deposition. One of the problems with this type of contamination is that it contaminates herbage and food animals, and so it leads to prolonged effects on the environmental exposure, particularly via diet. It has been estimated that the dose over 50 years caused by the accident is less than 2% of the average dose from all sources received each year.*

Radiological protection and monitoring

The principal organization responsible for setting standards relating to radiological protection is the International Commission on Radiological Protection (ICRP), which is a non-governmental scientific organization. In the UK, the National Radiological Protection Board (NRPB) advises the government on the suitability of proposed standards, and the current ICRP recommendations have been adopted by the UK government. There are three central requirements in the ICRP recommendations:

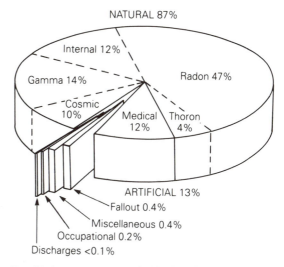

Fig. 39.1 Average annual effective dose equivalent to the population of the UK, 2.5 mSv. (Source: National Radiological Protection Board (1989) *Living with Radiation*, HMSO, London.)

1. No practice shall be adopted unless its introduction produces a positive net benefit.
2. All exposures shall be kept as low as reasonably achievable (ALARA), economic and social factors being taken into account.
3. The dose equivalent to individuals shall not exceed the limit recommended for the appropriate circumstances by the ICRP.

The current recommendation in relation to the dose achieved by a member of the public is as follows (although ICRP recommendations are currently under review):

'The average annual effective dose equivalent over a lifetime (assumed to be 70 years) shall not exceed the principle limit of 1 mSv per annum, however certain years are permitted at 5 mSv provided that the overall average for a lifetime does not exceed 1 mSv per annum.'

This standard excludes the contribution from natural radiation, that is, it is over and above background concentrations, and does not include exposure from medical procedures. Fig. 39.1 illustrates the source of the average annual effective dose equivalent to the population of the UK,

---

* Nevertheless, in the UK in 1995 there are still restrictions in some areas on the movement and use of food animals arising from the 1986 incident.

Table 39.2 Average annual risk of death in the UK from some common causes

Cause	Risk of death per year		
Smoking 10 cigarettes a day*	1 in 200	or 500	$\times 10^{-5}$
Natural causes, 40 years old	1 in 700	140	$\times 10^{-5}$
Accidents on the road	1 in 10 000	10	$\times 10^{-5}$
Accidents in the home	1 in 10 000	10	$\times 10^{-5}$
Accidents at work	1 in 50 000	2	$\times 10^{-5}$
Most exposed from nuclear effluents† (0.3 mSv)	1 in 70 000	1.4	$\times 10^{-5}$
All causes	1 in 80	1200	$\times 10^{-5}$

*For smoking, the risk indicated here includes all the adverse effects of smoking: for lung cancer only the risk is about halved.
†Estimated, not observed.
Source: National Radiological Protection Board (1989) *Living With Radiation*, 3rd edn, HMSO, London.

which is approximately 2.5 mSv, of which approximately 1% is due to discharges to the environment and 12% from medical exposure, the remainder being natural source radiation. In order to illustrate the level of risk, Table 39.2 compares calculated risks for death in the UK from some common causes.

Legal controls
There are principally two control organizations who enforce radiological protection legislation relating to environmental releases. HMIP is responsible for enforcement of the Radioactive Substances Act 1993. In addition, discharges from certain nuclear sites require authorization from MAFF (see Chapter 30 for controls over occupational exposure).

The principal requirements of the Radioactive Substances Act 1993 are that all static and mobile radioactive substances are registered, and that accumulations of waste prior to disposal, and disposal of such waste, are authorized.* The authorizations detail discharge limits, and monitoring requirements, and compliance with these authorizations is checked by HMIP.

Monitoring
The Chernobyl disaster illustrated that an overseas radiological incident could have an effect on the UK and that in these circumstances the national response plan in place for accidents arising within the UK was not suitable. As a result, the Department of the Environment has developed **RIMNET (Radioactive Incident Monitoring Network)**, which is a series of automatic gamma ray dose rate monitoring stations throughout the UK. This will provide an independent warning of any overseas accidents; a monitoring data base upon which to judge the impact of elevated levels; and a monitoring network and information handling network to measure and determine effects of such accidents. It involves coordination to ensure proper interpretation of data collected and provide central guidance on the necessary actions.

Also, as a result of the Chernobyl incident, a large number of local authorities have now instigated environmental radiation monitoring programmes. The majority of these rely on periodic gamma ray dose rate monitoring by portable instruments, although some more detailed strategies do exist involving sampling and analysis of water, soil and food. In order to ensure that data obtained by local authorities are quality assured and are also fed into the network of RIMNET in the case of an accident, the local authority associations have formed **LARRMACC (Local Authorities Radiation and Radioactivity Monitoring Advice and Collation Centre)**. This organization is responsible for providing guidance on monitoring protocols and also for collating local authority monitoring data and coordinating its input into the central government data base.

The NRPB also publishes guidance on **derived emergency reference levels (DERLS)** [8], which are for use in the case of an accident to assess the results of environmental measurements and determine necessary emergency actions. DERLs have been evaluated for a range of radionuclides for a number of exposure pathways, and also for individual foodstuffs and water.

A useful booklet on RIMNET has been produced by the Department of the Environment

* These procedures are analysed in *Environmental Health Procedures* 4th edn, W.H. Bassett (1995), Chapman & Hall.

Table 39.3 Typical UK waste generation

Waste type	Generation (million tonnes)
Radioactive waste	
low level	1.0
intermediate	0.16
high level	0.004
Hazardous industrial waste	5 to 10 per year
Coal mining spoil	50 per year
Refuse (England and Wales)	20 per year

Radioactive waste figures are the estimated total to 2000.
Source: Radiological Protection Board (1976) *Living With Radiation*, 3rd edn, HMSO, London.

(1993 HMSO) and this also outlines the National-Response Plan for dealing with overseas nuclear accidents, including the role of local authorities.

As part of the National Response Plan lead local authority environmental health departments have been designated and these will be the channel through which information is made available to all local authorities in an emergency. Lead authority arrangements are described in a paper RIMNET – Lead Local Authority Arrangements, issued by the Local Authority Associations in March 1994 and is available through the associations.

Radioactive waste disposal

One of the most complex problems arising out of the use of radioactive materials is the disposal of waste generated. In order to put radioactive waste generation into perspective, Table 39.3 compares radioactive waste generation in total to the year 2000, with the typical annual arisings of other types of waste.

There are two main options for radioactive waste disposal:

1. Containment: waste is held in shielded containers remote from high population and is held until the radioactivity has decayed to safe levels.
2. Dispersal: the material is diluted with ordinary waste until the average activity is low enough for conventional disposal.

At the present time, low-level waste is generally diluted and disposed of by landfill, while most medium-level, and all high-level waste is stored until it has decayed to a level at which it can be regarded as low-level waste.

There are a number of problems with repository storage of radioactive waste which affect the options for disposal as follows:

1. Certain radioisotopes have very long half lives (a thousand years plus), therefore the storage container needs to remain intact for extremely long periods.
2. No-one can with any certainty predict the behaviour of any building materials over long periods.
3. Continual inspection of storage systems will be required to detect leakage.
4. The choice of construction material and site location is very difficult. It must provide the necessary shielding and corrosion resistance, and it also needs to consider actions of decay products which may have different chemical characteristics to the original waste.
5. Liquids are more difficult than solids as intimate contact with containers may cause accelerated corrosion. In addition, if the container leaks the liquid will escape more rapidly than solid waste.
6. The choice of suitable disposal sites is affected by the ability to predict geological activity over the time scales necessary for a certain impact assessment for a long-term storage site. Perhaps one of the most difficult problems of all is the public pressure and objection to the thought of containment of high-level radioactive wastes near to their homes (the NIMBY – not in my back yard syndrome).

The current research programme into radioactive waste disposal has suggested that the most acceptable option is deep burial. For high-level wastes this would involve vitrification of the waste and disposal inside a stainless-steel cylinder. The cylinders would be stored in cooling ponds until a disposal route was available. The preferred option appears to be deep burial in sound geological strata where long-term geological stability has been modelled and demonstrated, and with minimal ground water flow around the storage site. In the UK, Nirex (Nuclear Industry Radioactive Waste Executive) has been undertaking detailed research, particularly into the disposal of intermediate and low-level wastes [9].

There are a number of options for deep disposal including under land, disposal under the sea-bed with access from the coast, and disposal under the sea-bed with access from the sea. Each of these options has both advantages and disadvantages, and research is currently being undertaken by the government to determine the most scientifically acceptable method of disposal.

FUTURE POLICIES IN ENVIRONMENTAL PROTECTION

'Pollution control and environmental policy generally should be accorded the priority and resources adequate for their integration into the National decision making process so that their potential benefits can be realised to the full and at the least cost.'

This was one of the conclusions of the Royal Commission on Environmental Pollution in their tenth report, *Tackling Pollution – Experience and Prospects* [4]. Environmental protection measures have often been fragmented and have not been an integral part of government or industrial decision-making processes. The government, on 25 September 1990, published a White Paper entitled *This Common Inheritance – Britain's Environmental Strategy* [1]. This is the first comprehensive white paper on the environment and is very wide ranging including pollution control, heritage, planning and countryside matters. Although the white paper was the subject of some criticism from a number of bodies, it does lay out some important strategies for future environmental protection measures. This final section of this chapter will examine two of the major global environmental problems, the steps proposed to meet the recommendations of the Royal Commission's tenth report outlined above and will examine three potential future environmental problems.

Environmental management

There has been an increase in the corporate awareness of environmental issues in industry. The development of the BS5750 quality management approach has been extended to consider environmental performance and propose management systems for taking account of environmental issues.

This lead to the introduction of a British Standard BS7750 on environmental management systems. This standard was established to help organizations establish management systems to review and improve environmental performance and to allow verification and audit of these activities.

The introduction of the EC Eco Audit in 1993 heralded an important step in EU policy with the establishment of a system of control based upon industry self-assessment. There is now development of this approach to establish an international standard for assessment of environmental performance throughout Europe and the rest of the world.

Sustainable resource management

Perhaps one of the most important aspects of the new wave of environmental concern, is the recognition that environmental protection, or perhaps more properly environmental management, is about defining strategies and implementing steps to ensure that words are put into action. The concept of sustainable management stems from the sustainable development theory outlined above, and recognizes that environmental resources are limited and that depletion will seriously degrade future environmental quality as well as prosperity.

Sustainable resource management is concerned primarily with good stewardship of environmental resources by a better understanding of the interrelationship between man's activities and environmental systems. Sustainable resource management includes, for example, the establishment of air quality standards and water quality objectives, to identify potentially unacceptable environmental releases which may have long-term impacts on the environment or, indeed, harm health. It also includes actions to ensure recycling of resources and protection of environmentally sensitive resources, such as tropical rain forests.

The term 'management' is very important when considering the concept of sustainable resources. It is concerned with achieving a balance between the environmental objectives and costs, and the economic and social costs involved in achieving these objectives. Environmental protection is not by any means a cheap option, and it is unrealistic to apply a rigorous, environmentally-biased perspective to resources and development. However, it is possible by careful planning and management of the environment to continue with industrial activities. but taking into account their effect on the environment to achieve a realistic balance between both concerns. While many current concerns are global problems, unless there is commitment at national level, the prospects for international collaboration to tackle these problems would not be encouraging.

The white paper [1] does outline steps to achieve better management of environmental resources applying the sustainability concept. These include:

1. the formation of an expert committee to establish air quality standards;
2. active encouragement for recycling operations;
3. establishing water quality objectives; and
4. instigating better handling and treatment of waste waters to protect bathing and drinking water standards.

In future it is likely that, following initial assessment of the most effective measures, the role of economic measures in environmental protection will increase.

Trans-boundary pollution

Trans-boundary pollution is a simple enough concept; pollution knows no boundaries. Global warming, the greenhouse effect and stratospheric ozone depletion, while being extremely complex environmental problems. are now becoming part of everyday vocabulary. The threat of irrecoverable damage to the environment and the potential

impact of this to future life styles does tend to focus the attention. Photochemical oxidation reactions which produce ozone are currently seen as a local problem, although trans-boundary movement of these pollutants does occur.

The only successful way to tackle trans-boundary pollutants is by international agreement and collaboration to ensure that control measures are taken on a worldwide basis, particularly as the economic effect of taking these measures could cause significant commercial and market distortions. It is recognized that in relation to ozone depletion control of, and in some cases the ban of, ozone depleting substances, such as chlorofluorocarbons (CFCs), is necessary. In relation to the greenhouse effect and global warming, it is recognized that an energy and transportation policy in relation to the generation of pollutants capable of causing global warming, such as carbon dioxide, will be needed to achieve the necessary reductions in pollutant loads. In the case of photochemical oxidants, the control of nitrogen oxides and volatile organic compounds will have to take the effect of stringent reductions in order to achieve the existing and proposed air quality standards for nitrogen oxides and ozone respectively.

The Convention on Climate Change ratified at the 1992 Earth Summit by over 150 countries is an example of the international efforts to deal with trans-boundary pollution.

Integrated environmental policy

The white paper [1] recognizes the need to integrate environmental concerns into all government policies. In particular, energy and transportation policy need careful reconsideration in light of environmental concerns. This is likely to lead to a push for greater energy efficiency, to reduce the generation of environmentally harmful pollutants, and to meet the objectives of sustainable resource management. In addition, the role of non-fossil fuel energy production methods is likely to attract further investigation and development. It is essential that environmental costs are applied when considering energy generation programmes, and that the best practicable environmental option is adopted. This will lead to more diversity in energy production methods, and with clear environmental cost being reflected in energy prices, will make the renewable energy options, such as wind power and tidal power, more economically attractive.

One of the main criticisms of the government's white paper was the failure to adopt the so-called carbon tax on fossil fuels. This is seen as a method of reducing energy consumption by applying a taxation levy on fossil fuels which are provided for combustion and energy production. This point again reinforces the need to consider environmental measures along with economic and social implications. The concept of a carbon tax appears to have received widespread support. However, unless the approach is adopted internationally, this will lead to higher energy production costs and eventually higher industrial and manufacturing costs, which will have significant impacts on the import and export markets for UK produced goods. This is one area where clear international collaboration is necessary to achieve the desired effect, as unilateral action could be economically and commercially catastrophic.

Transport policy is another area where environmental concerns will have far-reaching effects. There has to be a move towards more efficient transportation methods e.g. more efficient motor cars running on cleaner fuels. The EU has instigated measures to require cleaner motor vehicle engines, including, for example, the fitting of catalytic converters to reduce motor vehicle pollution. It is perhaps a reflection on society that speed and power in motor vehicles are often demanded by the public in preference to better fuel efficiency. The public acceptance of more fuel-efficient motor vehicles, perhaps at the cost of power and speed, is a true test for environmental education and 'green consumerism'. The other aspect of transportation is the balance between road building and investment in public transport. A number of UK cities are already looking at rapid transit links as a more efficient method of public transport, although it is widely accepted that a good public transportation policy relies upon diversity of transport modes.

Integrated pollution prevention and control

The EU has introduced a new proposed Directive to implement the Integrated Pollution Control (IPC) approach developing in the UK across Europe. The draft Integrated Pollution Prevention and Control (IPPC) Directive is based upon the principles of IPC in the Environmental Protection Act 1990, namely prior authorization of releases to the environment as a whole. One of the major developments in the draft Directive is the proposal to replace the EU control system based upon BATNEEC with a new system based upon Best Available Techniques (BAT).

This is accompanied by a revision of the definition of BAT to include:

1. techniques must be industrially feasible in the relevant sector from both a technical and economic point of view.
2. Available includes techniques developed on a scale which allows implementation in the relevant industrial context under economically viable conditions.

These revisions take account of the deletion of the NEEC element.

Environmental quality standards

There is an expansion in the use of environmental standards for determination of authorization conditions. The UK is currently developing a number of air quality standards beyond those contained in the EC Directives, these will augment the water quality standards currently used for assessment of river water and sea water quality.

In the proposed IPPC Directive, there is much greater emphasis placed upon the use of environmental quality standards to the point that if environmental quality standards are possibly going to be breached by a process, even if the application of BAT has been secured, the process should be refused authorization. This approach seeks to tie together the control of releases at source by application of control systems with the need to achieve certain levels of environmental quality.

Future environmental problems

Perhaps the most important challenge for environmental protection in the short term is to ensure that all of the current and proposed control mechanisms and philosophies are implemented effectively and efficiently. The new concept of integrated pollution control must be shown to work in order to encourage our international colleagues that integrated pollution control and BPEO approaches are the best future methods of environmental protection.

Two particular forms of pollution which are likely to receive more public and regulatory interest in the short- to medium-term future are genetically modified organisms and contaminated land.

Genetically modified organisms.

The public perception of genetically modified organisms (GMOs), known by such other terms as biotechnology or genetic engineering, immediately strikes a note of concern in the general populous. The public seem to imagine scientists in laboratories working on new forms of germ warfare or genetically engineering new forms of animal life. In reality, the majority of genetically modified organisms are put to much more beneficial use, e.g. the development of new varieties of crops with improved disease resistance or yield, or the use of bacteria which have been modified to produce human insulin for use by diabetics.

After initial research, it is necessary to release genetically modified organisms into the environment to carry out a detailed investigation of their interaction and development in conditions outside a laboratory. This process may involve certain risks, such as:

1. unexpected side effects;
2. cross fertilization of certain characteristics from the introduced organism to a wild variety; and
3. a new organism may be excessively competitive and therefore disturb the balance of current ecosystems.

In order to control the release into the environment of GMOs, the Environmental Protection Act 1990 requires that anybody working with such organisms carries out a full assessment of environmental risks and, in some cases, obtains consent from the Secretary of State, and that all involved with GMOs use BATNEEC to prevent environmental damage. In addition, the Act gives the Secretary of State powers to appoint inspectors and enforce the controls.

Contaminated land

The contamination of land resulting from its previous use has become a complex and important issue. Contamination may arise from previous waste disposal activities, e.g. the generation of landfill gas from landfill operations, or may relate to previous industrial activities on the site, e.g. old gas works where the contamination may include heavy metals or cyanide. The result of a House of Commons Select Committee on the Environment into the subject of contaminated land was published in January 1990 [10]. The committee concluded that 'there is land in the United Kingdom which is contaminated and which is a threat to health and to the environment both on site and in the surrounding area'. There has never been a concerted effort to identify contaminated land within the UK, but it has been estimated that there are up to 100 000 contaminated sites, covering up to 120 000 acres (which is 0.4% of the total land area of the UK). In addition, it was estimated that there are 1400 former waste tips now generating methane at potentially dangerous levels.

The existing legislation on the control of contaminated land is imprecise, and as a consequence the problem is normally only addressed when land is proposed for redevelopment and conditions are imposed under the controls of the Town and Country Planning Act 1990. The assesssment of when land is contaminated is aided by guidance notes produced within the Department of the Environment by the Interdepartmental Committee on the Redevelopment of Contaminated Land (ICRCL), which in particular provides guidance on 'trigger concentrations'. The concept of trigger concentrations is designed for use only at the planning stage for new development, and as a guide to necessary remedial works prior to development.

The Select Committee Report and the government's response, published in July 1990 [11] raise the following issues for further consideration:

1. The Environmental Protection Act 1990 provides power for the Secretary of State to make regulations relating to local authorities producing and maintaining registers of contaminated land. (DoE July 1991.)
2. More consideration of the leachate and ground water problems relating to contaminated land and better interface between local authorities and the National Rivers Authority.
3. A possible duty on vendors to declare all information in their possession relating to potential contamination.
4. The production, along with large land owners and statutory undertakings, of a code of practice for the preparation of contaminated land for sale and the conditions that should be placed on that sale.
5. The establishment of statutory liability for damage caused by contaminated land, particularly to adjacent property.
6. More research into the long-term effectiveness of clean-up measures.
7. Study into the BPEO for contaminated land treatment.

There is no specific power available in existing legislation to take action where contamination is identified on land. There is some suggestion that the statutory nuisance provisions of Part III of the Environmental Protection Act 1990 might be suitable for use in these circumstances. It appears that currently reliance will be placed upon dealing with contaminated land at the planning stage, and using planning conditions to enforce adequate clean-up meaures to alleviate the contamination to meet the standards appropriate for that particular form of redevelopment.

Despite several government proposals, legislation to implement the introduction of registers of contaminated land has not yet been implemented.

There are serious reservations, as any land being included on such a register would almost certainly become blighted in relation to sale and development. A further review was issued in 1994, *Paying for our Past*, which proposes a number of measures and sought comment on a number of central issues:

1. What should the objectives be of a contaminated land policy?
2. What should be the relationship between common law and statutory law?
3. Should there be an extension of strict liability?
4. Who should pay for putting right environmental damage?
5. How should markets be provided with information?
6. What roles should the public sector bodies have?

These questions are fundamental to any policy development in regard to contaminated land, and it can be expected that having canvassed views, the policy is likely to be developed based upon the comments received to this document.*

There is also an EU green paper relating to environmental liability which provides an insight to possible future EU Directives on the subject of liability for environmental damage and the provision of insurance against such damage.

CONCLUSION

The environmental 'band-wagon' moved along gathering pace in the 1980s and has now resulted in major environmental initiatives in the early 1990s. The first step must be to ensure that these new systems and strategies are effectively implemented so that the predicted environmental gains can be achieved into the next century. More information is now available concerning the environmental impact of man's activities, and further steps will need to be taken to implement policies, particular to deal with global pollution issues. The economic effects of environmental

* In November 1994 the DoE published a further paper 'Framework for Contaminated Land'. This will be based on a 'suitable for use' approach to the control and treatment of existing contamination. It is likely that the new Environment Agency will take the lead role. Provisions are also contained in the Environment Bill due to be enacted in 1995.

protection actions are now more clearly understood, and it is likely that in future economic control measures may also be implemented, although it is essential that an effective regulatory system and enforcement programme remains. There is currently a lot of activity in the development of environmental strategies, but they only become effective in achieving environmental protection if they are carefully and effectively implemented with the support of the government, industry and the general public. Environmental protection is the responsibility of everybody.

REFERENCES

1. Government White Paper (1990) *This Common Inheritance – Britain's Environmental Strategy*, HMSO, London.
2. Royal Commission on Environmental Pollution (1988) *Best Practicable Environmental Option*, 12th report, HMSO, London.
3. Royal Commission on Environmental Pollution (1976) *Air Pollution Control: An Integrated Approach*, 5th report, HMSO, London.
4. Royal Commission on Environmental Pollution (1984) *Tackling Pollution – Experience and Prospects*, 10th report, HMSO, London.
5. Royal Commission on Environmental Pollution (1985) *Managing Waste: The Duty of Care*, 11th report, HMSO, London.
6. Department of the Environment (1988) *Environmental Assessment*, Circular 15/88, HMSO, London.
7. Department of the Environment (1989) *Environmental Assessment – A Guide to the Procedures*, HMSO, London.
8. National Radiological Protection Board (1986) *Derived Emergency Reference Levels*, HMSO, London.
9. United Kingdom Nirex Limited, *The Way Forward – A Discussion Document*, HMSO, London.
10. House of Commons Select Committee on the Environment (1990) *Contaminated Land*, HMSO, London.
11. Department of the Environment (1990) *Government's Response to the First Report from the House of Commons Select Committee on the Environment – Contaminated Land*, Cmnd 1161, HMSO, London.

FURTHER READING

Department of the Environment (1986) *Assessment of Best Practicable Environmental Options for Management of Low and Intermediate Level Solid Radioactive Wastes*, HMSO, London.

Haigh, N. (1989) *EEC Environmental Policy and Britain*, Longman Group, London.

HM Inspectorate of Pollution (1989, 1990) *First and Second Annual Report*, HMSO, London.

Institution of Environmental Health Officers (1989) *Contaminated Land*, Aspinwall and Co. for IEHO, London.

Miller, C. and Wood, C. (1983) *Planning and Pollution*, Oxford University Press, Oxford.

National Radiological Protection Board, *Living With Radiation*, 3rd edn, HMSO, London.

National Society for Clean Air (1990) NSCA Pollution Handbook, NSCA, Brighton.

Pearce, D. *et al.* (1989) *Blueprint for a Green Economy*, Earthscan, London.

Wood, C. (1989) *Planning Pollution Prevention*, Heinmann Newnes, Oxford.

World Health Organization (1987) *Air Quality Guidelines for Europe*, European Series No. 23, WHO Regional Office for Europe, Geneva.

40 Noise

John F. Leech and Michael Squires

INTRODUCTION

The problem of noise pollution has been recognized since Roman times and should not be considered solely as a problem of our mechanized age. However, over the last 10 years there has been a significant increase in the number of complaints received by local authorities (Table 40.1).

This is due in part to the continuing growth of public sensitivity to noise and a change in the public's attitude to the environment generally.

The Wilson Committee Final Report published in 1963 [1] can still be considered to be the most comprehensive study of noise in society in the UK. The Committee was appointed in April 1960,

'to examine the nature, sources and effects of the problem of noise and to advise what further measures can be taken to mitigate it.'

Much of what was recommended by the Committee later became incorporated in BS4142:1967 [2] which was revised in 1990. The report highlighted road traffic, railways, aircraft, construction and entertainment/advertising as the sources responsible for the majority of unwanted sound affecting the population. Noise from road traffic was considered to be the prime source of noise affecting people. The Wilson report [1] also provides the widely accepted definition of noise: 'sound which is undesired by the recipient'.

A number of surveys have been undertaken to determine noise levels in the UK and the effects of environmental noise on people at home.

Table 40.1 Noise complaints received by environmental health departments under the Control of Pollution Act 1974 (sections 58 and 59)

Year	Total (England and Wales)
1982/3	52 678
1983/4	66 552
1984/5	74 475
1985/6	81 777
1987/8	91 578
1989/90	97 798
1990/91	123 859

Source: Institution of Environmental Health Officers (1982–1990/91) *Environmental Health Reports*, CIEH, London.

The most recent survey undertaken to determine noise levels in the UK was carried out by the Building Research Establishment (BRE) in 1990 [3]. The survey involved measuring noise levels over a 24-hour period outside 1000 dwellings in England and Wales. In addition to the measurement of sound levels, the survey also recorded the sources of noise identified at each site.

Data published in 1993 indicated that 7% of the dwellings were exposed to noise levels above 68 dB $L_{A10\ 18h}$, the level above which sound insulation compensation must be paid in the case of new road developments. Furthermore at over 50% of the sites the daytime levels ($L_{Aeq\ 16h}$) exceeded 55 dB(A). WHO [4] has suggested that general daytime outdoor noise levels of less than 55 dB L_{Aeq} are desirable to prevent any significant

Table 40.2 Noise sources outside dwellings: England and Wales, 1990

Noise source	Percentage of sample sites at which noise source was recorded
Roads	92
Aircraft	62
Animals and birds	57
Trees rustling	18
Children	18
Domestic	16
Railways	15
Farm equipment	10
Construction work	5
Industry	4
Motorways	2

Source: Sargent, J.W. and Fothergill, L.C. (1993) A survey of environmental noise levels in the UK. *Proceedings of Noise 93*, **7**, 161–6.

community annoyance. The main source of noise identified at the sample sites was road traffic noise, which was noted at 92% of the sites (Table 40.2).

A noise attitude survey [5] was carried out in 1991 by the BRE as part of the Department of the Environment's noise research programme. One adult from each of 2373 randomly selected households was surveyed. The results of the survey indicate that road traffic noise (28%) is the most widespread form of noise disturbance, followed by neighbour noise (22%), aircraft noise (16%) and train noise (4%). This survey has been considered to have produced responses which, for the first time, fully reflect the extent and nature of the adverse consequences of noise.

The degree to which noise affects people depends on a number of factors:

1. Frequency. Generally the higher the frequency the greater the annoyance.
2. Loudness. Generally the louder the noise the greater the nuisance, and it has been found that dislike of noise is more related to loudness than to any other easily measured characteristic.
3. Time of day. Sounds acceptable at 6 pm may not be acceptable at 6 am.
4. Unexpectedness. The effect of this is more apparent on some than on others, but all the evidence points to the effect being of short duration.
5. Uncertainty of direction and unfamiliarity. It is a natural reaction to experience a sense of unrest until the direction and source of a noise is established.
6. Irregularity and duration. Continuous impulsive or rhythmic noise is more irritating than a 'smooth' noise: with intermittent noise much will depend on the frequency of the repetition, e.g. a noise four times a day is not so annoying as one heard 40 times a day.
7. Necessity. If the noise generating activity is trivial or thought, by the complainant, to be unnecessary, his or her annoyance is increased.
8. General state of health, sensitivity and emotional attitude of a person towards noise. Poor health or emotional instability lowers the tolerance level of acceptability.
9. Level of background noise. The difference in the loudness between a noise and the background noise is very important. The greater the difference the greater is the annoyance likely to be – BS4142: 1990 refers [2].
10. Economic link. A factor which might also affect a person's reaction to a noise is their involvement with the source of the noise. It is noticeable that when investigating complaints of noise arising from a factory, those that work there or occupy houses belonging to the company are much less voluble in their complaints. This may also explain why only a few isolated complaints are sometimes received in respect of noise which can rightly be regarded as a serious nuisance.

These factors indicate that the assessment of noise is subjective, sound on the other hand can be measured objectively (see below). The effects of noise on people are various and often inter-related, and will vary from person to person.

Noise can induce acute physiological responses, such as increases in blood pressure and pulse rate. The quality of the noise seems to be of importance: uncontrollable noise from a neighbour's voice is reported as being more irritating than impersonal sounds, such as traffic and machine noise [6]. There is evidence that the adverse effects of noise depends, to some extent, on individual characteristics that have been termed 'sensitivity' and predisposition to 'annoyance'.

Nuisance from noise is much more likely when sound insulation is inadequate, and is, therefore, commonly found in low-cost housing [7]. Moreover, there is evidence which suggests that self-reported nervousness, irritability and poor concentration are related to exposure to traffic noise [8]. Noise at night interferes with sleep patterns, shortens the time spent in deep sleep and reduces REM sleep [9]. This pattern, if prolonged, can give rise to anxiety, headaches, irritability and chronic fatigue [10]. Moreover, day-time fatigue can impair motor co-ordination [6].

LEGAL FRAMEWORK

Prior to 1960, in order to deal with noise control local authorities had to rely on local Acts and bye-laws made under the Local Government Act 1933 and on common law. The findings of the Wilson Committee [1] resulted in the passing of the Noise Abatement Act 1960. This Act stated that noise or vibration which was a nuisance should be a statutory nuisance for the purposes of Part III of the Public Health Act 1936. Furthermore, restrictions of operations on highways, etc. of loudspeakers were introduced.

Concern about noise problems continued to develop rapidly during the 1960s, and in 1970 the government formed the Noise Advisory Council (NAC) with a brief:

'to keep under review the progress made generally in preventing and abating the generation of noise, to make such recommendations to Ministers with responsibility in this field and to advise on such matters as they refer to council'.

NAC was formed to keep under review the noise abatement activities of central and local government. In order to help NAC achieve its aim, working groups concentrating on different aspects of noise abatement policy were set up.

NAC was disbanded in 1981 but it produced a number of reports and publications some of which will be referred to later. The work of NAC assisted the government in drawing up Part III of the Control of Pollution Act 1974, which repealed the Noise Abatement Act 1960. The 1974 Act formed the main framework of noise control legislation and provided powers for dealing with noise from construction sites, noise in streets and for drawing up codes of practice on particular noise problems such as burglar alarms (see below). It also empowered local authorities to set up noise abatement zones (see below).

The noise nuisance provisions of the Act, although still applicable in Scotland, are in England and Wales now covered by Part III of the Environmental Protection Act (EPA) 1990 (see Chapter 7). The Noise and Statutory Nuisance Act 1993 amends the EPA and extends the duties of local authorities to deal with noise nuisance in the street, introduces discretionary powers to allow the operation of loudspeakers in the street and provides adoptive powers relating to the control of the installation and operation of burglar alarms (see below). The Health and Safety at Work, Etc, Act 1974 generally covers occupational noise by requiring employers to provide a safe place and safe system of work (see below).

As with other areas of environmental health work, the EU has adopted directives relating to noise abatement which the UK must implement. Directives stating maximum permitted noise levels for motor vehicles, construction plant and subsonic aircraft and detailing measurement procedures for all these sources have been adopted. The Noise at Work Regulations 1989 implemented Directive 86/188/EEC on the protection of workers from the risk related to exposure to noise at work. A list of directives and EU measures relating to noise are listed in Table 40.3.

THE NOISE REVIEW WORKING PARTY

Even though controls exist to deal with noise there is still a major problem. In December 1989 the Secretary of State for the Environment announced a review of the controls of environ-

Table 40.3 Directive and EC measures relating to noise

Number	Title	Date adopted	brought into force	OJ no. and date	Purpose
Vehicles/construction/plant/aircraft					
70/157	Directive on the approximation of laws in the member states relating to the permissible sound level and the exhaust system of motor vehicles	06.02.70	10.08.71	L42 23.02.70	To fix the permissible limits for the sound level, the equipment, conditions and methods for measuring this level
73/350	Directive adapting 70/157 to technical progress	07.11.73	01.03.74	L 321 21.11.73	To prescribe measures for exhaust systems
77/212	Council amendment to 70/157	08.03.77	01.04.77	L 66 12.03.77	(Now superseded by Directive 84/424)
84/424	Council amendment to 70/157	03.09.84	06.09.84	L 238 06.09.84	Amends noise limits set in 77/212; buses and lorries under 3.5 tonnes are categorized together, and those over categorized by horsepower
92/97	Amendment to 70/157	10.11.92	01.07.92	LO 371 19.12.92	Reduces noise limits for cars, buses and HGVs by between 2 and 5 dB(A)
78/1015	Directive relating to the permissible sound level and exhaust system of motorcycles	23.11.78	01.10.80	L 349 13.12.78	To fix the permissible limits for the sound level, the equipment, conditions and methods for measuring this level; to prescribe measures for exhaust systems
87/56	Amendment to Directive 78/1015	18.12.86	01.10.88	L 24 27.01.87	To modify the test procedure
89/235	Modification of Directive 78/1015 on sound levels of motorbikes	13.03.89	01.10.90	L 98 11.04.89	To lay down common technical standards for exhaust systems; to provide a model EC type approval certificate
74/151	Directive relating to certain parts and characteristics of wheeled agricultural or forestry tractors	04.03.74	07.04.75	L 84 23.03.74	To fix the permissible limits for the sound level, the equipment, conditions and methods for measuring this level
80/51	Directive relating to the limitation of noise emission from subsonic aircraft	20.12.79	21.06.80	L 18 24.01.80	To make it compulsory for the member states to apply annex 16 to the Chicago Convention on Subsonic Aircraft to establish mutual recognition of validity certificates; to determine exemptions
83/206	Amendment to 80/51		26.04.84	L 117 04.05.83	To ensure that aircraft landing in the EC since 21.04.84 respect standards laid down by ICAO Chicago Convention

Table 40.3 continued

Number	Title	Date adopted	brought into force	OJ no. and date	Purpose
89/629	Directive limiting noise emissions from subsonic aircraft	04.12.89 13.12.89		L 363	To prohibit registration after 01.11.90 of aircraft unable to meet specific noise limits
92/14	Directive limiting aircraft noise	02.03.92		L 76 23.03.92	To ban all aircraft unable to meet chapter 3 standards from operating into or out of EU after 01.04.95 and all chapter 2 aircraft after 01.04.92
79/113	Directive on the approximation of the laws of the member states relating to the determination of the noise emission of construction plant and equipment	19.12.78	21.06.80	L 33 08.02.79	To define the sound level for construction plant and equipment: to define the criteria to use for expressing results, equipment and conditions for carrying out measurements and calculation method
81/1051	Amendment to 79/113	07.12.81	14.06.83	L 376 30.12.81	To determine the noise emitted to the operator's position by all categories of machines
84/532	Directive relating to common provisions for construction plant and equipment – 'framework' directive.	26.09.84	26.03.86	L 300 19.11.84	To establish a framework for avoiding barriers to trade for construction plant and equipment
84/533	Directive on the limitation of the noise emitted by compressors	17.09.84	26.09.89	L 300 19.11.84	To lay down maximum permissible values for sound levels and to prescribe methods of measurement of that sound
84/534	Directive on the approximation of the laws of the member states relating to the permissible sound level for tower-cranes	17.09.84	26.09.89	L 300 19.11.84	To lay down maximum permissible values for sound levels and to prescribe methods of measurement of that sound (amended 22.09.86, No. 86/491)
84/535	Directive on the approximation of the laws of the member states relating to the permissible sound power level of welding generators	17.09.84	26.09.89	L 300 19.11.84	To lay down maximum permissible values for sound levels and to prescribe methods of measurement of that sound
84/536	Directive on the approximation of the laws of the member states relating to the permissible sound power level of power generators	17.09.84	26.09.89	L 300 19.11.84	To lay down maximum permissible values for sound levels and to prescribe methods of measurement of that sound
84/537	Directive on the approximation of the laws of member states relating to the permissible sound power level of powered hand-held concrete-breakers and picks	17.09.84	26.09.89	L 300 19.11.84	To lay down maximum permissible values for sound levels and to prescribe methods of measurement of that sound

Table 40.3 continued

Number	Title	Date adopted	Date brought into force	OJ no. and date	Purpose
86/662	Directive on the limitation of noise emitted by hydraulic and rope-operated excavators and by dozers and loaders	22.12.86	26.09.89	L 384 31.12.86	See title
89/392	Directive on approximation of laws on machinery (amended by 91/368)			L 183 29.06.89	See title
Lawn mowers					
84/538	Directive on the approximation of the laws of the member states relating to noise emitted by lawn mowers	17.09.84	01.07.87	L 300 19.11.84	To lay down maximum permissible values for sound levels and to prescribe methods of measurement of that sound
88/180 and 88/181	Directive modifying Directive 84/538 on noise levels of lawnmowers	22.03.88		L 81 26.03.88	To harmonize the legislation of the member states on permitted noise levels for lawnmowers
Household appliances					
86/594	Directive on airborne noise emitted by household appliances	01.12.86	04.12.89	L 344 06.12.86	To harmonize the methods of measuring the noise, arrangements for checking, general principles for publishing information on the noise emitted by these appliances
Protection of workers					
86/188	Directive on the protection of workers from the risks related to exposure to noise at work	12.05.86	01.01.90	L 137 24.05.86	To protect workers from risks to hearing by setting limits on noise levels at which preventative action is required

mental noise. In February 1990 the Noise Review Working Party was formed with the following terms of reference:

The noise review will consider aspects of noise control, with particular reference to Part III of the Control of Pollution Act 1974. Topics of interest will be burglar and car alarms, traffic noise, noise and planning (with reference to DOE Circular 10/73) and neighbourhood noise. The review will consider the possible need to increase the powers of local authorities to deal with noise nuisance. There will also be an examination of the current state of research regarding measurement of noise and its effects. (The review was extended to include aircraft noise.)

The Working Party Report [11] was published in October 1990 and made 53 recommendations, some of which in relation to noise nuisance have been included in the Environmental Protection Act 1990 (section 79) and others which were incorporated in the Government's white paper on the environment [12] published in September 1990. The recommendations and the Government's response to them are considered in the relevant sections later in the chapter.

SOUND AND VIBRATION

Characteristics of sound and units of measurement

Sound is propagated by a source vibrating, which causes any elastic medium such as air to fluctuate. If a stone is thrown into a pond, waves can be seen radiating outwards across the surface of the pond. Sound propagates in three dimensions not just two as with the water.

The sound waves which travel outward from the source are really minute positive and negative fluctuations of pressure caused by the air being alternatively compacted and rarefied by the source vibrating. The lowest pressure difference detectable by the average person is 0.00002 Newtons per metre squared (2×10^{-5} N/m^2 [Pa]), while the largest pressure difference detectable without pain is 20 N/m^2 (Pa).

A sound level meter is a sound pressure meter measuring these fluctuations in pressure. Because the range of pressures detectable by the ear is so great, i.e. 20 Pa is one million times greater than 2×10^{-5} Pa, a logarithmic scale is used for convenience. The decibel (dB) is the unit used to measure the sound pressure variation; it is a ratio of measured pressure squared to a reference pressure squared:

$$\log_{10} \frac{(\text{pressure})^2}{(2 \times 10^{-5})^2} \text{ bels}$$

or

sound pressure level (SPL)

$$= 10 \log_{10} \frac{(\text{sound pressure})^2}{(\text{reference pressure})^2}$$

where reference pressure = 2×10^{-5} N/m^2.

Decibels, being logarithmic, cannot be added or subtracted arithmetically, i.e. two noise sources each producing 80 dB do not combine to produce 160 dB but 83 dB. The addition of SPLs is indicated in Table 40.4.

Table 40.4 Addition of sound pressure levels

Difference in dB between two sources	0	1	2	3	4	5	6	7	8	9	10
Add to high level	3	2.5	2	2	1.5	1	1	1	0.5	0.5	0

If the difference between two sources is 10 dB or more, then the SPL remains that of the higher. Some examples of sound pressure levels are shown in Table 40.5.

Table 40.5 Typical sound pressure levels

Sound pressure (n/m^2)	Sound source	SPL (dB)
0.00002	Silence (threshold of hearing)	0
0.0002	TV studio	20
0.002	Soft whisper	30
	Public library	40
0.02	Normal conversation at 1 m	60
	Radio set (loud)	70
0.2	Small car at 7.5 m	80
	Heavy lorry at 7.5 m	90
2.0	Pneumatic chipper	100
20.0	Boilermakers' shop	120

Frequency

Having considered pressure waves moving out from the source, frequency or the rate of repetition needs to be understood. With a continuous sound, a succession of air compactions will pass out from the source and the distance between each compaction will be the same – this is called the wavelength. The velocity of sound in air at sea level and at 20°C is 340 m/sec. If we take this figure as a working figure then we can see that:

$$\text{frequency} = \frac{\text{speed of sound (C)}}{\text{wavelength}}$$

or

$$\text{speed of sound} = \text{wavelength} \times \text{frequency}$$

It is of interest to note that the velocity of sound is dependent on the medium through which it travels (Table 40.6) and it can be shown that it

Table 40.6 Velocity of sound in various materials

Material	Approximate velocity of sound (m/sec)
Air	340
Lead	1220
Water	1410
Brick	3000
Wood	3400
Steel	5200

is dependent on the medium's modulus of elasticity (Young's modulus [E]) and its density.

The human perception of sound is dependent upon the frequency of the sound and the ear's best response is between 1000 and 4000 Hz. Generally, in noise control we are looking at a combination of frequencies rather than a single frequency or pure tone. For ease of measurement the frequency spectrum can be divided into octave or one-third octave bands. Octave bands are ranges of frequency, each octave is designated by a number which is the square root of two multiplied by the lower frequency, i.e. 88–176 Hz has a centre frequency of 125 Hz.

One-third octave bands are exactly that, i.e. each band is a third of an octave band. Acoustic engineers involved in the design of silencing for a factory may well need to measure frequency by narrow band analysis in which band widths can be much smaller, to identify particular problems.

'A' weighting

An A-weighting filter is incorporated into sound level meters allowing direct measurement of this parameter. The A-weighted frequency response follows approximately the 40 phon equal loudness curve and correlates closely with people's subjective response to noise. A-weighting is now used internationally in standards to rate noise (Fig. 40.1). There are other weighting curves B, C, D and E, but all have specialized uses, the A weighting being by far the most frequently used.

Sound power level

Sound power level (SWL) is a measure of the total energy of the source; it is independent of the

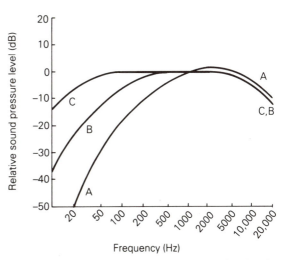

Fig. 40.1 International standard A, B and C weighting curves for sound level meters.

environment. The sound pressure level can be calculated at any distance from the source if the SWL of the source is known:

$$\text{Sound power level (SWL)} = \frac{\text{(Sound power)}}{\text{(reference power)}} \text{ dB}$$

Convention is to use sound intensity rather than pressure, and intensity is expressed in watts per square metre. The reference sound power is 10 watts.

Sound pressure is related to unit area, therefore to determine the SWL, the sound pressure over a total area enclosing the source has to be found.

Therefore $\quad$ SWL = SPL + 10 $\log_{10}$ A dB
where A is the area in metres squared.
We know that A $\quad = 4\pi r^2$
where r is the distance from the source in metres.
So $\quad\quad\quad$ SWL = SPL + 10 $\log_{10}$ 4πr^2
$\quad\quad\quad\quad\quad\quad = $ SPL + 20 $\log_{10}$ r+11.

Loudness

Loudness is a subjective characteristic of sound, i.e. a listener's impression of the amplitude of

Table 40.7 Relationship between phons and sones

Phons	Sones
40	1
50	2
60	4
70	8
80	16
90	32
100	64
110	128
120	256

sound. Loudness is primarily related to sound pressure, but sound of a constant pressure can be made to appear louder or quieter by changing its frequency. In practice, an increase in noise level of 10 dB(A) at any point in the decibel scale approximates to a doubling of loudness. The unit used to indicate loudness is the phon which is defined in BS 3045:1981 [13] as a dimensionless unit used to express the given loudness of a sound or noise.

The loudness level in 'x' phons is judged by the average person to be equal in loudness to 'x' decibels at 1000 Hz, e.g. any sound judged to be equal in loudness to a pure tone of 50 dB at 1000 Hz has a loudness level of 50 phons. The phon scale is logarithmic. As phons are dimensionless units which allow for variation of the sensitivity of the ear with frequency, they do not give a direct indication of a change in loudness level, e.g. a sound of 60 phons is not generally twice as loud as a sound of 30 phons. The sone scale of loudness gives a direct relationship between different loudness levels.

The sone is defined in BS 3045:1981 [13] as 'a unit of loudness on a scale designed to give scale numbers approximately proportional to the loudness'.

The relationship between phons and sone is shown in Table 40.7.

A noise of 64 sones (100 phons) is twice as loud as a noise of 32 sones (90 phons). Units of loudness do not usually feature in noise control measures.

NOISE MEASUREMENT

Noise indices

In practice in the real environment, noise levels are almost always fluctuating widely, are often multi-sourced, and the sources are often transient or mobile and a simple instantaneous measurement is meaningless. As a result of these technical and social difficulties, surveys have been made to quantify the relationship between noise and its effect on the quality of life.

Different indices are used for different noise sources; they all relate the noise to time either directly or statistically. The indices most likely to be used by environmental health staff are $L_{Aeq,T}$, $L_{EP,d}$, L_{A10}, L_{A90} and $L_{Ar,T}$. Others sometimes used include noise and number index (NNI) and traffic noise index (TNI).

$L_{Aeq,T}$ (A-weighted equivalent continuous sound level with respect to time)

This is a measure of energy of the noise. It is defined as 'the value of the A-weighted sound pressure level in decibels of continuous steady sound that within a specified time interval, T, has the same mean-square sound pressure as a sound that varies with time.

$$L_{Aeq,T} = 10 \log_{10} \left\{ 1/T \int_{t1}^{t2} (PA^2(t)PO^2)dt \right\}$$

This index is now widely used for environmental measurement, being quoted in BS4142:1990 [2] as well as in the Health and Safety at Work Act 1974. It is also increasingly being used for aircraft noise and railway noise.

$L_{EP,d}$

The $L_{EP,d}$ is the index used in the Noise at Work Regulations 1989 (SI 1989 No. 1790) and is the 'daily personal exposure to noise'. It is arrived at by measuring the A-weighted sound pressure level and the duration of exposure. One method of measurement is by using an integrating sound level meter complying with BS6698: 1986 (IEC804: 1985) [14] and measuring the L_{Aeq}. It can also be measured on a simple sound level meter and calculated using the nomogram shown in 'Noise at work, noise assessment, information and control, Noise guide 3'.

L_{A10} (18 hour)

This index of traffic noise is used as the basis for measurement in the Noise Insulation Regulations 1973 and 1975 (SI 1977/1763) made under the Land Compensation Act 1973. It is the sound level in dBA exceeded for 10% of the time worked on an hourly basis from 6 am to midnight (18 hours) on a normal weekday.

$L_{A90,T}$ (background noise level)

The $L_{A90,T}$ is the A-weighted sound pressure level of the residual noise in decibels exceeded for 90% of a time 'T'. It is the level quoted in BS4142: 1990 [2] for background noise.

$L_{Ar,T}$ (rating level)

The $L_{Ar,T}$ is the equivalent continuous A-weighted sound pressure level in decibels at the measurement position produced by the specific noise source under investigation over a given reference time interval plus any adjustments for the character of the noise. It is quoted in BS4142: 1990 [2].

Noise and number index (NNI)

This index of aircraft noise measurement is based on the combined effect of the loudness of individual aircraft and the number of flights in a specified period. The NNI is not relevant to airports with less than 80 aircraft per day, each of which needs to produce an average peak noise level of more than 80 PNdB. NNI was introduced following a survey at Heathrow Airport; it has now been superseded by $L_{Aeq,T}$.

Traffic noise index (TNI)

This index resulted from a survey of noise levels and annoyance in Greater London in 1966 [15]. It is based on A-weighted sound pressure levels:

$$\text{TNI} = L_{A90} + 4(L_{A10} - L_{A90}) - 30.$$

Noise monitoring equipment

Sound level meters

A sound level meter is an instrument designed to measure sound pressure in an objective, reproducible manner, and consists of a microphone, a processing unit and visual display or read-out facility (Fig. 40.2).

The microchip and digital technology has moved the meter forward great distances over the last few years. Sound level meters can now be programmed to carry out complex statistical measurements including all the indices discussed in this chapter.

The results of extended measurement periods can be saved within the meter or down loaded to a computer for analysis at leisure in the office. Specially written software allows many statistical indices to be measured simultaneously with small portable battery-powered meters.

In the future sound intensity measurement may well become widely used if the instrumentation becomes competitive with existing equipment both in price and portability and the higher level of expertise needed to carry out the measurements can be accommodated. This will provide a very powerful tool allowing directional readings and making calculation far more provable. Sound measuring equipment must currently meet the following standards:

1. BS5969: 1981 [16] (specification for sound-level meters) (IEC651; 1979).
2. BS6698: 1986 [14] (integrating/averaging sound-level meters (IEC 804: 1985).

The standards specify four degrees of precision for sound-level meters:

1. Type 0 (intended as a laboratory reference standard).
2. Type 1 (for laboratory and field use where the acoustic environment can be closely specified and/or controlled).
3. Type 2 (for general field applications).
4. Type 3 (for field noise surveys).

Many of the regulations made under legislation enforceable by environmental health departments specify equipment complying with type 2 or better. BS4142: 1990 [2] in a footnote states. 'Use

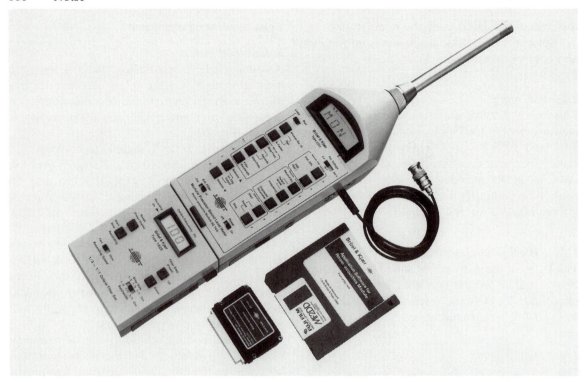

Fig. 40.2 Precision sound level meter and octave filter set. (Courtesy of Brüel & Kjaer (UK) Ltd, Harrow Weald Lodge, 92 Uxbridge Road, Harrow, Middlesex HA3 6BZ.)

of equipment with performance equivalent to that of sound level meters complying with type 1 of BS5969 [16] is preferred'.

Environmental noise analysers

An alternative method of making long-term environmental noise surveys is to use either the environmental noise analyser (Fig. 40.3) or graphic recorder. These instruments are self-contained, reasonably robust and by the use of microprocessor control can be programmed for prolonged hands-off monitoring in the field. Noise analysers will produce a complete written history of statistical parameters over the measurement period, while a graphic recorder will let the operator have a analogue trace of the time/noise signal in addition to the ability to produce sequential set period L_{Aeq} bar charts.

Computers and sound level measurement

All the major producers of sound measurement equipment have meters available which can be used as stand-alone instruments or as part of sophisticated systems linked into computers and capable of producing comprehensive information.

Hand-held meters will measure a frequency spectrum in octave or third octave in real time making the measurement of sound much easier and quicker (Fig. 40.4)

Frequency analysis allow the identification of a particular source from many potential sources and real time measurement makes this a far more realistic option.

Computers are reducing in size, the laptop, the notebook and the notepad, whilst the storage capacity and ability to run complex software has increased. The environmental health officer going forth to monitor a night-long noise event no longer has to look like a christmas tree or feel that he needs a pantechnicon to transport the hardware.

Sound measurement equipment manufacturers also provide the necessary software to integrate their equipment with the computer allowing the

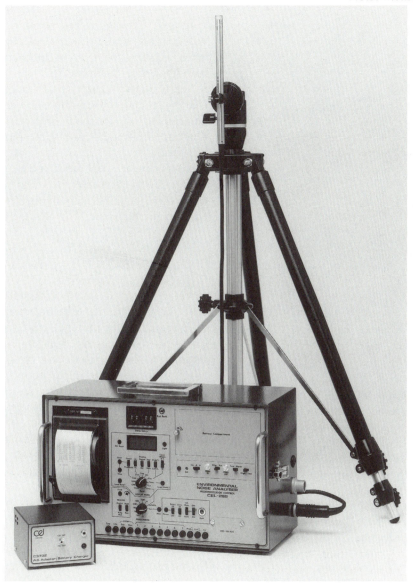

Fig. 40.3 Environmental noise analyser. (Courtesy of Lucas CEL Instruments Ltd, 35–37 Bury Mead Road, Hitchin, Herts SG5 1RT.)

control, storage and transfer onto commercially available spreadsheets.

Once the data are put onto a spreadsheet they can be manipulated, and the presentation of the information that can be gleaned from it becomes an artform in its own right.

Dedicated software
Programmes in a variety of languages to assist the acoustician in road noise, railway noise, industrial noise, building acoustics, aircraft noise and propagation with barrier effects are available from specialist software houses. In fact the tool to design a sound environment.

This software allows the acoustician access to computer-aided noise solution modelling which will be invaluable in project design. It also allows the production of both grid and contour noise maps in graphical form ideal for planning meetings.

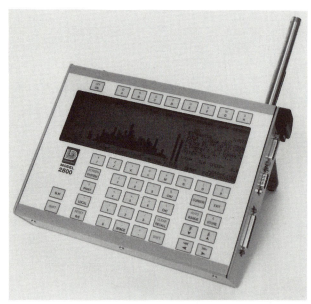

Fig. 40.4 Sound level meter and real time frequency analyser. (Courtesy of Larson Davis Ltd, 16 Scardale Crescent, Scarborough, North Yorkshire YO12 6LA.)

Calibration of noise monitoring equipment

All sound-measurement equipment should be calibrated before and after each series of measurements using a calibrator or pistonphone complying with class 2, BS7189: 1989 [17]. If carrying out prolonged measurements, intermediate checks on calibration should be made.

Every 2 years, all equipment should be sent to an accredited laboratory for a compliance test; calibrators and pistonphones must comply with BS7189: 1989 [17], and other equipment with BS6698: 1986 [14] or BS5969: 1981 [16] type 1 or 2.

VIBRATION

The Environmental Protection Act 1990 Part 3, section 79 (statutory nuisances and clean air) defines noise as including vibration. Vibration is the movement of a solid body about an axis. A metal sheet oscillating can be seen to display three physical properties: first, it moves over a distance which is called its displacement; second, it has a velocity which is at its peak as it crosses its axis and is zero at its point of maximum deflec-

tion; and, thirdly, it has positive and negative acceleration. These three physical properties are linked mathematically, and can each be measured individually or together.

There are two main types of vibration: deterministic and random. Deterministic vibration can be determined by mathematical formulae, while random vibration has to be determined by statistical means.

Generally, the root mean square (RMS) values are used for measurement as these reflect the time history and peak measurements reflect an instantaneous moment only.

$$X_{rms} = \sqrt{1/T} \int_0^{At} X^2(t)dt.$$

Investigating officers may wish to measure vibration to determine whether possible damage may arise, or if a nuisance is being caused (Fig. 40.5). Measurements for nuisance confirmation are likely to be taken within a building, and it is worth noting that the worst effects will normally be felt at mid-floor spans on upper floors. BS6472: 1984 [18] specifies the measurements that should be made to determine human reaction to vibration.

As with noise there is now available a wide range of microchip-controlled computer-compatible equipment; it is now easy to acquire data, the expertise comes in interpreting it once it has been obtained.

NOISE CONTROL TECHNIQUES

Attenuation

Sound propagates outwards from its source; if the source is comparatively small in relationship with the distance to the receiver it can be considered a point source. Large sources, such as factories, listened from close to, or sources, such as roads, are considered as line or plane sources.

With a point source the intensity of sound is inversely proportional to the square of the distance from the source to the receiver (Fig. 40.6). In the case of a line source, the intensity is inversely proportional to this distance.

A point source gives an attenuation of 6 dB(A) per doubling of distance. A line source gives an attenuation of 3 dB(A) per doubling of distance.

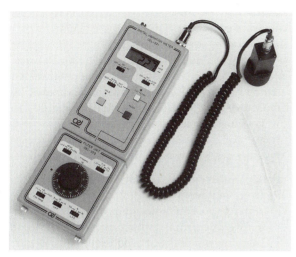

Fig. 40.5 Vibration analyser. (Courtesy of Lucas CEL Instruments Ltd, 35–37 Bury Mead Road, Hitchin, Herts SG5 1RT.)

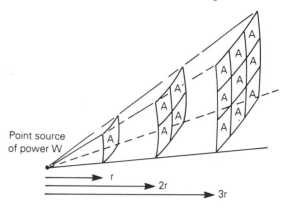

Fig. 40.6 The dispersion of sound from a sound point. It can be seen that the intensity is inversely proportional to the square of the distance between source and receiver, i.e. it attenuates 6 dB per doubling of distance. (Courtesy of Brüel & Kjaer (UK) Ltd, 'Acoustic Noise Measurement'.)

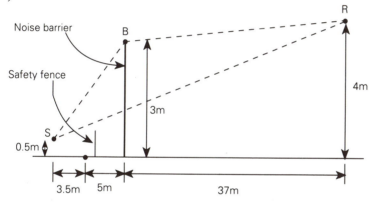

Fig. 40.7 Path of noise transmission. S = source; B = barrier; R = reception point. (Courtesy of the Department of Transport and the Welsh Office, 'Calculation of Road Traffic Noise', HMSO, London.)

In practice quite large sources can be treated as point in origin.

In addition to the attenuation due to distance, many other factors can alter the sound level between the source and receiver. Meteorological changes, such as temperature gradient and wind, can play a part, and so it is recommended that no readings are taken with a wind speed above 24 kph (15 mph). The ground surface also plays an important part in altering the sound level – soft, absorbent vegetation attenuates sound quicker than hard concrete surfaces.

Barriers are often introduced primarily to reduce noise, this technique is often used where motorways pass through noise-sensitive areas (Fig. 40.7).

Mass law

Within a building the air-borne sound insulation offered by a wall is quoted in terms of the sound reduction index (SRI), which is dependent on the transmitted sound power and the incident sound power:

$$\text{SRI} = \frac{\text{Wi}}{\text{Wt}}$$

Wi = incident sound power and Wt = transmitted sound power.

The mass law states that within the mass controlled region, the SRI increases by 6 dB(A) for each doubling in frequency or given mass per unit area, or for each doubling of mass (thickness) at a given frequency.

$$SRI = 20 \log_{10} (fM) - 47 \text{ dB}.$$

where f = frequency of the incident sound in Hz and M = mass per unit area of the wall in g/m².

Noise in buildings

Sound generated within a room reaches the listener both directly from the source, and also from reflections from the walls and furniture of the room. A room with hard surfaces readily reflects sound, and the reflections or echo take a comparatively long time to die away. This is a reverberant or live room. A room with many absorbent surfaces is quiet, the sound dying away quickly. It is an acoustically dead room.

Reverberation time (RT) is the time it takes for the sound level within a room to decrease by 60 dB. Sabines formula shows the relationship between the absorption of a given room and the RT.

$$RT = \frac{0.161V}{Sa}$$

where V = the room's volume, S = the room's total surface area, and a = the absorption coefficient.

The Building Regulations 1991
Approved document E (1992 edition, took effect on the 1 June 1992) – Resistance of passage to sound – has replaced the 1985 edition.

The requirements have been extended to cover material change of use to a dwelling so it can now be used for conversion of a building to flats.

The walls separating a kitchen from other rooms within a dwelling not used exclusively by that dwelling are now also covered.

The requirements for floors is now specified to also include stairs where they are part of the separation between dwellings. The guidance for new dwellings has been improved, a higher

standard of performance for different types of construction is now sought. A particular recommendation is to increase the mass of certain precast separating floors and concrete block walls. Section 6 of the document describes methods of gaining approval for construction treatments by laboratory or field testing. Part E of Schedule 1 to the Building Regulations 1991 requires:

AIRBORNE SOUND (WALLS) E1. – A wall which –

(a) separates a dwelling from another building or from another dwelling, or
(b) separates a habitable room or kitchen within a dwelling from another part of the same building which is not used exclusively as part of the dwelling,

shall resist the transmission of airborne sound.

AIRBORNE SOUND (FLOORS AND STAIRS) E2. – A floor or a stair which separates a dwelling from another dwelling, or from another part of the same building which is not used exclusively as part of the same dwelling, shall resist the transmission of airborne sound.

IMPACT SOUND (FLOORS AND STAIRS) E3. – A floor or a stair above a dwelling which separates it from another dwelling, or from another part of the same building which is not used exclusively as part of the dwelling, shall resist the transmission of impact sound.

Enclosures
Noisy machines or activities can often be installed, or carried out, in enclosures or partial enclosures. BS5228: 1984 [19] Part I gives examples of the use of enclosures on construction sites. Enclosures used in factories nearly always have to have openings for access or ventilation but, even then, using sheet material with a weight of 10 kg/m² lined with 25 mm absorbent lining, it is possible to achieve a reduction in noise of about 20 dB.

AV mounts
The mounting of machinery on anti-vibration mounts can have a positive effect in reducing structure-borne noise. Care must be exercised in

the choice of mounts as vibration produced by a machine at a lower frequency than its mounted resonant frequency will not be isolated. Vibrations at the resonant frequency may be amplified. Mountings should have internal damping. The displacement of all mounts must be equal to avoid the machine starting to rock.

Examples of practical noise control

Noise reduction at source is always the best answer when possible. The ideal solution is to stop making the noise. Is there a quieter way of doing the job? Is maintenance up to scratch? Blunt saws, worn bearings or transmissions can increase noise from a machine. Where two gear wheels of the same diameter, one with twice as many teeth as the other, are operating at the same rotational velocity, the one with twice the number of teeth will produce its noise at twice the frequency of the other because the source of the noise is a succession of impacts as the teeth mesh.

Machines can be enclosed or screened; in general, the closer the screen is to the machine, the greater the reduction in noise. Machines can be re-sited indoors or behind a building. An enclosure should be air tight and made of a heavy material which has stiffness designed into it. The more expensive commercially available machine enclosures often make use of a composite material made up of a dense material between steel. The inside of an enclosure should be lined with an acoustically absorbent material to reduce reflections and thus lower the internal noise levels.

Fan noise is a frequent source of complaint. If the noise is tonal in character, it can be beneficial to operate a large diameter fan at a slower speed. However, because the noise now generated will be at a lower frequency, it will travel further away and may widen the area of complaint. A better solution may be to install a silencer behind the original fan.

PLANNING AND NOISE

The right to enjoy the environment without being subjected to excessive noise intrusion has been established at common law. Obviously, prevention is better than cure and, therefore, consideration should be given to the likely effects of noise at the development control stage.

In order to address the issue of planning and noise and provide guidance for local authorities the Government introduced Department of the Environment Circular 10/73 [20]. This circular was directed primarily at the control of development and acknowledged that a great deal could be achieved by positive planning to reduce the risk of noise disturbance. It emphasized the need for close cooperation between planning, environmental health and highways authorities in the control of developments to contain and, where possible, reduce the impact of noise.

The Circular gave guidance to local authorities on the use of their planning powers, and stated that new noise-sensitive development should not be allowed in areas exposed to unacceptable levels of noise. For example, the Circular presumed that sites were not suitable for residential development if they were subjected to a traffic noise in excess of 70 dB(A) on the $L_{10(18 \text{ hour})}$ scale unless the properties were screened from the noise, or sound insulated to the standard prescribed in the Noise Insulation Regulations 1975 (SI 1989 No. 1790). It also made references to noise from roads, aircraft and industry, and suggested criteria upon which local authorities should base their policies.

The Noise Review Working Party Report 1990 [11] considered the issue of planning and noise and the following recommendations were made:

1. Circular 10/73 should be revised as quickly as possible to include areas of concern such as aircraft noise including helicopters, noise from railways, sporting activities, recreation and entertainment. It should also distinguish between industrial noise from fixed installations, and noise from mineral workings and waste disposal facilities. Furthermore it should make a requirement that all applications except for housing should include information relating to the possible noise implications of the project.

2. The establishment of action levels to assist in the assessment for noise-sensitive developments.
3. BS4142: 1990 should be more extensively revised to take account of peaks of noise and of noisy events of short duration, particularly at night.
4. More research in respect of community response to various types of industrial noise is required.
5. The provisions of section 60 of the Control of Pollution Act 1974 should be extended to mineral extraction sites, oil and gas sites and waste disposal sites in conjunction with a specific code of practice for these sites.

The Government has now issued PPG 24 'Planning and Noise (1994)' and this replaces circulars 10/73 and 1/85. The PPG takes on board the comments and recommendations of the Working Party and provides more comprehensive guidance about a wider range of noise sources, namely noise from traffic, aircraft, railways, industrial and commercial developments, construction and waste disposal sites, sporting, entertainment and recreational activities. Furthermore in order to assist local authorities in the appraisal of new, noise sensitive, developments adjacent to a noise source the concept of noise exposure categories has been introduced. Four categories have been introduced and recommended noise limits for each category for the development of dwellings and schools exposed to the various noise sources are detailed in an appendix to the document. The categories are:

A. For proposals in this category, noise need not be considered as a determining factor in granting permission, although the noise level at the high end of the category should not be regarded as a desirable level.
B. In this category authorities should increasingly take noise into account when determining planning applications, and require noise control measures.
C. There should be a strong presumption against granting planning permission for proposals in this category. Where permission is given, i.e.

if no other suitable quieter sites are available, conditions should be imposed to ensure an adequate level of insulation against external noise.
D. For proposals in this category planning permission should normally be refused.

Where a planning authority is disposed to give planning permission for a noisy development, conditions should be attached to any permission granted. Local authorities should refer to the model conditions detailed in PPG 24.

Local authorities should only impose conditions where they are satisfied that they are:

1. necessary;
2. relevant to planning;
3. reasonable;
4. enforceable;
5. relevant to the development;
6. precise.

In April 1993 the Department of the Environment published the Mineral Planning Guidance Note 11 (MPG 11) [23]. This provides advice for both mineral planning authorities and the industry on how the planning system can be used to keep noise emissions from surface mineral workings within environmentally acceptable limits without imposing unreasonable burdens on the minerals operators. The main provisions of MPG 11 can be summarized as follows:

1. Recommends the use of a modified form of BS5228 [19] on the prediction of noise emissions. The model takes into account barrier and soft ground attenuation, weather condition, noise reflection and mobile plant.
2. Recommends two methods for setting noise limits for mineral sites. One method is based on BS4142 [2] the other on absolute noise limits – these noise limits can be incorporated into planning conditions.
3. Provides advice on how to effectively monitor noise levels from surface mineral sites.
4. Advises on noise abatement methods which can be the subject of planning conditions and/ or incorporated into good practice by the operator.

Rating noise

BS4142: 1990 [2] provides a method for rating industrial noise affecting mixed residential and industrial areas. This should be used for assessing the calculated or measured noise levels from new or modified premises, or the measured noise levels from existing premises. This is a useful method when considering the likely environmental effects of new or modified industrial developments.

The revised standard recommends the use of $L_{Aeq,T}$ as the specific noise level of the noise source under investigation, and $L_{A90,T}$ for background noise levels. The method is not applicable for assessing noise where background noise levels are below a sound pressure level of 30 dB(A), or for assessing noise levels measured inside buildings. An assessment of the noise for complaint purposes is made by subtracting the measured background noise level from the rating level ($L_{Ar,T}$), which is the specific noise level plus any adjustment for the character of the noise. A difference of 10 dB or more suggests that complaints are likely. As the difference decreases the likelihood of complaint diminishes; at a difference of −10 dB there is a positive indication that complaints are unlikely. The 1990 Standard is currently under revision.

ENVIRONMENTAL ASSESSMENT (EA)

The Town and Country Planning (Assessment of Environmental Effects) Regulations 1988 implement the requirements of EC Directive 85/337/EEC on environmental assessment (see Circulars 15/88 [24] and 24/88 [25]). The background to the Directive was that in Europe not all countries had a system which provides for detailed, case-by-case scrutiny of new development proposals. In the UK, the existing development control systems ensure that the objectives of the Directive are met in most cases.

An EA is a technique for gathering expert quantitative analysis and qualitative assessments of a proposed development's likely environmen-

tal effects. Information including a description of the project and measures to be taken to minimize any adverse effects on the environment, including for example a noise assessment, might be required by the planning authority when considering applications to which these regulations apply. An EA is mandatory for projects listed in Schedule 1 to the 1988 Regulations, e.g. large power stations, chemical installations, toxic waste facilities and asbestos plants. Projects listed in Schedule 2 may require an EA if the planning authority considers that the proposal by virtue of its size, nature and location is likely to have significant environmental effects. The required content of the statement is set out in Schedule 3.

Environmental health departments have an important role to play in advising planning departments and their committees. Equipment should be available within the department to predict, monitor and assess the likely environmental effects of proposed developments. Where possible, one officer from the department should liaise with the planning department, all applications should be screened and comments conditions considered necessary forwarded to the planning department as quickly as possible. A representative from the department should also attend and advise at committee meetings where planning decisions are taken.

NEIGHBOURHOOD NOISE

This term can be used to describe noise from a number of sources, e.g. industrial noise, transport noise, entertainment noise, noise in the street and noise from neighbours. The 1991 BRE survey [5] indicated that 22% of the adult population are bothered by neighbourhood noise or more precisely by neighbour noise. Neighbour noise complaints generally relate to hi-fi equipment, barking dogs, DIY activities, voices, car repairs and domestic activities.

Neighbourhood noise is not a problem solely confined to large towns and cities. In the country, people can be affected by various noise sources, e.g. from industrial operations such as quarrying, agricultural activities, and leisure activities such as clay pigeon shooting. In towns and the country alike, noise from such sources as well-established industry or agricultural activities is often tolerated until new residents, with higher environmental expectations, move into the area.

Noise nuisance arising from fixed premises can be dealt with by the nuisance procedures of the Environmental Protection Act 1990, except in Scotland where sections 57–59 of the Control of Pollution Act 1974 still apply. The above Acts have been amended by the provisions of the Noise and Statutory Nuisance Act 1993. This new Act extends the list of statutory nuisances to include 'noise that is prejudicial to health or a nuisance and is emitted from or caused by a vehicle, machinery or equipment in the street'. The aim of the new Act is to control nuisances caused by vehicle repairs, persistent DIY, vehicle alarms and noise from refrigeration units and generators on stationary vehicles. It is a defence against a statutory nuisance action to prove that the 'best practicable means' has been employed to control the noise, this is defined in section 79 of the Environmental Protection Act 1990 and section 72 of the Control of Pollution Act 1974 (see Chapter 7). This defence is only available in the case of the new provisions where the vehicle, equipment or machinery is used for industrial, trade or business purposes. In the case of entertainment noise where, for example, a public entertainment licence is required, local authorities may, when issuing the licence, attach noise conditions. In these cases, nuisance action can still be taken if necessary.

The Noise and Statutory Nuisance Act also amends section 62 of the Control of Pollution Act 1974. This section of the Act bans the use of loudspeakers in streets between 9 pm and 8 am, except for emergency use by the fire, police and ambulance services. The Environmental Protection Act is amended to give discretionary power to local authorities to consent to the operation of loudspeakers for non-advertising purposes during the prohibited hours. It is suggested that this will allow charitable and other entertainment events to operate loud speakers after 9 pm with

the approval of the local authority. The use of loudspeakers in the street for advertising, entertainment, business or trade is not allowed at any time, except in the case of vehicles selling perishable foodstuffs, which may use loudspeakers between noon and 7 pm. The EPA is also amended to enable the Secretary of State to alter these times should he so choose.

Section 71 of the 1974 Act empowers the Secretary of State to issue codes of practice or approve codes produced by other bodies for minimizing noise. For example, BS5228: 1984 [19], which deals with the control of noise from construction sites (see below) was prepared by the British Standards Institution and approved by the Secretary of State. Codes of practice on noise from ice cream chimes, the control of noisy parties, burglar alarms and model aircraft have been produced by the Department of the Environment. Work has been done on producing codes for clay pigeon shooting, pop concerts, motorbike scrambling, power boats, water skiing and audible bird scarers. The Noise Review Report [11] considers that codes of practice are of great importance as a means of providing advice and guidance for those involved in the control of environmental noise. It is important to remember that any code produced, while it may be taken into account by the courts, does not have the force of regulations.

As mentioned above the Department of the Environment have issued a Code of Practice dealing with noise from burglar alarms. The Noise and Statutory Nuisance Act provides an adoptive power, for local authorities, which introduces controls over the installation and operation of these types of alarms. There is no specified date when these provisions will come into force, the Secretary of State is given the power to make a Commencement Order and issue regulations to bring them into force.

The Noise Review Report [11] considered neighbourhood noise and made a number of recommendations, one of which suggested the establishment of neighbourhood noise watch schemes, modelled on existing neighbourhood watch schemes. The government has suggested that they will sponsor a pilot quiet neighbourhood scheme, probably in one of the London boroughs.*

CONSTRUCTION SITES

Part III of the Control of Pollution Act 1974 (sections 60 and 61) gives local authorities the power to exercise certain controls over noise emanating from construction and demolition sites. The Act recognizes the need to protect residents and people working in the vicinity of these sites.

Local authorities may, regardless of whether a statutory nuisance has been caused or is likely to be caused, serve a notice on a developer or contractor requiring the implementation of measures to control noise from on the site. These powers remain the same irrespective of the character of the area. However, local authorities will temper any conditions they impose to take account of the locality.

The conditions imposed could include limitation of hours worked per day, the positioning of noisy machinery on the site, the designation of vehicular access routes about the site, and the provision of enclosures for noisy machinery or operations. The local authorities should also ensure that best practicable means are employed by the contractor.

A developer or contractor can also apply to the local authority for a prior consent for their proposed works, and the developer or contractor can appeal against any notice served by the local authority or against the failure to agree the details of a prior consent.

Once a prior consent is agreed or a notice served, it is a defence for a developer or contractor to prove he or she was complying with the conditions therein in any subsequent nuisance action. These procedures are detailed in *Environmental Health Procedures* [26].

BS5228: 1984 [19] was produced to give guidance to local authorities in the methods of predicting, measuring and assessing noise on construction and open sites and its impact on those exposed to it. The standard is in four parts:

1. **Part 1**.Code of practice for basic information and procedures for noise control.
2. **Part 2**.Guide to legislation for noise control applicable to construction and demolition, including road construction and maintenance.
3. **Part 3**.Code of practice for noise control applicable to surface coal extraction by opencast methods.
4. **Part 4**.Code of practice for noise control applicable to piling operations.

In setting noise conditions the local authority should take into account:

1. The site location: proximity of noise sensitive premises.
2. Existing ambient noise levels: the larger the increase in noise over the ambient noise level, the more likelihood of complaints.
3. Duration of site operations: the longer the perceived duration of site operations the more likely noise is to provoke complaint. Residents may be willing to accept higher noise levels if they can anticipate an early cessation of activity on the site.
4. Hours of work: residential property and offices may have different priorities regarding the times when noisy work should be carried out on a site. Night-time work would keep domestic residents awake. However, the same activity in the day may interfere with speech in a nearby office. Noise conditions imposed on evening work may need to be much stricter than daytime limits – BS5228: 1984 [19] suggests as much as 10 dB(A) less. Night-time work would necessitate very careful consideration; the times at which people are getting to sleep and just before they rise appear to be particularly sensitive.
5. Attitude of the site operator: local people will be more amenable to noise if they consider that the site operator is, in his planning and management, doing all he can to keep noise to a minimum.
6. Noise characteristics: the presence of impulsive noise or noise with tonal characteristics may be less acceptable than actual sound level readings would lead one to believe.

* The police role in respect of noise complaints is examined in 'A Review of Police Core and Ancillary Tasks: Interim Report', October 1994, Home Office.

NOISE ABATEMENT ZONES (NAZ)

The Noise Advisory Council (NAC) in a report published in 1971 [27] was critical of the nuisance approach to the abatement of noise. The Noise Abatement Act 1960 did not give local authorities the power to prevent noise, only to deal with noise nuisance. A later report from the NAC [28] further emphasized this point.

These issues were addressed by The Control of Pollution Act 1974 (sections 63–67) which gave local authorities the power to establish NAZ in order to control noise increases and to achieve noise reductions in existing noisy situations, as well as preventing the increase in background noise due to new developments.

Under the Act, local authorities can designate all or part of their area as a NAZ. The Local Government Planning and Land Act 1980 repealed the requirement that the Secretary of State should confirm a noise abatement order.

The order will specify classes of premises to which it applies, e.g. industrial premises, places of entertainment, commercial premises, etc. In practice there is no reason why named premises could not be included in the schedule. Once the order has been implemented, the local authority is obliged to measure noise levels from the specific premises along the perimeter of the premises. The Control of Noise (Measurement and Register) Regulations 1976 make provision with respect to the methods to be used by local authorities when measuring noise levels, and the maintenance of a public register. Detailed guidance on the introduction of such areas may be found in DOE Circular 2/76 and in Building Research Station Digests Nos. 203 and 204.

While these sections of the Act gave local authorities the power to control noise increases within the community, it is a power which is not widely used. It is very time consuming and labour intensive to collect the initial noise data and also to maintain the public register in which the measured noise levels must be recorded.

The Government recognized these problems and in its white paper on the environment [12] stated its intention to devise simpler and more practical procedures for dealing with NAZ. The

Noise Review Report [11] recommends that the system could be simplified by using procedures issued in a code of practice rather than under the existing legislation. Such a method would allow local authorities to adjust the requirements to local circumstances, and it is felt that this may result in a revival of NAZs.

In response to the recommendation of the Noise Review Working Party the Department of the Environment requested the BRE to undertake a review of the NAZ system which was completed during 1992. The BRE surveyed local authorities and found 37 local authorities had designated a total of 58 NAZs [29]. However, of these only 28 of the zones had complete Noise Level Registers and 40 of the NAZs were now either inactive or abandoned. Whilst the survey concluded that NAZs were unpopular it also indicated that they could be of use for preventing excessive noise from a small number of premises.

As yet there have been no new policy developments in response to the findings of this report.

RAILWAY NOISE

Generally speaking, complaints relating to noise from this source are less common than those relating to other noise sources. The 1991 BRE Survey [5] indicated that 4% of the adult population are bothered by railway noise. This is somewhat surprising when one considers that the noise generated can often be higher than levels from sources which frequently give rise to complaint. This could be due to the fact that the public tend to tolerate noise from this source and believe that nothing can be done to reduce the levels of noise. Furthermore, by comparison, far less people live adjacent to railways than, for example, next to major roads.

However, many local authorities are faced with the increasing demand for housing land such that locations adjacent to existing railway lines are now being considered for housing use. The increased use of existing lines and the construction of new routes suggest that railway noise is more likely to cause more widespread annoyance in the future. The opening of the Channel Tunnel will have a major effect in this respect in the south-east.

A national survey of the community response to railway noise was undertaken by Fields and Walker of the Institute of Sound and Vibration Research (Southampton University) [30]. This study combined a social survey (1453 respondents) and a noise measurement survey in 75 study areas in the UK. The study concluded that railway noise is a problem for those living adjacent to railway lines, and this was quantified further to suggest that 2% of the nation's population are bothered by noise from this source. Furthermore, the equivalent continuous noise level over a 24-hour period ($L_{Aeq,24h}$) closely related to people's reaction to railway noise; more so than any other accepted noise indices examined. It further concluded that approximately 170 000 people are exposed to railway noise above 65 dB(A)$L_{eq,24h}$, and that maintenance noise is rated as a bigger problem than passing train noise. Above 45dB(A)$L_{eq,24h}$ there was found to be a steady increase in annoyance with increasing $L_{Aeq,24h}$. There is no simple threshold below which people were not annoyed.

In the absence of any statutory guidelines various standards have been adopted by local authorities when considering the development of land adjacent to railway lines, in some cases a 24-hour L_{eq} is set, while in others separate daytime and night-time levels are set. For example, some authorities prohibit noise sensitive development where the 24-hour L_{eq} level exceeds 60 dB(A), while others may require noise insulation double glazing.

In March 1990 the Government set up an independent committee to recommend a noise insulation standard for dwellings near new railway lines. The Mitchell Committee published its report in February 1991. In November 1991 the Minister for Public Transport confirmed that noise insulation regulations for new railway lines would be issued.

In October 1993 draft regulations – The Noise Insullation (Railways and Other Guided Transport Systems) Regulations 1993 – and a Technical Memorandum describing the procedures for predicting and measuring noise levels from moving railway vehicles were issued for consultation. The purpose of the regulations is to introduce provisions for new railway lines similar to those contained in the Noise Insulation Regulations 1975 (as amended).

The regulations will only apply when it is not possible to reduce noise below the trigger levels (see below), initially it will be expected that bodies constructing new railway lines will take all the necessary steps to reduce noise by careful design and the use of screens and landscaping.

Eligible properties, dwellings or other residential properties, which will be entitled to noise insulation treatment must satisfy the following conditions:

1. are within 300 metres of the new or altered system; and
2. are subject to a noise increase of at least 1 dB(A) as a result of vehicles using that new system; and
3. are subject to noise levels from vehicles using the new, altered and any relevant existing system of not less than 68 dB $L_{Aeq\ 18h}$ between 06.00 and midnight or 63 dB $L_{Aeq\ 6h}$ between midnight and 06.00; and
4. the railway noise level has increased the noise level by at least 1 dB(A).

The regulations confer duties or powers on railway authorities to carry out insulation work or pay grant, set out the machinery for offering and accepting insulation work or grant payment, specify the extent of insulation work that should be carried out and detail appeal procedures. The Technical Memorandum is divided into three main sections: a general method of predicting noise levels at a distance from a railway; procedures to deal with the prediction of railway noise in situations such as stations and sidings; and procedures and requirements for the measurement of railway noise where prediction is not possible. Although the consultation period for the draft regulations ended in December 1993 no timetable has been set for laying them before Parliament.

Table 40.8 Maximum noise limits for motor vehicles

Vehicles	Current (db(A))	Proposed (dB(A))
Goods vehicles over 3.5 tonnes		
Over 150 kW engine power	84	80
75–150 kW engine power	83	78
Below 75 kW engine power	81	77
Good vehicles below 3.5 tonnes		
Goods vehicles 2–3.5 tonnes	79	77
Goods vehicles below 2 tonnes	78	76
Buses		
With over 9 seats, over 3.5 tonnes GVW and over 150 kW engine power	83	80
With over 9 seats, over 3.5 tonnes GVW but below 150 kW engine power	80	78
With over 9 seats, but below 3.5 tonnes GVW	78–79	
Cars	77	74

Table 40.9 Motorcycle noise limits

Engine capacity (cc)	1st stage (dB(A))	2nd stage (dB(A))	Date of entry for type 1st stage	Date of entry for type 2nd stage
<80	77	75	1.10.88	1.10.93
80–175	79	77	1.10.89	31.12.94
>175	82	80	1.10.88	1.10.93

Note: Stage II limits reduce these limits by a further 2 dB and are intended to become effective from 1995–6.

ROAD TRAFFIC NOISE

The noise limits for road-going motor vehicles are prescribed in regulations made under the Road Traffic Act 1972, the Motor Vehicle (Construction and Use) Regulations 1986 (as amended) and the Motor Vehicle Type Approval (Great Britain) Regulations (Table 40.8). The Motor Vehicle Type Approval Regulations reflect EEC Directives and have been amended to encompass 92/97/EEC. This reduces the current limits for new vehicles, cars, dual purpose, and light goods vehicles with petrol engines from the 1 October 1995 and to all new vehicles from 1 October 1996 subject to ratification by the European Commission. The Commission will introduce proposals by 31 March 1994 for further reductions.

Motorcycles

Motorcycle noise is controlled in the UK by the Road Vehicle (Construction and Use) (Amendment No.3) Regulation 1989 and The Motorcycles (Sound Level Measurement Certificates) (Amendment) Regulations 1989. These Regulations implement EC Directive 78/1015/EEC as amended by 87/56/EEC. The effect of these Regulations is to control noise from motorcycles in two stages (Table 40.9).

Local authority involvement in road traffic noise

The local authority responsible for highways in an area may, using the Road Traffic Regulation Act 1967 reroute through traffic out of a residential area, and this could overcome a particular noise problem.

The Heavy Commercial Vehicles (Controls and Regulations) Act 1973 requires the highway authority to prepare written proposals for the management of lorries. This allows the introduction of improved traffic schemes.

The Land Compensation Act 1973 Part II enables householders to claim a grant from the highway authority to provide noise insulation if they experience significantly increased noise levels from a new or substantially improved road. The avenue which opens the possibility of noise insulation is set out in the Noise Insulation Regulations 1975 (as amended) for England and Wales (similar legislation/regulations apply in Scotland).

The Noise Insulation Regulations 1975 make grants available for secondary glazing of habitable rooms of a dwelling if it is estimated that the L10 (18 hour) will be raised to above 68 dB(A) due to a new road or substantially-improved road during the 15 years following its opening (this is taken to mean at least the addition of a new carriageway), with a contribution of least 1 dB(A) from traffic using the new road or 5 dB(A) from improvements to an existing road. Grants are not available to provide insulation where the new or increased noise is due to a traffic management scheme. The Noise Insulation Regulations 1975 refer to the Department of Transport and Welsh Office publication, *Calculation of Road Traffic Noise* [31].

The Noise Review Working Party [11] considered transportation noise and made a number of comments and recommendations. These included whether the current standard of 68 dB(A) L10 (18 hour) for noise insulation work remains appropriate and the possible extension of the existing rights to compensation against increased traffic noise to include those affected by permanent traffic management schemes.

In response to this report, the government has stated that it is considering covering noise in the annual MOT test, and will seek to tighten international noise regulations for vehicles. Furthermore, consideration will be given to the extension of compensation to those affected by permanent traffic management schemes and to an examination into improved design and specification in road construction to reduce traffic noise.

AIRCRAFT NOISE

According to the BRE survey [5], 16% of the adult population are bothered by aircraft noise, this compares with 28% who are bothered by road traffic noise. Aircraft engines are very noisy, especially jet engines, and even though much work continues to be done to reduce sound levels by, for example, producing quiet-engined aircraft, an acute problem still exists for many people.

Powers available to control environmental noise in the Control of Pollution Act 1974 and Environmental Protection Act 1990 deal with noise from fixed sources, and specifically excludes noise from aircraft, the exception being noise from model aircraft. Section 76 of the Civil Aviation Act 1982 exempts aircraft from statutory action being taken in respect to noise nuisance. Sections 78 and 79 of this Act provides power for

the Secretary of State for Transport to apply operational controls and enforce noise standards on aircraft and give directions to airport owners in relation to noise insulation grant schemes. For example, operational restrictions relating to night flights are applied at Heathrow, Stansted and Gatwick airports, and similar restrictions apply between April and October at Manchester and Luton airports.

Standards set by the International Civil Aviation Organization are enacted in the UK, and the Air Navigation (Noise Certification) Order 1986 implements the most recent international recommendations in respect of the control of aircraft noise at source.

The noise and number index (NNI) (see page 665) was formulated and adopted as an index of disturbance from aircraft noise. There was considerable support for the replacement of the NNI, and the government changed the index for measuring aircraft to L_{eq} (16 hr) db(A) based on measurements over 16 hrs between 0700 and 2300.

In recent years, there has been a considerable increase in the number of non-commercial flights. There are in the region of 7000 British-registered general aviation aircraft flying from about 280 small airfields in the UK; these aircraft are generally used for private flying. This, together with the increased use of helicopters, which can land and take off from very small areas, has created a new aircraft problem. This problem was identified by the Noise Review Working Party [11], and in response to this report the government has confirmed that it intends to examine the need for further action on controlling noise from helicopters landing outside airfields, and from light or recreational aircraft.

In August 1991 the Department of Transport issued a consultation paper [32] which set out the Government's proposal on the above issues. In March 1993 the Department of Transport published the Government's conclusions [33] following the responses to the consultation paper. The new system will build on the existing, mainly voluntary, scheme of control at most civil airports and airfields. The main points in the Governments proposals are:

- to commission and consult on guidance to create a national framework to assist preparation of noise amelioration schemes.
- to encourage aerodromes to review existing noise amelioration measures and their enforcement, and arrangements for local accountability.
- to open discussions with BAA and local consultative committees about making Heathrow, Gatwick and Stansted airports more responsible and locally accountable for their noise control measures.
- to introduce a new enabling power for aerodromes to establish and enforce noise control arrangements, including for ground noise.
- to introduce a new power of designation to replace existing sections 5 and 78–80 of the Civil Aviation Act 1982.
- designated aerodromes to prepare a noise amelioration scheme, consult locally and agree it with the 'lead' local authority – disputed points to be settled by the Secretary of State.
- to introduce new powers of enforcement to enable local authorities to take action against designated aerodromes who do not enforce schemes.
- introduce a 'call-in' power for the Secretary of State to approve schemes.
- these new powers to be capable of being applied to all aerodromes from the largest airports to the smallest private sites, including those used by helicopters.

Primary legislation will be required to introduce the new designation power. The timetable for this legislation has not been set out as yet.

OCCUPATIONAL NOISE (also see Chapter 26)

The Noise at Work Regulations 1989, came into force on 1 January 1990 and are designed to protect people at work from suffering damage to their hearing. These regulations implement the requirements of EC Directive 86/188/EEC. The regulations stipulate three 'action levels':

1. a first action level of 85 dB(A);
2. a second action level of 90 dB(A)
3. a peak action level of 200 pascals (equivalent to 140 dB ref. μPa).

If the noise level in a workplace is above the first action level, then the employer shall ensure that a 'competent' person makes a noise assessment which is sufficient to:

1. identify which of the employees are so exposed; and
2. provide them with such information with regard to the noise to which those employees may be exposed as will facilitate compliance with the duties under the Health and Safety at Work, Etc, Act 1974 and the Noise at Work Regulations 1989.

When the level lies between the first and second action level, the employer must provide suitable and sufficient ear protectors to employees who ask for them. These must be maintained by the employer in good condition. However, there is no duty either on the employer or the employee to ensure they are worn.

Where the exposure is above the second action level, the employer must provide suitable and sufficient ear protectors capable of keeping risk down to no more than that expected from the action levels. Employers and employees have a duty to ensure they are worn.

Areas in the workplace that are identified as being above the second action level must be identified and designated an 'ear protection zone'. These zones should be clearly marked with signs complying with BS5378: 1980 [34] and it should be ensured that everyone entering the zones is wearing ear protection.

The peak action level is most likely to be encountered where cartridge operated tools, shooting guns or similar loud, explosive noisy devices are used, and workers exposed above this level will also be exposed to levels above 90 dB(A) $L_{EP,d}$.

A 'competent person' does not have to be a qualified acoustic engineer. However, he should be capable of working unsupervised and have a good basic understanding of what information needs to be obtained and how to make the necessary measurements.

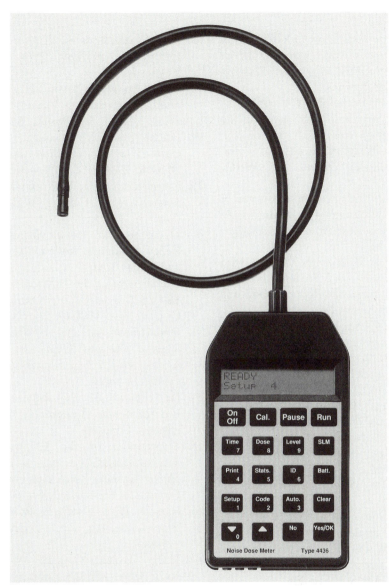

Fig. 40.8 Noise dose meter. (Courtesy of Brüel & Kjaer (UK) Ltd, Harrow Weald Lodge, 92 Uxbridge Road, Harrow, Middlesex HA3 6BZ.)

The Institute of Acoustics (IoA) provides training courses leading to the Certificate of Competence in Work-Place Assessment. Training on noise is also available in modular form as part of more general courses, i.e. National Diploma in Occupational Safety and Health of the National Examination Board in Occupational Safety and Health (NEBOSH), the Certificate of Operational Competence in Comprehensive Occupational Hygiene of the British Examining and Registration Board in Occupational Hygiene (BERBOH), and the IoA Diploma in Acoustics and Noise Control. One method of measuring personal exposure to workplace noise is by the use of a noise dose meter (Fig. 40.8).

REFERENCES

1. Wilson, A. (1963) *Noise, Final Report*, HMSO, London.

2. British Standards Institution (1990) *Method For Rating Industrial Noise Affecting Mixed Residential And Industrial Areas*, BS4142: 1990, BSI, Milton Keynes.

3. Sargent, J.W. and Fothergill, L.C. (1993) A Survey of Environmental Noise levels in the UK. *Proceedings of Noise 93*, **7**, 161–66.

4. World Health Organization (1980) *Noise: environmental health criteria 12*, WHO, Geneva.

5. Grimwood, C.J. (1993) A national survey of the effects of environmental noise on people at home. *Proceedings Institute Of Acoustics*, **15**, (Part 8) 69–76.

6. Mant, D.C. and Muir Gray, J.A. (1986) *Building Regulation and Health. Building Research Establishment Report*, Building Research Establishment, Watford.

7. Gray, P.G. and Cartwright, A. (1958) Noise in Three Groups of Flats with Different Floor Insulations, Res. Paper No 27, Nat. Build. Stud. HMSO, London.

8. Ising, H. *et al.* (1980) Health effects of traffic noise. *International Archives of Occupational and Environmental Health*, **47**, 179.

9. Gloag, D. (1980) Noise and health: public and private responsibility. *British Medical Journal*, **281**, 1404.

10. Oswald, I. (1975) *Sleep*, Penguin Books, Harmondsworth

11. Report of the Noise Review Working Party (1990) HMSO, London.

12. Government White Paper (1990) *This Common Inheritance – Britain's Environmental Strategy*, HMSO, London.

13. British Standards Institution (1981) *Method of Expression of Physical and Subjective Magnitude of Sound or Noise in Air*, BS3045: 1981, BSI, Milton Keynes.

14. British Standards Institution (1986) *Integrating/Averaging Sound Level Meters*, BS6698: 1986 (IEC804: 1985), BSI, Milton Keynes.

15. Greater London Council (1966) *Traffic Noise Survey*, GLC, London.

16. British Standards Institution (1981) *Specification for Sound Level Meters*, BS5969: 1981 (IEC651: 1979), BSI, Milton Keynes.

17. British Standards Institution (1989) *Sound Calibrators*, BS7189: 1989, BSI, Milton Keynes.

18. British Standards Institution (1984) *Guide to Human Exposure to Vibration in Buildings*, BS6472: 1984, BSI, Milton Keynes.

19. British Standards Institution (1984) *Noise Control on Construction and Open Sites*, BS5228: 1984, BSI, Milton Keynes.

20. Department of the Environment (1973) *Planning and Noise*, Circular 10/73, HMSO, London.

21. Department of the Environment, Planning Policy Guidance Note (PPG) 24, Planning and Noise, HMSO, London.

22. Department of the Environment (1985) *The Use of Conditions in Planning Permission*, Circular 1/85, HMSO, London.

23. Department of the Environment (1990) *Mineral Planning Guidance: the control of noise at surface mineral workings*. (MPG 11), HMSO, London.

24. Department of the Environment (1988) *Environmental Assessment*, Circular 15/88, HMSO, London.

25. Department of the Environment (1988) *Environmental Assessment of Projects in Simplified Planning Zones and Enterprise Zones*, Circular 24/88, HMSO, London.

26. Bassett, W.H. (1995) *Environmental Health Procedures*, 4th edn, Chapman and Hall, London.

27. Noise Advisory Council (1971) *Neighbourhood Noise*, HMSO, London.

28. Noise Advisory Council (1974) *Noise in the Next Ten Years*, HMSO, London.

29. Grimwood C. (1992) Noise abatement zones – A method of preventing deterioration in environmental noise levels? *Proceedings of the Institute of Acoustics*, **14**, part 4.

30. Fields, J.M. and Walker, J.G., The response to railway noise in residential areas in Great Britain., *Journal of Sound and Vibration*, **85**, (2), 177–255.

31. Department of Transport and Welsh Office (1988) *Calculation of Road Traffic Noise*, HMSO, London.

32. Department of Transport Consultation Paper: Control of Aircraft Noise, August 1991.

33. Department of Transport, Review of Aircraft Noise Legislation, Announcement of Conclusions, March 1993.

34. British Standards Institute (1980) *Safety Signs and Colour Specification for Colour and Design, BS5378: 1980, BSI, London.*

FURTHER READING

Penn, C.N. (1979) *Noise Control*, Shaw and Sons, London.

Sharland, I. (1972) *Woods Practical Guide To Noise Control*, Cambridge University Press, Cambridge.

National Society For Clean Air And Environmental Protection (1994) *1994 Pollution Handbook*, NSCA, Brighton.

Open University, The Control of the Acoustic Environment, OU, Milton Keynes.

Health and Safety Executive (1990) *Noise at Work Assessment, Information and Control*, Noise Guides 3–8, HMSO, London.

Williams, Dr M. (1988) *Noise and Vibration Measurements for Environmental Health Officers*, Brüel and Kjaer (UK) Ltd, Harrow.

41 Air pollution

Michael J. Gittins

INTRODUCTION

It has long been recognized that there is an association between atmospheric pollution and health. John Evelyn, the diarist, was one of the first to observe the link between coal smoke and the ill-health of Londoners. Writing in 1661, he said

> Her inhabitants breathe nothing but an impure and thick Mist, accompanied with a fuliginous and filthy vapour, which renders them obnoxious to a thousand inconveniences, corrupting their Lungs, and disordering the entire habit of their Bodies; so that Catharrs, Phthisicks, Coughs, and Consumptions rage more in this City, than in the whole Earth besides.

His observations, although profound, were largely ignored.

It was not until 1953, following an episode when some 4000 excess deaths were associated with a long-lasting smog in London, that any serious attempt was made to consider the problem. A committee on air pollution was established, the Beaver Committee [1], which was required to 'examine the nature, causes and effects of air pollution and the efficacy of the present preventative measures; to consider what further preventative measures are practicable; and to make recommendations'. After due deliberation, the production of two reports, and considerable parliamentary debate, the Clean Air Act 1956 was enacted. As a result, England benefited from measures designed to reduce the worst effects of coal smoke on the urban population.

The striking feature of this example is that the pollution was obvious, but that it took a significant event to cause the government to investigate the relationship between cause and effect in order to determine the need for preventative measures.

It is generally the case that legislative reform is triggered by disasters; the most effective catalyst to any bureaucracy appears to be excess civilian deaths.

Pollution is not always visible; nor are its effects always apparent in the immediate vicinity of the point of discharge. It is possible, under certain local atmospheric conditions, for ground-level concentrations of gases to cause physical discomfort. There is growing concern that there is an association between the presence of small suspended particles (PM 10s) and oxides of nitrogen in the atmosphere, and the increased incidence of asthma, especially in young children. (Both of these pollutants are particularly associated with vehicle emissions.) In contrast ozone, as a natural component of the upper atmosphere, is being depleted by emissions of CFCs; the fate of the ozone layer has become a matter of international concern.

Even if emissions are controlled in an adequate manner during the normal operation of plant, there is always the possibility of massive release of toxic or flammable gas as a result of bad management, or poor pollution-control practices. Examples have been seen at Flixborough, England, when an explosion devastated a chemical plant causing loss of life and millions of pounds of damage; in Seveso, Italy, when the local population suffered the consequences of a massive release of dioxin; and in Bhopal, India, where countless deaths were caused by emissions from a chemical plant.

There has recently been a move towards a more proactive approach based on the concept of sustainable development. This approach was the foundation of the United Nations Conference on Environment and Development, popularly known as the **'Earth Summit'**, held in Rio de Janeiro in June 1992. One of the principal outcomes of that conference was the establishment of a Commission on Sustainable Development to monitor progress in the implementation of the agreements reached at Rio. Another was a general endorsement of **Agenda 21**, a comprehensive and forward looking action plan for the next century. Agenda 21 calls on governments to prepare national strategies for sustainable development. It is important to bear in mind that pollution control policies are only a part of sustainability, and that Agenda 21 requires the comprehensive consideration of all issues which have an effect on the state of the environment, both now and in the future. Although this chapter is limited in its scope, the broader strategy must be borne in mind.

It follows that policies to control air pollution must relate to the entire spectrum of emissions, both the obvious and the invisible. Processes must be understood so that account can be taken of intermediates as well as feedstock and end-products. While there is sometimes a case for the dilution and dispersion of exhaust gases, their final environmental fate must be determined. Account must also be taken of the worst case – plant failure – in addition to emission limits associated with normal operation.

Enforcement is not merely the adoption of appropriate technology, it is also the consistency of approach. Local authorities should establish adequate quality control systems, so as to ensure that their policies are implemented in a consistent manner. Attention must also be paid to the way in which quality assurance can be achieved nationally, within the context of a large number of local authorities not, necessarily, operating to the same objectives.

Monitoring of air quality must be seen as a procedure based on the current needs of the community and the changing recognition of the importance of various pollutants. It is arguable that the technology of the British Standard volumetric method of measurement of smoke and sulphur dioxide is not an adequate basis for all aspects of information gathering or decision making. It has its place, of course, in the foundation of a network of monitors measuring pollutants most closely associated with the combustion of fossil fuel, but there are now other issues which have to be recognized, and considered on a regular basis when investigatory activities are considered.

The concept of the authority being proactive, not reactive, has long been a foundation in public health, but application of this approach has not always been fully honoured. In the broadest sense, districts have not always been inspected, 'from time to time, for the presence of nuisance'. Monitoring programmes do not always reflect the needs of the day; it is therefore important that a regular programme of review is operated as part of management procedures.

The investigation of complaints forms the third component of service delivery. There should be few complaints if potential emitters are kept under regular scrunity and if the authority is aware of all significant discharges to the atmosphere. It would be naive to suppose that such a situation could be met in practice. Even if all scheduled works comply fully with the use of 'best available technology' to control pollution, smoke control is properly enforced and there is an adequate monitoring programme, there will still be occasions when justified complaints require action. Procedures for the organization of investigation and for the communication of findings have to be clearly established. Evidence has to be collected and reviewed in an impartial manner, making the best use of existing information bases where appropriate. Prosecution is usually the last resort, but cannot be avoided where genuine problems have been identified; indeed there is a danger that the local authority could be found guilty of maladministration if it fails to bring proceedings once convinced that a nuisance exists or that an offence is being committed. One of the greatest problems in the investigation procedure would seem to be the inability of the investigators to make decisions. Another is that local authorities do not have prosecution policies.

As important as the implementation of policy is the need to communicate information to a public who have an ever increasing interest in environmental matters. This is not always easily done, and it is not always possible to satisfy the expectations of some pressure groups. Such problems should not stop the presentation of the results of monitoring together with adequate supplementary information to allow interpretation. The need for freedom of information is generally accepted, but not yet adequately addressed.

SUSTAINABLE DEVELOPMENT
(also see Chapter 39)

Sustainable development was defined in the Report of the World Commission on Economic and Environmental Development – The Bruntland Report – as '**development that meets the needs of the present without compromising the ability of future generations to meet their own needs**'. This concept is not entirely new to the UK, in 1989 a report 'Sustaining our Common Future', was published by the Government, which set out policy aims and measures for the UK specifically directed towards sustainable development. The theme was also incorporated into the white paper on the environment 'This Common Inheritance [2], published in 1990.

A Commission on Sustainable Development, under the aegis of the United Nations, was established in 1993, as an outcome of the Rio Earth Summit, to monitor progress in the implementation of the agreements reached at Rio. Also agreed in 1993 was **Agenda 21**, a comprehensive and forward looking action plan for the next century, which required national strategies for sustainable development.

Agenda 21 must be seen as a global plan which recognizes the different needs of developed and developing countries. Because economic development in one nation will affect the economy of other countries it is necessary to consider the impact of home policy and practice on other parts of the world. This will include the impact which the UK has on the developing world and on other areas such as Central and Eastern Europe and the Former Soviet Union. The UK Strategy for Sustainable Development will also take into account, where appropriate, the action envisaged in the EC's Fifth Environmental Action Programme.

It has to be recognized that many people aspire to economic development, with rising living standards of living, and to a safe and pleasant environment. They wish to pass these on to future generations. Economic development is needed to raise the living standards of the present population and of future generations alike. It is important to recognize that there are many ways of combining economic activity with environmental protection. They include energy efficiency measures, improved technology and techniques management, better product design and marketing, waste minimization, environmentally sensitive farming practices, sound decisions on land planning, improved transport efficiency, informed choices by consumers and changes in lifestyles.

Decisions about levels of protection should be based on the best possible economic and scientific analysis. Where appropriate actions should be based on the so called '**precautionary principle**'. The processes of public decision making, in central and local government, and by other public bodies should provide a proper assessment of the issues and for environmental appraisal before action is taken; the balance of likely costs and benefits must be established. Where quantifiable measurements are not available the next best analysis must be made: implicitly, values are placed upon aspects of the environment when, for example, measures are taken to reduce threats to global atmosphere or to avert threats to health.

It is also important that the private sector takes full account of environmental costs – the 'polluter pays principle'. (see Chapter 39). Economic instruments are designed to achieve environmental objectives by making true costs of action transparent to decision makers.

There is also a need to encourage individuals to better understand the principles of sustainable development and to take account of environmental costs in their private lives. Increasingly people are aware of this need and committed to it, but they often need better information.

In considering sustainability, the main effects, in relation to air quality are controlling emissions of harmful substances, particularly those produced by road traffic, and protecting ecosystems by continuing the reduction of emissions which cause acid rain. The Strategy will need to consider the potential impact of air borne pollution not only in the UK, but also through trans-boundary movements in other countries, such as the Scandinavian bloc.

Air pollution can affect health and damage material, as indicated later in this chapter. The level at which the ecosystems are judged to be at risk is called the '**critical load**'. The Department of the Environment has formed a Critical Loads Advisory Group which has produced maps of critical loads for soils and fresh waters. Further study is necessary to relate ecosystems' response to measured acid depositions.

Many polluting emissions from homes and industry have reduced over the last 20 years. Since 1970, emissions of sulphur dioxide, the main contributor to acid rain, have fallen by 45%, and 'black smoke' emissions by almost 70%. They will fall further over coming years as implementation of existing UK and EU controls is completed. The UK is committed under EU legislation to reduce sulphur dioxide emissions from large combustion plant by 60% by 2003, compared with the 1980 level. Emissions from large combustion plant in 1993 accounted for 83% of the total emission. By 1991, a 23% reduction has been achieved. Under the most recent scenario the 2003 target will be met. Longer term objectives for sulphur dioxide emissions are under review in the negotiations to revise the Long Term Transboundary Air Pollution Agreement for Europe.

Although industrial and domestic air pollution has declined there has been a substantial growth in air pollution from road traffic.* For example emissions of oxides of nitrogen and smoke have both increased by over 70% since 1980. Tighter standards introduced in 1993 for new vehicles, particularly those with petrol engines, together

with tighter checks for older ones, should help to reverse this trend. Government has projected that there may even be a steady improvement in air quality by the end of the century and beyond. There will still, in the foreseeable future, be a strong likelihood of episodes of high air pollution levels in cities because catalytic converters on cars are not effective until they warm up – in winter temperature inversions can trap pollution close to the ground leading to a gradual build up of products of combustion. There will be some summer days when high ozone concentrations are detected; diesel smoke is likely to remain a year-round problem.

Looking further ahead the introduction of new, cleaner power generation technology should have dealt with the main sources of acid rain within the next 10–20 years. This will leave a few highly sensitive, naturally acidic uplands in Northern England, Scotland and Wales still at risk according to current projections. New technology, coupled with measures to reduce the impact of traffic, especially in urban areas, will be required to avoid renewed growth of our most polluting emissions towards the end of the period covered by the Strategy.

EFFECTS

Background

Although some of the effects of air pollution are well understood there are issues, especially those related to human health, where the picture is far from complete. Continuing research identifies new associations – what is emerging is an ever increasingly complex series of relationships. The principal issues have been summarized by the Department of the Environment in its publication, *The Monitoring of the Environment in the United Kingdom* [3] as follows:

1. harmful gases or particles may be inhaled by people or animals, or may attack the skin, causing ill health or death;
2. gases may damage leaves and shoots of plants, reducing amenity and the yields of crops and trees;

---

* These issues and the need for an integrated strategy for the management and improvement of air quality are discussed in 'Air Quality: Meeting the Challenge' [14]. Also see 'Transport and the Environment, 18th Report of the Royal Commission on Environmental Pollution', Cmnd 2674, HMSO.

3. particles of substances which settle out onto soil or vegetation may cause damage or contaminate human or animal food;
4. air pollution can screen out sunlight, corrode structures and be a nuisance in many ways, especially through smells and the settlement of air-borne dust.

Traditionally, problems have most closely been associated with the inefficient combustion of coal, but other issues are now being recognized. Increasingly, interest is growing in the use of small population health statistics to enable perceived worries to be critically analysed and quantified. Investigations must be based on properly designed projects if useful information is to be obtained (see Chapter 19).

Effects on humanity

Although it is generally agreed that air pollution has a detrimental effect on health,* its actions are generally insidious. In only a limited number of cases does it produce a specific disease or symptoms, photochemical smog can cause eye irritation in some major cities, e.g. Los Angeles; chest diseases can be associated with occupational exposure to dust. Epidemiological studies show connections between air pollution and morbidity and mortality in chronic bronchitis sufferers, there is a demonstrable association between atmospheric sulphate levels and ill health and there is growing concern at the perceived increase in child asthma. Many factors contribute to this relationship: it is impossible to consider any one in isolation. Effects will depend upon:

1. the general health of the subject;
2. the duration of the exposure;
3. the concentration of the pollutant;
4. the nature of the pollutant.

Physiological effects

Defences exist in the nose and respiratory tracts which facilitate the removal of particulates. Further cleaning of air is achieved by the complex structure of the nasal cavity and upper respiratory tract,

which causes heavier particles to be deposited by impact. The body readily removes these materials.

Particles less than 10 μm may pass deeply into the lungs to be deposited in the alveoli. In low concentrations, such particles may be removed to lymph nodes where they cause discoloration of tissue and, possibly, the formation of nodules. Large concentrations of mineral material, such as silica or asbestos, produce the industrial diseases pneumoconiosis and asbestosis respectively. It is the particle size or falling velocity which determines the depth of penetration.

Exposure to oxidant gases, such as sulphur dioxide, causes constriction of the airways with an associated cough reflex and reduction or reversal of mucous transfer. Energetic coughing, to remove phlegm, may not only be exhausting but can be fatal to a patient with reduced lung capacity and heart or chest disease.

Limited information is available to allow the production of safe exposure limits for the range of chemicals which may be discharged to the atmosphere. One approach has been to use the occupational exposure levels (OELs), published by the Health and Safety Executive, as the base, reducing values by the use of correcting factors. Values of between a twenty-fifth to a fortieth of the OEL have been postulated, but there is no clear scientific basis for this approach. (Indeed the basis of certain OELs have been called into question as they appear to be founded on limited animal research.) Upper and lower limits are being determined by the DoE.

Synergistic effect is of particular concern in a human or animal health context. Two substances may each, independently, have little effect, but can act together to produce a significant reaction. Limited information is available on synergism.

Effects on animals

Effects of air pollution on animals are similar to those on humans, at least in those cases where there is a common physiology. Of particular interest is the effect of fluorine on herbivores, as there is no parallel mechanism for human expos-

---

* See the Committee on the Medical Effects of Air Pollutants: Report May 1992–December 1993 and the Advisory Group on the Medical Aspects of Air Pollution Episodes: Activities Report 1990–1993, Department of Health.

ure. The main source of fluoride emission is from processes which involve the heating of minerals, e.g. the firing of heavy clay, manufacture of glass, burning coal or aluminium smelting. Fluorine is a protoplasmic poison with an affinity for calcium – it interferes with the normal calcification process. Symptoms are hypoplasia of dental enamel and, at higher levels of exposure, abnormal growth rate of bones (which can cause lameness). Advanced fluorosis in cattle is indicated by anorexia, diarrhoea, weight loss, low fertility and reduction in milk production.

Effects on vegetation

Deposition has the effect of reducing the rate of photosynthesis by reducing the amount of light reaching leaves. Stomata and folial pores can be obstructed reducing transpiration. Oxidant gases can cause leaf collapse, chlorosis, growth alterations or a reduction in nitrogen fixing. It is possible to diagnose possible sources of damage to plants by a careful study of foliage, but due account must also be taken of frost or insect damage, drought, mould or disease.

Effects on materials

The principal mechanisms which cause damage are abrasion, deposition and removal (the damage caused by regular cleaning), direct chemical attack or electrochemical corrosion. The rate at which damage is caused will be influenced by moisture, temperature, sunlight, air movement and the chemical nature of the pollutant. Moisture encourages oxidation, permits electrolytic action and accelerates chemical action. The rate of chemical action is temperature dependent, but the significance of water accumulation, which occurs when surfaces fall below dew point, must not be ignored. Sunlight is itself damaging and aids the formation of photochemical oxidants.

Particular chemicals in the atmosphere will cause particular effects on materials. Carbon dioxide, in solution, will dissolve limestone, but has little effect on sandstone because of the less reactive nature of silica. Most metals are vulnerable to acid attack, particularly in the presence of moisture. Textiles suffer soiling effects, but other materials, e.g. leather and paper, can be embrittled by the absorption of sulphur dioxide from the atmosphere. Rubber is particularly affected by ozone at levels as low as 0.02 ppm.

Atmospheric effects

In recent years, emphasis has shifted from the local level to matters of global concern, causing a redirection in the foundations of policy making. Three strategic issues have been identified which seem to have worldwide implications; global warming brought about by the accumulation of 'greenhouse gases' in the atmosphere; damage to the ozone layer caused by the interaction of chlorofluorocarbons in the stratosphere; and acid rain linked to the long distance transport of oxides of sulphur and nitrogen, which are finally deposited with precipitation. None of these subjects can be resolved by local action; progress will be determined by the extent to which governments are capable of agreeing international initiatives. The prospect of solutions to the problems is not eased by the apparent gap between scientific need and political expediency!

Research and information

It is important that use is made of existing research and published information at the earliest stage in the design of an investigation. One criticism of local authorities is their reluctance to acknowledge or utilize work previously carried out. While there is a limit to the resources available to local government for research activities, there is opportunity for collaborative studies with other agencies, such as universities and health authorities. There is also a growing number of publications which review recent research in a critical manner.

Of particular relevance is the 'Environmental Health Criteria' series published by the World Health Organization in collaboration with the United Nations Environment Programme and the International Labour Organization. This runs into 180 titles at the time of writing. The main objective of this series is to carry out and disseminate evaluations of the effects of chemicals on health and on the quality of the environment. Supporting activities include the development of epidemiological, experimental laboratory, and risk assessment methods that could produce internationally compatible results, and development of expertise in the field of toxicology.

The format of these studies is uniform; a review of physical and chemical properties, analytical method, sources of human and environmental exposure, environmental transport and distribution, environmental levels, human exposure, effects on organisms in the environment, metabolism, effects on experimental animals, effects on humans and evaluations of health and environmental risks. Each study is comprehensively referenced. A major risk assessment of some 10 000 chemicals is being undertaken in the EU.

BACKGROUND TO LEGISLATIVE CONTROLS

From the time that public health legislation was first enacted, the thrust of control has been directed towards the abatement of nuisance. It is for this reason that, generally, action has only been taken to control emissions when they have become the subject of complaint. Despite any duty to inspect the district, 'from time to time', many local authorities have either been restrained, or have restrained themselves, from taking action until there has been a reasonable body of evidence to support the existence of nuisance. This has lead to accusations that controls have not been applied uniformly across the country.

An exception to this generalization relates to the control of smoke. It has long been realized that smoke can be offensive. Initially, the concerns were associated with coal smoke. The London smog of 1952 triggered the first of two Clean Air Acts (1956 and 1968). At that time much domestic and industrial heating was provided by the combustion of coal. The 1956 Act introduced the concept of domestic smoke control by following the pioneering work of a few far-sighted councils who had introduced their own smokeless zones. Industrial emissions, largely associated with hand-fired boilers, were limited by restrictions on the periods during which smoke could be emitted and the density of such smoke.

Powers were also provided to limit grit and dust emissions from furnaces, although regulations related to coal-fired boilers were never extended to other plant, such as incinerators or cupolas.

It was not until the Environmental Protection Act 1990 came into force that specific powers to control processes were given to local authorities.

Almost all areas of the country which have previously been recognized as having poor air quality have been made subject of smoke control orders. The procedure necessary to establish an order is complex, it is unlikely that further orders will be declared in the light of Government policy. For this reason it is not proposed to provide here information on this aspect of the subject. Some information is provided on enforcement action and on the implications of smoke control orders to commercial and industrial premises.

It is important that anyone involved in pollution control work is able to make observations of dark and black smoke, but such activities are more likely to be associated with the burning of trade or industrial waste than emissions from chimneys serving conventional furnaces. The convenience of gas has seen a massive change in fuel utilization over the last 20 years. This practice has made its own contribution to the reduction in the concentration of particulates in the atmosphere. The wisdom of burning natural gas in large combustion plants, such as power stations, is open to question.

While there is a need to be familiar with different boiler types, this information is no longer the highest priority. The enactment of the Environmental Protection Act 1990 has focused interest on the uniform control of a wide range of other furnaces. It is now as important to understand the principles of metal melting, glass manufacture and mineral processing. These subjects are considered here, but reference to contemporary specialist works is necessary to achieve an adequate comprehension of the relevant technology.

ENVIRONMENTAL PROTECTION ACT 1990

The 1990 Act lays down new procedures for the application of integrated pollution control (IPC), to a range of processes which have considerable pollution potential, and a new approach to air pollution control to be implemented by local authorities. Plant is required to apply the best available technique not entailing excessive costs (BATNEEC) to control emissions. From April 1991, all new and substantially changing major installations were subject to IPC. Existing plant has been brought under IPC in a phased programme, starting with large combustion plants in 1991–2. Similarly, the local authority control was introduced on a phased basis: new and existing processes are required to comply with the BATNEEC conditions contained in the relevance guidance rate. All existing plant should, by now, have been granted an authorization to an interim standard and a timetable has been agreed for upgrade to meet the final operating conditions.

Definitions

Section 1 of the Act provides a series of definitions relevant to the interpretation of Part I. These are set out below:

Environment consists of all, or any, of the air, water, and land; and the medium, air, includes the air within buildings and the air within other natural or man-made structures above or below ground (section 1(2)).

Pollution of the environment means pollution of the environment due to the release (into any environmental medium) from any process of substances which are capable of causing harm to man or to any other living organism supported by the environment (section 1(3)).

Harm means harm to health of any living organisms or other interference with ecological systems of which they form part and, in the case of man, includes offence caused to any of his or her senses or harm to his or her property; and harmless has a corresponding meaning (section 1(4)).

Process means any activities carried on in Great Britain, whether on premises or by means of mobile plant, which are capable of causing pollution of the environment and 'prescribed processes' means a process prescribed under section 2(1).

In the context of substances:

1. **activities** means industrial or commercial activities or activities of any other nature whatsoever (including, with or without other activities, the keeping of a substance);
2. **Great Britain** includes so much of the adjacent territorial sea as is, or is treated as relevant territorial waters for the purposes of Chapter I of Part III of the Water Act 1989 (now the Water Resources Act 1991) or, as respects Scotland, Part II of the Control of Pollution Act 1974; and
3. **mobile plant** means plant which is designed to move or to be moved whether on roads or otherwise.

The **enforcing authority** in relation to England and Wales, is the chief inspector or the local authority by whom, under section 4, the functions conferred or imposed by this Part . . . are for the time being exercized in relation respectively to releases of substances into the environment or the air; and **local enforcing authority** means the local authority (section 1(7)). Subsection (8) of section 1 defines the enforcing authority in relation to Scotland.

Authorization means an authorization for a process (whether on premises or by means of mobile plant) granted under section 6; and a reference to the conditions of an authorization is a reference to the conditions to which at any time the authorization has effect (section 1(9)).

A substance is **released** into any environmental medium whenever it is released directly into that medium whether it is released into it within or outside Great Britain and release includes:

1. in relation to air, any emission of the substance into air;
2. in relation to water, any entry (including any discharge) of the substance into water;
3. in relation to land, any deposit, keeping or disposal of the substance in or on land; and for this purpose **water** and **land** shall be construed in accordance with subsection (11) and (12).

For the purpose of determining into what medium a substance is released:

1. any release into
   (a) the sea or the surface of the sea-bed,

(b) any river, watercourse, lake, loch or pond (whether natural or artificial or above or below ground) or reservoir or the surface of the river-bed or of other land supporting such waters, or

(c) ground waters;

2. any release into
   (a) land covered by water falling outside paragraph (1) above or the water covering such land; or
   (b) the land beneath the surface of the sea-bed or other land supporting waters falling within paragraph (1a) above is a release onto land; and

3. any release into a sewer (within the meaning of the Water Industry Act 1991); shall be treated as a release to water. But a sewer and its contents shall be disregarded in determining whether there is pollution of the environment at any time.

In subsection (11) **ground water** means any waters contained in underground strata or in:

1. a well, borehole or similar work sunk into underground strata, including any adit or passage constructed in connection with the well, borehole or work facilitating the collection of water in the well, borehole or work; or

2. any excavation into underground strata where the level of water in the excavation depends wholly or mainly on water entering it from the strata.

Substance shall be treated as including electricity or heat (section 1(13)).

Prescribed substance means any substance of a description in regulations made under section 2(5), or in the case of a substance of a description prescribed only for release in circumstances specified under section 2(6)(b) means any substance of that description which is released in those circumstances.

INTEGRATED POLLUTION CONTROL
(See also Chapter 39)

The concept of integrated pollution control was developed by the Royal Commission on Environmental Pollution in its fifth report **Air Pollution Control: an Integrated Approach** [4]. In essence, the best practicable environmental option (BPEO) has to be applied to the control of solid, liquid or gaseous wastes. Where choice exists as to the sector of the environment into which waste should be discharged, a decision has to be made on the means by which environmental damage can be minimized.

In the case of larger works, control is executed by Her Majesty's Inspectorate of Pollution (HMIP), who consider the most appropriate abatement technology on the basis of integrated pollution control. Process specific guidance notes have been produced, in the name of the Chief Inspector.

It is anticipated that by 1996 HMIP will be working with the National Rivers Authority, and the Waste Regulation Inspectorate as the Environmental Agency. At the time of writing it is not envisaged that local authority air pollution work will be transferred to this Agency.

Local authorities are only required to consider issues related to air pollution. They are required to have regard to guidance, in this case published by the Department of the Environment, in the name of the Secretary of State for the Environment, which determine BATNEEC for particular processes. Expert groups have been established comprising representatives from industrial interests and the enforcement agencies who will continue to keep the advice under review and arrange revision on a programmed basis. This framework of information should lead to a uniform application of control across the country.

Section 2 of the Act enables the Secretary of State for the Environment to prescribe, by regulation, the processes which will require authorization.

The Secretary of State for the Environment is empowered to prescribe substances which may be released to the environment. Regulations may:

1. prescribe the substance which may be released, subject to control, to each environmental medium; and

2. prescribe the concentrations, periods of release and other limitations.

The Secretary of State may also make regulations establishing standards, objectives or requirements in relation to particular prescribed processes or substances:

1. in relation to releases from prescribed processes into any environmental medium, prescribe standards for:
   (a) the concentration, amount or the amount in any period of that substance which may be so released; and
   (b) any other characteristic of that substance in any circumstances in which it may be so released;
2. prescribe standard requirements for the measurement or analysis of, or release of, substances for which limits have been set under paragraph (1) above; and
3. in relation to any prescribed process, prescribe standards or requirements in relation to any aspect of the process.

This approach is in keeping with the pollution control philosophy of the EU and contrasts with some previous UK practice.

Power is given to the Secretary of State to make plans for:

1. establishing limits for the total amount, or the total amount in any period, of any substance which may be released into the environment;
2. allocating quotas as respect the releases of substances to persons carrying on processes in respect of which such limit is established;
3. establishing limits of the descriptions above so as to progressively reduce pollution of the environment;
4. the progressive improvement in the quality objectives and quality standards established by regulation.

AUTHORIZATIONS

Section 6 of the 1990 Act requires that no prescribed process can operate without an authorization. Prescribed processes are defined in section 2(1) of the Act and in part B of the Environmental Protection (Prescribed Processes and Substances) Regulations 1991 (as amended 1994) as follows:

* PG refers to the appropriate Process Guidance Note reference.

Combustion

PG* 1/1 Waste oil burners, less than 0.4 MW net rated thermal in-put (nrti).
PG 1/2 Waste oil or recovered oil burners, less than 3 MW nrti.
PG 1/3 Boilers and furnaces, 20–50 MW nrti.
PG 1/4 Gas turbines, 20–50 MW nrti.
PG 1/5 Compression ignition engines, 20–50 nrti.
PG 1/6 Tyres and rubber combustion processes between 0.4 and 3 MW nrti.
PG 1/7 Straw combustion processes between 0.4 and 3 MW nrti.
PG 1/8 Wood combustion processes between 0.4 and 3 MW nrti.
PG 1/9 Poultry litter combustion processes between 0.4 and 3 MW nrti.
PG 1/10 Waste derived fuel burning processes less than 3 MW nrti.

Non-ferrous metals

PG 2/1 Furnaces for the extraction of non-ferrous metal from scrap.
PG 2/2 Hot dip galvanising processes.
PG 2/3 Electrical and rotary furnaces.
PG 2/4 Iron, steel and non-ferrous metal foundry processes.
PG 2/5 Hot and cold blast cupolas.
PG 2/6 Aluminium and aluminium alloy processes.
PG 2/7 Zinc and zinc alloy processes.
PG 2/8 Copper and copper alloy processes.
PG 2/9 Metal decontamination processes.

Mineral processes

PG 3/1 Blending, packing, loading and use of bulk cement.
PG 3/2 Manufacture of heavy clay goods and refectory goods.
PG 3/3 Glass (excluding lead glass) manufacturing processes.
PG 3/4 Lead glass manufacturing processes.
PG 3/5 Coal, coke and coal product processes.
PG 3/6 Processes for the polishing or etching of glass or glass products using hydrofluoric acid.
PG 3/7 Exfoliation of vermiculite and expansion of perlite.
PG 3/8 Quarrying processes including roadstone plants and the size reduction of bricks, tiles and concrete.

PG 3/9 Sand drying and cooling.
PG 3/10 China and ball clay.
PG 3/11 Spray drying of ceramic materials.
PG 3/12 Plaster processes.
PG 3/13 Asbestos products.
PG 3/14 Lime slaking processes.

Incinerators
PG 5/1 Clinical waste incinerators processing under 1 tonne/hr.
PG 5/2 Crematoria.
PG 5/3 Animal carcass incinerators processing under 1 tonne/hr.
PG 5/4 General waste incinerators processing under 1 tonne/hr.
PG 5/5 Sewage sludge incineration processes under 1 tonne/hr.

Other industries
PG 6/1 Animal by-product rendering.
PG 6/2 Manufacture of timber and wood-based products.
PG 6/3 Chemical treatment of timber and wood based products.
PG 6/4 Processes for the manufacture of particle-board and fibreboard.
PG 6/5 Maggot breeding processes.
PG 6/6 Fur breeding establishments.
PG 6/7 Printing and coating metal packaging.
PG 6/8 Textile and fabric coating and processing.
PG 6/9 Manufacture of coating processes.
PG 6/10 Coating manufacturing processes.
PG 6/11 Manufacture of printing ink.
PG 6/12 Production of natural sausage casings, tripe, chitterlings and other boiled green offal products.
PG 6/13 Coil coating processes.
PG 6/14 Film coating processes.
PG 6/15 Coating in drum manufacturing and re-conditioning processes.
PG 6/16 Printworks.
PG 6/17 Printing of flexible packages.
PG 6/18 Paper coating processes.
PG 6/19 Fish meal and fish meal processes.
PG 6/20 Paint applications in vehicle manufacture.
PG 6/21 Hide and skin processing.
PG 6/22 Leather finishing processes.
PG 6/23 Coating of metal and plastic.
PG 6/24 Pet food manufacturing processes.

PG 6/25 Vegetable oil extraction and fat and oil refining processes.
PG 6/26 Animal feed compounding processes.
PG 6/27 Vegetable matter drying processes.
PG 6/28 Rubber processes.
PG 6/29 Di-isocyanate processes.
PG 6/30 Production of compost for mushrooms.
PG 6/31 Powder coating processes, including sheradizing.
PG 6/32 Adhesive coating processes.
PG 6/33 Wood coating processes.
PG 6/34 Respraying of road vehicles.
PG 6/35 Metal and thermal spraying processes.
PG 6/36 Tobacco processing.
PG 6/37 Knackers yards.
PG 6/38 Blood processing.
PG 6/39 Animal by-product dealers.
PG 6/40 Coating and recoating of aircraft and aircraft components.
PG 6/41 Coating and recoating of rail vehicles.
PG 6/42 Bitumen and tar processes.

Authorizations can only be issued in response to an application made under section 6(2). An authorization must not be granted to an operator if the local authority considers that the applicant would not be able to operate the process in compliance with the conditions imposed under section 7. Authorizations should be granted to a named operator, but can be transferred to any other person, without prior approval. Section 9(2) requires the transferee to notify the local authority of the transfer within 21 days of it taking place. This is an anomaly which is difficult to understand; the initial application requires the operator to demonstrate not only that suitable plant is to be used, but also, where appropriate, that suitable personnel are available to control the process. A change of ownership implies other changes; it does not seem unreasonable to expect prior notification and to expect there to be some review of operations before a transfer of operator authorization is made. While legal action could be taken if authorization conditions were found to have been breached, it would allow for better control if the Act had accepted the concept of approval, not only being personal, but also the valid subject of scrutiny before transfer.

Section 7(2) requires the authorization to contain the following:

1. any conditions which the local authority considers appropriate in order to meet the objectives in section 7(1);
2. any conditions which the Secretary of State directs are to be included under his powers (section 6(5)); he may also direct that certain conditions are not to be included (section 7(7));
3. any other condition which the local authority considers appropriate.

The objectives of section 7(2) are set out below:

1. to use BATNEEC to prevent or minimize the release of substances prescribed for air in regulations made under section 2(5) of the Act and to render harmless releases of all substances, whether or not prescribed, which may be released into the air;
2. to comply with any directions the Secretary of State issues to local authorities for the purposes of implementing the EC Treaty or international law obligations which relate to environmental protection;
3. to comply with any limits or requirements and to achieve any quality standards or quality objectives which the Secretary of State has set down in regulations made under section 2 of the Clean Air Act 1968, section 2 of the Health and Safety at Work Act 1974, Parts II–IV of the Control of Pollution Act 1974, Part III of the Water Act 1989 (now the Water Resources Act 1991) and section 3 of the Environmental Protection Act 1990;
4. to comply with any relevant requirements in a plan made by the Secretary of State under section 3(5) of the Act.

Section 7(4) imposes two general conditions in all authorizations:

1. for preventing the release of substances prescribed for any environmental medium into that medium or, where that is not practicable by such means, for reducing the release of such substances to a minimum and for rendering harmless any such substances which are so released; and
2. for rendering harmless any other substances which might cause harm is released into any environmental medium.

These general conditions place the operators under an obligation to use BATNEEC to prevent or minimize pollution. In accordance with section 7(6) these conditions apply only to those parts of the process not regulated by specific conditions which have been included in the authorization. Section 25 places the onus on the operator to prove in court that there has been compliance with general conditions. For specific conditions, it is for the local authority to prove that there has not been compliance.

Section 7(8) allows conditions which limit the amount or composition of any substance produced by or utilized in the process, or which require advanced notice of proposed change in the operation of the process. General Guidance Note No. 2 [5] contains suggestions on the way in which conditions should be drafted, including some 70 examples.

No condition can be imposed if it is solely designed to protect the health and safety of people at work (section 7(1)). Section 28(1) prevents the imposition of conditions designed to impose the final disposal of waste to landfill. If there is a conflict of interest between requirements of registration or authorization under the Radioactive Substances Act 1993 and Part I of the Environmental Protection Act 1990, the former shall have precedence.

There is no prescribed form of the issue of authorizations. They should contain the following information:

1. details of the operator;
2. a description of the process;
3. specific conditions preferably grouped in a structured manner, e.g. emission limits and controls; monitoring, sampling and measurement of emissions; operational plant; details of chimneys, vents and process exhausts [6].

General Guidance Note No. 2 [5] also contains an example of the lay-out of an authorization.

Detailed conditions should achieve three objectives:

1. make plain to the operator the standards of control which must be met;
2. be more readily enforceable than the general conditions;
3. provide more comprehensive information to the public who may wish to consult the register.

Local authorities who wish to draft their own conditions must ensure that they satisfy four critical tests:

1. enforceability;
2. clarity for both industry and public;
3. relevance to air pollution control;
4. workability.

In order to achieve the necessary level of consistency it is important that the local authority gives the most careful consideration to the adequacy of the specimen conditions suggested by the Secretary of State. This is of particular importance if there are a number of operators carrying out similar activities within the district. Conditions can be varied, but consistency both within a local authority, and nationally is important.

APPLICATIONS AND REGISTRATIONS*

The Secretary of State has issued clear guidance on the way in which local authorities are to process applications and establish public registers [5]. As a general principle, applications should not be determined until the authority is satisfied that all necessary information has been considered. Paragraphs 1(3) and 1(4) of Schedule 1 to the Act enable additional information to be sought. Clearly, delays should not be deliberately caused by unnecessary requirements. There is advantage in informal discussions prior to the submission of an application so that the scope of its content may be agreed.

Information to be provided by the applicant is set out in the Environmental Protection (Applications, Appeals, and Registers) Regulations 1991. Regulation 2(4)(b) requires three copies of an application to be submitted. The application should contain:

1. details of the operator and the location of the process;
2. a description of the process and the proposed techniques to prevent or minimize emissions to air of prescribed substances and to render harmless emissions to air of all substances;

3. details of the source, nature and amount of current and/or anticipated air emissions from the process;
4. proposals for monitoring, sampling and measurement of air emissions;
5. assessment of the likely effect of emissions to air on the environment.

Applicants should ensure that information is included on the way in which the process will comply with the BATNEEC requirements of the Act (sections 7(2) and 7(4)). The General Guidance Note No. 3 [6] contains a proposed application form, but regulations do not require the use of prescribed forms.

It is clear that in order for an adequate appraisal to be made of proposals, the detail given by the applicant must be comprehensive. In appropriate cases, it will include details of the process, from receipt of raw materials to despatch of wastes and finished products; and calculations of chimney heights and the qualifications of operational staff. Drawings and plans of the plant should be provided together with diagrams of the process in complex cases.

There are circumstances where the applicant can be required to justify the proposals. Examples include:

1. where there are a number of alternative means of minimizing air pollution;
2. where the proposals differ from published process guidance notes;
3. where the process is in a sensitive area, e.g. a Site of Special Scientific Interest (SSSI);
4. where the process is to be located in an area which already suffers high levels of air pollution, particularly if approaching or exceeding air quality standards.

All applications must include the necessary fee† which is determined under section 8 of the Act. Terms are to be set out by circular.

Applications must be advertised, subject to certain exemptions, and placed on a public register.

Statutory consultees are prescribed in the regulations. The Health and Safety Executive must be

---

* These regulations are under review in order to improve application and appeal administration, public access to information on potentially polluting processes, the consultation requirements and HSE and authorities' requirements, DoE 1994.
† See the Local Enforcing Authorities Air Pollution Fees and Charges Scheme (England and Wales) Revision 1994.

agricultural activities, and leisure activities such Countryside Commission in Wales) must be consulted on applications which affect SSSIs, except oil burners less than 0.4 MW.

A timetable has been laid down for the processing of applications. In the case of waste oil burners less than 0.4 MW, this is 2 weeks (it will therefore be necessary for officers to be delegated power to approve in this, if not all, circumstances), and in other cases 4 months.*

Application (except small oil burners) must be advertised by the applicant for at least 1 week in one or more newspapers circulating in the locality. In the case of mobile plant, the locality would be the area of the principal place of business. The content of the advertisement is determined. It must include:

1. the name of the applicant;
2. the address of the premises where the process will be carried out or the principal place of business in the case of mobile plant;
3. a brief description of the process;
4. details of the place where the application can be considered (the local authority must determine the arrangements which it proposes to make prior to approach by an applicant);
5. a statement of the need for responses to be submitted to the local authority within 28 days of the first notice;
6. the date of the first notice;
7. the address to which submissions must be made.

The advertisement must not be placed until 2 weeks after submission of the application to the local authority to allow an initial check to be made and for a copy to be placed on the public register; this determines the priority that will have to be given to the processing of applications. Consideration should also be given to the establishment of a mechanism to advise ward councillors of applications at this time. Generally, the latest date for the placement of the advertisement is 2 months. Determination of matters of commercial confidentiality may delay matters. Failure to advertise would invalidate the application.

Consultees must be sent a copy of the application within a month of receipt. In order to ensure that their views are taken into account, they must respond within 28 days. Similarly, representations made by the public within 28 days of the appearance of the advertisement must be considered. There is no legal reason why submissions received after that period should not also be considered. These requirements necessitate the operation of effective procedures to ensure the timely dispatch of relevant information and the dating of submissions received. It is important to ensure that all submissions are considered and that there is evidence that that consideration has taken place; if the decision-making process is to be undertaken by members, they should be provided with either copies of full submissions or abstracts.

Confidential information

General guidance on the information which should be treated as commercially confidential is contained in General Guidance Note No. 1 [7]. The guiding principle is that, wherever possible, information should be freely available to the public. Section 22(3) of the Act allows operators to apply for certain information to be kept from the public register for reasons of commercial confidence. If an application is made under the above provision, the local authority has 14 days from receipt for determination. If no decision is made in that period of time, the information is treated as being confidential. The onus is therefore clearly with the authority to have clear mechanisms for the processing of such applications – delegation may be necessary; local authority procedures associated with the calling of committee meetings take time – within the 2 weeks available for consideration it will not be easy to fit in member participation on a formal basis. This does not mean that consultation should not take place.

If the authority does not support the view that information is of a commercially confidential nature, the operator is to be advised in writing. (There is no public right of appeal against decisions that information should be withheld.) In such cases, the existence of the application should not be advertised, nor may it be sent to the statutory consultees until 21 days after notifi-

---

* For processes transferred to LA authorization by the 1994 Amendment Regulations the specified period is 9 months.

cation. In these circumstances, the authority would be advised to consider the use of a postal service which records the dispatch and receipt. If the operator appeals within the 21 days, the application must not be advertised nor sent to other interested parties until the appeal has been determined. In such cases, the decision period will begin from the date that the appeal is determined.

Under section 22(7), the Secretary of State has power to direct that information is included on the register, but it is unclear how this provision will operate.

Exclusion of information from the register is time limited; it is regarded as losing its commercial confidentiality after a period of 4 years unless otherwise determined. It is for the operator to apply for its renewal of the status of confidentiality – when appropriate the local authority should time monitor registers and ensure that additional information is included as and when appropriate.

Provision exists (section 22(4) and (5)) for the local authority to include information in an authorization or notice which may be commercially confidential, but this is not likely to happen often. Operators are given similar opportunities to those outlined above to object to the inclusion of such information to be kept secret. This is a difficult concept to come to terms with; if the authority does not consider the information as sensitive it is unlikely that it would first consult with the operator. Clear advice on the relevant criteria may not emerge until precedents have been established. It is stressed that even where an authorization contains commercial information, it is relevant for enforcement purposes. In the event of proceedings being taken, it is presumed that some mechanism would be devised for the case being heard in a closed court.

Operators can also claim (under section 21), that information be excluded from the register because its publication 'would be contrary to the interests of national security'. It is difficult to imagine any process in part B which would fit such criteria.

Variation of Authorizations

Section 11 of the Act allows an operator to apply for a change in the conditions of operation. Such changes are made by variation notices (section 10). Information to be provided includes:

1. the name and address of premises or principal place of operation as before;
2. a description of the proposed change with all relevant details, e.g. changes in emissions, techniques, environmental consequences, monitoring, and compliance with section 7(2) objectives;
3. details of the variation required under section 11(3)b or 11(4)b;
4. details of the variation required under section 11(6) [7].

If applications for variation are of a substantial nature, they will be subject to the same procedures for advertising and consultations as set out above. There is no time limit on the period for the determination of variations which do not entail substantial change; the reason for this is to encourage a prompt response rather than suggest that the full consultation period be utilized.

Registers

Registers should include the following information, taking account of the issue of confidentiality:

1. a copy of the application and supplementary information provided under Schedule 1, paragraph 1(3) of the Act;
2. a copy of the authorization;
3. copies of any variation, enforcement, prohibition or revocation notices; copies of applications for variations under section 11(4)(b) and notices requiring compliance with variation orders under section 10(5);
4. an individual copy of any relevant directions issued by the Secretary of State;
5. copies of any notices of appeal made under section 15, and appeal decision letters issued by the Secretary of State together with the inspector's report;
6. monitoring information, whether obtained by the local authority or supplied to it in compliance with condition of authorization. Note

that unless there is a requirement for information to be kept on the register, it cannot be so used;

7. identification, where necessary, that monitoring data is being withheld on grounds of commercial confidentiality. It is appropriate, and necessary, to report whether relevant conditions within the authorization have been met in relation to monitoring.

Local authorities are required to keep all monitoring data on register for minimum of 4 years. They are similarly required to keep all of the details set out in (1) to (7) above for the same period, or until superseded, whichever is the longer.

Registers must be available for public inspection at all reasonable times, and facilities should be available for copies to be made of register entries. Access to the register is free, but a reasonable charge may be made for providing copies of information.

Section 20(2) of the Act requires the local authority to hold copies of entries for all processes controlled by HMIP which are located within the district of the authority. HMIP is responsible for sending details on a regular basis, it should be expected to achieve the same response times as the local authorities themselves.

Monitoring

Guidance on monitoring for processes prescribed for local authority air pollution control are contained in a joint IEHO/Warren Spring Laboratory publication in two volumes [8,9] obtainable through CIEH.

Implications

In order to satisfy the various requirements in relation to publication of information, decisions have to be made on where the register is to be kept, and how the material which it contains is to be arranged.

Certain information may be excluded from public access on the grounds of commercial secrecy. This arrangement is subject to review every 4 years. It would be prudent to build into forward planning a system which brings time-lapsed information onto the public record unless an application is made by the operator. It does not seem necessary for the operator to be reminded of the need to reassess opinion on confidentiality, the responsibility is clearly with the company.

Consideration should be given to the means by which information on the public register can best be interpreted. It seems quite reasonable for the local authority to provide supplementary information of the significance of particular pollutants and guidance, where available, on general environmental levels.

As society becomes more concerned about the state of the environment, and hungry for information, consideration should be given to the incorporation of monitoring data in computer-based form which could be given 'read-only' public access. This would require participation from education and/or library facilities, but it could be a worthwhile exercise in the fostering of understanding.

SMOKE EMISSIONS

In 1993 the previous legislation relating to clean air was consolidated in the Clean Air Act of that year. It updated measures contained in the 1956 and 1968 Clean Air Acts, part of the Control of Pollution Act 1974 and various other provisions.

It should be noted however that repeal of sections 4–13 of the 1993 Act, i.e. those provisions dealing with the approval of smoke control equipment for new furnaces, fitting of approved plant to arrest emissions of grit and dust from furnaces, limits upon the rates of such emissions and their measurement has been proposed.

The proposal for the repeal of those longstanding provisions was based upon the proposition that they were originally introduced to control smoke and sulphur dioxide emissions from coal burning whereas modern furnaces increasingly use cleaner fuels. Larger furnaces would still be controlled under the authorization of processes under the Environmental Protection Act (see above) and local authorities could still act under Part 3 of that Act (see Chapter 7) to prevent smaller furnaces causing nuisance.

If this repeal is agreed by Parliament, the remainder of this section still needs to be interpreted accordingly.

Clean air legislation currently imposes limits on the emission of smoke by prescribing limits for dark and black smoke, and establishing a procedure for smoke control based on defined geographical areas.

Smoke observations

Provisions of the 1993 Act are not proposed for repeal to restrict emissions of dark and black smoke. The method used for the assessment of the intensity of the shade of a smoke emission is simple: it is based on comparison with a shaded chart. The Ringelmann Chart is described by BS2742: 1969 [10]. It comprises a white card on to which are printed, in black, grids which proximate to shades of obscuration. The 20% shade is represented by a grid in which the ratio of printing ink to plain card is 1:4. Similarly the 40%, 60%, and 80% shades are represented by print to paper ratios of 2:3, 3:2 and 4:1. These relationships are approximate as they were based on the assumption that the printing ink was truly black and the paper truly white; neither material can meet this standard in practice. It is important to recognize the possiblity that the characteristics of the chart could be influenced by the fading of the ink or the discoloration of the paper, whether by soiling or tinting caused by protective film.

Clear guidance is given in the Standard on the way in which the chart should be used. The position from which the observation is made should be carefully chosen. The chart should be used in daylight conditions and held in a vertical plane facing the observer. Where possible, it should be in line with the point of emission and so placed that the chart and smoke have similar sky backgrounds. The chart must be at a sufficient distance from the observer that the lines appear to merge until each square is a uniform shade of

grey; for most observers this distance is in excess of 18 m.

Observations should be carried out, as far as practicable, under conditions of uniform illumination from the sky. If the sun is shining it should be at right angles to the line of vision, not in front or behind the observer. The white square provides a useful indication of illumination of the chart; it also enables soiling of the paper to be recognized. Observations at steep angles should be avoided. The darkness of the smoke, at the point where it leaves the chimney or bonfire, should be compared with the chart; the number of the shade which appears to most closely match the darkness of the smoke determined, and the duration of the emission measured. The darkness of smoke which is intermediate between two shades may be estimated to the nearest quarter Ringelmann number in favourable conditions. In order to use the chart, it seems necessary to use at least two people: one to support it and the other to make the observation. This has resource implications.

A miniature chart has been produced (BS2742: 1969) [10] to the same precision as the Ringelmann chart. Hatching has been replaced by shades of grey colour, similar to those used on paint colour charts. It is designed to be used about 1.5 metres from the observer's eye; conditions for observation are as previously described. As the chart is printed on slightly translucent card, it should be backed with a sheet of white opaque material or inserted in a holder.

Dark smoke is defined in section 3 of the 1993 Act, as smoke which, 'if compared in the appropriate manner with a chart of the type known at the date of the passing of the Act as the Ringelmann Chart, would appear to be as dark as or darker than shade 2 on that chart'. Black smoke is defined in the Dark Smoke (Permitted Period) Regulations 1958 (SI 1958 No. 498) as smoke which, 'if compared . . . with . . . the Ringelmann Chart, would appear to be as dark as or darker than shade 4 on the chart'.

Section 3(2) of the Clean Air Act 1993 continues, 'for the avoidance of doubt it is hereby declared that . . . the court may be satisfied that smoke is or is not dark . . . notwithstanding that there has been no actual comparison with a

Ringelmann Chart'. This does not seem to suggest that any officer can stand up in court testifying the intensity of a smoke emission without having carried out the necessary comparison; some familiarity with the procedure is necessary.

There was a time when day-to-day opportunities to make smoke observations would be an adequate foundation for experience. Arguably, this is no longer the case. The duty would seem to rest with the local authority to find opportunities to enable its staff to view smoke emissions under controlled conditions and make assessments which could be compared between the various members of the group, at that time. By use of either the full-size chart or the miniature version, it should be possible to rapidly acquire a visual memory of the levels of obscuration which could be relied upon for future action.

It is possible to check individual performance in group tests; a regular practice of enforcement agencies in the USA. Obviously, there is no absolute right measurement – assessment is by comparison; but no individual who is to be used as an expert witness could differ by more than one shade when group assessments were being carried out. Perhaps the most difficult component of this concept of qualitative assessment would be the identification of a chimney which smoked with such consistent reliability that it could become the target of programmed staff training.

Emissions of dark or black smoke from chimneys

Section 1 of the Clean Act 1993 (not proposed for repeal) prohibits, subject to conditions, emissions of dark and black smoke from chimneys serving boilers and industrial plant. Details of the restrictions are determined by the Dark Smoke (Permitted Period) Regulations 1958 (SI 1958 No. 498). Two separate circumstances are considered: continuous and intermittent emissions. The limit for a continuous emission of dark smoke, caused otherwise than soot-blowing, is 4 minutes.

The determination of intermittent emissions is limited to aggregate emissions for a period of up to 8 hours. In the case of one chimney, emissions of dark smoke shall not exceed 10 minutes in the aggregate period of 8 hours or, if soot-blowing is carried out, for not longer than 14 minutes in aggregate in that period. The periods of 10 and 14 minutes shall increase in the case of a chimney serving two furnaces to 18 and 25 minutes respectively; in the case of a chimney serving three furnaces 24 and 34 minutes respectively; and in the case of a chimney serving four or more furnaces 29 and 41 minutes respectively. The maximum aggregate emission of black smoke is 2 minutes in any period of 30 minutes. Aggregate emissions are considered by carrying out an observation over a period of time and accumulating incremental emissions.

In any proceedings taken under this legislation, account must be taken of the statutory defences contained in section 1. They are as follows:

1. that the contravention complained of was solely due to the lighting up of a furnace which was cold, and that all practicable steps had been taken to prevent or minimize the emission of dark smoke; or

2. that the contravention complained of was solely due to some failure of a furnace or the apparatus used in connection with a furnace, that that failure could not have been foreseen, or, if foreseen, could not have been provided against, and that the contravention could not reasonably have been prevented by action taken after the failure occurred; or

3. that the contravention complained of was solely due to the use of unsuitable fuel, that suitable fuel was unobtainable, that the least unsuitable fuel which was available was used, and that all practicable steps had been taken to prevent or minimize the emission of dark smoke as the result of the use thereof; or

4. that the contravention complained of was due to a combination of two or more of the causes specified in paragraphs (1) to (3) above and that the other conditions specified in those paragraphs are satisfied in relation to those causes respectively.

When considering the defences it is important to bear in mind the date of the primary legislation. In the mid-1950s coal was the most widely used industrial fuel, hence the allowance made for furnaces being lit from cold, the emphasis on the availability of suitable fuel and the generous periods allowed for emission. If the 1958 Regulations had been updated, it would have been reasonable to have imposed more stringent standards which reflected contemporary combustion technology.

When an emission of dark smoke is observed, it is necessary to advise the owner of the boiler in plant 'as soon as may be', and confirm the fact, in writing, before the end of 4 days of becoming aware of the offence in accordance with section 51 of the 1993 Act.

While procedures for notification are not prescribed, it is apparent that certain information must be obtained at the earliest opportunity after the alleged offence has been observed. Immediate examination of the plant is vital in order that comprehensive evidence can be gathered of the likely cause of the emission, and the possible relevance of the statutory exemption. It is for individual local authorities to determine the way in which investigations should be carried out, and to balance the competing pressures between requiring the investigation officer to seek immediate contact with senior management, a time consuming exercise in a large organization, and the immediate visit to the boiler-house or furnace.

Familiarity with plant and the fundamental principles of combustion technology are important. It seems reasonable to begin an investigation by identifying the particular boiler or furnace which was causing the emission. Details should be recorded of the description of the plant and the fuel used to fire it. An attempt has to be made to gather concise information of the operating cycle, the nature of the fuel and the condition of the fuel and combustion air supplies. Not only is it important to take into account information on the possibility of there having been a break down, but also on the immediate and longer term steps taken to mitigate the problem. What is the general state of maintenance? Does there appear to be a planned programme of maintenance, or does it seem that mechanical and electrical engineering works are only undertaken when absolutely necessary? These factors are important in determining the relevance of defences. While information can be considered during the preliminary stages of an investigation, in an informal manner, it is necessary to issue a caution when it has been decided that there has been an offence, and to limit the use of statements to information obtained after the caution was given. Evidence must be based on contemporaneous notes.

Provisions, similar to those related to industrial boilers and furnaces, restrict emissions from vessels, provided that they are in waters as defined by section 44 of the Clean Air Act 1993. Details are beyond the scope of this chapter, but are to be found in the Dark Smoke (Permitted Periods) (Vessels) Regulations 1958 (SI 1958 No. 878).

New plant

Section 4 of the 1993 Act requires all new furnaces (other than domestic boilers rated at less than 16 kW) to be, so far as practicable, capable of operating continuously without emitting smoke when burning the fuel for which they were designed. (This is proposed for repeal – see note on page 699.)

'Furnace' is nowhere defined in the Act, but can be interpreted as any enclosed or partially enclosed space in which solid, liquid or gaseous fuel is burned, or in which heat is produced.

Section 4 also requires that the local authority be advised of proposals to install new furnaces, other than domestic boilers. If requested, the local authority can be required to consider whether the unit is capable of substantially smokeless combustion; there are few circumstances when an application cannot be approved. Unless the officer has delegated authority, the decision has to be made by the authority.

Investigation and research

Section 45 of the 1993 Act enables the local authority to give whole or partial exemption from provision of the Act. If an application is made but not determined to the satisfaction of the applicant, appeal may be made to the Secretary of State for the Environment.

Industrial bonfires

Section 2 of the Clean Air Act 1993 (not proposed for repeal) prohibits emissions of dark smoke from trade or industrial premises. Subject to specific exemptions for prescribed matter, the prohibition is absolute: no permitted periods are provided. 'Industrial or trade premises' are defined, in subsection (6) as 'premises used for any industrial or trade purpose or premises not so used on which matter is burnt in connection with any trade or industrial process'. This legislation is used to control smoke emissions from 'bonfires', including those on demolition sites.

Materials conditionally exempt from the provisions of this legislation are detailed in the Clean Air (Emission of Dark Smoke) (Exemption) Regulations 1969 (SI 1969 No.1263) as follows:

1. Timber and any other waste matter (other than natural or synthetic rubber or flock or feathers) which results from the demolition of a building or clearance of a site in connection with any building operation or work of engineering construction (within the meaning of section 176 of the Factories Act 1961). (Conditions A, B and C.)
2. Explosive (within the meaning of the Explosives Act 1875) which has become waste; and matter which has become contaminated by such explosive. (Conditions A and C.)
3. Matter which is burnt in connection with:
   (a) research into the cause or control of fire; or
   (b) training in fire fighting.
4. Tar, pitch, asphalt and other matter which is burnt in connection with the preparation and laying of any surface, or which is burnt off any surface in connection with resurfacing, together with any fuel used for any such purpose. (Condition C.)
5. Carcases of animals or poultry which:
   (a) have died, or are reasonably believed to have died, because of disease;
   (b) have been slaughtered because of disease: or
   (c) have been required to be slaughtered pursuant to the Diseases of Animals Act 1981. (Conditions A and C, unless the burning is carried out by or on behalf or an

inspector (within the meaning of the Diseases of Animals Act 1981)).
6. Containers which are contaminated by any pesticide or by any toxic substance used for veterinary or agricultural purposes; and in this paragraph 'container' includes any sack, box, package or receptacle of any kind. (Conditions A, B and C.)

The three conditions are as follows:

1. Condition A: that there is no other reasonably safe and practicable method of disposing of the matter.
2. Condition B: that the burning is carried out in such a manner as to minimize the emission of dark smoke.
3. Condition C: that the burning is carried out under the direct and continuous supervision of the occupier of the premises concerned or a person authorized to act on his or her behalf.

As in the case of emission of smoke from chimneys, it is necessary to investigate the circumstances of the emission immediately after completing the investigation so as to be able to test the relevance of the exemptions.

Several issues arise from the exemptions which are worthy of brief consideration. There is growing concern about the way in which material is squandered; while it may be permissable to burn waste from building and demolition operations, more thought needs to go into finding methods of reusing such materials. While the legislation permits the burning of contaminated containers, it does not authorize smoke emissions associated with the burning of pesticides or similar hazardous substances. The disposal of such material should be carried out in an environmentally responsible manner and in accordance with the COSHH requirements (see Chapter 28). Exemptions are not available for emissions of dark smoke produced for effect purposes associated with film making or other 'entertainment' activities.

Smoke nuisances

Details of procedures which enable action to be taken in respect of statutory nuisances from smoke, etc. are contained in Part III of the Environmental Protection Act 1990 (see Chapter 7).

Smoke control areas

Sections 18–22 of the 1993 Act lay down the procedures under which local authorities may establish and enforce the provisions of smoke control orders. The concept of smoke control is to prohibit the emission of smoke from domestic and industrial chimneys. The measure was introduced to remedy serious problems largely associated with the domestic combustion of coal. It has had a profoundly beneficial effect on air quality throughout the country, although it is arguable that similar improvements may have taken place in response to other social pressures, such as the widespread switch to gas-fired domestic heaters and boilers. It was never envisaged that the entire nation would be covered by smoke control orders – almost all of the areas where poor air quality has been reported have been made the subject of orders; where they have not, the procedure to introduce them is largely under way. For this reason, a detailed description of the steps to be taken to introduce an order is not provided here.

Owners or occupiers of private dwellings within a smoke control area may recover seven-tenths of the 'reasonable costs' of conversion of all fireplaces normally used to burn coal. Guidance of 'reasonable costs' is published in circulars by the Department of the Environment. Discretionary powers exist to enable the payment of additional monies, up to the full 'reasonable costs' and to assist charities and other religious buildings. Originally, the local authority recovered a portion of its expenditure directly from the treasury; now the government contribution is included within the Housing Investment Programme (HIP) allocation. Financial contributions have never been available to industrial or commercial premises to enable them to meet the terms of an order.

Subsection (2) of section 20 of the 1956 Act states, subject to exemption and limitation 'if, on any day, smoke is emitted from a chimney of any building within a smoke control area, the occupier of the building shall be guilty of an offence'.

At any time that an order is made, certain buildings or classes of fireplaces may be exempt from the terms of the order, but the local authority has no power to exempt other buildings, at a later date, unless a new order is made. The effect of this is of particular significance to industrial and commercial plant. Coal, oil, and wood cannot be burnt unless on an exempt fireplace – exempt fireplaces consist of either generic plant, such as 'any fireplace specifically designed or adapted for the combustion of liquid fuel', or an appliance named in one of the Exempted Fireplaces Orders, made by regulation, under section 21 of the Act.

The use of statutory instruments to define appliances is a clumsy and inappropriate approach; although the only option allowed by the Act – each statutory instrument defines not just the appliance but the manner in which it is operated – it follows that compliance with the manufacturer's instructions is necessary, but that the relevant instructions are those produced at the time of the passing of the statute. This does not allow documentation to keep up to date with technical progress.

Few incinerators have been the subject of statutory exemption; it is unlikely that incineration plant currently in use in premises is the subject of specific exemption unless the order was recently made, or is vague in its wording. It follows that almost all incinerators within a smoke control area must meet the 'no smoke' standard.

Although smoke control deliberately sought to prohibit the combustion of coal on open domestic fires, it can still be used on a small number of 'exempt fireplaces'. Use of other solid fuel was encouraged, with a recognition that smokeless combustion could not always be achieved. For administrative simplicity 'smokeless fuel' can be used, regardless of any possible emission, provided that it is specifically identified, by regulation, as an authorized fuel. The lists of exempted fireplaces and authorized fuels continue to grow – for this reason details must be obtained from an examination of current legislation.

If a chimney is observed emitting smoke, notification must be made within 4 days as previously described. Investigation should be undertaken to make sure that the appliance does not enjoy the benefit of an exemption or that the fuel use has not been authorized.

Both acquisition and delivery of fuel, other than authorized fuel, in a smoke control area is illegal under section 27 of the Clean Air Act 1993 – this does nothing to stop the retail sale of coal and other unauthorized fuels – a significant loophole in the legislation.

GRIT AND DUST EMISSIONS

The need to control grit and dust emissions from combustion plant has long been recognized. Whilst the authorization procedure under the EPA 1990 brought such process plants under control, most boilers are still subject to the controls of the Clean Air Act 1993. However these are proposed for repeal – see note on page 699.

Definitions

Grit is defined by the Clean Air (Emission of Grit and Dust from Furnaces) Regulations 1971 as particles exceeding 76 μm in diameter, dust by BS3405: 1983 [8] as particulates between 1 and 75 μm in diameter, and fume by the Clean Air Act 1956, section 13, as air-borne solid matter smaller than dust.

Control (proposed for repeal)

Section 6 of the Clean Air Act 1993 requires that new furnaces are provided with plant for the arresting of grit and dust which has been approved by the local authority. The plant to which this provision applies is as follows:

1. furnaces which burn pulverized fuel; or
2. furnaces which burn solid matter at a rate of more than 45.4 kg an hour; or
3. furnaces which burn liquid or gaseous fuel at a rate equivalent to 366.4 kilowatts or more.

Section 5 provides for regulations to be made limiting emission of grit and dust from furnaces. The only regulations so far enacted are the Clean Air (Emission of Grit and Dust from Furnaces) Regulations 1971 which apply to:

1. boilers;
2. indirect heating appliances (in which combustion products are not in contact with the material being heated);
3. furnaces in which the combustion gases are in contact with the material being heated but the material does not contribute to grit and dust emissions.

The Regulations lay down the permitted limits based on heat output and heat input depending on the type of furnace under consideration.

Section 7 allows certain exemptions to the general requirements. The minister can make regulations, and has made the Clean Air (Arrestment Plant) (Exemption) Regulations 1969 (SI 1969 No. 1262). They must be referred to for definitive information; in general they exclude mobile plant, temporary sources of heat and power, and a range of mechanically fired furnaces which burn less than 1 ton an hour, with the exception of incinerators. The local authority is empowered, on application, to exempt specific furnaces if it is satisfied that the emission will not be prejudicial to health or a nuisance.

Measurement of grit and dust

Section 10 provides for the measurement of grit and dust. The provision is restricted to those classes of plant referred to in section 3 of the 1968 Act as referred to above. If the local authority is satisfied that there are grounds for concern, it may serve a notice requiring measurements to be made. If the plant burns less than 1 ton an hour (other than pulverized fuel), or less than 8.2 MW liquid or gaseous fuel, the operator can, and probably will, serve a counter notice requiring the authority to carry out the tests at its own expense, and to repeat the measurements 'from time to time' until the counter notice is withdrawn. This is a curious concept in the light of policy broadly accepting that the 'polluter must pay'. Section 12 enables a notice to be served requiring information on fuel or waste burned on furnaces in relation to this provision.

Procedural details are contained in the Clean Air (Measurement of Grit and Dust from Furnaces) Regulations 1971 (SI 1971 No. 162). The

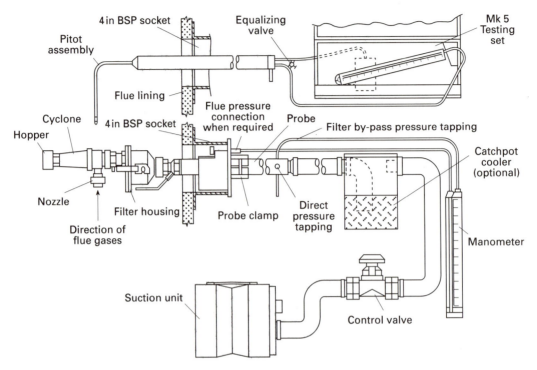

Fig. 41.1 Schematic arrangement of BCURA sampling train. (Source: IEHO/Warren Springs Laboratory (1993) *Emission Monitoring*, Vol.2, IEHO, London.) Reproduced by kind permission of the IEHO.)

local authority must give at least 6 weeks' notice requiring adaptations to be made to the chimney and the provision of necessary equipment to enable measurements to be made, in accordance with the method described in BS3405: 1983 [1]. Once the stack has been adapted the local authority may require, giving at least 28 days' notice, tests to be carried out in accordance with the method set out in *Measurement of Solids in Flue Gases* [12].

Before making the measurements, the operator of the plant must give the local authority at least 48 hours' notice of the date and time of the commencement of the tests. The local authority may be present while testing is taking place. Results must be sent to the local authority within 14 days in a report which includes the following information:

1. the date of test(s);
2. the number of furnaces discharging into the stack at that time;

3. the results of the measurements.

Further tests may be required to be made if the local authority is of the opinion that true emission levels cannot otherwise be determined, but not at intervals of less than 3 months.

Even if the plant is of sufficiently limited capacity for the operator to serve a counter notice on the local authority, it is still necessary for scaffolding and services to be provided at the expense of the operator. Measurements must be made by the authority, or by consultants acting on its behalf. Details of the method of measurement are summarized below.

Apparatus used in the measurement of grit and dust emissions.

The most widely used apparatus is the BCURA cyclone probe described in Emission Monitoring Guidance Manual [8]. Fig. 41.1 shows the schematic arrangement of the BCURA Sampling Train.

The method of operation is relatively simple. A sample of the flue gases is drawn through the sample nozzle, which faces upstream in the flue. Grit and dust particles are removed by centripetal action and driven into a detachable hopper. This has a cut-off rate of about 5–10μm, particulates below this size can be collected on a filter section packed with silica wool. The pump is protected against excess heat by the insertion of a water catch-pot between it and the gas stream, if the sampling temperature is likely to exceed 100°C.

The apparatus was originally designed to measure emissions from coal-fired boilers, cement works, etc., where a significant particulate burden could be anticipated. It has been used to monitor oil-fired boilers, but a sampling period of 2 to 3 hours may be necessary to collect 0.5 to 1.0 g of solids.

As this is a gravimetric method, accurate balances are required to determine small differences in the weight of the collecting hoppers, and the filter before and after sampling. Often sampling is required to be carried out at heights of over 20 m above the ground. Although a safe means of access has to be provided by the operator of the plant, there are clearly identifiable difficulties in the operation of this sampling procedure. The equipment is heavy; the environment in which sampling takes place may be hostile; and speed is essential – weight gain due to moisture absorption must be avoided.

Before sampling begins it is important to ensure the suitability of the sampling points by reference to BS3405: 1983. Flue gas velocity is determined by making a number of measurements of gas pressure in the system using a pitot tube and a manometer. The location of the points in the stack is dependent on the internal diameter of the flue; this should be measured by probe as drawings may be inaccurate. Gas has to be collected by the sampling head in isokinetic conditions; the gas velocity at the nozzle must equal the velocity of the surrounding gas stream. (Sample at too fast a flow rate and the sample will contain excess fine material; too slow and the smaller particles will escape capture.) Essentially, the correct sample velocity is achieved by the use of a suitably sized nozzle and regulation of the rate of flow through the pump, using the valve. As sampling continues, the valve may need to be adjusted to allow for the increased pressure drop across the system, caused by the clogging of the filter.

Sampling periods are largely determined by experience. A significant mass of dust, at least 0.5 g, has to be collected. This could take between 5 minutes to 3 hours. Ideally, sampling should be carried out during steady state conditions of operation, but this is difficult to achieve in many types of plant. Given good conditions and experienced staff, the method is only accurate to ±25%.

CHIMNEY HEIGHT (proposed for repeal – see note on page 699)

Control of chimney height for all significant combustion plant under local authority control is contained in provisions of section 14 of the 1993 Act. It applies to boilers and plant which:

1. burns pulverized fuel; or
2. burns solid matter at a rate of 45.5 kg/hour; or
3. burns liquid or gaseous matter at a rate of 366.4 kilowatts.

may not be used unless the height of the chimney has been approved by the local authority. Details of the proposals are to be sent to the local authority and must be adequate to allow the necessary calculations to be carried out. The local authority has 28 days in which to determine the application. If it is anticipated that it will take a longer period, there must be agreement between the two parties. Failure to determine the application, and to convey the decision in writing to the applicant within 28 days, will allow approval to be assumed on the basis of the application, without conditions; it is important that the procedure associated with the processing of applications be well managed and that regard be taken of the resolutions of the authority in relation to delegated power of officers.

A chimney height shall not be approved unless the local authority is satisfied that it is sufficient to prevent, so far as is practicable, the smoke, grit, dust, gases or fumes becoming prejudicial to health or a nuisance having regard to:

1. the purpose of the chimney;
2. the position and description of buildings near it;
3. the levels of the neighbouring ground;
4. any other matters requiring consideration in the circumstances.

A simple method for the calculation of chimney heights is provided in *Chimney Heights, Third Edition of the 1956 Clean Air Act Memorandum* [13]. Its relevance is limited to chimneys serving plant with a gross heat input of between 0.15 MW to 150 MW, including stationary diesel generators. It does not deal with direct fired heating systems which discharge into the space being heated, gas turbines or incinerators (which require separate treatment depending on the pollutants to be emitted).

The method first provides an uncorrected chimney height based on gross thermal input, in the case of low sulphur fuels, or sulphur dioxide emission, in other cases. Adjustment is made based on the district in which the development is taking place, and the need to increase the height to correct for effects of surrounding buildings. The method must be treated with some caution. The Memorandum made it clear that there will cases in which local knowledge and experience suggests that the results obtained for the calculations should be varied.

Although the intermediate stages of the calculation should be performed with a reasonable degree of accuracy, the final result should be rounded to the nearest metre. In circumstances where the Memorandum will not provide adequate guidance, e.g. where a chimney discharges through a roof with complicated structures, or in difficult topography, specialist advice should be sought.

Discharge for Fan Diluted Systems

The 3rd edition Memorandum, referred to above, also gives guidance on the location of outlets for fan-diluted emissions. Discharges at the uncorrected chimney height (U), are acceptable, even if below the roof level of the building, subject to conditions:

1. the emission velocity must be at least 75/F m/s, where 'F' is a the fan dilution factor. F = V/Vo, where V is the actual volume of flue gas and Vo is the stoichiometric combustion volume. For natural gas Vo is $0.26 \ Q \ M^3$/s.
2. The outlet must not be within 50 U/F of a fan assisted inlet (except for intakes of combustion air).
3. The outlet must not be within 20 U/F of an openable window on the emitting building.
4. The distance to the nearest building must be at least 60 U/F.
5. The lower edges of all outlets must be at least 3 m above ground level, with the exception of inputs of less than 1 MW where 2 m is permissible.
6. The outlets must be directed at an angle above the horizontal – preferably 30 – and must not be under a canopy.
7. Flue gas should not be emitted into an enclosed, or almost totally enclosed, well or courtyard.

Under certain circumstances, defined in the Clean Air (Heights of Chimneys) (Exemption) Regulations 1969 (SI 1969 No. 411), it is not necessary to apply for approval for a chimney. The provisions largely relate to the use of temporary plant.

If a building is erected which over-reaches the chimney of an adjoining building, there is provision for the height of the chimney to be raised within section 73 of the Building Act 1984. Part J of the Building Regulations 1985 provides for the design of flues for smaller capacity plant, not covered by the chimney height memorandum. Heating appliances are divided into two categories:

1. solid fuel and oil-burning appliances with a rated output of up to 45 kW; and
2. gas-burning appliances with a rated capacity of up to 60 kW.

Approved document J indicates that such installations will meet the required regulations if so installed as to:

1. receive sufficient air for proper combustion of the fuel and operation of the flue;
2. be capable of normal operation without the products of combustion becoming a hazard;
3. be capable of normal operation without causing damage by heat or fire to the fabric of the building.

ENVIRONMENTAL MONITORING

Local authorities are to be given a statutory duty to monitor air quality and establish air quality action areas when needed. They will also be required to establish Air Quality Management Areas to tackle poor air quality. The proposals are contained in a DoE paper: 'Air Quality: Meeting the Challenge' [14].

This would require consultation with other local interests, and with the Environmental Agency. If a problem extended beyond the boundaries of a single authority, a broader strategy would be necessary. Unless local authorities demonstrate their ability to co-ordinate actions there is a strong likelihood that Central Government will take on the responsibility.

Air pollution monitoring must be undertaken, in a structured manner, to determine the levels of particular contaminants, and to allow comparisons to be made between data, on a temporal and spatial basis. Correct technique is important to enable causal relationships to be investigated between levels of specified pollutants and effects under investigation. A study may be simple or complex depending on the nature of the substances under investigation and the possible effects. Some cause and effect relationships are well understood e.g. the damage of vegetation by oxidant gases or the soiling caused by particulates. Others are not yet fully researched, e.g. the exact relationship between sulphur dioxide and particulate levels and ill health is yet to be determined.

Surveys can be designed to establish 'background levels', where measurements are made remote from individual sources, and hot-spot monitoring where the purpose is to find out information on the levels around defined sources. A number of networks are currently in operation, designed to provide different types of information.

The largest and best known is the **smoke and sulphur dioxide** monitoring, which is considered in detail below. The individual sites provide information which is relevant to policy making, but can hardly be regarded as having a role in immediate health protection because of the time which is taken to produce results.

The method is supposed to measure suspended particulates and sulphur dioxide – it does neither of these things. Levels are inferred by the use of reasonable approximations on the basis that the technology is both robust and inexpensive to operate.

A known volume of air is passed through a filter to remove particulate matter, then through a solution of hydrogen peroxide to absorb sulphur dioxide. Certainly, the filter removes particulates, but although results are expressed gravimetrically, they are based on an estimate of the mass of material collected assessed by the darkness of the stain on the filter. Light reflectance is not, necessarily, associated with mass; it correlates to particle size and colour. The assumption that urban air particulates are of a uniform nature throughout the country is not wholly sustainable – gravimetric techniques are expensive to operate and subject to their own operational difficulties. There is justification in the current method so long as its limitations are recognized. (It must be borne in mind that capture of a significant amount of white dust would not be revealed by the reflectometer.) Sulphur dioxide is not measured; the liquid in the bubbler will react with any gas – acid or alkaline; carbonic acid produced by dissolving carbon dioxide may not be important, but results can be significantly influenced by emissions of ammonia, whether of biological or chemical origin.

While detailed consideration of the weaknesses of the volumetric instrument as described in BS1747: 1969 (Parts 2 and 3) [15] is not of direct relevance to this text, it is a useful demonstration of the difference between the perception of what is being measured and what is represented as being measured.

Although the method has a number of weaknesses, it can be demonstrated to have provided a reasonable representation of pollution throughout the country at a critical time in policy development.

In recent years, concern has switched to the need for information on levels of **oxides of nitrogen and ozone**. The Royal Commission on Environmental Pollution [16] highlighted the paucity of information on this subject in their tenth report. A network has now been established which collects information from some 17 sites throughout the country. In addition to oxides of nitrogen and ozone, measurement is made of sulphur dioxide and PM_{10}s. Instrumentation is fully automatic, transmitting results by telephone lines to enable instant collation. Calibration is carried out automatically on a daily basis to monitor the quality of performance. In addition to the long-term output from this instrumentation, the information is available for use on a daily basis to supplement weather forecasts with reports on air quality. A similar network has been established as part of the research programme into acid deposition. It is likely that this network will be extended to 36 sites.

Three EU Directives on air quality exist; *nitrogen dioxide* (85/203/EEC), *smoke* (80/779/EEC) and *sulphur dioxide and lead* (82/884/EEC). There are discussions in progress in relation to benzene.

Attention is now being turned on emission control as a means of reducing levels of pollution to the atmosphere. In this context, a range of controls are being implemented which relate to stationary plant and vehicle emissions.

There is particular concern about oxides of nitrogen and hydrocarbons. The use of diffusion tubes to determine oxides of nitrogen has been widely established. Hydrocarbons are a precursor, with oxides of nitrogen, for the production of acid rain. A limited network, which will measure volatile organic compounds, in the range C2–C6, is in the process of being established. It is envisaged that future monitoring will focus on the following substances: sulphur dioxide, nitrogen dioxide, particulates, polycyclic aromatic hydrocarbons, lead, benzene, ozone, 1-3-butadiene and carbon monoxide.

The proper design and implementation of environmental surveys is important if adequate use is to be made of the findings. Some understanding of analytical techniques is necessary, as is the confidence limits of the technique being used but of fundamental importance are the basic principles of planning and operation.

In selecting the most appropriate way to conduct an investigation, the following factors must be taken into account:

1. the purpose of the exercise;
2. the methodology;
3. the siting of equipment;
4. timing and period of measurement;
5. interpretation of results.

Purpose of the survey

Surveys may be carried out for a number of reasons: to assist in the investigation of a complaint; to relate pollution levels to ill health; to associate emissions with sources; to make comparisons between data sets; to assist with modelling; or to determine priorities.

Complaints range from general to specific. In some cases, such as the deposition of acid smuts, the mechanism causing the phenomenon is understood; the survey will be designed to allow the identification of the source. On other occasions, particularly associated with damage to plants or ill-health, the nature of the mechanism causing the damage may have to be determined before the monitoring can begin.

The effect of air pollution on human health is normally insidious; it rarely causes acute illness. In extreme cases, there may be an association with local and significant emissions of toxic substances or prolonged exposure to high levels of pollution which should be obvious. The use of air monitoring in the UK has been mainly directed towards the collection of information for eventual analysis. In other countries, notably the USA and Japan, monitoring has been used to give advance warning of possible health hazards and, in extreme circumstances, to order the shut-down of industry or the management of road traffic. Results of the Extended UK Network are beginning to be applied in a similar manner.

The difficulty in determining the relationship between emissions and sources should not be underestimated. In all but the simplest case, local meteorology must be taken into account. Gases do not follow uniform patterns of movement; local turbulence causes considerable displacement and will produce significant variations in ground level concentrations, assuming constant emission rate, if measurements are made in real time. A further difficulty is the association of the determinant with the source – often there are several potential sources of emission of a single substance within close proximity of an area of interest. Difficulties will remain in identifying the contribution which a smelter may make to ground level concentrations of lead, while petrol engine exhaust continues to be a significant source of emission. Analysis which not only identifies elements but provides details on the compounds is sometimes possible, but is extremely expensive.

Consideration of the results of a survey necessitates the examination of the findings in the widest context. Measurement can be made at a single site over sufficient periods to allow trends to be studied. Comparisons may be diurnal or seasonal. Comparisons can also be made between the area under study and other locations, provided similar methods of measurement have been adopted.

In the past, air pollution was measured in circumstances where levels of pollution were unsatisfactory in order that improvements could be recorded. The number of stations which report to the national survey have been much reduced as the effects of smoke control programmes and the reduction in the use of coal have been recognized. It is important that trends continue to be monitored at a representative range of urban sites, in addition to those areas which are near the limits imposed by air-quality criteria, to ensure the comprehensive nature of national environmental monitoring.

Monitoring provides the foundations for modelling techniques, and subsequently allows the validation of models. Currently, limited use appears to be made of modelling in the determination of emission control limits, but it is likely that this attitude will change as attention is given to the imposition of overall emission limits within specified areas.

Information on pollution levels allows the most effective use to be made of resources. At national, regional and local levels, it is important to take account of existing levels and trends, and use the results to plan further strategies based on sound assessment of priorities.

Methodology

The selection of survey equipment may be determined by the nature of the investigation. The following points should be considered:

1. the nature of the pollutant, solid, liquid or gaseous: will it settle under normal atmospheric conditions or remain in suspension?;
2. the need to identify the source of emission;
3. the instrumentation available;
4. the resources available.

In considering the method, consideration should be given to all reasonable alternatives. This information should be included in any report of the findings. At this stage, the protocol of the survey should be agreed for subsequent reference.

Choice of instruments

SIMPLE COLLECTORS OF DEPOSITED MATTER. Particulate matter can be collected by a variety of receptors allowing crude comparisons to be made between the mass collected at different sites under similar conditions. The following collectors are in general use:

1. adhesive plastic sheets mounted horizontally or vertically;
2. greased glass plates;
3. petri-dishes;
4. other receptacles, such as plastic washing-up bowls.

Physical examination of the material may provide information on the source. It is possible to develop considerable expertise if particles are examined under an optical microscope, particularly if it is possible to use polarized light. Multi-volume catalogues of photographs of magnified particles are available which can be used for comparison. Alternatively, particles could be collected from various local emitters to build up a library of reference material. This is a time consuming exercise which is only likely to be appropriate in a limited number of cases.

DEPOSIT GAUGES. Various deposit guages have been developed to carry out long-term assessment of deposited matter. They are of limited value as collectors, and in all cases collect precipitation, which may influence the nature of the deposited matter. Their main contribution is for the examination of long-term trends. The following are in general use:

1. the British Standard deposit gauge (BS1747: 1969, Part 1) [15];
2. the ISO deposit gauge;
3. the CERL directional deposit gauge consists of four vertical pipes mounted on a frame. Each pipe has a rectangular opening cut into its wall. The upper end of each pipe is closed whilst the lower discharges into a receptacle. The stand is so arranged that openings face to the cardinal points or towards, away and at right angles to a suspect source;
4. frisbees.

SIMPLE SMOKE/SULPHUR DIOXIDE ASSESSMENT. The following instruments are used for this purpose:

1. The daily volumetric instrument (BS1747: 1969, Parts 2 and 3) comprises one filter and one Dreschell bottle. It requires daily servicing.
2. The eight port volumetric instrument is a set of eight filters and eight Dreschell bottles. Gas is directed to one sample set by the use of an automatic valve. The equipment can operate for a week without attention. Gas volumes are metered weekly and averaged for daily results.

3. The sequential particulate sampler is a single filter through which passes a paper strip which can be advanced on a regular, programmed basis allowing capture of series of stains.
4. Directional samplers are two or more volumetric instruments driven by an anemometer and a wind vane. One measurement channel can be assigned to low wind speed, another to come into operation when air movement is from a sector of interest; an additional set can operate when air movement is from any other sector.

GAS DETECTION TUBES. A number of companies manufacture gas detection tubes which can be used for the detection and measurement of specific gases in the atmosphere. A range of detector tubes are produced, each being sensitive to a single chemical or range of chemicals. The tubes are sealed at either end and not exposed to the atmosphere until ready for use. A known volume of gas is aspirated through the tube by the operation of hand-held bellows or a syringe. The air passes first through a pre-filter designed to remove other chemicals which would interfere with the reaction, then through sensitized crystals which undergo colour change proportional to the concentration of the subject gas. Concentration is assessed by the depth of penetration of the colour change and the volume of gas tested. Such equipment is robust and accurate, within defined ranges, provided that the tube used is within its 'shelf date'. Often this is the only technique readily available for local authority use for specific surveys.

Diffusion tubes can be used which allow the assessment of specific gases by a process of adsorption. They are left out for prolonged periods of time enabling investigation of particular substances without excessive expenditure. They have been used for the investigation of nitrogen dioxide in a number of cities enabling, for example, the production of NO_2 contours across London.

INSTRUMENTATION. There are a range of techniques available for the molecular analysis of gases, liquids and solids. It is not within the scope of this chapter to provide a comprehensive guide to the range of techniques which could be used. Arguably, the best introduction to this subject is to be found in *Undergraduate Instrumental Analysis* [17]. The following information summarizes the current situation:

1. **Gas chromatography** is used extensively for quantitative analysis, but it does not reveal the molecular structure or molecular weight of the sample. It is a method based on the retention time and the signature of the sample.
2. **The electron microscope** can be used on dusts and fibres.
3. **Emission spectrography** is used extensively for qualitative analysis – it can determine the concentration of metals down to fractional parts per million. For quantitative analysis, it is the best method for metals and metalloids. Flame photometry is a quantitative method and is used for the determination of alkaline metals and alkaline earths.
4. **Infra-red spectroscopy** is used routinely for quantitative analysis for organic compounds, mainly for liquid samples (it is less applicable for solids). It requires skill to get good results. For qualitative analysis, it distinguishes between aliphatic and aromatic compounds, identifies functional groups and presence of hetero elements, and except in exceptional cases does not give a sample's molecular weight or the position of functional groups.
5. **Mass spectrometry** is used extensively for quantitative analysis for the determination of the components of liquid and gas samples. For qualitative analysis it is used to identify molecular weight up to 1000, and can identify functional groups and the structure of molecules; it cannot identify the relative position of functional groups; it will confirm the presence of hetero elements.
6. **Nuclear magnetic resonance.** For quantitative analysis it is useful at high per cent concentrations but it is not considered as highly accurate. As a qualitative method it identifies hydrogen and carbon organic molecules, and gives an indication of hetero ele-

ments, such as sulphur, nitrogen, halides. It does not indicate the sample's molecular weight, but can reveal the relative position of functional groups.
7. **Radiotracer techniques** are used to investigate pathways in biological systems by the use of labelling compounds.
8. **Raman scattering.** Various laser-based devices have been developed based on Raman scattering. They are used for external atmospheric monitoring.
9. **Spectrophotometric** analysis is used extensively for quantitative routine anlysis. It is very sensitive.
10. **Ultra-violet absorption** is used routinely for quantitative analysis for unsaturated compounds; it has a limited application for trace analysis and spectral interference can be a problem. It is particularly useful as a qualitative method for identifying functional groups; it does not give an indication of molecular weight.
11. **Ultra-violet fluorescence.** For quantitative analysis, it is very sensitive but subject to interference. For qualitative analysis it is used for determining unsaturated compounds, particularly aromatics; it does not give an indication of molecular weight, but does give an indication of functional groups.
12. **X-ray absorption.** As a qualitative method it reveals contours and locations of high-atomic-weight elements in low-atomic-weight matrices.
13. **X-ray diffraction.** As a quantitative method it is used for the determination of the crystallinity of polymers and mixtures of crystals, soils and natural products. As a qualitative method it is used to measure crystal lattice dimensions.
14. **X-ray fluorescence** is used extensively for quantitative analysis of particularly high atomic weight elements; it is sensitive and reliable. As a qualitative method its procedures are elaborate.

CASCADE IMPACTORS. Characterization of the size of particles in the ambient air can be achieved by specialist equipment. This technique is rarely used in the UK. An example of the equipment is the Modified Anderton Cascade sampler. Particles pass through a series of jets with progressively smaller cross sections (sampling rate 5–6 cfm). At each jet a fraction of the particles is impacted on a collection plate; the range of particle sizes collected depends on the jet velocity at that stage, the jet-to-collection surface distance, and the collection characteristics of the previous stage. Particles not collected at the first stage follow the air stream over the collection plate until the jet velocity is sufficient for impaction. A collection filter can be installed instead of the sixth stage to collect small, unarrested particles. Measurement is gravimetric.

HIGH VOLUME SAMPLERS. These are widely used by the Environmental Protection Agency in the USA. Particulate matter is collected on a fibreglass filter; the measurement is gravimetric and chemical analysis of the sample is possible.

Location of the instruments

Sampling sites must be carefully selected so as to be representative of the area under consideration. Particular attention must be paid to the existence of local discharges which could influence results. The following factors should be considered:

1. accessibility;
2. protection from vandalism and extreme weather conditions;
3. the effects of turbulence from adjacent buildings or trees;
4. the height of the sampling receptor.

Timing and duration of the survey

The timing and duration of the survey can be either:

1. intermittent or continuous;
2. cumulative or instantaneous.

Cumulative sampling gathers the sample over a determined period before bulk analysis; instantaneous sampling enables a constant value of the pollutant. The latter technique produces considerable data. Use of a data logger to record output and allow subsequent statistical analysis is essential.

Interpretation of results

Care must be taken in the consideration of the results of a survey, and the conclusions which may safely be reached. It is essential that the limitations of the method are fully understood and that this information is included in any report.

Requirements for causal relationship

The requirements for the establishment of a causal relationship have been set down in the *Shorter Textbook of Medical Statistics* [18] (also see Chapter 19). The following factors must be considered:

1. **Strength of association.** Consider the relative incidence of the condition under study in the populations contrasted. For example, prospective enquiries have shown that the death rate from lung cancer in cigarette smokers is 9 to 10 times higher than in non-smokers; the death rate in heavy cigarette smokers is 20 to 30 times as great.
2. **Consistency of observed association.** Have similar findings been made by different observers in different places, different circumstances and time? Weight should be put on similar results reached in different ways.
3. **Specificity of association.** If the association is limited to specific groups and particular sites and types of disease, and there is no association between the exposure and other causes of effect, there is clearly a strong argument in favour of causation.
4. **Biological gradient or dose response curve.** A linear relationship between exposure and effect is suggestive of a cause and effect relationship.
5. **Biological plausibility.** It is helpful if the causation is biologically plausible. This is dependent on the current understanding of biological methodology.
6. **Coherence of evidence.** Cause and interpretation of the association should not seriously

conflict with general knowledge of the natural history and biology of the condition.

7. **The experiment.** It may be possible to appeal to experimental or semi-experimental evidence. Does preventative action influence the effect?

8. **Reasoning by analogy.** Does an exposure to another similar agent produce a recognized, similar effect?

None of the above tests can bring indisputable evidence for or against the cause and effect hypothesis. What they can do, with greater or lesser strength, is to help to answer two fundamental questions. Is there any other way to explain the set of facts under consideration? Is there any other answer equally or more likely than the cause and effect proposed?

AIR QUALITY GUIDELINES

Air quality guidelines, where established, can provide a background for defining emission standards, monitoring programmes, specifying priority remedial actions and obtaining assistance from international agencies. The concept of air quality guidelines has found favour in a number of European countries; Germany has used them as a base for mandatory control. WHO has recently published a comprehensive paper on the subject, *Air Quality Guidelines for Europe* [19]. The principal aim of air quality guidelines is to provide a basis for protecting public health from adverse effects of air pollution and for eliminating, or reducing to a minimum, those contaminants of air that are known to be hazardous to human health and wellbeing.

Guidelines are intended to provide background information to those involved in making risk-management decisions, particularly in setting standards, but their use is not restricted to this. They also provide an information base for everyone involved in air pollution control and the planning process. If guideline values are adopted, it does not follow that a national monitoring network has to be established to ensure compliance: it may be sufficient to carry out local measurements in locations of particular interest.

Guidelines cannot, however, be adopted blindly – consideration must be given to existing levels, and environmental, social and cultural conditions. In some cases, there may be valid reasons to pursue policies which will result in certain pollution levels being at or above the guideline values.

Ambient air pollution can cause nuisance, or acute and long-term toxic effects. Air quality guidelines either indicate levels and exposure times at which no adverse effect is expected in the case of non-carcinogenic substances, or provide an estimate of lifetime cancer risk from those substances which are human carcinogens.

It is important to note that guidelines have been established for individual chemicals. Mixtures of pollutants may have an additive, synergistic or antagonistic effect. However, knowledge of such interaction is rudimentary. WHO states that an adequate safety margin should exist between guideline values and concentrations at which toxic effects may occur.

Action limits

If Air Quality Standards are to be used it follows that action limits will have to be agreed in order to determine the circumstances under which particular advice is to be given. The Department of the Environment has begun to consider a formal framework for such action. Three threshold levels have been considered; alarm, long-term acceptable and background.

The **alarm** is the upper extreme, it is the level above which there is a serious risk of widespread adverse health effects on a significant proportion of the population. Effects would not necessarily be confined to particularly sensitively groups, although these might be the first to demonstrate effects.

Long-term acceptability is the equilibrium point beyond which further action to reduce pollution would not – given current circumstances and scientific knowledge – be sensible. For some pollutants, which have potentially serious effects on sensitive groups, it may be appropriate to set the threshold at or close to a 'no-effect' level. For certain types of carcinogenic substances, for which there is no safe level, the appropriate course may be to set it at a minimum risk level at which the risk of irreversible effects would remain but would be very low. For some other pollutant, however, where for example impacts are slight but costs of abatement strategies relatively high, it may be appropriate to set the acceptable threshold significantly above a no-effects level.

Policy should be informed by a **background** threshold. This would define the level of a pollutant which might be expected without human activity. Such background levels might differ from place to place, depending on factors such as local geography, geology, vegetation and weather conditions, but indicative levels should be identified for reference.

Obviously high, short-term concentration, which may result from accidental release, is not covered by guidelines.

At the time of writing, three air quality guidelines have been set by the EU; the pollutants dealt with are smoke and sulphur dioxide, nitrogen dioxide and lead. Table 41.1 indicates the reference values for smoke and sulphur dioxide – the inter-relationship between these two substances should be noted.

The Directive for nitrogen dioxide is less complicated; a limit value of 200 μg/m^3 is set based on the 98th percentile of mean values per hour recorded throughout the year.

In the case of lead, the Directive states that the annual mean concentration of lead in air should not exceed 2 μg/m^3. The DoE is proposing in its paper 'Air Quality: Meeting the Challenge' [14] to set standards for the range of substances to be monitored. So far the following air quality standards have been set:

> Benzene – upper limit 5 ppb annual average
> – lower limit 1 ppb annual average
> Ozone – upper limit 50 ppb 8-hour average
> 1-3-butadiene – 1 ppb annual average
> Carbon monoxide – 10 ppb 8-hour running
> average.

The upper limit (alert) is the level at which immediate action must be taken. The lower limit is a long-term target above which it is understood to be a significant health hazard.

Where it is found that the air quality in part of an area does not meet the prescribed limits,

Table 41.1 Air quality guidelines (Directive 80/729/EEC)

| Reference period | Limit values – air | |
	Smoke (μg/m^3)	Sulphur dioxide (μg/m^3)
1 year	80(68)	120 – if smoke, less than 40 (34)
(Median of daily values)		80 – if smoke, more than 40 (34)
Winter	130(111)	180 – if smoke, less than 60 (51)
(Median of daily values)		130 – if smoke, more than 60 (51)
(1 October–31 March) Year (peak)		
(98 percentile of daily values)	250(213)	350 – if smoke, less than 150 (128)
		250 – if smoke, more than 150 (128)

Note: The levels given above are based on the European method of measurement. In the UK, the values to be used, assuming that monitoring is carried out using the 'volumetric method', are shown in parentheses.

action has to be taken. Although, in the medium term, measures will have to be adopted to reduce emissions to an acceptable level, it may be necessary, in the short term, to exempt the problem area from the requirements of the legislation.

Of course, the application of air quality standards does not meet with universal acceptance. A study of air pollution levels and mortality rates within most of the major metropolitan areas of the USA revealed little association between specific pollutants and death rates [20]. The authors concluded that the statistics did not lend support to the use of air quality criteria. They found that there was little specific evidence that levels could be considered 'safe' or a level below which no health effects could be detected. They concluded that there was no air pollution standard which would 'protect the public health or welfare'. Instead, they argued that standards should simply be based on benefit-cost trade-offs. That is to say society should weight the cost and benefits of achieving various levels of air quality, and once a desired level has been selected, the standard corresponding to it should be determined. This issue will remain a matter of debate in public health circles.

INVESTIGATION OF COMPLAINTS
(also see Chapter 8)

There are four components to the investigation of complaints. They may seem obvious, but this procedure is not always recognized in practice:

1. determination of the alleged problem;
2. design of the investigation;
3. consideration of remedial action; and
4. execution.

It may be considered as stating the obvious to suggest that there is a particular need to identify the nature of a complaint, but this is vital if subsequent action is to be effective. It is not unknown for resources to be squandered on irrelevant issues. A carefully constructed interview with the complainant will ensure that the appropriate issues are identified from the first stage of the enquiry.

The design and implementation of investigations should always be considered, although many routine issues can be executed without the need for a significant level of preparation. In even the simplest case, there should be a procedure – a standard approach which has been laid down and is available to all staff in an organization. This does not imply that each action is the subject of a multi-page document, scripting the content of interviews, but there are clear advantages in management determining the manner in which they feel that the service should be delivered. This concept forms the basis of quality assurance and quality management. If implemented, it minimizes ambiguity within the organization. Staff have an absolute understanding of what is required of them; 'customers' receive a similar or identical service; all legislation is applied in an equitable manner. Once the concept of quality management is widely used by individual local authorities, it should be possible to extend the principles across authority boundaries so unifying

actions regionally and nationally. Within air pollution control, the foundations of such an approach have been set by BATNEEC notes; this is unquestionably the trend for the future.

An example of a procedure for complaint investigation is set out below. It relates to the action to be taken following a complaint that dark smoke is being emitted from the burning of industrial waste on a bonfire. The procedure is not cited as the ultimate response, but as a guide for the implementation of this approach.

1. Complaint recorded.
2. Complainant interviewed, preferably by telephone, within 3 working days. If contact is not made, a letter is sent indicating their need to contact the investigating officer. Details of the location of the problem, frequency and timing of emissions are obtained together with relevant information.
3. The property file for the subject site is checked for history, if any.
4. Visit to suspect premises within 7 working days. No more than three unsuccessful visits to be made without further contact with the complainant. Each observation to be of no less than 5 minutes duration unless emissions are detected.
5. Analysis of emissions of dark smoke are to be carried out formally using prescribed procedures. The smoke shade to be recorded is based on 15 second periods.
6. If there is clear evidence of dark smoke emissions, then there is an immediate visit to the site where contact is made with a senior representative of the organization.
7. Examination of the bonfire is made to establish the possible cause of the dark smoke. What was being burnt? What steps were taken to supervise the fire? What other means existed to dispose of waste? Other relevant information.
8. Decide if an offence has been committed. If so, caution the representative and continue the investigation in accordance with judges' rules.
9. Endorse the file including details of difficulties, e.g. threats and aggression.

10. Within 3 days, a letter is sent to the organization confirming the circumstances of the observations and warning of the possibility of legal action. A reply is invited.

11. Policy is that each organization is granted one formal warning. Any subsequent action will include legal proceedings. In the case of peripatetic operators, such as builders or demolition contractors, this policy relates to all their actions in the area of the authority.

12. Copies of correspondence, the statement and report is to go to the line manager within 2 weeks of the observation. All relevant documentation is to be with the prosecution solicitor within a further week.

13. If there is no evidence of an offence after the three visits a letter is sent to the organization indicating the concern and reminding it of its responsibilities.

14. If proceedings are taken, a letter is sent advising the complainant within 7 working days – a summary of the action for the information of the committee is sent within same period.

The steps set out above are not proposed as a 'right' policy but only a possible procedure. It would be reasonable to write to the organization who had been the subject of the complaint advising it of the law and the way in which it should dispose of waste. The use of a computerized data base allows steps to be integrated into the complaint procedure and for necessary correspondence to be generated as and when necessary. In also allows the work to be better monitored, including the time targets at various stages of the operation.

While activities associated with a simple example can be broken down into component activities, there are occasions when this approach is inappropriate. No management system is likely to anticipate every eventuality. In such circumstances, the need to define the objectives of the investigation is even more clearly identified. Before expending considerable time on the collection of information, it is worthwhile reviewing the possible remedies and available literature. Only by being aware of the final destination is it possible to sketch out the route.

If a problem is felt to affect a significant number of people, it may be necessary to carry out a survey in the community. An early decision to make is the advisability of seeking to interview all potential householders in the prescribed area of interest. To do so can lead to the accusation that concerns have been generated by local authority action; failure to do so results in biased evidence. In order for action to be justified, it is necessary to be able to demonstrate that there is a genuine effect. There is a tendency for the defence to balance the evidence of complainants with the opinions of other residents who have a comparable experience of a situation. Clearly it is possible to take into account the existence of economic ties – employees of an organization are genuinely more tolerant than others who have no direct involvement. The crucial issue is the proportion of the exposed population who can be regarded as independent witnesses who register the existence of a nuisance.

The use of diaries to enable complainants to record the timing of events is helpful, especially if both quantitative and qualitative information is required. Results can be collated to show spatial and temporal distributions. Meteorological information can be obtained to relate observation to possible sources. The use of local meteorological detail, including impressions from respondents, should not be overlooked, especially if the nearest meteorological observation point is distant from the area under study. Local topography can influence wind conditions. Collation should not only highlight contradictory statements, but also consider the possibility of collusion. There is a limit to the possibility of independent observers reporting identical timing for events or descriptions of experiences.

If questionnaires are to be used, much effort has to be invested in their design and content. There is considerable advice published on the way in which questions should be posed and responses invited. (If questionnaires submitted to local authorities by various researchers are typical, then the understanding of this science seems less than adequate.) Questions must be precise and umambiguous. The question setter must carefully consider the precise information needed before construction of a step-by-step model for its re-trieval. Questionnaires must be piloted, if only within a critical group of colleagues, to eliminate the worst errors or omissions.

There is continuing concern about the association between ill-health and air pollution. It is possible, using local health statistics, to consider the existence of a causal relationship [18], but the design of an epidemiological survey is a complex matter. Experts from the various relevant disciplines should be involved from the beginning; in addition to the need for medical expertise, assistance from a medical statistician can be invaluable. Guidelines on the design of such studies have been published by WHO [20]. A hypothesis has to be posed and the study designed to test it. The questions to be considered at the design stage are:

1. Who should be studied? Are particular sub-groups of the population at risk? How should control groups be selected?
2. Who should be measured? Can specific agents be measured? Is there a single pathway, e.g. via inhalation, or have several routes to be considered simultaneously? How are health effects to be assessed?
3. Where has the study to take place? Should geographic position, meteorology, etc., be taken into account when selecting the locality? Are there existing monitoring stations or sets of data relating to the environmental factors in question? Is there a need to involve other agencies?
4. When should the study be carried out? Are seasonal effects likely to be important? Is the available time span sufficient to provide a satisfactory estimate of long-term exposures? Should exposure be averaged over months or years, or are short-term peaks relevant in some cases?

Before a survey is begun, a clear protocol must be produced and agreed with all participating professionals to ensure the subsequent acceptability of findings.

There is no point in embarking on an investigation unless there is a clear outcome either in terms of informal intervention, statutory remedy or the production of useful data. This principle applies in relation to all aspects of work, from the most simple case of complaint to complex epidemiological research. It is equally important that the public, whether a single complainant, or a community, are made aware of actions and findings. Criticism frequently levelled against both local and central government is the needless way in which officials cling to the need for secrecy. Barriers are being broken down by progressive local authorities, pressure groups and even reported redirection of government policy. Information is best shared when the authority publicizes its activities. It is not sufficient to base a freedom of information policy on the principle that those seeking data will be satisfied – interested parties should be aware of the information which is held and, where necessary, advised without having to ask.

REFERENCES

1. Committee on Air Pollution (1954) *Final Report of the Committee on Air Pollution*, Cmnd. 9322, HMSO, London.
2. Department of the Environment (1990) *This Common Inheritance – Britain's Environmental Strategy*, HMSO, London.
3. Department of the Environment (1974) *The Monitoring of the Environment in the United Kingdom*, HMSO, London.
4. Royal Commission on Environmental Pollution (1976) *Air Pollution Control: an Integrated Approach*, 5th report, HMSO, London.
5. Department of the Environment (1991) *General Guidelines Note No. 2, Authorizations* (including detailed guidance on drafting conditions), HMSO, London.
6. Department of the Environment (1991) *General Guidelines Note No. 3, Applications and Registers*, HMSO, London.
7. Department of the Environment (1991) *General Guidance Note No. 1, Introduction to the System, etc.*, HMSO, London.
8. Institution of Environmental Health Officer and Warren Spring Laboratory (1993) *Emission Monitoring*. Volume 1. *General Aspects of Monitoring*, CIEH, London.

9. Institution of Environmental Health Officers and Warren Spring Laboratory (1993) *Emission Monitoring*, Volume 2. *Monitoring Methods and Specific Power Requirements*, IEHO, London.

10. British Standards Institute (1969) Notes on the Ringelmann and Miniature Smoke Charts, BS2742: 1969, BSI, London.

11. British Standards Institute (1983) *(Simplified) Method for Measurement of Particulate Emission Including Grit and Dust*, BS3405: 1983, BSI, London.

12. Hawksley, P.G.W., Badzioch, S. and Blackett, J.H. *Measurement of Solids in Flue Gases*, Institute of Energy (out of print).

13. Department of the Environment (1981) *Chimney Heights, Third Edition of the 1956 Clean Air Act Memorandum*, HMSO, London.

14. Department of the Environment (1995) *Air Quality: Meeting the Challenge – the Government strategic policies for air quality management.*

15. British Standards Institution (1969) Methods for the Measurement of Air Pollution, BS1747: 1969, BSI, London.

16. Royal Commission on Environmental Pollution (1984) *Tackling Pollution – Experience and Prospects*, 10th report, HMSO, London.

17. Robinson, J.W., *Undergraduate Instrumental Analysis*, Marcel Dekker, New York.

18. Hill, A.B. (1977) *Short Textbook of Medical Statistics*, Hodder and Stoughton, London.

19. World Health Organization (1987) *Air Quality Guidelines for Europe*, European Series No.23, WHO, Geneva.

20. World Health Organization (1983) *Guidelines and Studies in Environmental Epidemiology*, Environmental Health Criteria No.27, WHO, Geneva.

42 Radon in buildings

Alan Blythe

INTRODUCTION

Although radon was first discovered by the German physicist, Dorn, back in 1900, relatively modest importance was given to it in this country until 1984, when the tenth report of the Royal Commission on Environmental Pollution [1] recognized the serious threat posed to health from radon, and the International Commission on Radiological Protection (ICRP) published new principles [2] for limiting public exposure.

The results of the National Radiological Protection Board's (NRPB) national and regional surveys of radon in houses of 1984/85 [3, 4] prompted the government to issue a ministerial statement in January 1987 [5], which detailed an action plan for tackling domestic radon.

Radon had at last 'come of age' and many more surveys – including three organized by the then Institution of Environmental Health Officers (IEHO) – ensued. New, more exacting standards for public protection have been developed and radon now has a justifiably high profile in the indoor air pollution arena.

BASIC PROPERTIES

Radon is a tasteless, odourless, invisible, noble gas which can only be detected using specialized equipment. Together with thoron, radon contributes over half the average annual dose to the UK population from ionizing radiation sources (Fig. 42.1); in high radon areas this proportion may rise to a staggering 90%, or more, for exposures above the current action level' (see below).

SOURCES OF RADON

The element radon is a naturally occurring inert, but alpha-radioactive, gas produced within both the uranium 238 and thorium 232 radioactive decay chains (Fig. 42.2). ^{222}Rn, commonly known as radon, is produced from the decay of ^{226}Ra in the ^{238}U decay chain, and ^{220}Rn, commonly known as thoron, is produced from the decay of ^{224}RA in the ^{232}Th decay chain. The dispersion of these gases is quite different owing to their different half-lives, 3.8 days for radon compared with 55 seconds for thoron.

In contrast to thoron, radon is able to move considerable distances from its parent during its lifetime. It can diffuse readily out of surface soil into the atmosphere and into the basements and living areas of houses. For this reason, it is the ^{238}U decay chain and radon that are usually considered more important in terms of environmental alpha-radioactivity than the ^{232}Th decay chain and thoron.

Natural uranium also contains 0.7% of the isotope ^{235}U, which comprises a further decay chain in which an isotope of radon, ^{219}Rn, is produced. However, ^{219}Rn has a half life of only 4 seconds and, together with its very low natural abundance, means that it can be effectively ignored as a source of radon in the home.

As uranium is an essential constituent of around a hundred minerals, it is not surprising to

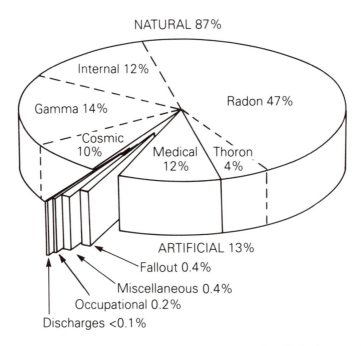

Fig. 42.1 Average annual effective dose equivalent to the UK population (2.5 mSv overall). (Courtesy of NRPB (1989) *Living with Radiation*, 4th edn, NRPB.)

find traces in diverse geological formations [7]. The more soluble forms, such as pitchblende, coffinite and uraninite, may be found in alluvial deposits and sediments, while in igneous rocks uranium occurs in accessory minerals, along grain boundaries and crystal lattice defects. Uranium is normally found at less than 1 ppm: where it has been leached and precipitated in a reducing environment, e.g in some sandstones and iron sulphites, it can attain concentrations of 0.05–0.2% uranium. Finer grain sediments, such as shales, concentrate uranium in organic matter at generally 30–60 ppm (much higher in some Upper Cambrian formations). Phosphatic sediments contain deposits of 10–60 ppm uranium, or more, while lignites formed under reducing conditions show greater variations in uranium content up to 1%. It should be remembered that uranium is mobile as organic complexed or colloidal particles, especially under oxidizing conditions in acid or carbonate rich waters. (See Table 42.1 for the content of uranium in different rock types.)

The element thorium is present both as the precursor in the ^{232}Th decay chain, and as intermediate nuclides in the ^{238}U decay chain. The long half-lives of these nuclides means that the geological behaviour of thorium must be taken into account.

All rocks and soils to a certain extent emit ionizing radiation through the alpha, beta and gamma emission nuclides within the two uranium decay series, the thorium decay series and the beta and gamma emissions of ^{40}K (radioactive potassium) [7].

Alpha particles are the least penetrating of all these emissions, the most energetic travelling only 10 cm in air. Beta radiation is absorbed by around 0.5 cm of rock or soil. Therefore, from the body of the earth itself and from within building materials it is only the gamma radiation that

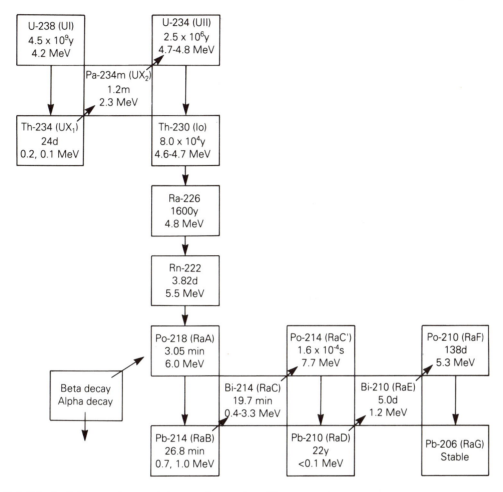

Fig. 42.2 Principal decay scheme of the uranium series. (Courtesy of Dr D. Henshaw, Bristol University.)

provides a background radiation dose to the occupants in houses, whereas gaseous radon diffuses into houses where it may be inhaled, providing an alpha-radiation dose to the body, chiefly the lungs.

Granites are by no means the most radioactive rocks, and some shales contain one hundred times more uranium than the most highly radioactive granites. Acid volcanics cover large areas and have equivalent uranium and thorium contents to granite. The highly evolved and fissured potassium-rich granites in Cairngorm and Etive in Scotland emit high levels of radioactivity, as do the granite areas of the Lake District and the south west of England. However, it should be appreciated that even higher levels of radioact-

ivity may be associated with sedimentary rocks, such as phosphatic limestone of lower carboniferous age, and the black shales and marine shale bands in the coal measures.

DISTRIBUTION OF RADON

Uranium that goes into solution is capable of migrating over long distances to be concentrated both in surface and ground waters, depending on the particular conditions that affect the rate of weathering. However, it should be appreciated that the important isotope ^{226}Ra radium is not as mobile in surface oxidizing conditions as uranium, but can go into solution and migrate

Table 42.1 Uranium contents and typical ranges in different rock types

Rock type	Mean (ppm)	Range
Igneous		
Mafic	0.8	0.1–3.5
Diorite and quartz diorite	2.5	0.5–12
Silicic	4.0	1.0–22
Alkaline intrusive		0.04–20
Sedimentary		
Shale	3.0	1–15
Black shale		3–1250
Sandstone	1.5	0.5–4
Orthoquartzite	0.5	0.2–0.06
Carbonate	1.6	0.01–10
Phosphorite		50–2500
Lignite		10–2500

Source: Bowle, S.H.V. and Plant, J.A. (1983) *Natural Radioactivity in the Environment* Academic, London.

significant distances before being absorbed into other oxides or clay minerals, such as iron and magnesium. Of course, bearing in mind the ^{238}U decay series means that wherever ^{226}Ra is found, its important immediate daughter product, ^{222}Rn (radon), will be produced. Since its half-life is only 3.8 days, it can diffuse easily through porous rocks, ground or surface waters, through faults and fissures and into thermal springs. As would generally be expected, radon levels generally relate to locally occurring radium levels, and the two are relatively inseparable in concentration apart, that is, from the diffusion of radon into houses [7]. (See Fig. 42.3.)

HEALTH EFFECTS AND RISKS

While the scientific community may dispute the relative severity of the various health effects from high radon inhalation rates, it remains clear that alpha particle irradiation of the bronchial epithelium through short-lived radon daughters is the most significant cause of radiation-induced lung cancer. Medical science has, however, fully accepted the synergistic link between radon and smoking in terms of enhanced risk to health which is demonstrated quite clearly from Tables 42.2 and 42.3.

The **whole** lifetime risk to persons exposed at the present radon 'action level' (see below) of 3% is a rationalized figure derived from combining the risk factor for smokers (10%) with the risk factor for non-smokers (1%). It may, therefore, be deduced that while the current action level for radon in homes may be quite acceptable in public protection terms for non-smokers, moderate smokers exposed to radon concentrations as low as 10% of the current action level (i.e. 1 mSv y^{-1}) could still run a lifetime risk of premature death equivalent to their chances of dying in a motor vehicle traffic accident (or more significantly, ten times that risk at the action level).

Perhaps this rather startling multiplicative effect (synergism) upon the smoking and radon risk factors should justify further special assistance and advice being offered to inveterate smokers in high radon areas.

However these risks are quantified, it is worth bearing in mind that they are calculated for **long-term** exposure at a time when most families rarely live in the same house for longer than an average of 7 years. Conversely, of course, they could conceivably move to a new house with relatively higher, or equivalent radon potential. Also the 'average concentration' figures given must apply over a 'lifetime', giving an effective dose equivalent (or just 'dose') of 1 mSv y^3 for every 20 Bq m^{-3} radon gas effectively measured.

MONITORING AND EXPOSURE MECHANISMS

Monitoring techniques

Direct 'active' instruments
These usually comprise sensitive electronic instruments which give a direct, almost instantaneous, reading, related to the ambient radon concentration obtained during the relatively short period of measurement.

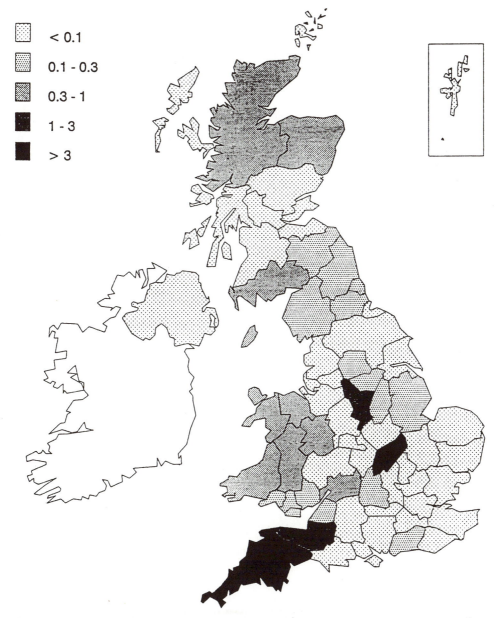

Fig. 42.3 Percentage of homes by county and region with radon concentrations above 200 Bq m^{-3} [8]. (Courtesy of NRPB, Clarke, R. and O'Riordan, M.C. (1990) Rumours of radon. *Science and Public Affairs*, **5**, (2), 25–36.)

Most incorporate a small air pump which draws air containing radionuclides through a filter where radon daughter products are deposited for counting as total alphas or determined by spectrometry techniques. Immediate results may also be obtained from zinc sulphide scintillators and diffused junc-tion devices. The radon 'working level' (see below) is determined by correlating the total alpha count with the airflow rate over the (short) monitoring period.

Such instruments are most often used in mines and caves to determine relatively short-term

Table 42.2 Lifetime risk of lung cancer from lifelong exposure to radon at home for various parts of the UK population

Average concentration (Bq m^{-3})	Lifetime risk (%)		
	Whole	Smokers	Non-smokers
20	0.3	1	0.1
100	1.5	5	0.5
200	3.0	10	1
400	6.0	20	2

Source: NRPB (1990) *Board Statement on Radon in Homes*, Vol. 1, No. 1, HMSO, London.

Table 42.3 Approximate lifetime risks of premature death from various causes including lung cancer from lifetime exposure to radon daughters in dwellings (revised 1990)

Cause	Risk %
Malignant neoplasms (all cases)	25
Radon daughters, 100 mSv y^{-1} (2000 Bq m^{-3})	30
Malignant neoplasms, bronchus and lung (all causes)	6
Radon daughters, 20 mSv y^{-1} (400 Bq m^{-3})	6
Motor vehicle traffic accidents	1
Radon daughters, 10 mSv y^{-1} (200 Bq m^{-3})	3
Accidents in the home and residential institutions	1
Motor vehicle traffic accidents involving collision with pedestrian	0.3
Radon daughters, 1 mSv y^{-1} (20 Bq m^{-3})	0.3
Conflagration in private dwellings	0.06

Source: National Radiological Protection Board (1987) *Exposure to Radon Daughters in Dwellings*, NRPB GS,b, HMSO, London.

occupational exposure, but could be misinterpreted to underestimate the long-term risk in houses.

There seems to have been a recent upsurge in interest in such rapid methods of determining radon concentration, usually by direct measurements of radon with electronic instruments or, alternatively, by charcoal canisters submitted for laboratory analysis. Where the sampling takes place over a few hours or even a few days, it again must be regarded as being highly speculative in terms of long-term radon concentration which is, after all, **the significant factor** we are seeking in trying to assess the health effects of long-term exposure, i.e. dose.

There can be no doubt, however, that in certain circumstances, e.g. the requirement for a quick assessment prior to, say, purchasing a potential property, short-term 'grab' sampling techniques can have a limited value. They cannot, however, in any way be expected to predict average long-term trends in radon evolution, which naturally varies both from day to night (diurnally) and from season to season. Such methods also fail to recognize that people's homes are used in different ways at different times of the year: in winter, heating systems generate a relatively high negative pressure inside living areas, which would tend to draw **comparably more** randon-laden air into the living areas from the ground, when tightly closed doors, windows and draught stripping systems are all working to optimum efficiency in reducing air change and thereby innocently enhancing radon concentrations. Thus, any radon concentrations would tend to be at their highest in winter when a short-term sample over this period would obviously give a false (high) result. Similarly, a short-term sample taken in spring or summer, when householders tend to open windows and doors and heating systems are not working at all – other than providing domestic hot water – again give a false (low) reading as little, if any, relative negative internal air pressure is likely and higher air change rates would dissipate any radon present to quite low levels and again give misleading results.

It is worth reiterating that the NRPB specify monitoring to a standard approved by them **for at least 3 months** before it will accept the reading as being valid to justify application of remedial measures, and the Department of the Environment's grant system, as embodied in the Housing and Local Government Act 1989 cites a similar 3-month period for testing before a grant may be approved for homes above the current action level. However, the NRPB has calculated reasonably accurate **seasonal adjustment factors** for the 3-month radon results taken at any time throughout the year, which may be utilized to obtain equivalent average concentrations during the winter months. Measured concentrations are multiplied by the appropriate factors, as detailed in Table 42.6.

It should also be appreciated that there are various firms operating (particularly in the south west) who are purporting to give householders an accurate reading of radon concentration over a weekend's electronic meter measurements, and it is highly likely that such readings could generate false positives and lead householders into unnecessary anxiety and expense, when long-term readings using properly calibrated passive radon detectors would given an accurate measure of **mean concentration** as opposed to **meaningless peak fluctuations**.

For all these reasons, it is **essential** that environmental health departments support the scientifically correct and accurate methods of radon measurement accredited by the NRPB, endorsed by the CIEH, and such other reliable laboratory services that may become available (NRPB accreditation is the crucial factor in determining choice).

Passive track-etch detectors
Originally manufactured from the proprietary alpha-senstive plastic CR-39, these essentially long-term monitors are now marketed by various companies and are currently recognized as the NRPB preferred method for accurately estimating radon exposure, and hence dose, over time. While the NRPB utilizes detectors of its own design and manufacture for its many surveys, the CIEH has specified 'Radosure' radon detectors made by Track Analysis Systems Ltd, at Bristol University and similar track-etch detectors manufactured by N.E. Technology Ltd of Reading to equivalent high-quality standards.

The complete detector comprises a small plastic pot containing a postage stamp-sized rectangle of radon-sensitive plastic – a polymer of diethylene glycol bis (allyl carbonate). The tightly-lidded pot protects the sensitive plastic from physical damage and allows radon to diffuse inwards; alpha particles produced from radon decay invisibly damage the detector sliver, which chemical etching later reveals as discrete pits in its surface (Fig. 42.4). The number of these alpha 'tracks' correlates directly with radon concentration over the period of detector exposure.

Ideally, measurements should be carried out for a minimum of 3 months and in different rooms in the house, so that natural habitual variations can be integrated into the calculation of mean radon concentration. However, as previously stated, the NRPB has advised correction factors for different exposure periods for readings taken at any time of year.

Diffusion-barrier activated charcoal detectors
Perforated canisters of activated charcoal (25–100 g) are exposed to radon-laden air for the measurement period, thereby 'trapping' radon which decays and deposits its daughter progeny in the charcoal. Indoor measurements usually vary over a relatively short period (2–10 days) which is strictly recorded for subsequent laboratory use.

The laboratory collates the gamma ray emissions from the progeny and thereby calculates the radon gas concentration. Recent research suggests very accurate correlation of charcoal canister results in comparison with the 'true' values obtained by the NRPB from alpha-spectrometric measurements of radon daughters (within 2.5% for 4-day measurements).

Whilst excellent 'rapid' screening results may be obtained with the method, charcoal canisters are not suitable for long-term mean concentrations and must be kept sealed and dry until opened for exposure.

Exposure mechanisms

The main factors affecting radon levels in buildings include varying combinations of the following:

1. The content of radon-producing uranium/radium in underlying ground: likely to be highest in fissured igneous rocks, such as granite, with porous rocks, such as limestone, or soil cover allowing variable diffusion rates the surface.
2. The presence of suitable routes for radon-laden air to seep into the building, e.g. cracks,

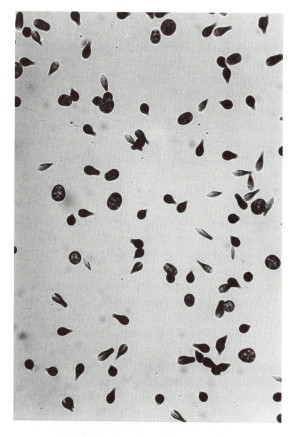

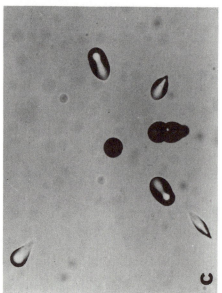

Fig. 42.4 Print of radon track – etch pits. (Courtesy of Dr D. Henshaw, Bristol University.)

service entry points, poor construction and joints.

3. The presence of sufficient negative pressure inside the building to 'suck' radon inwards – usually caused by heating, wind effects and inappropriate ventilation.

4. Restricted air change inside the buildings – energy conservation measures, such as double-glazing and draught stripping, fail to provide adequate dilution to dissipate incoming radon.

5. The habits of the occupants in terms of comfort standards and occupancy rates of different rooms in relation to the ground floor level.

6. The time of day (night) and season – relative radon levels are usually higher at night (early am) and during the winter months.

The prevalence of these factors, acting singly or in various combinations, can cause wide differences in measured radon concentrations within houses in the same area or even in the same street.

It can, therefore, never be assumed that single-point sampling in defined locations (town, village, hamlet or street) can be accepted as truly representative of **all** house or workplaces in that vicinity. The more tests undertaken, the more accurate the radon picture will become.

Radon surveys

Local authority monitoring

It should be borne in mind that the NRPB's current rules of confidentiality concerning radon surveys do prevent them from revealing particular results to third parties (unless previously agreed by the owner or occupier of the premises concerned). In formulating plans for future surveys, environmental health departments should seek guidance from the NRPB on how specific its information will be before contemplating whether or not to purchase detectors from an independent laboratory source where availability and access to results can be guaranteed to the local environmental health department. (See also 'Confidentiality' below.)

Bristol University-based Track Analysis Systems Ltd and Reading-based N.E. Technology

Ltd fulfil this latter criterion in terms of scientific credibility, quality and access to results.

Environmental health departments contemplating expansion of radon surveys in their districts should have full knowledge of the latest NRPB *Board Statement on Radon in Homes* [9], which gives the latest position with regard to assessment of risk and how that risk should be handled in terms of the varying radon concentrations encountered. This advice is absolutely critical in terms of balancing the need for any subsequent follow-ups and the sort of guidance that should be provided in order that householders and HSW managers can satisfactorily resolve their radon problems.

A preliminary survey of the local authority district should be conducted, either **randomly** or **targeted** upon either:

1. Likely radon-active areas based on the British Geological Survey, i.e. igneous rock, carboniferous limestone outcrops, (see the case history on the Northamptonshire approach to radon in the appendix to this chapter); etc.;
2. centres of population; or
3. various combinations of both.

To try and allay the possibility of initial public anxiety, many environmental health departments utilized staff or councillor homes as the starting point for their surveys, and these have already generated quite useful data, which although arguably not fully random in nature, is still likely to be sufficiently dispersed to give a measure of random spread across various districts.

Depending on the resources available to expand such surveys, and political awareness of the degree of risk perceived from elevated radon in a particular area, environmental health departments should seek to expand their knowledge of radon concentration across their districts in the following manner:

1. Previously revealed 'hot spots' (houses where radon exceeds the prevailing action level of 200 Bq m^{-3}) would justify a follow-up on the basis of trying to delineate the extent of the area of high radon concentration.
2. A personal approach by an officer well versed in radon is always best – someone who can talk easily about the possible ramifications of the test, and also the possibility of grant aid should testing prove radon concentrations above the action level.
3. Such surveys should be conducted on a next house or next but **n** house basis, where **n** is the number of houses missed between sample sites, ideally keeping the same interval between sample properties so that some degree of consistency can be claimed. It must be accepted that in field work this is impracticable and difficult to achieve, as very often the target properties cannot be surveyed due to reluctant householders, and it obvious that one can only site detectors where there is a degree of commitment from the householder to co-operate fully. The overall target should be to survey a reasonable number of homes in the vicinity of a hot spot, to get some idea of its likely extent.
4. The aim should be to spread detectors out from a preliminary hot spot on the basis of a dense inner circle of detectors being backed up with an outer circle of detectors spread more sparsely to try and discern a trend in radon concentration radiating out from the first focal hot spot, and discover from this information how far the hot-spot area extends.

Note that this approach is not foolproof due to the many variables affecting radon concentration such as specific underlying geology/differences in construction/differences in ventilation rates between (even) adjoining properties.

The Department of the Environment will only offer grants on houses that have been surveyed in accordance with the NRPB method, i.e. detectors should have been placed in living and bedroom areas over a minimum 3-month period and a representative reading calculated to decide if radon concentration is near or above the prevailing action level (see below).

The detectors should have been produced by a laboratory suitably accredited for that purpose, calibrated to a national standard (Track Analysis Systems Ltd of Bristol University; N.E. Technology Ltd of Reading or the NRPB can be used with confidence; with the developing interest in radon, other reputable commercial organizations may enter the field and obtain similar accreditation).

The NRPB is willing to accept high results obtained by local authorities in their screening measurements, i.e. samples where **preliminary results** have indicated radon concentrations at or above the action level. The NRPB would normally follow these up with a definitive 3-month survey utilizing two detectors, one in the bedroom and one in the living area, and apply a seasonal correction (Fig. 42.5). Thus it should be noted that single 3–6 months observations can only approximate an annual estimate of dose.

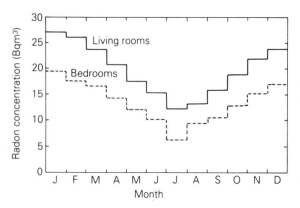

Fig. 42.5 Annual variation in radon including in ground floor living rooms and first floor bedrooms. (Source: Documents of the NRPB (1990), Radon affected areas: Cornwall and Devon, Vol.1, No. 4.)

Once the initial hot spots have been fully explored for extent and intensity, it would be necessary for most local authorities to look elsewhere to see if other areas of their districts need additional coverage. With limited resources this is arguably difficult to achieve, but many local authorities could well apply their scant resources wisely on the basis of the geological survey to determine which are the most likely areas of activity within the council's area to explore in greater detail.

In view of the foregoing, it is the CIEH view that radon is not simply a problem of the igneous/ granite rock areas of the south west of England,

parts of Derbyshire and the north east of Scotland, but, in fact, extends throughout the country as CIEH surveys have repeatedly proven, i.e. out of just under 5500 houses so far surveyed in 27 English counties and six Welsh counties, a significant number of homes have been detected as having radon above the current action level (Table 42.4.).

It is therefore essential that district council environmental health departments respond positively to any requests from householders who feel that they may be at some risk, or have expressed a need to know their own local radon concentrations. Such reactive work is very useful for discerning trends and should be acted upon as soon as possible to encourage a public perception that the environmental health department is not only the correct focal point to refer such enquiries, but that **professionally based, scientific surveys will ensue with confidential results and follow-up advice appropriate to the concentrations found**. A case study which details an investigation by environmental health departments in Northamptonshire is included in an appendix to this chapter.

Since all surveys of premises essentially depend upon good public relations between the environmental health department and the owner or occupier of such premises, be they dwellinghouses or workplaces, it is useful that maximum publicity is given to local surveys, but that **results are emphasized to be confidential to each individual property owner** (see 'Confidentiality' below). Note that workplace measurements must reference the Ionizing Regulations 1985 methodology and standards (see below).

In order to facilitate the expansion of district surveys, some form of basic promotion will have to take place, usually in the form of a circular with a reply slip so that householders are reassured as to the need for such surveys and can be encouraged to believe that not only will this usually be a free service, but also that there will be no release of results without permission of the individual who commissioned the survey. **It should, indeed, however, be emphasized that in order for this survey to be worthwhile to the local authority, the district council reserves the right to use the**

Table 42.4 Institution of Environmental Health Officers national radon surveys 1987/88, 1989, 1990 results

County	Counties containing homes above current action level (200 Bq m⁻³ – 10 mSv y⁻¹)						High	Total houses surveyed
	1st survey 1987/88		2nd survey 1989		3rd survey 1990			
	Sample size	No. above action level	Sample size	No. above action level	Sample size	No. above action level		
England								
Avon	144	3	74	4	14	4	1192	232
Berkshire					22	1		22
Cleveland	124	1			6			130
Cumbria	123	3	6	2			1251	129
Derbyshire			10	2			306	10
Devon			98				547	98
Dorset	58	1	29	1	21		582	108
East Sussex			25	3	25		332	50
Gloucestershire	59	3	27	3	15	1	432	101
Hereford & Worcester	6	1	40	1	54			101
Humberside	72	1			55	2		127
Kent	57		65		88	1		210
Lancashire	157	3	34	1	10	1	484	201
Leicestershire	196	1	10		25	1		231
Lincolnshire	50	1	35	1	35	1	929	120
Northamptonshire	12	3	77	11	255	34	1387	344
Northumbria			9		80	7		89
North Yorkshire	22		10		25	1		57
Oxfordshire	35	1						35
Shropshire			82	2	40	2		122
Somerset			5		61	1		66
Staffordshire	171	1	29		85		1360	285
Warwickshire	62	1	30					62
West Midlands	147	3					684	147
West Sussex	50	3	4		25	1	314	75
West Yorkshire	42	2	74	3	52	1	577	168
Wales								
Clwyd	48	6	25	6	21	1	891	46
Dyfed	59	2	9		5			73
Gwent	83	1			41	1		124
Mid Glamorgan	68	1			38	2	840	106
West Glamorgan					12	2		12
Powys					25	2		25
Total houses surveyed 1987/88 = 2583			1989 = 1355		1990 = 1556		Grand Total 5494	

Courtesy of CIEH and Dr M. Courtis.

information gained to mount further surveys in the vicinity.

It should be appreciated that such 'cold marketing' techniques may generate a very limited response unless there is some prior local anxiety about ambient radon levels in homes or businesses. It may well be possible to generate interest in such a survey (interest not anxiety!) by promoting the need for such surveys at committee/council meetings where the local media will readily pick up and report anything to do with radioactivity.

In an area suspected of elevated radon concentration where simple circulars have not had the desired response rate, it may be necessary to go onto house-by-house surveys by trained technical officers who, hopefully, will encourage householders to participate after explaining the objectives of the survey.

While this method is arguably very expensive and resource-intensive, it does tend to produce the best uptake, provided technical officers have been trained to the correct competence level and have a sufficient grasp of the subject to convince householders of the health department's scientific credibility in mounting such radon surveys.

NRPB surveys
Following on from its first national survey in 1984/85, involving 2309 randomly-selected houses by postcode, the NRPB mounted a selective regional survey of 700 homes, mostly in Devon, Cornwall, Derbyshire and Caithness.

The average radon concentration measured in homes across the UK was found to be around 20 Bq m^{-3}, but the selected, geologically radon-active regions produced a mean level of 200 Bq m^{-3}, with a 'high' of 8000 Bq m^{-3} [8].

The NRPB [10] has ascertained that so far approximately 17 700 homes suffer radon in excess of the current action level (200 Bq m^{-3}) from 191 000 tests completed; further results are awaited. It extrapolates these figures to estimate that nationally, out of a total housing stock of some 23 million houses, around 103 500 will be over the action level.

A similar exercise carried out by the IEHO on the basis of its first national survey in 1987/88, produced an estimate of 230 000 houses over the present action level – a factor of two difference [11].

STANDARDS – ACTION LEVELS AND AFFECTED AREAS FOR HOMES AND OTHER BUILDINGS

Various national governments and international agencies – most notably the International Com-

mission on Radiological Protection (ICRP) and WHO – have sought over the years to establish and revise radiological protection standards as the state of knowledge concerning risk has grown.

Existing homes

There are currently some ten different national/international recommendations for radon limitation in existing homes, ranging from a 'low' of 150 Bq m^{-3} (7.5 mSv y^{-1}) in the USA, to a 'high' of 800 Bq m^{-3} (40 mSv y^{-1}) in Norway, Sweden and Finland (soon to be revised) [9].

The UK's current action level of 200 Bq m^{-3} (10 mSv y^{-1}) for existing homes was adopted by the government in January 1990, after the NRPB had revised its assessment of risk in line with new experimental and epidemiological evidence from the ICRP, the US National Research Council (NRC) and the United Nations Scientific Committee on the Effects of Atomic Radiation (UNSCEAR). It seems highly likely that other countries will soon follow the US and UK lead towards lower limit values.

New homes

A narrower band of international recommendations applies to radon limitation standards for new homes, ranging from 140 Bq m^{-3} (7 mSv y^{-1}) in Sweden to 250 Bq m^{-3} (12.5 mSv y^{-1} in Germany.

The NRPB's current advice to the UK government reflects the widespread criticism levelled at its previous recommendation, which targeted new-build at one quarter the old action level for existing homes, i.e. 100 Bq m^{-3} (5 mSv y^{-1}) 'as the basis for implementing changes to building procedures in areas of the country where high levels of radon are likely' [12].

Thus the latest recommendation for new (and future) homes is that they 'should be so constructed that radon concentrations are as low as reasonably practicable and at least below 200 Bq m^{-3}' [9], i.e. **no more** than the action level for existing homes, and incidentally **double** the previous recommendation.

Department of the Environment interim guidance on the construction of new dwellings

When originally introduced in 1988, this enhancement and extension of the Building Regulations to require radon proofing measures to be incorporated in newbuild houses in certain high-risk areas of Cornwall and small parts of Devon was well received for specifying a (then) lower limit of 200 Bq m^{-3} (10 mSv y^{-1}) when the prevailing action level was twice that figure (Building Regulations 1985, Part C: Site Preparation and Resistance to Moisture).

However, the Department of the Environment's revision and expansion of the risk areas to include the whole of Cornwall, Devon and parts of Somerset, Derbyshire, Northamptonshire and the Scottish regions of Highland and Grampian, where significant radon hot spots have been found is to be applauded.

Affected areas

This concept was introduced early in 1990 by the NRPB in its *Board Statement on Radon in Homes* [9] 'so as to concentrate effort on radon where it is most needed'. While admitting that any such criteria are likely to be arbitrary, it suggested that affected areas would comprise a 1% probability of present homes, or of future homes **without** preventative measures, being above 200 Bq m^{-3} (10 mSv y^{-1}).

On 7 November 1990, Cornwall and Devon were formally declared affected areas based upon the results of over 8000 radon tests in the two counties [13]. This new status encourages all home-owners to have (free) radon measurements made, and requires builders and developers to incorporate radon-proofing measures in newbuild within certain worst-affected localities. Affected areas can only be defined by the NRPB, based upon the best available radiological evidence relative to geological or other physical phenomena.

It seems logical, therefore, to suggest that, for the 1% affected area criterion to be satisfied, **at least** 1½% of homes in a given study locality would need to be tested (as applied in Devon and Cornwall), to give a statistically significant sample on which to base assessment. Extended nationally, this would require pro rata tests, some 1 000 000, when only around 200 000 (<20%) have been carried out to date. As at April 1994, it was estimated that **only** around 2000 (11%) homes had been remedied out of 18 000 found to be above the current action level, which is, in turn, a paltry 1.9% of the NRPB's projected UK total of 105 500 houses affected, an insignificant 0.9% of CIEH's estimated 230 000 homes affected above the action level. We clearly have a long way to go down the survey route before we can be confident that we have truly grasped the reality of the national radon problem.

Occupational exposure

The Ionizing Radiation Regulations 1985 and its associated approved code of practice (ACOP) form the necessary backdrop to any assessment of risk and the formulation of protection standards against excessive radon exposure in the workplace.

The subsequent reassessment of risk estimates by the NRPB in November 1987 [14] (following the earlier ICRP 1987 Como Statement) lead to a recommendation that for the most exposed groups of workers, individual exposures should be so controlled as not to exceed an average dose of 15 mSv y^{-1}. While the legal dose limit for workers remains at 50 mSv y^{-1}, most industries rightly aim to keep doses to their employees as low as reasonably achievable, and the NRPB's 15 mSv y^{-1} has now become *de facto* the effective acceptable 'never exceed' standard.

In assessing occupational exposures, the term working level month (WLM) will be encountered, which is essentially a traditional American mining unit related to radon daughter exposure. One working level (WL) equates to the emission of 1.3 × 10^8 MeV of alpha energy from any combination of radon-222 short-lived decay products (daughters) in 1 m^3 of air. One WLM is the exposure resulting from a concentration of 1 WL for 170 hours.

The ACOP sets the practical annual limit (2000) hours for radon daughter exposure at 4

WLM, and categorizes workplace exposure at 0.1 WL (controlled areas; 8-hour radon gas concentration equivalent of 1000 Bq m^{-3}) and 0.03 WL (supervized areas; 8-hour radon gas concentration equivalent of 400 Bq m^{-3}). All controlled area employees must undergo personal dose assessment utilizing personal dosemeters (identical to standard domestic radon detectors and usually work on the safety helmet).

The Health and Safety Executive has published a detailed guidance circular on the application and enforcement of the Ionizing Radiation Regulations by local authority environmental health officers and others which, while providing valuable technical advice, was rightly criticized for being too traditionalist in its perception of risk areas [15], when first introduced.

The HSE's response, embodied in their Information Document HSE 560/20 of January 1992, widened their definition of 'Geographical Areas of Concern' into Derbyshire, Northamptonshire, Somerset, Grampian and the Highlands of Scotland.

It also, at last, referenced the synergistic link between smoking and radon, extolling the health benefits of restraint. **The inclusion of a suitable disclaimer and list of organizations known to supply dosimeters and provide a survey results analysis service was also welcomed.**

However, these limited initiatives were clearly still not properly addressing the perceived widespread risk of significant occupational exposure potential, particularly for workplaces within radon-affected areas.

Mounting pressure on HSE lead them into piloting a mailshot-based (passive) workplace radon survey protocol from their Plymouth Regional Office in February 1993, which was to be expanded nationally during 1994 as the recommended approach to workplace radon exposure.

This 'low-key', low-resource approach is certainly worthwhile, but has been criticized by the Association of District Councils (ADC) as lacking the necessary enforcement rigour that only a fully revised LA Advice Circular could properly address. Accordingly the following protocol for 'Radon in Workplace and Buildings: Measurement and Control' has been put forward by the

ADC and NRPB as a basis for future professional advice. It is currently being evaluated by the HSE.

1. All workplace buildings in Radon Affected Areas should be measured (Affected Areas as defined by the NRPB). At present they include Cornwall, Devon, Northamptonshire and parts of Somerset and Derbyshire. As other areas are likely to be identified through the UK, workplace measurements should extend on a priority basis accordingly.

2. Measurements should be made with track-etch detectors. These devices record the time-integrated concentration of radon during the period of deployment. NRPB operates a validation scheme for laboratories making measurements of radon in homes. These laboratories are also competent to make measurements in other buildings. (The current list is given in Table 42.5: it is updated regularly by NRPB.)

Table 42.5 Laboratories currently validated by NRPB for radon measurements in homes

Kodak	Radon Control
c/o Foxtrot Security Ltd	35 Exeter Street
7 De Vere Gardens	North Tawton
Kensington, London W8 4AR	Devon EX20 2HB
NE Technology	Siemens Plessey Controls Ltd
Bath Road	
Beenham	Sopers Lane
Reading RG7 5PR	Poole
	Dorset BH17 7ER
NRPB	TASL
Chilton	HH Wills Physics
Didcot	Laboratory
Oxon OX11 0RQ	Tyndalls Avenue
	Bristol BS8 1TL

3. Track-etch detectors should be deployed in rooms or similar parts of workplaces that are routinely occupied. Since radon comes into buildings mainly from the ground, the detectors should be deployed in ground floor or basement rooms as appropriate.

4. Detectors should be deployed in one-third of all such rooms with at least two detectors for each separate building and one for each 100 m² of floor space. They should be placed on convenient surfaces such as desks or shelves out of direct sunlight, heat and draughts and measures taken to ensure they are not disturbed.

5. Detectors should be left in place for any period of 3 months and then returned to the laboratory for assessment. The laboratory determines the concentration of radon recorded by each detector during the period of deployment. It then applies a seasonal adjustment to each value so as to calculate the concentration during winter months: adjustment factors recommended by NRPB are given in Table 42.6. (*Note*: measurements can thus be made at any time of year with a high degree of confidence.)

Table 42.6 Seasonal adjustment of 3-month radon results to obtain average concentrations during winter months

Period of deployment	Adjustment factor
January to March	1.00
February to April	1.14
March to May	1.32
April to June	1.58
May to July	2.00
June to August	2.25
July to September	2.18
August to October	1.75
September to November	1.42
October to December	1.21
November to January	1.04
December to February	1.00

Note: Measured concentrations are multiplied by the appropriate factor.

6. The laboratory reports the individual values of the adjusted concentrations in Bq m⁻³, the symbol for becquerel per cubic metre, which represents the activity concentration of radon gas in air.

7. Reported values above 400 Bq m⁻³ are *prime facie* evidence that the radon progeny concentration exceeds 0.03 WL during normal working hours. With a value of 0.4 for the equilibrium factor, 400 Bq m⁻³ corresponds to 0.043 WL: the margin allows for higher concentrations in non-working hours. WL is the symbol for Working Level in which the potential alpha-energy concentration of radon progeny is expressed.

8. When any reported concentration exceeds 400 Bq m⁻³, the employer should be advised to reduce radon below this value so as to avoid the need for compliance with the Ionising Radiations Regulations 1985.

9. If an employer challenges the assumption that an annual average of 400 Bq m⁻³ is more than 0.03 WL, he should be invited to determine radon progeny concentrations during normal working hours in winter. Measurements should be made for 20 consecutive work days under normal conditions in the room with the highest reported radon concentration. Instruments should be of suitable design with calibration at NRPB before and after the exercise.

10. If an employer chooses not to reduce the radon concentrations but to comply with the Regulations, he will need to meet certain requirements determined by the highest reported concentration. These are given in Table 42.7 for 400, 1200 and 4000 Bq m⁻³, which are deemed to correspond to 0.03, 0.1 and 0.3 WL during working hours. For the full requirements, reference should be made to the Regulations and the associated sub-regulatory documents.

Table 42.7 Requirements for compliance with the Ionising Radiations Regulations 1985 at various radon concentrations in buildings

Radon (Bq m⁻³)	Regulatory requirement
400–1200	Notification of circumstance Designation of supervised area
1200–4000	Designation of controlled area Investigation of circumstance
4000	Limitation of concentration

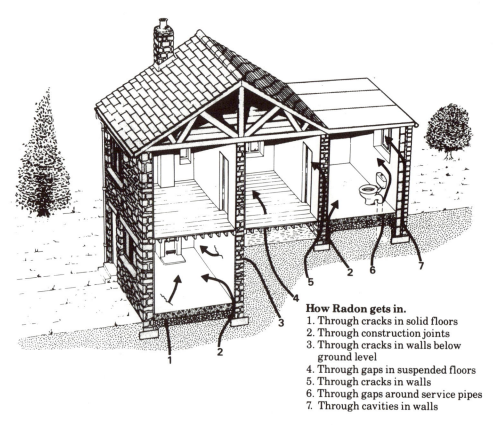

How Radon gets in.
1. Through cracks in solid floors
2. Through construction joints
3. Through cracks in walls below
   ground level
4. Through gaps in suspended floors
5. Through cracks in walls
6. Through gaps around service pipes
7. Through cavities in walls

Fig. 42.6 Entry of radon in buildings. (Source: Department of the Environment *The Householder's Guide to Radon*, 3rd edn, HMSO, London. Courtesy of the Controller of HMSO.)

11. Radon concentrations should be reduced as much as reasonably practicable below 400 Bq m^{-3}. There are a number of ways of doing so as shown in the Householders' Guide to Radon published by DOE. The most reliable and effective method is to create a slightly negative pressure under the floor with a low power fan. Reduction factors of an order of magnitude are readily achieved. Installation and running costs are not high. A list of organizations with a record of successful radon reductions is available from the local Council Environmental Health Department and many firms are now offering to guarantee their work as an added reassurance.

12. Radon measurements should be repeated for any workplace building in an Affected Area that has been extended or structurally modified to an appreciable extent, i.e. sufficient to justify planning approval. Buildings in which action has been taken to reduce radon concentrations should be re-measured every 2 years to ensure that the actions remain effective. Reduction methods that depend on mechanical devices should include monitoring arrangements such as simple manometers in the fan system. Repairs to reduction systems should be effected without delay.

REMEDIAL MEASURES AGAINST RADON INGRESS

The principal motive force behind radon ingress to buildings is the minute negative pressure differences inside caused by heating and/or wind effects, and usually comprises no more than a few pascals in magnitude.

Restricted ventilation (double glazing, draught stripping and sealed flues) in modern homes, to help conserve valuable heat, limits the ability of the small amounts of incoming fresh air to effect meaningful dilution and hence radiation concentrations increase. Radon is thus drawn inside buildings through a variety of entry routes as shown in Fig. 42.6.

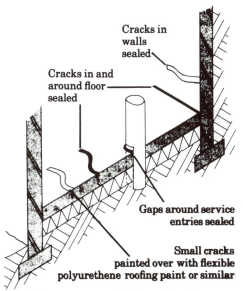

Painting over or sealing cracks and service entries in solid floors, and cracks in walls against the ground. It is important to achieve an airtight seal. Pay particular attention to cracks around the edges of rooms.

Fig. 42.9 Sealing cracks and service entry points. (Source: Department of the Environment, *The Householder's Guide to Radon*, 3rd edn, HMSO, London.)

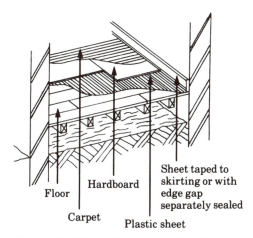

Suspended timber floor covered with a plastic sheet. A plastic sheet can also be used on solid floors (but not over wood block floors) as an alternative to sealing just the cracks. Edges should be well sealed.

Fig. 42.7 Simple DIY treatment. (Source: Department of the Environment: *The Householder's Guide to Radon*, 3rd edn, HSMO, London.)

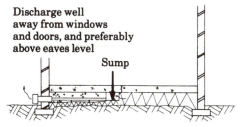

A radon sump beneath a solid floor with a fan to depressurise the soil.

Fig. 42.8 Increased sub-floor ventilation. (Source: Department of the Environment, *The Householder's Guide to Radon*, 3rd edn, HMSO, London.)

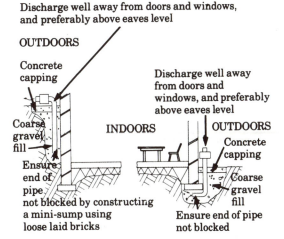

Fig. 42.10 Radon collection sump (side excavation). (Source: Department of the Environment, *The Householder's Guide to Radon*, 3rd edn, HMSO, London.)

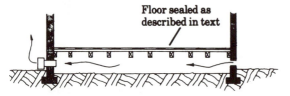

Enhancing ventilation under a suspended floor with an increased number of air bricks. A fan may also be fitted (see text).

Fig. 42.11 Sub-floor sump with fan. (Source: Department of the Environment, *The Householder's Guide to Radon*, 3rd edn, HMSO, London.)

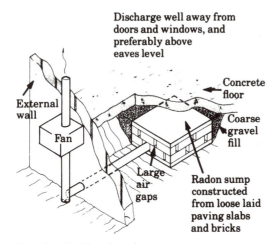

Fig. 42.12 Construction of a radon sump. (Source: Department of the Environment, *The Householder's Guide to Radon*, 3rd edn, HMSO, London.)

As radon enters as gas mixed with air, all remedial measures are geared up to prevent the gas penetrating living areas.

Most effective measures to keep radon out of buildings rely on a combination of preventative measures (Figs 42.7–42.12):

1. seal entry routes (above);
2. pressurize living areas (especially ground-floor rooms);
3. depressurize/extract air from sub floors/sub foundations;
4. provide dilution through excess ventilation of living areas.

In the latter respect (4), however, ventilation practices need to be carefully controlled, as tests have shown that an emphasis on ventilating upper floors and using open fires with unrestricted flues downstairs will tend to **increase** depressurization of ground-floor rooms and thereby exacerbate radon entry.

The Department of the Environment's *A Householder's Guide to Radon* [16] provides valuable information and comparable rough costings on radon proofing; it emphasizes the possibility of DIY remedies for the less technical and non-arduous tasks.* Whether carried out by the gifted amateur or reputable contractor, the essential element of all remedial work is that it must be performed to a high quality standard, as any shoddy workmanship would soon be revealed in a subsequent radon test, which is the only real way to check the effectiveness of radon-proofing measures. Also worth noting is that to qualify for a grant under the Housing and Local Government Act 1989 (see below), a subsequent test **must** prove that radon reduction to at least below the action level has been attained.

Remedial action timescales

Both the *Householder's Guide to Radon* [15] and the NRPB *Board Statement on Radon in Homes* [9] give similar suggested timescales for remedial action at various radon concentrations with the underlying exhortation that (the affected householder) 'should take action as soon as is reasonably practicable'.

Presumably, these tables relate directly to risk assessment, but take a median line covering households, including smokers and non-smokers. The graph at Fig. 42.13 depicts these median

---

* Also see Building Research Establishment Guides to Radon Remedial Measures in Existing Dwellings – these are aimed at builders who carry out remedial work and those competent at DIY.

values and **estimates** the effect of the **additional** risk to smokers – and, conversely, the **diminished** risk to non-smokers – in projections for their likely action timescales. Thus a smoker living in a house at the action level ought to install a remedy, ideally within 2¼ years; conversely, his or her non-smoking neighbour might not worry for 20 years, or more (but the overall timescale suggests 7½ years, so prudence dictates that this lower figure should be accepted for non-smokers, too). While this graphical exercise is meant to be scientifically definitive, it demonstrates again that perhaps habitual smokers in high radon areas warrant particular priority in terms of prompt assistance with remedial works for radon proofing (or, preferably, specifically targeted health education campaigning to encourage them to stop the habit for good).

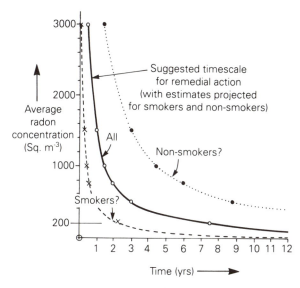

Fig. 42.13 Radon proofing. (Source: figures supplied by NRPB.)

RADON IN WATER SUPPLIES

Whilst it is well known that radon emanates from uranium-rich fissured rock strata and is highly soluble in toluene, its moderate solubility in water is a key transport mechanism for bringing radon to the surface, especially via cold ground water

which usually contains high ^{222}Rn concentrations. Therefore, the highest concentrations of radon usually emanate from deep ground water sources such as is found in deep wells and springs emerging from deep aquifers in areas of susceptible geology.

Whilst this water may be sufficiently aerated and freed from its radon burden if allowed to stand a while once drawn from the tap, it may be ingested immediately, when radon can diffuse through the stomach/intestine walls and be thence transported, via the bloodstream to the lungs, before being eventually exhaled. It has been calculated that the ingestion dose is approximately 10% of the inhalation dose, so in certain **affected areas** radon-rich water entering the home must first be purged before consumption. It has been estimated* that the following domestic processes release appropriate amounts of radon into the indoor atmosphere, which could equate to 1–2% (and normally not more than 10%) of the total radon entering the house.

Dish*/clothes washers	0.95	liberated in indoor air
Showering	0.66	"
Bath	0.42	"
Drinking	0.35	"
Toilet flushing	0.35	"

* Releases most entrained ^{222}Ru.

Generally speaking, it has been estimated that for each 100 Bq 1^{-1} of radon in water, there is an added 10 Bq m^{-3} of radon in air, which is equivalent to an annual dose of 0.5 mSv (50% of the principal ICRP dose limit).

Standards for radon in water

WHO guidelines on **committed effective dose** for radon in water ingestion equate to 50 mSv per year, which is equivalent to a referenced annual intake of 5000 Bq per year. However, it is significant to realize the WHO assumptions are based on an average intake per person of 2 litres a day, of which half should be via tap water and, in addition, water-based cold drinks will be consumed to the tune of approximately 0.12 litres per day (50 litres per year). It can thence be calculated that the (guideline) reference level should be set at approximately 100 Bq l^{-1}.

The normal radon concentrations in ground water are given in Table 42.8.

Table 42.8 Normal average radon concentrations in ground water

Surface waters (average)	= 0.5–1 Bq l^{-1}
Ground waters (average)	= 7.5–25 Bq l^{-1}
Ground waters (Devon/ Cornwall)	= 50–1000 Bq l^{-1}
Highest UK*	= 100 000 Bq m^{-3}
Highest USA	= >1 000 000 Bq m^{-3}

*Mine/cave water readings may reach *several* million Bq m^{-3} in Devon and Cornwall.

Sampling for radon in water

1. Bucket/well sample
Use kilner jars with a sealed lid.

Method:

(a) Draw a fresh quantity of water into a container. Fully immerse the lid and the jar. Remove lid under water and fill completely. Fit lid and seal *under* water.

2. Tap samples
Use a small vial.

Method:

(a) Remove any tap aerators that may be present.
(b) Run the water for approximately 10 minutes.
(c) Adjust flow to a slow run (no air bubbles apparent).
(d) *Completely* fill 2 small vials of water.
(e) Rapidly despatch all samples to the laboratory for analysis.

Basic laboratory techniques

The most common methods employed are:

1. **Gamma spectroscopy** usually employs a sodium iodide crystal or germanium lithium scintillator which counts the gamma radiation emitted by radon progeny.
2. **Direct liquid scintillation** – Water is injected into a glass scintillation vial and a toluene fluor added. Radon extracts into the toluene and the mixture separates to a transparent phase. The alpha particles 'flash' and light is emitted which is counted via a photomultiplier tube and suitable electronics.
3. **Alpha track detection** – In affected properties a rapid estimate of any ground water radon concentrations can be obtained using standard alpha-track polymer detectors installed in the WC system. An inverted cup at the water surface with alpha-track detector affixed at the top, is left in place for 3–6 months and returned to the supplier laboratory; the 'standard' method for etching and direct counting of alpha-tracks directly relates to radon concentration.

Other methods include extraction concentration count and alpha scinillation count.

Control methods

Three basic generic approaches are usually employed:

1. **Remove entrained radon after water has been drawn from the supply.** This method requires good ventilation of bathrooms, laundries, showers and kitchens and this is often sufficient in itself to prevent appreciable radon build up. However, depressurizing the house could increase the influx of soil gas and restrict proper ventilation.
2. **Remove radon from the water before it reaches the breathing zone of habitable areas:**
   (a) **Storage** – Store freshly drawn radon-laden water and leave for 13 days, which gives a 90% reduction. However, this is not a practical method for normal use and can only be employed where large capacity storage systems can be employed.
   (b) **Aeration and heating** – Aeration of water to purge radon is obtained by increasing the surface area through spraying into a vessel vented safely to atmosphere.

Alternatives utilize a compressed air treatment, a contraflow cascade (termed 'packed tower aeration') or heating elements.

3. **Filtration**. This is the most practical method often employed in domestic situations and utilizes an activated carbon absorption medium (granular activated carbon (GAC)).

ADMINISTRATIVE AND FINANCIAL ISSUES

Confidentiality

Whilst brief mention was made in the section headed 'Local Authority Monitoring' above, of the practical operational implications of the current NRPB policy on maintaining confidentiality of its test results only to participating householders (not to the local authority environmental health officer, unless by prior approval), it should be clearly understood that the utmost discretion should be exercised in respect of divulging results. For most people, their home is their biggest investment asset: they often rely on its growing collateral for future prosperity. Any threat to its ultimate sales potential through radon blight would be reprehensible, and environmental health officers involved in radon survey work should act accordingly. Results – particularly high ones – should only be made known to the householder concerned and officers on a 'need to know' basis: when not in use they should be locked away and not freely discussed in public.

However, having carried out a test at the local authority's expense, such results could and should form the basis for further surveys in the vicinity of a newly discovered hot spot, even if the original householder chooses not to act to remedy his or her property (in spite of the local environmental health officer's encouragement to do so).

The acid test for confidentiality vis-à-vis public protection comes at the time of sale or resale, particularly where vendors have failed to agree to environmental health officers revealing radon test results on solicitor's property searches. Clearly, legal advice should be sought from individual council solicitors, but the over-riding principle must lean towards public protection. The potential health risk posed to an innocent and possibly young family unknowingly exposing themselves to high radon levels is such that the test **occurrence** should first be revealed to the purchaser's solicitor with a view to direct enquiry of the vendor's solicitor of the actual result. If, in spite of exhortations, it is still not forthcoming, the environmental health officer's professional duty is clearly to reveal the test result to the purchaser's solicitor, after due legal consideration.

Until such time as a mandatory radon test certificate is built into conveyancing procedures – possibly incorporated within the much-vaunted 'house log-book' – this dilemma will remain with us.

House renovation grants

Under the provisions of the Local Government and Housing Act 1989, local authorities may approve an application for a renovation grant (see section 101(2)(a)) to ensure that the dwelling or building complies with such requirements with respect to construction or physical condition as may from time to time be specified by the Secretary of State for the purposes of this section (section 115(3)(f)).

The detailed guidance from the relevant Department of the Environment Circular [17] specifies in paragraphs 64 and 65 (and the Annex B, section 3, specification) that radon-proofing works necessary to reduce domestic radon levels below the prevailing action level will rank for discretionary grant, subject to a follow-up confirmatory test to a standard specified by the NRPB (essentially a 3–6 month passive trackctch detector screening test from an accredited laboratory).

Most unfortunately, the Department of the Environment's provisions to offer monetary aid for affected householders to combat radon could founder on the financial hardship 'test of resources' criteria ('means testing') intended to direct financial assistance to the most needy cases, In reality, the vast majority of house owners will have to find their radon proofing finances themselves – from perhaps a second mortgage or bank loan – unless they elect a DIY approach. However, people on income support or in receipt of housing benefit may still qualify for grant, if the local authority exercises its discretion favourably and annual Housing Investment Programme allocations are not fully/over committed elsewhere. It is significant that a mere handful of grants (less than 12) have been awarded for radon mitigation in England and Wales in the past 4 years – a clear indication of current Department of Environment policy which has been severely criticized by many leading authorities on the subject [18].

As a serious health threat has now been officially recognized in radon, it seems perverse to deny *mandatory* grant aid to all affected householders, so that we may quickly find and eradicate high radon from an NRPB estimated 0.5% of our national housing stock (or 230 000 homes/1% according to the CIEH).

NATIONAL AND REGIONAL REPRESENTATIVE BODIES DIRECTLY INVOLVED IN RADON

1. Government advisers
   (a) National Radiological Protection Board (NRPB), Chilton, Didcot, Oxon OX11 0LQ. Tel: 01235 831600.
   (b) Building Research Establishment (BRE), Garston, Watford WD2 7JR. Tel: 01923 664707.
   (c) Health & Safety Executive (HSE), Baynards Place, 1 Chepstow Place, London W2 4TF. Tel: 0171 243 6000.
2. Professional/trade representative bodies
   (a) Royal Institute of British Architects, 66 Portland Place, London W1N 4AD.
   (b) Federation of Master Builders, Gordon Fisher House, 14/15 St James Street, London WC1N 3DP.
   (c) Building Employers Confederation, 82 New Cavendish Street, London WC1N 3DP.
   (d) National House Building Council, 58 Portland Place, London W1N 4B6.
   (e) The Radon Council, PO Box 39, Shepperton, Middlesex TW17 8AD.
   (f) Chartered Institute of Environmental Health, Chadwick Court, 15 Hatfields, London SE1 8DJ.
   (g) South West Radon Committee, c/o Environmental Health Department, Teignbridge District Council, Forde House, Newton Abbot, Devon TQ12 4XX.
   (h) Northamptonshire Steering Group on Radon, c/o Borough Environmental Health Officer, Wellingborough Borough Council, 20 Sheep Street, Wellingborough, Northants NN8 1BL.

REFERENCES

1. Royal Commission on Environmental Pollution (1984) *Tackling Pollution – Experience and Prospects*. 10th Report, Cmnd 9149, HMSO, London.
2. International Commission on Radiological Protection (1984) *Principles for Limiting Exposure of the Public from Natural Resources of Radiation*, Pergamon Press/ICRP Publication 39 Ann ICRP, 14, No.1.
3. Green, B.R.M.G., Brown, L., Cliff, K.D., Bristol, C.M.H., Miles, J.C.H. and Wrixon, A.D. (1985) Surveys of natural radiation exposure in UK dwellings with passive and active measurement techniques. *Science of the Total Environment*, **45**, 459–66.
4. National Radiological Protection Board (1987) *Exposure to Radon Daughters in Dwellings*, NRPB GS, 6, HMSO, London.
5. *Hansard* (House of Commons), 27 January 1987, wls 189–97.
6. National Radiological Protection Board (1989) *Living with Radiation*, HMSO, London.
7. Edited extracts from Bowie, S.H.U. and Plant, J.A. (1983) *Natural Radioactivity in the Environment, Applied Environmental Geochemistry*, Academic Press. London.
8. Clarke, R. and O'Riordan, M.C. (1990) Rumours of radon. *Science and Public Affairs*, **5(2)**, 25–36.

9. Documents of the NRPB (1990) *Board Statement on Radon in Homes*, Vol. 1. No. 1, HMSO, London.

10. Kendall, G.M. *et al. NRPB – R272 Exposure to Radon in UK Dwellings*, HMSO.

11. Institution of Environmental Health Officers (1988) *Report of the IEHO Survey on Radon in Homes 1987/8*, IEHO, London.

12. National Radiological Protection Board (1987) *Exposure to Radon Daughters in Dwellings*, NRPB ASP 10, HMSO, London.

13. Documents of the NRPB (1990) *Radon Affected Areas: Cornwall and Devon*, Vol. 1, No. 4, HMSO, London.

14. National Radiological Protection Board, *Interim Guidance on the Implications of Recent Revisions of Risk Estimates and the ICRP Como Statement*, NRPB, 659, HSMO, London.

15. Health and Safety Executive (1989) *LAC Legal (L) 2/6/90 Ionizing Radiation Regulations 1985 (IRR 85) Exposure to Radon in Buildings*, HMSO, London.

16. Department of the Environment (1992) *The Householder's Guide to Radon*, 3rd edn, HMSO, London.

17. Department of the Environment (1990) *Local Government and Housing Act 1989 House Renovation Grants*, Circular 12/90, HMSO, London.

18. Department of The Environment (1993) *British Attitudes to Radiation and the Paradox of Radon*, Professor T. Lee, University of St Andrews.

APPENDIX

CASE STUDY: RADON, THE NORTHAMPTONSHIRE APPROACH

M. Jones

Borough Environmental Health Officer, Wellingborough Borough Council

There are seven district councils in Northamptonshire, but initially only two took part in the first IEHO national survey in 1987/88 each placing monitors in only six houses, for which 25% showed readings above the government action level of 200 Bq m^{-3}.

The high readings were unexpected, as there is no granite in the county of Northamptonshire. The other known geology to give elevated readings on occasions was limestone; however, from the geological maps the houses affected were not built on limestone, but on Northampton Sand ironstone bearing strata. For the second IEHO survey during the winter of 1988/89, a total of four local authorities in the county took part. Taking advice and looking to monitor dwellings built on Northampton Sand strata, all four local authorities found properties with high readings. Detectors in properties built on other geological strata showed no elevated readings.

By this time it was appreciated the problem was not peculiar to one local authority and an officer working party was set up with a representative from each district council and one from the county council to explore this phenomenon. It was agreed research was required to investigate the cause and extent of the problem via Leicester University Geological Department.

Fortuitous research for an environmental science student's degree thesis proved most interesting and showed that radon levels in soil gas varied considerably and indicated it could be linked closely to geology. It was realized that much more detailed research was needed and all district councils and the County Council agreed to fund a research assistant at Leicester University to carry out a study.

The questions environmental health officers needed answers to were:

1. What is the extent of the radon problem in Northamptonshire?
2. What is the cause of the radon?
3. Is it possible to predict radon potential in new buildings?

During the research a close working relationship developed between the Research Assistant, the British Geological Survey (BGS) and the National Radiological Protection Board (NRPB). The BGS advised on methodology for soil gas readings and NRPB for validation of the equipment.

The work involved using an Integrated Gamma-Spectrometer and a Portable Radiation Monitor (with Lucas Cell Adaptor) and a Passive Radon Gas Detector.

As the research developed it was felt the outcome could be a map of the county showing radon potential of the various soils, taking into account a number of factors including:

1. radon in soil gas;
2. porosity of soil, subsoil and underlying strata;
3. in-house radon results.

In the course of the research as many excavations as possible were examined, not only to obtain first hand information, but to confirm the strata accorded on published geological maps. There was also the need to identify the radon source. At the time the group were fortunate to have a number of major road works under construction and this enabled detailed examination to be made of vertical sections and strata as cuttings were formed. It soon became evident that the Northampton Sand strata was not only porous and fissured, but also contained, mainly near its base, a scattering of phosphatic nodules (pebbles). Specimens of these were taken to the University to analyse for uranium content and some nodules were found to exceed 50 ppm.

During the research project over 3500 soil gas radon readings were taken covering all the various geological deposits outcropping in the county. Median^{222}Rn values for each deposit were calculated.

A third consideration was the results of in-house monitoring for radon. Free access to these results was hampered because of the NRPB's unwillingness to divulge the result for any address other than to the occupier, because of confidentiality rules, and this study relied upon householders being prepared to inform local authorities of their results when they became available. However, over 1000 household results were able to be incorporated into the equation. This comparison has allowed a haphazard assessment to be made for each geological formation and deposit.

A Northamptonshire Radon Hazard Map has now been produced by Leicester University Geological Department based on digitized geological maps obtained from the BGS. The final map shows solid geology and drift, however solid and drift maps are also presented separately. Each geological deposit has been placed into one of four hazard groups on the map:

Group 1   Low hazard
Group 2   Slight hazard
Group 3   Moderate hazard
Group 4   Elevated hazard

The definitions of these hazards varies not only with the level of radon in the soil gas, but with the geological strata, i.e. porous or impervious and with the known in-house reading.

The Northamptonshire Radon Hazard Map shows what is most likely to occur under normal conditions. As more data become available some geological formations may move from one hazard group to another, but it is hoped it will facilitate better consideration of the need for precautions being taken when building new dwellings and commercial premises.

This research has been funded for almost 3 years and although there are still many questions left unanswered, the local authorities involved felt that, whilst they had sufficient basic information to enable them to carry out their environmental protection functions, the research had been very worthwhile at a cost of approximately £4000 to each authority.

43 Waste management

Jeff Cooper

INTRODUCTION

Unlike air and water pollution, national legislation to prevent pollution from solid wastes was only introduced in the twentieth century. Before the introduction of the Control of Pollution Act (COPA) in 1974, legislative provision was based on local Acts or permissive powers in legislation, normally covering other aspects of pollution or public health. Indeed, many sections of the Control of Pollution Act 1974 Part I, Waste on Land, were not implemented because the necessary regulations were not introduced for many years. Section 1, which placed a duty on each waste disposal authority (WDA) to arrange for the disposal of all controlled waste in its area, had never been implemented and now Part I of the 1974 Act has been superseded by Part II of the Environmental Protection Act 1990 (EPA).

One of the major influences on the way the UK government legislates for the control of solid waste is and increasingly will be the EU, together with its obligations under international treaties. These factors will become even more important as the 1990s progress, particularly when members of the EU ought to conform to uniform standards of solid waste pollution control in order to achieve market equality.

At present, the enforcement of such standards is weak and is likely to remain so for much of the decade until the EU-wide environmental protection agency becomes effective. Therefore, while Britain may not emulate the standards of solid waste management adopted by Germany, Denmark or the Netherlands due to difficulties with landfill, it will undoubtedly remain in advance of the southern Mediterranean countries for the rest of the century.

EARLY PROVISION OF WASTE DISPOSAL SERVICES (see also Chapter 1)

Legislative provision for the collection and disposal of waste in the UK before and during the nineteenth century was extremely patchy. Arrangements for the regular clearance of wastes from streets, privies, middens and ash pits was recognized as fundamental to improve the health of towns, but until late in the century these needs were met by the passage of private Acts of Parliament empowering individual towns to undertake these necessary measures.

Usually the privilege of collection and disposal of waste was sold to the highest bidder, in that in a largely agricultural country and with the majority of the waste being organic – from horse, human and food waste – the material was a valuable source of fertilizer, especially as it was frequently left *in situ* for weeks or months to mature. However, its quality could not always be guaranteed, as the following example from Windsor demonstrates:

'The ditches of which I have spoken are sometimes emptied by carts. And on the last occasion their contents were purchased for the sum of £15 by the occupier of land in the parish of Clewer, where meadows suffered from the extraordinary strength of the manure which was used without previous preparation.'[1].

The attempt made to provide a minimum level of cleansing provision through the Public Health Act 1848 failed because it was largely permissive, not compulsive. And although the Act was adopted by about 200 local authorities, this was inadequate given the need to establish minimum standards for public cleansing, especially after the repeal of the Corn Laws when waste became less valuable as competition from imported grain progressively impoverished the agricultural sector.

The multiplicity of bodies responsible for different aspects of public health and the continuing problem of, *inter alia*, poor waste collection and disposal practices led to the appointment of a Royal Sanitary Commission in 1869 to resolve the crisis. The resulting Local Government Act 1871 introduced sanitary districts throughout the country in 1872, and the appointment of a medical officer and an inspector of nuisances became obligatory for each district.

The Public Health Act 1875 thereafter consolidated, for areas outside London, the wide spread of laws relating to public health. This prescribed the duties of urban and rural sanitary districts which included, *inter alia*, responsibility for scavenging. Unlike the period before 1875, when appointed, the municipal scavengers were paid employees, and although clearance of waste was not always sufficiently frequent to avoid putrescible materials becoming a nuisance, the solid waste from houses was taken off by hand or horse-drawn cart to be disposed of, after any valuable components had been salvaged, by tipping or incineration.

BACKGROUND TO WASTE COLLECTION DISPOSAL AND ADMINISTRATION*

The collection of waste

Prior to the COPA, domestic solid waste was officially known as 'house refuse' for which there was no legal definition. However, it was accepted that it was the sort of refuse which arose from the ordinary domestic occupation of a dwelling. The main Act dealing with domestic refuse before COPA was the Public Health Act 1936. Under Section 72 a local authority could and, if required by the minister, had to undertake the removal of household refuse as respects the whole or any part of its area.

Surprisingly, perhaps, it was only with the introduction of the Collection and Disposal of Waste Regulations 1988, which enforced the provisions of sections 12–14 of COPA, that for the first time was every collection authority under a duty to collect household waste in its area.

The variation in the standards of refuse collection services provided by local authorities was examined in great detail in the Report of the Working Party on Refuse Storage and Collection [2] published in 1967, which revealed great diversity in the frequency of collection, types of material which were collected or not accepted for collection, and in the types of waste receptacle and equipment used for collection. Concern was also expressed about the lack of provision for the disposal of bulky waste, garden waste and cars, which were often disposed of in quiet country lanes, ditches or any other spot convenient for the increasingly affluent and mobile population.

The need for facilities for people to dispose of these types of waste was recognized by the introduction of a Private Member's Bill introduced by Duncan Sandys MP, which became the Civic Amenities Act 1967 subsequently revised as Refuse Disposal (Amenity) Act 1978. These Acts have permitted local authorities to establish civic amenity (CA) sites, more sensibly referred to as household waste disposal sites, tidy tips and by a number of other terms, including recycling centres, as the vast majority of sites now incorporates these facilities. Indeed, the duty to manage the site in return for salvage rights can be of financial advantage to the local authority. While most CA sites were managed by WDAs, section 51 of the EPA requires their management to be contracted out by the WDAs as well as the disposal of waste from these facilities.

---

* In January 1995 the Government announced that, for the first time, there should be a Waste Strategy for England and Wales. A consultation draft has been issued – 'A Waste Strategy for England and Wales. Consultation Draft 1995', DoE. This is essential background reading for the student.

The disposal of waste

Reports of the irresponsible disposal of toxic waste became steadily more prominent in the press during the 1960s, and the fear of contamination of water prompted government action. In 1964, the Minister of Housing and Local Government, together with the Secretary of State for Scotland, appointed the Technical Committee on the Disposal of Toxic Wastes. Its terms of reference were:

To consider present methods of disposal of solid and semi-solid toxic wastes from the chemical and allied industries, to examine suggestions for improvement, and to advise what, if any, changes are desirable in current practice, in the facilities available for disposal and in control arrangements, in order to ensure that such wastes are disposed of safely and without risk of polluting water supplies and rivers.'

The chairman of that Committee, Dr A. Key, had already chaired the Technical Committee on the Experimental Disposal of House Refuse in Wet and Dry Pits, which started work in 1953 and produced its report, *Pollution of Water by Tipped Refuse* [3] in 1961. Its terms of reference were:

'To define and generally guide experiments to be carried out at the Bushey Urban District Council's old sewage works on the tipping of household refuse of various categories under dry and wet conditions of deposit, with special reference to the pollution of underground water; to report on the results of the experiments; and to make recommendations as to their practical application.'

These early experiments confirmed the pollution potential of the percolate (now termed leachate) from freshly deposited refuse, but that this rapidly declined and that the use of sand and other materials placed at the base of landfills would considerably attentuate the pollution potential of household refuse.

The recommendations of the 1970 Key Report [4], the companion report of the Working Party on Refuse Disposal, produced in 1971 and the earlier Report on the Working Party on Refuse Storage and Collection 1967, were being incorporated into a comprehensive piece of environmental legislation when several incidents of fly-tipping of drums of toxic chemicals in the Midlands prompted a rapid legislative response.

The Deposit of Poisonous Waste Act 1972 was enacted in 20 days, and was the first piece of legislation worldwide to protect the environment from the dumping of hazardous waste. While it should have been repealed and replaced by COPA in 1974, the 1972 Act lasted until 1980 when the special waste consignment note system was brought in under the Control of Pollution (Special Wastes) Regulations 1980. These regulations were designed primarily to comply with internationally agreed obligations under the EC Directive on dangerous and toxic wastes (78/319/EEC). The consignment note system is similar to the notification requirements of the 1972 Act to provide cradle to grave notification, to ensure that Waste Regulation Authorities (WRAs) are able to monitor movements of special waste and the techniques of disposal.

The administration of waste disposal

Until 1965, responsibility for the disposal of house waste rested with the same authority which collected it, namely the metropolitan borough, county borough, or the urban or rural district council. However, this was recognized as increasingly unsatisfactory in metropolitan areas. Generally, waste disposal had to be undertaken through incineration, where standards of emission control were almost non-existent, or through the use of transfer stations where again spillage *en route* accounted for a proportion of the disposal.

In 1963, the London Government Act transferred responsibility for waste disposal to the Greater London Council (GLC) which effectively became the first WDA. The new and enlarged London boroughs retained responsibility for collection of house waste, but were directed by the GLC as to its ultimate destination by delivery to a landfill site, incinerator or transfer station.

Even after two decades, the establishment of an environmentally sound system of waste disposal had not totally been achieved.

This system for waste management was extended to the rest of England under the Local Government Act 1972, but in Wales, Scotland and Northern Ireland, responsibility for waste disposal remained with the much enlarged district councils rather than being transferred to the upper tier of local government administration. Under the Control of Pollution Act 1974 these new local government bodies and English county councils became waste disposal authorities (WDAs) after they came into existence on 1 April 1974.

In 1976 under COPA, for the first time a system of day-to-day regulation of waste disposal and waste transfer facilities was added to the planning conditions and Public Health Act powers which had been the only means of controlling waste disposal from 1947. Under the Town and Country Planning Act any change of land use, including use of land for disposal of waste required planning permission, although use of land for waste disposal prior to 1 January 1948, meant that land could continue to be used for disposal of waste. The local government bodies which administered these waste regulation duties were the new WDAs created under COPA.

The abolition of the metropolitan counties and the GLC in 1986 prompted a number of changes in the arrangements for waste disposal and waste regulation. Because there is a mix of voluntary and statutory arrangements, the administrative system for waste disposal and that for waste regulation became and continues to be complex.

The London Waste Regulation Authority has a London-wide responsibility. Waste disposal is organized on the basis of four statutory waste authorities: the West (six boroughs), East (four boroughs) and north (seven boroughs) London Waste Authorities and the Western Riverside Waste Authority (four boroughs) with each of the remaining 12 boroughs being responsible for their own disposal of waste, although in the case of Bexley this was undertaken in arrangement with Kent County Council. In Greater Manchester, while waste regulation is undertaken jointly for the area, Wigan Metropolitan District Council has responsibility for disposal of waste while the other nine MBCs use the services of Greater Manchester Waste Disposal Authority. On Merseyside the WDA has control of both disposal and regulation. The metropolitan district councils (MDCs) in West Yorkshire delegated all duties to the West Yorkshire Waste Executive in contrast to South Yorkshire, where only a small central advisory team provides site licensing guidance and administers the special waste regulations, and the main duties are undertaken by individual MDCs. Similar arrangements to the latter operate in the West Midlands and Tyne and Wear. These arrangements will be altered as the regulations under the EPA come into effect.

The two-tier system of local government in the non-metropolitan areas of England and in Wales and Scotland may lead to all waste management functions (except waste regulation) being concentrated within their local administration.*

EUROPEAN PERSPECTIVES

Increasingly, the EU will continue to influence the introduction of environmental legislation in the UK. However, it is commonly acknowledged that the first EU statement on waste management, the Framework Directive (75/442/EEC) – see DoE circular 11/94, was closely modelled on COPA. The Directive on dangerous and toxic wastes (78/319/EEC) was one of the first daughter directives to be formulated. Both these Directives have been amended, by 91/156/EEC and 91/689/EEC respectively. In addition there are several other directives affecting waste management in the UK:

1. disposal of PCBs (1976);
2. transfrontier shipment of hazardous waste (1984) (see page 750);

---

* Following review by the Local Government Commission, the two tier system in Scotland and Wales and in certain parts of England is to be replaced during 1996/97 by single tier government. One of the responsibilities for the new councils will be as WCAs and WDAs.

3. titanium dioxide (1989);
4. protection of groundwater (1980);
5. air pollution from municipal waste incinerators (1989);
6. environmental impact assessment (1985);
7. disposal of waste oils (1985 and 1987);
8. beverage containers (1985);
9. freedom of access to information on the environment (1990).

Article 1 of the 'Freedom of Access to Information on the Environment' (90/3/3/EEC) states:

'The object of this directive is to ensure freedom of access to and dissemination of information on the environment held by public authorities and to set out the basic terms and conditions on which such information should be made available.'

This will clearly have an impact on the way local authorities undertake all aspects of pollution monitoring work in the future.

Many elements of this European legislation can be clearly seen in many of the provisions of the Environmental Protection Act, which received Royal Assent on 1 November 1990.

THE ENVIRONMENTAL PROTECTION ACT 1990

Under COPA, responsibility for waste regulation and disposal of waste collected by local authorities rested with the WDA. The Environmental Protection Act 1990 has split the existing English and Welsh WDAs (county councils in the English non-metropolitan areas, district councils in Wales and a variety of arrangements for English metropolitan authorities (see section above)) into three bodies:

1. that part of the WDA which operates waste disposal facilities became a local authority waste disposal company (LAWDC), where the council did not decide to sell off whatever assets it held;
2. the regulatory aspects were taken on by the waste regulation authority (WRA); and
3. that part of the WDA arranging contracts for waste disposal retained the name of waste disposal authority.

The purpose of the new WDAs is to arrange for the disposal of any waste the collection authority has in its possession. District (and borough) councils will continue as waste collection authorities (WCAs), and will keep their function of collecting household waste, with discretionary power to collect other types of controlled waste.

These different authorities and the WCAs are defined in section 30 of the EPA, and the transition process to the new LAWDCs is outlined in section 32. Detailed guidance on the latter issue was provided by the Department of the Environment in February 1991, and each authority has an individually agreed timetable for setting up a LAWDC, or establishing a private company in partnership with an existing waste disposal contractor, or selling any waste disposal facilities the authority may own.

Section 31 provides powers for the Secretary of State to make two or more WRAs into a joint or regional authority. The main aim of this provision was to ensure consistency of regulatory standards over a wide area to avoid waste migrating to those areas which might have looser controls. In late 1990, recommendations for voluntary regional waste regulation bodies based on the existing standard BE regions were produced by the Department of the Environment, and by April 1991 all English WRAs were members of those new bodies in the groupings proposed by the Department.

The situation in Scotland is different in that district councils retain their existing responsibilities of collection, disposal and regulation.

Further changes in the organization of both waste disposal and waste regulation are inevitable as the reorganization of local government takes place and as the Environment Agency is formed (probably in April 1996). The responsibility for contracting for waste collection and disposal services will remain with the new local authorities.

The Environment Agency will bring together those fuctions performed by the National Rivers Authority (NRA), HMIP and the waste regulation responsibilities of local government within a non-departmental public body to provide a 'one-stop shop' for pollution prevention.

The duty of care

One of the fundamental changes introduced by the EPA is the concept of a duty of care under which 'it shall be the duty of any person who imports, produces, carries, keeps, treats or disposes of controlled waste, or, as a broker, has control of such waste, to take all such measures applicable to him in that capacity as are reasonable in the circumstances'. Waste producers and others responsible for waste have 'to prevent the escape of the waste' on to unlicensed land or in contravention of the conditions of a waste management licence. It also requires the holder of the waste to transfer it only to an authorized person such as:

1. the WCA;
2. the holder of a waste managment licence;
3. a registered carrier under section 2 of the Control of Pollution (Amendment) Act 1989.

Section 34 'does not apply to an occupier of domestic property as respects the household waste produced on the property'.

Guidance as to what actions are 'reasonable in the circumstances' are contained in a code of practice produced by the Department of the Environment issued in December 1991 [5] and see also DoE Circular 19/91, EPA 1990 sect. 34, 'The Duty of Care'.*

REGISTRATION OF CARRIERS OF CONTROLLED WASTE

The carriage of waste

The Control of Pollution (Amendment) Act 1989 (COP(A)A) enabled the Secretary of State to make regulations requiring any persons carrying controlled waste in the course of their business, or otherwise with a view to profit, to be registered.

The Controlled Waste (Registration of Carriers and Seizure of Vehicles) Regulations 1991, SI 1991/1624, came into force on 14 October 1991 and the initial application period for registration for existing carriers expired on 31 May 1992.

Those exempt from registration are:

1. WCAs/WDAs/WRAs.
2. People who carry only their own waste (except where building or demolition waste is concerned; all people involved in the carriage of waste from construction, building repair/ improvement or demolition must be registered).
3. British Rail, ferry operators, etc.
4. A charity or recognized voluntary body.

One of the aims of the registration of carriers is to curb fly tipping activities. Therefore to ensure compliance with the duty of care it is an offence to transfer controlled waste to an unauthorized person, an authorized person being a registered carrier for these purposes.

Registration for people and companies is with the Waste Regulation Authority where they have their principal place of business. A fee of £95 is payable with the application for registration which lasts 3 years, following which concurrent renewal costs £65.

The WRA must decide whether an applicant should be registered to carry controlled waste. It may refuse to register a carrier if the applicant (or an associate) fails to comply with the application requirements or has unspent convictions for prescribed offences. The prescribed offences relate primarily to environmental matters but also include the offence of non-possession of a vehicle operator's licence.

The WRA would check the conviction status of all applicant carriers against its own records of convictions and against those held by other WRAs in England, Wales and Scotland via the Co-ordinated Local Authorities Database of Waste Carriers (CLADWAC) computer database held by the London Waste Regulation Authority.

The registration may be revoked if the carrier commits a prescribed offence. Carriers whose applications are refused or whose registration is revoked may appeal to the Secretary of State for the Environment.

Carriers who are registered receive a Certificate of Registration which is standardized throughout Great Britain and bears a unique registration

---

* The Environment Bill, scheduled for enactment in 1995, contains provisions to make producers more responsible for their waste and to promote or secure an increase in the re-use, recovery or recycling of waste.

number. They may also purchase copies. Carriers stopped by the Police or by WRA officers may be required to produce documentary proof of registration within 7 days.

COP(A)A also empowers the WRA to seize vehicles suspected of being used for the illegal deposit of waste where it proves impossible to trace those in charge of the vehicle(s) at the time of the offence. If not claimed the vehicle and its load can be sold.

The Transfrontier Shipment of Waste Regulations 1994 provides a system of prior notification and authorization for the movement of waste consignments between states in the EU and in and out of the Union area. The Control of Pollution (Special Waste) Regulations 1980 are to be amended.

The definition of waste

One of the few aspects of COPA not changed by the EPA was the definition of controlled waste. The definition used under section 30 of COPA is re-stated in section 75 of EPA whereby:

'(2)' **Waste** includes –

(a) any substance which constitues a scrap material or an effluent or other unwanted surplus substance arising from the application of any process; and
(b) any substance or article which requires to be disposed of as being broken, worn out, contaminated or otherwise spoiled;

but does not include a substance which is an explosive within the meaning of the Explosives Act 1875.'

In addition, under section 75(3), 'Any thing which is discarded or otherwise dealt with as if it were waste shall be presumed to be waste unless the contrary is proved'.

Controlled waste comprises household, industrial and commercial waste 'or any such waste'.

Household waste means waste from:

1. domestic property, that part of building used wholly for the purposes of living accommodation;
2. a caravan;
3. a residential home;

4. a university school or other educational establishment;
5. a hospital or nursing home.

Industrial waste comes from:

1. any factory (within the meaning of the Factories (Act 1961);
2. premises connected with transport services;
3. premises used for gas, water, electricity or sewage services;
4. premises used for postal or telecommunications services.

Commercial waste means waste from premises used for trade and business or for sport, recreation or entertainment, but excludes household and industrial waste and mine or quarry waste or agriculture.

The Secretary of State has reserve powers to specify types of waste as falling into specific categories of waste, so that under the Collection and Disposal of Waste Regulations 1988, for example, clinical waste is classified as industrial waste (see below). The Controlled Waste Regulations 1992 (amended 1993 and 1994) provide descriptions of wastes which are to be treated as being (or not being) household, industrial or commercial waste and prescribes the cases in which a charge may be made for the collection of household waste. Certain types of agricultural and mining and quarrying wastes are expected to become controlled waste to meet the requirements of Directive 91/556/EEC.

Section 17 of COPA, which provides enabling powers to the Secretary of State to make regulations on special waste, is retained by section 62 of EPA. The control of special wastes is regulated by the Special Waste Regulations 1980, but the government is reviewing these, partly to accommodate changes in European legislation.

Article 1 of Directive 75/442/EEC provided that ' "waste" means any substance or object which the holder disposes of or is required to dispose of pursuant to the provisions of national law in force'. This provision was given effect in Great Britain by the definition of waste in section 30(1) of the Control of Pollution Act 1974 and the re-enactment in section 75 of the Environmental Protection Act 1990. These provisions do not define authoritatively what is and is not waste.

What they do is to include within the ordinary meaning of the word waste, certain substances about which there might otherwise have been doubt. Other Member States adopted their own national definition of waste.

The Government has decided that the application of a single definition of waste would best serve the interests of environmental protection and efficient waste management and the Control of Pollution Act and Environmental Protection Act definitions (see above) will be replaced by primary legislation when this becomes possible.

In the meantime only those substances/objects which are defined as waste in the Framework Directive will in the UK be subject to controls which apply to the collection, transport, storage, recovery and disposal of waste. This change is effected through the Waste Management Licensing Regulations 1994.

Pending the introduction of primary legislation to repeal the existing definition of waste in section 75(2) of the Environmental Protection Act, the practical effect of these modifications is to transpose into national legislation the Framework Directive's definition of waste; and to ensure that only 'Directive waste' is subject to control as household, industrial or commercial waste (i.e. as 'controlled waste').

Advance guidance on this position and on the new definition of waste was given by the Department of the Environment in DOE/WM5 under cover of a letter 3 December 1993 and DoE Circular 11/94, EPA 1990 Part 2, Waste Management Licensing in the Framework Directive on Waste, gives detailed guidance on the definition of waste and on its interpretation.

'Directive Waste' means any substance or object in the categories set out in Part 2 of Schedule 4 to the 1994 Regulations (see below) which the producer or the person in possession of it discards or intends or is required to discard but with the exception of anything excluded from the scope of the Directive by Article 2.

The Waste Management Licencing Regulations 1994, Schedule 4, Part II
Substances or objects which are waste when discarded etc.

1. Production or consumption residues not otherwise specified in this Part of this Schedule (Q1).
2. Off-specification products (Q2).
3. Products whose date for appropriate use has expired (Q3).
4. Materials spilled, lost or having undergone other mishap, including any materials, equipment, etc., contaminated as a result of the mishap (Q4).
5. Materials contaminated or soiled as a result of planned actions (e.g. residues from cleaning operations, packing materials, containers, etc.) (Q5).
6. Unusable parts (e.g. reject batteries, exhausted catalysts, etc.) (Q6).
7. Substances which no longer perform satisfactorily (e.g. contaminated acids, contaminated solvents, exhausted tempering salts, etc.) (Q7).
8. Residues of industrial processes (e.g. slags, still bottoms, etc.) (Q8).
9. Residues from pollution abatement processes (e.g. scrubber sludges, baghouse dusts, spent filters, etc.) (Q9).
10. Machining or finishing residues (e.g. lathe turnings, mill scales, etc.) (Q10).
11. Residues from raw materials extraction and processing (e.g. mining residues, oil field slops, etc.) (Q11).
12. Adulterated materials (e.g. oils contaminated with PCBs, etc.) (Q12).
13. Any materials, substances or products whose use has been banned by law (Q13).
14. Products for which the holder has no further use (e.g. agricultural, household, office, commercial and shop discards, etc.) (Q14).
15. Contaminated materials, substances or products resulting from remedial action with respect to land (Q15).
16. Any materials, substances or products which are not contained in the above categories (Q16).

(*Note*: the reference in brackets at the end of each paragraph of this Part of this Schedule is the number of the corresponding paragraph in Annex I to the Directive.)

Illegal deposit of waste (for other powers to deal with abandoned waste see Chapter 7)

The key section of the EPA is section 33. This section makes fly-tipping illegal and requires that any other waste disposal activity is undertaken only under and in compliance with, the conditions of a waste management licence. Section 33(1) states that:

'a person shall not –
(a) deposit controlled waste, or knowingly cause or knowingly permit controlled waste to be deposited in or on any land unless a waste management licence authorizing the deposit is in force and the deposit is in accordance with the licence:
(b) treat, keep or dispose of controlled waste or knowingly cause or knowingly permit controlled waste to be treated, kept or disposed of: –
  (i) in or on any land, or
  (ii) by means of any mobile plant except under and in accordance with a waste management licence;
(c) treat, keep or dispose of controlled waste in a manner likely to cause pollution of the environment or harm to human health.'

A contravention of the main offence under section 33(1), or a contravention of a condition of waste management licence, is an offence. Under COPA a breach of site licence conditions could be enforced only when a deposit of waste was witnessed.

Section 33 introduces the concepts of 'pollution to the environment' and 'harm to human health'. The definitions are given in section 29 and reiterate the definitions used in Part I of the Act with specific reference to waste on land. Penalties for offences under section 33 raise the maximum fine from £2000 under COPA to £20 000 and/or 6 months imprisonment on summary conviction and an indictment and unlimited fine and/or imprisonment for 2 years. For offences involving special waste the latter prison term is raised to a maximum of 5 years.

As with many other aspects of environmental legislation, anyone can initiate a prosecution for an offence under section 33, in that the previous COPA limitation restricting prosecution to either the Director of Public Prosecutions, through the Crown Prosecution Service, or the Waste Disposal (Regulation) Authority has been lifted.

Waste management licences (WMLs)*

The COPA provisions with respect to licensing waste disposal sites, sections 4–10, have been strengthened in sections 35–44 of the EPA. Waste management licences are granted by the WRA for facilities treating, keeping and disposing (including depositing) 'any specified description of controlled waste', and also includes the treatment and disposal of waste by mobile plant. Under the EPA the matters which a WRA must take into consideration before issuing a licence are different from COPA. The WRA has a duty not to reject a licence unless this action is necessary to prevent (section 36(3)):

1. pollution of the environment;
2. harm to human health; or
3. serious detriment to the amenities of the locality.

The last proviso applies only to land covered by established use certificates. These three reasons are very wide ranging and have replaced the two criteria used by COPA Part I, whereby a licence could only be refused 'for the purpose of preventing pollution of water or danger to public health'.

In addition to these criteria with respect to the site, the licence applicant also has to be assessed by the WRA as 'a fit and proper person' to hold such a licence. Guidance on this matter is provided by section 74. A person is judged on his ability both to carry out the activities authorized by the licence, and to fulfil the conditions of the licence. Also a person would fail this test on three counts:

---

* For the planning aspects of WMLs see Planning and Pollution Control PPG 23, 1994.

1. that he or another relevant person has been convicted of a relevant offence;
2. that the management of the site covered by the licence is not in the hands of a technically competent person;
3. that a licence applicant has no intention of making financial provision adequate to discharge the obligations arising from the licence.

The definition of a fit and proper person, however, is not absolute. The WRA is given some considerable discretion over whether the conviction by a person of relevant offence does or does not make a person 'fit and proper'. The WRA has the duty to have regard to guidance from the Secretary of State over this matter. This can include guidance on qualifications and experience that a licence holder requires. This would, for example, include the Certificate of Competence developed under the auspices of the Waste Management Industry Training Advisory Board (WAMITAB) (Regulations 4 and 5 of the 1994 Regulations – see below – deal with this.)

Prior to issuing the licence, an English or Welsh WRA must refer the proposal to the National Rivers Authority (NRA) and the Health and Safety Executive (HSE). However, the WCA no longer has to be informed. As with COPA, if the WRA and NRA fail to agree either on the granting of the licence or the proposed conditions, there is an appeal to the Secretary of State and his decision is binding on the WRA.

Licence modification, revocation and suspension

The power of the WRA to modify licence conditions under section 7 of COPA is continued under section 37 of the EPA. The holder of the licence can also apply for a modification. Under the EPA, the Secretary of State can also direct a WRA to modify licence conditions. This could, for example, be used to implement provisions of any new EC directive, such as a landfill directive. While modifications may be referred to the NRA and/or HSE, section 37(5)(b) allows the WRA to judge whether these consultees might be affected. If not, modification can proceed without consultation. Where an application to modify conditions is rejected or if the holder is unhappy about a modification imposed by the WRA, the holder can appeal to the Secretary of State.

Section 38 replaces section 7 of COPA permitting WRAs to revoke or suspend the licence or revoke certain parts of it. The latter may be needed at a landfill site, e.g. to retain in force conditions relating to gas and leachate management but prevent further tipping. There are two grounds for revocation under section 38(1):

1. that the licence holder has ceased to be a fit and proper person due to conviction for a relevant offence; or
2. that continuation of the activities authorized by the licence would cause pollution of the environment, harm to human health, or would be seriously detrimental to the amenities of the locality affected.

However there is the prerequisite that a revocation can only be made where the pollution, harm or detriment cannot be avoided by modifying the conditions of the licence.

Revocations under section 7(4) of COPA have been rare because of the onerous task of having to prove both that the damage was so serious that revocation was imperative, and that modification of condition would not have resolved the problem. Similar potential applies also to a new provision, suspension of licences under section 38(6) of the EPA, but oddly reference is made to **serious** pollution of the environment and **serious** harm to human health in that subsection.

Under COPA, the WDA could also revoke a licence under section 9. This power is contained by section 42 of the EPA. If it appears to the WRA that a condition is not being complied with, a compliance notice can be served on the holder. This specifies a time period for compliance which, unless fulfilled, enables the WRA to revoke the licence entirely, partially or suspend it.

Appeals and compensation

Under the provisions outlined above relating to licence modifications and revocations, the licence holder can appeal to the Secretary of State against the WRA's action (section 43). While the appeal is being determined, the WRA's action is held in abeyance.

WDAs were reluctant to use their immediate modification or revocation powers as they were concerned about the possibility of paying compensation. This reluctance was exacerbated by the outcome of several appeals which appeared bizarre, and given that appeals to the Department of the Environment in the late 1980s and early 1990s were taking 2 to 3 years to decide, the amounts payable as compensation could be considerable.

Surrender of licences

Section 39 provides for the surrender of a licence, but only if the surrender is accepted by the WRA. This is a change from COPA where an operator could surrender the licence whenever he or she felt like it, possibly leaving enormous problems with gas and leachate control, for example.

Under the EPA, when a licence holder wishes to surrender a licence the WRA has the duty to satisfy itself that the licensed site will not cause pollution of the environment or harm to human health. On the surrender of a licence, the WRA issues a certificate of completion. (See Waste Management Paper 26A – Landfill Completion).

Management of completed disposal facilities

The granting of a certificate of completion on the surrender of a licence, the WRA absolves the former licence holder of any further responsibility for the land. The liability for any further work needed will therefore fall on the WRA once the licence has been surrendered. Under section 61(9), should the WRA identify a site that has created a significant environmental problem but where it has already granted a certificate of completion, it can undertake remedial work but cannot attempt to recover the cost from the landowner, unlike all other circumstances. Given the fact that landfill gas emissions can continue for several decades and likewise leachate can cause problems for long periods, it is probable that WRAs will be reluctant to issue certificates of completion.

Faced with a refusal to issue a certificate of completion, the licence holder can appeal to the Secretary of State. A successful appeal against the wishes of the WRA may therefore hold considerable finance implications under section 61(9), noted above.

Fees and charges

Section 41 permits the Secretary of State to introduce fees and charges for applications for waste management licences and their retention. (See the Waste Management Licencing (Fees and Charges) Scheme 1994). Such fees would be charged by them and paid to the WRA. Indeed, under section 41(7), failure to pay the fees may render a licence holder liable to revocation of the licence. The WRA cannot set its own fees. While it is the duty of the Secretary of State to make regulations prescribing the fees and the charging scheme, it is 'with the approval of the Treasury' (section 41(2)).

The Waste Management Licensing Regulations 1994

These regulations bring into operation the new concepts of waste licensing introduced by the Environmental Protection Act and outlined above and became fully effective on 1 May 1994. Waste Management paper No. 4 Licensing of Waste Management Facilities and DoE Circular 11/94 Environmental Protection Act Part 2, Waste Management Licensing, the Framework Directive on Waste both give guidance on and support the new system. The Waste Management paper has been given statutory status and provides formal guidance to WRAs.

Removal of unlawful waste deposits (see also Chapter 7)

The WDA's power to require the removal of waste unlawfully deposited on land under section 16 of COPA is continued under section 59 of the EPA. It permits a WRA or WCA to serve notice on the occupier of any land to either remove a particular waste and/or to eliminate or reduce its consequences. However, the occupier can apply to the magistrates' court for the notice to be quashed within 21 days of the service of the notice. If the court is either satisfied that the appellant neither deposited nor caused or permitted the deposit of waste or that there is a material defect in the notice, the notice can be quashed.

There is also provision under section 59(7) and (8) for the WRA or WCA to remove the waste or reduce its consequences and then recover the cost by charging the person who deposited, knowingly caused or knowingly permitted the deposit of waste. Recouping costs where material is fly-tipped is clearly only possible when someone has been successfully prosecuted under section 33.

WRA's responsibilities for closed landfills

Section 61 provides for every WRA to locate closed landfills and evaluate them for gas and leachate emissions. Having found such sites, it is the duty of WRA to keep the situation under review and, where pollution to the environment and harm to human health is possible, the authority has the duty to rectify the problem. The WRA is then entitled to recover any costs from the owner of the land. (See Waste Management Paper 26 – Land filling wastes.)*

Waste disposal plans

The responsibility for production of a waste disposal plan under section 50 of the EPA rests with the WRA, while it was the WDA under COPA (section 2). WRAs must carry out a survey to decide what arrangements are needed to treat or dispose of controlled waste within their area. They must plan the arrangements made, and proposed, by waste disposal contractors for the treatment and disposal of waste in their area. However, while the COPA waste disposal planning system had some logic in that the WDA has responsibility for the disposal of WCA waste, the WRA has no operational control to influence treatment methods and disposal routes.

In preparing, or modifying, the plan, the WRA has to consult with the NRA and the WCAs in its area, other WRAs where waste is proposed to be exported beyond the WRA's boundaries, and other people who are likely to be undertaking the disposal or treatment of controlled waste in the area of the authority. (In Wales there is also need to consult the county council.)

As with COPA, having drawn up a draft plan the authority is required to 'provide members of the public with opportunities of making representations' and 'consider any representations'. The WRA has the duty to send a copy of the further draft to the Secretary of State (section 50(9)) to ensure that the WRA has adequately met the criteria outlined in section 50(3). Finally, the WRA must 'provide adequate publicity in its area' for the final plan and submit a copy to the Secretary of State.

WRA annual reports

The EPA in section 67 requires each WRA to prepare and publish an annual report on the discharge of its functions under Part II of the Act. The report covers details of all licences granted, modified and suspended, implementation of the waste disposal plan, the number and descriptions of all prosecutions, and the expenditure and income relating to functions under Part II. The report is required to be published within 6 months of the end of the financial year, and a copy sent to the Secretary of State. This will be used as part of HM Inspectorate of Pollution's (HMIP's) auditing procedure to check the effectiveness of WRAs.

Waste recycling plans (see also page 762)

The duties of WCAs regarding the reclamation of household and commercial waste arising in their area are outlined in section 49(1) of the EPA. The WCA is required:

'(a) to carry out an investigation with a view to deciding what arrangements are appropriate for dealing with the waste by separating, baling or otherwise packaging if for the purpose of recycling it;
(b) to decide what arrangements are in the opinion of the authority needed for that purpose;

---

* Section 61 has not yet been implemented and new provisions are under consideration through the Environment Bill, due for enactment in 1995.

(c) to prepare a statement ('the plan') of the arrangements made and proposed to be made by the authority and other persons for dealing with waste in those ways;

(d) to carry out from time to time further investigations with a view to deciding what changes are needed; and

(e) to make any modification of the plan which the authority thinks appropriate in consequence of any such further investigation.'

The target for this waste reclamation activity was set by the government in the white paper, *This Common Inheritance – Britain's Environmental Strategy* published in September 1990 [6]. Fifty per cent of household waste is reckoned to be recyclable, and of this the government requires 50% to be recycled by the year 2000, an overall waste reduction effect of 25% by waste reclamation actions, mainly undertaken through the auspices of local authorities.*

Although it is generally assumed that each local authority should be aiming to achieve the recycling target, the target is a national one, not one for every local authority to achieve because many will be too distant from market outlets even to make glass reclamation a resource efficient option. In addition, there is the problem that nowhere in section 49 is there reference to local authorities' role as purchasers of recycled materials or goods, clearly a prerequisite if the government target is to be achieved.

Having drawn up its draft plan, the WCA is required to submit a copy to the Secretary of State for him to ensure that the authority has fulfilled its requirement with regard to section 49(3), which specifies the type of information which is required to be included. Having complied with any directions which the Secretary of State may impose, the WCA has the duty under section 49(5):

'(a) to take such steps as in the opinion of the authority will give adequate publicity in its area for the plan or modification: and

(b) to send to the waste disposal authority and waste regulation authority for the area which includes its area a copy of the plan or particulars for the modification'.

Unlike the procedure with the waste disposal plan, there is no requirement for consultation with the public or any other authority prior to its production.

Despite the fact that the WCA must undertake the planning for waste reclamation, as with COPA, it is the WDA which retains the final say over recycling. Among its other duties, the WDA (EPA section 51(4)) 'shall give directions to the waste collection authorities within its area as to the persons to whom and places' at which the controlled waste they collect is to be delivered. In addition, section 48(4) requires that, 'where a waste disposal authority has made with a waste disposal contractor arrangements, as respects household waste or commercial waste in its area or any part of its area, for the contractor to recycle the waste, or any of it, the waste disposal authority may, by notice served on the waste collection authority, object to the waste collection authority having the waste recycled; and the objection may be made as respects all the waste, part only of the waste or specified descriptions of the waste'. There is no provision in the EPA for WCAs to appeal against an objection by the WDA. Therefore, were a WCA to produce a recycling plan incorporating source segregation, this could be overturned by the WDA.

A further barrier to waste reclamation is introduced under the EPA for those metropolitan authorities and Welsh districts which are both WCA and WDA. Specifically, under section 48(6) and (7) of the EPA:

'(6) A waste collection authority may, subject to subsection (7) below, provide plant and equipment for costing and baling of waste retained by the authority . . .

(7) subsection (6) does not apply to an authority which is also a waste disposal authority . . .'

Informal guidance provided by the minister when this restriction was debated during the third reading suggested that equipment beyond that normally associated with the fulfilment of a

---

* Also see 'A Waste Strategy for England and Wales – Consultation Draft January 1995', DoE and Welsh Office.

WCA's duties would be regarded as falling within the restriction of section 48(6) and (7).

A further complication with regard to waste reclamation exists with respect to the responsibilities of the WRA in drawing up its waste disposal plan, which requires (section 50(4)) that, 'it shall be the duty of the authority to have regard to the desirability, where reasonably practicable, of giving priority to recycling waste'. It is also its duty to consider (section 50(7)):

(a) what arrangements can reasonably be expected to be made for recycling waste; and
(b) what provisions should be included in the plan for the purpose'.

However, while there is a statutory requirement (section 50(a)(ii)) to consult the WCAs in its area, there is no requirement to consult the WDA(s) in the area.

While a timetable for the production of waste recycling, and waste disposal, plans is not given in the EPA, the Secretary of State retains the power to require them within a specified period of time. The Government requested the submission of recycling plans by 1 August 1992 and waste disposal plans by the end of 1994.

Guidance to WCAs in the preparation of waste recycling plans is available in the Waste Management Paper No. 28 produced in July 1991 [7], which lays down clear guidelines as to the authority's requirements with respect to the information to be included in this plan under section 49(3):

'(a) the kinds and quantities of controlled waste which the authority expects to collect during the period specified in the plan;
(b) the kinds and quantities of controlled waste which the authority expects to purchase during that period;
(c) the kinds and quantities of controlled waste which the authority expects to deal with in the ways specified in subsection (1)(a) above during that period;
(d) the arrangements which the authority expects to make during that period with waste disposal contractors . . .;

(e) the plant and equipment which the authority expects to provide . . .; and
(f) the estimated costs or savings attributable to the methods of dealing with the waste in the ways provided for in the plan'.

However, there is no duty for the WCA to enhance its current waste reclamation activities, where these exist.

One positive measure to encourage the reclamation of waste is contained in section 52(1), which provides that where a WCA undertakes such reclamation the WDA makes payments to WCA 'of such amount representing its net saving of expenditure on the disposal of the waste as the authority determines'. Guidance and regulations issued in February 1992 and March 1994 provide for the means of calculating the amount to be paid by WDA to WCA as from April 1992 and April 1994 when payments doubled. The basis of payment from April 1994 is the long-run marginal cost of each WCA's highest cost method of waste disposal. While payments between WDA and WCA are mandatory, those to others undertaking waste reclamation measures which make savings in waste disposal and/or collection costs are discretionary, although the Secretary of State can introduce regulations to make such payments obligatory (see DoE Circular 4/92. EPA (Waste Recycling Payments) Regulations and the Amendment Regulations of 1994).

This measure, which is an advance on the position under COPA and dealt with in the Department of the Environment Circular 13/88, was felt to be necessary because while most source segregation reclamation is undertaken by WCAs, the main benefit accrues to the WDA through savings in waste disposal costs.

Waste collection and waste receptacles

Sections 45–47 of the EPA largely replicate duties and powers of WCAs under sections 12–14 of COPA, the regulations for which were finally introduced as part of the Collection and Disposal of Waste Regulations 1988. The ability of WCAs to establish kerbside source segregation collection schemes, as opposed to the pre-1992 door-to-door schemes has been permitted under section 46(1), whereby 'the authority may . . . require the occupier to place the waste for collection' in receptacles of a kind and number specified. However, agreement has to be given by the highway or roads authority and provided that arrangements have been made as to the liability for any damage arising out of their being so placed' (section 46(5)(b)).

Under section 45, the WCA has a duty to arrange for collection of household waste except for premises which are isolated or inaccessible so that collection costs would be 'unreasonably high', and that adequate arrangements for its disposal can reasonably be expected to be made. There is also a duty for the WCA to collect or arrange collection of commercial waste when requested. As regards industrial waste, the WCA may arrange for its collection if requested by the occupier, but a WCA can only exercise this power with the consent of the WDA (section 45(2)). For commercial and industrial waste, the WCA has a duty to recover the costs for both its collection and disposal, 'unless in the case of charge in respect of commercial waste the authority considers it inappropriate to do so'. Section 45 also deals with the duties of WCAs with regard to the emptying of cesspools and privies.

While section 46 deals with the provision of receptacles for household waste, section 47 covers those for commercial or industrial waste. While the authority has considerable discretion as to the number and type of containers to be used and their positioning for the collection of waste and recyclables, under section 46(7) an occupier can appeal to a magistrates' court that the authority's request is unreasonable or that 'the receptacles in which household waste is placed for collection from the premises are adequate'. However, this appeal procedure must be initiated within 21 days of a notice being served on the occupier or the end of the notice period. A similar provision exists for receptacles from industrial and commercial premises, but the grounds for objection are different in that while the requirement of unreasonable provision is repeated the other ground is that 'the waste is not likely to cause a nuisance or

Table 43.1 UK average composition of household refuse

Screenings – 2 cm	10%
Vegetable and putrescible	20%
Paper and board	33%
Metals	8%
Textiles and man-made fibres	4%
Glass	10%
Plastics	7%
Unclassified	8%

Source: Department of the Environment (1991) *Waste Management Paper No. 28*, Recycling of Waste, HMSO, London.

be detrimental to the amenities of the locality' (section 47(7)(b)).

REFUSE ANALYSIS

The analysis of household waste is concerned with the physical characteristics and composition of that waste, e.g. its density, ouput per household and the amount of paper. Data obtained from such analyses helps to predict the changing nature of waste, and is a valuable aid in determining methods of collection, transportation and disposal.

Since 1974, the Department of the Environment has co-ordinated UK waste analysis data. Table 43.1 shows the national average composition of household refuse, although these may vary substantially between different Local Authority areas.

Reliable waste analysis can be used for organizing collection rounds, calculating storage requirements of blocks of flats, and long-term forecasting to enable strategies to be planned and research organized.

In seeking improved efficiency and higher standards of waste recycling, treatment and disposal, it is essential that reliable data are available on the raw material emanating from the waste industry. There are numerous examples of where waste analysis, correctly carried out, has enabled treatment and disposal plant design to be adequately assessed. Similarly, there are many cases of where lack of analysis data has not only lead to

Table 43.2 Distribution of waste disposal in the UK in 1990

Agricultural waste	80 m tonnes
Mining waste	51 m tonnes
Quarrying waste	57 m tonnes
Industrial waste	45 m tonnes
Municipal solid waste	35 m tonnes
Sewage sludge	36 m tonnes
Hazardous waste	4 m tonnes
Radioactive waste	0.02 m tonnes

under or gross over design, but also the wrong treatment system being selected.

Table 43.2 shows the distribution of waste disposed of the UK in 1990.

REFUSE STORAGE

It is important that during periods of storage, refuse of any type of premise should be kept dry. An accumulation of moist or wet refuse is not only offensive and difficult to remove, but forms an excellent breeding medium for flies.

Domestic storage

The vast majority of domestic residences now have one of two alternative types of refuse storage facility. The traditional galvanized and plastic dustbins are gradually being phased out and replaced by either plastic refuse sacks or 240 litre wheeled bins, again, manufactured from plastic materials (see Fig. 43.1).

With increasing concern over the dangers from needle stick injury and sharp, protruding refuse in a plastic sack, allied to the litter problems generated by such containers, the wheeled bin has become increasingly more popular. Although provision of such a receptacle usually requires the householder to place the bin at the curtilage of the property or at the kerbside, the merit of having almost three times the capacity of a traditional dustbin and nearly six times the capacity of a refuse sack is seen as a considerable advantage, both in containing waste generation in one place and dramatically reducing the litter problem.

High-rise flats

British Standard 5906 details the requirements for the gravity transport system of waste disposal in multi-storey buildings. It is specific on dimensions, materials, finishes and ventilation requirements. Waste is deposited on each floor in hoppers and transported via gravity chutes to containers in the basement. The British Standard gives information on these chutes and hoppers, and the location, dimension, construction, lighting, ventilation and cleansing of the storage chambers. Where there is likely to be excessive accumulations and bulk cylindrical containers are inadequate, a refuse compactor may be located to receive refuse in these situations.

Removal distances

Access for removal is very important, and consideration must be given to the distance of carry to the external removal point. According to BS5906, these distances should not be more than **25 m** or, when wheeling a container, not more than **10 m**. Care must be taken in the design of refuse storage areas, that the gradient from the storage point to the point of collection access should not **exceed 1:14**.

Commercial and industrial waste storage

Where there are large volumes of waste accumulations, refuse skips or bulk containers of 1100 l capacity and above are frequently used (Fig. 43.1). Where collection frequency is limited or where there is a problem of space, refuse compactors may be installed. These can reduce the volume of waste down to 20% of its original bulk, which also helps to control smell, litter and reduces fire risk. Waste, so compacted, is not likely to attract vermin and insects and gives lower transport costs. British Standard 5832 deals with the most popular type of compactor waste containers of 10 cu m capacity. Provision for the installation of the compactor should be made at the design stage so that space, electrical fittings and access to, plus removal of, compacted refuse is planned in. Compacted refuse is heavy and may need wheeled transport, and so the siting of the

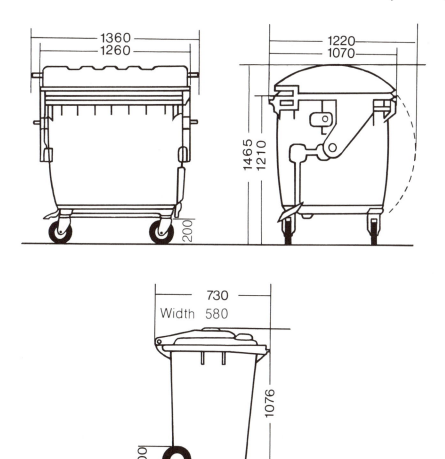

Fig. 43.1 240L (below) and 1100L (left and right above) wheeled refuse storage containers. (Courtesy of SSI Schafer.)

compactor must take into account steps and ramp access.

External storage

Sufficient storage capacity should be provided for the agreed span of time between collections, and consideration should be given to providing an enclosed compound for refuse containers, which encourages hygiene around the building, controls litter, discourages vandalism and helps to avoid the problem of flytipping. Enclosed refuse storage compounds must have natural and artificial lighting, appropriate ventilation, smooth, cleanable floor surfaces, hose points and drainage facilities, be easily accessible for deposit and removal of refuse, and have a lock-up entry. The containers must usually be accessible from the ground floor, with vehicular access not more than 25 m from the material without collectors having to pass through a building. Rear access is an advantage, especially in conditions where there are large amounts of traffic and parking problems.

All access roads for refuse vehicles must have suitable foundations and surfaces to withstand the maximum weights of the vehicles likely to be used. Manhole covers, gully gratings and the like, should be of a heavy duty construction; overhead service cables and pipes should be not less than 7 m from ground level; and there should be sufficient room to allow manoeuvrability of heavy goods vehicles in the 17 to 24 tonne range. If skips or large compactors are used, consideration must be given to high overhead clearance for the emptying of such equipment.

The screening of waste storage areas by planting creates a good impression. Landscaping should be practical with low maintenance requirements, and should be impact resistant.

RECYCLING

Recycling of waste is undertaken in order to:

1. provide a cheaper alternative to virgin raw materials in the manufacturing process;
2. ensure that rapidly diminishing natural resources are not used up;
3. reduce waste disposal costs; and
4. increase the life of diminishing waste disposal facilities.

The EPA imposes a duty on waste collection authorities to prepare 'recycling plans' accessible to the public, outlining what action the authority is taking in respect of recycling (see page 756). The government has indicated that in its view 50% of all waste is potentially recyclable and that by the year 2000 it is its hope that all councils will be recycling 50% of this fraction i.e. 25% of overall waste.

There are two methods of recycling currently operated in the UK: recycling at source, and recycling at the disposal point. Many local authorities base batteries of containers at strategic locations around their authority where members of the public can bring recyclable commodities, such as glass, cans, plastics and paper, to central collection points. Increasingly, a number of authorities are experimenting with second household waste receptacles on the doorstep where the resident can separate potentially recyclable materials.

This waste is then taken to a recycling centre where it can either be manually or mechanically sorted. In some authorities where recycling is not undertaken at source, facilities are available to extract certain materials at the waste treatment and/or disposal point, e.g. electromagnetic sep-

aration of steel cans. It is imperative that if recycling of household waste material is to become the preferred means for disposal of our waste, suitable markets for reclaimed waste must be found.

Wastepaper

There are many grades of wastepaper, the highest being produced by paper mills themselves, almost all of which is recycled. Publishers and printers also create waste, which is usually worthy of recycling. However, it is low grades of wastepaper which are normally created in the home and made available for local authority collection. Over half the paper and board produced in this country is made from wastepaper, and over three-quarters of it is used to make packaging such as cardboard boxes and cartons for cereals, soap powders and other products. Wastepaper is not used for cartons which come into direct contact with the food, because of possible hygiene problems.

Plastics

Recycling of plastics from household waste is still in its early states of development. The most commonly available material is polyethylene, which is sometimes recycled, especially from waste accumulations at supermarkets. It is used as a shrink wrapping for trays of packaged goods. Plastic bottles made from PVC for packaging mineral waters are also recycled, and are often chopped up to make things such as underwater drainage pipes and garden posts. Polypropylene, used in the making of crates and battery cases, can be recycling into drainage pipes, and PET which is used in the production of drinks containers, can be reused in the clothing industry and also for bottles for nonfood products. Mixed plastic waste can be reprocessed to make products such as road signs, motorway acoustic insulation walls, fencing pallets and outdoor furniture. Residual plastics, which are in such tiny quantities that it is not possible to collect, can be allowed to pass through the waste stream, where they may help to fire incinerators and, thereafter, the product can be reclaimed for use as heat or energy.

Ferrous metals

All ferrous metals are attracted by magnets and, therefore, it is not critical that this material is separated at source, if the waste is ultimately to go through an incinerator plant with overband electromagnetic separation. However, larger materials, i.e. white goods: fridges, cookers and washing machines, can normally be segregated at the disposal point for recycling. At the present time, about 90% of food and drinks cans are made of ferrous metal, and they are best extracted from mixed waste.

Aluminium

Much of the aluminium waste is obtained from old cars and white goods, with only very small quantities from household waste. Aluminium currently makes up less than 1% of household waste, and it is used for milk bottle tops, foil containers and about half of all drinks cans. In 1992 a £28 aluminium can smelting facility was opened in Warrington, which is capable of reclaiming 50 000 tones a year of all-aluminium cans.

Glass

Glass bottles have traditionally been refilled rather than recycled, e.g. door-to-door milk delivery, but inevitably there are casualties in this system. It is difficult to mechanically separate glass from other household waste, so it is best to keep it separate and deliver it to bottle banks. Glass is heavy and dense, and so needs to be collected in large quantities to be worth transporting to a treatment plant for cleaning and recycling. Most waste glass (cullet) can be recycled, and bottle banks are normally placed near shopping centres or household amenity centres. Every effort should be made to keep the colours of glass separate because in this country over two-thirds of the glass produced is clear and mixed cullet can only be used in considerable volumes in green glass furnaces.

Compost

The food and garden waste that ends up in household waste containers can be used to make compost. This waste makes up about one-fifth of all household waste, and is called the putrescible fraction. It may be separated either by the householder or at a treatment centre which makes compost for use as soil conditioner. Separation of the compostable fraction, which is currently not widely practised in the UK, has advantages in that the rest of the waste can be burned more efficiently, because much of the moisture is removed with the compostables, and even if the rest of the waste goes direct to landfill, such segregation helps to reduce the amount of landfill gas that is generated.

REFUSE COLLECTION

Organization

Labour

The collection of refuse from domestic, commercial and industrial premises is usually undertaken by the local authorities themselves, using their direct labour organizations or by commercial waste collection and disposal companies. There has been a significant increase in the involvement of the latter organizations since the introduction of compulsory competitive tendering to the UK waste management industry in the late 1980s (see Chapter 3).

Irrespective of the organization undertaking the work, the system universally favoured is the task system, where a defined number of premises are cleared each day and an incentive bonus is paid on top of the basic wage for completion of that day's work. The system is favoured to a continuous system in that with increasing concern over security of premises and linked properties, it is imperative that occupiers know precisely when they should make the receptacles available for collection. Rounds are routed to ensure the minimum of unproductive travel, usually geared to start and finish near to the depot and/or ultimate disposal point. Collection rounds are subject to periodic review, as the vehicles and equipment are constantly upgraded and to reflect any changes in the demographic nature of the authority, the working practices and population movement. There has been a move away from incentive bonus schemes, which have tended to encourage uncontrolled working practice, to ensure early finishes on each day. The implementation of compulsory competitive tendering has tended to load the working day in order to minimize the number of vehicles utilized on the service, thus reducing high capital cost elements for incorporation in tender bids. The system of task and finish is rapidly diminishing.

It is normal for household refuse to be collected once per week but, where authorities are currently experimenting with recycling schemes, there is some movement towards fortnightly collection of recyclable material and fortnightly collection of other waste. Such schemes have to be carefully monitored from an environmental point of view, to ensure that there is no public health risk or nuisance. The advent of the wheeled bin system, together with a kerbside collection scheme, has dramatically reduced the number of crew members on each vehicle. Future developments tend to suggest a move towards double shift working and 7-day collections in order to further reduce the number of high-cost vehicles incorporated into the service. Another advantage of the advent of the wheeled bin system is that the lifting device on the collection vehicles enables domestic waste and commercial waste to be collected at the same time, thus reducing the duplication of travelling time and overlapping of rounds when these services were segregated.

Transport

The traditional transport system for refuse collection is now compaction vehicles, ranging from 16-tonne single rear axle to 24-tonne twin rear axle vehicles. Where the geographical nature of the round is such that large vehicles cannot negotiate the area, then smaller derivatives are used, but in order to ensure maximum economic pay loads and work content, these should operate within a

short distance of the disposal point, or should have a transfer facility to ensure that there are no long, unproductive hauls to the tipping site. The optimum arrangement is to have two or, at the most, three trips to the disposal point, allowing rest periods and lunch breaks to coincide wherever possible, thus ensuring faster working when the work is resumed. The vehicles used tend to be compaction vehicles, with power-operated pressure plates producing compaction ratios in the region of 4:1. Typical payloads of a 17-tonne gross vehicle weight (GVW) vehicle would be in the order of 8 tonnes per load. Although there are few variations between the major manufacturers of refuse collection vehicles, there are specialist variants for unusual situations, i.e. a smaller, non-HGV type vehicle may be used in rural locations where there is considerable inter-premise travel, narrow-bodied vehicles are used in inner cities where access and manoeuvrability is limited, and some authorities are experimenting with one man crews using automatic lifting devices and/or side loading lifting devices on the vehicles. Fig. 43.2 shows the operation of a rotary drum compaction system capable of dealing with both sacks and wheeled bins.

Where it is impossible to operate close to a disposal point or a transfer station, a system known as the relay system of working is introduced (where there is a ratio of vehicles to gangs of men, in the order of 2:1 or 3:2). Drivers within the relay system are not considered part of the loading team, but as one vehicle moves out to make the journey to the disposal site, a new vehicle comes in to enable the crew to continue working. Starting and finishing times may have to be staggered to allow this system to work.

Where the wheeled bin system is in operation, a lifting rig is fitted to the rear of the vehicle with dust curtains, and the wheeled bins tip in behind the curtain, in an elevated state, producing a dust-free collection system. Other lifting devices can be fitted to the rear of large-capacity compression vehicles to enable them to lift refuse compactors, refuse skips and a variety of bulk containers. For certain industrial applications, front-end loading compression vehicles are used, where a pair of

METHOD OF OPERATION

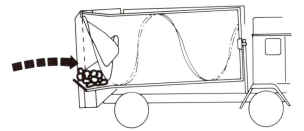

Refuse is loaded into the rear hopper.

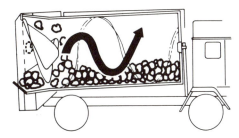

Refuse is carried foward, tumbled and broken down by drum rotation. Weight is always distributed along full length of drum.

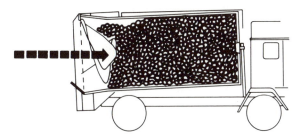

With all drum free space filled as loading continues, the load is compacted by the action of stationary helical compression cone against the rotating refuse.

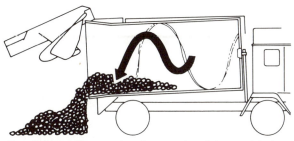

For discharge the rear door is opened and drum rotated in reverse direction to "screw-out" refuse.

Fig. 43.2 Rotary compaction refuse collection vehicle. (Courtesy of Laird (Anglesey) Ltd.)

forks operate hydraulically in front of the cab, lifting containers over the top of the vehicle and tipping the refuse into the roof of the body. These vehicles are often used where access is particularly difficult.

Health and safety in refuse collection

There are serious health and safety implications involved in the operation of refuse compaction vehicles. Between 1977 and 1984, 28 fatal and 64 major injuries and 320 accidents were notified to the HSE. Of these total accidents, 77% occurred during the collection round.

Guidance Note PM52, *Safety in the Use of Refuse Compaction Vehicles* [8], gives recommendations on the design and operation of vehicles, including operational controls and safe systems of work.

LITTER

In the UK the demand for action against litter is hardening as exemplified by its prominence in the waste management objectives detailed in the government's white paper *This Common Inheritance – Britain's Environmental Strategy*:

> 'The government aims to encourage the best use of valuable raw materials, and safe and efficient disposal of waste. This means:
> - minimizing waste
> - recycling materials and recovering energy;
> - tight controls over waste disposal: and
> - action against litter.'[6]

Britain is the only country to have a national anti-litter organization, the Tidy Britain Group, formerly called the Keep Britain Tidy Group but renamed to reflect reality. There remains the paradox that despite the increased funding for the Tidy Britain Group and ever widening legislative provision against littering in the early 1990s, most people perceive that the problem is becoming worse.

Although Part IV of the EPA does not repeal the whole of The Litter Act 1983, it does take over its main provision (section 1), creating an offence of leaving litter (section 87 of the EPA).* The 1983 Act itself consolidated the previous Litter Acts of 1958 and 1971, and repealed the Dangerous Litter Act 1971.

The essence of Part IV is provided in section 87:

(1) If any person throws down, drops or otherwise deposits in, into or from any place to which this section applies, and leaves anything whatsoever in such circumstances as to cause, or contribute to, or tend to leave to, the defacement by litter of any place to which this section applies, he shall, subject to subsection (2) below be guilty of an offence.

(2) No offence is committed under this section where the depositing and leaving of the thing was:
 (a) authorized by law, or
 (b) done with the consent of the owner, occupier or other person having control of the place in or into which that thing was deposited.'

The maximum fine for littering has been raised to £2500 from £400 under the 1983 Act, somewhat academic given that fines in 1993 averaged £48 although the level of costs was often greater. Section 88, however, extends the fixed penalty notice system to all litter authorities originally introduced by Westminster City Council through the City of Westminster Act 1988. These powers cannot be exercised by county councils (section 89(a)), except for areas designated by the Secretary of State, but does include National Park Committees and Boards and the Broads Authority which are not principal litter authorities under section 86(2). These provisions were introduced on 13 February 1991.

Members of the public can take court action to compel authorities to remove litter from public land in their control (section 91, see below), although the 5 days' notice requirement (section 91(5)) prior to the institution of proceedings does

provide ample time for remedial action to be undertaken. There is also encouragement to institute proceedings in that the authority would have to reimburse the expenses of the complainant in bringing the complaint and proceedings before the court where magistrates are satisfied that the complaint is justified.

Local authorities have the power to establish litter control areas under section 90, which would apply to private landowners subject to the Secretary of State setting the necessary regulations (sections 90(1)). Also street litter control notices can be issued by the local authority (section 93) on occupiers of premises to curb litter or refuse on the street or adjacent land.

The most significant change in litter control under the EPA is that local authorities have to reach a quality standard for cleanliness, or absence of litter, from an area (see 'The Code of Practice' below). This is in contrast to the traditional specification of service input for street cleansing and litter removal services (section 89(7)).

The final section of Part IV, section 99 gives district and borough councils powers with regard to abandoned shopping and luggage trolleys. The extent of their powers to curb the measure of abandoned trolleys is given in Schedule 4, which includes the power to seize and remove trolleys and to exact payment for their return or to arrange for their disposal after a period of 6 weeks.

The following information is extracted from the statutory *Code of Practice on Litter and Refuse* [9] issued within the powers given to ministers under section 89 of the EPA, and is reproduced by kind permission of the Controller of HM Stationery Office.

'The Code of Practice

The Environmental Protection Act places a new duty on the Crown, local authorities, designated statutory undertakers and the owners of some other land to keep land to

---

* The provisions of the EPA have been reassessed by the Advisory Group on Litter in 'Review of Litter Provisions of the EPA 1990 – Summary Report'. DoE and Welsh Office, July 1994.

which the public has access clear of litter and refuse, as far as is practicable. (In the case of designated statutory undertakers, the duty may apply additionally to land to which the public does not have access.) The duty also applies to the land of designated educational institutions. The Act requires the Secretary of State, under section 89(7), to issue a Code of Practice to which those under the duty are reqired to have regard.

The objective of this Code of Practice is

'to provide guidance on the discharge of the duties under section 89 by establishing reasonable and generally acceptable standards of cleanliness which those under the duty should be capable of meeting'.

It will immediately be apparent that this Code, in its approach to litter clearance, is innovative in at least two ways. Firstly, it attempts, by defining standards of cleanliness which are achievable in different types of location and under differing circumstances, to ensure uniformity of standards across Great Britain.

Secondly, the Code is concerned with **output standards** rather than **input standards** – that is to say, it is concerned with **how clean** land is, rather than **how often it is swept**. Indeed, this Code does not suggest cleaning frequencies at all – it simply defines certain standards which are achievable in different situations. This may mean that an area which all but escapes littering will seldom need to be swept whereas a litter blackspot may need frequent attention. It will be seen then, that the Code offers considerable scope for local authorities and others to target their resources to areas most in need of them, rather than simply sweeping a street because of the dictates of an arbitrary rota. Expressed in its simplest terms: 'if it isn't dirty, don't clean it'.

Statutory duties

Section 89(1) of the Act places on the Crown and (in England and Wales) county, district and London borough councils, the Common Council of the City of London, and the Council of the Isles of Scilly and (in Scotland) regional councils, district or island councils, joint boards (collectively known as 'principal litter authorities') a duty to ensure that all land in their direct control which is open to the air and to which the public has access is kept clear of litter and refuse, so far as is practicable. In addition, where the duty extends to roads, they must also be kept clean – again, as far so is practicable.

Section 86(9) transfers the responsibility for cleaning all roads except motorways (which remain with the Secretary of State) from the highways authorities to the district and borough councils.

A similar duty is placed on designated statutory undertakers. One difference between the duty as it applies to statutory undertakers and the duty applying to principal litter authorities is that the duty on the statutory undertakers might cover some land in the direct control of a statutory undertaker **to which the public has no right of access** (such as railway embankments).

The duty also applies to land in the open air and which is in the direct control of the governing body or local education authority of designated educational institutions.

Similar duties may be imposed by principal litter authorities (other than county councils, regional councils or joint boards) on owners of other land by designating their land as a 'litter control area'.

The Act allows the Secretary of State to specify descriptions of animal faeces to be included within the definition of refuse. He may also, by regulation, prescribe particular kinds of things which, if on a road, are to be treated as litter or refuse. (See The Controlled Waste Regulations 1992.)

Practicability

The caveat in the summary of the duty concerning practicability is very important. It is inevitable that on some occasions circumstances may render it impracticable (if not totally impossible) for the body under the duty to discharge it. It will be for the courts to decide, in all cases brought before them, whether or not it was impracticable for a person under the duty to discharge it but certain circumstances are foreseeable in which the discharge of the duty may be considered by the courts to be impracticable.

Enforcement

In the great majority of cases those under the duty will wish to achieve the highest possible standards of cleanliness. However, the Act makes provision for the occasion when a body under the duty may not discharge it adequately. Under section 91 a citizen aggrieved by the presence of litter or refuse on land to which the duty applies may, after giving 5 days' written notice, apply to the magistrates' court (or, in Scotland, the Sheriff) for a 'litter abatement order' requiring the person under the duty to clear away the litter or refuse from the area which is the subject of the complaint. Failure to comply with a litter abatement order may result in a fine (with additional fines accruing for each day the area remains littered). Any person contemplating enforcement action should not just consider the presence of litter but is advised to consider whether the body in question is complying with the standards in the Code before notifying them, since, under section 91(11) the Code is admissible in evidence in any court proceedings brought under that section.

Similarly, local authorities can act against any other body under the duty which appears to them to be failing to clear land of litter and refuse.

Cleanliness standards

This Code of Practice is based on the concept of four standards of cleanliness:

- no litter or refuse, known as grade A;
- predominantly free of litter and refuse apart from small items, known as grade B;

- widespread distribution of litter and refuse with minor accumulations, known as grade C; and
- heavily littered with significant accumulations, known as grade D.

Animal faeces, as prescribed by the Secretary of State in regulations, will not necessarily imply an area has fallen to a specific standard. They may be present where the cleanliness of the area has fallen to grade B, C, or to D, and must be considered alongside other litter and refuse.

Photographs showing examples of the various cleanliness standards in a variety of locations are included in the Code.

Zones

The Code has two key principles:

- areas which are habitually more heavily trafficked should have accumulations of litter cleared away more quickly than less heavily trafficked areas; and
- larger accumulations of litter and refuse should be cleared more quickly than smaller accumulations.

The Code therefore divides land types into 11 broad categories of zones according to land usage and volume of traffic. Within the broad descriptions of zones set out below it will be for the local authority or other body under the duty to allocate geographical areas to particular zones (including, where applicable, beaches for the purposes of Category 5 Zone, roads for Category 6 and 7 Zones, educational land for Category 8 Zone, railway embankments for Category 9 and 10 Zones and canal land for Category 11). This allocation must be given due publicity, not least to avoid unjustified complaints, although how it chooses to do so will be a matter for the individual body under the duty. Annotated maps in town halls, libraries and other central offices might be appropriate.

Section 95 requires cetain local authorities to keep a register on which are recorded details of land which has been designated a 'litter control area' and where street litter control notices have been issued. Bodies under the duty could use a similar arrangement to publicize their zonings.

In allocating geographical areas to the various zones the duty body will need to use its best judgement, possibly after a period of consultation. It is recognized that there is a level of detail below which it would not be practicable to allocate land to different zones. The duty body will want to avoid, for example, dividing a particular street into three different zones simply because it displays characteristics of each of those zones.

Categories

The concepts of standards of cleanliness, practicability and zonings are brought together in the Code which identifies, for different situations, practicable and achievable response times during which the duty body should restore the land in question to a particular condition.

It is stressed that the time periods given below are response times for cleaning an area which has become littered. They do not represent intervals between sweeps, which in many cases could be much longer.

Category 1 Zone

So far as is practicable, in town centres, shopping centres, shopping streets, major transport centres (including railway and bus stations and airports), central car parks and other public places where large numbers of people congregate, grade A should be achieved after cleaning. If this falls to grade B, it should be restored to grade A within 6 hours. If it falls to grade C it should be restored to grade A within 3 hours and grade D should be restored to grade A within 1 hour.

If the standard should fall to grade B or below during the period from 8 pm to 6 am, it should be restored to grade A by 8 am.

Category 2 Zone

So far is practicable, in high density residential areas (containing, for example, terraced houses and flats), land laid out as recreational areas where large numbers of people congregate, and suburban car parks and transport centres, grade A should be achieved after cleaning. If this falls to grade B, it should be restored to grade A within 12 hours. If it falls to grade C, it should be restored to grade A within 6 hours, and grade D within 3 hours.

Category 3 Zone

So far as is practicable, in low density residential areas (containing, for example, detached and semidetached houses), other public parks, other transport centres and areas of industrial estates grade A should be achieved after cleaning. If this falls to grade C, it should be restored to grade A within 12 hours, and if it falls to grade D it should be restored to grade A within 6 hours.

Category 4 Zone

So far as is practicable, in all other areas grade A should be achieved within 1 week of the standard falling to grade C, and 60 hours of the standard falling to grade D.

Category 5 Zone

Local authorities should identify those beaches in their ownership or control which might reasonably be described as 'amenity beaches'. Any assessment should take into account the level of use of the beach for recreational purposes.

As a **minimum** standard, all beaches identified by the local authority as amenity beaches should be generally clear of all types of litter and refuse between May and September inclusive. This applies to items or materials originating from discharges directly to the marine environment as well as discards from beach users. The same standard should apply to inland beaches where substantial numbers of bathers or other beach users may congregate.

Category 6 Zone – Motorways and strategic routes

On motorways and strategic routes (which may be the responsibility either of the Secretary of State or the local authority), and on associated lay-bys, grade A should be achieved after cleaning of paved areas, and grade B should be achieved after cleaning of verges. If the standard falls to grade C, the area should be restored to grade A (paved areas) or grade B (verges) within 4 weeks. If the standard falls to grade D, the area should be restored to grade A (paved areas) or grade B (verges) within 1 week.

In the case of central reservations these time limits shall not apply, but it might be practicable to restore them to grade A and grade B respectively when other work is carried out either on the central reservation itself or in a part of the carriageway immediately adjacent.

Category 7 Zone – Local roads

For local roads not falling within Zones 1 to 4, and on associated lay-bys, grade A should be achieved after cleaning of paved areas and grade B after cleaning of verges. If the standard falls to grade C, the area should be restored to grade A (paved areas) or grade B (verges) within two weeks. If the standard falls to grade D, the area should be restored to grade A (paved areas) or B (verges) within 5 days.

Category 8 Zone – Educational institutions

The aim when cleaning relevant land of designated educational institutions should be to remove all litter and refuse (grade A).

As a minimum standard during school, college or university terms, grade B should be achieved after cleaning on all relevant land of designated educational institutions. If the standard falls to grade C it should be restored to at least grade B within 24 hours (excluding weekends and half-term holidays). During other periods, if the land in question is used for a purpose authorized by the governing body or managers or the institution, it shall be restored to grade B within 1 week of it having fallen to grade C.

Out of term time, where the land in question has fallen to grade C, the governing body or managers shall ensure that it is returned to grade B as soon as is practicable.

Category 9 Zone – Railway embankments within 100 m of station platform ends

Grade B should be attained after clearance. If the standard falls to grade C, the area should be restored to grade B within 2 weeks. If the standard falls to grade D, the area should be restored to grade B within 5 days.

Category 10 Zone – Railway embankments within urban area (other than defined in Category 9 Zone)

Grade B should be attained after clearance. If the standard falls to grade C, the area should be restored to grade B within 6 months. If the standard falls to grade D, the area should be restored to grade B within 3 months.

Category 11 Zone – Canal towpaths, to which the public has right of access, in urban areas

On paved areas, grade A should be achieved after clearance. If the standard falls to grade C, the area should be restored to grade A within 2 weeks. If the standard falls to grade D, the area should be restored to grade A within 5 days.

On grassed or non-paved areas, grade B should be achieved after clearance. If the standard falls to grade C, the area should be restored to grade B within 4 weeks. If the standard falls to grade D, the area should be restored to grade B within 1 week.

The relationship between zone categories and cleansing standards is shown in Fig. 43.3. This diagram is taken from a publication of the Tidy Britain Group, *Guidelines for Category Zonation of Local Authority Land in Accordance with the Code of Practice on Litter and Refuse*. These guidelines, which outline zoning procedures and suggest ways in which these can be mapped, are obtainable from Keep Britain Tidy at The Pier, Wigan WN3 4EY.

The appendix to the litter code gives guidance (not as part of the statutory code of practice) to

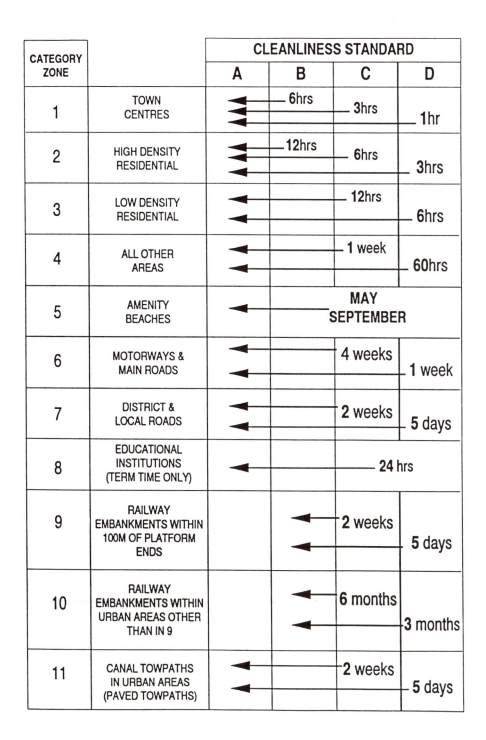

Fig. 43.3 Cleanliness standards. Summary of maximum time limits for restoring to an acceptable grade of cleanliness. (Reproduced by kind permission of the Tidy Britain Group.)

local authorities and other bodies with duties under the code on the ways of devising programmes to address the litter problem. It suggests that there are six main elements to such programmes:

1. **Appraisal**: a thorough examination of the nature, extent and cost of litter in the district. This should include a review of waste management practices including:
   (a) cleansing methods;
   (b) litter bin provision and servicing;
   (c) identification of those voluntary groups and commercial/industrial businesses who might help to resource the programme.
2. **Action**: this part of the programme should include:
   (a) consideration of the use of 'hit-squads' to deal with grade C and D conditions;
   (b) special arrangements to deal with litter from high litter production areas, e.g. markets;
   (c) supplementary servicing of litter bins;
   (d) street washing.

Action plans should be published and these should include identification of quality assurance monitoring and details of the zoning arrangements for the area.

3. **Campaigns:** full community involvement is to be encouraged and an effective public information campaign is essential.
4. **Education:** through the integration of environmental education into the curriculum, teachers and schools will have a vital part to play in shaping positive attitudes towards tidiness and litter abatement.
5. **Training:** the organization's own approach to litter control and waste management should stress the role of all individuals in that organization (including local authorities).
6. **Enforcement:** local authorities implementing the fixed penalty scheme for depositing litter and the discretionary powers relating to abandoned supermarket trolleys should discuss their plans with the police and clerk to the magistrates' court.

STREET CLEANSING

There are many differing types of street cleansing systems depending on the type of location, be it urban, rural, heavily industrialized, inland, seaside, seasonal population changes, etc. No particular system is either the wrong or the right system, it is very much a case of 'horses for courses', and tailoring the best option for each particular situation.

It is true to say that there has been a shift away from the manual emphasis in street cleansing towards mechanical systems in the last decade.

Street orderly

The simplest conventional form of street cleansing is the road sweeper with a street orderly barrow. This is unquestionably the most thorough method of cleansing, but by virtue of the considerable element of walking, and the limited capacity of the barrows involved, the distance travelled will not be great in a working day. The merits of this system are local knowledge, community identity and thoroughness.

Pedestrian-controlled electric vehicles

In inner town areas where access is restricted but where large accumulations of sweepings and waste are anticipated, pedestrian-controlled vehicles are often used. Their capacity may be as much as 8 × 4 cu ft, bins, or as an alternative a side-and-end-loading tipping body, and the facility exists for a crew to work in a gang of either three or four persons covering a larger area of work.

Cabacs

The next progression up the range is the cabac type vehicle, which comprises a similar body to the pedestrian controlled vehicle, but with a cab at the front. The cab will hold up to five drivers/sweepers. The range of these vehicles is considerably greater and speeds of up to 40 mph can be achieved. There are no exhaust emissions causing atmospheric pollution, and the vehicles are quiet in operation, which is particularly advantageous when working in residential areas early in the morning. Cabacs are also a useful mobile amenity block providing shelter from the rain, hand-washing facilities, clothes lockers and generally some shelter and warmth during other inclement weather. By virtue of their greater range to that of a pedestrian controlled vehicle and less likelihood of fatigue for the crew, they can be used to move between areas, particularly from shopping parade to shopping parade, and have a much wider range of options.

Mechanical/suction sweeping machines

The conventional mechanical sweeping vehicle is used extensively on trunk, principal and main arterial roads. The machines are available in single sweep or dual sweep options to cater for single carriageway and dual carriageway. The single version is left-hand drive to enable the driver to position himself or herself with good sight of the channel that he or she is sweeping. These machines sweep at between 2 and 5 mph. Smaller, scaled-down versions can be used on pedestrian precincts and areas of restricted manoeuvrability.

Miscellaneous vehicles

There are a number of miscellaneous vehicles which can be used for street cleansing purposes, e.g. refuse collection vehicles or light vans, once they have fulfilled their useful life on a regular round, can often be used to service manual street cleansing crews, picking up bags or emptying street cleansing bins from strategic locations. In some of the larger cities in the UK, street orderly boxes are set into the pavement, and sweepers are engaged in a practice which appears at first glance to be sweeping litter and detritus down a street gully. These boxes are often emptied by a night shift street cleansing crew.

Street washing is common in some large cities in the UK, and this can be undertaken by attachments fitted to mechanical sweepers or gully emptiers. It can also be used in connection with a bowser and a reel, or from stand pipes. This practice is, however, not as universal as it used to be 20 years ago, although open-air markets often still use this particular feature.

Seasonal variations

Winter brings snow, frost and ice as additional hazards, spring and summer the growth of weeds on footways and channels, and autumn leaf deposits.

Pavement gritters, knapsack and road sweepers, mounted weed control kits and pedestrian-operated or vehicle-mounted leaf blowing units are all recently developed equipment designed to improve operator performance in the field of street cleansing.

Other non-elemental factors that must be taken into account are tourism and student populations, often requiring seasonal staff to cope with fluctuating service demands and workload.

Street cleansing – prevention or cure?

The whole question of street cleansing and its 'bedfellow', litter abatement, hinges on the question, prevention or cure? Unquestionably, the cure is costlier to achieve, easier to manage, and simpler to perform. However, a radical new approach to the problem of an untidy Britain has emerged. The Tidy Britain Group's 'People and Places Programme' is aimed at increasing the awareness of all sections of the community to littering and its effect on the society in which we live. The programme is designed at changing attitudes towards the problem and promote a long-term systematic approach to litter abatement and environmental improvement. Nationally around 100 councils have adopted the programme.

WASTE DISPOSAL AND TREATMENT

The principal methods are:

1. incineration;
2. controlled landfilling; and
3. composting.

Considerations which influence the adoption of a particular method of disposal are:

1. the physical characteristics of the district;
2. the situation of disposal sites;
3. daily yield and average composition of refuse;

4. ultimate disposal of residual products;
5. capital outlay and running costs.

Incineration

Incineration is not now as popular as it was 20 to 30 years ago, losing favour mainly on the grounds of cost. However, because of lack of landfill space and increasing distances for haulage, some areas have adopted incineration as their means of disposal. Plant using the modern techniques for emission control should cause no nuisance. The limit on emission of pollutants are becoming more stringent under the EC directives, as now being implemented through Part I of the Environmental Protection Act 1990. This increases the cost of disposal by this method. It is likely that incineration will remain viable only when it is used to generate energy. Therefore after 1996 only those UK incinerators which reclaim energy from waste will continue to operate.

While in theory it is possible to utilize the ash from the incineration process, especially when the ferrous metal content has been removed by magnetic extraction, in normal circumstances it is of such poor quality that only a very small proportion is used as a low quality fill.

Until the commissioning trials started for the South East London Combined Heat and Power (SELCHP) plant in December 1993 there had not been a municipal waste incinerator built in the UK since 1978. Incinerators dealing with other types of waste, such as special and clinical wastes and sewage sludge, however, have continued to be constructed during that period. Also in 1993 a power plant fired by 60 000 tonnes a year of whole tyres started operating in Woverhampton and the year before a plant burning chicken litter was built in East Anglia. The SELCHP plant is illustrated in Fig. 43.4.

As with the SELCHP plant, the provision of enhanced payments for the electricity generated by these plants through the Non-Fossil Fuel Obligation payments system under the Electricity Act 1989 is a substantial additional inducement to the building of incinerators.

There are a variety of combustion systems used for waste incineration, with some more suited to liquid chemical wastes or sewage sludge and others most suited to municipal waste. The following main types in use, using the terminology from the 1993 Royal Commission on Environmental Pollution's (RCEP) Seventeenth Report, Incineration of Waste are [10]:

1. mass burn with excess air combustion;
2. ashing rotary kiln;
3. slagging rotary kiln;
4. fluidized bed;
5. pulsed hearth;
6. multiple hearth;
7. liquid injection.

The RCEP report suggested that the minimum economic threshold for development of a municipal solid waste (MSW) incinerator is around 200 000 tonnes a year. The SELCHP plant in Deptford, Lewisham has a capacity of 420 000 tonnes while the Coventry plant which also has energy recovery and was completed in 1976 has a capacity of 160 000 tonnes a year.

Mass burn incinerators

Mass burn incinerators are used to burn municipal solid waste but can also be used to burn suitable commercial and industrial wastes. The capacity of existing plants in the UK varies according to the number of furnace units incorporated in the design (up to 5) and the size of each unit can vary from around 10 tonnes per hour up to 30 tonnes per hour.

Waste is fed by crane from storage bunkers to the feed hopper, from where it flows down, usually aided by a mechanical stoker, into the combustion chamber. Air is introduced through a moving grate in the chamber which agitates the waste promoting thorough exposure of the waste to the air. Waste is fed onto the grate and during the initial drying stage, 50–100°C, volatile compounds are released. These burn above the grate, where secondary air is introduced to facilitate complete gas phase combustion. The remaining waste moves down the grate and continues to burn slowly and after about an hour the residues are discharged from the end of the grate, where they are usually quenched and in most cases the ferrous fraction is magnetically extracted prior to deposit.

POWER GENERATION

Steam leaves the boilers at a temperature of 395°C and 46 bar, and is fed directly to a single 32 megawatt [MW(e)] steam turbine generator in the Turbine Hall (15).

Steam from the turbine can be used to produce maximum electricity output; alternatively, some or all can be diverted to the steam/water heat exchangers to heat the future District Heating network. Steam is also used to preheat the combustion air for the refuse burning process in the Air Preheater (16).

As there is no source of cooling water on the site it has been necessary to provide a bank of air cooled condensers (17) to condense the exhaust steam from the turbine. They are forced draught units mounted on a steel structure and the fans are equipped with variable low speed drives to prevent audible noise emissions.

Electricity is generated at 11 kV and transformed up to 132 kV for export to the electricity supply system which passes very close to the plant.

HOW THE PLANT WORKS

Refuse collection vehicles (1) tip the solid waste - without pre-sorting into the storage pit (2) from where it is transferred by over-head cranes (3) to the feed hopper (4) of the stoker feed chute. Hydraulic ram feeders (5) provide controlled charging of refuse onto the surface of the Martin reverse-acting stoker grate (6).

The forced draught fan (7) supplies primary air via the under-grate air zones to the burning refuse layer on the stoker grate (6). This fan and the overfire air fan (8) draw the air from the refuse storage pit area thus preventing the egress of unpleasant odours from the plant.

The heart of the System for waste combustion is the stoker grate itself (6). The grate surface is sloped downwards from the feeder end towards the residue discharge end and is comprised of alter-nate steps of fixed and moving grate bars. The moving grate steps perform slow stirring strokes against the grate slope. This ensures that the burning refuse layer is continually rotated and mingled to form an even depth of bed and red hot mass is pushed back to the front end of the grate. In this way an intense fire builds up immediately at the front end of the grate, with all combustion phases (such as drying, ignition and combustion itself) taking place simultaneously.

Burned out residues are transferred at the bottom of the stoker grate, by an ash discharger (18) and by the residue handling sys-tem (19) and deposited in the residue pit (21). During the trans-fer, ferrous metals are removed by the magnetic separator (19).

The energy released by the process is recovered in the boiler. In this unit, the furnace walls and the division walls between the boiler sections (9) are of solidly welded membrane design. The superheater (10) is carefully sited in the multi-pass boiler whilst the economiser section (11) is in the fourth pass. The econo-miser is followed by the lime scrubber reactor (12) where a fine spray of a lime (from the lime storage silo (22)) and water mix-ture is introduced into the flue gases. This has the effect of neu-tralising acid gases contained in the flue gases and as the lime/salts cool, heavy metals condense onto the particulates. This particulate matter is removed from the gas stream by the bag-house filter (13) and the now clean and dedusted flue gases are ejected to atmosphere by the induced draft fan (14) via the 100 metre tall chimney.

Flue gas treatment residues are stored in the ash silo (23). Both these residues and the burned out ash residues and separated metals from the stoker grate are loaded onto transport within the building and removed from the site. Ash and flue gas treat-ment residues are landfilled and the metals are recycled.

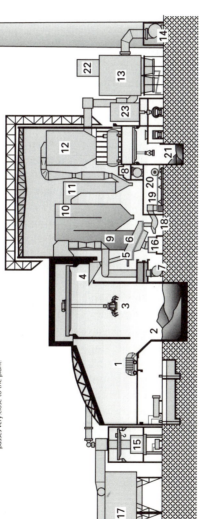

Fig. 43.4 Waste to energy plant, South East London Combined Heat and Power Ltd. (Diagram and description by courtesy of SELCHP, 7B Evelyn Court, Deptford Business Centre, London SE8 5AD.)

Although there are a considerable variety of designs for mass burn incinerators, the most efficient appear to be those with reciprocating or roller grates and the combustion chamber in the form of a vertical shaft.

Ashing rotary kiln

Ashing rotary kiln incinerators are used primarily to burn chemical waste. They are also suitable for the combustion of clinical waste and MSW but have not been used in the UK for disposal of MSW. Rotary kilns used for clinical waste range from around 1 to 3 tonnes per hour, for chemical waste up to 10 tonnes per hour and for MSW up to 20 tonnes per hour.

Waste is fed into a refractory-lined drum which acts as the grate surface in the primary combustion stage. The waste is ignited on entry to the drum and the rotating action of the drum mixes it with air supplied via nozzles in the furnace wall. A secondary combustion chamber is fitted with air inlets and after-burners, usually operating at 1100–1300°C, to complete the combustion of the gases.

Slagging rotary kiln

Slagging rotary kiln incinerators are most suitable for chemical waste. This type of incinerator is very similar in method of operation to the ashing rotary kiln but uses a higher combustion temperature (1400°C). This melts most inorganic waste and ash and therefore produces a liquid slag which traps particulate matter in the kiln before being solidified, usually in a quench tank but occasionally by air cooling. The vitrified slag has a very low leaching rate for heavy metals and organic compounds.

Fluidized bed

Fluidized bed incinerators are used in the UK mainly to burn dewatered sewage sludge cake, usually at about 3 tonnes an hour. They are also suitable for burning clinical waste, some chemical wastes and municipal waste which has been processed to effect size reduction. None of the units operational in the UK incinerates MSW.

Other systems

Multiple hearth, pulsed heath and liquid injection incinerators are not used for the incineration of MSW.

The essential elements of an incineration plant are shown in Fig. 43.5 and are:

1. **facilities for handling, storing and mixing feedstock** without creating a hazard or a nuisance. In the diagram vehicles enter the tipping hall (A) and unload waste into a bunker (B), from which a grab on a crane (C) transfers it to a hopper (D) leading to the grate.
2. **A combustion chamber** (F) which is designed to achieve very efficient combustion in both the solid/liquid (*primary*) and gas/aerosol (*secondary*) phases. In the plant illustrated the waste is agitated mechanically as it moves over the **grate** (E) in order to expose it to air and maintain a free flow through the grate bars.
3. **A heat recovery system** (G) for cooling the exhaust gases prior to cleaning them. This minimizes corrosion, thermal stress and the formation of undesirable compounds such as dioxins. It also opens up the opportunity of utilizing the energy recovered.
4. **A gas-cleaning system**, typically consisting of a scrubber (H) and an electrostatic precipitator (J).
5. **A fan** (K) to draw the cleaned gases out of the plant so that they can be dispersed from the **stack** (L).
6. Facilities for the collection, handling, and where necessary **treatment of solid residues**. Ash and clinker from the grate fall into a water-filled quench tank (M) and are moved by conveyor (N) to a bunker (P); and fly ash is collected from the electrostatic precipitator (S).
7. Facilities for the collection and **treatment of liquid effluents** (Q, R) from the scrubber and quench tank.

Controlled landfilling

The term 'controlled landfilling' describes a system of disposing of refuse by depositing in a methodical, as distinct from a crude or indiscriminate, manner. The greater part of all controlled

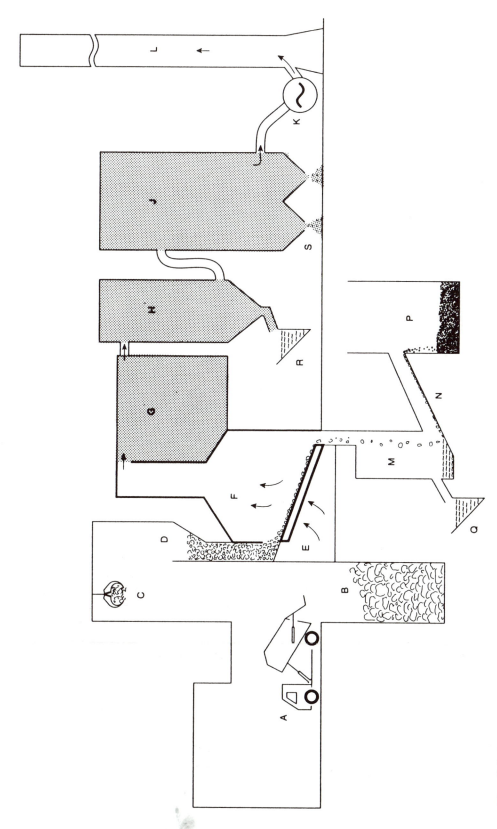

Fig. 43.5 An incineration plant for municipal waste (arrows indicate air or gas flow). (Source: Royal Commission on Environmental Pollution, 17th Report, Incineration of Waste.)

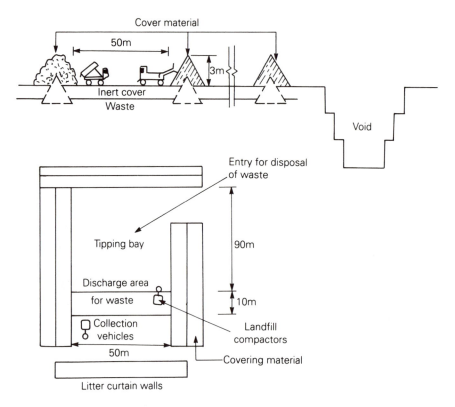

Fig. 43.6 Cell method of landfill operation. (Source: Department of the Environment (1986) *Landfilling Wastes*, Waste Management Paper No. 26, HMSO, London. Reproduced by kind permission of the Controller, HMSO.)

waste is disposed of in this manner and the system, if properly supervised, provides a satisfactory method of disposal. Mineral excavations or low-lying sites, as well as opencast sites, are selected for the purpose, and, by the utilization of refuse in the manner described below, are reclaimed for useful purposes. In many districts, on grounds of land reclamation alone, this method of disposal of refuse is justified. There has been a recent trend for disposal of waste over land, thus creating new, improved landform.

There are three methods of landfill operation:

1. Trench method: this involves the excavation of a trench (which may be very large) into which waste is deposited. The excavated material is then used as cover. This technique is a variation of the cell method described below. It should be distinguished from the construction of trenches into already deposited solid waste for the disposal of liquid wastes. The trench

method has found very limited application in the UK.

2. Area method: waste may be deposited in layers and to form terraces over the available area. However, with this type of operation, excessive leachate generation may occur unless high-waste inputs are maintained, thereby providing adequate absorptive capacity to account for rainfall. This method has been used widely in the UK, but is no longer favoured since operational control may be difficult.

3. Cell method: this method involves the deposition of waste within preconstructed bunded areas (Fig. 43.6). It is now the preferred method since it encourages the concept of progressive filling and restoration. It is a method which is beginning to have widespread application.

The main points about the deposition of the crude refuse are:

1. Where the base of the site cannot support the weight of vehicles, a preformed base is required.
2. Waste should be deposited at the top or base of a shallow sloping working face, and not over a vertical face. The face of the tip should slope at an incline of no greater than 1 in 3.
3. The deposit of waste should be in thin layers, and the use of a compactor enables a high density to be activated. Each layer should not exceed 0.3 m thickness.
4. At the end of the working day, all exposed surfaces should be covered with an inert material to a depth of at least 0.15 m.
5. The management and workforce should be fully aware of the site safety regulations and of the need to observe them.
6. An effective system of litter control is essential.
7. Measures need to be taken to control birds, particularly gulls and crows, where sites receive quantities of putrescible matter. Control measures include:
   (a) birdscarers
   (b) distress calls
   (c) falcons
   (d) nets.
8. Effective measures to ensure good pest control are necessary. Good compaction of the material will reduce the likelihood of infestation by both insects and rodents, as will the daily covering of waste. However, regular systems of both rodent and insect control need to be established on a programmed basis.
9. Waste should not be burnt on the landfill site.

Fig. 43.7 shows a typical operational plan for a landfill site.

The main elements of the site restoration plan following the cessation of landfilling are:

1. A plan for restoration should form an integral part of the landfill operation.
2. The intended final levels and contours should be indicated within the plan, as should the systems for leachate control.
3. There must be a clear and efficient system for the management of landfill gas.
4. Landfill site capping should be constructed of material having a permeability of 1×10^{-7} cm/s or less, and should extend over the whole site to increase water run-off. A basic aim of the cap is to minimize leachate production by minimizing water entry to the tipped area.
5. The cap should be covered with an appropriate thickness of soil to protect the cap from damage by, for example, agricultural machinery.

Fig. 43.8 shows a section through a landfill site situated on clay strata and indicates both completed and operational parts of the site. Department of the Environment Waste Management Paper No. 26, *Landfilling Wastes* [11], provides a most useful technical source of information on the problem and solutions in current day practice. Waste Management Paper No. 26A (1993) provides guidance on assessing the completion of licensed landfill sites. (See also Department of the Environment Waste Management Paper No. 27, HMSO.)

Types of landfill sites

There are two basic forms of landfill sites, dilute and disperse sites and containment sites.

Dilute and disperse sites

The dilute and disperse site is operated on the basis that leachate, that is generated slowly, migrates through unsaturated strata. During the passage, chemical, physical, biological and microbiological activity reduces the pollutants present. When this leachate comes into contact with water it is quite weak. Further dilution takes places in the aquifer, thus further reducing the polluting characteristics. This method has been used extensively in Great Britain.

In theory, the method appears to be safe, but there are a few cases of pollution of water from such practice which have been attributed to disposal of intractable industrial waste or improper geological situation for such a site.

There is an increasing reluctance by the NRA to allow such sites, as the risk to water resources from such sites, even though small, is unacceptable. Once an aquifer gets contaminated, then its 100% purification is almost impossible.

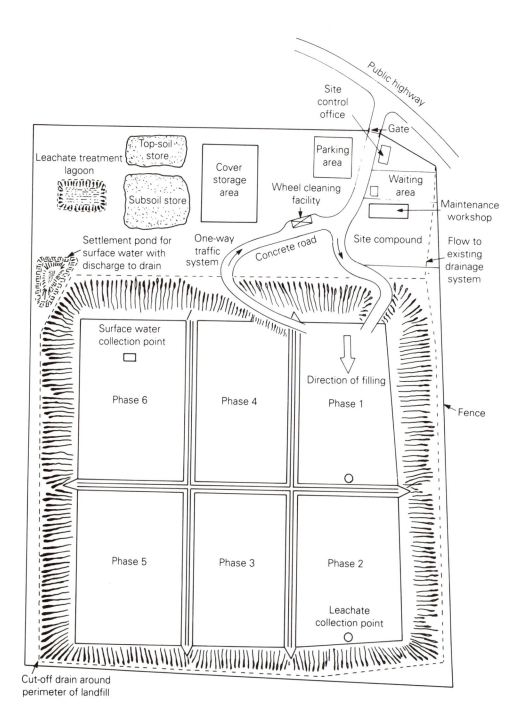

Fig. 43.7 Typical operational plan for landfill site. (Source: Department of the Environment (1986) *Landfilling Wastes*, Waste Management Paper No. 26, HMSO, London. Reproduced by kind permission of the Controller, HMSO.)

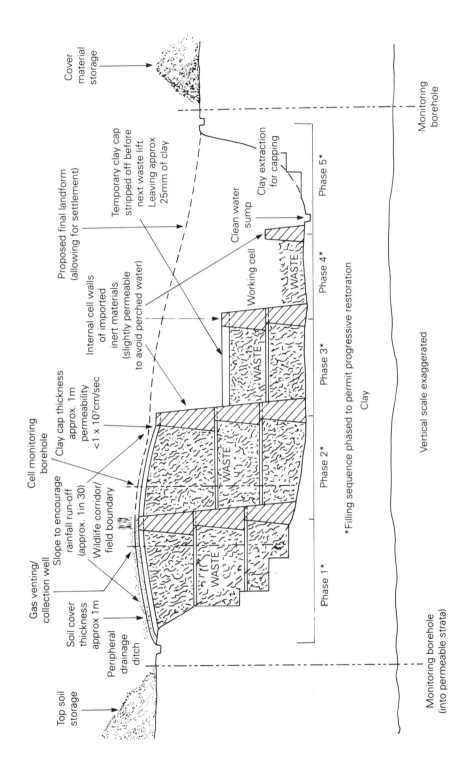

Top soil storage

Peripheral drainage ditch

Soil cover thickness approx 1m

Gas venting/ collection well

Slope to encourage rainfall run-off (approx. 1 in 30)

Wildlife corridor/ field boundary

Cell monitoring borehole

Clay cap thickness approx. 1m permeability <1 x 10⁷cm/sec

Proposed final landform (allowing for settlement)

Internal cell walls of imported inert materials (slightly permeable to avoid perched water)

Temporary clay cap stripped off before next waste lift. Leaving approx 25mm of clay

Cover material storage

Working cell

Clean water sump

Clay extraction for capping

Monitoring borehole

WASTE

Phase 1*   Phase 2*   Phase 3*   Phase 4*   Phase 5*

*Filling sequence phased to permit progressive restoration

Clay

Vertical scale exaggerated

Monitoring borehole (into permeable strata)

Fig. 43.8 Section through landfill situated on clay strata. (Source: Department of the Environment (1986) *Landfilling Wastes*, (1986) HMSO, London. Reproduced by kind permission of the Controller, HMSO.)

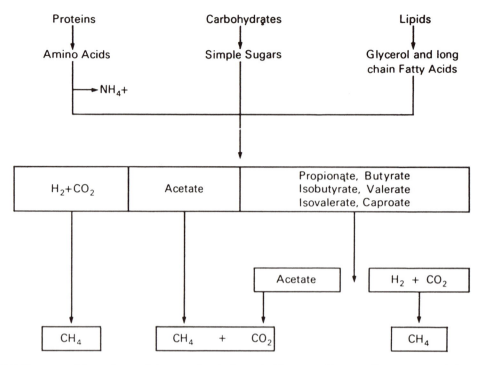

Fig. 43.9 Decomposition of materials occurring in household waste. (Source: Department of the Environment (1986) *Landfilling Wastes*, Waste Management Paper No. 26, HMSO, London.)

Containment sites

The containment site is a site where the base, sides and the top of the site (once landfilling finishes) is sealed with a suitable mineral or synthetic impermeable liner.

In this country, clay is extensively used to seal the site. In the USA and some European countries, synthetic plastic liners are used. Depending on the country and geology of the site, either a single liner, a composite liner or double liner is incorporated. Further research is needed to evaluate the advantages and disadvantages of various liners in different conditions.

Decomposition of household waste after landfilling

Within the landfill site aerobic conditions will initially prevail but anaerobic conditions are rapidly established. The biodegradation of various components of refuse in landfills is extremely complex but three main stages can be distinguished (Fig. 43.9).

In the first stage degradable waste is attacked by aerobic organisms present in the waste in the presence of oxygen in air trapped in the waste to form more simple organic compounds, carbon dioxide and water. Heat is generated and the aerobic organisms multiply.

The second stage commences when all the oxygen is consumed or displaced by carbon dioxide and the aerobic organisms die back. The degradation process is then taken over by organisms which can thrive in either the presence or absence of oxygen. These organisms can break down the large organic molecules present in food, paper and similar waste into more simple compounds such as hydrogen, ammonia, water, carbon dioxide and organic acids. During this stage carbon dioxide concentrations can reach a maximum of 90%, but usually reach about 50%.

In the third and final anaerobic stage species of methane-forming organisms multiply and break down organic acids to form methane gas and other products (Fig. 43.10).

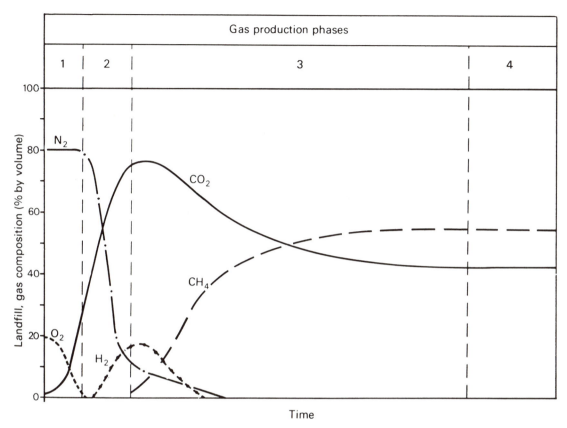

Fig. 43.10 Typical production pattern for landfill gas. (Source: Department of the Environment (1986) *Landfilling Wastes*, Waste Management Paper No. 26, HMSO, London.)

Composting

As a waste treatment technique in the UK composting was almost eliminated in the 1970s. Up to that time there were several schemes which were producing compost from a feedstock of ordinary household waste, usually using Dano drums or similar slowly rotating trommels where the waste was retained for between 2 days and a week before being placed in windrows for further processing.

The production of a growing medium from mixed refuse became increasingly difficult to market and the cost of this method of waste processing was considerably higher than the cost of landfill. In contrast, in most mainland continental counties the technique has continued to be used for treatment of up to 10% of household waste, although in most cases the resulting material has been used in land reclamation or as landfill cover.

While the average dustbin or black bag contains around 20% of putrescible, and largely compostable, waste there is an even greater amount of readily compostable material available from residents' gardens and the councils' parks departments, which although traditionally composted, until very recently increasing amounts were going to landfill for disposal.

Research carried out on pilot collections of source separated compostable waste in the UK suggest that at least half of the weight of compostable waste could be reclaimed. Monitoring of 4000 households which participated in Leeds City Council's split wheeled bin trial which started in December 1990 showed that of an estimated 4.4 kg of compostable waste produced each week by households, half was correctly separated for collection. Early results from East Hertfordshire District Council's 2200 household trial of brown wheeled 'bio-bins' showed a diversion rate of 40% but the scheme started during the growing season and there is a greater proportion of the population with gardens than in the Leeds initial trial area.

Therefore a national collection of compostable waste would yield around 1.5–2 M tpa of kitchen waste plus an equal amount of garden waste, currently brought to civic amenity sites.

The development of composting systems in the UK is taking two main forms: the centralized composting of green wastes and the promotion of home composting systems. The development of markets to accommodate increasing amounts of compost is an essential aspect of the development of centralized composting systems. The main priority of local authorities promoting home composting is the need for a comprehensive coverage of composting units in those areas chosen for this type of waste reduction strategy to ensure that there will be an effective diversion of the putrescible waste fraction.

In the early 1990s a number of green waste composting systems had been established, mainly using green wastes from parks departments and civic amenity waste disposal sites. In a limited number of cases selected commercial and industrial wastes have been used to improve the mix of materials composted. In only a small minority of cases have centralized composting systems incorporated kitchen waste materials because of the potential problems of attraction of vermin and the increased chance of odour. In several mainland European countries these difficulties have been overcome by the building of enclosed composting facilities which obviously increases the cost of this method of waste treatment.

The greatest barrier to the expansion of green waste composting schemes is the requirement to develop markets to take the growing media, mulches and chippings produced, and throughout the year, as the market is highly concentrated into the spring months.

In contrast, the establishment of home composting facilities attempts to effect the reduction of waste at source. By early 1994 around 25 UK local authorities had established home composting initiatives, each with more than 250 units. These varied from free or heavily subsidized provision of conventional garden composters, rotating units or Green Cone digesters. In a minority of instances wormeries have also been offered, but these have greater operational limitations than other types of unit.

One of the main difficulties in assessing the success of home composting schemes is that there is often little data on what proportion of the population is already practising composting at home and what proportion of the materials generated in the home are composted. How many more people therefore will be composting as a result of the provision of the new composting units?

To overcome some of these difficulties the London Borough of Sutton offered composters only in one collection round where the record of waste collected had been measured over several years and therefore the effect of provision of composters could be measured. Despite the generous discounts on the three types of unit offered the participation rate was too low to assess accurately the effect of the distribution of the composters.

To overcome this problem during 1994 the council planned to provide Green Cone digesters to all households in another part of the borough with people having positively to refuse to accept the unit. Whether this approach would produce a sufficient waste reduction effect to recoup the cost of the units, as has been claimed for some North American cities, is difficult at this stage to determine.

In some cases, such as in East Hertfordshire and Leeds, where there is separation of compostable material, alternate fortnightly collections of different fractions of household waste have been instituted. Potentially where very high coverage of home composting units has been achieved fortnightly collections might be considered in those circumstances. However many residents, councillors and local authority officers are rightly wary of instituting such a change of service provision. Where fortnightly collections have been instituted, almost always where wheeled bin collection systems have been instituted, very few operational problems have been experienced or complaints received.

Solid fuel substitutes

A fairly recent development has been the manufacture of a fuel derived from waste by the separation of materials and compressing the paper, cardboard and plastics hard enough to form them into pellets. They have half to two-thirds of the calorific value of coal.

There has been some doubt expressed as to its economical viability as well as its suitability due to the higher quality requirement on emissions of flue gases. The extensive use of the system is doubtful.

CLINICAL WASTE

General background

The following information is adapted from *Clinical Waste – an Appraisal* [12], published by the London Waste Regulation Authority, to whom we are grateful for permission to include it.

Internationally

The World Health Organization (WHO), the Commission of the European Communities and the United States Environmental Protection Agency (EPA), have all, in the course of the last few years, emphasized the need for clinical waste to be safely managed, from the point of production via various methods of movement to its final disposal. The concern expressed by these bodies reflects the growing awareness of the threat to public health that can arise from the improper handling and disposal of such wastes.

WHO in *Management of Waste from Hospitals* [13] (published in 1985 and reflecting the conclusions of a working party in the summer of 1983), classified health care waste into eight main categories, while the EPA in *Guide for Infectious Waste Management* [14] recommended that health care facilities should prepare an Infectious Wastes Management Plan outlining policies and procedures for the management of infectious wastes, which it divided into six main categories plus four 'optional' categories. Details of these categories are included in *Clinical Waste – an Appraisal* [12].

Nationally

In the UK, the same concern about the need for the safe management of clinical waste has been expressed by the Department of the Environment, the Department of Health, the Health and Safety Commission (HSC) and the Royal Commission on Environmental Pollution.

National awareness of the need for tighter control and regulation of clinical wastes increased at the beginning of the 1980s. Prior to this, items had been washed and cleaned or sterilized after use, but there was now a major conversion to the use of one-trip plastics and disposable materials. Disposable syringes, catheters, probes, urine bags and special clinical packs, together with one-use and discarded protective clothing, linen and dining equipment, became the accepted substitute for much of the long-life equipment previously used in the medical and clinical field.

This trend, coupled with the switch to waste disposal in plastic bags in a whole range of colours, gave rise to a marked increase in the output of clinical wastes. The casual manner in which these wastes were mixed with general waste disposal streams also gave cause for concern and in 1982 the HSC issued a guidance document entitled *The Safe Disposal of Clinical Waste* [15]. This defined and categorized clinical waste and gave advice on its handling, transport and disposal.

The HSC's definition of clinical waste, which has been generally accepted in the UK, runs as follows:

'Waste arising from medical, nursing, dental, veterinary, pharmaceutical or similar practice, investigation, treatment, care, teaching or research which by nature of its toxic, infectious or dangerous content may prove a hazard or give offence unless previously rendered safe and inoffensive. Such waste includes human or animal tissue or excretions, drugs and medicinal products, swabs and dressings, instruments or similar substances and materials.'

The HSC document divided clinical waste into the following five categories:

1. **Group A:**
   (a) soiled surgical dressings, swabs and all other contaminated waste from treatment areas;
   (b) material other than linen from cases of infectious disease;
   (c) all human tissues (whether infected or not), animal carcases and tissues from laboratories, and all related swabs and dressings.
2. **Group B:**
   discarded syringes, needles, cartridges, broken glass and any other sharp instruments.
3. **Group C:**
   Laboratory and post-mortem room waste other than waste included in Group A.
4. **Group D:**
   certain pharmaceutical and chemical waste.
5. **Group E:**
   used disposable bed-pan liners, urine containers, incontinence pads and stoma bags.

In 1983 the Department of the Environment published *Clinical Wastes: a Technical Memorandum on Arisings, Treatment and Disposal* [16] including a code of practice which estimated that the amount of clinical waste arisings from National Health and private hospitals in Great Britain in 1980 was some 33 000 tonnes. A comparable estimate was not available for clinical waste arisings from community health service practices, but the paper suggested it could be as much as 15% of clinical wastes arisings at hospitals. It stated that waste from home treatment would in total represent the largest arisings of clinical wastes, but as individual arisings were usually small and irregular in time a precise figure could not be given, though three to five times the amount arising in hospitals was thought probable. It was noted that about 1.7 million cat and dog carcases were also disposed of each year.

The paper stressed that the segregation of clinical waste from all other wastes was the key to proper disposal. It suggested that the segregation system set out in the HSC document should be adopted as a national standard and urged hospitals to ensure that their management structures for waste disposal were adequate, and that a

waste disposal policy was formulated and implemented. It was emphasized that packaging for clinical wastes should be of a high integrity.

In 1987, the British Standards Institution adopted a classification for the analysis of hospital wastes in its BS3316:1987 Part 4 [17] and grouped hospital waste in six categories.

The Royal Commission on Environmental Pollution in its eleventh report *Managing Waste: The Duty of Care* [5] recommended that all regional health authorities should prepare and implement waste disposal plans that matched the arisings and the disposal facilities in health care establishments. It also recommended that publicity should be given by government health departments through health authorities to the guidelines and code of practice prepared by the HSC and the Department of the Environment on the disposal of clinical waste so that community health care establishments were made aware of good practices, which could then be enforced. It was urged that publicity material prepared by the health departments should be made available for doctors and nurses in the community to give to patients who might have to dispose of clinical waste. It also recommended that Crown immunity should cease to apply to the National Health Service (NHS) and that incineration and other waste disposal facilities operated by or on behalf of the NHS should, in consequence, be subject to exactly the same controls and standards as similar facilities operated by other organizations.

In its response to the Royal Commission (July 1986), the government expressed its own concern about reported standards of waste handling within the NHS and stated that, while it had no current plans for removing Crown immunity, the situation would be kept under review. They considered it unnecessary for regional health authorities (RHAs) to duplicate, in effect, the work of the Waste Disposal Authorities (WDAs) in preparing waste disposal plans, but urged the RHAs to co-operate with the WDAs in making their information available. The government also made it clear, in separate pronouncements, that it expected the NHS to meet and maintain the standards required by the Control of Pollution

Act 1974, the Clean Air Acts and supporting regulations and that responsibility for emissions from NHS hospital chimneys would be considered as part of a forthcoming review of air pollution control (now see Part I of the Environmental Protection Act 1990).

It will be clear from the foregoing that the 1980s heralded a heightened national awareness of the potential dangers from the mismanagement of clinical waste from all sources and saw the emergence of a new determination to tackle the problem.

Legislation

The general framework for the control of waste including clinical waste is included earlier in this chapter. However, there are specific requirements which need to be considered.

The Controlled Waste Regulations 1992

These Regulations, applicable to both England and Wales, contain a legal definition of clinical waste. Clinical waste means:

1. any waste which consists wholly or partly of human or animal tissue, blood or other body fluids, excretions, drugs or other pharmaceutical products, swabs or dressings, or syringes, needles or other sharp instruments, being waste which unless rendered safe may prove hazardous to any person coming into contact with it; and
2. any other waste arising from medical, nursing, dental, veterinary, pharmaceutical or similar practice, investigation, treatment, care, teaching, or research, or the collection of blood for transfusion, being waste which may cause infection to any person coming into contact with it.

Certain classes of waste are prescribed so that charges can be made for their collection and disposal. The Regulations define clinical waste and then distinguish between the two basically different sources from which it emanates: clinical waste from a private dwelling or residential home (Schedule 2), which is categorized as household waste for which a charge for collection may be made, and clinical waste from any other source (Schedule 3), which is categorized as industrial waste.

Thus, a local collection authority has a duty to collect clinical waste in the first category if requested to do so, but has the power to make a charge for this service. The Department of the Environment has stressed that it expects the collection authorities to take account of the social benefits, and the obvious undesirability of discouraging occupants from making the desired special arrangements, before deciding to make a charge. It also stresses that the Regulations are not intended to disrupt existing arrangements, i.e. collection by health authorities, where those are satisfactory and that the primary objective of the prescription is simply to promote public safety (Department of the Environment Circular 13/88).

All other clinical waste, i.e. that which does not emanate from a private dwelling or residential home, is categorized as industrial waste. The local collection authority does not have any duty to collect it, but may if requested to do so, and then only after first obtaining permission from the disposal authority. A disposal authority in England where it is separate from the collection authority may also collect clinical waste where it is prescribed as industrial waste. The collecting authority has a duty to make a reasonable charge for its collection and disposal.

All other waste from a hospital, unless otherwise prescribed, falls into the category of household waste. This means that the local collection authority has a duty to collect it free of charge.

Health and Safety at Work, etc. Act 1974

This Act applies to all health care activities in the UK and thus its provisions apply in requiring the safe handling, storage, transportation and disposal of clinical waste arising from those activities. Briefly, the relevant sections of the Act require that a safe system of work (which should be in writing) exists, which is monitored to ensure that proper and adequate resources, training, equipment and information are provided to ensure the minimization of risk to health or safety of employees and public alike.

Table 43.3 Recommended colour coding for containers for clinical waste

Colour of bag	Type of waste
Black	Normal household waste: not to be used to store or transport clinical waste
Yellow	All waste destined for incineration
Yellow with a black band	Waste, e.g. home nursing waste, which preferably should be disposed of by incineration, but which may be disposed of by landfill when separate collection and disposal arrangements are made
Light blue or transparent with light blue inscriptions	Waste for autoclaving (or equivalent treatment) before ultimate disposal

Source: Health and Safety Commission (1982) *The Safe Disposal of Clinical Waste*, HMSO, London.

Segregation of waste

The HSC's *Safe Disposal of Clinical Waste* [15] recommends that the identification of various kinds of waste for disposal in a particular manner is best achieved by the use of easily identifiable colour-coded containers. Care should be taken to avoid confusion with other sorting systems which may be colour coded, e.g. for soiled, foul and infected linen in hospitals and other health care premises. All organizations involved with handling clinical waste are therefore strongly advised to adopt the colour coding given in Table 43.3.

Disposal

Taking into account the conclusions of the Department of the Environment's guidance document, Waste Management Paper No. 25 [16] recommends that incineration should be the preferred disposal route for the following clinical wastes whether they arise in the community or medical and veterinary establishments:

1. Group A: human tissues, limbs, placentae and infected carcasses and dialysis waste;

2. Group B: all sharps;
3. Group C: all pathology wastes unless they have been effectively autoclaved and are suitable for treatment and disposal by this method (Howie Code);
4. Group D: small amounts of solid medicines and injectables (but not large arisings of pharmaceuticals whose disposal should be on the advice of the Waste Disposal Authority, the National Rivers Authority or River Purification Board and the Pharmaceutical Society of Great Britain. Waste Management Paper No. 19 also provides advice).

The guidance document also expresses a preference that the following materials are incinerated, but notes that other disposal methods could be acceptable: Group A: soiled surgical dressings, swabs and other contaminated wastes.

It is now accepted that clinical waste should, wherever possible, be incinerated in incinerators designed to destroy all grades of clinical and special waste.

In practical terms, landfill should only be used as an emergency back-up to incinerators, and even then only for certain types of non-infectious clinical waste. The dangers of infection from hepatitis B, and more recently HIV, and the anxiety surrounding these matters has meant that the use of landfill for the disposal of clinical waste, even under carefully controlled conditions, has virtually ceased, because of stringent restrictions on site licensing.

The third report of the Hazardous Waste Inspectorate in June 1988 drew attention to the unsatisfactory performance of some NHS incinerators, which operate at too low temperatures to achieve totally sterile residues. For the future, in addition to maceration and high temperature incineration, there are other methods for the disposal of clinical waste so as to render them non-hazardous and harmless. In Germany, a process is in operation whereby clinical waste is treated at the site of production, it is shredded, making the waste unrecognizable, then subjected to microwave treatment, which results in thermic disinfection. It is able to handle all types of clinical waste, including hypodermic needles, bandages, dialysis filters, etc., and the resulting disinfected granules can then be compacted into a container for shipment to a licensed landfill site for final disposal. The control of atmospheric emissions from hospital incinerators, including those handling clinical waste, is now exercised through the authorization procedures of Part I of the Environmental Protection Act 1990.

STORAGE, COLLECTION AND DISPOSAL OF OTHER HAZARDOUS WASTE

Storage

There are only a small number of licensed facilities in the country for disposal of hazardous waste, and the cost of transport and disposal of hazardous waste has increased severalfold in recent years. This has resulted in the increasing number of storage facilities within the premises of the waste producers, as well as installation of transfer station and bulking stations, being licensed for this purpose by waste regulation authorities, so that economical loads are transported for disposal.

Under the Control of Pollution (Special Waste) Regulations 1980 the deposit, on the premises on which it is produced, of special waste, pending its disposal elsewhere requires a licence, other than in the following quantities:

1. liquid waste of a total volume of not more than 23 000 l deposited in a secure container or containers; and either;
2. non-liquid waste of a total volume of not more than 80 m³ deposited in a secure container or containers; or
3. Non-liquid waste of a total volume of not more than 50 m³ deposited in a secure place or places.

These regulations are under review.

A secure container or place is one designed or adapted so that as far as it is practicable, waste cannot escape from it, and members of the public cannot have access to the waste contained within it.

This means that safe storage of all hazardous waste is essential, even when the quantities are below the licensable limits. This is achieved by the proper segregation and labelling of all containers, and storing them in bunded areas or impervious areas so that no risk to water resources exists. The site is made secure by providing proper fencing and lockable gates.

Collection

The collection of hazardous waste is, and must be, carried out by operators who have knowledge of the properties of the waste and have experience of handling such waste so that they know what equipment and vehicles should be used. It is essential that two or more consignments of hazardous waste are not mixed during transportation unless it is clear that the materials are fully compatible. These have been serious incidents when two wastes, upon mixing, have resulted in a dangerous chemical reaction.

Some waste authorities provide a specialist collection service for small quantities of hazardous chemicals. The advantage of such a service is that hazardous chemicals are not so liable to be dumped in the dustbins, streams or lay-bys where the risk to people is high.

Disposal

The following methods are used for disposal of hazardous waste:

1. Landfilling. A significant number of hazardous waste are disposed of by co-disposal with household waste.* It is, however, essential that disposal takes place in a properly engineered site so that leachate is not able to pollute the water resources.
2. Incineration. Incineration of organic hazardous waste is the best method of disposal provided the incinerator is capable of destroying such chemicals by proper design in terms of temperature, retention time and oxygen intake, and the operation is well controlled.
3. Chemical fixation. Hazardous waste, particularly inorganic waste, is capable of being mixed with suitable chemicals, such as cement, so that the polluting waste is bound chemically

* See Draft Waste Management Paper No. 26F – Landfill Co-disposal, October 1994, DoE.

or physically within them so that no polluting leachate is generated.

4. Co-disposal with sewage. Certain chemical waste can be treated by controlled feeding into the flow of sewage works. The rate of deposit is controlled in such a manner that it does not kill micro-organisms in the treatment works. The micro-organisms then degrade these wastes into harmless components.

REFERENCES

1. Poor Law Commissioners (1842) *Report on an Enquiry into the Sanitary Condition of the Labouring Population of Great Britain*, HMSO, London, p. 14.
2. Report of the Working Party on Refuse Storage and Collection (1967), HMSO, London.
3. Technical Committee on the Experimental Disposal of House Refuse in Wet and Dry Pits (1961) *Pollution of Water by Tipped Refuse*, HMSO, London.
4. Report of the Technical Committee on the Disposal of Toxic Waste (1970), Key Report, HMSO, London.
5. *Waste Management – The Duty of Care: a code of practice* (1991) HMSO, London.
6. Government White Paper (1990) *This Common Inheritance – Britain's Environmental Strategy*, HMSO, London.
7. Department of the Environment (1991) *Waste Management Paper No. 28*, Recycling of Waste, HMSO, London.
8. Health and Safety Executive *Safety in the Use of Refuse Compaction Vehicles*, Guidance Note PM52, HMSO, London.
9. Department of the Environment (1991) *Code of Practice on Litter and Refuse*, HMSO, London.
10. Royal Commission on Environmental Pollution (1993) *Seventeenth Report, Incineration of Waste*, HMSO, London.
11. Department of the Environment, *Landfilling Wastes*, Waste Management Paper No. 26, 1986 revised 4th impression 1990, HMSO, London.
12. London Waste Regulation Authority (1989) *Clinical Wastes – an Appraisal*, LWRA, London.
13. World Health Organization (1985) *Management of Waste from Hospitals*, WHO, Geneva.
14. United States Environmental Protection Agency (1986) *Guide for Infectious Waste Management*, EPA.
15. Health and Safety Commission (1982) revised 1994 *The Safe Disposal of Clinical Waste*, HMSO, London.
16. Department of the Environment (1983) *Clinical Wastes: a Technical Memorandum on Arisings, Treatment and Disposal*, Waste Management Paper No. 25, revised 1995, HMSO, London.

FURTHER READING

London Waste Regulation Authority (1989) *Guidelines for the Segregation, Handling and Transport of Chemical Waste*, revised 1994, LWRA, London.

Environmental Health Procedures, 4th edn (1995), Bassett, W.H., Chapman & Hall, London.

44 The water cycle

Edward Ramsden

INTEGRATED WATER MANAGEMENT

The integrated system of water management, introduced by the Water Act 1973, set up ten public authorities in England and Wales, which combined both the utility and regulatory functions relating to water supply and sewage disposal for the first time. Overall management of the water cycle, comprising the river basins, catchment areas and other water resources, through the supply and distribution chain, is the basic principle involved. Usage as well as the final disposal of waste water are also important parts of the cycle. (See Fig. 44.1.)

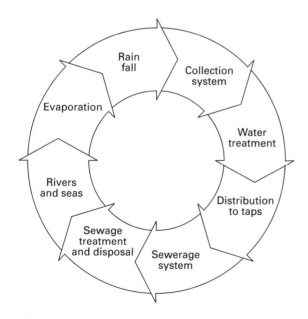

Fig. 44.1 The water cycle.

The Water Act 1989 (now consolidated into the Water Industries Act 1991 and the Water Resources Act 1991), while ostensibly embodying the same principle of managing the water cycle, did so by separating and privatizing the water supply utility and the disposal of sewage. The Act made the regulatory functions and river basin management in England and Wales the responsibility of the National Rivers Authority (NRA).

Under the Act, the utility assets of the ten former water authorities were taken into the ownership of the ten water companies (plcs), set up under the Act. The 29 statutory water companies, already existing, were retained, but gained the power to become public companies. Responsibility was given to the NRA for control of water pollution, management of water resources, fisheries, flood defence and land drainage, as well as navigation functions.

Originally, it was intended that the then existing water authorities should be privatized intact [1]. However, this idea was thought to be contrary to EU pollution control legislation and liable to be challenged in the European courts. As a consequence, the privatization of the water industry was delayed until after the 1987 General Election [2]. Pollution control and environmental management and river basin regulation functions were, as a response to European legislative requirements, separated from the utility management functions and made the responsibility of the new NRA.

It is anticipated that the NRA will form an important constituent part of the national Environmental Protection Agency, which is due to be established in 1996. Two further national Government bodies assist with the regulation of the water industry, the Office of Water Services (OFWAT) and the Drinking Water Inspectorate (DWI).

The Director General of OFWAT has duties with respect to the economic and performance standards of the water industry. Each water service company has allocated to it, by the director general, a customer service committee, to protect the interests of consumers and potential customers. Both the Secretary of State and the director general are given power, by section 18 of the Water Industry Act 1991, to enforce the provisions upon the water undertakers, both of the Act and its regulations.

Concurrent powers are given to serve enforcement orders, although the bulk of the requirements, including the Water Supply (Water Quality) Regulations 1989 (amended 1990) are to be enforced by the Secretary of State. Failure to comply with an order (either provisional or final) may be followed by a 'special administration order', issued by the High Court under section 24, or by civil proceedings.

The water undertakers have a general duty to develop and maintain an efficient and economical system of water supply within their areas. They also have a duty to maintain a supply of water of adequate pressure for domestic purposes, subject to certain conditions, to premises which are connected to the mains supply. Provision of water which is unfit for human consumption by a water undertaker is an offence, although prosecutions may only be instituted by the Secretary of State or the Director of Public Prosecutions.

Public water supplies must comply with the standards laid down in the Water Quality Regulations. Power is available under the 1989 Regulations for the Secretary of State to grant relaxations of the drinking water standards. Details of the relaxations are to be sent to the relevant local authorities, who are free to make objections [3]. The relaxations will in any case require improvement of the supply by a definite date.

Local authorities have a general duty to take all steps to keep themselves informed about the wholesomeness and sufficiency of all water supplies in their districts. If the local authority is aware of a public supply which is, or is likely to become, unwholesome or insufficient, they have a duty to notify the water undertaker. If the undertaker fails to take satisfactory action then, in turn, they must notify the Secretary of State.

In respect of private supplies, local authorities have specific responsibility for monitoring and, where private supplies are unwholesome or insufficient, they have the power to require improvements by service of notice on the owners and occupiers of the premises [3]. **'Wholesomeness'** of water is now established in England and Wales by the 1989 regulations. Section 79 of the Water Industry Act 1991 gives them wide powers to tailor their actions to the circumstances of particular supplies. Under Regulation 8 of the 1989 Regulations, local authorities also have a complementary power to grant relaxations for certain parameters, provided no public health risk is involved [3].

In order to carry out their duties under the regulations and the Water Industry Act 1991 (England and Wales) central advice has been made available to local authorities. Ministers have given advice in Circular 24/91 (England), 68/91 (Wales) and 20/1992 (Scotland) and have also published the *Manual on Treatment of Private Water Supplies*.

In England and Wales, house plans which are deposited with a local authority under the Building Regulations must be rejected, unless satisfactory arrangements are made for a water supply (section 25 of the Building Act 1984). It should be noted, however, that the building regulations themselves do not apply to cold water supplies, and reference should be made to the relevant water bye-laws for installation standards. In addition, the local authorities have powers to require a satisfactory water supply in an occupied house (section 69 of the Building Act 1984) [3].

Provision of an adequate systems of drains and sewers is fundamental to the effective drainage of an area. The duty of providing sewerage services was originally given to local authorities and, subsequently, passed to the water authorities set up in 1973. Finally, this duty passed to the sewerage undertakers established by the Water Act 1989, which are effectively the statutory water and sewerage utility companies set up under that Act. Thus, for the first time in Britain, provision of an adequate public sewerage and sewage disposal system became the responsibility of the private business sector.

Disposal of waste water and effluent resulting from the use of water, including sewage, is also subject to a network of legal controls. Principal among these is Part III of the Water Industry Act 1991, but some of the powers under the Public Health Acts 1936 and 1961, the Building Act of 1984 and the Public Health (Drainage of Trade Premises) Act 1937, as well as other, associated legislation, remains in force. Much of Part IV of the Water Industry Act 1991 is to be implemented by regulations, which in turn are subject to the influence of the requirements of EC legislation.

While the disposal of sewage is the responsibility of the water utility companies, a number of important powers and duties are also held by the NRA and Her Majesty's Inspectorate of Pollution (HMIP) as well as the local authorities. The water utilities have the duty, as sewerage undertakers, to provide, improve and extend a system of public sewers, ensuring the effective drainage of their area. They are also required to provide sewage disposal facilities, including trade effluent.

Responsibility for disposal of effluent and sewerage is thus largely divided between the three main public and private organizations: the NRA, the water utility companies, acting as 'sewerage authorities', and the local authorities.

Control of effluent discharges to the natural water environment is regulated by the NRA established under the Water Act 1989. The NRA operates on a strongly regional basis and the Act provides for regional river advisory committees in England and Wales. In addition, an advisory committee for Wales is established to advise the Secretary of State on matters relating to the NRA functions in Wales. It is proposed that the NRA should become an integral part of a unified national Environmental Protection Agency in 1996.

The basis of the new system introduced by the Water Act 1989 and now contained in the Water Resources Act 1991 is the establishment of statutory water quality objectives. Section 82 of the 1991 Act gives power to the Secretary of State to establish classification standards for all 'controlled waters', which includes boreholes into ground water, inland waters, rivers, watercourse, docks, coastal waters and territorial waters. Classification of waters by the Surface Water (Classification) Regulations 1989 (SI 1989, No. 1148) under Section 104 do not, in themselves, create operational standards. Service of a notice under section 105 of the Act by the Secretary of State on the NRA triggers the standards by requiring their implementation by a specified date on particular waters.

In turn, the NRA has a general duty to achieve and maintain the objectives, including monitoring the extent of pollution in controlled waters. Clearly in exercising this duty there is a need for a close relationship with both the water utility companies (sewerage undertakers) and the local authorities. In the latter case, there is a particular need to ensure that any controlled waters abstracted for domestic use as private supplies comply with the water quality objectives in the 1989 classification regulations, as well as the 1989 water quality regulations.

Control powers over pollution are given to the NRA, in the form of a prohibition under Section 86 of the Water Resources Act 1991, against the discharge of polluting matter into controlled waters, which either had been prohibited by notice or 'contains a prescribed substance or a prescribed concentration of such a substance or derives from a prescribed process . . . which exceed the prescribed amounts'. In addition, by Section 87 of the 1991 Act, it is given power to consent to discharges and issue disposal licenses, although not for any of the substances prohibited under Section 86.

It is the NRA's duty to comply with surface water quality objectives, coupled with its power to limit discharges from sewage works, industrial sources and individual polluters which, for the first times, creates a framework for the incremental improvement of the natural aquatic environment. It is open to the Secretary of State to progressively introduce more stringent water

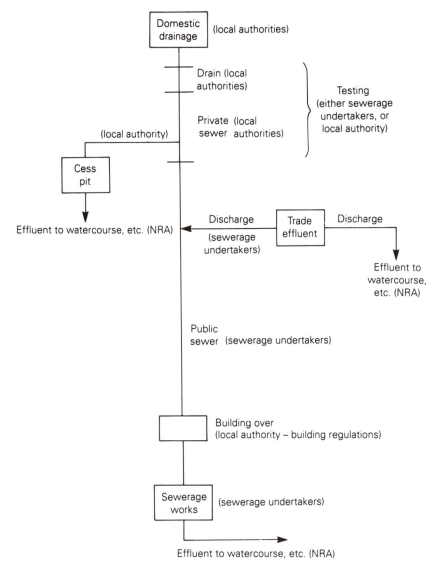

Fig. 44.2 Responsibility for control of the drainage sector of the water cycle.

quality objectives, which in turn will result in greater use of control powers by the NRA.

It is now an essential principle of the water cycle that local authorities are responsible for private drainage, including cesspits, sewerage undertakers are responsible for public sewers and sewage disposal works, and the NRA controls final discharges to watercourses etc. (see Fig 44.2) Thus, if trade effluent is discharged to a public sewer the discharge requires the consent of the sewerage undertakers, while if it is the discharged direct to a natural water course, it is subject to control by the NRA.

Precipitation, abstraction and use of water, followed by discharge of waste water into the sewerage system, disposal of sewage and trade effluent is concluded with the controls over purity of discharges. This completes the 'water cycle'. It is subject to a complex and interrelated legal code, some of which originates in the last century, and involves the complementary activities of both private water utility companies and public authorities.

It is against the background of these legislative arrangements, in England and Wales, that the water cycle should be considered.

WATER COLLECTION

Physical Properties of Water

Pure water is colourless, tasteless, odourless and of neutral reaction, i.e. neither acid nor alkaline. It is practically incompressible; the density of water is taken as the standard of comparison for all liquids and solids.

Water is one of the greatest solvents known to science, and for this reason is never found pure in nature. The term 'pure' water is accepted as meaning water which is dietetically pure. For practical purposes it may be regarded as water which complies with the standards laid down in the Water Supply (Water Quality) Regulations 1989 (amended 1990). Water will dissolve and take into solution all gases. Most solids are acted upon by water to some extent if contact is of sufficiently long duration. Its high solvent properties must be remembered by all who have duties relating to its storage and distribution.

Sources of Water Supply

Constant evaporation of water exposed to the air, the diffusion of water vapour throughout the atmosphere, with its subsequent condensation and descent in the form of rain, hail or snow, constitutes a circulation of water which is continuous over the surface of the earth. Of the precipitation which reaches the earth, part percolates into the ground until it reaches an impermeable stratum above which it accumulates; part flows away and forms rivers and lakes; part is absorbed by the soil itself and supports plant life; and the remainder is evaporated. Condensed water from the atmosphere is thus the primary source of all water supplies.

The sources from which it is practicable to derive water for public and domestic purposes are:

1. Surface water: lakes, rivers, etc;
2. Underground water: springs, wells and boreholes;
3. Rainwater (for isolated dwellings);
4. Seawater: by de-salination (not usual in the UK).

Supplies are broadly classified as either:

1. **public supplies**, distributed by statutory water supply companies; or
2. **private supplies** to a single user, or a small group of users.

Rainwater

In open and upland districts, rainwater may be used for domestic purposes, provided it is not contaminated by improper methods of collection and storage. As a practical source of domestic supply, its use is limited since particular care is required to be given to the method of collection, generally as roof water, in an effort to reduce any pollution from extraneous sources such as bird droppings. Where it is the sole source of supply, allowance must be made in storage capacity to overcome any long period of drought.

Rainwater falling upon a roof after periods of drought is liable to be highly polluted, and care is needed to prevent use of the first flushing. In any case, arrangements should be made for suitable treatment, to comply with the EC Directive 80/778/EEC relating to the quality of water intended for human consumption.

Surface water

Surface water supplies arise from rivers and lakes and man-made reservoirs. For supply purposes, these can be considered as two different types of source. Reservoirs and lakes store water for many months, during which time considerable changes may occur in its quality.

Bacterial decay occurs and the time available for settlement permits a reduction in suspended material and other constituents. On the other hand, algae growth may give rise to treatment problems. In particular, warm, stable weather conditions have caused the growth of **toxic blue-green algae**, which is a risk to animals or humans ingesting the untreated water. The algae grow below the surface, but each cell has built-in flotation capacity. When the conditions are right for growth, the algae rise to the surface to form a layer of distinctive blue/green scum.

Algal toxins are of three main types:

1. neurotoxins which damage the nervous system;
2. hepatotoxins which damage the liver;
3. lipopolysaccharides which irritate the skin.

Half to two-thirds of blue/green algal blooms are toxic, although toxicity varies from day to day. While small animals have died from ingesting water containing the blooms and cases of human illness are known, there have been no confirmed reports of human deaths recorded in the UK. Because of the dilution factors and water treatment, carry-over of the toxins into the main supply is unlikely, but not thought to be impossible. Little is yet known of this risk, nor specific protective treatment for the water, although chlorination is thought to be effective.

Under certain conditions, impounded water may become stratified leading to high levels of oxygen in the upper layers of water, but **oxygen deficiency** near the bottom of the reservoir allows chemical reduction and the dissolution of various metals and other contaminants which may render the water difficult to treat.

The huge volume of water held in reservoirs, however, may act as an effective buffer against accidental pollution by affording dilution and, by good management, the quality of water abstracted from reservoirs tends to be reasonably constant in quality.

Water abstracted from rivers varies in quality depending upon rainfall and the possibility of accidental, or even deliberate, pollution by irresponsible industrialists and/or the agricultural community must be borne in mind. To meet these two aspects, it is imperative that sufficient treatment plant is installed, to enable compliance with both the compositional and microbiological EC standards (Directive 80/718/EEC).

Table 44.1 Table of hardness

Water type	Hardness (mg/l CaCO₃)
Soft	0–50
Moderately soft	50–100
Slightly hard	100–150
Moderately hard	150–200
Hard	200–300
Very hard	Over 300

Acid rain and other atmospheric pollutants in water

An important contaminant of most natural waters is carbon dioxide (CO_2). This gas, resulting from atmospheric pollution as a consequence of the combustion of hydrocarbon fuel, is dissolved by rain falling through the atmosphere. In passing over and through earth covered with vegetation, a complex interaction takes place, which is of crucial importance. The resultant run off may be strongly acid, the so called 'acid rain' which has been damaging to forests, herbage, natural lakes and wildlife.

Hardness

Normally passing through more than one layer of soil before entering feeder streams, the nature of the soil, as well as the particular chemical reaction which results, are crucial to the final composition of the water. In its simplest form, the dilute solution of carbonic acids increases the solvent properties of the water and enables it to dissolve calcium and magnesium from limestone or chalk strata, and to hold them in solution as bicarbonates. Water in which these salts are dissolved is described as being 'hard'.

Hardness, or the soap destroying power of water, is generally described as of two kinds: temporary hardness, due to the presence of bicarbonates of calcium and magnesium; and permanent hardness, due to the sulphates of these salts. It is conventional practice to express both types of hardness as milligrams per litre (mg/l) of calcium carbonate $CaCO_3$. Table 44.1 lists the commonly accepted levels of hardness in public water supplies, against their content of calcium and magnesium salts expressed as $CaCO_3$.

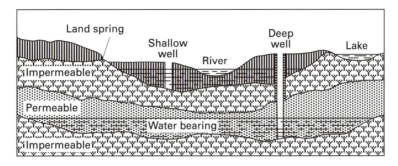

Fig. 44.3 Surface and underground water supplies.

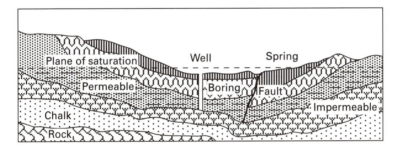

Fig. 44.4 Artesian water supplies.

Groundwater

Water sources are basically of two forms: either from lakes, rivers or streams (surface waters), or, in the case of water which has percolated into the earth, they are available from springs, or wells of different kinds. Whilst subsequent treatment of the water supply may make it suitable for delivery to the consumer's tap, its initial condition is the major factor which influences the eventual quality and safety of the supply. Surface water, from lakes, reservoirs and rivers, often provides a more consistent and manageable source for public supply, it is subject to greater risk of contamination and requires careful and suitable treatment. Ground water, particularly from deep sources, often provides a far better, though possibly less consistent source of supply. As a result, surface water should only be considered for a private supply, in circumstances where no adequate ground water supply exists:

1. **Springs** – may take the form of a main spring, an intermittent spring, or an artesian supply.
2. **Wells** – Shallow well, deep well or bore-hole (including artesian wells; see Fig. 44.3).

Artesian wells result from the underground pressure in an aquifer being released through a natural fault, or a borehole, so that water is forced to the surface of the ground (see Fig. 44.4).

Underground water from deep boreholes is normally considered to be the most palatable and safest water, since the passage through the ground acts as a natural filtration process. Shallow wells and springs are liable to local contamination and surface waters generally require treatment to ensure their suitability for drinking purposes. Since 1975, the EC Directive 75/440/EEC relating to the quality of surface water to be used for the abstraction of drinking water has been in force (see also below). Such water may also be suitable for recognition as a natural mineral water (see the Natural Mineral Waters Regulations 1985).

Springs

A land spring is a simple outcropping of water which has percolated into a permeable subsoil and followed the first impermeable stratum to a point at which it reaches the surface, as shown in Fig. 44.3. Such a spring is generally intermittent and will vary in volume with the rainfall of the immediate neighbourhood. It is obviously liable to organic and other pollution by direct percolation through the top soil. As a result, it is often little better than land drainage in quality and whilst it may be possible, after careful investigation, to authorize its use as an acceptable private supply, all too often such sources are unsatisfactory due to agricultural pollution. Quite different is a spring supply issuing from deep, water-bearing strata which can produce both a consistent volume and high quality supply.

Wells

Subsoil water is held above the first impermeable stratum, the soil above which becomes water bearing. A well should be situated above, and not below, possible sources of pollution. A well that taps water above the first impermeable stratum is known as a **shallow well** (Fig. 44.3) – the term 'shallow' in this connection having no definite relation to the actual depth expressed in terms of measurement, but an indication of the stratum from which it is abstracted.

Deep ground water supplies are those derived from water-bearing strata below at least one impervious stratum. Such water is frequently under pressure, owing to the fact that the plane of saturation may be much above the lowest level of the impervious stratum by which the water is contained. A deep well is one that taps the deep supply, as shown in Fig. 44.3, and must be constructed so as to exclude subsoil water. It should be water tight down to a point slightly below the level of the deep supply.

Water will rise in any well up to the level of the plane of saturation, which may be actually above the surface of the ground (Fig. 44.4). If a well or boring is driven through the impermeable stratum by which a supply is retained, water will rise to or above the surface under its own 'head'. This is known as an **artesian supply**.

Similarly, a natural fault in the impounding stratum may give rise to a deep or artesian spring, as shown in the diagram.

The practice of obtaining water from wells is universal and of great antiquity. Well water is an important source of supply in all countries.

The necessity for care in the location and construction of wells can hardly be exaggerated. When water is being extracted from a well sunk into any but the most open water-bearing subsoil, e.g. gravel, the surface of the water about it will fall more or less in the shape of an inverted cone, and this cone of depression may assist the ingress of pollution matter during pumping. To prevent this, protection of the source is needed by, for example, excluding animals from the vicinity. (See Figs. 44.5 or 44.6).

The extent to which it is necessary or advisable to fence in the area round a shallow well as a protection against surface contamination is dependent upon the hydrographical conditions, the porosity and filtering efficiency of the soil, and upon the extent to which the water in the well is liable to fall when ordinary pumping is in progress. Lowering of the water below the ordinary plane of saturation sets up conditions favourable to contamination from polluted air, as well as polluted soil. A grass crop on the protected area about a well, if practicable, is desirable, as the roots form a filtering mat, and the grass tends to prevent surface drying and consequent cracking of the soil, which would permit seepage of contaminated surface water. Careful assessment of the supply should include taking microbiological and chemical samples in accordance with the Private Water Supplies Regulations.

Most of the old wells met with in practice are roughly lined with open jointed brickwork which permits water to enter from the top and sides as well as from the bottom. This is frequently a means of pollution. The compulsory closing of a well is a serious matter for those dependent upon it. In many cases, this step may be avoided at

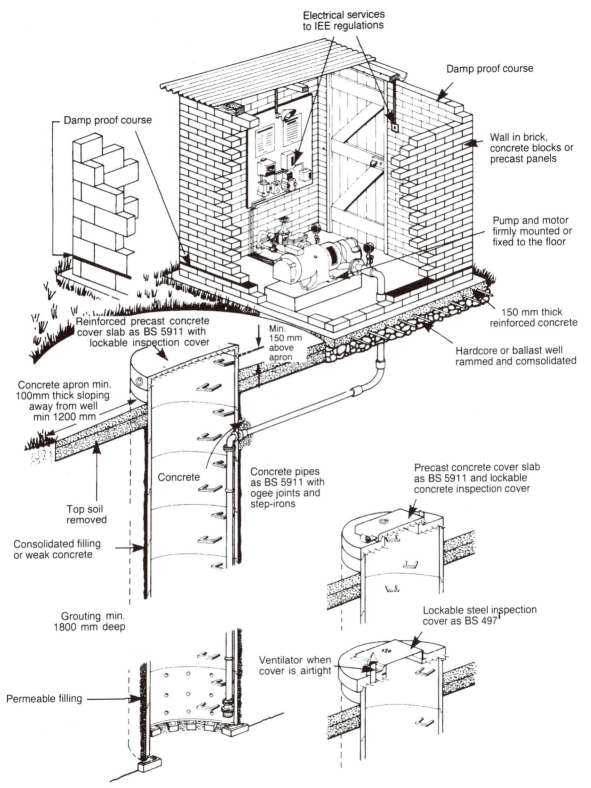

Fig. 44.5 Well and pump installation – typical arrangements to exclude pollution from surface sources. (Source: *Manual on Treatment of Private Water Supplies*, HMSO, London.)

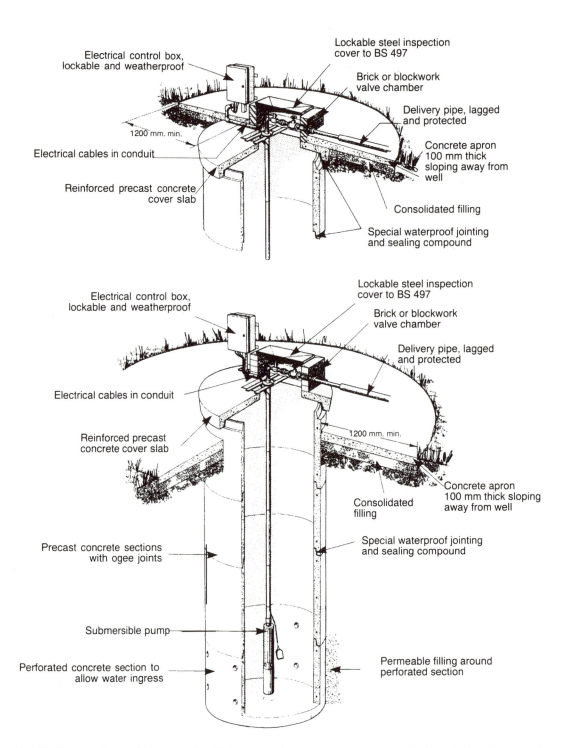

Fig. 44.6 Well and submersible pump installation – typical arrangements to exclude pollution from surface sources. (Source: *Manual on Treatment of Private Water Supplies*), HMSO, London.)

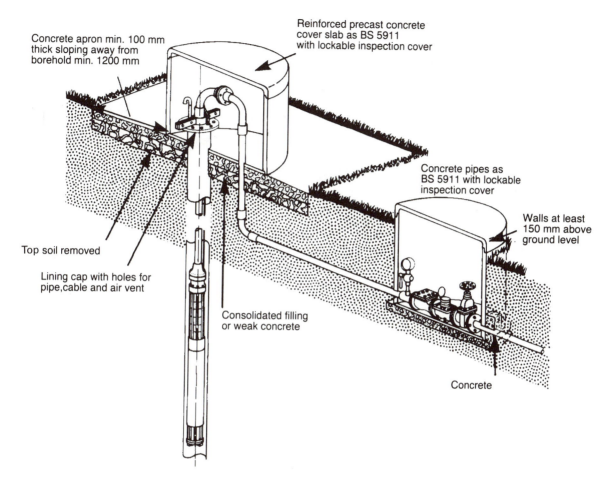

Fig. 44.7 Borehole well headworks. (Source: *Manual on Treatment of Private Water Supplies*), HMSO, London.)

reasonable expense by lining the well with concrete pipes grouted in cement or clay.

Provided this is combined with modern headworks and an adequate concrete apron to prevent contaminating percolation, it may be possible to rehabilitate an old well in this way (Figs 44.7 and 44.8). However, it must be clearly established that contamination is the result of the inadequate construction of the well, as no re-construction will improve an inadequate, shallow supply which is contaminated by some other means, such as a leaking cesspool, or silage pit.

Where no public supply is available, construction of new wells should have regard to the guidance given to local authorities in the *Manual on Treatment of Private Water Supplies* [25]. In many cases, where a suitable water-bearing substratum is available, a simple bore-hole with an electric pump may provide an adequate supply for a single household. In all cases of new construction particular care must be taken to protect the source by lining it, to prevent percolation from surrounding ground at a shallow level, and provision of an impermeable apron.

WATER TREATMENT

Contamination of public supplies

It depends both on the original quality and also how water is protected at source, in transit, in storage, and in distribution as to whether or not

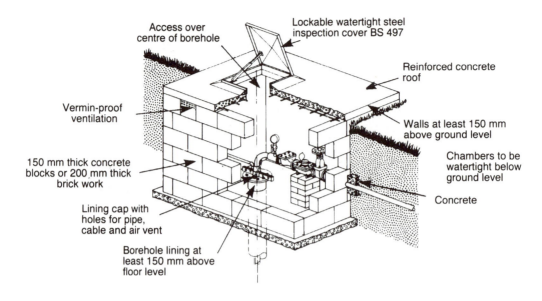

Access over
centre of borehole

Lockable watertight steel
inspection cover BS 497

Reinforced concrete
roof

Vermin-proof
ventilation

Walls at least 150 mm
above ground level

Chambers to be
watertight below
ground level

150 mm thick concrete
blocks or 200 mm thick
brick work

Concrete

Lining cap with
holes for pipe,
cable and air vent

Borehole lining at
least 150 mm above
floor level

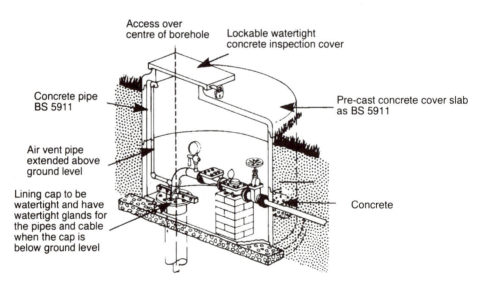

Access over
centre of borehole

Lockable watertight
concrete inspection cover

Concrete pipe
BS 5911

Pre-cast concrete cover slab
as BS 5911

Air vent pipe
extended above
ground level

Lining cap to be
watertight and have
watertight glands for
the pipes and cable
when the cap is
below ground level

Concrete

Fig. 44.8 Borehole well headworks. (Source: *Manual on Treatment of Private Water Supplies*), HMSO, London.)

water will reach the consumer in pure condition. Heightened public concerns over environmental pollution generally has increasingly focused on drinking water quality. Both run off from surfaces and percolation through sub-soil as well as exposure of open bodies of water in streams, rivers, reservoirs, ponds and lakes exposes water to additional contamination risks.

The main sources of potential contamination are industrial, agricultural and sewage. EC Directive 80/778/EEC lists some 62 parameters for water, of which a number relate to each source of contamination. In addition to obvious toxic substances, such as heavy metals, there are increasingly recognized risks associated with such things as nitrate and nitrite levels, organic solvents, aluminium and hydrocarbons.

Nitrates

Increased use of artificial nitrogen fertilizers has raised the level of nitrate run off from farm land. As a result, the levels of nitrates in water supplies have increased, particularly in those parts of the UK subject to intensive arable farming. Elevated levels of nitrates may cause **methaemoglobin-aemia** or **'blue baby syndrome'**, a rare blood condition affecting, particularly, bottle-fed babies. There is thought to be an elevated risk of cancer due to high levels of nitrates, but epidemiological studies have failed to support this contention.

Metals

There is increasing concern over elevated levels of aluminium as it has been associated with **Alzheimer's disease**, a condition with symptoms of progressive dementia. While there is still some doubt about its effect, increased public concern, coupled with EU requirements, have highlighted this contaminant. It occurs naturally in many waters, and also results from some treatment methods.

Lead is a recognized toxic water pollutant, from ancient times. Acute lead poisoning from water, with its immediate neurological effects, anaemia and muscle cramps, is a thing of the past. Recent concerns have focused on the problem of sub-clinical lead poisoning, with some contention over the perceived symptoms of a shift in educability of the very young and hyperactive behaviour. It is important to remember that lead has long-term cumulative effects and, as a consequence, is a multi-source problem, of which water is but one component.

While other metals, such as iron and manganese, may cause discoloration in the water, at the levels found in Britain they do not pose a risk to human health.

Industry

Industrial sources of pollution may include consented discharges into water courses, leaching of substances from contaminated land or licensed industrial tips, and illegal dumping of industrial waste on land or into water sources. Agricultural sources of contamination include foul silage effluent and nitrates and nitrites from land drainage.

Sewage discharges and Cryptosporidium

The final discharges from sewage works into fresh water, even if meeting laid down standards, may contaminate water supplies. This is of particular importance if river abstraction takes place close to the point of discharge. There is also the risk of contamination by microorganisms from sprayed or injected sewage sludge onto agricultural land. In addition, improperly controlled drainage from animal husbandry or silage may contaminate water sources, notably private supplies.

Whilst chlorination is important to eliminate viruses which may survive the filtration process, adequate filtration is the crucial step in controlling the chlorine-resistant parasite *Cryptosporidium* [4]. It is important, in the case of river or surface water abstraction, that specific allowance is made for this risk in any water treatment process. About 2% of the cases of acute diarrhoea in Britain are caused by *Cryptosporidium*, although the majority of these are due to direct infection from animals, including man and farm animals, or other sources. It was the subject of the first major report of the National Water Advisory Group (Badenoch Report – published 1990) [4], which concluded that although *Cryptosporidium* is often present in Britain's drinking water supplies, mains water is generally safe to drink.

Normal levels of chlorination are ineffective against *Cryptosporidium*, and the principal means of control at the treatment stage is filtration. Slow sand filters seem to be the most effective means for the removal of *Cryptosporidium* oocysts, the effectiveness of other filters depending upon their filter medium and pore size. Infection of water supplies is usually from agricultural sources, due to sewage contamination, often as a result of periods of heavy rain. Operational failures include failure to effectively back-wash filters and by-passing slow-sand filters.

Contamination of private supplies

The operators of private wells need to be aware of possible hazards associated with their use. These may be of two forms, microbiological and chemical.

Microbiological

Microbiological contamination may arise from improper construction and use or from the unobserved seepage of farm drainage or septic tank effluent. Regular testing for the **coliform** group of indicator organisms is necessary to ensure that wells remain satisfactory, and that no harmful organisms are gaining access.

Chemical

Chemical contamination may involve nitrates from excessive fertilizer use in the vicinity, pesticides from agriculture and a variety of other chemicals. Occasional analyses should be undertaken to ensure that no increase in levels of chemical constituents in the water is occurring. A particular concern with many small domestic supplies is the pick-up of lead from old lead piping since, in many cases, shallow wells and springs are soft and acidic in nature, and the resultant water plumbo-solvent.

Monitoring

Responsibility for monitoring public water supplies is placed on the statutory water undertakers in England and Wales, by the Water Supply (Water Quality) Regulations 1989 [5] (amended 1990). Water companies must also determine, in respect of each of their supply zones, sufficient suitably located sampling points, to enable a representative sampling pattern for each of the laid down parameters. Standard arrangements for patterns and numbers of samples are also laid down in the Regulations.

Water undertakers must notify local authorities and district health authorities of the results of monitoring, by the 30 June in the following year, and must inform them of any event which gives

risk to the health of persons living in that local authority area. Local authorities have power to require information about any such incident and may also have their own sampling arrangements.

While sampling frequencies are laid down for water undertakers under the Regulations, local authorities are given discretion to make their own arrangements to check public supplies. They are free to take such samples of water in their area as they reasonably require, although by Department of the Environment Circular 20/89 implementing the Water Act 1989, the Secretary of State did not expect any increase in sampling, in view of the availability of information from water undertakers.

Private water supplies, including the maintenance of sampling programmes, are the responsibility of district councils. This is usually undertaken by the environmental health department, who must identify private suppliers in their district, carry out the necessary sampling and, where required, provide advice on improving the supplies to achieve the standards required by the directive. The Private Water Supplies Regulations 1991 specifies the information which local authorities in England and Wales are able to obtain about private supplies, specifies classification of supplies, and the parameters in the 1989 Regulations which are to be applied, and prescribe monitoring frequencies and charges.

Private supplies to be identified include rural supplies, bottled water, which is not 'natural mineral water', and water supplies in food production undertakings, which are not direct from the public main. This may include transport catering in long distance buses or trains. Powers exist within section 140 of the Public Health Act 1936, in England and Wales, to cut off polluted private water supplies from wells, tanks, or other sources of supply. Similarly, storage wells, tanks, or water butts which are liable to contamination, may also be dealt with by powers contained in section 141 of the same Act [3].

Sampling techniques

Under Regulation 21 of the Water Supply (Water Quality) Regulations 1989 (amended 1990) water undertakers must apply 'the appropriate requirements' when taking samples. Similarly, by Regulation 33, local authorities are required to follow the same procedure. Steps should be taken during the taking, handling, transporting, storing and analysing of water (or causing to be analysed), to ensure that the sample is:

1. representative of the quality of the water;
2. not contaminated when being sampled;
3. kept at such a temperature and in conditions which will ensure there is no material change in the sample;
4. analysed as soon as possible:
5. analysed by a laboratory with a proper, verified quality control system.

In practice, sampling for chemical analysis is a relatively simple procedure, and only requires a fairly large but properly representative quantity of water in a 1 or 2 litre bottle. Microbiological samples, on the other hand, should be taken with care, to avoid contamination of the sample. The water should first be run off, to ensure the sample is taken from the mains supply, and the tap then 'flamed' for a minute or so with a portable gas blowlamp, provided that the tap is metal. Subsequently, the water should be further run for 2–3 minutes before taking the sample.

Care should be taken to prevent the water becoming contaminated by the neck of the bottle. This is achieved by only opening the flow to a fine stream, which can be directed into the bottle without touching the neck. The ground glass stopper should only be held by the rim, avoiding touching the actual surface with the fingers, before replacing immediately the bottle is full.

All sample bottles should contain a small quantity of sodium thiosulphate, to dechlorinate the water and stabilize any coliform organisms in the sample.

Water quality standards

Public health objectives for analysis of water samples are mainly (1) to determine its suitability, particularly for domestic purposes and, (2) to ensure the maintenance of required standards of purity, notably those laid down in European legislation. In particular in the food industry, the standards apply, if the wholesomeness of the finished product may be affected by the quality of the water used. Examples of situations where food or drink may be affected by water are where water is:

1. used as an ingredient;
2. otherwise used in the course of preparing food;
3. used for washing of equipment, etc, or the personal cleanliness of food handlers.

Water must be of the necessary standard when it arrives at food premises; if it is mains water, this is the responsibility of the water undertakers. If it is a private supply, the local authority is responsible. In either case, thereafter it is the responsibility of the local authority to ensure its quality.

It is important to remember that results from any single sample only indicate the condition of the water at the particular time the sample was taken. It is only by regular, systematic sampling and maintenance of a database of results over a period of time that a clear picture of water quality may be identified. In particular, this allows identification of variations from the norm, enabling assessment and investigation.

EC directives now cover (1) quality requirements of surface water for the abstraction of drinking water (Directive 75/440/EEC), and, (2) water for human consumption at the consumer's tap (Directive 80/778/EEC). Both directives utilize 'guide' values, which are preferred levels, as well as maximum admissible concentrations, known in one case as 'I' values, and in the other as 'MACs'. Similarly, in respect of softened water, intended for human consumption, values have been fixed for certain parameters which must be equal to minimum required concentrations, 'MRCs'.

Quality of surface water
The surface water Directive (75/440/EEC) sets values for each of the different categories of water from the purest upland source (A1) to lowland polluted river supplies (A3), and in addition indicates the treatment requirements for each.

Table 44.2 EU requirements for abstracted surface water (intended for human consumption)

Parameter	A1	A2	A3
Coloration (mg/l Pt Scale)	20	100	200
Temperature (°C)	25	25	25
Nitrate (mg/l NO_3)	50	50	50
Fluoride (mg/l F)	1.5	–	–
Dissolved iron (mg/l Fe)	0.3	2	–
Copper (mg/l Cu)	0.05	–	–
Zinc (mg/l Zn)	0.05	0.05	0.1
Arsenic (mg/l As)	0.05	0.05	0.1
Cadmium (mg/l Cd)	0.005	0.005	0.005
Total chromium (mg/l Cr)	0.05	0.05	0.05
Lead (mg/l Pb)	0.05	0.05	0.05
Selenium (mg/l Se)	0.01	0.01	0.01
Mercury (mg/l Hg)	0.001	0.001	0.001
Barium (mg/l Ba)	0.1	1	1
Cyanide (mg/l Cn)	0.05	0.05	0.05
Sulphates (mg/l SO_4)	250	250	250
Phenols (mg/l C_6H_5OH)	0.001	0.005	0.1
Dissolved or emulsified hydrocarbons (mg/l)	0.05	0.2	1
Polycyclic aromatic hydrocarbons (mg/l)	0.0002	0.0002	0.001
Total pesticides (mg/l)	0.001	0.0025	0.005
Ammonia	–	1.5	4

Table 44.2 gives the 'I' values which are mandatory only for the three types of water, A1, A2 and A3. Directive standards are applied by the statutory water undertakers and monitored by the NRA.

Quality of drinking water

After abstraction and treatment, water intended for human consumption in England and Wales is subject to the drinking water directive (80/778/EEC), which in turn was implemented by the Water Act 1989, its Regulations and associated circulars. The Water Industry Act 1991 requires local authorities to keep themselves informed about the quality of water supplies in their area. In practice this is generally satisfied by a sampling programme, including access to information on water quality held by the Water Service Company concerned. Water supplied for human consump-

tion must be 'wholesome', defined by reference to the standards set in the Water Supply (Water Quality) Regulations 1989, which in turn incorporates the relevant elements of the EC Directive.

The Directive requirement covers the following water supplies:

1. water for human consumption supplied by a statutory undertaker as a 'public supply';
2. water for consumption supplied by a non-statutory water undertaker, including private supplies and bottled water not covered by the exclusions;
3. water supplied for use in food production undertakings.

Exclusions from the Directive are, broadly, bottled natural mineral waters, medicinal waters and non-potable use of water in food production undertakings.

To comply with the 1989 Regulations, steps must be taken to ensure that drinking water supplies meet the requirements of all 56 parameters. The requirements (see Table 44.3) are in the form of either MAC values, or MRCs. The Regulations make no requirements in respect of guide level values (GLs) which are included in the Directive standards.

Patterns of sampling and frequency of analyses are also laid down in the Directive and subsequently Regulations, as are the reference methods of analysis.

Natural mineral waters

Before exploitation and bottling of natural mineral waters is permitted, it must satisfy laid down quality criteria (the Natural Mineral Waters Regulations 1985). The waters may then be 'officially recognized', and are subject to specific requirements over treatment and bottling (EC Directive 80/777/EEC).

The Drinking Water in Containers Regulations 1994 implement Directive 80/778/EEC by prescribing quality standards for drinking water sold in bottles, closing the legislative loophole for products such as bottled water. They do not apply to natural mineral waters nor medicinal products.

Among the maximum values (see Table 44.3) are:

1. temperature – 25°C;
2. colony counts – 100 per ml at 22°C and 20 per ml at 37°C, within 12 hours of bottling;
3. absence of faecal coliforms and faecal streptococci.

The major enforcement provisions and defences of the Food Safety Act 1990 apply.

Purification of water

Methods employed for water purification depend upon the volumes to be treated and the source of the water, hence the degree of purification necessary. Where underground supplies are involved which are already of good quality, simple treatment is used consisting of chlorination, pH correction and, occasionally, filtration. Surface supplies usually require more extensive treatment, including several of the processes of storage, screening, aeration, coagulation, settlement, filtration, pH correction and chlorination. For some waters, additional processes such as softening, activated carbon filtration, micro-straining or ozonization are employed. Where the local health authority has requested it, fluoridation may also be used.

Treatment processes

STORAGE Storage of polluted waters in reservoirs has been a recognized treatment process for many years. By complex natural means, during long periods of storage, bacteria decay to relatively low numbers and suspended matter settles out, often carrying with it harmful metals and other substances. A significant reduction in nitrate levels may occur by the action of bottom muds, and hardness values change. A disadvantage may be the growth of algae giving problems at the treatment, settlement and filtration stages of treatment, or imparting tastes and odours to the water – the use of algicides, such as copper sulphate, is not always successful. If the water is eutrophic, due to organic impurities in the incoming water, concentrations of iron, manganese and phosphates may increase and the water deoxygenate due to bacterial activity; aeration of supplies is used occasionally to counteract this effect.

Mixing devices are installed in some reservoirs to overcome this problem. These may be aeration devices at the reservoir bottoms or pumps fitted with jetting nozzles to induce turbulence. High manganese content may be counteracted by dosing with potassium permanganate.

SCREENING Virtually all intakes to water supply systems are screened, varying from simple bar types to complex micro-strainers. The nature of the screening is at least partly determined by the nature of the raw water entering the treatment works.

SLOW SAND FILTRATION Although largely superseded by chemical coagulation and sedimentation treatment in more recently constructed works, a large proportion of water supplied by the water industry is still subjected to this process, which was one of the earliest devised. Slow sand filters consist of large, open filter beds constructed with impermeable walls and floors, containing about 1 m of fine sand laid on 0.3 m of shingle with suitable drainage tiles at the bottom. Filters work under a head of 1 m of water, percolating through at the rate of 13 litre/m²/hr. The bed acts partly as a fine strainer, but most of the purification occurs by biological action, involving the formation of a gelatinous film on the surface of the sand (the 'schmutzdecke'), which contains a variety of micro-organisms. The film slowly builds up in thickness during a filter run until the rate of filtration is retarded below a practical limit when the filter is cleaned by removing the top 10 cm of sand; this sand is cleaned by washing with water and returning to the bed. Filters may be returned to use with or without replacement of the top layer, but will not reach full purification efficiency until the schmutzdecke has reformed and the quality of filtered water must be monitored carefully during this initial phase to ensure its safety.

In many works, raw water is passed first through primary filters to reduce suspended matter and hence the load on the slow sand filters, permitting an increased time between cleaning.

COAGULATION, FLOCCULATION AND SEDIMENTATION Coagulation, flocculation and sedimentation is the

Table 44.3 Water Supply (Water Quality) Regulations 1989, the Private Water Supplies Regulations 1991, and the Drinking Water in Containers Regulations 1994

Parameter	Units of measurement	Concentration of value (maximum unless otherwise stated)
Organoleptic		
1. Colour	(mg/l Pt/Co scale)	20
2. Turbidity (including suspended solids)	Formazin turbidity units	4
3. Odour (including hydrogen sulphide)	Dilution number	3.0 at 25°C
4. Taste	Dilution number	3 at 25°C
Physico-chemical		
5. Temperature	°C	25
6. Hydrogen ion	pH value	9.5
		5.5 (minimum)
7. Sulphate	mg SO_4/l	250
8. Magnesium	mg Mg/l	50
9. Sodium	mg Na/l	150
10. Potassium	mg K/l	12
11. Dry residues	mg/l	1500 (after drying at 180°C)
Undesirable substances		
12. Nitrate	mg NO_3/l	50
13. Nitrite	mg NO_2/l	0.1
14. Ammonium (ammonia and ammonium ions)	mg NH_4/l	0.5
15. Kjeldahl nitrogen	mg N/l	1
16. Oxidizability (permanganate value)	mg O_2/l	5
17. Total organic carbon	mg C/l	No significant increase over that normally observed
18. Dissolved or emulsified hydrocarbons (after extraction with petroleum ether); mineral oils	μg/l	10
19. Phenols	μg C_6H_5OH/l	0.5
20. Surfactants	μg/l (as lauryl sulphate)	200
21. Aluminium	μg Al/l	200
22. Iron	μg Fe/l	200
23. Manganese	μg Mn/l	50
24. Copper	μg Cu/l	3000
25. Zinc	μg Zn/l	5000
26. Phosphorus	μg P/l	2200
27. Fluoride	μg F/l	1500
28. Silver	μg Ag/l	10 (note: if silver is used in a water treatment process, 80 may be substituted for 10)
Toxic substances		
29. Arsenic	μg As/l	50
30. Cadmium	μg Cd/l	5
31. Cyanide	μg CN/l	50
32. Chromium	μg Cr/l	50
33. Mercury	μg Hg/l	1
34. Nickel	μg Ni/l	50
35. Lead	μg Pb/l	50
36. Antimony	μg Sb/l	10

Table 44.3 continued

37. Selenium	μg Se/l	10	
38. Pesticides and related products:	μg/l	0.1	
(a) individual substances			
(b) total substances	μg/l	0.5	
39. Polycyclic aromatic hydrocarbons (μg/l)	μg/l	0.2	
Microbiological parameters			
40. Total coliforms	number/100 ml	0	
41. Faecal coliforms	number/100 ml	0	
42. Faecal streptococci	number/100 ml	0	
43. Sulphite reducing *Clostridia*	number/20 ml	1 Multiple tube method	
44. Colony counts	number/1 ml at 22°C or 37°C	No significant increase over that normally observed	
Other parameters (the maximum concentrations are average values or concentrations over the preceding 12 months)			
45. Conductivity	μS/cm	1500 at 20°C	
46. Chloride	mg Cl/l	400	
47. Calcium	mg Ca/l	250	
48. Substances extractable in chloroform	mg/l dry residue	1	
49. Boron	μg B/l	2000	
50. Barium	μg Ba/l	1000	
51. Benzo 3,4 pyrene	ng/l	10	
52. Tetrachloromethane	μg/l	3	
53. Trichloroethene	μg/l	30	
54. Tetrachloroethene	μg/l	10	
Additional parameters for desalinated or softened waters			
55. Total hardness	mg Ca/l	60	
56. Alkalinity	mg HCO$_3$/l	30.0	

Table 44.4 Optimum coagulation pH over alkalinity values

Alkalinity (CaCO$_3$)	Optimum coagulation pH
Soft waters <50 mg/l	5.0–5.5
Medium hard waters 50–200 mg/l	60.–7.2
Hard alkaline waters >200 mg/l	6.0–7.5

main process now used for the removal of impurities. Coagulation is the process of aggregation of the colloidal-sized particles which comprise the natural colour and turbidity of the water. It is brought about by the addition of coagulants, such as aluminium or ferric sulphate.

The effectiveness of the process is dependent on pH over a range of values of alkalinity, as given in Table 44.4.

Coagulation is followed by the process of flocculation, which is the growth in size of the coagulated particles over a period of time. The end result of this process is a relatively dense precipitate known as a floc, which will settle readily or be removed effectively by filtration.

Sedimentation is achieved in tanks, of which there are many designs. Most designs ensure that the floc remains in contact with the water stream for a long period of time. This is achieved by preventing immediate settlement and by continuously removing only a proportion of the floc as a sludge, since the floc is an efficient absorber of many impurities such as trace metals, bacteria, etc.

Most tanks work on an upward flow principle, water entering the tank at its base, rising through a 'blanket' of floc, and clarified water being removed via decanting troughs from the top of

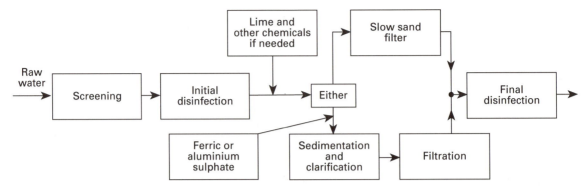

Fig. 44.9 Schematic – water treatment process.

the tank. Upflow rates vary from 1 to 3 m/hr, but higher rates can be used with some designs.

RAPID SAND FILTRATION Sedimentation is usually followed by rapid sand filtration to ensure removal of any floc carried through with the decanted water. Rapid gravity filters are normally used, employing filtration rates of 6 m/hr although modern designs may operate at 20 m/hr with peak flows as high as 50 m/hr.

The filter normally consists of a large open tank containing a bed of sand 1 to 1.2 m deep supported on layers of coarse sand and gravel. Water is fed onto the top of the sand and removed through drains in the floor of the filter. The difference in level between water in the tank and the filtered water channel provides a 'head' to force the water through the filter. As solids are removed, the filter becomes clogged and the head loss across it increases. When this reaches a maximum, usually when the bed has increased to 2 m, or alternatively when break-through of suspended material occurs, the filter is backwashed using various combinations of clean water to expand the sand bed and the injection of compressed air to break up the aggregates in the sand (Fig. 44.9).

PRESSURE FILTERS There are a number of different forms and designs of pressure filters, with various filter mediums. They are used where it is undesirable to break the pressure after pumping, e.g. from a borehole. These perform in the same way as a rapid gravity filter, but the filter shell is a pressure vessel, usually cylindrical in shape. The head available for flow through the filter is the drop in pressure between filtered and unfiltered water. Somewhat higher head losses can be allowed to develop before backwashing of this type of filter is required.

Disinfection

Chlorine is used almost universally in the water industry as a disinfectant to ensure that water is free from harmful bacteria. It is added either as a gas or as a solution of sodium hypochlorite, the latter being the norm for small supplies. When the source is very pure, e.g. borehole water, the dose rarely exceeds 0.5 mg/l and the process is known as **marginal chlorination**. For most other supplies, **breakpoint chlorination**, or **super-chlorination** and dechlorination, are used.

Most natural waters contain oxidizable material and ammonium salts and these exert a **chlorine demand** which must be satisfied if **free chlorine**, which is the most bactericidal form of chlorine, is to remain in the water. It is usual, therefore, to add sufficient chlorine just to overcome the chlorine demand and to maintain a small free-chlorine residual. This is known as breakpoint chlorination. Super-chlorination is the name given to the process of adding excessive chlorine so that the breakpoint is well exceeded and, in this case, the residual is controlled by the addition of a dechlorinating agent, sulphur dioxide.

In addition to maintaining chlorine in its most effective bactericidal state, a free residual should leave no taste in the water.

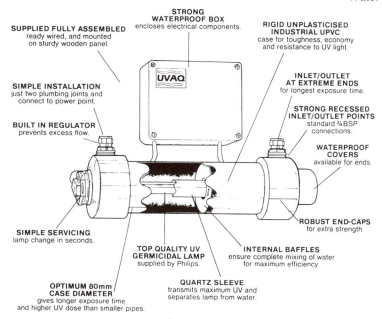

Fig. 44.10 Ultra-violet light sanitizers unit. (Courtesy of UV A Q, Unit 2, Mills Road, Chilton Industrial Estate, Sudbury, Suffolk.)

Ultra-violet irradiation

Short wave ultra-violet radiation at around 254 nm in the short wave UVC region, which is the most effective against micro-organisms, may also be used to disinfect water supplies. This spectrum is also harmful to the eyes and skin, and manufacturers' safety precautions must be adhered to. UV treatment has no residual effect and it is usually applicable to localized supplies. Of particular importance in the control of legionella and other organisms within recirculating water systems.

Ultra-violet light sanitizing units (Fig. 44.10) are usually in the form of a tubular enclosing water jacket unit with a central, low-pressure mercury vapour discharge lamp UV emitting element, fitted into a tubular quartz sleeve, surrounded by the water supply. In line water flows through the unit, from one end to the other, contact time being maintained by a flow regulator device. The mercury tube gradually deteriorates and must be replaced every 6–12 months; the unit must be maintained in a clean condition to ensure effectiveness.

OZONIZATION Ozone, the triatomic modification of oxygen, was first produced in large quantities by Von Siemens in 1857 utilizing an electrical discharge tube. Over the years, this process has been improved and it is now possible to produce small quantities of ozone economically. Water treatment plants throughout Europe have used this process extensively for bacterial purification, but its use in Britain has been limited.

This method of purification is relatively expensive when compared with chlorination, but has several advantages:

1. ozone is a good bactericide and is probably a better viruscide than chlorine;
2. it can be very effective in removing colour from moorland waters;
3. certain tastes and odours are removed;
4. there is no smell associated with the treated water.

ACID WATERS The addition of coagulants and chlorine to water tends to make it acidic. In addition, many upland waters are naturally acidic due to the presence of natural substances, such as fulvic acid. Such waters are often soft. Treatment is required to prevent acidic waters corroding either iron or galvanized pipes, giving rise to discoloration ('red water'); or copper pipes giving blue staining on ceramic ware, or lead pipes which may lead to an increase in lead intake by the consumer (plumbo-solvency).

Acidity is normally corrected by dosing the supply with lime, either as a slurry or as a solution prepared in lime saturators, although the former is the most common. Occasionally, sodium hydroxide (caustic soda) or sodium carbonate are used as alternatives to lime. A pH value above 8.0 is normally recommended for soft supply waters.

Other treatments

MANGANESE Depending upon the source of the water and the resulting level of contaminants it contains, other treatment may well be necessary. For instance, high manganese levels may sometimes occur in upland surface waters, particularly in dry weather conditions. Addition of potassium permanganate, followed by effective filtration, if necessary in two stages, is used to ensure effective reduction of the manganese levels.

TASTES AND ODOURS These may be reduced by aeration, or by the use of granular activated charcoal. The aromatic materials adhere to the charcoal and may be removed by subsequent filtration.

FLUORIDATION Sodium fluoride is added to the public supply at the request of the health authority, in order to reduce the incidence of dental caries. This models the effect which has been demonstrated in those areas where fluoride, in the form of calcium fluoride, exists naturally. It must be said that the addition of fluoride to public water supplies is contentious and has been debated by Parliament on a number of occasions. It is principally controlled by the Water (Fluoridation) Act 1985.

WATER DISTRIBUTION

Distribution and use of public water supplies is generally governed by the Model Water Byelaws

1986,* made by the water utility undertakers and private water companies. In the UK a Byelaws Guidance Panel has been formed and has produced a guide to the model bye-laws [5] as a means of assisting water inspectors, manufacturers, architects, consultants, merchants, installers and consumers. A British Standards code of practice, BS6700: 1987 [6], gives general guidance on water installations to buildings and their curtilages. Classified lists of accepted fittings [7] are made available from the Water Byelaws Advisory Service (WBAS), who make provision for the assessment and testing of water fittings.

In general, pipes laid underground must be protected from damage, permeation by gas or passage through sources of pollution, and not be constructed from materials which can themselves cause contamination. As a principle, this means that the line of the pipes should avoid passing through drainage manholes, cesspits, or similar, and any alignment with gas mains should be carefully assessed. The distribution system itself is not to be made from any material or substance which could contaminate the water supply. As a principle, back syphonage of water from installations, hoses and the like is to be avoided by the use of check-valves, pipe interrupters, vacuum breaks, or air gaps between the mains supply and the point of use.

Storage cisterns

Domestic supplies of cold water for drinking purposes should, ideally, be taken direct from the water main, via a service pipe, to the domestic taps from which drinking or cooking water is obtained. There are circumstances in which it is necessary, or desirable, to have a domestic storage cistern, for instance, where mains supplies are intermittent, or in the case of a pumped private supply.

In addition, potable supplies to the food or other industries, where large quantities of process water are needed, may require a storage cistern. In each of these cases, it is necessary to have a covered cistern, protected against ingress of

---

* In January 1995 the DoE issued a consultation paper 'Replacing the Water Byelaws'. The paper discusses the need for such controls and what the most appropriate form of legislation might be.

insects and with an adequate overflow warning pipe [5].

Where an underground or partially below ground storage tank for potable water is required, this should be constructed of waterproof concrete. It must be designed, constructed and tested in accordance with BS8007: 1987 [8].

Water supply pipes

Pipes used for water distribution may be made from a variety of materials, including ductile iron, steel tube, wrought steel, asbestos cement or concrete. In the case of iron or steel pipes, these must be protected both internally and externally, in accord with BS534: 1990 [8], although internal linings containing coal tar are now prohibited. Service pipes are usually of copper, plastic or, occasionally, stainless steel. Lead, which was formerly used, is now prohibited from installation. Copper pipes may not be connected to, or incorporated into, any lead pipe, unless it is protected from galvanic action. To achieve this, copper should not be connected, or inserted 'upstream' of lead pipework.

DOMESTIC FILTRATION AND PURIFICATION

Although water supplied by the statutory undertakers is usually sufficiently pure, circumstances sometimes arise, particularly in the case of private supplies, which make some form of additional domestic treatment either necessary, or desirable. Of the various forms of treatment available, filtration is the most common, on an ongoing basis. This may be particularly useful in the case of private supplies, in addition to other steps, to ensure that the source is pure. It is important that filtration should be related to the contamination which is desired to be removed, as filter mediums vary in their effectiveness at removing particular substances.

Distillation and reverse osmosis

Distillation or reverse osmosis units may be used to desalinate seawater or brackish waters to produce freshwater. Distillation units may be fitted on the cold water supply, under the sink, and consist of a boiling unit with either water or air cooling for the condensation stage. They are very effective at removing impurities, but have a slow flow rate and sometimes produce warm drinking water. Air cooling units may be noisy or if water-cooled expensive in water usage.

Distillation may carry over light fractions, in the case of contamination by organic substances. These may be removed by an additional activated carbon filter. The resultant unit may be bulky and will certainly be expensive to run and maintain.

Reverse osmosis units are essentially filters with a semi-permeable membrane. Filtration is achieved by the differential pressure on each side of the membrane. Sometimes the units are combined with other types of filter or trap, to produce a complete system that is very effective at removing contaminants. Flow rates of the water is low and a lot of water is wasted, typically only 25% of the water being available, the rest running to waste. High water pressures are required to make the system work effectively.

Filtration

A wide variety of water filters are available (Fig. 44.11) for domestic use and their effectiveness is variable. They are basically of two configurations: on-tap fittings, and under-sink arrangements. On-tap filters may either fit directly onto the tap, in which case the limited size affects flow rate and effectiveness, or the filter stands on an adjacent work surface. Under-sink units are permanently plumbed into the cold water feed and provide filtered water via a separate tap.

Generally, filtration units are fitted with replaceable, or cleanable, cartridges. Filter mediums may be of various materials, including plastic materials, metal gauzes and discs, unglazed porous ceramic, ion exchange resin, activated carbon and silver.

Unglazed ceramic cartridges, modelled on the older, on tap, Pasteur-Chamberlain filter, are effective at filtration, but require frequent cleaning and a high water pressure to produce even a low rate of flow. The fine pores of ceramic

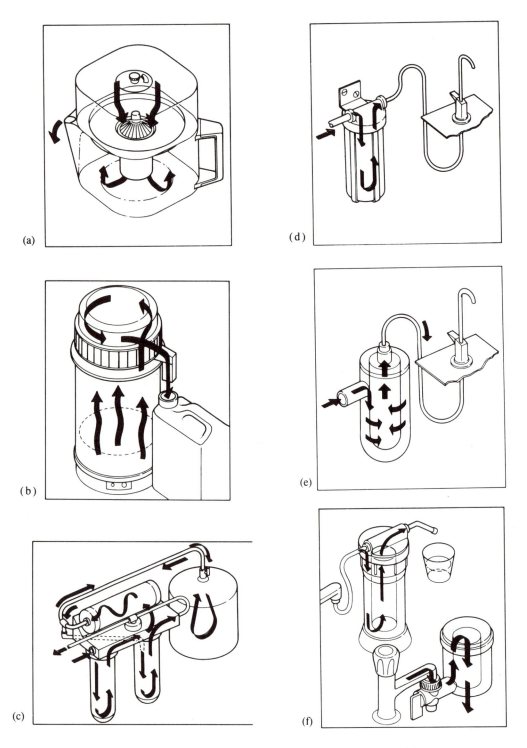

Fig. 44.11 (a) Jug filter. (b) Distillation unit. (c) Reverse osmosis under-sink filter. (d) Activated carbon under-sink filter. (e) Ceramic filter. (f) On-tap filters. (Reproduced with kind permission of the Consumers' Association Ltd. Source: 'Water Filters', *Which?*, August 1990.)

material are effective at mechanical filtration, cleaning being achieved by scrubbing the cartridge with a stiff brush and immersion in boiling water. They also often contain activated carbon, to improve filtration, and the addition of silver to reduce micro-organisms.

Activated carbon filters are the most popular type of domestic filter, and are often combined with silver to reduce bacterial growth. Numerous fine channels through the medium allow effective filtration, by the contaminating substances attaching to the carbon material, and a reasonable flow rate. However, they do not remove all impurities and are ineffective at removing hardness.

All filters should conform to BS6920 and should be installed in accordance with the water bye-laws, including a non-return valve, to prevent contamination of the mains supply. Cartridges need changing regularly, and units should be thoroughly cleansed, to prevent build up of bacteria, which can recontaminate the water.

Other methods of domestic purification

The best method of dealing promptly with drinking water suspected of spreading disease is by boiling. Statutory water undertakers will issue 'boiling orders' where there is a short-term risk from the mains supply. It is a primary means of protection in the case of a suspect supply, and if a boiling order is in force, its importance should be impressed on all concerned. It is not a practical proposition for any length of time and is difficult to implement with a considerable population. As a result, other means of treatment must be used for sanitizing water on a regular basis.

Chemical treatment by chlorination, or ultraviolet light treatment are effective means of reducing micro-organisms in water. Chlorine is readily available as a solution of sodium hypochlorite, containing about 10% available chlorine or, occasionally, as calcium hypochorite (bleaching powder), containing about 33% available chlorine. Both tend to decay and lose chlorine over a period of time and should be kept in air tight containers, although any deficiency in strength may be counteracted by an increased dose.

An effective sanitizing strength will achieve at least 1 ppm free chlorine in the water supply, although this will result in taste effects. A solution prepared from 31 g of bleaching powder, or 100 ml of sodium hypochlorite, to 1 litre of water will be sufficient to treat 10 000 litres of water.

If the water is very impure, discoloured, or contains much suspended matter, it will reduce the effectiveness of the chlorine and it should first be clarified. This may be achieved by the addition of equal parts of alum and powdered chalk, and allowed to stand before decanting to a separate tank for chlorination. It should be allowed a contact time of at least 4 hours before consumption.

If primary filtration is carried out, particularly slow sand filters, this should precede chlorination, although on-tap or under-sink filtration may follow the process. In the case of heavily polluted water, it is important to make sure that free chlorine is available after addition of the solution to the water.

Testing for chlorine

A variety of tests have been used over the years to test for residual chlorine, including the addition of potassium iodide and the use of orthotolidine. The latter test is still a standard method in the USA but has largely been supplanted in Britain by the use of Dr Palin's DPD (NN-Diethylparaphenylene diamine) test method.

By using a standard Lovibond comparitor, DPD tablets and appropriate comparison discs, estimates can be made of free and combined residual chlorine, as well as total residual levels. It is particularly useful to estimate chlorine levels at the same time as taking micro-biological samples.

THE SEWERAGE SYSTEM

Introduction

Provision of an adequate system of drains and sewers is fundamental to the effective drainage of an area. The duty of providing sewerage services was originally given to local authorities and, subsequently, passed to the water authorities set up in 1973. Finally. this duty passed to the sewerage undertakers established by the Water Act 1989 and which now operate under the framework of the Water Industry Act 1991. Thus, for the first time in Britain, provision of an adequate public sewerage and sewage disposal system became the responsibility of the private business sector.

Drains and sewers

It is important to an adequate understanding of the principles of drainage that the difference between 'drains' and 'sewers' should first be considered. The various definitions are contained in section 343 of the Public Health Act 1936 and section 219 of the Water Industry Act 1991. Effectively a **drain** is a single pipe from either one building or a number of buildings 'within the same curtilage'. The meaning of curtilage is sometimes subject to fine legal interpretation, and a regard for the precise circumstances of a particular case (see, for example, *Cook v Mignion* (1979) JPL 305 and *Weaver v Family Housing Association* (1975) 74 LGR 255), but broadly the words mean the boundary or fence of a particular property.

A **sewer** generally is a pipe taking drainage from a number of drains. Such a sewer may be a **public sewer** where it is 'vested' in a sewerage undertaker by the various powers under the two Acts. In other cases, where drains have been connected together to form a sewer (in order to simplify drainage, but the overall ownership remains conjointly with the property owners), the sewer is a **private sewer**, being constructed solely for the use of those properties. In exactly the same way as a drain, it is to be maintained by, and at the expense of, the person or persons to whom it belongs. Private sewers and drains are generally laid in the gardens, courts, or yards of the various premises to which it belongs. However, they remain private up to the point of connection with the public sewer, even where it runs under public pavements and the public highway.

Provision of sewerage

Under section 94 of the Water Industry Act 1991, sewerage undertakers must 'provide, improve

and extend . . . a system of public sewers'. They must also maintain and cleanse the sewers, as well as provide disposal facilities, including sewage disposal works. Their duty extends to making provision for trade effluent discharged under the powers of Part 3 of the 1991 Act. This duty, to provide sewerage for their districts, is similar to that placed upon the predecessor authorities, but with the significant introduction of enforcement orders under section 18 of the Water Industry Act 1991. In addition, regulations, made under section 95 of the same Act, may prescribe performance standards – see the Sewerage Servies (Customer Service Standards) Regulations 1989.

Connections to sewers

Owners and occupiers of premises are given the right, by section 34 of the Public Health Act 1936, subject to certain restrictions, to drain into public sewers. The actual connection to the sewer may be made by the sewerage undertakers if they elect to do so, under section 36 of the same Act, or otherwise it may be made by the owner or occupier themselves. In the latter case, they must give 'reasonable notice' to the statutory undertaker, who may supervise the works. In either case, and subject to appeals, the sewerage undertaker may refuse to allow the drain to communicate with the public sewer if 'the mode of construction or condition of the drain or (private) sewer is such that [it] would be prejudicial to their sewerage system'. Sewerage undertakers may also, at their expense, alter the existing drainage system of premises where the drainage is sufficient for the premises, but is, 'not adapted to the general sewerage system'. This is subject to giving adequate notice, the provision of 'equally effectual' drainage and rights of appeal to a magistrates' court [3].

Sewer Requisition

Section 98 of the Water Industry Act 1991 provides requisitioning arrangements for public sewers, similar to those first introduced by the Water Act 1973. Essentially this allows owners, occupiers or local authorities (including new towns and development corporations) to serve a notice on the appropriate sewerage undertaking company, requiring it to provide a public sewer for domestic purposes in a particular area. In these circumstances, section 99 of the 1991 Act requires the person or authority to pay the capital costs over a period of 12 years. In the absence of regulations, there is no clear indication of precisely the circumstances under which sewerage undertakers must comply with their general duty to provide sewers at their own expense, as opposed to waiting for the use of requisitioning powers (including the attendant cost penalty) by individuals or communities.

Agency arrangements

The relationship between sewerage undertakers and local authorities is reinforced by section 97 of the 1991 Act, which allows them to carry out sewerage functions on behalf of the sewerage undertakers. Clearly, where agency agreements exist, the operational arrangements and the various powers are consolidated within one authority, which eases the making of local decisions. While formerly the water authorities had a duty to enter into such agency agreements with local authorities, this has been replaced by the discretionary power given to the statutory undertakers. In the longer term, it is likely that a decline in the number of agency arrangements will result from at least some of the sewerage undertaking companies taking commercial decisions to carry out their own operations, or make them subject to competitive tender.

Miscellaneous provisions

Power is also given, by section 21 of the amended Public Health Act 1936, to enable sewerage undertakers to use highway drains and sewers for sanitary purposes, by agreement with the highways authority. This power is also actionable by the local authorities. The Public Health Act 1936 powers over adoption of sewers (sections 17 and 18), construction standards (section 9), purification of sewage (sections 30 and 31), rights of owners and occupiers to drain into public sewers

(section 34), power to alter the drainage system of premises (section 42) and the power to make corrections to public sewers (section 36) were unaltered by the Water Act 1989 or that of 1991, except they are also exercised by the sewerage undertakers.

Local authority powers

For a detailed description of local authority powers in relation to sewers and drains together with flow diagrams, see *Environmental Health Procedures* [3].

New drains and sewers

Provision of drainage in new buildings is controlled by section 21 of the Building Act 1984. When plans of a building or an extension are deposited with a local authority, under the Building Regulations 1991, they must be rejected if the arrangements for drainage, where necessary, are not satisfactory. Proposals for provision of drainage must include proper connection to the public sewer, cesspool or some other place, as required by the local authority or, on appeal, by the magistrates' court. Connection to a public sewer cannot be required unless the sewer is within 30.5 m (100 ft) and the owner is entitled to construct a drain through the intervening land. A local authority may, however require a building to be drained into a sewer that is more than 30.5 m distance, if it bears the cost of construction and maintenance of the drain, from the sewer up to the point within that distance of the building.

Section 22 of the Building Act 1984 gives the local authority power to require construction of a private sewer to new buildings, where they 'may be drained more economically or advantageously in combination'. Clearly, if there is to be any expectation that a private sewer is to be adopted as a 'public sewer', by the sewerage authority, it should accord with any constructional standards laid down by the sewerage authority. The maintenance of private sewers is likely to cause interowner disputes and legal difficulties, particularly if large numbers of properties are connected. For this reason, developers should be encouraged to enter into a formal adoption agreement, under section 18 of the Public Health Act 1936, ensuring that the sewer will be adopted, provided it is constructed to the standard agreed.

The Building Regulations 1991 require that 'any system which carries foul water from appliances within the building to a foul water outfall shall be adequate'. The Regulations make similar provision for roof water. The specific requirements are contained in approved document 'H', made under the Regulations, with foul drainage dealt with under H1 and rainwater drainage under H3.

Section 60 of the Building Act 1984 makes a specific requirement, enforceable by local authorities, for the provision of ventilation to a soil pipe serving a WC. The same section also places a prohibition on the use of rainwater pipes from a roof as soil pipes, or the use of surface water drains as a ventilation shaft for foul drainage.

If it is proposed to erect a building or extension over a drain, public sewer or disposal main, section 18 of the Building Act 1984 requires the local authority to reject any plans submitted under the 1991 Regulations if maintenance or access to the drain, sewer, etc. is to be interfered with. ('Disposal main' means an outfall pipe from a sewage works which is not a public sewer.) Consent may be given to erect a building under these circumstances, and the plans passed, provided the authority is satisfied that it may 'properly consent'. Approval of such a construction may be subject to conditions and specific constructional requirements.

Plans which are deposited, showing a proposal to build over a drain, sewer or disposal main, must be notified to the sewerage undertaker by the council concerned. In turn, the undertaker may specify to the council 'the manner in which [it is] to exercise [its] functions' under section 18. In practice this means that it will either require the local authority to reject the plans, or specify the conditions and/or constructional standards required. Clearly, where the local council is itself acting as agent for the sewerage undertaken under section 21, it may determine these matters on behalf of the undertaker. The powers relating to rejection of plans also applies to an 'initial notice' given by an approved inspector under the Building Regulations 1991.

Defective drainage

Three main powers are given to local authorities to deal with defective existing private sewers and drains:

1. Under section 17(3) of the Public Health Act 1961 they may serve a 48-hour notice to deal with a **stopped up drain, private sewer**, etc. If the notice is not complied with, they may carry out the necessary work themselves and reclaim the expenses from the persons concerned. This is subject to rights of appeal, particularly over the cost of the works and the apportionment of the costs if more than one property is concerned.

2. Under section 17(1) of the Public Health Act 1961, they may serve a 7-day notice of their intention to deal with a **drain, private sewer etc., that has not been maintained** and **kept in good repair**, and can be repaired for less than £250. They may recover the expenses from the 'person concerned' but, on appeal to the courts, will be required to justify their conclusion that the pipe or appliance was not properly maintained. The court may also enquire into the apportionment of the costs charged to the person or persons on whom the notice was served and make an order concerning the expenses or apportionment (section 17(7)).

3. Section 59 of the Building Act 1984, which replaced the almost identical powers formerly contained in section 39 of the Public Health Act 1936, gives local authorities the duty of serving a notice in a wide variety of situations concerning existing **defective private drainage**. This applies to virtually all pipes and appliances, including cesspools, other than public sewers. The period allowed for appeal against notices served under this section is 21 days. As a consequence, a longer period, often 28 days, must be allowed for compliance. This delay may cause difficulty where a serious risk to public health exists.

Section 22 of the Public Health Act 1961 gives local authorities power to **cleanse or repair defect-**

ive drainage etc., at the **request of an owner or occupier** and at his or her expense. In practice, this is a useful alternative to service of a notice, carrying out work in default and recovering the expenses, where the owner or occupier is willing to carry out the work. Indeed, many local authorities enclose a 'request authority' with the service of notice, to offer the opportunity of early remedy for what is often a serious public health problem.

Any **court, yard, etc., which is inadequately surfaced** so that surface water drainage is unsatisfactory, may be dealt with by the local authority serving a notice on the owner under section 84 of the Building Act 1984. This provision only applies in relation to a yard or court which is common to two houses, or a house and a commercial or industrial building. It does not apply to highways maintained at public expense.

In addition, powers contained in the 1936 Act to deal with overflowing and leaking cesspools (section 50) and care of sanitary conveniences (sections 51 and 52) are similarly enforced by local authorities (district councils) serving notice on owners, or occupiers, as appropriate.

Testing of drains or private sewers which are thought to be defective is an important prerequisite for serving notice to repair or cleanse them. Power to carry out tests is contained in section 48 of the Public Health Act 1936, and is given to the 'relevant authority', which in the case of drains or sewers communicating with a public sewer means the sewerage undertakers. It is not clear whether this restricts local authorities to testing drains and sewers which communicate with private disposal facilities, or whether it simply limits their ability to test the final run of drainage which connects to the public sewer. The different wording of sub-section (1) of section 48 should be noted, which refers to 'a drain or private sewer communicating directly or indirectly with a public sewer'. Once again, where an agency agreement exists between a local authority and the relevant sewerage undertaker, the matter is simplified.

It is not always necessary to expose and examine the drains to check for defects and, initially, the application of a non-pressure smoke test or colour test is sufficient. At the least, this will give

an indication of any break in the drains and its approximate location. If necessary, remote television probes may be used to examine the interior of drainage systems, and it is now rarely necessary to expose drains before the nature and location of the defect has been established. Water tests, under pressure, should only be applied to new drainage systems, where prescribed by the Building Regulations 1991. (See 'Drain testing' below.)

If alterations or repairs are carried out to underground drains, other than in an emergency, the person carrying out the work must give the local authority at least 24 hours' notice, by section 61 of the Building Act 1984. If any work involves the permanent disconnection or disuse of any drains, they must, by section 62 of the same Act, be sealed off 'at such points as the local authority may reasonably require'. Section 63 of the 1984 Act also requires that a water closet, drain or soil pipe should be properly constructed or repaired. If conditions prejudicial to health or a nuisance are caused by such works, then the person carrying them out is guilty of an offence.

Local authorities are authorized, by section 67 of the Building Act 1984, to **loan temporary sanitary conveniences** where works on drainage etc., necessitates disconnecting WCs etc. They may make charges for the loan, provided it exceeds 7 days and is not a result of work made necessary by a defect in a public sewer.

TRADE EFFLUENT

Section 27 of the Public Health Act 1936 places a general prohibition on passing any matter into a drain or public sewer which is harmful to it, or might interfere with the disposal of sewage. There are also specific prohibitions on the discharge of chemical waste, steam, high-temperature liquids, petroleum and calcium carbide. This is particularly important when considering means of arresting materials before they enter the drainage system (see below).

The Public Health (Drainage of Trade Premises) Act 1937, originally enforced by local authorities, is now the responsibility of the sewerage undertakers and its provisions have been consolidated in the Water Resources Act 1991, part 4. Before discharging trade effluent into a public sewer, the occupier or owner of the trade premises concerned must seek a consent from the undertakers under section 118. The application must be in writing and state:

1. the nature or composition of the effluent;
2. The maximum quantity to be discharged in any one day; and
3. the highest rate at which it is to be discharged.

Copies of any consents given must be kept available for public inspection at the offices of the undertaker.

Important changes have been made to the 1937 Act provisions by section 138 of the Water Industry Act 1991. This section makes provision for 'prescribed substances' present in the effluent in 'prescribed concentrations' and effluent derived from a 'prescribed process', or involving use of 'prescribed substances' in specified quantities or amounts. Regulations made under this section, the Trade Effluents (Prescribed Processes and Substances) Regulations 1992, have 'prescribed' the substances contained in list 1 of EC Directive 76/464/EEC, on pollution caused by certain substances discharged into the aquatic environment. In addition, the Regulations prescribe effluents derived from five types of process including asbestos processes, giving effect to Article 3 of EC Directive 87/217/EEC, on the prevention and reduction of environmental pollution by asbestos.

Section 130 of the Water Industry Act 1991 requires the sewerage undertakers to refer any applications for consent, or any proposal to make an agreement to discharge trade effluent, to the Secretary of State. It is for him to determine whether the operation should be prohibited, or any conditions to be applied to a consent or agreement. Appeals by aggrieved persons are to be made to the director general of water services. These are important modifications of the 1937 Act, foreshadowing an evolving policy to protect the aquatic environment.

Drainage systems

Two main systems of drainage are employed to dispose of sewage, trade effluent and surface-water run off from roofs and hard surfaces. In the one case, rain or surface-water drainage is kept separate from soil and waste drainage, and the two are conveyed by separate drains to separate outfalls. Surface water is conveyed direct to a natural watercourse and foul sewage to a disposal works. This is known as the **separate** or, occasionally, the dual system of drainage.

Where surface water and foul water are conveyed together, this is referred to as **combined drainage**. Combined drainage has the virtue of simplicity but requires pipework of much larger capacity to deal with storm water. The need to allow for smaller and therefore cheaper, capacity sewerage systems often leads to the construction of **storm-water overflows**. Storm-water overflows are usually constructed as part of an inspection chamber and vary in design; essentially they provide an overflow from the system at a high level, usually connecting with a natural watercourse.

At one time, it was thought that the effluent was graduated at times of storms, with freshwater flowing over the top of the foul sewage, and the discharge was thought to consist almost entirely of rainwater. It is now accepted that this is not the case, and the overflows at times of storm are of highly diluted sewage. This in turn introduces the risk of contamination of water-courses by overflows. This problem can be particularly serious in the case of sewer blockages, which can lead to the discharge of large volumes of undiluted sewage through storm-water overflows.

The advantage of separate drainage is the avoidance of surcharging of sewers by vast volumes of surface water during storms. This in turn allows the construction of smaller capacity drains and sewers to deal only with foul drainage. In practice, however, truly separate drainage is difficult to maintain, and is often confusing, leading to wrong connections being made by developers. The contamination by tar used in roads and domestic driveways and, more particularly, by increasing amounts of oil and other deposits from motor vehicles, are rendering this system of drainage less and less effective as a means of preventing contamination of the natural water environment. In towns, often the only water sufficiently clean for direct discharge into a river is water from roofs. The essential principles of separate drainage require that this should be conveyed through pipes and gullies used exclusively for the purpose. In some instances there is a combination of the two systems called **partially separate**, when some rainwater is allowed into the foul water system. On balance, despite higher construction costs, the separate system should be favoured.

The discharge of foul water into a sewer provided for surface water or, except with the approval of the sewerage undertaker, the discharge of surface water into a sewer provided for foul water, is prohibited by section 34 of the Public Health Act 1936 (as amended). The connection of a waste pipe from a lavatory basin or a WC, for example, to a rainwater pipe, discharging into a sewer provided for surface drainage only, would be an offence under this section and may also be an offence under part 'H' of the Building Regulations 1991.

Separate drainage should always be adopted in connection with any individual house or premises which drains into a cesspool or private sewage disposal plant. Rainwater pipes from roofs and gulleys (provided only for surface drainage), may be made to discharge into prepared soakaways in the gardens, etc., subject to consent from the NRA. In premises where sewage treatment is carried out on site, drains conveying surface water may discharge into the outlet of the purification plant, provided this also is agreed with the NRA.

Drainage – design and construction

Drainage should generally be in accordance with approved document 'H' of the Building Regulations 1991, which includes appropriate references to British Standards Institute documents. Part 'H1' deals with sanitary pipework and drainage; part 'H2' deals with cesspools and tanks; and part 'H3' deals with rainwater drainage. Enforcement of the 1991 Regulations is the responsibility of either the local authority or, in the case of self-certification, of the approved inspector.

New drainage within a building should be

capable of withstanding an air or smoke test of at least 38 mm water gauge for at least 3 minutes, although smoke testing is not recommended for uPVC pipes. New drains and private sewers, carrying either foul or surface water, should be capable of withstanding a water test with a pressure equal to 1.5 M of head, and measured from the invert of the pipe at the head of the drain. Alternatively, an air pressure test, with a maximum loss of head on a manometer of 25 mm in a period of 5 minutes for 100 mm gauge or 12 mm for a 50 mm gauge, may be applied.

The performance of new drainage should minimize the risk of blockage or leakage, prevent foul air entering the building, ensure effective ventilation of the system and be accessible for clearing blockages. Cesspools should have sufficient holding capacity and, in particular, septic tanks and settlement tanks should be large enough to enable breakdown and settlement of solid matter. Cesspools, septic tanks and settlement tanks should be watertight, adequately ventilated and not located so as to risk public health or the contamination of water supplies. They should also be accessible for emptying. Rainwater drainage systems should carry rainwater from the roof to either a surface water or combined sewer, a soakaway or a watercourse.

Materials for drainpipes
The most important part of any sewage collecting system is the pipe. Various types of pipe are now available for the conveyance of sewage and surface water. Subject to the pipe, bedding, and jointing material being chemically inert in their surroundings and content, the following are acceptable (they should conform to the relevant British Standard):

1. vitrified clay pipes (BS 65: 1981);
2. concrete (BS 5911: 1982–9)
3. cast iron (BS 416: 1973; BS 437: 1978);
4. galvanized steel (drainage stacks) (BS 3869: 1973);
5. asbestos cement pipes (BS 3656: 1981);
6. unplasticized PVC (BS 4514: 1983; BS 4660: 1973; BS 5481: 1977).

Table 44.5 Recommended minimum gradients

		Foul drainage	
Peak flow (litres/sec)	Pipe size (mm)	Minimum gradient (1 in . . .)	Maximum capacity (litres/sec)
<1	75	1:40	4.1
	100	1:40	9.2
>1	75	1:80	2.8
	100	1:80*	6.3
	150	1:150†	15.0

*Minimum of 1 WC.
†Minimum of 5 WCs.

Drainage design

SIZE AND FALL Drainage is made self-cleansing by ensuring that the velocity is within a range that is neither too fast, nor too slow (the **self-cleansing velocities**). If the flow is too slow, solid material and detritus will settle out and accumulate, while an over-rapid flow results in the water elements leaving the solid material behind as deposits. The capacity of the system should be large enough to carry the expected flow and this, in turn, will determine both the diameter and gradient of the pipework in the system (see Building Regulations 1991 approved document 'H').

The layout of a drainage system should be as simple as possible, changes of direction should be minimized and the gradient, or fall, should be adequate and uniform. The flow depends upon the number and type of appliances connected, and the capacity upon the size and gradient of the pipes. (See Table 44.5.)

Drains carrying soil water or trade effluent should have a minimum diameter of at least 100 mm, while waste water only may be carried in pipes with a minimum diameter of 75 mm. The capacity of pipe-work carrying both rainwater and sewage should allow for the increased peak flow at times of storm. It should not be forgotten that both the size and the fall of drainage has a direct effect upon the cost of construction, and that flat topography sometimes makes achieving an adequate gradient difficult.

MEANS OF ACCESS Any drainage system should have adequate means of access to clear blockages which cannot be reached by any other means. The Building Regulations 1991 prescribe provisions that allow for normal means of rodding from either:

1. rodding eyes;
2. access fittings;
3. inspection chambers;
4. manholes.

Access points should be provided at the following points:

1. at or near the head of each drain run;
2. at a bend or change of gradient;
3. at a change of pipe size;
4. at a junction, unless each run can be cleared from some other access point;
5. in long, straight runs of drainage.

JUNCTIONS Any junction between pipes in a drainage or sewerage system should be made so that the tributary drain or sewer discharges its contents into the other drain or sewer obliquely in the direction of flow.

VENTILATION An essential of a good drainage system is the maintenance of a free passage of air throughout each part of the system. Permanent openings are required at the lowest and highest points, and careful consideration needs to be given to air discharge points in order to prevent odour nuisance. Except under special conditions, the use of intercepting traps should now be avoided, but these will often be found in older systems.

Soil pipes, waste pipes and ventilation pipes

Building Regulations 1991 provisions are contained in approved document 'H', and require that the capacity of the system should be large enough to carry the expected flow. The document should be referred to for minimum guidance on the size and gradient of pipe, together with the appropriate British Standard reference.

The essential principles for a drainage system within a building are the same as those for an overall drainage or sewerage system. The system should:

1. convey the waste to disposal, e.g. a foul drain or sewer;
2. minimize risk of blockage or leaking;
3. prevent foul air from entering the system;
4. be ventilated;
5. be accessible for clearing blockages.

To achieve these objectives requires the system to be constructed in accordance with the approved document 'H', part 1 and the British Standards codes to which it refers. The system normally consists of a central, ventilated stack pipe within the building, which is connected to individual sanitary appliances by branch discharge pipes.

Rainwater gutters and pipes

As with foul drainage, the basic requirements for rainwater drainage are that the system should be capable of carrying rainwater from the roof of a building to an outfall, sewer, soakaway, or a watercourse. In addition, the system should minimize the risk of blockages and be accessible for clearing blockages.

The specific requirements are contained in Part 3 of approved document 'H' under the 1991 Regulations. This lays down provisions for calculation of the area drained, gutter sizes and outlet sizes, as well as general arrangements for freshwater drainage. Reference is also made to relevant British Standards codes of practice, as an alternative, or to supplement the requirements of the approved document.

Approved document 'H' assumes that rainfall is to be at a rate of 75 mm an hour, and makes no provision for roofs less than 6 m^2. It is important that rainwater, or surface water, is not drained to a cesspool or septic tank.

Interception of oil and petroleum

The prevention of the entry of oil and petroleum spirit into drains and sewers is a matter of increasing importance as motor vehicle traffic continues to increase.

Drains provided for the floors and washing spaces of garages, filling stations and similar premises where petroleum spirit is used should be constructed as entirely separate systems, and made to discharge into a suitable petrol interceptor before joining a sewerage system.

DRAIN TESTING

The smoke test

This test is usually applied to existing drains, with a view to revealing and locating leakage and detecting defects, which may be connected with rat infestations. It may be applied by the use of a smoke 'rocket' or by a specially constructed machine.

A smoke 'rocket' is essentially a large, smoke-generating firework and its value is very limited. No pressure can be applied, and its main use is for tracing connectings and demonstrating the presence or absence of obstruction, rather than as a test for soundness.

One of the best-known smoke-testing machines and the method of applying a smoke test is illustrated in Fig. 44.10. The apparatus consists of a double-action bellows and a smoke box, which is enclosed by a light copper dome working in a water seal. More compact and lightweight apparatus is also available, which includes a vertical pump connected to the smoke chamber and a manometer to indicate pressure.

Smoke-producing material, such as a specially prepared paper or oily cotton-waste, is placed in the smoke box and lighted. By slowly working the bellows, large volumes of pungent smoke are produced, and this is conveyed by means of a flexible tube into the drain through a gully, WC or access chamber, whichever is convenient, but preferably at the low end of the system.

In order to ensure that the drain is filled with smoke and not merely air locked, traps should be emptied and resealed one by one as the smoke appears through them. The last openings to be sealed are those of the ventilating pipes. When these are sealed, a slight pressure may be set up in the drain. The copper dome rises with the action of the bellows, and if the drain is quite sound, is maintained in a slightly elevated position.

Considerable care is needed in the application of this test. If any pressure, however slight, is exerted in excess of that which can be resisted by the head of the water seals of traps when depressed, smoke is forced through into the building and the test may be rendered misleading and therefore useless.

The coloured-water test

This test is useful for tracing drain connections, leakages and gradients. A drain that is sound under a pressure test is not necessarily a good drain. The joints may contain cement on the inside – a common defect in stoneware drains laid by unskilled persons. The fall may be insufficient or may even be in the wrong direction. These are serious defects and may be detected and, to some extent, measured by the coloured-water test. The test should be applied to the drain in sections, each section being first washed out with clean water.

Coloured water, produced by the use of a dye sachet, is poured into the drain in small measured quantities with intervals of time between each. Any water retained by obstructions or improper levels is displaced by the coloured water, and the amount of this which it is found necessary to add before the first trace of it is discharged at the outlet represents approximately the amount of water normally retained by the drain.

The coloured-water test is also useful for determining the source of water which may be causing a nuisance, e.g. water percolating through a basement wall which is normally dry. A drain passing near the wall may be suspected. For this purpose a solution of fluorescein is poured into the drain. This chemical when added to water possesses a bright green fluorescence, which is unmistakable and easily discerned even though it may be very highly diluted.

The air test

This is a very convenient and useful test for soil and waste pipes. The application of the test to a soil pipe is illustrated in Fig. 44.12. All plugs used in the test must be water-sealed, in order that any leakage of air through them may be detected.

The test is delicate, and the pressure obtainable limited by the depth of water seals in the traps. A valuable and important feature of the test is that by its use the weakest water seal in connection with a pipe under test is indicated. A pressure equal to 38 mm water gauge is usually applied and this should remain constant for 3 minutes.

The test may also be used for drains before they are submerged in water or the trench filled in. Junctions are sealed off and expanding plugs screwed into each end of the length to be tested. The 'U' tube is connected to the plug at one end of the drain, and air pumped through the other until 100 mm water pressure is indicated. The cock at the pump is turned off and if the water pressure drops by more than 25 mm in 5 minutes for a 100 mm gauge, the drain is unsatisfactory. A maximum drop of 12 mm is allowed for a 50 mm gauge (after allowing a suitable time for stabilization of the air temperature).

Unlike the water test, the air test is of equal severity regardless of the length of the drain tested. An objection sometimes raised against the test is that while it may indicate leakage, it does not locate it. This is only partially true. If leakage is indicated, suspected joints should be coated with a soap solution. By this means, escaping air is easily discerned.

The water test

The Building Regulations 1991 require that drains should be watertight and tested by either a water test or an air test as prescribed for new drainage systems.

The lower end of the drain is plugged by means of an expanding rubber stopper or, if this is difficult, by a flexible pneumatic stopper. A 1.5 m head of water, above the invert of the pipe, at the top end of the pipe line, is used to create the pressure, and this can be obtained by temporarily jointing a 90 degree bend and a straight pipe of the same diameter as the pipeline, to the head of the line and filling with water. Care must be taken to prevent airlocks in unventilated branches. This is done either by emptying the traps or by passing a ventilated pipe through the water seals. Arrangements for carrying out the test are con-

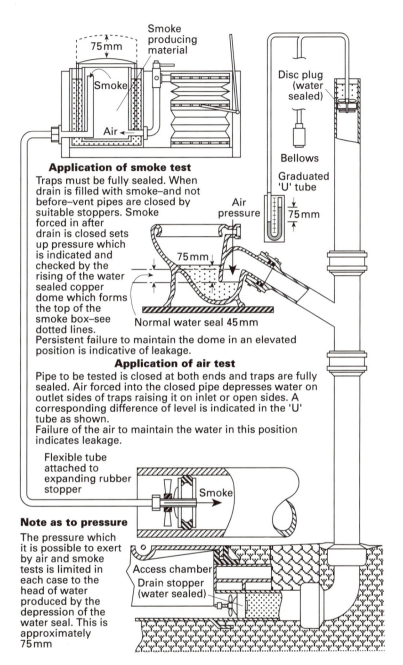

Fig. 44.12 Application of smoke test and air test.

tained in approved document 'H' of the Regulations.

The section of drain should be filled and allowed to stand for 2 hours, before being topped up. The leakage over 30 minutes should be measured by adding water up to the original level, and should not be more than 0.05 litres for each metre run of drain, for a 100 mm diameter drain, equal to a 6.4 mm/m drop in water level. In the case of a 150 mm diameter drain the loss should not exceed 0.08 litres/m run, or 4.5 mm/m drop in water level.

To prevent damage, the head of water to the lower end of the drain should not exceed 4 m and it may be necessary to test the system in sections.

Television surveys

Increasingly, testing of drains and sewers is being replaced by use of internal inspection, using specialized closed circuit television systems (CCTV). As a result, it is now rarely necessary to expose drains or sewers, before the precise nature and location of any defect has been established. Special cylindrical video cameras of stainless steel construction, watertight to over 100 psi, are used to examine the interior of pipes from as small as 50 mm through to 600 mm in diameter. They may be mounted on appropriately sized skids, which are pushed, or pulled through the pipe with rods. Alternatively, the camera may be mounted on an electrically driven tractor unit, which can crawl along the pipe interior. The camera transmits an image to a closed-circuit monitor, usually in a vehicle, where defects can be detected and noted. Video tapes and photographs may also be produced.

In its simplest form, CCTV pipe inspection units provide monochrome pictures, from a single angle. A cable meter indicates the position of the defect by measuring the length which has been inserted into the drain or sewer. Other units may be highly sophisticated, providing high definition colour video reproduction, with a wide variety of control and measuring facilities, including the ability to negotiate acute bends. Pan, tilt and zoom facilities may be available on the lens, as well as an on-line computer analysis of the video signal to provide text data on the pipe dimensions and levels. As a result, use of such complex equipment is largely confined to specialized contractors, who may be hired to carry out specific surveys. However, increasing availability of cheaper equipment, capable of providing sufficient information for most purposes, provides the opportunity for local authority's to acquire their own CCTV systems.

The Cleansing and repair of Drains and Sewers

Methods available to cleanse and repair underground pipework and remove blockages, include the following:

1. **Rodding.** Rodding is still a widely used method and is particularly applicable to the smaller pipes. Clearance of the blockage is attempted by bringing the end of a flexible rod into contact with the material responsible for the obstruction. Various devices are available for use at the tip of the rod, including spirals and rubber plungers, the latter using air compression in addition to mechanical pressure. The material responsible for the obstruction is not, however, removed, but is merely transported along the drainage system, and for this reason large quantities of water are required for flushing.

2. **Flushing.** The routine flushing of sewers and drains which are not laid to a self-cleansing velocity is essential and flushing of other sewers may be necessary from time to time in order to remove sludge and grit. Flushing devices are constructed as part of some systems, as with the automatic syphon which is fed by mains water and discharges by syphonic action. Where such systems are not installed, flushing can be accomplished by the use of hydrant water supplies via 100 mm diameter hoses, or with mobile flushing tanks.

3. **Hydraulically propelled devices.** Water is discharged into the sewer behind a sewer ball or jetting ball, which is slightly smaller in diameter than the pipe. The flow behind the device is driven through the gap between the device and the pipe wall at a high velocity, and a scouring action results. The method is used for dislodging sludge and grit.

4. **Winched devices.** This system can be used to remove debris and roots but access via two manholes is required. A bucket or similar device is winched through the sewer by hand or power and the debris collected and removed.

5. **Jetting.** This is most effective in pipes between 150–375 mm in diameter. Water under pressure is fed through a hose to a nozzle contain-

ing a rosette of jets, and is sufficient to dislodge material on the pipe walls and debris lying along the invert. The system uses a purpose-built vehicle incorporating a water tank and including a suction unit for gully cleansing.

6. **Repairs**. As an alternative to conventional repairs to underground pipes by excavation and replacement of damaged sections, new, *in situ* repair systems are now available. Essentially, the commercially available systems consist of installing a liner to the damaged pipe(s) and subsequent internal remotely controlled cutting of lateral connections. Steps involved include use of CCTV cameras to carry out a preliminary survey of the pipe, to prepare the interior for the insertion and to control the installation. Pipe liners currently available include those made of preformed stainless steel or polyethylene. Alternatively, *in situ* linings may be formed by use of polyester and polyurethane felt tubing impregnated with thermosetting resin, cured on site by use of hot water. In this latter case, internal patches up to 3 metres long, may also be applied to pipe defects, using the same technology, controlled by CCTV monitoring.

THE NATURE OF SEWAGE

Sewage is a cloudy, aqueous solution containing mineral and organic matter as particles floating and, in suspension, colloidal material and substances in true solution. It also contains living organisms, particularly very large numbers of bacteria, viruses and protozoa. Its nature may be altered by rainwater gaining access to the sewerage system by design (combined system), or by infiltration through the pipe joints. Trade wastes also alter its composition. (See Table 44.6.)

TREATMENT OF SEWAGE

Inland sewage disposal works usually provide full primary and secondary treatment, with discharge

Table 44.6 Typical chemical composition of a dry weather domestic sewage

Mineral content dissolved and suspended	420 mg/l
Organic matter dissolved and suspended	620 mg/l
Total solids	1040 mg/l
5-day bio-chemical oxygen demand	310 mg/l

of final effluent mainly into rivers. Sewage from some coastal towns is still discharged directly into the sea, without treatment. Sometimes the sewage is screened and macerated before discharge in order to hasten its breakdown by the salt water, wave action and sunlight. Provided the outfall is sufficiently long, and has a properly designed terminal diffuser, giving sufficient opportunity for the natural action of the sea on organic material, it has been argued by the British Government in the past that this can prove an effective method of disposal. However, the implementation of the Urban Waste Water Treatment directive (91/271/EEC) [11] will effectively put an end to this method.*

Disposal schemes

The basic principles underlying the conventional treatment of sewage are physical and biological. In the case of public sewage disposal works, operated by statutory sewerage undertakers, the treatment may be extensive.

Fig. 44.13 shows in schematic form sewage treatment processes.

Physical
This involves the removal of solids usually by screening followed by detritus and sedimentation tanks. Screens may be fixed or moving. Fixed screens may be vertical or inclined at an angle and, in the larger works, are mechanically raked. Moving screens may be an endless belt of wire mesh or perforated plate, or a revolving drum where the sewage passes into the drum and out through the sides which are perforated.

Grit, sand, etc., is removed by passing the sewage through a settlement tank (grit chamber), or sometimes by passing the sewage through a channel at a constant velocity.

* See the Urban Waste Water Treatment (England and Wales) Regulations 1994.

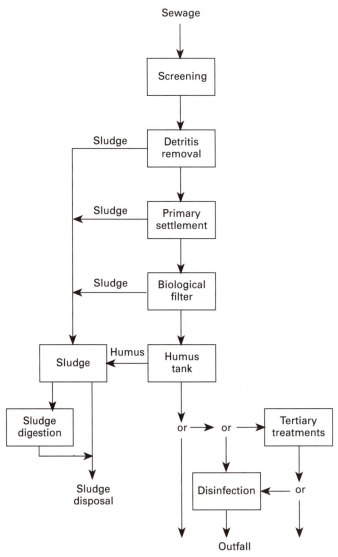

Fig. 44.13 Schematic – sewage treatment process.

This is followed by sedimentation, allowing much of the suspended solids to settle, by passing the sewage slowly through tanks. These may be circular, or rectangular with a horizontal flow, or square with an upward flow. The solids settle as a sludge, and with a properly designed system, consists of 60 to 80% of the solids originally contained in the sewage. The sludge from the rectangular tanks may be cleared manually by suction or mechanical scraper, and the vertical flow tank is mechanically scraped and discharged under hydrostatic head.

Biological
This consists of the oxidation of the organic matter left in the sewage after settlement, and is effected primarily by the action of bacteria. This part of the treatment may be achieved by:

1. running the liquor over the land;

2. filtration; or
3. the activated sludge process.

LAND TREATMENT This method has almost totally fallen into disuse, except for small communities. The two systems used were surface irrigation and sub-surface irrigation.

In the first system, the sewage from settlement tanks is distributed over the area by a system of channels or carriers. Handstops are necessary to control the distribution and to ensure that parts of the site are periodically rested. A porous or underdrained soil is necessary, and this should be turned over at yearly intervals. The area of land required will depend on its nature, and with gravel or sand 60 m² (70 sq yd) per house may be sufficient, but in the case of heavy soils, e.g. clay, 167 m² (200 sq yd) may be necessary.

The second method also requires a fairly porous soil, but should not be adopted if the level of the water table in winter is less than 1.8 m (6 ft). The system consists of a system of irrigation trenches fed from either: (1) a main distribution centre, (2) a central open channel running at right angles to the irrigation trenches, or (3) a central drain feeding subsidiary distribution channels at the intersection of the irrigation trenches.

This system is not generally recommended and should only be used if the construction of a filter is not practicable.

FILTRATION The use of the word filtration is rather misleading as the function of the filter is not to filter out suspended solids but to bring the sewage, after settlement, into contact with a durable medium, such as hard clinker or broken stone or plastic, on the surfaces of which develops a film containing micro-organisms which feed on or oxidize the impurities in the sewage. The process is assisted by the action of worms, insects, algae, etc. The micro-organisms are aerobic so that the filter bed must be adequately ventilated to ensure their activity. The media making up the filter beds should conform with BS1438: 1971 [10] and is usually of 50 mm nominal size except for the bottom 150 mm which is 100–150 mm. The tanks may be either rectangular or circular and

vary from 1.4 m to 3.0 m in depth, although 1.4 m is essential. Some mechanical means is provided for the dispersion of the liquor over the surface of the filter and, in the case of rectangular beds, this is usually a tipping trough with channels; and in the case of a circular bed, a rotary distributor fed via a dosing chamber and syphon. The dosing chamber balances the variation in flow and ensures a head sufficient to operate the rotary arms otherwise ponding will result. The filter material is usually supported on perforated tiles or pipes to ensure aeration of the lower media.

The amount of liquor which can be treated on the filter (the dosing rate) is determined by the strength of the liquor, but will usually be about 547–780 litres/cu metre per day.

Another system aimed at the same effect is the alternating double filtration (ADF) system where settled sewage is applied at a high rate to one filter and, afterwards, pased over a second one. Periodically (weekly or even daily) the order of the filters is reversed.

Another form of biological treatment is the rotating disc filter, which uses a medium in the form of discs or random elements packed in a perforated drum. This is finding favour in small treatment works, particularly for local communities (see below).

ACTIVATED SLUDGE PROCESS When large volumes of sewage have to be treated, the biological breakdown is achieved by the activated sludge process. In this process the sewage, after settlement, is aerated in tanks by compressed air being blown into the sewage through porous plates or pipes at the bottom of the tank or, alternatively, the sewage takes up atmospheric oxygen by being continually agitated by agitators rotating on or near the surface of the sewage. For small works, an oxidation ditch may be used as an alternative to tanks.

A further development of the activated sludge process is the deep-shaft process. The system incorporates a deep shaft (usually the deeper the better), which is divided into down-flow and up-flow sections. After coarse screening and grit arrestment, the sewage or industrial effluent enters the shaft continuously and is circulated around the sections of the shaft many times before overflowing into a flotation tank where the solids settle.

Compressed air is introduced into the shaft to ensure the circulation of the effluent and provide the conditions suitable for the health and activity of the aerobic bacteria which purify the liquid.

Due to the turbulence caused at the bottom of the shaft and the long time the bubbles are in contact with the liquor while rising to the surface, the oxidation process is very efficient and high rates of treatment are possible.

The shaft can also be used for aerobic digestion of sludge, which is considerably less than with the conventional activated sludge process. The conventional sewage works need large, open tanks for aeration of the sewage, and also tanks for the anaerobic digestion of the sludge, so that the deep-shaft system is much more acceptable environmentally, uses far less land and produces less sludge with the consequent saving in the cost of its disposal. It is also possible to locate variations of the process underground, making for even greater acceptability.

Humus

The film which forms on the media in the biological filter becomes detached periodically, and this, together with other fine particles still in suspension in the sewage, is allowed to settle in humus tanks. After passing through these tanks, the effluent should be fairly clear and innocuous, and suitable for discharge into a watercourse, although it will have a relatively high biological oxygen demand (BOD), and some organisms will have survived the process. Alternatively, the humus can be removed by passing the liquid over land.

Tertiary treatment

When very high standards of purification are necessary, a third stage is adopted in which there is further sedimentation or filtration. The methods used include irrigation over grass plots, slow or rapid sand filtration, retention in lagoons, micro-straining or upward-flow clarifiers.

A final sterilization process may also be used at this stage, usually by the addition of chlorine,

although use of ultra-violet filters is now seen as a more environmentally acceptable alternative.

Micro-straining by use of Continuous Membrane Filtration (CMF) results in a large reduction in both bacteria and viruses. The technology has largely been developed in Australia, although pilot plants do exist in both the USA and in Britain. CMF is capable of producing a very high effluent, but its application has so far been confined to small scale sewage disposal works.

Sludge

The solids deposited in the settlement tanks is known as sludge. It is a thickish, offensive-smelling liquid with a very high water content, and various ways have been devised to eliminate much of the water. One of the greatest problems with sewage disposal is getting rid of the sludge. The principal methods adopted are:

1. **Barging to sea**. This is a cheap process often used in coastal areas, or where a navigable river provides access to the sea. Disposal of sludge to sea has been banned by the EU from 1998, and alternative methods will now have to be adopted for those places still disposing of sludge in this way.

2. **Land disposal**. Running wet sludge onto flat land or into trenches allows the material to dry, and the land can then be ploughed and used for crops. This has the problem of large land usage, and causes considerable smell and insect problems. The method depends heavily on the quality of the land and the soil drainage, which together with the other inherent defects has led to its virtual disuse.

3. **Lagooning or air drying**. The sludge is drained into shallow tanks, the bottom of which is covered with a 150 mm layer of clinker or ashes. Over a period of months, the moisture drains and evaporates until the sludge is sufficiently dry to dig out. It may be used as a fertilizer, but it does not break down readily in soil and is not popular with farmers. While it is cheap, the absence of a ready market, together with the problems of nuisance from smell and flies, has reduced its popularity.

4. **Direct spraying or injection on agricultural land**. Tankers of liquid sludge may be sprayed directly onto agricultural land, where it breaks down readily and has the virtue of cheapness. Objections to the smell problems associated with sludge spraying may be overcome by direct injection into the soil. However, there are concerns over infectious organisms carried by spray drift, as well as the environmental effect of run off, particularly close to beaches and estuaries. While the method is popular at the time of writing, environmental concerns make it undesirable.

5. **Incineration**. Increasingly incineration is being used for sludge disposal, particularly in European countries. It has a number of advantages, but there are concerns over the dispersion of industrial contaminants, such as heavy metals or chlorinated organic compounds.

6. **Anaerobic digestion**. Sludge is stored in closed tanks and heated to 35°C for several weeks. Anaerobic bacteria thrive under these conditions, and bring about biochemical changes which reduce the volume of the sludge and render it inoffensive. During the process, CO_2 and methane are given off. The methane may be used for heating the tanks and buildings, or for electricity generation.

Digested sludge is a good soil conditioner in addition to containing nitrogen and phosphorus. Provided it does not contain excessive toxic waste arising from trade processes, it is a useful fertilizer.

Smell nuisance

Sewage disposal works, sewers and pumping stations have been a consistent source of smell nuisance to their neighbours and have caused considerable offence to residential areas in particular. As a result the planned location, particularly of large works, is likely to be a source of considerable sensitivity. As a result of the EC Urban Waste Water directive, there is likely to be a considerable increase in applications for new works, by the ten regional water companies, each of which will be subject to full environmental impact assessments. Odour control will be an important part of those assessments and is best built in to the new plants, which will need careful consideration at the design stage. Modern plants, designed to minimize or eliminate smell, are capable of being fully enclosed, often underground, which provides an ideal opportunity to control ventilation of odours (e.g. by carbon adsorption). Use of bio-filters and bio-scrubbers also helps to reduce odours at their source, with claimed reduction efficiencies in the range 94–99%.

Small sewage disposal schemes

The attainment of a satisfactory standard of purification is possible if the plant is properly constructed and designed to meet the requirements of each particular case. Size, shape, and construction are all important. Size must be relative to the strength and amount of crude sewage to be dealt with: these depend upon the number of persons occupying the building and the amount of water likely to be used by each. Where an adequate supply of water is available, a sewage flow of 120 litres per head per day may be taken as the average to be dealt with.

A high degree of purification must be the prime object of any disposal scheme, and to be efficient, it must be automatic, require a minimum of attention, and be free from objection, either of sight or smell. The design should be in accordance with BS6297: 1983 [12]. The principal points of construction and use of the several units are described below.

Septic tank

The purpose of this unit is to retain crude sewage until the soluble solids liquify, and the insoluble solids precipitate as sludge. During decomposition, solids float to the surface, forming a scum which should be removed only when necessary.

1. Capacity. In BS6297: 1983 [12] total capacity, where desludging is carried out at not more than yearly intervals, is given for general purposes by the formula:

$$C = (180P + 2000) \text{ litres.}$$

Where C is the capacity of the tank (in litres), with a minimum value of 2720 and is P the design population with a minimum of 4.

2. Design. The tanks should be in series, either one tank divided into two by a partition or two separate tanks. The length of the first tank or section should be twice its width, and provide about two-thirds of the total capacity. For populations of over 60 persons, duplicate tanks, operated in parallel, are recommended, so that while one unit is in use the other can be desludged.

3. Inlets and outlets. These should be so designed that the discharge of sewage into the tank and the decanting of the clarified sewage is done with the minimum disturbance of the scum or sludge in the tank. For tanks up to 1200 mm wide, 'dip' pipes, with the bottom arms about 450 mm below liquid level, are satisfactory. For tanks wider than 1200 mm, two dip pipes fed from a trough inlet are recommended, with a full width weir acting as an outlet. It is customary to have a scum board fixed about 150 mm from the weir, the board should stretch the full width of the tank and be about 450 mm wide, 300 mm of this being below the water level.

4. De-sludging. The design should include facilities for desludging, and the floor of the tank should slope towards the inlet, providing a 'well' for the collection of the sludge as it is being pumped out or, if the site is sloping and makes it impossible, discharged by gravity through a valve.

5. Covers. These are unnecessary from the point of efficient working of the plant, but should be provided to small tanks purely as a safety precaution. Larger tanks can be surrounded by a fence.

Settlement tanks

A primary settlement tank, if properly designed and maintained, will produce a more highly clarified tank effluent than that produced from the conventional two-chamber brickwork or concrete septic tank. Settlement tanks may be of the horizontal-flow or upward-flow type. Laboratory and field trials demonstrated that the three-stage vertical chamber principle produces a tank effluent which can be readily dispersed through land drains laid in suitable porous subsoils, or filtered biologically where this form of secondary treatment is necessary, or where for a variety of reasons disposal by land treatment is not desirable or permissable.

Tanks are also available in either precast concrete or fibreglass reinforced plastics, in a range of capacities from 2750–18 000 litres, as standard prefabricated tanks or in larger capacities when required.

The principal function of the tank is to effectively produce quiescent conditions by reducing upward flow velocities between chambers, thus permitting the maximum retention of sludge in the base.

Biological filter

The principles for biological treatment are the same as in large public sewage disposal schemes. In very small schemes, the filtration process is very much simplified. Care should be taken to ensure that distribution of sewage over the surface of the filter is even, or the effluent will form defined channels and purification will be proportionately incomplete. The design of the distributor is an important factor in the success or failure of a plant [12].

Humus or secondary settlement tank

The design should be similar to that of the septic tank, with weir inlet and outlet with baffle and scum boards. The capacity should be not less than that suggested in BS6297: 1983 [12].

It may be desirable to make secondary tanks equal in size to primary tanks, otherwise the formulae for calculating is as follows:

Horizontal flow tanks: $C = 135P^{0.85}$

where C is the gross capacity of the tank (in litres); and P is the design population with a minimum value of 4.

Upward flow tanks: the gross capacity should not be less than that determined by the formulae above, and the surface area should not be less than:

$$A = 3/40 \; P^{0.85}$$

where A is the minimum area (in m^2) of the tank at the top of the hopper, and P is the design population with a minimum value of 4.

Outfall

Purified sewage effluents may be disposed of by surface or subsoil irrigation or, subject to consent by the NRA, by discharge into a stream. Such a consent will prescribe conditions as to the quality and quantity of the discharge, and may include provisions relating to the siting and construction of the outlet, sampling point etc. Rain and surface water should be kept separate from sewage where purification has to be effected on site, but a drain conveying this water may with advantage join the outlet from the humus tank.

There are also now available prefabricated 'packaged' sewage disposal units for small communities. An example of this is the Klargester Ames Crosta BioDisc, which is a complete self-contained sewage treatment plant, designed for small communities in a range of sizes to serve from 5 to 150 persons. Larger communities can be accommodated by arranging units in parallel. The complete treatment process is carried out in one totally enclosed compact unit.

The units are fabricated in fibreglass and may be installed either above or below ground. Crude sewage is piped direct to the BioDisc entering the baffled primary settlement zone via a deflector box which stills the flow. The heavier solids sink to the bottom of the compartment to disperse into the main sludge zone. any floating solids will be retained by means of a baffle. The effluent, with lighter solids still in suspension, passes into the 'bio zone', which comprises a chamber with transverse baffles arranged so that the liquid must follow a serpentine path from zone inlet to outlet. The baffles also separate a series of slowly rotating circular discs into banks, so that the sewage passes through each bank in turn. Micro-organisms naturally present in the sewage adhere to the partially immersed discs to form a biologically active film, feeding upon the impurities and rendering them inoffensive. The organisms feed and multiply very rapidly in the presence of an ample supply of oxygen, and as each portion of the film on the rotating discs is alternately in contact with settled sewage and atmospheric oxygen, conditions are ideal for efficient purification.

The sludge from the primary and bio zones collects and consolidates in the base of the unit. The unit can accommodate a large quantity of consolidated sludge before desludging is necessary, say, every 4–6 months, and this can be done by a gully emptier or similar suction unit.

Effluents – analyses and interpretation of reports

Sewage effluents discharging into streams must normally conform to standards set by the NRA usually based upon the recommendations of the Royal Commission on Sewage Disposal. These most frequently refer to biochemical oxygen demand (BOD) and suspended solids. The values achievable by a well-run works are fractions of the plant design capacity. These and other constituents have been interpreted as follows:

The Royal Commission on Sewage Disposal

A maximum BOD level of 20 mg/l in effluents was recommended, where the dilution in the river was at least 8:1. Although this value is now varied according to circumstances by the NRA, the majority of works have been designed to produce an effluent reaching this standard.

The BOD test is essentially a measure of biodegradable material present in an effluent and is dependent upon the conditions under which the test is applied. Furthermore, under the original conditions of the test, the result included the oxygen demand of nitrogenous materials. To overcome this, an allylthiourea is added to suppress nitrogenous oxidation.

Total oxygen demand and chemical demand are two further tests and differentiate oxidizable organic and inorganic matter present.

In the case of suspended matter a limit of 30 mg/l was recommended, where the dilution was 8:1, but in a similar manner to BOD, this value is now varied to suit the circumstances. Suspended solids are normally determined as total and volatile.

Sewage always contains chloride to an extent depending upon the strength of the sewage, the presence of trade wastes and the content of the water supply. It remains unaltered through the treatment process. Medium sewage contains up to 100 mg/l of chloride whereas a strong sewage may contain up to 500 mg/l.

Nitrogen is present in a number of forms, particularly ammonia, nitrite and nitrate representing different oxidation states.

Ammonia arises from the aerobic or anaerobic decomposition of nitrogenous organic matter and, since it is extremely toxic to fish and interferes with the chlorination of drinking water, it is undesirable in effluents discharged to these waters. Nitrates represent the final oxidation stage of ammonia and its presence indicates a well-run plant. When a plant is operating ineffectively, there is likely to be oxygen deficiency at, for example, an overloaded filter, and the oxidation of ammonia may only proceed to the nitrite stage. Thus a trace of nitrate may indicate imperfect treatment.

For activated sludge plants, it has been considered uneconomic to carry the purification process beyond the clarification stage and little or no nitrate may be produced, yet the effluent may be well clarified with low BOD and suspended matter.

EC Urban Waste Water Standards*

Royal Commission standards, as interpreted, will be largely replaced by the requirements of directive 91/271/EEC [11] as the compliance dates are arrived at. In each case the directive lays down sampling frequencies, technical compliance standards for discharges and percentage of failed samples allowable, as follows (also see Tables 44.7 and 44.8).

The minimum annual number of samples shall be determined according to the size of the treatment plant and be collected at regular intervals during the year:

2000–9999 pe†	12 samples during the first year, four samples in subsequent years, if it can be shown that the water during the first year complies with the provisions of the Directive: if one sample of the four fails, 12 samples must be taken in the year that follows:
10 000–49 999 pe†	12 samples
50 000 pe† or over	24 samples

For full details of sampling methodology and standards, consult Annexe I of Council Directive 91/271/EEC [11].

Conservancy

The term 'conservancy' is used to describe those systems of sanitation in which faecal matter is retained in some form or other of closet apparatus, and is not carried away by water through a proper drainage system. So far as towns are concerned, very little conservancy takes place and has been almost universally replaced by water carriage. Conservancy is, however, the only practicable system in sparsely populated districts.

Conservancy and water supply are closely associated. Absence of an adequate public water supply necessitates recourse to private means of supply; it also necessitates conservancy. There is thus produced the double public health problem of, firstly, insufficient safe water for domestic purposes, and, secondly, adequate disposal of sewage, frequently on sites not suitable for a septic tank system of disposal.

Provided they are properly sited and installed under skilled supervision and are properly maintained, conservancy systems do not necessarily imply a lowering of normal standards of hygiene. Nevertheless, such systems must always be regarded as potential dangers to health, e.g. to water, by contamination of the earth, and to food, through contamination by flies.

---

* Also see the Urban Waste Water Treatment (England and Wales) Regulations 1994.
† pe = population equivalent.

Table 44.7 Requirements for discharges from urban waste water treatment plants subject to Articles 4 and 5 of the Directive. The values for concentration or the percentage of reduction shall apply

Parameters	Concentration	Minimum percentage of reduction	Reference method of measurement
Biochemical oxygen demand (BODS) at 20°C without nitrification	25 mg/l O$_2$	70–90 40 under Article 4(2)	Homogenized, unfiltered, undecanted sample. Determination of dissolved oxygen before and after 5-day incubation at 20°C ± 1°C, in complete darkness. Addition of a nitrification inhibitor.
Chemical oxygen demand (COD)	125 mg/l O$_2$	75	Homogenized, unfiltered, undecanted sample. Potassium dichromate
Total suspended solids	35 mg/l (optional) 35 under Article 4(2) (more than 10 000 pe)† 60 under Article 4(2) (2000–10 000 pe)†	90 (optional) 90 under Article 4(2) (more than 10 000 pe)† 70 under Article 4(2) 12 000–10 000 pe)†	Filtering of a representative sample through a 0.45 μm filter membrane. Drying at 105°C and weighing. Centrifuging of a representative sample (for at least 5 minutes with mean acceleration of 2800 to 3200 *g*), drying at 105°C and weighing

Table 44.8 Requirements for discharges from urban waste water treatment plants to sensitive areas which are subject to eutrophication as identified in Annex IIA(a). One or both parameters may be applied depending on the local situation. The values for concentration or for the percentage of reduction shall apply

Parameters	Concentration	Minimum percentage of reduction (in relation to the influent)	Reference method of measurement
Total phosphorus	2 mg/l P (10 000–100 000 pe)† 1 mg/lP (more than 100 000 pe)†	80	Molecular absorption spectro-photometry
Total nitrogen	15 mg/l N (10 000–100 000 pe)† 10 mg/l N (more than 100 000 pe)†	70–80	Molecular absorption spectro-photometry

Cesspools

Cesspools are the cheapest and therefore the commonest means of storage of sewage outside a sewered area. A cesspool is not a means of disposal of storage, it is merely a means of storing sewage until it can conveniently be disposed of. A drain discharging into a cesspool should be reserved for foul water only, and should be 'disconnected' by means of an intercepting trap and chamber. Surface drainage should be treated separately, e.g. by discharge into soakaway pits.

Cesspools should be constructed in accordance with BS6297:1983 [12]. The cesspool should be on sloping ground, lower than nearby buildings, and regard should also be had to the prevailing winds. There should be no risk of pollution, particularly of water supplies and the tank should be at least 15 m from any inhabited building.

Cesspools should have a minimum capacity of 18 000 litres (18 m³) (Building Regulations 1991 approved document 'H') and preferably not less than 45 days usage for the buildings it serves. Regard should be had for the means of emptying, before a decision is made over the capacity or, indeed, whether to use a cesspool at all.

Cesspools must be watertight and may be made of a variety of materials. Factory made cesspools are available in glass reinforced plastics (GRP), polyethylene or steel. Prefabricated tanks should have a British Board of Agreement (BBA) certificate.

Under the Building Regulations 1991, cesspools have to be constructed to enable access for emptying and also to avoid contamination of water supplies. An existing cesspool which does leak or overflow is subject to the requirements of section 50 of the Public Health Act 1936, and the service of a notice by the local authority. It can specify the works to be done to deal with any soakage or overflow. This includes regular emptying [3].

The emptying of cesspools by contractors or local authorities, rather than by individuals, enables the use of gully emptiers, or cesspool emptiers, as part of the public cleansing service. A cesspool emptying vehicle has a closed steel tank of about 4500 litres capacity, and is fitted with a 15 cm inlet valve. It should be provided with armoured rubber pipe of sufficient length to connect the tank with cesspools in the neighbourhood. The engine produces a vacuum equal to 50 cm in the cylinder. The valve is then opened and the contents of the cesspool are transferred through the pipe into the cylinder, by the pressure of the atmosphere. The pipe should extend to the bottom of the cesspool so that the sludge is first removed and followed by the liquid sewage above it. There is no agitation of the sewage; the whole proceeding should be inoffensive and may be carried out at any time of the day. The tank should be either discharged at a sewage disposal works, or into a large capacity public sewer, through a proper disposal chamber. Indiscriminate disposal onto land is not acceptable.

Earthclosets
These are now little used and depended upon the power of dry earth to neutralize faecal matter. The receptable is essentially a stout, galvanized iron bucket, which in order to ensure frequent emptying should not be of more than 55 litres capacity. It should be movable, but held in position by a suitable guide, and fitted closely into a suitable enclosure. The earth should be clean, dry, fertile top-soil sifted to a 6 mm mesh. Sand or ashes are not suitable for the purpose.

The fitness standard laid down in the Local Government and Housing Act 1989 requires the provision of a water closet. Any property provided with dry conservancy, including earth closets, is unfit and should be subject to action under housing legislation (see Chapter 20).

Chemical closet
Chemical closets have greatly improved in appearance over the years, although they are now more generally used for camping, caravanning and boating. They all operate with a deodorizing, liquefying or sterilizing liquid being basically a solution of formalin. Some manufacturers claim that waste matter, treated with their chemicals, can be safely disposed of down a drain, but unless there are specific disposal points as on camp sites, marinas, etc, the views of the controlling authority should be sought beforehand.

The closets are usually constructed of strong plastic or fibreglass, and range from an enclosed bucket to semi-permanant recirculating units with filtration units and electric 'flushing' pumps. Similar built-in units are used in aircraft, long-distance motor coaches and Channel Tunnel trains.

Treatment and Disposal of Farm Wastes

The development of intensive farming practices together with increasing urbanization and rising expectations for the environment, have lead to increased complaints of smell. Farming is an industry in its own right, and produces a volume of trade waste which must be disposed of without a risk of nuisance or danger to public health.

Character of the waste

Animal excreta is the main problem, and it has been estimated [13] that the total volume of excreta from all livestock (June 1987 Census) (cattle, pigs, sheep, poultry) is 121 000 000 tons. Also the demand by multiple stores for pre-packed washed vegetables has led to a big increase in this work at farms (it has been stated that washed carrots require 12 000 gallons of water per acre (22 079 litres/ha of crop), so that large quantities of polluted water have to be dealt with.

Methods of disposal

The seven usual methods adopted are:

1. **Dry handling**. The aim is to keep manure as dry as possible and the excreta, mixed with bedding, is taken to a midden or store with walls of earth, railway sleepers or maybe concrete. The depth of the manure is restricted to 1–1.5m to help evaporation, and retained for 6–9 months before distribution on the land. The bedding absorbs much of the liquid, and some drains from the store into channels or pipes and is dealt with separately.
2. **Semi-dry handling**. The excreta is kept apart from any bedding; faeces and urine are mixed to give a slurry which is spread on the land.
3. **Semi-liquid handling**. The procedure initially is as for (2) above, but is mixed with water (1 part water to 1 part manure) to enable it to be spread by vacuum tanker.
4. **Irrigation**. The solid and liquid manure are washed down by water to a storage tank with enough water to give a mixture of 1 part manure to 2 parts water. Some system of agitation in the tank is required, and the liquid manure is spread on the land by pump, pipes or rain gun. The tank should be large enough to hold 10–14 days diluted effluent.
5. **Discharge to sewers**. Being a trade waste, farm effluent could, subject to the consent and conditions laid down by the sewerage under-taker, be discharged into a public sewer. Regard would have to be had for the 'strong' nature of the effluent and its effect upon any sewage treatment works.
6. **Oxidation in lagoons**. Unfortunately, due to the low temperature usually experienced in this country, this has not proved very success-ful. The best results are obtained by having as large an area as possible with the slurry not at a depth greater than 1.5 m. If the slurry is too deep, anaerobic action commences with the creation of offensive smells.
7. **Soakaways**. Provided the soil is suitable and there is no danger of polluting underground water supplies, soakaways or blind ditches can be used for draining off the liquor, the de-posited solid matter being removed periodic-ally. The consent of the NRA is required for this.

Camp Sanitation

Among the public health problems associated with the use of camps of all kinds, none is more important than the provision of sanitary accommodation.

Large, permanent camps require piped water supplies; they also need a water-carriage system of drainage. Where, in addition, a sewage disposal plant is necessary, the types of plant already described are suitable and can be adapted to all purposes.

In small camps and those of a temporary character, some form of conservancy system alone is practicable. In open-air conditions, the provisions described below can be quite satisfact-ory, but in every case they must be sited, con-structed, and maintained under the direction and supervision of the environmental health officer of the district concerned. All latrines must be fitted with seats and covers and otherwise made fly-proof.

Earth latrines

The simplest method of disposing of human excrement in non-sewered districts is by returning it directly to earth, but it is necessary to ensure that all danger of spreading disease is minimized. Surface pollution must be avoided. The most suitable provision is a dug latrine.

Earth latrines, soakaways, etc, may be used with safety only where pollution of the subsoil water is not a risk. Faecal organisms reaching the ground water from a point source, e.g. a latrine, do not travel evenly in all directions, but are carried only with the ground-water flow. In a careful investigation in the USA, pollution was found to travel to a distance of between 25–30 m 'with the stream', but did not reach 3 m in any other direction. Usually, the groundwater is flowing in a definite direction, and provided the direction is known, an earth latrine or a soakway can be safely located. In ordinary soils, it may be assumed that the area outside a radius of 6 m, and extending round one-half of a circle 'up stream' or above the latrine, is safe from danger of pollution. In chalk and similar formations, however, the water is in fissures which form subterranean streams running long distances in all directions. No earth latrine may be used with safety in such formations.

The deep trench
In temporary camps where field sanitation alone is practicable, an earth latrine, properly constructed and supervized, is a sanitary and satisfactory provision. The latrine in most common use is of the deep trench type which, owing to its size, is generally arranged for communal use, and because of that, is open to many objections.

The trench latrine should be 1 m in width and not less than 2.5 m in depth. It should be provided with a well-constructed riser or seat, the openings of which should be arranged over the lateral centre of the trench, the front and back being constructed to prevent the ingress of surface water. Self-closing covers should be provided to the openings, and all necessary measures should be taken to render the trench fly-proof when it is closed.

The contents of a deep trench latrine should at frequent intervals be covered with about 75 mm of fertile topsoil (not the sterile earth previously dug out). The nitrifying organisms in top soil rapidly neutralize and break down faecal solids and render them innocuous. The action is biological and quite efficient. Only where a latrine is sunk into dense, water-tight earth, and contains foul liquid matter, should a disinfectant be used.

The bored-hole latrine
This simple form of the earth latrine has been adopted with marked success in the tropics, but is equally suitable for use elsewhere. By means of a hand-operated land auger of simple design, a hole 400 mm in diameter is bored in the earth to a depth varying from 4.5–6 m. The walls of the hole being circular and undisturbed are, in ordinary soil conditions, self-supporting.

Container closets
The best of these are the earth closet and the chemical closet already described; they are both suitable for camp purposes.

Sullage water
On no account should crude sullage be discharged into a river, stream, ditch, or lake, or over unprepared ground. The simplest means of disposal is by soil absorption through a soakage pit. Even in the most favourable formations, the ability of the soil to absorb sullage water is lessened as time goes on, and it may be reduced to a point at which complete disposal is not possible. In order to preserve soil absorptivity, grease and soap curd should be removed by passing sullage water through a grease-trap, before it is discharged into a soakage pit.

For field use, a grease-trap is designed to ensure that sullage water passing through it has a long journey at low velocity between inlet and outlet, so that grease and soap curd may separate from the water and float to the surface, where they are retained. Two 'baffles' only are necessary, one to form the inlet and the other the outlet chamber; these should pass down to two-thirds the depth. The trap should be deep rather than shallow and long and narrow rather than square. A length to breadth proportion of 3 to 1 is desirable. A capacity of 225 litres is suitable for general purposes.

Soakage pits
The purpose of a soakage pit is to receive waste liquids as and when they are produced, and to act as a reservoir from which they may soak continuously into the surrounding ground. The pit should be filled with coarse rubble to support the sides

and cover – but leaving the maximum of voids – and covered with earth at least 300 mm in depth. Apart from geological conditions, efficiency is dependent upon two factors: water content and the extent of the soakage surface. Generally, the water content should be equal to 1 day's production of sullage. Soakage surface is represented by the perimeter plus the base; the shape should provide the maximum perimeter by comparison with the volume, e.g. rectangular rather than square. Where the surface stratum is dense, it should if possible be pierced, and a more permeable stratum brought into use. A form of vertical drainage – useful for both sullage and surface water – is thereby obtained.

Chemical precipitation

In large camps, or where the soil is or has become non-absorbent, sullage must be purified, or more correctly clarified; it may then be disposed of in the same way as ordinary surface water.

A simple method of purification, used in military camps, consists in treating sullage with two simple chemicals – ferrous sulphate and hydrated lime. The quantities required vary with the sullage, but in ordinary conditions, for every 250 gallons of sullage, 1 lb of ferrous sulphate (427 mg/l) and 1–1½ lb of lime (427–1641 mg/l) are required. Effective precipitation depends upon obtaining a correct alkalinity; the lime is used for this purpose. A pH of 9 is suitable; this turns phenolphthalein pink.

The sullage is collected into a tank. The ferrous sulphate, after being dissolved in water, is then added; the lime is similarly dealt with, and the whole contents of the tank are thoroughly agitated. A heavy floc results which precipitates rapidly, forming a closely packed sludge and leaving the supernatant water clear. The process does not completely remove grease; water from a cookhouse should therefore be passed through a grease-trap before treatment. The clarified water is comparable to an ordinary purified sewage effluent, except that the 'oxygen-absorbed' figure is high – about 10 parts per 100 000. This can be corrected by aeration, e.g. by causing the effluent to pass through an open channel and, if possible, over weirs before discharging into a stream.

A sullage purification plant is easily constructed. Two precipitating tanks are usually necessary, to be used in rotation; they can be formed from precast concrete rings or pipes placed on end in a suitable excavation, the bottoms being concreted in the form of an inverted frustum of a cone, into which the sludge can gravitate. The outlet for clarified effluent is fixed not less than 300 mm above the bottom of the tank and at a level from which the effluent can gravitate to a suitable place of disposal. Two outlets fixed at different levels, afford useful flexibility of working.

Sludge is dealt with on shallow lagoons. It is usually at too low a level to run by gravity to these; the hydraulic head provided by the supernatant water when the tank is full is utilized to eject and lift it to the required level. It dehydrates rapidly, forming an innocuous residual which may be disposed of on land.

The ferrous sulphate and lime contained in the sludge produced from the first two or three charges is used to assist in the precipitation of subsequent charges. For this reason desludging is carried out only when the sludge level rises to within a few inches of the clear water outlet.

DISPOSAL OF EFFLUENT TO RIVERS AND THE SEA

The final stage in the water cycle is the drainage of water from the land environment to the sea. Sources of drainage include:

1. Natural drainage from hard surfaces and land.
2. Fresh water drains.
3. Storm water overflows.
4. Final effluent, either treated, or untreated, from sewerage systems.

Drainage may be either via the rivers and their tributaries, or direct to sea, but eventually all drainage is resident in the ocean. In UK an as yet incomplete network of statutory standards, voluntary standards and information, influences both the quality of drainage and the resultant river and sea water.

Rivers

During the course of water privatization, powers were included in the Water Resources Act to enable OFWAT to declare statutory water quality objectives (SWQOs). It was intended that they would replace the non-statutory river quality objectives (RQOs), which were mostly adopted in the period between 1979 and 1981 by the former water authorities.

If river water quality needs to be improved to comply with RQOs, action will be required to regulate, or prohibit individual discharges into the receiving waters. Possibly because, even at the beginning of 1994, large numbers of sewage treatment works still needed to be improved to achieve the non-statutory RQOs, the new system of SWQOs still had not been introduced at that time.

In effect, the Urban Waste Water directive [11] allows for two options to regulate discharges from sewage works:

1. Uniform discharge limits for suspended solids, biological oxygen demand (BOD) and chemical oxygen demand (COD).
2. Minimum percentage reduction in the values of the parameters during the treatment process.

Generally, the view has been taken that the second method is more difficult to enforce, requiring monitoring of both the influent and the effluent. However, in December 1993, the Department of the Environment decided that the percentage reduction method was to be adopted as the basis for implementing the muncipal waste water directive in the UK. Resultant safeguards over river water quality, by using this method, do not necessarily provide the power to achieve the RQOs. Consequently SWQOs continue to be delayed, despite original stated intentions.

Although inland sewage disposal works usually provide full primary and secondary treatment, with discharge of final effluent mainly into rivers, sewage from many coastal towns is still discharged directly into the sea, without treatment. Sometimes the sewage is screened and macerated before discharge in order to hasten its breakdown by salt water, wave action and sunlight. It has been argued by the British Government in the past that this can prove an effective method of disposal, provided the outfall is sufficiently long and has a properly designed terminal diffuser, giving sufficient opportunity for the natural action of the sea on the organic material. However, the implementation of the Urban Waste Water Treatment Directive (91/271/EEC) [11] will effectively put an end to this method at bathing beaches and within estuaries.*

As from certain dates, being either 2000 or 2005, depending upon the size of their population, all towns and villages with a 'population equivalent' (pe) of over 2000, will have to subject their 'Urban Waste Water' (Sewage) to specified treatment requirements. In general terms this will mean both primary and secondary treatment, but in the case of discharges to particularly sensitive areas, specific tertiary treatments will also be required.

Even those communities which are too small to be required, by the terms of the directive, to install full secondary systems, must still provide 'appropriate' methods of treatment to ensure that they comply with the quality objectives laid down. Annex I to the directive lays down emission limit values, sampling patterns and methodology together with the percentage reductions to be achieved. The directive also requires controls over the disposal of sewage sludge by 1998, which will require a phasing out of sludge dumping at sea by that date.

These requirements should have a marked effect upon coastal waters, although the British Government continued to negotiate over derogations in the run up to implementation, because of the short timescale to implement major capital investment. A House of Lords Select Committee also expressed reservations about the use of uniform limit values and proposals for sludge disposal. Whilst their report [14] was not published until after the directive was agreed, it suggested that the use of environmental quality objectives, rather than discharge limit values, was

---

* Now see the Urban Waste Water Treatment (England and Wales) Regulations 1994.

more suitable for sewage disposal and also expressed concern over the environmental costs of landfill or incineration of sewage sludge.

One source of more detailed information on the contamination of water is the NRA Water Quality Series, e.g. No. 15 *Contaminated Land and the Water Environment* and No. 15 *Abandoned Areas and the Water Environment*, both published in 1994.

The sea

The sea is the final stage of the water cycle, within man's control, before natural evaporation and the climate takes over. Disposal of sewage outfall effluent to sea, either directly, or as a result of drainage from rivers has caused concern for three main reasons:

1. Effects upon bathing beaches and other recreational uses.
2. Impact upon the sea environment and its ecosystems.
3. Concentration of polluting substances into the food chain of animals and man, through the 'Silent Spring' [15].

Increased use of sea water for recreational purposes has lead to the first of these being of greatest concern.

Natural bathing water quality
Council Directive (76/160/EEC) [16] concerning the quality of bathing water, commonly referred to as the bathing water directive, was adopted by the Council of the European Communities in December 1975. Principle objectives of the Directive are to protect both human health and the environment by maintaining the quality of bathing waters. This Directive does not apply to swimming pools or waters intended for therapeutic purposes, but to those fresh or saline open waters, where bathing is explicity authorized by the competent authorities, or is not prohibited, and is practised by a large number of bathers.

In Britain, the term 'bathing water' is taken by the Department of the Environment to mean an area where bathing is traditionally practised by a large number of people as defined by the directive. Examples are sites with lifeguards, or where changing huts, car parks or chalets are provided on a substantial scale for bathers. There was no definition in the legislation as to what might constitute large numbers of bathers, resulting in wide divergence within the European community over implementation. 'Bather' appears to be interpreted rather narrowly in Britain, to mean swimming, and the bathing season is taken as being from May to September.

Because of their responsibilities for controlling water pollution, the NRA have been designated as competent authorities by the Department of the Environment. In turn, the NRA are required to identify bathing waters for sampling and monitoring and to ensure that the waters comply with standards set by the Directive. Results of the sampling programme undertaken by the NRA at all EU designated beaches during the bathing season are supplied to the coastal local authorities.*

With respect to coastal water quality, the local authority role is to advise the public of any health concern which could arise as a result of use by bathers. In 1990, the Minister of State for the Environment and Countryside announced, in response to the House of Commons Environment Select Committee report on pollution of beaches, that local authorities were to be encouraged to display bathing water quality information on beaches and other prominent sites around resorts.

Standards set by Directive 76/160/EEC [16] have been subject to considerable controversy and there have been calls for new imperative standards (especially in relation to viruses) to be put into effect. In its fourth report, *Pollution of Beaches* [17], the House of Commons Environment Committee added to the call for a review of the EU directive standards, in light of the then current epidemiological and viral scientific research.

Quality requirements for bathing water are detailed in the annexe to Directive 76/160/EEC [16] (see Tables 44.9–44.11). Some 19 physical, chemical and microbiological parameters are

---

* The NRA publish an annual report on bathing water quality in England and Wales.

listed, of which 13 are 'I' (imperative) values and/ or 'G' (guide) values. Coliform counts are valuable indicative values, although regarded by some researchers as too fragile to reflect survival rates of pathogens in sea water. Only in exceptional circumstances have derogations been permitted to the standards. To conform, 95% of samples for parameters where an 'I' value is given must meet the values set and 90% of samples in other cases. Waivers may be granted because of exceptional weather or geographical conditions etc. Minimum sampling frequencies are laid down and the Directive specifies how and where samples are to be taken, but it does not specify handling procedures for samples before analysis. The **streptococci and salmonella** parameters only have to be checked when there is reason to suppose the presence of these organisms, although a proposed amendment by the Commission early in 1994, will introduce standards for **faecal streptococci**. Based upon the established 95% pass results, they are an 'I' standard of 400 organisms per 100 ml of water and a 'G' standard of 100 per 100 ml.

Directive 76/160/EEC [18] has been partially implemented in the UK by the Bathing Waters (Classification) Regulations 1991 which are enforceable by the NRA.

Health risks from bathing water
There was for many years a view in the UK that sewage-contaminated bathing water did not represent a serious risk to public health. This was fostered to a large extent by a Public Health Laboratory study [18] and a Medical Research Council report [19], both of which concluded in 1959 that infection from seawater bathing could be discounted for all practical purposes, unless the pollution was so gross as to be aesthetically revolting.

The tenth report of the Royal Commission on Environmental Pollution, *Tackling Pollution – Experience and Prospects* [20], published in 1984, showed that many bathing waters and beaches in the UK suffered from an undesirable degree of contamination by sewage. It confirmed that the risk of infection by serious disease is small, but the visible presence of faecal and other offensive materials leads to a serious loss of amenity and

Table 44.9 Quality requirements for bathing water: microbiological parameters

Microbiological parameters	G	I	Minimum sampling frequency
Total coliforms per 100 ml	500	10 000	Fortnightly (1)
Faecal coliforms per 100 ml	100	2000	Fortnightly (1)
Faecal streptococci per 100 ml	100	–	(2)
Salmonella per litre	–	0	(2)
Entero viruses PFU 10 l	–	0	(2)

Notes: G = guide; I = mandatory
(0) Provision exists for exceeding the limits in the event of exceptional geographical or meteorological conditions.
(1) When sampling taken place in previous years produced results which are appreciably better than those in this annexe, and when no new factor likely to lower the quality of the water has appeared, the competent authorities may reduce the sampling frequency by a factor or two.
(2) Concentration to be checked by the competent authority when an inspection in the bathing area shows that the substance may be present, or that the quality of water has deteriorated.
(3) These parameters must be checked by the competent authorities when there is a tendency toward the eutrophication of the water.
Source: Council Directive of 8 December 1975 Concerning the Quality of Bathing Water (76/160/EEC).

is unacceptable. Royal Commission evidence included that obtained from the Department of Health and Social Security which did not rule out the possibility that sewage contamination of bathing waters and beaches could be associated with an increased risk of travellers' diarrhoea and similar complaints. Views expressed by WHO [21], the US Environmental Protection Agency [22] and the European Commission confirmed opinions that there is potential risk to health from bathing in sewage-contaminated sea water. In *The State of the Marine Environment* [23], an Environmental Programme Report published in 1990, the United Nations also supports this view. In a section dealing with human health effects, the report concludes that:

Gastro-intestinal infection due to swimming in sewage polluted sea water is the most wide-

Table 44.10 Quality requirements for bathing waters; physiochemical parameters

Physiochemical parameters	G	I	Minimum sampling frequency
pH	–	6–9 (0)	(2)
Colour	–	No abnormal change in colour	Fortnightly
Minerals oils (mg/l)	–	No film visible on the surface of the water and no odour	Fortnightly (2)
Surface-active substances reacting with methylene blue (mg/l)	≤0.3 –	No lasting foam	(2) Fortnightly
Phenols (mg/l) (phenol indices)	≤0.3 – ≤0.005	– No specific odour ≤0.05	(1) (2) Fortnightly (1) (2)
Transparency (m)	2	1 (0)	Fortnightly (1)
Dissolved oxygen (% saturated O_2)	80–120	–	(2)
Tarry residues and floating materials as wood, plastic articles, bottles, containers of glass, plastic, rubber or any other substance. Waste or splinters	Absence		Fortnightly (1)
Ammonia mg/l NH_4			(3)
Nitrogen Kjeldahl mg/l N			(3)

Notes and source as in Table 44.9.

Table 44.11 Quality requirements for bathing water; other parameters

Other substances regarded as indicators of pollution	G	I	Minimum sampling frequency
Pesticides (mg/l) (parathion, HCH, dieldrin)			(2)
Heavy metals (mg/l) such as: Arsenic (As) Cadmium (Cd) Chrome VI (VI) Lead (Pb) Mercury (Hg)			(2) (2)
Cyanides (mg/l C)			
Nitrates and phosphates (mg/l NO, PO_4)			(2)

Notes and source as in Table 44.9.

spread health effect in estuarine and of the coastal areas with high population densities. Recent epidemiological studies in the USA and in the Mediterranean have cast new light on the causal relationship between bathing in sea water contamined with pathogens of faecal origin and disease among the bathers. The relationship is particularly strong in the case of children under five. Earlier views that there is no demonstrable link between human disease and bathing in sea water, can no longer be supported.

By 1990, the Department of the Environment had designated 44 beaches in the UK as 'bathing waters'. There remain, however, large areas of water which are used extensively for recreational activities, including swimming, canoeing and windsurfing, which have not been designated. Most of these activities involve immersion in water and must represent a risk to health, if the water is polluted. There is as yet no standard available to define acceptable limits for recreational water quality.

Bathing water studies
In the search for a definitive 'health' standard for bathing water, a number of studies have taken place, notably those of Cabelli in the USA, in which large numbers of bathers and non-bathers

at seaside beaches were questioned and subject to a follow-up questionnaire. Cabelli's conclusions were that sea bathing in modestly polluted waters produced a significant elevation of minor infections of the ear, nose and throat, as well as gastrointestinal infections, in bathers compared with non-bathers. During the period 1989 to 1993 a UK national study into the health effects of sea bathing was carried out by the Water Research Centre (WRC) on contract to the Department of the Environment. Two complementary methods were used in a total of 14 separate, although interrelated, studies involving over 17 000 people. The methodology employed was first tested in two pilot studies conducted at Langland Bay in 1989 and reported in 1991, whilst the final report to the Department of the Environment was published in 1994 [10].

Conclusions included a noted increase in minor symptoms, after contact with sea water, which were not related to the microbiological quality of the water. However, relative increases in diarrhoea seemed to be related to the mean counts of coliforms and enteroviruses. In the case of the controlled clinical trial, symptoms of gastroenteritis in bathers were related to the counts of **Faecal streptococci** in the water at about chest level. Overall, the report concludes, '. . . findings suggest that activity in sea water meeting these Imperative standards does not pose any significant risks to health'. It is worth noting that separately published results from the randomized clinical trials conclude:

1. Categorical and multiple logistic regression procedures were used to identify relationships between water quality and gastro-enteritis and to assess the validity of pooling the data from all four studies.
2. A significant dose response relationship was identified between faecal streptococci (per 100 ml) measured at chest depth and gastroenteritis (p<0.001). The relationship was independent of site studied.
3. Non-water-related risk factors did not confound the relationship and no significant interaction between the confounders and the water quality index was found.

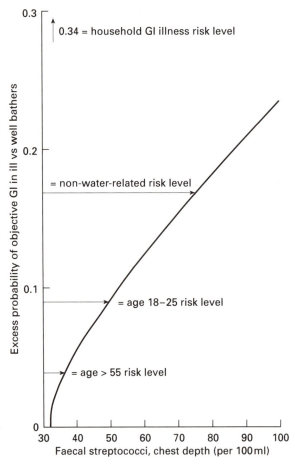

Fig. 44.14 Policy implications. 1. The model allows the prediction of the probability of gastroenteritis (i.e. the risk of illness) at a given faecal streptococci level. This probability can be compared with the risk of illness attributable to the other risk factors such as household illness. 2. The results clearly indicate that the current mandatory standards specified in Directive (76/160/EEC) may not be appropriate. Consideration should be given to changing both the recommended sampling depth and the microbial indicators used to assess compliance of EC marine waters. 3. The results provide the necessary scientific information of the construction of standards or objectives for marine recreational waters as used by 'normal' adult bathers. (Source: Kay, D., *The Health Effects of Sea Bathing*, Results of the UK Randomized Clinical Trial Experiments.)

4. The threshold of risk was objectively defined as 32 faecal streptococci per 100 ml at chest depth. The resulting model (p = 0.012) is shown above (in Fig. 44.14) [24].

Clean beaches campaign

Blue Flag awards for clean beaches is a European campaign initiated by the Foundation for Environmental Education in Europe (FEEE) to reward efforts that meet the standards of the Blue Flag charter. The four basic categories of criteria for entry include water quality, beach cleanliness and management, as well as provision of environmental education and information.

Water quality criteria are met by full compliance with EU bathing water imperative and guideline standards, with no industrial or sewage discharges. Recommended emergency plans and monitoring regimes are included. There must be no gross pollution of beaches by faeces or other wastes and no litter or oil pollution. Banning dogs, together with monitoring, are also criteria for determining beach quality.

Environmental education is achieved by the provision of current information on water quality, which must be published and updated regularly. It is also required that immediate public warning is given if, for any reason, the beach is unsafe, or is grossly polluted.

Beach management and safety criteria are to include the provision of adequate litter bins, which are regularly maintained and emptied, beach clean ups after peak days, no driving or camping on beaches, no dumping and safe access. There are also recommended standards for sanitary facilities, beach guards and first aid facilities and telephones.

REFERENCES

1. Department of the Environment and Welsh Office (1986) *The Water Environment: the Next Steps*, consultation paper, HMSO, London.
2. Department of the Environment, Ministry of Agriculture, Fisheries and Food, and Welsh Office (1987) *The National Rivers Authority: the Government's proposals for a regulatory body in a privatised water industry*, HMSO, London.
3. Bassett, W.H (1992) *Environmental Health Procedures*, 3rd edn, Chapman & Hall, London.
4. Report of the Group of Experts (1990) *Cryptosporidium in Water Supplies*, Chairman Sir John Badenoch, HMSO, London.
5. Water Research Centre, Ellis Horwood Ltd, *Water Supply Bylaws Guide*.
6. British Standards Institute (1987) *Design, Testing and Maintenance of Services Supplying Water for Domestic Use within Buildings or their Curtilages*, BS6700:1987, BSI, London.
7. Water Bylaws Advisory Service, *Water Fittings and Materials Directory*, WBAS, Slough.
8. British Standards Institute (1987) *Code of Practice for the Design of Concrete Structures for the Retaining of Aqueous Liquids*, BS8007:1987, BSI, London.
9. British Standards Institute (1990) *Specification for Steel Pipes, Joints and Specials for Water and Sewerage*, BS5534:1990, BSI, London.
10. *Health Effects of Sea Bathing* (WM1 9021) Final Report to the DoE by the WRc, DoE 3412/2 January 1994
11. Council Directive of 21 May 1991 Concerning Urban Waste Water Treatment (91/271/EEC). *Official Journal of the European Communities* **(O.J.) L135**; 30 May.
12. British Standards Institute (1983) *Design and Installation of Small Sewage Treatment Works and Cesspools*, BS6297: 1983, BSI, London.
13. Riley, C.T. and Jones, K.B.C (1970) *Origins and Nature of Farm Wastes*, Symposium on Farm Wastes, University of Newcastle upon Tyne.
14. House of Lords' Select Committee on the European Communities (1991) *Municipal Waste Water Treatment*, 10th Report 1990–91, HMSO, London.
15. Carson, R. (1956) *Silent Spring*, Hamish Hamilton, London.
16. Council Directive of 8 December 1975 Concerning the Quality of Bathing Water (76/160/EEC)
17. House of Commons Environment Committee (1990) *Pollution of Beaches*, 4th Report, HMSO, London.
18. *Public Health Laboratory Service (1959)* Sewage contamination of coastal bathing waters

in England and Wales. *Journal of Hygiene*, **57**.

19. Medical Research Council (1959) *Sewage Contamination of Bathing Beaches in England and Wales*, Memorandum No. 37, HMSO, London.

20. Royal Commission on Environmental Pollution (1984) *Tackling Pollution – Experience and Prospects*, Comnd 9149, HMSO, London.

21. WHO (1989) *Microbiological/Epidemiological Studies on the Correlation between Coastal Recreational Water Quality and Health Effects*, Revised Protocol submitted by WHO Secretariat ICP/CEH083/10, WHO, Geneva.

22. US Environmental Protection Agency (1986) *Ambient Water Quality Criteria for Bacteria*.

23. United Nations Environment Programme (1990) *The State of the Marine Environment*.

24. Kay, D. *The Health Effects of Sea Bathing*, Results of the UK Randomized Clinical Trial Experiments.

25. *Manual on Treatment of Private Water Supplies – DWI*, Department of the Environment/Welsh Office/Scottish Office: HMSO, London.

FURTHER READING

Dawson, A., West, P. (1993) (eds) *Drinking Water Supplies: A Microbiological Perspective*, HMSO, London.

Appendix

CONSTRUCTION TECHNOLOGY

Detailed technical information about building construction techniques, defects and their remedies is not included in this edition. This is not only because of limitations of space by the inclusion of a wide range of new material, but also because of the availability of comprehensive information on these subjects elsewhere.

Building Research Establishment

One such source on building defects and their remedies is the Building Research Establishment (BRE) which produces a wide range of publications of interest to those involved with environmental health. Of particular interest are:

1. **Digests**. A comprehensive series of almost 350 separate publications covers practically every aspect of building technology, including the main defects to be found in houses and their remedies, e.g. dampness including condensation, lighting, heating, ventilation, sanitary pipework and defects in timber.
2. **Defect action sheets (DASs)**. Currently extending to over 140 separately published sheets, these describe common faults in housebuilding, how to avoid them and specifications for remedial action. The material is again wide ranging and includes defects in substructure, walls, roofs and services.
3. **Technical notes (TNs)**. This is a series of practical notes on timber and timber-related subjects, including defects caused by timber pests and fungal growth.
4. **Reports (BRs)**. These are detailed accounts of research findings providing in-depth information for building and associated professionals.
5. **Information papers (IPs)**. These deal with research results in relation to construction and how to apply them.
6. **Video cassettes**. These include cassettes on condensation in the home, giving simple explanations to householders of its causes and remedies, and traffic noise and sound insulation, explaining the L_{10} noise index and methods of insulating buildings against noise.
7. **Packages** – which include literature and audio-visual presentations and are available for condensation, designing for natural and artificial lighting and noise for neighbours which deals with poor sound insulation between dwellings and the source of one of the commonest complaints to environmental health departments.
8. **Update** – a monthly package of information on construction, e.g. materials profiles, building techniques, research findings, technical reviews, practical guidelines and changes in legislation. Annual Subscription £75.

A full list of BRE publications is available annually at £5. Leaflets listing the currently available BRE reports and books, information papers, digests, defect action sheets, and audio-visual material and packages are available free from:

BRE Bookshop
Building Research Establishment
Garston
Watford
WD2 7JR

Building Regulations

In relation to the constructional aspects of new buildings, the reader is referred to the Building Regulations 1991 and their supporting documents. *The Manual to the Building Regulations* published by HMSO for the Department of the Environment sets out the Regulations and includes both explanatory notes for each and references to the appropriate approved documents.

Approved documents, which are published separately, give practical guidance about the ways of meeting the requirements of the Regulations, and describe particular methods of construction, give reference to other publications and give acceptable levels of performance. They include a wide range of explanatory diagrams.

The complete set of volumes of these documents including the manual, mandatory rules and the approved documents is also available from the Building Research Establishment.

Chartered Institution of Building Services Engineers (CIBSE)

Although publishing a wider range of material, there are a number of CIBSE publications which are of particular value to those involved in environmental health:

1. *CIBSE Guide A – Design Data*. This brings together information required for the design of heating, ventilation and air-conditioning systems. It is split into nine sections which are available separately; of special use is section A1: 'Environmental Criteria for Design' which indicates the thermal, acoustic and visual factors to be taken into account in relation to thermal environment, ventilation, lighting, sound and vibration to produce a satisfactory work or leisure environment.
2. *CIBSE Guide B – Installation and Equipment Data*. This compromises 16 sections which are not available separately, but includes section B2, 'Ventilation and Air Conditioning Requirements', and section B8, 'Sanitation and Waste Disposal'.
3. *CIBSE Code for Interior Lighting* (1994). This gives the Institution's recommendations on all aspects of interior lighting and includes illuminance and glare standards.

These publications and a full publications list is available from:

Publications Sales Department
CIBSE
Delta House
222 Balham High Road
London SW12 9BS

Defects in Buildings

This extensive reference volume by the Property Services Agency and the Department of the Environment (1989) *Defects in Buildings*, HMSO, London deals with the diagnosis and cure of defects over the whole range of buildings, and is a valuable guide to staff in environmental health departments. After dealing generally with the causes of deterioration, durability of materials, principles of diagnosis and investigation techniques, each main building element is analysed in relation to:

1. symptoms of defects;
2. investigation of those symptoms;
3. diagnosis and cure.

Each description for all defects in each element contains a reference to the appropriate BRE publication, BS codes of practice and other sources of information.

FURTHER READING

Further information may be gained from the following books published by E. and F.N. Spon, London.
Curwell and March (1986) *Hazardous Building Materials* (ISBN 0419 137 408).
Ranson (1987) *Building Failures* (ISBN 0419 142 606).
Richardson (1990) *Defects and Deterioration in Buildings* (ISBN 0419 201).
Singh (1994) *Building Psychology: management of decay and health in buildings* (ISBN 0419 190 201).

Index

Page references in *italics* refer to Figures; those in **bold** refer to Tables.